Aravind
FAQs in
Ophthalmolo

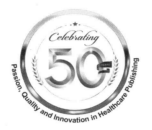

Aravind
FAQs in
Ophthalmology

SECOND EDITION

N Venkatesh Prajna DNB FRCOphth

Director-Academics
Aravind Eye Hospital
Madurai, Tamil Nadu, India

JAYPEE BROTHERS MEDICAL PUBLISHERS
The Health Sciences Publisher

New Delhi | London | Panama

Jaypee Brothers Medical Publishers (P) Ltd

Headquarters

Jaypee Brothers Medical Publishers (P) Ltd
4838/24, Ansari Road, Daryaganj
New Delhi 110 002, India
Phone: +91-11-43574357
Fax: +91-11-43574314
Email: jaypee@jaypeebrothers.com

Overseas Offices

J.P. Medical Ltd
83 Victoria Street, London
SW1H 0HW (UK)
Phone: +44 20 3170 8910
Fax: +44 (0)20 3008 6180
Email: info@jpmedpub.com

Jaypee-Highlights Medical Publishers Inc
City of Knowledge, Bld. 235, 2nd Floor
Clayton, Panama City, Panama
Phone: +1 507-301-0496
Fax: +1 507-301-0499
Email: cservice@jphmedical.com

Jaypee Brothers Medical Publishers (P) Ltd
Bhotahity, Kathmandu, Nepal
Phone: +977-9741283608
Email: kathmandu@jaypeebrothers.com

Website: www.jaypeebrothers.com
Website: www.jaypeedigital.com

Aravind FAQs in Ophthalmology

First Edition: 2013
Second Edition: **2019**

ISBN 978-93-86261-09-0

Printed at Rajkamal Electric Press, Kundli, Haryana.

Preface to the Second Edition

The first edition of this book has received an overwhelming response, both nationally and internationally. I have especially been enthused by the generous feedback from the student community, who felt that this book is a very useful tool for their examination preparation. As a continuation, the second edition has been planned to be even more comprehensive. Additional topics have been included in the existing chapter and additional newer chapters have been created. The chapter on the management summary of commonly kept examination cases would serve as an invaluable tool for the students to confidently present before the examiner. I would like to reiterate that this book should be seen as an adjunct and not as a replacement to the existing excellent textbooks in ophthalmology.

N Venkatesh Prajna

Preface to the First Edition

The specialty of ophthalmology has developed by leaps and bounds in the recent past. Excellent, comprehensive books are being brought out at regular intervals, which help an ophthalmologist to keep abreast with the times. In my 15 years experience as a residency director, I have often found the need for a concise, examination-oriented ready-reckoner, which would be of use to the postgraduates to answer specifically to the point. This book aims to fill this gap and serves as a compilation of the frequently asked questions (FAQs) and the answers expected in a postgraduate clinical ophthalmology examination. This book should not be misconstrued as a replacement to the existing standard textbooks. These questions have been painstakingly gathered over a 10-year period from the collective experience of several senior teachers at Aravind Eye Hospital, Madurai, Tamil Nadu, India. Apart from the examination-oriented questions, this book also contains examples of case sheet writing and different management scenarios, which will help the students to logically analyze and answer in a coherent manner. I do sincerely hope that this book helps the postgraduate to face his/her examination with confidence.

N Venkatesh Prajna

Acknowledgments

I have received tremendous support from all the faculty and students of the entire Aravind Eye Care System (AECS) in improving the existing popular edition of the FAQ's in Ophthalmology. Without their help and insights, it would not have been possible to bring out a revised edition. I would also like to thank the student community from across the country, who continue to give their feedback and their appreciation through emails and letters, which have encouraged me to think of ways and means to expand the scope of this book. I would also like to sincerely acknowledge and thank the secretarial help rendered for me by Mrs Uma Devi, from the central office of the AECS, who patiently helped in editing the book and making sure that all changes are incorporated. I am very grateful for the management of the AECS for giving me unlimited time and support for making this exercise possible. I would also like to acknowledge the tremendous support of my immediate family for patiently supporting my professional career. My parents, Dr Namperumalsamy and Dr Natchiar were excellent teachers in their own right and I have learnt a lot from them. My wife, Dr Lalitha and my children Dr Meera Lakshmi and Aravind Krishna have been a source of joy and pride in my professional journey. I do sincerely hope that this book takes the fear factor out of the examinations.

I especially appreciate the constant support and encouragement of Mr Jitendar P Vij (Group Chairman) and Mr Ankit Vij (Managing Director) of M/s Jaypee Brothers Medical Publishers (P) Ltd, New Delhi, India, in publishing the book and also their associates particularly Ms Chetna Malhotra Vohra (Associate Director—Content Strategy) and Ms Nikita Chauhan (Senior Development Editor) who have been prompt, efficient and most helpful.

Contents

CHAPTER
1

Introduction

1.1. VISUAL ACUITY

1. **Define visual acuity.**

   Visual acuity is defined as the reciprocal of the minimum resolvable angle measured in minutes of arc for a standard test pattern.

2. **Define visual angle.**

   It is the angle subtended at the nodal point of the eye by the physical dimensions of an object in the visual field.

3. **What are the components of visual acuity?**

   Visual acuity has three components:

   i. *Minimum visible*: Detection of presence or absence of stimulus.
   ii. *Minimum separable*: Judgment of location of a visual target relative to another element of the same target.
   iii. *Minimum resolvable*: Ability to distinguish between more than one identifying feature in a visible target. Threshold is between 30 seconds and 1 minute of arc.

4. **What are the components of measurement of vision?**

   i. Visual acuity
   ii. Field of vision
   iii. Color vision and
   iv. Binocular single vision.

5. **Who developed classic test chart?**

   Professor Hermann Snellen in 1863.

6. **What is the testing distance? Why do we check at that distance?**

   The testing is done 6 m (20 ft) away from the target. At this distance, divergence of rays that enters the pupil is so small that rays are considered parallel. Hence, accommodation is eliminated at this distance.

7. **Describe about the Snellen's chart.**

The letters are:

   i. It consists of series of black capital letters on a white board arranged in lines, each progressively diminishing in size.

   ii. Lines comprising letters have such a breadth that they will subtend at an angle of 1 minute at the nodal point of the eye at a particular distance.

   iii. Each letter is designed such that it fits in a square.

   iv. The sides of the letter are five times the breadth of constituent lines.

   v. At given distance, each letter subtends at an angle of 5 minutes at the nodal point of the eye.

8. **What does normal 6/6 visual acuity represent?**

It represents the ability to see 1 minute of arc which is close to theoretical diffraction limits.

9. **Explain LogMAR charts.**

   i. Used for academic and research purposes.

   ii. This is a modification of Snellen's chart, where each subsequent line differs by 0.1 log unit in the minimum angle of resolution (MAR) required for that line.

   iii. They have equal number of letters in each line.

   iv. Used at a distance of 4 m.

10. **What is the procedure of testing visual acuity (VA) using Snellen's chart?**

   i. Patient is seated at a distance of 6 m from the Snellen's chart because at this distance the rays of light are practically parallel and patient exerts minimal accommodation.

   ii. Chart should be properly illuminated (not less than 20 ft candle).

   iii. Patient is asked to read with each eye separately.

   iv. Visual acuity is recorded as a fraction.

     – Numerator: Distance of the patient from the chart.

     – Denominator: Smallest letters read accurately.

   v. When the patient is able to read up to 6 m line, the VA is recorded as 6/6—normal.

   vi. Depending on the smallest line patient can read from distance of 6 m VA is recorded as 6/9, 6/12, 6/18, 6/24, 6/36 and 6/60.

   vii. If the patient cannot see the topline from 6 m, he/she is asked to walk toward the chart till one can read the topline.

   viii. Depending on the distance at which patient can read the topline, the VA is recorded as 5/60, 4/60, 3/60, 2/60 and 1/60.

ix. **Finger counting:**
If patient is unable to read topline even from 1 m, he/she is asked to count fingers (CF) of the examiner, the VA is recorded as CF-3', CF-2', CF-1' or CF close to face depending on the distance (in meters) at which the patient is able to count fingers.

x. **Hand movements (HM):**
When the patient fails to count fingers, the examiner moves his/her hand close to patient's face. If the patient can appreciate the hand movements, the VA is recorded as HM positive.

xi. **Perception of light (PL):**
When the patient cannot distinguish HM, examiner notes if the patient can perceive light or not. If the patient can perceive light, then it is recorded as PL+ and if the patient cannot perceive light, then it is recorded as P.

xii. **Projection of rays (PR):**
If PL is +ve, then PR should be checked by shining light in all four directions and patient is asked whether he/she is able to recognize the direction of light rays that is shown and is recorded in all four quadrants.

11. How is a decimal notation represented?

It converts Snellen fraction to a decimal.
For example: Snellen 20/20—decimal 1.0
Snellen 20/30—decimal 0.7
Snellen 20/40—decimal 0.5.

12. How is near vision tested?

i. Near acuity testing demonstrates the ability of a patient to see clearly at a normal reading distance.

ii. Test is usually performed at 40 cm (16″) with a printed, handheld chart.

iii. The following charts are used:
   - Jaeger's chart
   - Roman test types
   - Snellen's near vision test types.

13. Explain Jaeger's chart.

i. Jaeger, devised it in 1867.

ii. It consisted of ordinary printed fonts of varying sizes used at that time. Various sizes of modern fonts that approximate the original chart is used.

iii. In this chart, prints area marked from 1 to 7 and accordingly patient's acuity is labeled as J1 to J7, depending upon the print one can read.

14. What is Landolt's testing chart?

   i. It is similar to Snellen's chart, except instead of letter, broken circles are used.

   ii. Each broken ring subtends an angle of 5 minutes at the nodal point.

   iii. It consists of detection of orientation of the break in the circle.

15. What is Vernier acuity?

   i. It is the smallest offset of a line which can be detected.

   ii. It is measured using a square wave grating.

   iii. Offset of 3–5 seconds of an arc is normally discernible.

   iv. It is less than limit of Snellen VA and is therefore called as hyperacuity.

16. What are potential acuity testing?

These tests are used to assess the visual acuity of eyes in which it is not possible to see the macula because of cataract.

   i. Pinhole test

   ii. Bluefield entopic phenomena: Ability to see moving white dots when blue light diffusely illuminates the retina. It represents light transmitted by WBCs in the perifoveal capillaries.

   iii. Interferometers: It projects laser light from two sources on to the retina. Interference occurs when two sources meet. It is seen as Sine wave Grating if macula is functioning.

17. What are Roman test types?

   i. Devised by the Faculty of Ophthalmologist of Great Britain in 1952.

   ii. It consists of "Times Roman" type fonts with standard spacing.

   iii. Near vision is recorded as N5, N6, N8, N10, N12, N18, N36, and N48.

18. Explain Snellen's near vision test types.

   i. Snellen's equivalent for near vision was devised on the same principle as distant types.

   ii. Graded thickness of letters of different lines is about 1/17th of distant vision chart letters.

   iii. Letters equivalent to 6/6 line subtend an angle of 5 minutes at an average reading distance (35 cm/14″).

19. What is the procedure of testing near vision?

   i. Patient is seated in a chair and asked to read the near vision chart kept at a distance of 25–35 cm with a good illumination thrown over his or her left shoulder.

   ii. Each eye should be tested separately.

   iii. Near vision is recorded as the smallest type that can be read completely by the patient.

iv. A note of approximate distance at which the near vision chart is held should be made.

v. Thus, near vision is recorded as:

NV = J1 at 30 cm (in Jaeger's notation)

NV = N5 at 30 cm (in Faulty's notation)

Feet	Meters	LogMAR
20/20	6/6	0.00
20/30	6/9	0.18
20/40	6/12	0.30
20/60	6/18	0.48
20/80	6/24	0.60
20/120	6/36	0.80
20/200	6/60	1.00

20. What is the principle of pinhole?

Pinhole admits only central rays of light, which do not require refraction by the cornea or the lens. Patient can resolve finer detail on the acuity chart in this way, without use of glasses.

21. What do we infer from pinhole testing?

i. If the pinhole improves VA by two lines or more, then there is more likely a chance of refractive error.

ii. If the pinhole does not improve vision, then other organic causes should be looked for.

22. What is the size of pinhole?

1 mm/1.2 mm

23. What are the types of pinhole?

i. Single—no more than 2.4 mm in diameter is used.

ii. Multiple—central opening surrounded by two rings of small perforation.

24. How is the pinhole testing performed?

i. Position the patient and occlude the eye not being tested.

ii. Ask the patient to hold the pinhole occluder in front of the eye that is to be tested. The habitual correction should be worn for the test.

iii. Instruct the patient to look at the distance chart through the single pinhole.

iv. Instruct the patient to use little hand or eye movements to align the pinhole to resolve sharpest image on the chart.

v. Ask the patient to begin to read the line with the smallest letters that are legible as determined on the previous vision test without the use of pinhole.

25. What are the variables used in visual acuity measurements?

The conditions that may cause variability in acuity measurements for both near and distance are:

External variables:

i. If lighting level is not constant during testing.

ii. Variability in contrast: Charts with higher contrast will be seen more easily than those with lower contrast.

iii. If chart is not kept clean, smaller letters will become more difficult to identify.

iv. When projector chart is used, cleanliness of projector bulb and lens and condition of projecting screen will affect the contrast of letters viewed.

v. The distance between projector and chart will affect size of letters.

vi. Sharpness of focus of projected chart.

vii. Incidental glare on the screen.

Optical considerations:

i. If patient is wearing eye glasses, be sure the lenses are clean. Dirty lenses of any kind, whether trial lenses or contact lenses, will decrease visual acuity.

ii. Effects of tear film abnormalities, such as dry eye syndromes, can be minimized by generous use of artificial tear preparation.

iii. Corneal surface abnormalities produce distortions and must be addressed medically.

iv. Corneal or lenticular astigmatism may necessitate use of special spectacle or contact lens.

Neurologic impairments:

i. Motility defects such as nystagmus or any other movement disorder which interferes with the ability to align the fovea will lower the acuity measurement.

ii. Visual field defects

iii. Optic nerve lesions

iv. Pupil abnormalities

v. Impairment by drugs, legal or illicit.

26. What are the causes of poor near acuity than distance acuity?

i. Presbyopia/premature presbyopia

ii. Undercorrected/high hyperopia

iii. Overcorrected myopia

iv. Small, centrally located cataracts

v. Accommodative effort syndrome

vi. Drugs with anticholinergic effect

vii. Convergence insufficiency

viii. Adie's pupil

ix. Malingering/hysteria.

27. How to test the vision in infants?

i. Blink response—in response to sound, bright light/touching the cornea.

ii. Pupillary reflex—after 29th week of gestation.

iii. Fixation reflex—usually present at birth. It is well developed and well elicited by 2 weeks to 2 months.

iv. Follow movements—following horizontally moving targets. It is seen in full term newborn and is well developed by first month. Vertical tracking is elicited by 4–8 weeks.

v. **Catford drum test:**
   - It is based on the observation of pendular eye movement that is elicited as the child follows an oscillating drum with dots.
   - Test distance: 60 cm (2 ft)
   - Displayed dot size: 15–0.5 mm
   - Dot represent 20/600 to 20/20 vision.
   - Smallest dot that evokes pendular eye movement denotes acuity.
   - Disadvantage: Overestimate of vision by 2–4 times. It is unreliable for amblyopia screening.

vi. **Preferential looking tests (PLT):**
   - The principle is based on the behavioral pattern of an infant to prefer to fixate a pattern stimulus rather than a blank stimulus both being of the same brightness.

vii. **Teller acuity card test:**
   - It is a modification based on PLT designed for a simpler and rapid testing.
   - It has 17 cards, each of 25.5 × 51 cm. 15 of these contain 12.5 × 12.5 cm patches of square wave gratings.
   - Cycle consists of 1 black and 1 white stripe and an octave is halving or doubling of spatial frequency.
   - Testing distance: Infants up to 6 months of age—38 cm
                           7 months to 3 yr of age—55 cm
                           Later—84 cm
   - Advantage: Very useful quick test for infants and preschool children up to 18 months.
   - Disadvantage: It tests near acuity, not distance acuity. It measures resolution acuity not recognition acuity. It overestimates VA.

viii. **OKNOVIS:**
   - Principle: Based on the principle of arresting an elicited optokinetic nystagmus by introducing optotypes of different sizes.
   - Portable handheld drums moving at 12 rpm with colored pictures to elicit an optokinetic nystagmus.

- Testing distance: 60 cm
- Optotypes of different sizes are then introduced to arrest OKN.

ix. **Cardiff acuity cards:**
- Principle: Based on the principle of preferential fixation on cards which have picture optotype and a blank located vertically.
- Child identifies picture by verbalizing, pointing or fixation preference.

x. **Visually evoked response (VEP):**
- It records the change in the cortical electrical pattern detected by surface electrodes monitoring the occipital cortex following light stimulation of the retina.
- Two types of stimuli:
  Pattern—checker board or stripes
  Flash—unpatterned
- Preferred is pattern reversal type.
- Can be recorded in two modes: Transient or steady state.

28. How do you infer visual acuity from fixation pattern?

Fixation pattern	Visual acuity
Gross eccentric fixation	<CF 1 m
Unsteady central fixation	<6/60
Steady central fixation but not maintained	6/60–6/36
Central steady fixation, can maintain but prefers other eye	6/24–6/9
Central steady fixation, free alternation or cross fixation	6/9–6/6

To call it as good fixation, it should be central, steady, and maintained. Preference of fixation in one eye denotes that poor vision in non-fixating eye.

29. How is vision tested in infants aged about 1–2 years?
i. **Boeck candy test (Cake decoration test):**
- Initially child's hand is guided to the bead and then to his mouth.
- Each eye is alternatively covered and the difference is noted.

ii. **Worth's ivory ball test:**
- Ivory balls 0.5″ to 1.5″ of diameter are rolled on the floor in front of the child
- Asked to retrieve each
- Acuity is estimated on the basis of the smallest size for the test distance.

iii. **Sheridan's ball test:**
- These are Styrofoam balls of different sizes rolled in front of the child
- Quality of fixation for each size is assessed

- Same can be used as mounted balls used at 10 ft distance against black screen. Fixation behavior for each ball is observed by the examiner hidden behind the screen.

30. How is vision tested in children of around 3 years of age?

  i. **Miniature toy test:**
   - A component of STYCAR test
   - Pair of miniature toys are used
   - Test distance is 10 ft
   - Child is asked to name or pick the pair from an assortment.

  ii. **Coin test:**
   - Coins of different sizes at different distances are shown
   - Child is asked to distinguish between the two faces of the coin.

  iii. **Dot VA test:**
   - In a darkened room, the child is shown an illuminated box with printed black dots of different diameters
   - Then, smaller dots are shown
   - Smallest dot identified correctly twice is taken as acuity threshold.

31. How is vision tested in children aged 3–5 years?

  i. Vision test using pictures, symbols or even letters become applicable in this age group.

  ii. Training by mother at home is helpful
   - Illiterate E-cutout test
   - Tumbling E test
   - Isolated hand figure test
   - Sheridan–Gardiner test
   - Lippmann's HOTV test
   - Pictorial vision test
   - Broken wheel test
   - Boek candy bead test
   - Light home picture cards.

  iii. **Illiterate E-cutout test:**
   - Child is given a cutout of an E and asked to match this with isolated E's of varying sizes
   - When child starts understanding orientation of E, VA chart consisting of E's oriented in various directions are used.

  iv. **Tumbling E test:**
   - Preferred for mass screening in preschool children
   - Consists of different sizes of E, in one of the four positions—right, left, up, or down
   - Distance: 6 m
   - Each eye is tested separately.

    v. **Landolt's C:** Similar to the E test.
   vi. **Sheridan's letter test:**
- Uses five letters H,O,T,V, and X in five-letter set
- A and V are added in seven-letter set
- C and L are also added in nine-letter set
- Testing distance is 10 ft (3 m)
- Child is expected to name the letters/indicate similar letter on the card in hand

  vii. **Lippman's HOTV test:**
- Uses only four letters H,O,T,V at test distance of 3 m
- Simpler version of Sheridan test.

32. What is hyperacuity?

The human eye is capable of seeing more than the ability of the retinal cones to resolve. This ability is called hyperacuity. It is due to the involvement of higher cortical centers in the parietal cortex, for example:
  i. Vernier acuity
 ii. Stereo acuity

Vernier acuity:

This is the ability to discern the Vernier separation between two lines not in perfect alignment. It is in the range of 10–20 seconds of an arc.

Stereoacuity:

This is the ability to perceive a separation in the three-dimension (3D) depth perception.

33. What is Stiles–Crawford effect?

Stiles and Crawford have shown that pencils of light entering the eye obliquely are less effective as stimuli, compared to those entering the pupil centrally. They pointed out that this effect is not due to aberrations in the optical system but is most likely related to the orientation of the receptors in the retina. This directional sensitivity of the retina is referred to as the Stiles–Crawford effect.

1.2. COLOR VISION

1. **How will you test color vision by Ishihara chart?**
    i. Room should be adequately lit by daylight
    ii. Nature of the test should be explained to the patient
    iii. Full refractive correction is worn
    iv. It is preferable to do the test before pupillary dilatation
    v. One eye is first occluded and the other eye is tested
    vi. The plates are kept at a distance of 75 cm from the subject with the plane of the paper at right angle to the line of vision
    vii. The standard time taken to answer each plate is 3–5 seconds.

2. **Explain about Ishihara chart.**
    i. Designed to provide a test which gives a quick and accurate assessment of color vision deficiency of congenital origin
    ii. It consists of a total of 25 plates.

Plate number	Normal	Points with red-green defects		Inference
1	12	12		Both subjects with normal and defective color vision read plate 1 as 12.
2	8	3		
3	6	5		
4	29	17		
5	57	35		Subjects with red-green defects read these plates as those in abnormal column. Totally color blind are unable to read.
6	5	2		
7	3	5		
8	15	17		
9	74	21		
10	2	X		Majority of subjects with color vision deficiency read these plates incorrectly.
11	6	X		
12	97	X		
13	45	X		
14	5	X		Subjects with normal color vision do not see any number. Those with red-green deficiency read the numbers given in the abnormal column.
15	7	X		
16	16	X		
17	73	X		
18	X	5		
19	X	2		
20	X	45		Subjects with protanopia read these plates as given in abnormal column (1), those with deutranomaly read them as given in column (2).
21	X	73		
		Protan	Deutran	
22	26	6	2	
23	42	2	4	
24	35	5	3	
25	96	6	9	

3. **Classify color blindness.**

  i. **Congenital color blindness:**

    X-linked recessive inherited affecting predominantly males

    Types:
    – Dyschromatopsia:
      Anomalous trichromatic color vision:
      a. Protanomalous: defective red color appreciation
      b. Deuteranomalous: defective green color appreciation
      c. Tritanomalous: defective blue color appreciation
    – Dichromatic color vision:
      a. Protanopia: Complete red color defect
      b. Deutranopia: Complete green color defect
      c. Tritanopia: Complete blue color defect
    – Achromatopsia:
      a. Cone monochromatism—presence of only one primary color
      b. Rod monochromatism

  ii. **Acquired color defects:**
    – Type I red-green defects—similar to protan defects
      Seen in progressive cone dystrophies
      a. Stargardt's disease
      b. Chloroquine toxicity
    – Type II red-green defects—similar to deutran defects
      Seen in optic neuropathies, Leber's optic atrophy, ethambutol toxicity
    – Type III tritan defects
      Seen in progressive rod dystrophies, peripheral retinal lesions, macular edema.

4. **What are the difference between congenital and acquired color blindness?**

Congenital	Acquired
Present at birth	Present after birth (3 months)
Type and severity constant	Can change with time
Type of deficiency can be diagnosed precisely	Can show combined color vision deficiency features
Both eyes are equally affected	Very rarely both eyes are equally affected
Visual fields and visual acuity are usually normal	Commonly there is a reduced visual acuity with field changes
Predominantly are red-green defects	Most commonly are tritan defects
Higher incidence in male population	Equal incidence in both sexes

5. **What are the theories of color vision?**

   i. **Trichromatic theory of Young and Helmholtz:**

      It postulates the existence of three types of cones, each with a different photopigment maximally sensitive to either red, green, or blue. The sensation of any given color is determined by relative frequency in pulse from each of the cone systems.

   ii. **Opponent color theory of Hering:**

      It states that some colors appear to be mutually exclusive, for example, reddish green.

6. **Mention the genes associated with color vision defects:**

   Gene for rhodopsin—chromosome 3
   Gene for red and green cones—"q" arm of X chromosome
   Gene for blue cone—chromosome 7.

7. **Explain about the neurophysiology of color vision.**

   i. **Genesis of visual signals in photoreceptors:**

      Photochemical changes in cone pigments followed by a cascade of biochemical changes produce visual signal in the form of cone receptor potential.

   ii. **Processing and transmission of color vision signals:**

      The action potential generated in photoreceptors is transmitted by electrical induction to other cells of retina across the synapses if photoreceptors, bipolar cells, and horizontal cells and then across synapses of bipolar cells, ganglion cells, and amacrine cells.

   iii. **Processing of color signals on lateral geniculate body (LGB):**

      All LGB neurons carry information from more than one cone cell. Color information carried by ganglion cells is relayed to parvocellular portion of LGB.

      Spectrally non-opponent cells (30%) give same type of response to any monochromatic light.

      Spectrally opponent cells (60%) are excited by some wavelengths and inhibited by others.

      Four types:
      – Cells with red/green antagonism
         a. $+R/-G$
         b. $+G/-R$
      – Cells with yellow/blue antagonism
         a. $+B/-Y$
         b. $+Y/-B$

   iv. **Analysis of color signals in visual cortex:**

      Color information from parvocellular portion of LGB is relayed to layer IVc of striate cortex in area 17. From here it passes to blobs in

Layers II and III. It is relayed to thin strips in usual association area and then to lingual and fusiform gyri of occipital lobe (specialized area concerned with color).

8. **What are the tests for color vision apart from Ishihara chart?**

    i. **Hardy–Rand–Rittler**
       – It is also a pseudoisochromatic chart test. Useful to identify protan, deutran, and tritan defects. It consists of 24 plates with vanishing designs containing geometric shapes. Four plates are introductory plates, 6 are for screening (4 for protan and deutran, 2 for tritan), 10 are for grading severity of protan and deutran defect and last 4 are for grading tritan defect.
   ii. **The Lantern test:** The subject has to name the various colors shown to him using a lantern. He is judged based on this.
       – There are three types: Edrige Green, Holmes Wright Types A and B.
  iii. Farnsworth Munsell 100 hue test is a spectrographic test where colored chips are arranged in ascending order.
   iv. City University color vision test is also spectrographic test where the central colored plate is matched to its closest hue from four surrounding color plates.
    v. **Nagel's Anomaloscope test:** The observer is asked to mix red and green colors in a proportion to match the given yellow color hue. It detects red-green deficiency.
   vi. **Holmgren's wool test:** The subject is asked to make a series of color matches from a selection of colored wools.

9. **What are the causes of acquired blue-yellow defects?**

   Glaucoma, retinal detachment, pigmentary degeneration of retina, ARMD, vascular occlusions, diabetic, hypertensive retinopathy, pappiloedema, central serous retinopathy, chorioretinitis.

10. **What are the causes of acquired red-green defects?**

   Optic neuritis, toxic amblyopia, Leber's optic neuropathy, Best's disease, optic nerve lesions, pappilitis, Stargardt's disease.

1.3. ANATOMICAL LANDMARKS IN EYE

CORNEA

1. Dimensions of cornea
   Horizontal diameter—11.75 mm
   Vertical diameter—11 mm
   Posterior diameter—11.5 mm
2. Endothelial cell count
   At birth—6000 cells/mm^2
   In young adults—2400–3000 cells/mm^2
   Corneal decompensation—cell count less than 500/mm^2
3. Thickness of cornea
   Center—about 0.52 mm
   Periphery—about 0.67 mm
4. Refractive index of cornea—1.37
5. Surgical limbus—2 mm wide
   Anterior limbal border—overlies termination of Bowman's membrane
   Mid-limbal line—overlies termination of Schwalbe's line
   Posterior limbal border—overlies sclera spur
   Preferred site for incision—mid-limbal incision.

SCLERA

1. Forms posterior five-sixth of eye ball
2. Thickness
   Posteriorly—thickest 1 mm
   Thinnest at insertion of extraocular muscles—0.3 mm
3. Vortex vein—passes through middle apertures 4–7 mm posterior to equator.

UVEA

1. Average diameter of iris—12 mm
2. Average thickness—0.5 mm
3. Thinnest part of iris—at the root
4. Pupil diameter—3–4 mm
5. Pars plicata—2–2.5 mm wide
6. Pars plana—5 mm wide temporally and 3 mm wide nasally
7. Ciliary processes 70–80 in number
8. Short posterior ciliary arteries—from ophthalmic artery, 10–20 branches
9. Long posterior ciliary arteries—2 in number
10. Anterior ciliary arteries—7 in number.

AQUEOUS HUMOR

1. Ciliary body—site of aqueous production
2. Posterior chamber—0.06 mL of aqueous
3. Anterior chamber—0.25 mL of aqueous
4. Depth of anterior chamber—3 mm in the center.

LENS

1. Diameter of lens
   i. 6.5 mm at birth
   ii. 9–10 mm in second decade
2. Thickness of lens
   i. 3.5 mm at birth
   ii. 5 mm at extreme age
3. Weight of lens—135–255 mg
4. Refractive index—1.39
5. Lens capsule thicker anteriorly than posteriorly.

VITREOUS HUMOR

1. Weight—4 g
2. Volume—4 cc, 99% water
3. Anterior hyloid membrane starts from approximately 1.5 mm from ora serrata
4. Vitreous base—4 mm wide, 1.5–2 mm area of pars plana anteriorly and 2 mm of adjoining peripheral retina posterior to ora serrata.

RETINA

1. Retinal surface area—266 mm^2
2. Macula lutea—5.5 mm in diameter
3. Fovea centralis
   i. 1.85 mm in diameter
   ii. 5° of visual field
4. Foveola
   i. 0.35 mm in diameter
   ii. Situated 3 mm from temporal edge of optic disk to 1 mm below horizontal meridian
5. Parafoveal area—0.5 mm in diameter
6. Perifoveal area—1.5 mm in diameter
7. Ora serrata—2.1 mm wide temporally and 0.7–0.8 mm wide nasally
8. Number of rods about—120 million
9. Number of cones—6.5 million

10. Highest density of cones at fovea—199,000 cones/mm^2
11. Each rod—40–60 μm long
12. Each cone—40–80 μm long.
13. Foveal avascular zone—500 μm in diameter
14. Optic disk—1.5 mm in diameter
15. Length of optic nerve—47–50 mm
    Intraocular—1 mm
    Intraorbital—30 mm
    Intracanalicular—6–9 mm
    Intracranial—10 mm

16. **Difference between retinal artery and vein.**

Characteristics	Artery	Vein
Color	Bright red	Dark red
Size	Thin	Thick
Central light reflex	Wide	Narrow
Spontaneous pulsation	Always absent in normal individuals	Can be present in 80% of normal cases

MUSCLES OF THE EYE

1. Extraocular and intraocular muscles of the eye.

Extraocular	**Intraocular**
Superior rectus	Ciliary muscles
Lateral rectus	Sphincter pupillae
Inferior rectus	Dilator pupillae
Medial rectus	
Superior oblique	
Inferior oblique	
Levator palpabrae superioris	

2. Six extraocular muscles—4 recti and 2 oblique.
3. Origin of recti—common tendinous ring (from the limbus) attached at the apex of orbit.
4. Insertion of recti:
   Medial rectus—5.5 mm
   Inferior rectus—6.5 mm
   Lateral rectus—6.9 mm
   Superior rectus—7.7 mm.
5. Superior oblique muscle—longest and thinnest of all extraocular muscles
   i. 59.5 mm long
   ii. Arises from body of sphenoid
   iii. Inserted on to the upper and outer part of sclera behind the equator.

6. Inferior oblique muscle—shortest of eye muscles
    i. 37 mm long
    ii. Arises from orbital plate of maxilla
    iii. Inserted in the lower and outer part of sclera behind the equator.

LACRIMAL APPARATUS

1. Lacrimal gland situated in lacrimal fossa formed by orbital plate of frontal bone.
2. Lateral horn of levator muscle aponeurosis divides the gland in two parts.
3. Upper and lower lacrimal puncta lie about 6 mm and 6.5 mm lateral canthus, respectively.
4. Canaliculi
    i. 0.5 mm in diameter
    ii. 10 mm in length, vertical 2 mm, and horizontal 8 mm
5. Lacrimal sac lies in lacrimal fossa formed by lacrimal bone and frontal process of maxilla.
6. Lacrimal sac is 15 mm in length and 5–6 mm in breadth.
7. Volume of sac—20 mm.
8. Nasolacrimal duct opens in—inferior meatus of nose
    i. 18 mm in length (12–24 mm)
    ii. Intraosseous part 12.5 mm and intrameatal part 5.5 mm
    iii. 3 mm in diameter.

EYELIDS

1. Upper eyelid—covers one-sixth of cornea.
2. Lower eyelid—just touches the cornea.
3. Palpebral fissure—horizontally 28–30 mm and vertically 9–11 mm.
4. Levator palpebrae superioris:
    i. Origin from lesser wing of sphenoid above annulus of Zinn.
    ii. Inserts on to septa between orbicularis muscle, pretarsal skin of eyelid, anterior surface of tarsus.
5. Length of LPS:
    i. Fleshy part 40 mm long.
    ii. Tendinous aponeurosis 15 mm long.
6. Tarsal plates—29 mm long, 1 mm thick.

ORBIT

1. Lateral wall of each orbit lies at an angle of 45° to the medial wall.
2. Lateral wall of two orbits are 90° to each other.

3. Depth of orbit—42 mm along medial wall, 50 mm along lateral wall.
4. Base of orbit—40 mm in width, 35 mm in height.
5. Volume of orbit—29 mL.
6. Ratio between volume of orbit and eyeball is 4.5:1.
7. Optic canal—length 6–11 mm, lateral wall shortest and medial wall longest.
8. What are the lymphatic drainage of the ocular structures?

   The lymphatics of the ocular appendages and conjunctiva follow the given route:

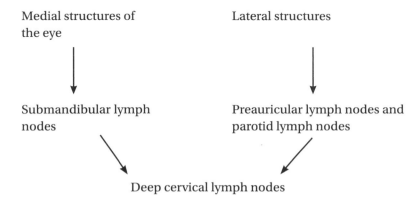

   Medial structures of the eye

   Lateral structures

   Submandibular lymph nodes

   Preauricular lymph nodes and parotid lymph nodes

   Deep cervical lymph nodes

9. **The vascular supply of orbit:**

   Ophthalmic artery: First major branch of internal carotid artery

   Enters the orbit: Within the dural sheath of the optic nerve and passes through the optic canal, below and lateral to the nerve.

   In the orbit: Emerges from the meningeal sheath, runs inferolateral to the optic nerve for a short distance, then crosses over it to run along the medial wall.

   Termination: Just posterior to the superior orbital margin, gives the terminal branches, the supratrochlear and dorsonasal arteries.

10. **Branches of ophthalmic artery:**
    i. Central retinal artery
    ii. Lacrimal artery
    iii. Ciliary arteries
    iv. Ethmoid arteries
    v. Supraorbital artery
    vi. Muscular branches
    vii. Medial palpebral arteries
    viii. Supratrochlear artery
    ix. Dorsonasal artery

MAIN SUPPLY to the orbit and adnexal structures with few supplementary branches from external carotid artery.

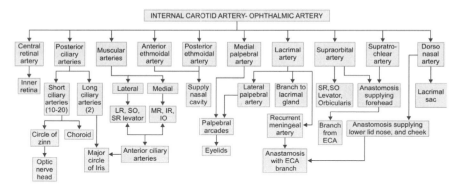

1.4. EMBRYOLOGY

1. **What is the embryologic derivation of ocular structures?**

    Surface ectoderm gives rise to:

    i. Lens
    ii. Corneal epithelium
    iii. Conjunctival epithelium
    iv. Epithelium of eyelids and cilia, Meibomian glands, and glands of Zeiss and Moll
    v. Epithelium lining nasolacrimal system

    Neural ectoderm gives rise to:

    i. Retinal pigment epithelium
    ii. Neural retina
    iii. Optic nerve fibers (optic nerve, optic chiasm, optic tract)
    iv. Epithelium of ciliary body
    v. Epithelium of iris
    vi. Iris sphincter and dilator muscles

    Mesoderm: Extraocular muscles

    i. A part of choroid
    ii. A part of corneal stroma

    Neural crest gives rise to:

    i. Corneal stroma (which gives rise to Bowman's layer)
    ii. Corneal endothelium (which gives rise to Descemet's membrane)
    iii. Most (or all) of sclera
    iv. Trabecular structures
    v. Uveal pigment cells
    vi. Uveal connective tissue
    vii. Ciliary muscle
    viii. Meninges of optic nerve
    ix. Vascular pericytes.

1.5. PHARMACOLOGY

ANTI-INFECTIVE DOSAGE

ANTIBIOTICS

TOPICAL

Cefazolin	- 5%
Ceftriaxone	- 10%
Penicillin	- 100,000 units/mL
Ticarcillin	- 0.6%
Ciprofloxacin	- 0.3%
Ofloxacin	- 0.3%
Moxifloxacin	- 0.5%
Gatifloxacin	- 0.3%
Polymyxin B	- 50,000 units/mL
Vancomycin	- 2.5–5%
Tobramycin	- 1–1.4%
Gentamicin	- 0.3–1.4%
Amikacin	-1–2.5%
Chloramphenicol	- 0.5%

FORTIFIED TOPICAL

Cefazolin	- 50 mg/mL or 133 mg/mL
Ceftriaxone	- 50 mg/mL
Cefamandole	- 50 mg/mL
Penicillin	- 1,00,000 units/mL
Methicillin	- 50 mg/mL
Ampicillin	- 50 mg/mL
Moxalactam	- 50 mg/mL
Carbenicillin	- 4 mg/mL
Ticarcillin	- 6 mg/mL
Bacitracin	- 10,000 units/mL
Polymyxin	- 50,000 units/mL
Vancomycin	- 50 mg/mL or 25 mg/mL
Gentamicin	- 14 mg/mL or 20 mg/mL
Tobramycin	- 14 mg/mL
Amikacin	- 10 mg/mL
Chloramphenicol	- 5 mg/mL

SUBCONJUNCTIVAL

Cefazolin	- 100 mg
Ceftriaxone	- 100 mg
Penicillin	- 0.5 million units

Polymyxin B	- 10–25 mg
Vancomycin	- 25 mg
Tobramycin	- 20–40 mg
Gentamicin	- 20–40 mg
Amikacin	- 25–50 mg
Chloramphenicol	- 100 mg

INTRAVITREAL

Cefazolin	- 2.25 mg/0.1mL
Ceftriaxone	- 3 mg
Penicillin	- 1000–5000/unit
Ciprofloxacin	- 0.1 mg
Ofloxacin	- 0.1 mg
Vancomycin	- 1 mg/0.1 mL
Tobramycin	- 0.2 mg/0.1 mL
Gentamicin	- 0.1 mg/0.1 mL
Amikacin	- 0.2–0.4 mg/0.08 mL

INTRAVITREAL INJECTION

VANCOMYCIN (1 mg in 0.1 mL)

– 500 mg powder—add 10 mL of Ringer lactate (RL) → 50 mg/mL
– 2 mL of above and add 8 mL of RL → 10 mg/mL
– Take 0.1 mL of above for injection → 1 mg in 0.1 mL

CEFAZOLIN (2.25 mg in 0.1 mL)

– 500 mg powder—add 10 mL of RL → 50 mg/mL
– 1 mL of above and add 1.2 mL of RL → 22.7 mg/mL
– Take 0.1 mL of above → 2.27 mg

CEFTAZIDIME (2.25 mg in 0.1 mL)

– 500 mg powder—add 10 mL of RL → 50 mg/mL
– 1 mL of above and add 1.2 mL of RL → 22.7 mg/mL
– Take 0.1 mL of above → 22.7 mg

AMIKACIN (0.4 mg in 0.1 mL)

– Use 100 mg vials   Take 0.8 mL of drug (40 mg)
– Add 9.2 mL of RL   (40 mg in 10 mL)
– Take 0.1 mL   0.4 mg in 0.1 mL

AMPHOTERICIN B (0.005–0.01 mg)

– 50 mg vial   Add 10 mL of water (5 mg/mL)
– Take 1 mL of above   Add 10 mL of water (0.5 mg/ mL)
– Take 1 mL of above   Add 10 mL of water (0.1 mg/ mL)
– Inject 0.1 mL of above (0.01 mg/ mL)

ANTIFUNGAL

Amphotericin B	- 1–10 mg/ mL drops, 2.5% ointment
Natamycin	- 5% suspension
Miconazole	- 1% drops, 2% ointment
Ketoconazole	- 1.5%
Fluconazole	- 0.2–2%
Flucytosine	- 1%

ANTIVIRAL

5-iodo-2-deoxyuridine	- 0.1% drops, 0.5% ointment
Trifluorothymidine	- 1% drops
Adenine arabinoside	- 3% E/o
Acyclovir	- 3% E/o

ANTI-INFLAMMATORY DRUGS

I. **Nonsteroidal anti-inflammatory drugs**

   A. *Topical*

	Generic name	Concentration (%)	Normal dosage
1.	Ketorolac tromethamine	0.5%	qid
2.	Flurbiprofen	0.03%	tid to qid
3.	Diclofenac sodium	0.1%	qid
4.	Indomethacin	1%	4–6 times/day
5.	Suprofen	1%	qid

   B. *Systemic*

	Generic name	Concentration (%)	Normal dosage
1.	Aspirin	300–600 mg	bd,tds,qid
2.	Acetaminophen	325 mg, 500 mg	bd,tds,qid
3.	Phenylbutazone	100 mg	tds to qid
4.	Oxyphenbutazone	100 mg	tds to qid
5.	Indomethacin	50 mg	tds
6.	Diclofenac sodium	25 mg, 50 mg	bd,tds,qid
7.	Ibuprofen	300–800 mg	tds,qid
8.	Ketoprofen	25 mg, 50 mg, 75 mg	tds,qid
9.	Flurbiprofen	500 mg	bd,tds
	Generic name	Concentration (%)	Normal dosage
10.	Naproxen	250 mg, 500 mg	bd,tds,qid
11.	Etodolac	200 mg, 300 mg	bd,tds,qid
12.	Ketorolac tromethamine	10 mg	qid

II. Corticosteroids

A. *Topical*

	Generic name	Concentration (%)
1.	Prednisolone acetate suspension	1%
2.	Prednisolone sodium phosphate solution	1%
3.	Fluorometholone suspension & ointment	0.1%
4.	Dexamethasone phosphate solution	0.1%
5.	Dexamethasone phosphate ointment	0.05%
6.	Hydrocortisone acetate suspension	0.5%
7.	Hydrocortisone acetate solution	0.2%
8.	Hydrocortisone acetate ointment	1.5%
9.	Betamethasone sodium phosphate solution	0.1%
10.	Betamethasone sodium phosphate ointment	0.1%
11.	Loteprednol etabonate	0.5% or 0.2%
12.	Rimexalone	1%
13.	Medrysone	1%

B. *Periocular*

1.	Methylprednisolone acetate (Depo-Medrol)	Depot preparation
2.	Triamcinolone acetonide (Kenalog)	Depot preparation
3.	Triamcinolone diacetate (Aristocort)	Depot preparation
4.	Hydrocortisone sodium succinate (Solu-cortef)	Solution
5.	Betamethasone (Celestone)	Solution

C. *Intraocular*

1.	Triamcinolone acetonide	4 mg in 0.1 mL
2.	Flucinolone acetonide	Slow release implants
3.	Dexamethasone	Slow release implants

D. *Systemic*

i. Oral

1.	Prednisolone (5 or 25 mg tablet)	1–2 mg/kg/day

ii. Intravenous

1.	Prednisolone	1–1.5 mg/kg/day
2.	Triamcinolone	
3.	Dexamethasone	200 mg/day
4.	Methylprednisolone	250–1000 mg in 100 mL Normal saline for 3 days

III. Immunomodulators
A. *Antimetabolites*

1.	Methotrexate	7.5–25 mg/week
2.	Azathioprine	100–250 mg/day
3.	Mycophenolate mofetil	1–3 g/day

B. Inhibitors of T-cell lymphocytes:
i. Oral

1.	Cyclosporine	2.5–5 mg/kg/day
2.	Tacrolimus	0.1–0.2 mg/kg/day

ii. Intravenous

1.	Sirolimus	Loading dose 6 mg/day, Maintenance dose 4 mg/day

C. Alkylating agents

1.	Cyclophosphamide	1–2 mg/day
2.	Chlorambucil	2–12 mg/day

ANTIGLAUCOMA MEDICATIONS
I. Cholinergic drugs
A. *Parasympathomimetics*

	Generic name	Concentration (%)	Normal dosage
1.	Pilocarpine	2%	od to qid
2.	Carbachol	0.75%, 1.5%, 2.25%, 3%	up to tid

B. *Anticholinesterases*

	Generic name	Concentration (%)	Normal dosage
1.	Echothiophate iodide	0.03%, 0.06%, 0.125%, 0.25%	od to bd
2.	Physostigmine	0.25%	od to tid
3	Demecarium	0.125%, 0.25%	bd

II. Adrenergic agents
A. *Sympathomimetics*
i. Nonselective

	Generic name	Concentration (%)	Normal dosage
1.	Epinephrine	0.25%, 0.5%, 1%, 2%	od to bd
2.	Dipivefrin	0.1%	bd

ii. **Selective (alpha 2 agonists)**

	Generic name	Concentration (%)	Normal dosage
1.	Brimonidine	0.2%	bd
2.	Apraclonidine	1%	od

B. *Beta-blockers*

   i. **Nonselective**

	Generic name	Concentration (%)	Normal dosage
1.	Timolol	0.5%	bd
2.	Carteolol	1%, 2%	bd
3	Levobunolol	0.5%	od
4	Metipranolol	0.1%, 0.3%	bd

   ii. **Selective**

	Generic name	Concentration (%)	Normal dosage
1.	Betaxolol	0.5%	bd

   iii. **Prostaglandin analogs**

	Generic name	Concentration (%)	Normal dosage
1.	Latanoprost	0.005%	od
2.	Travoprost	0.004%	od
3.	Bimatoprost	0.03%	od
4.	Tafluprost	0.0015%	od
5.	Unoprostone	0.12%	od

   iv. **Carbonic anhydrase inhibitors**

   a. *Topical*

	Generic name	Concentration (%)	Normal dosage
1.	Dorzolamide	2%	bd or tid
2.	Brinzolamide	1%	bd or tid

   b. *Systemic*

	Generic name	Concentration (%)	Normal dosage
1.	Acetazolamide	250 mg	bd to qid (available as tablet, sustained release capsule and powder for injection)
2.	Dichlorphenamide	50 mg	bd to tid
3.	Methazolamide	50 mg	bd to tid

v. **Hyperosmotic agents**
   a. *Oral:*

	Generic name	Concentration (%)	Normal dosage
1.	Glycerol	50%	2 mL/kg body wt
2.	Isosorbide	45%	2 mL/kg body wt

   b. *Intravenous:*

	Generic name	Concentration (%)	Normal dosage
1.	Mannitol	20%	5 mL/kg body wt over 30–60 minutes
2.	Urea	45%	

vi. **Neuroprotectors (Experimental)**
   a. NMDA receptor antagonists:
      1. Memantine
   b. Nitric oxide synthase inhibitors:
      1. Aminoguanidine
   c. Beta 2 adrenergic agonists:
      1. Brimonidine
   d. Calcium channel blocker:
      1. Nimodipine
   e. Neurotrophic factors:
      1. Neurotrophin 3
   f. Apoptosis inhibitors:
      1. Cytochrome C release inhibitors
      2. Caspase inhibitors
   g. Reactive oxygen species scavenger.

NEWER OCULAR HYPOTENSIVE AGENTS (The dosages of these drugs have not been given since it is currently experimental in nature)

I. **Natural products**
   A. Cannabinoids
      i. Topical CB1 agonists
      ii. WIN 55212-2

II. **Activators of extracellular matrix hydrolysis**
   A. Matrix metalloproteinases
   B. Inducers of matrix metalloproteinases
      i. Tert-butylhydroquinone
   C. Activator of glycosaminoglycan degradation compounds
      i. AL-3037A (Sodium ferri ethylenediamine tetra-acetate)

III. Protein kinase inhibitors
    A. Broad spectrum kinase inhibitors
        i. H-7
    B. Inhibitors of protein kinase C
        i. GF109203X
    C. Rho-associated coiled coil-forming kinase (ROCK) inhibitors
        i. Y-27632
        ii. H-1152
IV. Cytoskeleton modulator
    A. Ethacrynic acid
    B. Latrunculin B
    C. Swinholide A
V. Compounds that increase cyclic GMP
    A. Cyclic GMP analogs
    B. Nitric oxide donors
        i. Nitroglycerin
        ii. Isosorbide dinitrate
        iii. Sodium nitrite
        iv. Hydralazine
        v. Minoxidil
        vi. Sodium nitroprusside
    C. Natriuretic peptides
        i. Atrial natriuretic peptide (ANP)
        ii. Brain-derived natriuretic peptide (BNP)
        iii. C-type natriuretic peptide (CNP)
    D. Compounds that increase natriuretic peptides
        i. Candoxatril.

1.6. MICROBIOLOGY

Culture Media

1. **Classify culture media.**

   Based on the nutrient requirements:

   i. Simple media
   ii. Complex media—added ingredients brings out some special features
   iii. Enriched media—egg or blood is added to basal media
   iv. Enrichment media (liquid media)—to selectively enhance the growth of certain bacteria in a mixed culture
   v. Selective media (solid media)—inhibiting substance is added which inhibits other bacteria and enhances growth of a particular bacteria
   vi. Indicator media—changes color when there is a particular bacterial growth
   vii. Differential media—brings out differential characters in bacteria.

   Based on oxygen requirement:

   i. Aerobic media
   ii. Anaerobic media.

   Based on consistency:

   i. Solid media
   ii. Liquid media
   iii. Semi-solid media.

2. **How are ocular specimens collected for analysis?**

Site	Method
Conjunctiva	Dry sterile swab is used
Corneal ulcer	Scraping the edge and the base of the ulcer with a Kimura spatula
Lacrimal sac	Specimen is collected in a sterile container and processed within half-an-hour
AC tap, vitreous	Specimen collected using sterile syringe and immediately sent to lab
Orbital tissue	Specimen collected in a sterile container and immediately sent to lab

Staphylococcus aureus

1. **Describe the morphology of S. *aureus*.**

   They are gram-positive, spherical, aerobic, nonmotile, non-capsulated and non-sporing organisms.

2. **What are the infections caused by staphylococci in the eye infections of the eye?**
    i. Hordeolum internum
    ii. Hordeolum externum
    iii. Chalazion
    iv. Dacryocystitis
    v. Bacterial keratitis
    vi. Periorbital cellulitis
    vii. Orbital cellulitis
    viii. Endogenous endophthalmitis.

3. **Why *Staphylococcus* infection is considered as a major ocular hazard?**
   Resistance to antibiotics (MRSA) and common disinfectants make them a potential ocular hazard especially post-surgery.

4. **How will you diagnose *S. aureus* infection in lab?**
   Specimen: Pus from suppurative lesion
   Swab from conjunctiva/cornea is smeared for the identification of the organism
   Methods: Gram staining
   Coagulate test
   Culture and sensitivity

5. **What are the culture characteristics?**
    i. Growth in a wide temperature range in solid and liquid media.
    ii. Commonly used media are blood agar, nutrient agar, and MacConkey agar.
    iii. On nutrient agar colonies are large, circular, convex, smooth, shining, opaque, and easily emulsifiable.
    iv. On MacConkey agar, they produce small, pink, lactose fermenting colonies.

6. **What antibiotics are used in *S. aureus* infections?**
   Antibiotic treatment has to be started according to cultures and sensitivity reports. Empirical treatment includes the use of penicillinase resistant penicillin (like methicillin), first generation cephalosporin, etc.
   Drug of choice for MRSA - Vancomycin
   Drugs for VRSA - Daptomycin, linezolid, telavancin, quinopristin, dulfopristin

7. **What are the virulence factors and toxins of *S. aureus*?**
   Virulence factor: Coagulase, protein A, lipase, hyaluronidase, nuclease
   Toxins: α, β, γ, δ hemolysin, leucocidin, enterotoxin, Toxic shock syndrome toxin (TSST), exfoliative toxin.

Streptococcus pneumoniae (pneumococci)

1. **Describe the morphology and habitat.**

   They are gram-positive diplococci, arranged in pairs or short chains, aerobic, facultatively anaerobic, fastidious in growth requirement (growth enhanced by 5–10% (O_2). They are nonmotile and capsulated.

2. **What are the cultural characteristics?**

   On blood agar, they form small round colonies, surrounded by a zone of alpha hemolysis. The colony appearance is described as draftsman colonies. Capsulated strains produce mucoid colonies on blood agar.

3. **What are the ocular infections caused by pneumococci?**
   - i. Dacryocystitis—acute and chronic
   - ii. Corneal ulcer
   - iii. Conjunctivitis
   - iv. Endophthalmitis

4. **Lab diagnosis of pneumococci**
   - i. Grams staining
   - ii. Quellung reaction
   - iii. Culture on blood agar
   - iv. Animal inoculation

5. **Treatment of pneumococcal infection**

   Penicillin is the drug of choice. Other drugs include erythromycin, tetracycline, chloramphenicol

Neisseria Species

1. **What are the *Neisseria* species of ocular importance?**
   - i. *N. gonorrahoeae*
   - ii. *N. meningitides*

2. **Describe the morphology and cultural characteristics.**

   Gonococci—kidney shaped diplococci
   Meningococci—diplococci with flat surface facing each other
   Cultural characteristics: Chocolate agar and 10% CO_2 enhances their growth whereas toxins in medium inhibits its growth. In chocolate agar/modified Thayer martin medium they form 1–5 mm tiny, transparent, convex, glistening, mucoid colonies

3. **Ocular infections of *Neisseria* species**

   Gonococci: i. Ophthalmia neonatorum
   ii. Conjunctivitis in adults

Meningococci: i. Conjunctivitis
ii. Ulcerative keratitis
iii. Endophthalmitis

4. **How will you differentiate *N. gonorrhea* from *N. meningitides*?**

   N. meningitides gives positive reaction with maltose whereas *N. gonorrhea* does not.

5. **Lab diagnosis of *Neisseria* infection**

   Gram staining
   Culture in modified Thayer martin medium
   Serology: ELISA, FIA, immune blotting, latex agglutination

6. **Treatment of *Neisseria* infection**

Meningococcus:	Penicillin
	Chloramphenicol
	Cephalosporines
Gonococcus:	Tetracycline
	Erythromycin
	Cefoxitin
Ophthalmic neonatorum:	0.5% erythromycin ointment
	1% tetracycline

Hemophilus Influenzae

1. **Describe the morphology and cultural characteristics.**

   Morphology: Small, gram-negative, nonmotile, non-sporing organism exhibiting pleomorphism

   Cultural characteristics: Mostly aerobic but can grow anaerobically also. It requires factor V and factor X for its growth. When *S. aureus* is stretched across the blood agar plate inoculated with *H. influenzae*, the growth of *H. influenzae* will be large and well developed near *S. aureus* colonies than those further away from it. This phenomenon is called satellitism which shows that *H. influenzae* is dependent on factor V for its growth which is provided by *S. aureus*.

   Other culture media: Fildes agar, Levinthal medium

2. **What are the diseases caused by *H. influenzae*?**

   Ocular: i. Keratitis
   ii. Periorbital cellulitis
   iii. Orbital cellulitis
   iv. Endophthalmitis

   Systemic: i. Meningitis
   ii. Laryngoepiglottitis

    iii. Conjunctivitis
    iv. Pericarditis
    v. Pneumonia
    vi. Arthritis
    vii. Endocarditis
    viii. Otitis media
    ix. Sinusitis
    x. Bronchitis keratitis, endophthalmitis, orbital and periorbital cellulitis

3. **Is there any other importance regarding _H. influenzae_ related to eye?**

Yes. It can penetrates intact cornea

Pseudomonas Aeroginosa

1. **Describe the morphology and culture characters.**

Gram-negative rod, motile, non-capsulated but many strains have mucoid layer; non-sporing bligate aerobe, can grow anaerobically if nitrate is available. In ordinary media, colonies are large, opaque, irregular with distinctive, musty odor.

2. **What do you know about the resistance of _P. aeroginosa_?**

The bacillus is heat resistant; resistant to common antiseptics and disinfectants like chloroxylenol and hexachloroplane. It is sensitive to acids, glutaraldehyde, silver salts, and strong phenolic disinfectants.

3. **What are the antibiotics effective against _P. aeroginosa_?**

    i. Penicillines—piperacillin, bicarcillin, azlocillin,
    ii. Fluoroquinolone—ciprofloxacin, ofloxacin
    iii. Aminoglycosides—gentamicin, amikacin
    iv. Third, fourth, fifth generation Cephalosporins
    v. Newer drugs—imipenem and aztreonam

4. **How will you diagnose _P. aeroginosa_ in laboratory?**

Grows in most of the media like MacConkey agar, blood agar. Oxidate reaction is positive in case of mixed infections. Isolation can be done using cetrimide agar on which only _P. aeroginosa_ can grow. They produce a characteristic greenish blue color due to the presence of pyocyanin, pyoverdin and pyorubin pigments.

Nocardia Species

1. **What are the characteristic features?**

They are weakly gram-positive, acid-fast, catalase positive, rod shaped bacteria with beaded branching filamented.

2. **What are the culture characteristics of *Nocardia*?**

Colonies have varied appearance, most species have aerial hyphae. They are strictly aerobic, can grow slowly on nonselective culture media, on a wide temperature range.

3. **Describe the virulence of the organism.**

They have a low virulence but can cause serious opportunistic infection in immunocompromised. The virulence factors are enzymes catalase, superoxide dismutase, and cord factor.

4. **What is its ocular importance?**

It is the most common acid-fast organism causing bacterial keratitis in India.

5. **Describe about lab diagnosis of *Nocardia* keratitis.**

Specimen: Corneal scraping from the edge and base of the ulcer (without touching the ocular adnexa). Isolation is done using BCYE medium. Serological and cutaneous testing are not available.

6. **Discuss about the drug sensitivity.**

Amikacin remains the treatment of choice. Other drugs include aminoglycosides, sulfonamide, minocycline, imipenem, linezolid, etc.

7. **What infections can it cause in the eye?**

i. Keratitis
ii. Scleritis, sclera abscess
iii. Dacryocystitis
iv. Endophthalmitis
v. Subretinal abscess.

Corynebacterium Diphtheriae

1. **Describe the morphology of *C. diphtheriae***

Morphology and characteristics of *C. diphtheriae* are as follows:
i. Gram-positive, nonmotile, non-sporing, non-capsulated
ii. Slender nods with clubbing at one on both ends
iii. Shows pleomorphism
iv. They contain volutin or Babes–Ernst granules
v. Cells are arranged as pairs on groups. The arrangement being called Chinese letter pattern on calciferous arrangement.

2. **What are the cultural characteristics in various media?**

Media	Characteristics
Loeffler's serum slope	Small, grayish white, opaque colonies
Blood agar	Small, grayish white, opaque, non-hemolytic colonies
Potassium tellurite (selective media)	Black colored colonies

3. **What are the ocular infections caused by *C. diphtheria*?**
   i. Membranous conjunctivitis
   ii. Extraocular muscle palsy
   iii. Ciliary muscle palsy leading to paralysis of accommodation.

4. **Describe about the prophylactic measure.**
   i. Active, passive, and combined immunization is available.
   ii. Active immunization consisting of giving diphtheria toxoid along with tetanus toxoid and pertussis vaccine @ 6, 10, and 14 weeks of life and booster doses at 1½ years and 4–6 years.

5. **How will you treat membranous conjunctivitis?**
   i. Any case of membranous conjunctivitis should be treated as diphtheria with proven otherwise
   ii. Treatment includes
      – Antitoxic therapy +
      – Antibiotic therapy
   iii. Antitoxin
      – Moderate cases: 20,000 units diphtheria toxin intramuscular
      – Severe cases: 50,000–100,000 units—half IM, half IV dose
      – Antiserum instillation into the eye.
   Antibiotics include penicillin and erythromycin to be given both topically and systemically.

Mycobacterium Tuberculosis

1. **Describe the morphology of *M. tb*.**
   They are straight or slightly curved rods, occurring singly or in pairs or small clumps. They are acid-fast, nonmotile, non-sporing, non-capsulated, aerobic bacteria.

2. **Describe the cultural characteristics of *M. tb*.**
   Colonies take 2 weeks to appear. Solid medium most commonly used is Lowenstein–Jensen medium. *M. tb* forms day, rough, raised, irregular creamy white colonies with wrinkled surface which are not easily emulsifiable. In liquid media (Middlebrooke medium) growth begins at the bottom, creeps to the sides forming surface pellicle.

3. **Ocular manifestations of the infection.**
   i. Tuberculous ulcer of lid margin
   ii. Tuberculous nodule of the lid
   iii. Primary Tb of conjunctiva
   iv. Tuberculous dacryocystitits
   v. Phlynctenular keratoconjunctivitis

vi. Salzmann nodular degeneration
vii. Interstitial keratitis
viii. Scleritis
ix. Granulomatous uveitis
x. Tuberculous choroiditis
xi. Eales' disease
xii. Tb of orbital bone.

4. **Describe about the lab diagnosis of Tb.**
    i. Acid-fast staining
    ii. Culture
    iii. PCR-based ELISA
    iv. Western blot
    v. Animal inoculation
    vi. Cell culture
    vii. BACTEC
    viii. Mantoux test.

5. **Describe the treatment of Tb.**
    ATT is the treatment of choice consisting of isoniazid, rifampicin, etham-butol, streptomycin, pyrazinamide. The duration of treatment depends on the primary site of infection as well as the sensitivity of organisms to these first line drugs.

M. leprae

1. **What are the ocular manifestations of leprosy?**
    i. Thickened eyelids
    ii. Facial nerve palsy
    iii. Conjunctivitis
    iv. Interstitial keratitis
    v. Corneal ulcer/scarring
    vi. Iritis, scleritis, or episcleritis
    vii. Chronic granulomatous uveitis.

Chlamydia trachomatis

1. **What are the characteristic features of chlamydia species?**
    They are obligate intracellular gram-negative bacteria
    Three species of medical importance are;
    i. *Chlamydia trachomatis*
    ii. *Chlamydia psittaci*
    iii. *Chlamydia pneumonia.*

2. **What are diagnostic tests for *Chlamydia*?**

Demonstration of inclusion bodies (Halberstaedter–Prowazek bodies) in conjunctival smears using Giemsa stain and direct immunofluorescence

   i. **Cytology:** mixed neutrophilic mononuclear infiltrate is characteristic
   ii. **Isolation:** using conjunctival scrapings, M-coy cells treated with cycloheximide HeLa cell lines
   iii. **Serology:** complement fixation test, microimmunofluorescent antibody test
   iv. ELISA
   v. DNA PCR.

3. **How will you treat chlamydial infection?**

Chemotherapy using tetracycline (in adults) and erythromycin (in children).

Adenovirus

1. **Describe the morphology of adenovirus.**

It has a space vehicle appearance. The capsid consists of capsomeres arranged in an icosahedral pattern.

2. **Discuss about the adenovirus of ocular importance.**

Epidemic pharyngoconjunctival fever—3,4,7,14,21 (types)
Follicular conjunctivitis—1,2,3,5,6,7
Epidemic keratoconjunctivitis—8,19,37

3. **Lab diagnosis of adenovirus**
   i. Electron microscopy
   ii. Viral isolation using primary human embryonic kidney cells human epithelial cells and MRC-5 cells
   iii. Serology—complement fixation test—ELISA
   iv. DNA PCR.

Herpes Simplex Virus

1. **What are the ophthalmic infections caused by HSV?**
   i. HSV keratitis
   ii. Acute keratoconjunctivitis
   iii. Follicular conjunctivitis
   iv. Chorioretinitis
   v. Acute necrotizing retinitis.

2. **Explain about the lab diagnosis of HSV.**
   i. Microscopy—Tzanck smear
   ii. Antigen detection—fluorescent antibody technique
   iii. DNA PCR

iv. Viral isolation—human diploid fibroblast

v. Serology—ELISA, neutralization test, complement fixation tests.

3. **What is Tzanck smear?**

Swab/smears are stained with 1% aqueous toluidine blue 'O' for 15 seconds. Positive smear shows multinucleated giant cells with faceted nuclei and homogeneously stained "ground glass" chromatin.

4. **What are the drugs active against HSV keratitis?**

   i. Acyclovir

   ii. Idoxuridine

   iii. Foscarnet.

Rubella

1. **What are the clinical manifestations of congenital rubella syndrome?**

The triad of CRS consists of:

   i. Congenital heart disease

   ii. Cataract

   iii. Deafness.

Apart from the above, other features may include

Ocular: Glaucoma

                Chorioretinitis

Systemic: Hepatosplenomegaly

                Thrombocytopenia

                Mental retardation

                Myocarditis

                Osteitis

Cytomegalovirus

1. **What are the ocular involvement of congenital CMV infection?**

   i. Cataract

   ii. Glaucoma

   iii. Chorioretinitis

   iv. Microphthalmia.

2. **How will you differentiate chorioretinitis of CMV, toxoplasmosis?**

CMV retinitis	Congenital toxoplasmosis
Multiple foci of involvement	Solitary lesion
Involves periphery mostly	Involves posterior pole
Less destructive chorioretinal lesion	More destructive lesion

3. **What are the features of acquired CMV in the eye?**
    i. Retinal detachment (mostly bilateral)
   ii. Optic atrophy
  iii. Chorioretinitis.

HIV-AIDS

1. **What are the ocular manifestations of AIDS?**

    Anterior segment:
      i. Kaposi sarcoma
     ii. Herpes zoster ophthalmicus
    iii. Herpes simplex keratitis
     iv. Fungal keratitis
      v. Uveitis.

    Posterior segment:
      i. Manifestations due to HIV infection itself—HIV retinopathy
     ii. AION
    iii. Optic atrophy
     iv. Manifestations due to opportunistic infections like:
        – CMV retinitis
        – *Toxoplasma* retinochoroiditis
        – *Cryptococcus* chorioretinitis
        – Pneumocystic choroiditis
        – *Candida* endophthalmitis
        – Acute retinal necrosis.

2. **What are the features of HIV retinopathy?**
      i. Noninfectious microvascular disorder.
     ii. Features include cotton wool spots, microaneurysms, retinal hemor-rhages, vascular telangiectasias, and areas of capillary non-perfusion.
    iii. Most common manifestation is the microvascular changes whereas the earliest and most consistent finding in the cotton wool spots.
     iv. Retinal artery and vein occlusion occurs rarely. Thus a case of unexplained retinal artery on vein occlusions should be screened for HIV.

Candida Albicans

1. **Describe the morphology *C. albicans* and its habitat.**

    C. albicans in a yeast, round or ovoid, producing pseudomycelia. They are normal commensals of oral cavity, lower gastrointestinal tract, and female genital tract. It causes opportunistic infections in human being.

2. **Diagnosis of candida infection**
    i. Microscopy: Wet films
    ii. Gram staining
    iii. Culture: SDA—colonies are creamy white, smooth, with a yeasty odor
    iv. Corn meal agar forms chlamydospores

3. **What is Reynold–Braude phenomenon?**
    It is a rapid method of identifying *C. albicans*, when incubated in human serum at 37°C, *C. albicans* forms germ tubes within 2 hours.

4. **What is the treatment of *Candida* infection?**
    Since *Candida* mostly cause opportunistic infections, eliminating or reducing the predisposing risk factor in important. Local infections— topical nystatin eye drops 5% is used titrating according to response. For systemic infection—amphotericin B, 5 F-U clotrimazole can be used.

5. **What are the ocular manifestations of *candida*?**
    i. Lid candidiasis
    ii. Pseudomembranous conjunctivitis
    iii. Keratitis
    iv. Endophthalmitis.

Aspergillus Fumigatus

1. **Discuss its morphology and habitat.**
    A. fumigatus is a saprotroph found in soil and decaying organic matter. The fungal colonies produce conidiophore from which minute conidia are disseminated. The spores are found ubiquitously.

2. **Describe the pathogenesis of keratitis by *A. fumigatus*.**

Spores found ubiquitously dispersed
|
Accidental injury to the cornea by vegetative matter
or
Cow tail injury
|
Enters corneal stroma
|
Conidia germinate and hyphae penetrates the stroma
|
Tips of hyphae have multiple proteases which facilitates migration of hyphae throughout corneal stroma

3. **What are the ocular manifestations of *Aspergillus* infection?**
   i. Keratitis
   ii. Endophthalmitis.

4. **How will you diagnose *Aspergillus*?**
   i. By the clinical appearance of a fungal corneal ulcer.
   ii. Direct examination of fungal hyphae in freshly prepared 10% KOH mount, periodic acid Schiff, methanamine silver.
   iii. Culturing in Sabouraud's dextrose agar, potato dextrose agar—culture mount with lactophenol cotton blue reveals septate hyphae, conidiophores, sterigmata bearing conidial chains.

Fusarium Species

1. **What are the risk factors for *Fusarium* infection?**
   People engaged in agricultural work are more prone to have infection with *Fusarium* species. Microtrauma to the corneal epithelium leads to direct implantation of fungal spores into the corneal stroma.

2. **What are the toxins produced by *Fusarium*?**
   i. Moniliformins
   ii. Fusarins
   iii. Fumronisins.

Toxocara Canis

1. **What are the definitive and intermediate host?**
   i. Definite host: Dog
   ii. Intermediate host: Man

2. **What are the ocular lesions caused by *Toxocara canis*?**
   i. Diffuse chorioretinitis
   ii. Vitreous abscess
   iii. Peripheral retina and vitreous involvement with vitreous membrane formation
   iv. Posterior pole involvement with preretinal membrane formation
   v. Chronic endophthalmitis

3. **Lab diagnosis and treatment?**
   i. Eosinophilia in peripheral smear
   ii. ELISA
   iii. Histopathology
   iv. ELISA
   v. Western blot
   vi. PCR
   vii. Animal inoculation
   Treatment: Thiabendazole and diethylcarbamazine is effective.

Toxoplasma Gondii

1. **What is the definitive host and intermediate host?**
   i. Definitive host—cat (enteric cycle takes place)
   ii. Intermediate host—man (extra intestinal or tissue phase).

2. **Mode of transmission of infection**
   i. Consumption or handling of infected meat
   ii. Contact with car farces
   iii. Vertical transmission from mother to fetus.

3. **What are the ocular lesions of *Toxoplasma gondii*?**
   i. Retinochoroiditis
   ii. Retinal vasculitis
   iii. Retinal iridocyctitis
   iv. Vitritis.

4. **Lab diagnosis of toxoplasmosis**
   i. Sabin–Feldman dye test
   ii. Complement fixation test
   iii. Rapid agglutinations test
   iv. Indirect hemaggultination test
   v. Indirect immunofluorescence test.

5. **What is the basic pathology behind *Toxoplasma* lesions?**
   Hypersensitivity and autoimmune reaction is the basis.

6. **Treatment of toxoplasmosis**
   i. Sulfomethoxazole + pyrimethamide combination
   ii. Clindamycin
   iii. Atoraqueous
   iv. Clarithrombocycin
   v. Spiramycin (pregnancy).

Microsporidia

1. **Describe the morphology and habitat of microsporidia.**
   They are ubiquitous, intracellular, spore forming protozoans. The spores are double layered with thick cell wall. It encloses two nucleus, a polaroplast, a vacuole, and a coiled polar tubule. This coiled polar tubule is the characteristic feature.

2. **What are the ocular diseases caused by microsporidia?**
   i. Stromal keratitis
   ii. Keratoconjunctivitis
   iii. Corneal punctate epithelial keratopathy

3. **What are the methods to diagnose microsporidia in lab?**
   i. Electron microscopy
   ii. Direct microscopy using Gram's stain

4. **How will you treat microsporidia keratitis?**
   Antifungals like fluconazole or voriconazole can be used. Instillation of 0.1% Propamidine isetionate has been recommended.

Pythium Insidiosum

1. **Describe the morphology and habitat.**
   Class: Oomycota
   Genus: Pythium
   Species: Insidiosum
   i. Mainly found in stagnant fresh water
   ii. It is a pathogen of mammals causing pythiosis.

2. **Describe about pythiosis in humans.**
   Four forms of the disease is recognized:
   i. Subcutaneous
   ii. Disseminated
   iii. Ocular
   iv. Vascular.

3. **What is ocular pythiosis?**
   i. Ocular pythiosis is the only forms to infect an otherwise healthy human.
   ii. Predisposing factors include contact lens use while swimming in infected fresh water.
   iii. It can cause keratitis and periorbital cellulitis.
   iv. Prognosis is poor and majority of the cases may require a corneal transplantation or enucleation.

1.7. GENERAL PATHOLOGY

General Definitions

Hypertrophy

Hypertrophy is the increase in the size of individual cells, fiber, or tissues without an increase in the number of individual element.

Hyperplasia

Hyperplasia is the increase in number of individual cells in a tissue. This growth eventually reaches on equilibrium and is never indefinitely progressive.

Aplasia

Aplasia is the lack of development of a tissue during embryonic life (e.g., Aplasia of optic nerve).

Hypoplasia

Hypoplasia is the arrested development of a tissue during embryonic life (e.g., aniridia).

Metaplasia

Metaplasia is the transformation of one type of adult tissue into another type.

Dysplasia

Dysplasia is an abnormal growth of tissue during embryonic life.

Atrophy

Atrophy is the diminution of size, shrinking of cells, fiber, or tissues that previously had reached their full development.

Neoplasia

Neoplasia is a continuous increase in number of cells in a tissue caused by unregulated proliferation and in some cases failure of mechanisms that lead to cell death.

1. **What are the common fixatives used in ophthalmic pathology?**

Fixative	Use
10% neutral buffered formalin (NBF)	Routine fixation of all tissues (e.g., eyelid, conjunctiva, globe, orbit)
Bouin solution	Small biopsies (e.g., conjunctiva)
Absolute ethanol or methanol	Crystals (e.g., corneal urate crystals)
Cytology fixative (ethanol, methanol)	Liquid specimen or smears (e.g., vitreous, aqueous, fine needle aspirates, corneal smears)
Glutaraldehyde	Electron microscopy (corneal microsporidia)

(*Continued*)

(*Continued*)

Michael or Zeus transport medium	Immunofluorescence (e.g., conjunctival biopsy for mucous membrane pemphigoid)
Rosewell Park Memorial Institute (RPMI) house culture medium	Tissue culture (e.g., orbital humor for cytogenetics or flow cytometry)

2. What are the stains commonly used in ophthalmic pathology?

Stain	Material stained	Example of use
Hematoxylin–Eosin	Nucleus—blue Cytoplasm—red	General tissue stain
Periodic acid Schiff (PAS)	Glycogen and proteoglycans	Descemet's membrane, lens capsule, goblet cells
Alcian blue	Acid mucopolysaccharide	Cavernous optic atrophy
Alizarin red	Calcium	Band keratopathy
Colloidal iron	Acid mucopolysaccharide	Macular dystrophy
Congo red	Amyloid	Lattice corneal dystrophy
Massone Trichrome	Collagen/hyaline	Granular corneal dystrophy
Perls' Prussian blue	Iron	Fleisher ring
Oil Red O	Fat	
von Kossa	Calcium phosphate salts	Band keratopathy
Giemsa	Some bacteria and parasites	*Chlamydia* and *Acanthamoeba*
Grams stain	Bacteria	Bacterial infection
Gomori or Gorcott Methenamine silver stain	Fungal elements	*Fusarium*
Ziel-Neelsen	Acid-fast organisms	*Mycobacterium tuberculosis*

SQUAMOUS CELL CARCINOMA (SCC)

1. What are the sites involved?

   i. Conjunctiva (most common)

   ii. Eyelids

   iii. Lacrimal sac

2. What are the predisposing factors?

   i. Fair skinned individual

   ii. UV light exposure

   iii. HPV 16 infection

3. What are types of SCC?

   i. Squamous cell carcinoma in situ

   ii. Invasive SCC

4. **What are the clinical types of SCC of eyelid?**
   i. Nodular SCC—hyperkeratotic nodule with crusting and erosion
   ii. Ulcerating SCC—ulcer with red base and sharply defined indurated and everted border
   iii. Cutaneous horn

5. **What are the histopathology of squamous cell carcinoma?**
   Histology shows atypical squamous cell (with prominent nuclei and abundant eosinophilic cytoplasm) that form nests and strands that extent beyond the basement membrane into the dermis and incite a fibrotic tissue reaction. Well differentiated humors show characteristic keratin pearls and intercellular bridges (desmosome)

6. **What is the treatment for SCC?**
   i. Treatment of SCC is with surgical excision with adequate tumor clearance
   ii. Frozen section can be done
   iii. MOHS micrographic surgery—involves layered excision of the tumor

7. **What are the variants of SCC?**
   i. Bowens disease—indolent solitary (or multiple) erythematous sharply demarcated patches
   ii. Adenoacanthoma—rare pseudoglandular form of SCC.

BASAL CELL CARCINOMA (BCC)

1. **Which is the most common malignant tumor of eyelids?**
   BCC

2. **What are the sites of involvement in order of decreasing frequency?**
   Lowerlid > medial canthus > upperlid > lateral canthus

3. **What are the predisposing factors?**
   i. Sunlight
   ii. Genetic factor
   iii. Fair skinned individuals

4. **What are the clinical types of BCC?**
   i. Nodular BCC—most common
      – Slowly growing, slightly elevated pearly nodule with overlying dilated blood vessel
   ii. Noduloulcerative—centrally ulcerated with pearly raised rolled edges and dilated telangiectactic vessels over lateral margin
   iii. Sclerosing/morpheic—flat or slightly depressed pale yellow indurated plaque
      – This is infiltrative and extent is difficult to determine clinically.

5. **What is the histopathology of BCC?**
   i. BCC originates from the stratum basale of the epidermis and the outer root sheath of the hair follicle
   ii. Tumor cells have a relatively bland monomorphous nuclei and high N:C ratio
   iii. BCC forms cohesive bands with nuclear palisading of peripheral layer
   iv. In morphea variant, thin cords and strands of tumor cells are seen in fibrotic stroma.

6. **What is the treatment of BCC?**
   i. Treatment is complete excision with surgical margin control
   ii. Margin control is achieved with frozen sections or MOHS micrographic surgery.

7. **What is Gorlin syndrome/Basal cell nevus syndrome?**
   i. Autosomal dominant inheritance
   ii. Defect in tumor suppress gene PATCHED in chromosome 9q
   iii. Consists of multiple BCC of skin, odontogenic cyst of jaw, bifid rib, and vertebral anomalies and keratinizing pits on palms and soles.

MALIGNANT MELANOMA

1. **What are the common site of involvement?**
   i. Eyelids
   ii. Conjunctiva
   iii. Uveal tract

2. **What is the common age group affected by choroidal melanoma?**
   i. Median age group with 55 years
   ii. Males > females

3. **What is the most common primary intraocular malignancy in adult?**
   Ciliary body and choroidal melanoma

4. **What are the predisposing condition for uveal melanoma?**
   i. Fair skin
   ii. Lighter iris color
   iii. Numerous atypical cutaneous nevi
   iv. Iris and choroidal nevi
   v. Nevus of Ota
   vi. Uveal melanocytoma

5. **How does choroidal melanoma appear clinically?**
   i. It appears as a subretinal gray-brown dome-shaped lesion

    ii. As they grows, they break through the Bruch's membrane acquiring a mushroom or collar button shape

    iii. Less commonly diffuse pattern is also seen.

6. **What are the histologic types of choroidal and ciliary body melanoma?**

    i. Spindle cells—tightly arranged fusiform cells with indistinct cell membranes and slender or plump oval nucleus.

      – Consists of a mix of spindle A and spindle B cells arranged in bundles

      – Better prognosis

    Epithelioid melanoma—large pleomorphic cells with distinct cell membranes, large vesicular nuclei with prominent nucleoli and abundant cytoplasm

      – Cells lack cohesiveness and has worst prognosis

        a. Mixed cell type.

7. **What is ring melanoma?**

It is the diffuse variant of melanoma in ciliary body in which tumor extent for the entire circumference of the ciliary body.

8. **What are the important histologic variables associated with survival?**

    i. Size of tumor in contact with sclera

    ii. Tumor cell type

    iii. Extraocular extension

    iv. Ciliary body involvement

9. **What is the most common site of metastatic?**

Liver

10. **What are the genetic predispositions for uveal melanoma?**

    i. Mutations in GNA Q and GNA 11

    ii. Monosomy of chromosome 3

    iii. Trisomy of chromosome 8

11. **What are the treatment options available for choroidal melanoma?**

    i. Brachy therapy—for tumors <20 mm in basal diameter and up to 10 mm thick

    ii. External beam radiotherapy—for posterior tumor

    iii. Transpupillary thermotherapy (TTT)—for treating small tumor when radiotherapy is inappropriate

    iv. Enucleation—in case of large tumors, optic disc invasion, extensive involvement of ciliary body or angle and irreversible loss of useful vision.

RHABDOMYOSARCOMA

1. **What is the most common primary malignant orbital tumor in children?**

   Rhabdomyosarcoma

2. **What is the most common age group affected?**

   7–8 years

3. **What are clinical features?**
   i. Sudden onset proptosis
   ii. Reddish discoloration of eyelid
   iii. Grape like submucosal cluster in conjunctiva (Botyroid variant)

4. **What are the histologic types?**

   Rhabdomyosarcomas arise from primitive mesenchymal cells that differentiates toward skeletal muscle.
   Histological types are:

   i. Embryonal (most common)
      - Spindle cell are arranged in loose syncitium with occasional cells bearing cross striation usually showing frequent mitotic figures
      - Electron microscopy—typical sarcomeric banding pattern seen

   ii. Differentiated (least common)
      - Best prognosis
      - Feature numerous cells with striking cross striation

   iii. Alveolar
      - Worst prognosis
      - Tumor has distinct alveolar pattern

4. **What is the role of immunohistochemistry in rhabdomyosarcoma?**

   Immunohistochemistry is positive for desmin, vimentin, muscle specific actin, and myogenin

5. **What is the treatment for rhabdomyosarcoma?**
   i. Commonly used guidelines well produced by Inter group Rhabdomyosarcoma Study Group
   ii. Treatment comprises of combination of radiotherapy, chemotherapy, and surgical debulking.

1.8. SLIT LAMP BIOMICROSCOPE

1. **Who discovered the slit lamp?**

   On August 3, 1911, Alvar Gullstrand presented the first rudimentary model of slit lamp and explained its optics and refraction.

2. **Who coined the term slit lamp biomicroscopy? Why is it called so?**

   The term biomicroscopy was coined by Mawas in 1925. We call the instrument slit lamp biomicrosope as they identify these basic components:

   Slit lamp—focal narrow beam of light

   Microscope—for stereoscopic magnified observation

   Biomicroscopy—as it is helpful in examination of living eye

3. **List the various steps for carrying out the slit lamp examination.**
   i. Examination should be carried out in a semi-dark room so that the examiner's eyes are partially dark adapted.
   ii. Both the patient and the examiner must be seated in comfortable adjustable chairs.
   iii. Slit lamp table—must be stable and flat so that the slit lamp does not slide during the examination and the table should be mounted on a swinging arm or rolling table so that it is adjustable in height.
   iv. Adjust the patients chair high enough so that the patient naturally leans forward with the chin and forehead pressed firmly against the chinrest and headrest without stretching.
   v. With the patients' forehead and chin firmly in place the height of the chinrest can be raised or lowered by means of a nearby knob. In this way the patients' eye is brought level with the black demarcation line on one of the supporting rods of the patient positioning frame just below the level of forehead strap.
   vi. Adjust the settings on the slit lamp so that the patient is not initially subjected to uncomfortably bright light when the instrument is turned on. This can be accomplished by setting the instrument to provide a very narrow beam of light or by diminishing the light source if it is to provide diffuse illumination.
   vii. Oculars of the slit lamp are to be adjusted for the examiners interpupillary distance.

4. **What are the basic principles of slit lamp illumination?**

   There are three specific principles of slit lamp illumination:
   i. Focal illumination
   ii. Oblique illumination
   iii. Optical section

5. **Describe the principles.**

    i. Focal illumination—achieved by narrowing the slit beam horizontally or vertically. It permits isolation of specific areas of cornea for observation without extraneous light outside area of examination.

    ii. Oblique illumination—light beam is projected from an oblique angle. It is useful for detecting and examining findings in different layers of the cornea.

    iii. Optical section—this is the most important and unique feature of slit lamp achieved by making a narrow slit beam. Uses include determining depth or elevation of a defect in cornea, conjunctiva, or locating the depth of opacity within the lens, etc.

6. **What are the types of illumination used for examination?**

The different illumination in the sequence in which they are used are:

    i. Diffuse illumination

    ii. Sclerotic scatter

    iii. Direct focal illumination

    iv. Broad tangential illumination

    v. Proximal (indirect) illumination

    vi. Retroillumination from the iris
        – Direct
        – Indirect

    vii. Retroillumination from the fundus

    viii. Specular reflection

7. **What is meant by diffuse illumination?**

Diffuse illumination—also known as wide beam illumination.

    i. Principle—a wide unnarrowed beam of light is directed at the cornea from an angle of approximately 15–45°

    ii. Settings—microscope is positioned directly in front of the eye and focused on the anterior surface of the cornea
        – Magnification used is low to medium
        – Illumination is kept at medium to high

    iii. Uses
        – Gross inspection of any corneal scar, irregularities of lid, tear debris, etc.—mainly for obtaining an overview of ocular surface tissues (e.g. bulbar and palpebral conjunctiva)
      – It can be used with cobalt blue or red free filters.
      Cobalt blue—introduction of cobalt filter without fluorescein will cause corneal iron rings to appear black, so is useful in detecting subtle Fleischner ring in early keratoconus. The cobalt blue filter produces blue light in which the fluorescent dye fluoresces with yellow green color used for evaluating fluorescein staining of ocular surface tissues or the tear film or during Goldmann applanation tonometry.

Red free filter—produces light-green light for evaluation of rose Bengal Staining. Also used to evaluate nerve fiber layer.

8. **What is sclerotic scatter?**

i. Principle—the optical principle is based on fiberoptics—the total internal reflection of light
   - The slit beam is directed at the limbus. The opaque sclera scatters the light and some of the light is directed into the stroma where it travels through the entire cornea by repeatedly reflecting from its anterior and posterior surfaces.
   - In normal cornea—it creates a glowing limbal halo but no stromal opacity is visible.
   - When opacity is present—the internally reflected light is scattered back to the observer outlining the pattern as in Reis-Bucklers dystrophy.

ii. Settings—slit lamp is about 15° from the microscope.
   Slit beam is decentered if full view of cornea is desired.
   Slit height is set at full and slit width at medium broad.

9. **What is direct focal illumination?**

It is of two types:

i. **Direct focal illumination with broad beam**
   - Principle—slit lamp light is focused directly on an area of interest. Wider the slit beam, less information is presented to the examiner.
   - Settings—slit beam is approximately 30° from microscope.
     Slit height is full and slit width is medium broad.
   - Uses—crumb like deposits of granular stromal corneal dystrophy, stand out in direct focal illumination as they are white, reflect light, have sharp margins, and are embedded in clear cornea.

ii. **Direct focal slit illumination with a narrow beam**
   - Principle—slit lamp is placed obliquely and the slit beam is narrowed. The focused slit creates an optical cross-section of the cornea allowing the examiner to localize the level of opacities within the cornea and to determine corneal thickness.
   - Settings—slit lamp is positioned 30–45° from microscope
     Slit height is full and slit width is narrow.
   - Movement—moving the narrow slit systematically across the cornea allows to view serial optical sections and to construct a mental picture of corneal pathology.
   - Uses—moderately thin slit is used to identify the pigmentation of Krukenberg's spindle on the posterior surface of cornea.

The narrow slit beam localizes

- The net like opacity in Reis–Buckler's dystrophy to subepithelial area.
- Extreme thinning in area of descemetocele in cases of herpes simplex keratitis.
- Focal central thinning of cornea in cases of post keratitis scarring, and keratoconus.

10. What is broad tangential illumination?

   i. Principle—the examiner focuses the microscope on an area of interest and swings the slit beam far to the side at an extremely oblique angle so that the light sweeps tangentially across the surface of cornea. This enhances surface details by shadowing.

  ii. Settings—slit beam is 60–90° from microscope.
Slit height is narrow to one half and slit width is very broad.

 iii. Uses –
- Highlights irregularities on anterior corneal surface
  a. Corneal intraepithelial neoplasia
  b. Sterile stromal ulcers
  c. Calcific band keratopathy with holes
  d. Diffuse punctate epithelial keratopathy
- Highlights irregularities on posterior corneal surface, e.g. folds in Descemet's membrane.

11. What is proximal (indirect) illumination?

It combines features of both sclerotic scatter and retroillumination:

   i. Principle—a moderately wide slit beam is decentered and placed adjacent to an area of interest. Light travels through corneal stroma by internal reflection as it does in sclerotic scatter and accentuates the pattern of opacity.

  ii. Settings—slit lamp is about 15° from microscope.
Slit height is full and slit width is moderate.

 iii. Uses—highlights the internal structures of corneal opacity.
Enables the identification of details within the opacity, e.g. small foreign body within an area of corneal inflammation.
Also useful for observing iris sphincter.

12. What is retroillumination of iris? Give its uses.

Retroillumination of the iris can be of two types:

   i. **Direct retroillumination of the iris**
- Principle—the slit beam reflects from the surface of the iris and illuminates the cornea from behind and accentuates the refractive properties of corneal pathology.

It allows detection of abnormalities not apparent in direct illumination. For example, epithelial basement membrane fingerprint lines
- Settings—slit lamp is separated by 15–30° from microscope. Slit height is reduced and slit width is medium.

ii. **Indirect retroillumination of the iris**
- Principle—the slit beam is decentered so that it hits the iris near the pupil adjacent to the area of interest in the cornea.
  Microscope is adjusted so that the area of interest is viewed at the edge of the path of light reflected from iris (marginal retroillumination) or against the adjacent black pupil (indirect retroillumination).
- Settings—the beam can be decentered to allow viewing of object of interest over dark edge of pupil.
  Slit height is reduced to eliminate background scatter and slit width is narrow to medium.

13. **What is retroillumination from fundus?**
    i. Principle—slit beam is placed nearly coaxial with microscope and rotated slightly off axis so that it shines in through margin of pupil. this allows the red light reflected from the ocular fundus to pass through cornea to microscope.
    ii. Settings—slit lamp is aligned coaxial with microscope, then decentered to edge of pupil.
       Slit height is reduced to one-third to avoid striking the iris.
       Slit width is medium and curved at one edge to fit in the pupil.
    iii. Uses—the following abnormalities are seen:
       - Lattice dystrophy
       - Pseudoexfoliation
       - Keratic precipitates
       - Corneal scars
       - Meesmann's dystrophy
       - Map-dot fingerprint dystrophy
       - Lens vacuoles
       - Cataract
       - Corneal rejection lines.

14. **What is specular reflection?**
    i. Principle—it is based on Snell's law. When angle of incidence of slit beam equals the angle of observation of microscope, the reflected light from epithelial and endothelial surfaces are viewed.
    ii. Settings—beam height is full and beam width is narrow.
       Microscope and slit beam are 45–60° apart.

iii. Movement—place the slit beam adjacent to reflection of slit lamp filament from surface of cornea (corneal light reflex).
Slit beam is moved laterally until it overlaps corneal light reflection. Beam is moved further laterally to edge of corneal light reflection and focus on posterior corneal surface to visualize the paving stone like mosaic of endothelial cells.

15. What specialized examinations can be carried out with the help of slit lamp?

Diagnostic examinations:
   i. Gonioscopy
   ii. Fundus examination with focal illumination
   iii. Pachymetry
   iv. Applanation tonometry
   v. Ophthalmodynamometry
   vi. Slit lamp photography
   vii. Laser interferometry
   viii. Potential acuity meter test.

Therapeutic uses:
   i. Contact lens fitting
   ii. Yag capsulotomy
   iii. Delivery system for argon, diode, and YAG laser as for retinal lasers, peripheral iridotomy, ALT, synechiolysis, suturolysis
   iv. Corneal and conjunctival foreign body removal
   v. Corneal scrapings
   vi. Intraoperative slit lamp illumination:
      There is less risk of phototoxicity because a slit light at 5°, focused on the macula, provides a fixed illumination of 7000 lm, the same as with an intraocular fiber placed at 17 mm from the macula.

16. Describe optics of slit lamp.

Composed of two optical elements:
   i. Objective
   ii. Eyepiece

Objective lens consists of two planoconvex lenses. With their convexities put together providing a composite power of +22D. Eyepiece has a lens of +10D.

For good stereopsis tubes are converged at an angle of 10° to 15°.

Microscope uses a pair of prisms between objective and eyepiece to re-invert the inverted image produced by compound microscope.

Most slit lamps provides a range of accommodation from X6 to X40.

Modern slit lamps use one of the following three systems to produce a range of magnification:

i. Czapskiscope with rotating objectives:
   - Oldest and most frequently used.
   - Different objectives are placed on a turret type of arrangement that allows them to be fairly rapidly changed during examination.
   - Haag–Streit model, Bausch and Lomb, Thorpe model.
ii. Littmann–Galilean telescope principle:
   - Developed by Littmann.
   - Sits between objective and eyepiece lenses and does not require either of them to change.
   - Provide range of magnification typically 5.
   - It is called Galilean system because it utilizes Galilean telescopes to alter magnification.
   - Two optical components are positive and negative lens.
   - Zeiss, Rodenstock, American optical slit lamp.
iii. Zoom system:
   - Allows continuously variable degree of magnification.
   - Nikon slit lamp contains zoom system within objective of microscope and offers a range of magnification from X7 to X35.

17. How to evaluate tear film with evaluation with the help of slit lamp?

Examination of inferior marginal tear strip can yield information about volume of tears. The tear strip is a line just above lower lid. It is normally 0.5 mm in width and has a concave upper aspect. When thin or discontinuous, it is an evidence of deficient aqueous tear volume. The following are the parameters:

i. Beam angle   60°
ii. Beam height   Maximum
iii. Beam width   Parallel piped
iv. Filter   None
v. Illumination   Low or ambient lighting only
vi. Magnification   10–16X
vii. Another feature seen in dry eye is increased debris in tear film. Bits of mucus, sloughed epithelial cells—suggestive of delayed tear clearance.
viii. Alteration in morphology of conjunctiva—conjunctivochalasis.
ix. Pathologic signs of meibomian gland disease—ductal orifice pout or metaplasia (white shafts of keratin in orifices), reduced expressibility, increased turbidity, and viscosity of secretions.

18. How to measure lesions with slit lamp?

   i. Brightness—lowest intensity setting.

  ii. Slit lamp beam—slightly thicker than optical section.

 iii. Illuminating arm directly in front of viewing arm.

 iv. Focus vertically oriented beam on the lesion to be measured.

  v. Vary height of beam till it equals height of lesion. Read the scale.

 vi. Rotate the bulb housing 90° to orient the beam horizontally and repeat measurement by varying height of beam to measure horizontal dimensions of lesion.

vii. The bulb housing may be rotated less than 90° to perform diagonal measurement.

1.9. DIRECT OPHTHALMOSCOPE

1. **Who invented direct ophthalmoscope?**

   Invented by Von Helmholtz in 1850.

2. **Explain the procedure for examining with a direct ophthalmoscope.**
   i. It is ideally performed in a dimly lit room.
   ii. Patient is asked to look straight ahead at a distant object.
   iii. Examiner should be on the side of the eye to be examined.
   iv. Patient's right eye to be examined by the examiners right eye and scope to be held in right hand and vice versa.
   v. Examiner should first examine at an arm's distance.
   vi. Once the red reflex is appreciated, the examiner should move close to the patient's eye and focus on the structures to be examined.

3. **Explain the optics of direct ophthalmoscopy.**

   Principle—in emmetropic patients, the issuing rays will be parallel and will be brought into focus on the retina of the observer.
   Hence, light from the bulb is condensed by a lens and reflected off a two way mirror into patient's eye. The observer views the image of patient's illuminated retina by dialing in the required focusing lens.

4. **At what distance is distant direct ophthalmoscopy performed?**

   Performed at 2 ft (one arm's distance)

5. **What are the applications of distant direct ophthalmoscopy?**
   i. To diagnose the opacities in refractive media.
      – Exact location of the opacity can be determined by parallactic displacement.
      – Opacities which move in direction of movement are anterior to pupillary plane and those behind will move in opposite direction.
   ii. To differentiate between a hole and a mole of iris Mole looks black but a red reflex is seen through hole in iris as in iridodialysis.
   iii. To recognize the detached retina or a tumor arising from fundus.
   iv. Bruckners test: In children, refractive error can be assessed by dialing the lens, the power of which will help us focus on the retina clearly.

6. **What are the different reflexes seen on distant direct ophthalmoscopy?**
   i. Red reflex: normal
   ii. Grayish reflex: retinal detachment
   iii. Black reflex: vitreous hemorrhage
   iv. Oil droplet reflex: keratoconus

    v. White reflex (leukokoria):
- Retinoblastoma
- Retinopathy of prematurity
- Congenital cataract
- Toxocariasis
- Persistent primary hyperplastic vitreous
- Retinal dysplasias
- Coats' disease
- Choroidal coloboma.

7. What are the factors determining the field of vision in direct ophthalmoscopy?

    i. Directly proportional to the size of pupil.

    ii. Directly proportional to the axial length of the observed eye/refraction of the patient. Larger area with least magnification is seen in hyperopes and smaller area with maximum magnification is noted in myopes.

    iii. Inversely proportional to distance between observed and observers eye.

    iv. Smaller the sight hole of the ophthalmoscope, the better the field of vision.

8. What are the parts of direct ophthalmoscope?

    i. On/off rheostat

    ii. View aperture

    iii. Lens power indicator (Rekoss disk)

    iv. Pupil size—large/small

    v. Auxiliary controls—red-free filter, fixation target, slit beam, etc.

9. What is the therapeutic use of direct ophthalmoscope?

For xenon laser delivery.

10. How will you quantify disk edema using direct ophthalmoscope?

The direct ophthalmoscope is first focused on the surface of the disk. The dioptric power by which the disk focusing is clearly noted. Then the ophthalmoscope is used to clearly focus on the adjacent retina. The dioptric power for this maneuver is then noted. The difference between the dioptric powers gives the amount of elevation of the disk, i.e. every addition of +3D equals to 1 mm elevation of disc (phakics) 2 mm elevation of disc (aphakics).

In emmetropic eye each diopter of change of focus is equivalent to an axial length of 0.4 mm or a difference in focusing of 3D indicates a difference in level of 1 mm whereas in aphakics, 3D indicates a difference in level of 2 mm.

11. What are the characteristics of the image formed?

    i. V—virtual

    ii. E—erect

    iii. M—magnified.

12. What are the drawbacks of direct ophthalmoscope?
    i. Lack of stereopsis
    ii. Small field of view
    iii. No view of retinal periphery.

13. What is the magnification of direct ophthalmoscope?
Magnification is 15X.

14. What are the advantages of direct ophthalmoscope?
    i. Safe
    ii. Portable
    iii. Screening tool
    iv. Easy technique.

15. What are the uses of auxiliaries in direct ophthalmoscopy?
    i. Full spot-viewing through a large pupil
    ii. Small spot-viewing through a small pupil
    iii. Red-free filter change in retinal nerve fiber layer (RNFL) thickness
    iv. Identifying microaneurysms and other vascular abnormalities
    v. Slit-evaluating retinal contour
    vi. Reticule/grid-measuring vessel caliber or small retina lesions
    vii. Fixation target-identifying central/eccentric fixation.

16. How do you find patient's point of preferred fixation?
    i. Reduce illumination intensity and dial in fixation target
    ii. Ask patient to look into the light in center of target
    iii. Determine whether the test mark falls on the central foveal reflex or at an eccentric location
    iv. Ask patient whether the fixed object is seen as straight ahead off or center.

17. List the differences between direct ophthalmoscope (DO) and indirect ophthalmoscope (IO).

	Points	DO	IO
1.	Stereopsis	Absent	Present
2.	Magnification	15X	3–5X
3.	Static field of view	2 disk diameter	8 disk diameter
4.	Dynamic field of view	Up to equator	Up to ora serrata
5.	Retinal image	Virtual, erect	Real, inverted
6.	Technique	Easy	Difficult
7.	Illumination	Good	Excellent
8.	Uses	Diagnostic mostly	Diagnostic and therapeutic, e.g. PRP, barrage

1.10. INDIRECT OPHTHALMOSCOPE

1. **Who invented indirect ophthalmoscope (IO)?**

   Nagel in 1864.

2. **What is the principle behind indirect ophthalmoscopy?**

   Works on the principle similar to astronomical telescope.

   The principle is to make the eye highly myopic by placing a strong convex lens in front of the patient's eye.

   The emergent rays from an area of the fundus is brought to focus in between the lens and observer's eye as a real inverted image.

3. **What are the different types of condensing lens used in indirect ophthalmoscopy?**

   i. Planoconvex lens

   ii. Biconvex lens

   iii. Aspheric lens.

4. **What are the advantages and disadvantages of different type of lens?**

   i. **Planoconvex lens**

   Advantage: causes less reflex during examination

   Disadvantage: plane surface of the lens causes troublesome reflexes when held facing the observer, so convex side should face toward the observer.

   ii. **Biconvex lens**—both surface has +10D

   Advantage: either way it can be held

   Disadvantage: reflexes are more as compared to planoconvex lens.

   iii. **Aspheric lens**—lenses of greater power (30D/40D)

   Advantage:

   – Helps to obtain less magnification and greater field

   – Minimize aberration

   – Can be used with small pupil and extremely

   – Complicated retinal topography.

5. **What are the different power of the lenses which could be used as condensing lenses?**

   The various lenses used are:

   i. 15D (magnifies ×4: field about 40°)

   It is used for examination of the posterior pole.

   ii. 20D (magnifies ×3: field about 45°)

   It is commonly used for general examination of the fundus.

   iii. 25D (magnifies ×2.5: field is about 50°)

   iv. 30D (magnifies ×2: field is 60°)

It has shorter working distance and is useful when examining patients with small pupil.

v. 40D (magnifies ×2: field is 60°)

It is used mainly to examine small children.

6. **What is the power of accommodation during the examination?**

    i. The working distance is approximately one-third of a meter. This setup enables emmetropic observer to use only 1D of their accommodation to view the image in the condensing lens.

    ii. Myopes can increase or decrease their plus power to suit their refraction.

    iii. Presbyopes will need the equivalent of an immediate range add or their addition for near.

    iv. Hypermetropes will need their distance correction.

7. **Where is the image formed in IO?**

    It is formed between the condensing lens and the observer.

8. **Compare between different condensing power.**

Features	+14D	+20D	+30D
Distance from eye (inches)	3	2	1.5
Magnification	4–5×	3×	2×
Field	30	50	60
Stereopsis	Normal	¾ normal	½ normal
Illumination	Low	Medium	Bright

9. **What are the advantages of indirect ophthalmoscopy?**

    i. Larger field of retina can be seen

    ii. Lesser distortion of the image of the retina

    iii. Easier to examine if patient's eye movements are present or patients with high spherical or refractive power

    iv. Easy visualization of retina anterior to equator

    v. It gives a three-dimensional stereoscopic view of the retina

    vi. Useful in hazy media because of its bright light and optical property.

10. **What are the disadvantages of indirect ophthalmoscopy?**

    i. Magnification in IO is five times using a +20D lens. This is very less when compared to DO which is 15 times.

    ii. Indirect ophthalmoscopy is difficult to perform with small pupil.

    iii. Uncomfortable for the patients due to intense light and scleral indentation.

    iv. The procedure is more cumbersome, requires extensive practice both in technique and interpretation of the image visualized.

    v. Reflex sneezing can occur due to exposure to bright light.

11. Discuss the relative position of the image formed in emmetropic, myopic, and hypermetropic eyes.

    i. Emmetropia—the emergent rays are parallel and thus focused at the principal focus of the lens.

    ii. Hypermetropia—the emergent rays are divergent and are therefore focused farther away from the principal focus.

    iii. Myopia—the emergent rays are convergent and are therefore focused near the lens.

12. What are the color coding for fundus drawing?

For example:

i.	Optic disk	— Red
ii.	Arteries	— Red
iii.	Veins	— Blue
iv.	Attached retina	— Red hatching outlined in blue
v.	Detached retina	— Blue
vi.	Retinal tear	— Red with blue outline
vii.	Lattice degeneration	— Blue hatchings outlined in blue
viii.	Retinal pigment	— Black
ix.	Retinal exudates	— Yellow
x.	Choroidal lesions	— Brown
xi.	Vitreous opacities	— Green
xii.	Drusen	— Black
xiii.	Nevus	— Black
xiv.	Microaneurysms	— Red

13. How to perform indirect ophthalmoscopy?

    i. Explain the procedure to the patient.

    ii. Reassure him/her of the brightness of the light.

    iii. The patient should be lying flat on a stretcher without flexion or extension of the neck in a dark room.

    iv. The examiner throws light into patients dilated eye from an arms distance.

    v. Binocular ophthalmoscope with a head band or that mounted on a spectacle frame is employed.

    vi. Keeping eyes on the reflex, the examiner then interposes the condensing lens in path of the beam of light close to the patient's eyes and then slowly moves the lens away from the eye until image of the retina is clearly seen.

    vii. Use patients own hand/finger as target. Patients with sight will then use visual stimuli from his hand for fixation in addition to proprioceptive impulse. This is important in case of blind, monocular or uncooperative patients.

viii. The examiner moves around the head of the patient to examine different quadrants of the fundus.

ix. He has to stand opposite to the clock hour position to be examined. For example, to examine inferior quadrant (6 o'clock), the examiner should stand toward patient's head (12 o'clock).

x. The whole peripheral retina up to the ora serrata can be examined by asking the patient to look in extremes of gaze and using a scleral indentor.

14. **How to use scleral indentor?**

 i. It consists of a small curved shaft with a flattened knob like tip mounted on a thimble.

 ii. It can be held between the thumb and the index finger or it can be placed upon the index or middle finger.

 iii. The examiner should move the scleral depressor in a direction opposite to that in which he wishes the depression to appear.

 iv. Should be rolled gently and longitudinally over the eye surface.

15. **What is role of scleral indentation in examination of fundus?**

 i. Make visible the part of the fundus which lies anterior to the equator.

 ii. Making prominent the just or barely perceptible lesions of peripheral retina.

16. **What are the factors affecting the field of view?**

 i. Patient's pupil size

 ii. Power of the condensing lens

 iii. Size of condensing lens

 iv. Refractive error

 v. Distance of the condensing lens held from the patient's eye.

17. **How to calculate the magnification of image?**

$$\text{Simple magnification} = \frac{\text{Power of the eye}}{\text{Power of condensing lens}}$$

If power of the eye = 60 D
If condensing lens power = 20 D
Then magnification = 60/20 = 3 times.

1.11. X-RAYS IN OPHTHALMOLOGY

1. **What is the advantage of X-ray skull in ophthalmology?**

   The advantages of plain X-ray skull when compared to other investigations like CT scan are:

   i. Low cost
   ii. Easy availability and usage
   iii. Preliminary test to detect gross abnormality.

2. **What are the important structures in X-ray skull to be looked for in ophthalmology?**

   Most important structure to be looked for is the base of the skull. In this the pituitary fossa is the most important structure. Other land marks are the

   i. Anterior clinoid process
   ii. Planum sphenoidale
   iii. Chiasmatic sulcus
   iv. Tuberculum sellae
   v. Floor of the pituitary fossa
   vi. Dorsum sellae and
   vii. Posterior clinoids.

   Occasionally the pituitary fossa is deep and extend more in the vertical direction than in the anteroposterior direction and this has been termed the J-shaped sella and has no pathological significance.

3. **When do normal vascular markings of the skull become prominent?**

   Arterial markings in the skull are usually visible as thin wavy lines and may become marked when the external carotid branches supply a vascular lesion like a meningioma or an arteriovenous malformation.

4. **What are the abnormalities to be looked for in plain X-ray skull?**

   i. Fracture
   ii. Bone erosion: Local, e.g. pituitary fossa; generalized, e.g. Paget's disease
   iii. Abnormal calcification: Tumors, e.g. meningioma, craniopharyngioma, and aneurysm
   iv. Midline shift: If pineal gland is calcified
   v. Signs of raised intracranial pressure: Erosion of posterior clinoids.

5. **What are the causes of normal calcification in the X-ray skull?**

   i. Structures in the midline that produce calcification are:
   - Pineal body
   - Falx cerebri
   - The pacchionian granules
   - The labenular commissure.

ii. The normal structures away from midline that produce calcification are:
- Choroid plexus
- Petroclinoid ligament
- The lateral edge of diaphragma sellae
- The carotid artery.

6. **What are the abnormal calcifications seen on X-ray skull?**

Abnormal calcifications seen are:

i. Tuberculomas may show calcification in 6–7% cases
ii. The shape and size of the calcification may be diagnostic as in the case of double line wavy (rail road calcification) in Sturge–Weber syndrome
iii. To position and shape as in the case of supraseller area or speckled calcification (egg shell) seen in craniopharyngioma
iv. Meningioma
v. Retinoblastoma
vi. Pituitary adenoma
vii. Mucocele
viii. Phlebolith
ix. Other lesions are—tuberous sclerosis, toxoplasmosis, oligoden dro-glioma, aneurysmal sac, subdural hematoma, dermoid, cysticerco-sis, etc.

7. **What are the signs of raised intracranial tension (ICT) in children?**

i. There is increased separation of the sutures
ii. Increased convolutional markings
iii. Thinning of the bone
iv. Silver beaten appearance—due to pressure of sulci and gyri
Sutures beyond 2 mm is suspicious of raised ICT and sometimes this may be seen even in young adults up to 20 years. Conversely premature fusion of the sutures is seen in craniosynostosis.

8. **What are the signs of raised intracranial tension (ICT) in adults?**

In adults, there is full ossification of the skull bones and the sutures are possibly or fully closed and so sutural separation does not occur. Similarly abnormal convolution markings are also not seen.

The changes that occur in the sella turcica, constitute the most important signs in raised ICT.

i. In the earliest phase there is demineralization of the cortical bone leading to loss of the normal "lamina dura" (white line of the sellar floor).
ii. This is followed by thinning of the dorsum sellae and the posterior clinoid processes. The dorsum sellae becomes shortened and pointed resulting in a shallow sella turcica.

iii. In extreme cases, the sella becomes very shallow and flattened anterior wall gets demineralized and the floor and dorsum sellae are destroyed.

iv. Alternately, the pituitary fossa may enlarge in a balloon like fashion due to internal hydrocephalus. In such cases the enlarging III ventricle acts like an expanding intrasellar lesions (empty sella syndrome).

9. How is X-ray skull lateral view taken and what are the important structures seen in it?

With the patient erect or prone the head is turned with the affected side toward the film. The head is adjusted to true lateral position with the median plane parallel to the X-ray plate and the interorbital line at right angles to the film.

The important structures seen are:

   i. Sella turcica

   ii. Pterygopalatine fossa

   iii. Hard palate

   iv. Anterior and posterior walls of frontal sinus.

10. What is Caldwell view and how is it taken?

It is a posteroanterior (occipitofrontal) view angled 15° caudal to the canthomeatal line, the nose, and forehead touching the X-ray film, with orbitomeatal line perpendicular to the film. It is the best view for frontal sinus.

It shows:

   i. Shape and size of the orbits

   ii. Superior orbital fissure

   iii. Floor of the sella

   iv. Lamina papyracea.

11. What is Water's view and the structures seen on it?

It is a posteroanterior (occipitomental) view inclined with the tragocanthal line forming an angle of 37° with central ray, and the X-ray plate touching the chin.

It is the best view for maxillary sinus. It shows:

   i. Roof of the orbit

   ii. Superior and inferior orbital rims

   iii. Maxillary antrum

   iv. Ethmoidal air cells.

12. What is base view and the structures seen on it?

   i. Submentovertical view.

   ii. With the patient erect or supine, the head is hyperextended touching the vertex to the couch and shoulders raised. The film is placed lengthwise with its lower border just below the occipital protuberance. The baseline and the film are parallel. The central ray passes submentally and perpendicular to the X-ray plate and the tragocanthal line.

iii. Structures seen on it are:
  - Anterior wall of middle cranial fossa
  - Posterior wall of maxillary antrum
  - Basal foramina
  - Petrous temporal bones
  - Posterior wall of orbit
  - Foramen ovale and spinosum.

13. What is Rheese view and the structures seen on it?

i. In posteroanterior position, chin is raised till orbitomeatal line is 40° to the film. Then the head is rotated 40° away from the side to be X-rayed.

ii. Also called the optic foramen view as it shows:
  - Optic foramen
  - Superior orbital fissure
  - Lacrimal fossa.

14. What is Towne's projection and the structures seen on it?

i. In supine position the canthomeatal line and the median sagittal line is perpendicular to the film (frontooccipital/half axial).

ii. With the patient erect or supine, and the chin well down on the chest, the head is adjusted so that the radiographic baseline is at right angles to the film. The film is placed lengthwise with its upper border 5 cm above the vertex.

iii. This view not used commonly because of increased X-ray radiation to the eyes.

iv. Structures seen are:
  - Infraorbital fissure
  - Superior orbital fissure.

15. What is orbitomeatal line?

It is the line drawn from the lower margin of the orbit to the superior border of the external auditory canal.

16. What is the significance of optic foramen?

i. Seen in Rheese view

ii. Lies in the posteroinferior quadrant of the orbit

iii. Average normal diameter of the optic canal is 6–7 mm (< 2 mm and > 7 mm are pathological)

iv. Both optic canals have to be taken always for comparison. Difference greater than 1.5 mm is significant.

17. What are the causes of small optic canal?

    i. Congenital
    ii. Inflammatory—osteitis
    iii. Dysostosis like fibrous dysplasia, Paget's disease.

18. What are the causes of optic canal expansion?

    i. Raised intracranial tension
    ii. Vascular—AV malformation
    iii. Inflammatory—arachnoiditis, sarcoid granuloma, tuberculoma
    iv. Tumors—meningioma, neurofibroma, retinoblastoma.

19. What are the causes of optic canal erosion?

Medial wall

    i. Carcinoma
    ii. Mucocele
    iii. Granuloma of the sphenoid sinus.

Lateral wall

    i. Pituitary tumors
    ii. Craniopharyngioma
    iii. Roof—tumor of anterior cranial fossa.

20. What are the normal dimensions of the sella turcica?

Anteroposterior diameter: 4–16 mm. Average—10.5 mm
Depth: 4–12 mm. Average—8.1 mm.

21. What is the most common lesion causing enlargement of the sella?

Pituitary adenoma.

22. X-ray finding in chromophilic adenoma?

    i. Enlargement of the sella
    ii. Erosion of the floor of sella
    iii. Erosion of the under margins of the anterior clinoid process.

23. What is meant by double flooring of the sella?

Irregular and asymmetrical enlargement of the fossa mainly in posterior sellar lesions giving the appearance of double flooring on X-ray skull lateral view.

24. How is calcification in sella best seen?

X-ray skull lateral view

25. What is the commonest cause of calcification in midline?

Craniopharyngioma

26. Enumerate causes of calcification in and around sella.

    i. Atheroma
    ii. Meningioma

iii. Arterial aneurysm
iv. TB meningitis
v. Optic disk glioma.

27. What is empty sella syndrome?

It is an asymmetric enlargement of the sella due to downward herniation of the subarachnoid space into sella due to raised intracranial tension.

28. Enumerate causes of enlarged sella.

i. Chromophobe adenoma and other pituitary tumors
ii. Gliomas
iii. Teratomas
iv. Craniopharyngiomas
v. Empty sella syndrome
vi. Arachnoid cyst
vii. Ectopic pinealomas.

29. What is the most common cause of suprasellar calcification?

Craniopharyngioma

30. Name some common views used in orbital diseases.

i. Caldwell's view—supraorbital rim and medial orbital wall
ii. Water's view—roof and floor of the orbit
iii. Lateral view—face and orbits
iv. PA view—paranasal sinuses
v. Towne's view—supraorbital fissure.

31. What is oblique orbital line?

It is a roentgenographic structure formed by junction of medial and lateral portions of the greater wing of sphenoid.

32. Enumerate the causes of small orbit.

i. Anophthalmos
ii. Post-enucleation
iii. Microphthalmos
iv. Mucocele.

33. Enumerate the causes of large orbit.

i. Pseudotumor
ii. Tumors in muscle cone
iii. Congenital serous cysts
iv. Dysplasia.

34. Enumerate causes of bare orbits.

This is seen in X-ray orbit PA view

i. Due to hypoplasia of the lesser wing of sphenoid
ii. Seen in neurofibroma.

35. **What is blowout fracture?**

Fracture of the infraorbital plate without the fracture of the infraorbital rim.

36. **What is the view used to diagnose blowout fracture?**

Water's view

37. **What are the X-ray findings on Water's view in blowout fracture?**

   i. Fragmentation of the orbital wall
   ii. Depression of the bone fragments and prolapse of orbital soft tissue into the maxillary sinus—trap door deformity
   iii. Opacification of the maxillary antrum due to—hemorrhage, emphysema.

38. **What is the most common site of blowout fracture?**

Posteromedial portion of the orbital floor medial to the inferior orbital fissure.

39. **In what view can superior orbital fissure be best seen?**

Towne's projection.

40. **Name some conditions in which superior orbital fissure is widened?**

   i. Pituitary adenoma
   ii. Intracavernous aneurysm
   iii. Carotid-cavernous fistula
   iv. Mucocele of the sphenoid sinus
   v. Backward extension of intraorbital mass
   vi. Forward extension of intracranial mass.

41. **Enumerate some causes of narrowing of superior orbital fissure.**

Diseases causing increased density and thickness of bone like
   i. Fibrous dysplasia
   ii. Paget's disease.

42. **Enumerate some causes of hyperostosis of the orbit.**

   i. Acromegaly
   ii. Osteopetrosis
   iii. Anemia in childhood
   iv. Sphenoid ridge meningiomas
   v. Craniostenosis
   vi. Paget's disease.

43. **Name some causes of diffuse osteolysis of the orbit.**

   i. Hyperparathyroidism
   ii. Osteomyelitis
   iii. Wegener's granulomatosis
   iv. Malignant neoplasms invading the bone, etc.

44. What are the causes of bone destruction with clear cut margins?

   i. Dermoid cyst—most common

  ii. Histiocytosis

 iii. Meningioma.

45. Enumerate some causes of enlargement of the orbit.

   i. **Symmetrical**
- Congenital myopia
- Buphthalmos
- Mass in muscle cone
- Optic nerve glioma
- Optic nerve meningioma
- Neurofibroma.

  ii. **Asymmetrical**
- Hemangioma
- Lacrimal gland tumor
- Dermoid cyst
- Schwanomma.

46. What are the causes of intraorbital calcification?

   i. Ocular causes
- Retinoblastoma—most common
- Meningioma
- Hemangioma
- Phlebolith
- Dermoid cyst
- Cataract.

  ii. Ocular manifestation of systemic diseases
- Toxoplasmosis
- von Hippel–Lindau disease
- Tuberous sclerosis
- Sturge–Weber syndrome.

1.12. COMPUTED TOMOGRAPHY AND MAGNETIC RESONANCE IMAGING

1. Who invented computed tomography (CT)?

GN Hounsfield invented CT in 1972. It was initially known as EMI (electrical and musical industries) scan.

2. What is the principle of CT?

X-ray tube of CT machine emits a thin collimated beam of X-rays
↓
Attenuated as they pass through the tissues
↓
Detected by an array of special detectors
↓
X-ray photons within detectors generate electrical signals
↓
Electrical signals converted into images.

High density areas are depicted as white and low-density areas as black.

3. What is the radiation dose used in CT?

The X-ray dose for a standard CT is 3–5 rads and for high resolution CT is 10 rads.

4. What are all the different types of orbital planes employed during CT?

  i. Axial plane: Parallel to the course of the nerve
 ii. Coronal plane: Showing age, optic nerve, and extraocular muscles
iii. Sagittal plane: Parallel to the nasal septum.

5. What influences the resolution of CT?

Spatial resolution of a CT scan depends on slice thickness.
Thinner the slice, higher the resolution, require higher radiation dose.
2 mm cuts are optimal for the eye and orbit. In evaluation of orbital apex 1 mm slice is more informative.

6. What are the indications of CT?

    i. Palpable orbital mass
   ii. Unexplained proptosis, ophthalmoplegia, or ptosis
  iii. Preseptal cellulitis with orbital signs
   iv. Orbital signs associated with paranasal sinus disease
    v. Unexplained afferent dysfunction
   vi. Ocular surface or lid tumor with suspected orbital spread
  vii. Intraocular tumor with proptosis
 viii. Orbital trauma
   ix. When MRI is contraindicated.

7. **What is Reid's baseline?**

Line extending from inferior orbital rim to upper margin of external auditory meatus.

8. **What view best depicts optic canal?**

The plane inclined at 30° to the orbitomeatal line depicts the optic canal and the anterior visual pathway.

9. **What are Hounsfield units?**

Hounsfield units represent a scale of radiation attenuation values of tissues. The number assigned is called as Hounsfield number. This number can range from −1000 to +1000 HU or above. Higher the number, greater the attenuation of X-rays and higher the tissue density.

10. **What is contrast enhancement?**

A contrast enhancing lesion is one which becomes bright or more intense after contrast medium infusion. An increase in its Hounsfield value is a more reliable indicator of contrast enhancement than increase in brightness.

11. **What are the views for evaluation of bony orbit?**

Axial view: Lateral and medial wall, superior orbital fissure, optic canal. Coronal view: Orbit floor and roof.

12. **What are the causes of enlargement of superior orbital fissure?**

   i. Optic nerve meningioma with intracranial extension
  ii. Carotid-cavernous fistula
 iii. Infraclinoid aneurysm.

13. **What are the causes of extraocular muscle enlargement?**

Type of involvement	Common causes
Unilateral, single muscle involvement	▪ Thyroid ophthalmopathy ▪ Primary and secondary orbital tumors ▪ Myositis
Unilateral, multiple muscle involvement	Symmetrical ▪ AV shunts ▪ Vascular engorgement ▪ Thyroid ophthalmopathy Asymmetrical ▪ Myositis ▪ Metastatic tumors ▪ Thyroid ophthalmopathy
Bilateral, single muscle involvement	▪ Thyroid ophthalmopathy ▪ Metastatic tumors ▪ Myositis
Bilateral, multiple muscle involvement	▪ Thyroid ophthalmopathy ▪ Metastatic tumors ▪ Cavernous sinus thrombosis

14. Which part of optic nerve is readily visualized?

Optic chiasma is readily visualized because it is surrounded by cerebrospinal fluid in the suprasellar region.

15. Which part of optic nerve is poorly visualized?

Intracanalicular portion of optic nerve is poorly imaged on CT due to absence of intrinsic contract material and partial volume averaging from the adjacent bone.

16. What is the diameter of optic foramen?

Optic foramen is about 3 mm in diameter.
Anterior part of the optic canal—vertically oval in shape
Middle part of canal—round; Posterior part of canal—horizontally oval.

17. What are the causes of increase or decrease in size of optic foramen?

Enlargement of the optic canal—tumors of intracanalicular part of optic nerve—glioma, meningioma.

Decrease in diameter—fibrous dysplasia
  i. Paget's disease
 ii. Hyperostosis secondary to meningioma.

18. Differentiate between optic nerve glioma and meningioma.

	Glioma	Meningioma
Origin	Neoplasm of astrocytes	Neoplasm of meningothelial cells
Age	Children	Middle age
Sex	No prediction	More in females
Clinical features	Vision loss ↓ Proptosis	Proptosis ↓ Vision loss
CT scan	Intraconal fusiform enlargement of optic nerve	Tubular enlargement of optic nerve Tram track appearance
MRI	No calcification	Calcification may be seen
T1	Hypo- to isointense	Hypointense
T2	Variable intensity	Hyperintense

19. What are the features to be evaluated in case of orbital mass?

Following aspects should be evaluated on CT to aid diagnosis:
  i. Assessment of proptosis: using a mid-orbital scan, a straight line is drawn between the anterior margins of the zygomatic processes. Normally it intersects the globe at or behind the equator. The distance between the anterior cornea and the interzygomatic line is 21 mm normally. If greater than 21 mm or asymmetry greater than 2 mm—proptosis.
 ii. Size, shape, and site of the tumor

iii. Circumscription of the tumor
iv. Margin of the tumor—smooth (benign) or irregular (malignant)
v. Effect on surrounding structures—fossa formation (benign) or hyperostosis
vi. Internal consistency—homogeneous (benign) or heterogeneous (malignant).

20. Which is the most common site of bony metastasis?

The greater wing of sphenoid is the most common site of bone metastasis in orbit.

21. What are the CT findings in Graves' ophthalmopathy?

Graves' ophthalmopathy typically shows unilateral or bilateral involvement of single or multiple muscles causing fusiform enlargement with smooth muscle borders, especially posteriorly. Tendons are usually spared.

22. What are the factors to be assessed in case of an orbital trauma?

i. Evaluation of fractures.
ii. Number, location, degree, and direction of fracture fragment displacement.
iii. Evaluation of soft-tissue injury: muscle entrapment, hematoma, emphysema, etc.
iv. Presence and location of foreign bodies.

23. Where is "empty delta sign" seen?

Sigmoid sinus thrombosis.

24. What are the causes of ring-enhancing lesions?

i. Cysticercosis
ii. Tuberculoma
iii. Toxoplasmosis
iv. Metastasis
v. Abscess.

25. How does blood appear in CT?

Acute bleeding (< 6 h)—hyperdense
Subacute bleeding—isodense with brain (intraparenchymal changes)
Chronic (> 2 weeks)—hypodense.

26. What are the conditions where CT is preferred over magnetic resonance imaging (MRI)?

i. Acute trauma
ii. Bony lesions
iii. Metallic foreign body.

27. What are all the recent advances in CT scanning?

i. Spiral or helical CT scanner
ii. Three-dimensional CT.

28. What is the principle of MRI?

MRI depends on the rearrangement of hydrogen nuclei when a tissue is exposed to a strong electromagnetic pulse. When the pulse subsides, the nuclei return to their normal position, reradiating some of the energy they have absorbed. Sensitive receivers pick up this electromagnetic echo. The signals are analyzed, computed, and displayed as a cross-sectional image.

29. What are the imaging parameters?

T1 → longitudinal or spin–lattice relaxation.

T2 → transverse or spin–spin relaxation.

30. What is the basis of T1 and T2 imaging?

When the radiofrequency pulse is switched off, the T1 increases and T2 decreases.

T1

   i. Depends on the tissue composition, structure, and surroundings.
   ii. It is an expression of the time it takes for the energy imparted by the RF pulse to be transferred to the lattice of atoms that surround the nuclei.
   iii. T1 weighted images are good for delineating ocular anatomy.
   iv. Contrast weighted images are done with T1.

T2

   i. Comes about when the protons go out of phase due to in homogenicity of the external and internal magnetic field.
   ii. T2 weighted images are best to discern pathology.
   iii. The difference in the brightness seen on T2 images can be helpful in differentiating melanotic lesions and hemorrhagic process

31. List some T1 and T2 characteristics of some common tissues.

	T1 signal	T2 signal
Air Bone Dense calcification	Dark (hypointense)	Dark (hypointense)
Water, edema, CSF Vitreous	Dark	Bright
High protein Paramagnetic substances (gadolinium, melanin)	Bright	Dark
Fat	Bright	Dark
Gray matter	Dark gray	Light gray
White matter	Light gray	Gray

32. What are the strengths of magnets used in MRI?

0.3 tesla, 0.5 tesla, 1 tesla, 3 tesla, and 5 tesla.

33. What is gadolinium?

Gadolinium is a paramagnetic substance (unpaired electrons) that shortens the relaxation time of T1 and T2 weighted sequences. Administered intravenously it remains intravascular unless there is a breakdown of blood–brain barrier. It is visualized only in T1 weighted images appearing bright.

34. What are the structures that enhance with gadolinium?

Enhancement of tissues typically occurs with blood–brain barrier breakdown, which is caused by a neoplasm, infection or inflammation. The pituitary gland, extraocular muscle, choroids plexus, and nasal mucosa normally lack a blood–brain barrier, hence they enhance with gadolinium.

35. What are fat-suppression techniques?

Fat-suppression techniques are applied for imaging the orbit. It eliminates the bright signal of orbital fat and delineates normal structures (optic nerve and extraocular muscles), tumors, inflammatory lesions.

36. What are the types of fat-suppression techniques?

i. T1 fat saturation (used with gadolinium)
ii. Short T1 inversion recovery.

37. What is STIR?

STIR is short T1 inversion recovery. It is considered as optimal sequence for detecting intrinsic lesions of the intraorbital optic nerve (e.g. optic neuritis). STIR images have very low signal from fat but have high signal from water.

38. What is FLAIR?

FLAIR is fluid attenuated inversion recovery. This method eliminates bright signal from fluid, allowing a strong T2 weighted image to remain, which is useful for identifying multiple sclerosis plaques and ischemia. CSF looks dark (unlike in typical T2), allowing bright MS plaques to be visualized better.

39. What is diffusion-weighted sequence (DWI)?

This sequence is used to image acute cerebral infarctions within the first hour of stroke. Ischemia looks bright on DWI. These abnormalities are not detected on other MRI sequences or CT scan.

40. List few indications of MRI.

    i. Optic nerve lesions-intraorbital part of optic nerve and intracranial extensions of optic nerve tumors.

    ii. Optic nerve sheath lesions (e.g. meningioma)

    iii. Sellar masses

    iv. Cavernous sinus pathology

    v. Intracranial lesions of the visual pathway

    vi. Intracranial aneurysm.

41. What are the contraindications of MRI?

    i. Presence of metal (aneurysm clips, cochlear implants, pacemakers)

    ii. Cardiac bypass surgery patients (up to 1 month following surgery as there may be local bleeding at the site of metallic materials)

    iii. Claustrophobic patients (difficult to perform).

42. Differentiate between CT and MRI.

CT	MRI
▪ Better for bony lesions	▪ Better for soft-tissue delineation
▪ Sensitive to acute hemorrhage	▪ Insensitive to acute hemorrhage
▪ Posterior fossa degraded by artifact	▪ Posterior fossa well visualized
▪ Poor resolution of demyelinating lesions	▪ Demyelinating lesions well seen at all stages
▪ Degraded image of orbital apex because of bony artifact	▪ Good view of orbital apex
▪ Metal artifacts	▪ Ferromagnetic artifacts
▪ Axial and coronal images	▪ Axial, coronal, sagittal, and angled images
▪ Iodinated contrast agent	▪ Paramagnetic contrast agent
▪ Risk: ionizing radiation	▪ Risk: magnetic field
▪ Less claustrophobic	▪ More claustrophobic
▪ Less expensive	▪ More expensive

43. What structures are better delineated on MRI than CT?

    i. Distinction between optic nerve and its surrounding subarachnoid space

    ii. Intracanalicular optic nerve

    iii. Contents of superior orbital fissure

    iv. Intraorbital branches of cranial nerves

    v. Lens, choroids, and ciliary apparatus.

44. What is the finding in pituitary macroadenoma?

A classic "snow-man" or "figure of eight" appearance of pituitary macro-adenoma is seen in gadolinium enhanced T1 weighted image as it passes through the diaphragma sella to extend into suprasellar cistern.

45. How do you differentiate optic neuritis and optic nerve meningioma in MRI?

Optic nerve enhancement (T1 with gadolinium) can differentiate between optic nerve sheath meningioma and optic neuritis. In optic neuritis, gadolinium enhancement is transient, remitting in days, whereas the optic nerve enhancement in optic nerve sheath meningioma persists.

46. What is MR angiography?

MR angiography is a noninvasive method of imaging intra and extracranial carotids and vertebrobasilar circulation to demonstrate stenosis, dissection, occlusion, arteriovenous malformations, and aneurysms.

47. What are the advantages and disadvantages of MR angiography over CT angiography?

Advantage: Does not require contrast.

Disadvantage: Small aneurysms and thrombosed aneurysms may be missed.

Cornea

2.1. KERATOMETRY

1. **Define keratometry.**

    It is the measurement of the curvature of the anterior surface of the cornea across a fixed chord length, usually 2–3 mm, which lies in the optical spherical zone of the cornea.

2. **Who first invented the keratometer?**

    Helmholtz in 1854. He called it ophthalmometer. His instrument was made of two glass plates.

3. **Who modified Helmholtz's instrument for clinical use?**

    Javal and Schiotz.

4. **Explain the optical principle of the keratometer.**

    The principle of the keratometer is based on the geometry of a spherical reflecting surface. The anterior surface of the cornea acts as a convex mirror and the size of the image formed (first Purkinje image) varies with its curvature—inversely.

    An object of known size and distance is reflected off the corneal surface, and the size of the reflected image is determined with a measuring telescope. From this, the refracting power of the cornea can be calculated on the basis of an assumed index of refraction.

5. **What is the principle of visible doubling? Why is it necessary to have double images?**

    The image formed on the corneal surface is made to double using prisms. The keratometric reading is calculated by adjustment such that the lower edge of one image coincides with the upper edge of the other. From the amount of rotation needed to coincide the edges, the image size is measured by the instrument, and thereby the corneal curvature can be calculated.

It is necessary to have double images to overcome the problem of movement of the eyes during measurements. If the eye moves, both images move together and equally.

6. **How is doubling achieved in Javal–Schiotz keratometer?**

In Javal-Schiotz keratometer, doubling is achieved by a Wollaston prism which is incorporated in the viewing telescope. A Wollaston prism consists of 2 rectangular quartz prisms cemented together. Quartz being a doubly refractive substance, it splits a single beam of light to form two polarized light beams.

7. **Name some keratometers.**
   i. Helmholtz keratometer (not used now)
   ii. Reichert (Bausch and Lomb keratometer)—constant object size, variable image size
   iii. Javal–Schiotz keratometer—variable object size, constant image size.

8. **What is the relationship between the radius of curvature and dioptric power of the cornea?**

$$D = (n - 1)/r$$

where D is the dioptric power of the cornea
n is the index of refraction of the cornea
r is the radius of the cornea in meters
n is usually taken as 1.3375.

9. **What range of corneal curvature can be measured by keratometry?**

The Bausch and Lomb keratometer measures radius of curvature from 36.00D to 52.00D.

10. **What are the keratometric findings in spherical cornea?**

There is no difference in power between the two principal meridia. The mires are seen as a perfect sphere.

11. **What are the findings in astigmatism?**

In astigmatism, there is a difference in power between the two meridia. With The Rule (WTR) corneal astigmatism—mires will be vertically oval. Against The Rule (ATR) corneal astigmatism—mires look like a horizontal oval.
Oblique astigmatism—the principle meridia are between 30–60° and 120–50°. Irregular astigmatism—mires are irregular or doubled.

12. **What are the keratometric findings in keratoconus?**

Pulsating mires are indicative of keratoconus.
   i. **Early signs:**
      Inclination and jumping of mires (while attempting to adjust the mires, the mires jump. If an attempt is made to superimpose the plus mires, they will jump above and below each other).

ii. **Other signs:**
Minification of mires: In advanced keratoconus (K > 52D), the mires begin to get smaller, due to increased amount of myopia.
Oval mires: Occur due to large amount of astigmatism, mires are normal size and distinct borders. This is also called as egg-shaped mires.
iii. **Distortion of mires:** The mire image is irregular, wavy, and distorted.

13. Give some clinical uses of keratometry.
  i. Objective method for determining curvature of the cornea
  ii. To estimate the amount and direction of corneal astigmatism
  iii. The ocular biometry for the IOL power calculation
  iv. To monitor pre- and post-surgical astigmatism
  v. Differential diagnosis of axial versus refractive anisometropia
  vi. To diagnose and monitor keratoconus and other corneal diseases
  vii. For contact lens fitting by base curve selection
  viii. To detect rigid gas permeable lens flexure.

14. What are the sources of error in keratometry?
  i. Improper calibration
  ii. Faulty positioning of the patient
  iii. Improper fixation by patient
  iv. Accommodative fluctuation by examiner
  v. Localized corneal distortion, excessive tearing, abnormal lid position
  vi. Improper focusing of the corneal image.

15. What are the new types of keratometers?
  i. **Automated keratometer:** The reflected image is focused onto a photodetector, which measures image size, and then the radius of curvature is computed. Infrared light is used to illuminate the mires, as well as in the photodetector.
  ii. **Surgical/operating keratometer:** Keratometer attached to the operating microscope.

16. Name other methods of studying corneal curvature.
  i. Placido disk
  ii. Corneal topography.

17. What are the limitations of keratometry?
  i. The keratometer assumes that the cornea is a symmetrical spherical or spherocylindrical structure with two principal meridia separated by 90°, whereas in reality, the cornea is an aspheric structure.
  ii. The refractive status of only a very small central area of the cornea is measured, neglecting the peripheral zones.
  iii. Inaccurate for very flat or very steep corneas, i.e. effective only for a certain range of corneal curvatures.
  iv. Ineffective in irregular astigmatism, thus, cannot be used corneal surface irregularities.

2.2. CORNEAL VASCULARIZATION

1. **What are the factors that make a normal avascular cornea vascular?**

   Anything that breaks the normal compactness of cornea:
   i. Trauma
   ii. Inflammatory
   iii. Toxic
   iv. Nutritional
   v. Presence of vaso-formative stimulus.

2. **Classify corneal vascularization according to depth of involvement.**

   Superficial: Originates from superficial limbal plexus.

   Interstitial: Derived from anterior ciliary arteries.

   Deep or retrocorneal pannus: Seen in syphilitic cause of interstitial keratitis.

3. **What is pannus?**

   It is growth of fibrovascular tissue between the epithelium and Bowman's layer. It literarily means cloth. It can be degenerative or inflammatory.

   There are four types of pannus:
   i. Pannus trachomatous
   ii. Pannus leprosus
   iii. Pannus phlyctenulosus
   iv. Pannus degenerativas: associated with blind eyes like in bullous keratopathy.

4. **What is micropannus and what are the causes for the same?**

   When vascularization extends beyond 1–2 mm from the normal vasculature. Causes are:
   i. Inclusion conjunctivitis
   ii. Vernal conjunctivitis
   iii. Superficial limbic keratoconjunctivitis
   iv. Staphylococcal blepharitis
   v. Childhood trachoma
   vi. Contact lens wear.

5. **What is gross pannus and what are the causes for the same?**

   When vascularization extends beyond >2 mm from the normal vasculature. Causes are:
   i. Trachoma
   ii. Staphylococcal blepharitis
   iii. Atopic keratoconjunctivitis
   iv. Rosacea
   v. Herpes simplex keratitis

6. **What is progressive pannus and what is regressive pannus?**

   i. Progressive pannus: Infiltration is ahead of vascularization

  ii. Regressive pannus: Vascularization is ahead of infiltration.

7. **How do you treat corneal vascularization?**

   i. By treating acute inflammatory cause if any, vascularization decreases.

  ii. Radiation: Applicable to destruction of superficial rather than deep vessels.

     It acts by causing development of end arteritis resulting from trauma to endothelium.

 iii. Surgery:

    – **Peritomy:** removal of an annulus of conjunctival and subconjunctival tissue dissected outwards from limbus for 3–4 mm.

    – **Superficial keratectomy:** when vascularization is superficial or circumferential.

    – **Argon laser photocoagulation.**

8. **How do you differentiate between superficial and deep vessels?**

   i. Superficial vessels are usually arranged in arborizing pattern, present below the epithelial layer and their continuity can be traced with the conjunctival vessels. They are dark red in color and they branch dichotomously.

  ii. Deep vessels are usually straight, lie in the stroma, not anastomosing and their continuity cannot be traced beyond the limbus. They are pink in color.

9. **How are deep vessels arranged?**

They may be arranged as:

    i. Terminal loops

   ii. Brush

  iii. Parasol

  iv. Umbel

   v. Network

  vi. Interstitial arcade.

10. **What is the role of anti-VEGF in corneal neovascularization?**

The anti-VEGF will act on newly formed endothelial buds without pericytes. These drugs are tried in diabetic neovascularization. In corneal vascularization, once the vessels become mature with pericytes, these drugs are of limited value. Subconjunctival injections are tried to prevent new vessel formation after keratoplasty in highly vascularized corneas.

2.3. CORNEAL ANESTHESIA

1. **What is the nerve supply of cornea?**

   Long ciliary nerve, a branch of nasociliary nerve, which is a branch of ophthalmic division of trigeminal nerve, supplies the cornea.

2. **What are the branches of nasociliary nerve?**

   Nasociliary nerve, a branch of ophthalmic division of trigeminal nerve has the following five branches:

   i. Nerve to ciliary ganglion
   ii. Long ciliary nerves
   iii. Anterior ethmoidal nerve
   iv. Posterior ethmoidal nerve
   v. Infratrochlear nerve.

3. **How is the cornea innervated?**

   Myelinated and nonmyelinated axons distribute radially around periphery of cornea

   ↓

   Enter substantia propria of stroma in a radial manner and branch dichotomously (loose myelin sheath)

   ↓

   Preterminal fibers form a plexus in midstroma

   ↓

   Subepithelial plexus formed

   ↓

   Epithelial plexus formed where the axons are devoid of Schwann cells

4. **Which part of cornea is more sensitive?**

   Innervation density is more at center and decreases fivefold toward limbus.

5. **How much time does it take for nerves to regenerate?**

   By 4 weeks normal innervation pattern is seen, though neural density may be less. Center of the wound is devoid of sensation for more than 2 weeks.

6. **With which instrument can you measure corneal sensations?**

   This can be tested using a wisp of cotton. In order to quantitate, one can use an instrument called esthesiometer.

   Esthesiometer: Nylon monofilament of 0.08–0.12 mm diameter covers 4–10 corneal epithelial cells. Thus, it stimulates one sensitive nervous unit.

7. **What are the neurotransmitters that play a role in corneal sensations?**
   i. Substance P for pain
   ii. Calcitonin gene-related protein
   iii. Catecholamines—loss of this may lead to epithelial breakdown like that in neurotropic keratitis
   iv. Acetylcholine—levels related to corneal sensations.

8. **What are the physiological variations in corneal sensations?**
   i. Most sensitive at apex, least at superior limbus.
   ii. Sensitivity lowest in morning and highest in evening.
   iii. Sensitivity decreases with age.

9. **What are the conditions that affect corneal sensitivity?**
   i. **Congenital:**
      - Congenital trigeminal anesthesia
      - Corneal dystrophies—lattice dystrophy, Bassen–Kornzweig syndrome, Pierre–Romberg syndrome, iris nevus syndrome.

   ii. **Acquired:**
      - Diabetes mellitus: reduces sensitivity
      - Herpes simplex keratitis
      - Leprosy
      - Adie's tonic pupil: lesion is in ciliary ganglion or short ciliary nerves, where the nerves serving corneal sensations and those supplying the iris sphincter run side by side
      - Myasthenia gravis
      - Toxic corneal hypoesthesia: Carbon disulfide, hydrogen sulfide used as pesticides.

   iii. **Physiological:**
      - Iris color—lighters the iris color, more the sensitivity
      - Gender—more sensitive in males than females
      - Eyelid closure: decreases sensitivity. This is due to depressed acetylcholine levels with lid close. This is the reason for low corneal sensitivity in morning after a night's sleep.

   iv. **Pharmacological:**
      - Surface anesthetics like 4% lignocaine, 0.5% proparacaine
      - Beta blockers—temporary decrease
      - Sodium sulfacetamide—30% solution decreases sensitivity
      - Atropine—decreases sensitivity after 10 minutes of instillation This is due to decreased acetylcholine.

   v. **Hormonal:**
      - Preovulatory reduction in corneal sensations due to estrogen rise
      - Decreased corneal sensitivity during pregnancy.

vi. **Mechanical:**
- Contact lens: decreases corneal sensitivity. This may be attributed to the decrease in oxygen pressure at epithelial level.

vii. **Surgical:**
- Limbal incisions—after cataract surgery upper half of cornea may have decreased sensitivity for more than a year
- Corneal grafts: sensitivity may recover within 2 years
- Refractive surgeries: LASIK decreases sensations
- Other procedures: photocoagulation and retinal detachment surgeries
- Trigeminal denervation: decreases sensitivity.

10. When will you suspect corneal anesthesia?

i. Persistent non-healing corneal defect

ii. Symptoms are very less as compared to the epithelial defect.

11. How will you treat corneal anesthesia?

i. A central tarsorrhaphy may be necessary to promote healing.

ii. Corneal grafting will give disastrous results in the presence of corneal anesthesia.

2.4. CORNEAL DEPOSITS

1. **What are the causes of superficial corneal deposits?**
   i. **Pigmented:**
      - Iron lines
      - Spheroidal degeneration
      - Adrenochrome
      - Pigmented (non-calcified) band keratopathy
      - Cornea verticillata
      - Epithelial melanosis
      - Drugs—amiodarone, phenothiazines, epinephrine
      - Metals—iron, gold, copper
      - Blood
      - Bilirubin
      - Corneal tattooing
   ii. **Non-pigmented:**
      - Calcific band keratopathy
      - Subepithelial mucinous dystrophy
      - Coats' white ring
      - Drug deposits—amiodarone
   iii. **Refractile/crystalline:**
      - Meesmann's dystrophy
      - Superficial amyloid
      - Tyrosinemia
      - Intraepithelial ointment
      - Gout.

2. **What are the causes of stromal deposits?**
   i. **Pigmented:**
      - Blood staining
      - Siderosis
      - Bilirubin
      - Ochronosis
   ii. **Non-pigmented:**
      - Granular dystrophy
      - Macular dystrophy
      - Fleck dystrophy
      - Lipid deposition
      - Mucopolysaccharidosis
   iii. **Refractile/crystalline:**
      - Lattice dystrophy
      - Schnyder's dystrophy
      - Bietti's crystalline dystrophy.

3. **Which are the various iron lines?**
   i. **Stocker's line**: at head of pterygium
   ii. **Hudson–Stahli's line**: in palpebral area seen in old age
   iii. **Ferry's line**: at the border of a filtering bleb
   iv. **Fleischer's ring**: surrounding cone in keratoconus
   v. Between radial keratotomy incisions
   vi. Adjacent to contour changing pathology, like in Salzmann nodular degeneration.

4. **What is the reason for iron staining?**
   Tear pooling at the site of contour change will cause iron deposition.

5. **At what level of cornea is spheroidal degeneration located?**
   Bowman's layer and anterior stroma.

6. **What are the deposits in spheroidal degeneration?**
   Protein-rich matrix containing tryptophan, tyrosine, cystine, cysteine.

7. **What kinds of deposits are seen with epinephrine eye drops in glaucoma?**
   Adenochrome deposits.

8. **When does blood staining of cornea occur?**
   It occurs in presence of hyphema due to two reasons:
   i. Rise in intraocular pressure
   ii. Compromised endothelium

   Initial appearance of yellow granules within the posterior stroma is sign of need of evacuation of hyphema.

9. **How does blood staining in cornea clear?**
   It clears from the periphery to center due to the scavenging action of leucocytes which are present in perilimbal blood vessels.

10. **Where is Hudson–Stahli line found?**
    The most common iron line, located in lower third of cornea in the epithelium
    i. Usually run horizontally, higher nasally lower temporally
    ii. Typical bilateral and symmetric
    iii. Altered by various factors like corneal scar and contact lens wear
    iv. It increases in length and density with time
    v. Seen in as young as 2 years and increases with age up to 70 years.

11. **In which condition is Kayser–Fleischer ring seen?**
    i. It is seen in Wilson's disease (hepatolenticular degeneration) which is a condition of altered copper metabolism
    ii. It is seen before any nervous symptoms develop
    iii. It is a yellow-brown or green ring seen in the peripheral cornea

iv. Deposit is at level of Descemet's membrane

v. When chelating agents are given line disappears.

12. How do you differentiate between a picture of arcus senilis and Kayser–Fleischer (KF) ring?

Arcus has a clear intervening space between the limbus and line called the clear zone of Vogt, whereas as the KF ring comes from copper from peri-limbal blood vessels. There is no intervening space between limbus and line.

13. What are causes of epithelial melanosis?

  i. **Congenital:** Nevi.

  ii. **Sequelae of trachoma and other inflammations** due to migration of conjunctival melanoblasts from limbus.

  iii. **Striate melanokeratosis of Cowen:** Normally occurs in darkly pigmented individuals. Pigmented lines located in epithelium extend from limbus to central cornea. Probably result from migration of pigmented limbal stem cells onto the cornea.

14. What are causes of endothelial melanosis?

  i. **Congenital senile degenerative**: Myopia, diabetes senile cataract, chronic glaucoma.

  ii. **Mosaic pigmentation of Vogt:** outlines the endothelial cells.

  iii. **Turk's line:** due to convection current in anterior chamber.

  iv. **Krukenburg's spindles:** accentuation of general atrophic process in which pigment derived from uveal tract is deposited on corneal endothelium and aggregated in shape of spindle. Seen in pupillary axis.

2.5. BACTERIAL AND FUNGAL CORNEAL ULCERS

1. **What are the organisms capable of penetrating intact cornea?**
    i. *Neisseria gonorrhoeae*
    ii. *Haemophilus influenzae*
    iii. *Corynebacterium diphtheriae*
    iv. *Listeria*

2. **What are the common bacteria causing keratitis in India?**
    The most common causes of bacterial keratitis in our country are:
    i. Gram-positive organism:
       – *Streptococcus pneumoniae*
    ii. Gram-negative organism:
       – *Pseudomonas aeruginosa*
    iii. Acid-fast organism:
       – *Nocardia.*

3. **What are the common predisposing factors to keratitis?**
    i. Trauma
    ii. Contact lens wear
    iii. Preexisting corneal diseases—trauma, bullous keratopathy, and decreased corneal sensation.
    iv. Other factors—chronic blepharoconjunctivitis, dacryocystitis, tear film deficiency, topical steroid therapy, hypovitaminosis A.

4. **Which is the commonest organism causing keratitis in patients with chronic dacryocystitis?**
    Streptococcus pneumoniae.

5. **Which is the commonest organism among contact lens wearers?**
    Pseudomonas aeruginosa.

6. **What are the typical features of bacterial keratitis?**
    i. Symptoms are more than the signs and there will be lot of conjunctival congestion, discharge, and chemosis
    ii. Sharp epithelial demarcation with well-defined borders
    iii. Underlying dense, suppurative stromal inflammation.

7. **What are the characteristic features of specific bacterial keratitis?**
    i. Gram-positive cocci (such as *S. pneumonia*) cause localized, round, or oval ulcerations with distinct borders
    ii. Ulcus serpens or serpiginous keratitis also caused by *S. pneumoniae*
    iii. Gram-negative bacilli such as *Pseudomonas* cause a rapid fulminating ulcer with lot of suppuration and discharge and produce hour glass appearance in a matter of days

    iv. *Moraxella* causes indolent ulcers in debilitated individuals

    v. *Nocardia* typically causes a wreath-shaped ulcer which is superficial spreading.

8. **How do you do microbiology investigations in a case of corneal ulcer?**

    i. Proparacaine is used as the topical anesthetic of choice, since it has the fewest inhibitory effects on the recovery of microorganism

    ii. Corneal scraping should be performed along the edges and the base of the ulcer. For example, *S. pneumoniae* is recovered from the edges while *Moraxella* is recovered from the base

    iii. Avoid touching the conjunctiva and eyelashes

    iv. A Kimura spatula can be routinely used. A calcium alginate swab is supposed to give better recovery rates

    v. Smears can be placed on the central part of the slide in an area marked on the reverse

    vi. Culture plates are streaked using a C-shaped design.

9. **Name commonly used stains.**

    i. Gram stain

    ii. Acridine orange

    iii. Calcofluor–white

    iv. Giemsa.

10. **Which stains require fluorescence microscopy?**

Acridine orange, calcofluor–white.

11. **What are the steps in Gram stain?**

    i. Fix the slide in methyl alcohol

    ii. Flood the slide with crystal gentian violet for 1 minute

    iii. Rinse and flood with Gram's iodine for 1 minute

    iv. Rinse and decolorize with acid alcohol for 20 seconds

    v. Counterstain with dilute carbol fuschin (safranin) for 1 minute.

12. **What is the principle behind Gram stain?**

Gram-positive organisms have thicker peptidoglycan layer in cell wall which makes them more permeable to primary stain than gram-negative organisms. Gram-positive bacteria retain the gentian violet-iodine complex and appear purple. Gram-negative bacteria lose the gentian violet-iodine complex with the decolorization step and appear pink when counterstained with safranin.

13. **What is the use of Giemsa's stain?**

Apart from distinguishing between bacteria and fungi, Giemsa helps to understand the normal and abnormal cellular morphology (such as inflammatory cells).

14. Name common antibiotics active against gram-positive bacteria.

    i. Cefazolin (50 mg/mL)

   ii. Chloramphenicol (5–10 mg/mL)

  iii. Moxifloxacin

  iv. Vancomycin (15–50 mg/mL)

15. Name common antibiotics active against gram-negative bacteria.

    i. Tobramycin (3–14 mg/mL)

   ii. Gentamicin (3–14 mg/mL)

  iii. Amikacin (20 mg in 0.5 mL)

  iv. Ceftazidime

   v. Ciprofloxacin (3 mg/mL)

  vi. Levofloxacin (3 mg/mL)

 vii. Ofloxacin (3 mg/mL).

16. How do you make fortified antibiotics?

    i. **Gentamicin:** Add 2 mL of injectable gentamycin to 5 mL of commercial topical preparation.

5 mL commercial preparation has	— 15 mg
Added drug 2 mL	— 80 mg
Total in 7 mL	— 95 mg
1 mL contains	— 13.5 mg

   ii. **Cefazolin:** Add 5 mL or 10 mL distilled water or sterile saline to 500 mg vial of cefazolin to obtain 10% or 5% solution.

  iii. **Vancomycin:** Add 10 mL of distilled water or saline to 500 mg vial of vancomycin and obtain a 5% solution.

  iv. **Amikacin:** Add 10 mL of distilled water to 100 mg of amikacin to get 1% solution.

17. What are the typical features of fungal keratitis?

    i. Signs more than symptoms

   ii. Feathery margins

  iii. Raised dry surface

  iv. Satellite lesions

   v. Endothelial plaques

  vi. Cheesy hypopyon

 vii. Gritty texture while scraping.

18. Classify fungi.

    i. **Yeast** (e.g. *Candida, Cryptococcus neoformans,* Rhinosporidium)

   ii. **Filamentous**—septate and nonseptate

     Septate:

     Fusarium, Aspergillus, Curvularia

Nonseptate:

Mucor, Rhizopus

iii. **Dimorphic:**

Histoplasmosis.

19. **What are the most common fungi infecting the cornea?**

  i. *Fusarium*
  ii. *Aspergillus flavus*
  iii. *Aspergillus fumigatus.*

20. **How to differentiate *Nocardia* from fungal filament in KOH mount?**

Nocardia is slender, branching, and thinner than fungal hyphae.

21. **Name common media used for fungal culture.**

  i. Sabouraud's dextrose agar
  ii. Potato dextrose agar
  iii. Brain–heart infusion
  iv. Blood agar.

22. **Classify antifungals.**

  i. *Polyenes*
    – Larger molecular weight:
      Amphotericin, nystatin
    – Smaller molecular weight:
      Natamycin
  ii. *Azoles*
    Clotrimazole, Voriconazole, miconazole, ketoconazole, econazole.
  iii. *Antimetabolites*
    Flucytosine.

23. **What is the drug of choice in filamentous fungal infection?**

Natamycin 5% suspension (especially for *Fusarium*)

24. **What is the mechanism of action of amphotericin?**

Amphotericin is effective against *Aspergillus*. It selectively binds to sterol present in plasma membrane of susceptible fungi and alters membrane permeability.

25. **What is the dose of amphotericin?**

Topical: 0.1–0.2% hourly initially
Anterior chamber irrigation: 500 µg in 0.1 mL of normal saline.
Intravitreal: 5 µg in 0.1 mL of normal saline.

26. **How is amphotericin available?**

It is available as 50 mg dose in vial. It has to be stored in dark colored bottles to avoid exposure to light.

27. What is the mechanism of action of imidazoles?

At lower concentration it inhibits ergosterol synthesis and at higher concentration it causes direct damage to fungal cell membrane.

28. What are the indications of oral antifungals?

   i. Deeper ulcers not responding to topical therapy

  ii. Ulcers involving the limbus and extending to the sclera

In such cases ketoconazole tablets (200 mg bd) can be used, after assessing for liver function tests.

29. What are the complications of corneal ulcer?

    i. Descemetocele

   ii. Perforation

  iii. Anterior synechiae

  iv. Secondary glaucoma

   v. Cataract

  vi. Purulent iridicyclitis

 vii. Endophthalmitis.

30. What is the difference between hypopyon in bacterial and fungal corneal ulcer?

Hypopyon in bacterial ulcer	Hypopyon in fungal ulcer
Sterile (bacteria cannot invade intact Descemet's membrane	Infective
Fluid, move according to head posture	Thick and immobile

31. Write briefly on voriconazole.

It is a new azole derived from fluconazole. It is active against *Aspergillus, Fusarium, Candida*. It inhibits cytochrome P450 dependent 14 sterol demethylase, an enzyme responsible for conversion of lanosterol to 14-demethyl-lanosterol.

32. What are the signs to know whether the ulcer is healing?

    i. Blunting of the edges of perimeter of stromal infiltrate.

   ii. Decreased density of stromal infiltrate.

  iii. Decrease in stromal edema and endothelial plaque.

  iv. Decrease in anterior chamber reaction and reduction in the size of hypopyon.

   v. Re-epithelization.

  vi. Cessation in corneal thinning.

33. What are the indications for keratoplasty in infective keratitis?

   i. Perforated corneal ulcer

  ii. Impending perforation

   iii. Non-healing corneal ulcer in spite of appropriate and adequate antimicrobial therapy.

   iv. Ulcer threatening to involve the limbus

34. What are the principles in doing therapeutic keratoplasty?

   i. The aim is to control and eliminate the infection

   ii. The infected tissue along with 1 mm of uninvolved corneal tissue is removed

   iii. A peripheral iridectomy is performed

   iv. Interrupted sutures are used so that selective suture removal can be performed in indicated cases

   v. Postoperatively antibiotics are used for ulcers caused by bacteria and antifungals for fungal ulcers. Topical steroids are contraindicated in therapeutic keratoplasty done for fungal keratitis.

35. How do you treat non-healing corneal ulcers?

   i. First step is to reculture to identify/confirm the initial organism

   ii. Recheck adnexal structures, especially for dacryocystitis

   iii. Intrastromal injection of antimicrobials may be tried

   iv. Tarsorrhaphy.

36. What are the results of the mycotic ulcer treatment trial (MUTT)?

Natamycin is better than Voriconazole in treating filamentary fungal keratitis especially for keratitis caused by *Fusarium*.

2.6. *ACANTHAMOEBA* KERATITIS

1. **What is *Acanthamoeba*?**

    It is a freely living protozoa commonly found in soil, dust, fresh or brackish water, and upper respiratory tract in humans.

2. **What are the different species of *Acanthamoeba*?**

    They have been classified on basis of their cyst morphology and isoenzyme into eight species out of which two of them namely *A. castellani* and *A. polyphaga* are implicated in causing corneal infections.

3. **What is different forms/life cycle of *Acanthamoeba*?**

    i. Cystic (dormant) form
    ii. Trophozoite (active) form.

4. **What is the cause of *Acanthamoeba* keratitis (AK)?**

    A. Western world: It is commonly associated with contact lens wear.

    Contact lenses
    i.   Contact lens users (extended wear CL users are at a greater risk)
    ii. Homemade saline as a substitute for CL solution
    iii. CL wears in contaminated waters like swimming with CL

    B. Indian scenario: Commonly associated with contaminated water

    Trauma
    Exposure to contaminated water or soil (agricultural population)
    Tanker-fed water at home, cooling towers, air filters

    Surgery
    Penetrating keratoplasty
    Radial keratotomy.

5. **Why is so much of importance given to contact lenses in evaluating a case of *Acanthamoeba* keratitis?**

    This is because AK can spread in numerous ways in relation to contact lenses
    i.   Use of tap water in making CL solutions
    ii. Swimming in a swimming pool/sea (contaminated)
    iii. Shower while wearing lenses
    iv. Minor corneal damage or abrasion which can happen with CL use itself can cause AK.

6. **What is the pathogenesis of *Acanthamoeba* keratitis?**

    Upon binding to the mannose glycoprotein of the corneal epithelium, *Acanthamoeba* secretes proteins which are cytolytic to the epithelium as well as proteases, which causes further penetration.

7. **What is the presenting symptom in AK?**

The common symptoms are disproportionate pain compared to the signs associated with blurred vision.

8. **What is the reason for pain in AK?**
   i. Radial keratoneuritis
   ii. Limbitis
   iii. Scleritis.

9. **What are the signs of AK?**

The signs mimic a viral keratitis in many ways;
they are classified as early and late.

Early
   i. Epithelial irregularity (dirty looking, stippled unhealthy epithelium)
   ii. Pseudodendrites
   iii. Radial keratoneuritis
   iv. Stromal infiltration
   v. Satellite lesions
   vi. Disciform lesion

Late
   i. Ring infiltrate (oval shaped which is characteristic of this disease)
   ii. Stromal opacification
   iii. Scleritis
   iv. Descemetocele formation.

10. **What are the investigations done in AK?**

Noninvasive:
   i. Confocal microscopy

Invasive:
   i. Gram and Giemsa stain
   ii. Calcofluor white stain
   iii. 10% KOH mount
   iv. Acridine orange
   v. Immunofluorescent antibody stain
   vi. PAS and methenamine silver
   vii. Phase contrast microscope
   viii. PCR
   ix. Corneal biopsy.

11. **How is *Acanthamoeba* grown in a microbiological environment?**

The *Acanthamoeba* organism grows well on non-nutrient agar with *Escherichia coli* overlay. The organism creates a track by feeding on *E. coli*.

12. **What are the extracorneal complications of AK?**
    i. Scleritis
    ii. Cataract
    iii. Peripheral ulcerative keratitis
    iv. Glaucoma
    v. Iris atrophy
    vi. Chronic inflammation
    vii. Vascular thrombosis
    viii. Intraocular infection
    ix. The exact etiology of these complications is not known but likely to be due to drug toxicity (biguanides) or immune response of the body itself.

13. **What are the differential diagnoses of AK?**
    The main differential diagnosis is herpes simplex keratitis (both epithelial and stromal keratitis) and fungal keratitis.

14. **What is the treatment of AK?**
    It can be classified as:

    Medical
    i. **Biguanides**
       – Polyhexamethylene biguanide (PHMB) (0.02–0.06%)
       – Chlorhexidine 0.02–0.2%
    ii. **Diamidines**
       – Hexamidine 0.1%
       – Propamidine 0.1%
    iii. **Imidazole and triazole antifungals**
    iv. **Aminoglycosides (AMG)**
    v. **Polymyxins**

    Surgical
    i. Epithelial debridement
    ii. Cryotherapy
    iii. Deep anterior lamellar keratoplasty
    iv. Penetrating keratoplasty.

15. **What are the goals of treatment?**
    i. Eradication of trophozoites and cysts
    ii. Rapid resolution of immune response
    iii. Prevent recurrence
    iv. Prevention of complications.

16. **What is the mechanism of action of biguanides?**
    Biguanides interact with cytoplasmic membrane resulting in loss of cellular components and inhibition of respiratory enzymes.

17. **What is the mechanism of action of diamidines?**

It causes structural membrane changes affecting cell permeability. When the molecules enter amebic cytoplasm, denaturation of cytoplasmic proteins and enzymes occur. Hexamidine is a faster amebicidal drug than propamidine against trophozoites and cysts.

18. **Which is used as first-line of treatment between the two of the above classes of drugs?**

Biguanides have shown less toxicity compared to diamidines, so biguanides are used as a first line, but both can be combined in a severe case of AK. It is believed to have an additive or synergistic effect.

19. **How would you prepare a 0.02% solution of PHMB?**

The 20% parent solution is diluted 1000 times with saline or sterile water.

20. **What is a major side effect of PHMB?**

Vascularization of the cornea.

21. **How would you treat a case of limbitis and scleritis in a case of AK?**

Both can be a cause of significant pain. It is due to severe posterior segment inflammation. Limbitis is an early as well as a late finding. It occurs commonly. It is treated with flurbiprofen 50–100 mg 2–3 times a day.

Scleritis: less common. Responds well to NSAIDs. If not then systemic steroids are added.

22. **How would you treat a case of persistent epithelial defect?**

To exclude superficial bacterial infection which is very hard to distinguish in presence of severe AK. Topical therapy should be discontinued and non-preserved prophylactic broad spectrum antibiotic should be given to prevent bacterial super infection. After signs of improvement are seen anti-amebic therapy is reintroduced.

23. **How does an epithelial debridement help?**

It helps in the following ways:
   i. It serves as a therapeutic and diagnostic tool
   ii. It helps in better drug penetration.

24. **How is cryotherapy done?**

It kills only the trophozoites but not cysts.

A retinal cryoprobe is taken and a freeze-thaw method is used until a ball of ice forms near the applicator in the stroma. In this manner whole of the cornea is treated. Endothelial failure is a side effect.

25. **When would you perform keratoplasty?**

It is not required in most of the cases as medical therapy would suffice but is indicated in patients with—
   i. Non-healing ulcer in spite of appropriate anti-amebicidal therapy

ii. Corneal perforation that does not respond to corneal gluing

iii. Fulminant corneal abscess

iv. Intumescent cataract.

Many of these eyes will have associated limbitis and scleritis so must be started on prednisolone (1 mg/kg/day) or cyclosporine (3.5–7.5 mg/kg/day) which is tapered in post-graft period.

26. What are the newer modes of keratoplasty useful in AK?

In the initial stages, the disease is fairly superficial and, hence, a lamellar keratoplasty or deep anterior lamellar keratoplasty can be used to considerably shorten the course of the disease.

2.7. VIRAL KERATITIS

1. What are the common viruses causing keratitis?

  i. Adenovirus
 ii. Herpes simplex virus
iii. Herpes zoster

2. What are the types of herpes simplex keratitis?

Primary infection is extremely rare and almost all the cases which are seen are due to recurrent infections.

  i. *Epithelial keratitis:*
    a. Superficial punctate keratitis
    b. Dendritic keratitis
    c. Geographic keratitis
 ii. *Subepithelial keratitis:*
    a. Neurotrophic keratitis
iii. *Stromal keratitis:*
    a. Necrotizing keratitis
    b. Nummular keratitis
    c. Disciform keratitis
 iv. *Endothelium:*
    Endothelitis.

3. What are the differential diagnoses of dendritec keratitis of herpes simplex?

  i. Herpes zoster
 ii. Healing corneal abrasion
iii. *Acanthamoeba* keratitis
 iv. Toxic keratitis due to topical drugs
  v. Contact lens induced abrasions
 vi. Neurotrophic keratopathy.

4. What are the characteristics of a herpes simplex dendrite?

It is usually central, slender, arborizing lesion with terminal end bulbs. The base of the ulcer stains with fluorescein (due to loss of cellular integrity) while the terminal end bulbs stain by rose bengal (due to lack of mucin binding by the cells).

5. How will you treat dendritic keratitis?

  i. *Debridement:* Helps by removing viral laden cells and can be done for dendritic keratitis. It is not of any value for geographic keratitis.
 ii. *Topical acyclovir:* 3% ointment administered five times daily for 2 weeks or topical trifluridine 1% solution eight times daily for 2 weeks.

6. **What are the features of neurotrophic keratitis?**

It is also called as metaherpetic keratitis and is characterized by:

   i. Non-healing epithelial defect after appropriate and adequate antiviral therapy
  ii. Raised margins
 iii. Underlying gray and opaque stroma

   Treatment is to stop antivirals and to use lubricants. In nonresponsive cases, it may be treated with bandage contact lenses or temporary tarsorrhaphy.

7. **What are the features of disciform keratitis?**

This condition causes defective vision and presents as fusiform stromal edema associated with keratic precipitates underlying the zone of the edema. Few inflammatory cells in the anterior chamber may be seen.

8. **What are the features of necrotizing keratitis?**

This type of viral stromal keratitis mimics a bacterial or fungal suppurative infection. A previous history of recurrence of infection and the presence of corneal vascularization will help in the diagnosis.

9. **What are the findings of HEDS (Herpetic eye disease study)?**

   i. Topical corticosteroids given together with a prophylactic antiviral improves the outcome of stromal keratitis.
  ii. There is no benefit of using oral acyclovir in treating stromal keratitis.

10. **What are the features of a herpes zoster dendrite?**

   i. They are pseudodendrites
  ii. They are shorter, stockier, and elevated
 iii. They do not stain with fluorescein, but stain with rose bengal.

11. **What are the features of herpes-zoster ophthalmicus (HZO)?**

   i. *Lids:*
      a. Scarring
      b. Trichiasis
      c. Marginal notching
      d. Cicatricial ectropion or entropion
  ii. *Conjunctiva:*
      a. Ischemia with necrosis
      b. Circumcorneal congestion
 iii. *Cornea:*
      a. Punctate keratits
      b. Dendritic keratitis
      c. Stromal keratitis
      d. Corneal anesthesia

    iv. ***Iris:***
        Sectoral iris atrophy
    v. ***Anterior chamber:***
        Hemorrhagic hypopyon
    vi. ***Retina:***
        a. Focal choroiditis
        b. Occlusive retinal vasculitis
        c. Retinal detachment
    vii. ***Orbit:***
        a. Ptosis
        b. Orbital edema
        c. Proptosis in some cases
    viii. ***Central nervous system:***
        a. Papillitis
        b. Cranial nerve palsies (commonly third nerve involvement).

12. What is the treatment for HZO?

    i. Oral acyclovir 800 mg five times daily for 10–14 days
    ii. There is no use for topical antivirals
    iii. Topical steroids can be used for stromal keratitis
    iv. Oral corticosteroids can be used to reduce zoster pain especially in older individuals
    v. Lubricants
    vi. Tarsorrhaphy in severe cases of neurophic keratitis

13. How will you treat postherpetic neuralgia?

    i. Capsaicin cream applied to the skin
    ii. Low doses of amitriptyline or carbamazepine
    iii. Oral gabapentin.

2.8. INTERSTITIAL KERATITIS

1. What is interstitial keratitis?

Vascularization and nonsuppurative infiltration affecting the corneal stroma, usually associated with a systemic disease.

2. What are the causes of interstitial keratitis (IK)?
   i. Congenital syphilis
   ii. Acquired syphilis
   iii. Tuberculosis
   iv. Leprosy
   v. Onchocerciasis
   vi. Infectious mononucleosis
   vii. LGV—segmental and highly vascularized
   viii. Cogan's syndrome
   ix. Herpes zoster
   x. Herpes simplex
   xi. Mumps—diffuse rapid involvement of whole cornea, D/D from all others by the rapidity with it clears
   xii. Rubeola
   xiii. Vaccinia
   xiv. Variola
   xv. Leishmaniasis
   xvi. Trypanosomiasis
   xvii. Hodgkin's disease (rare)
   xviii. Kaposi's sarcoma (rare)
   xix. Mycosis fungoides (rare)
   xx. Sarcoid (rare)
   xxi. Incontinentia pigmenti
   xxii. Toxicity to drugs, such as arsenic
   xxiii. Influenza (rare).

3. What are the nonsystemic conditions that may result in interstitial keratitis?
   i. Chemical burns
   ii. Chromium deficiency.

4. What is the most common cause of interstitial keratitis?

The most important cause is syphilis. Of this, 90% is due to congenital syphilis and rest is due to acquired syphilis.

5. When does interstitial keratitis develop in congenital syphilis?

It usually occurs about the age of 5 years to early teen and is bilateral in 80%.

6. **When does the interstitial keratitis occur in acquired cases?**

It occurs within few days after the onset of infection, but generally occurs 10 years later. The majority of the disease is unilateral.

7. **What are the stages?**
    i. Progressive stage: with pain, photophobia cloudy cornea, iridocyclitis
    ii. Florid stage: Acute inflammation of the eye with deep vascularization of cornea
    iii. Regressive stage: Clearing starts from periphery. Ghost vessels may be present.

8. **What are the complications of IK?**
    i. Splits in Descemet's membrane
    ii. Band keratoplasty
    iii. Corneal thinning
    iv. Lipid keratoplasty
    v. Salzmann degeneration
    vi. Glaucoma.

9. **What are the systemic features of congenital syphilis?**
    i. History of previous stillbirths
    ii. Frontal bossing
    iii. Overgrowth of maxillary bones
    iv. Hutchinson's teeth—small band-shaped central permanent incisions
    v. Rhagades
    vi. Saber shins
    vii. Congenital deafness.

10. **What is Hutchinson's triad?**
    i. Hutchinson's teeth
    ii. Deafness
    iii. Interstitial keratitis.

11. **What is Cogan's syndrome?**

Non-syphilitic interstitial keratitis, which is bilateral and painful, with vestibuloauditory symptoms.

12. **What are the other causes of IK?**
    i. Tuberculosis   Sector-shaped sclerokeratitis
    ii. Leprosy   May be associated with pannus.

2.9. MOOREN'S ULCER

1. **Define Mooren's ulcer.**

   Mooren's ulcer is an idiopathic, painful, peripheral ulcerative keratitis (PUK).

2. **What are the other names of Mooren's ulcer?**
   i. Chronic serpiginous ulcer
   ii. Ulcus rodens.

3. **What are the symptoms of Mooren's ulcer?**
   a. Severe pain out of proportion to the size of the ulcer
   b. Decreased visual acuity due to
      i. Central corneal involvement
      ii. Irregular astigmatism
      iii. Associated uveitis
      iv. Perforation.

4. **Who described Mooren's ulcer?**

   Mooren's ulcer was first described by Bowman in 1849, and then by McKenzie in 1854 as "chronic serpiginous ulcer of the cornea or *ulcus roden.*" Mooren's name, however, became attached to this rare disorder because of his publication of cases in 1863 and 1867. He was the first to clearly describe this insidious corneal problem and define it as a clinical entity.

5. **Describe the clinical presentation of Mooren's ulcer.**

   The initial presentation is a stromal infiltration of the peripheral cornea. The limbus is involved in contrast to the other PUK's caused by rheumatoid arthritis and SLE.

   The clinical course of the ulcer is as follows:

   Stromal infiltration of the peripheral cornea
   (usually starts in the interpalpebral region)
   ↓
   Superficial ulceration
   ↓
   Peripheral spreading and deeper ulceration
   ↓
   Continued circumferential spreading
   ↓
   Hour glass cornea (contact lens cornea)

6. **Define Peripheral ulcerative keratitis.**

   Destruction of juxta-limbal cornea characterized by crescent-shaped destructive inflammation of corneal stroma associated with an epithelial defect, presence of stromal inflammatory cells and progressive stromal degradation and thinning.

7. **Describe the two clinical types of Mooren's ulcer.**

   Type 1:
   i. Occurs in older individuals
   ii. Unilateral
   iii. Mild to moderate symptoms.

   Type 2:
   i. Occurs in younger individuals, usually common among the black population
   ii. Bilateral and associated with worm infestation
   iii. Generally responds poorly to therapy.

8. **Watson classification of Mooren's ulcer**
   i. Unilateral Mooren's
   ii. Bilateral Aggressive Mooren's
   iii. Bilateral indolent Mooren's.

9. **What are Watson's criteria for Mooren's ulcer?**
   i. Presence of crescent-shaped peripheral corneal ulcer
   ii. Presence of extensive undermining of central edge of ulcer
   iii. Dense corneal infiltrates along the leading edge
   iv. Absence of scleritis
   v. Absence of detectable systemic disease.

10. **What are the clinical features of peripheral ulcerative keratitis?**
   i. Pain, epiphora, photophobia
   ii. Decreased visual acuity which can be sudden or gradual
   iii. Crescentic, juxta-limbal epithelial defect
   iv. Stromal yellow-white infiltrates
   v. Stromal thinning
   vi. Circumferential/central spread
   vii. Leading edge of ulcer shows infiltration

11. **What are the anatomic and physiological differences between the center and the periphery of the cornea?**

Central cornea	Peripheral cornea
Avascular	Close to limbal vessels
No inflammatory cells	Inflammatory cells like Langerhans cells are present
More prone for infectious disorders	More prone for inflammatory and immune-mediated disorders

12. **Describe the entities associated with Mooren's ulcer.**

Different entities have been described in association with Mooren's ulcer but none of the lesions have been proved to have causal relationship with Mooren's ulcer. Mooren's ulcer is seen associated with

  i. Helminthiasis
  ii. Hepatitis C infection
  iii. Herpes zoster
  iv. Herpes simplex
  v. Syphilis
  vi. Tuberculosis
  vii. Corneal trauma
  viii. Foreign bodies
  ix. Chemical trauma
  x. Surgical procedures like cataract extraction and PKP.

13. **Name few differential diagnoses for Mooren's ulcer (or PUK).**

  i. **Autoimmune disorders** like
    a. Rheumatoid arthritis
    b. Wegener's granulomatosis
    c. Polyarthritis nodosa
    d. Inflammatory bowel disease
    e. Giant cell arthritis.
  ii. **Collagen vascular disorders** like
    a. SLE
    b. Relapsing polychondritis
    c. Systemic sclerosis.
  iii. **Corneal degenerative conditions** like
    a. Terrien's marginal keratitis
    b. Pellucid marginal degeneration.
  iv. **Infectious causes** like
    a. Herpes simplex keratitis
    b. *Acanthamoeba* keratitis
    c. Bacterial keratitis.

14. **How do we differentiate Mooren's ulcer and PUK caused by rheumatoid arthritis?**

Rheumatoid arthritis is a frequent cause of PUK. The clinical picture of PUK in RA is not characteristic to RA but frequently it is associated with scleritis. Other associated ophthalmic findings include keratoconjunctivitis sicca (the most common ophthalmic finding), episcleritis, and sclerosing keratitis. Advanced systemic involvement is usually apparent at time of ocular involvement. The patient's clinical profile and positive serologic studies, in particular rheumatoid factor, will help establish the appropriate diagnosis.

15. **What are the ocular conditions associated with peripheral ulcerative keratitis?**

    i. Posterior scleritis
    ii. Retinal vasculitis
    iii. Elevation in intraocular pressure
    iv. Keratoconjunctivitis sicca-decreased Schirmer's measurement

16. **Describe the ophthalmic manifestations of Wegener's granulomatosis.**

    Wegener's granulomatosis is a rare multisystem granulomatous necrotizing vasculitis with upper and lower respiratory tract and renal involvement. Ocular involvement may be seen in upto 58% of patients, including proptosis due to orbital involvement, scleritis with or without PUK, PUK alone, uveitis, and vasculitis. Orbital involvement and scleritis are the most common ophthalmic manifestations. Prompt diagnosis is imperative because the initiation of immunosuppressive therapy, such as cyclophosphamide, can be both sight and lifesaving. Serum antinuclear antibody titers are raised in cases of Wegener's granulomatosis.

17. **How are Terrien's marginal degeneration and other corneal degenerations differentiated from Mooren's ulcer?**

    Terrien's marginal degeneration differs from Mooren's ulcer in that it is typically painless, does not ulcerate and is usually noninflammatory. The disease is usually bilateral but may be asymmetrical. Terrien's degeneration usually begins in the superior cornea, in contrast to Mooren's ulcer, which typically begins in the interpalpebral region as a fine, punctate, stromal opacity. A clear zone exists between the infiltrate and the limbus, which becomes superficially vascularized. Slowly progressive thinning follows. The thin area has a sloping peripheral border and a sharp central edge that is highlighted by a white lipid line. The epithelium remains intact, although bulging of thin stroma causes significant astigmatism.

18. **How is pellucid marginal degeneration differentiated from Mooren's ulcer?**

    Pellucid degeneration causes bilateral, inferior corneal thinning that leads to marked, irregular, against-the-rule astigmatism. Pain and inflammation are lacking and the epithelium is intact, thus differentiating it from Mooren's ulcer.

19. **Describe the pathophysiology of peripheral ulcerative keratitis.**

    i. Any inflammatory stimulus in peripheral cornea results in local cellular and humoral response
    ii. Which activates complement system, which in turn increase vascular permeability
    iii. Increase in neutrophils and release of proteolytic, collagenolytic enzymes (proteases and collagenases) occur which lyses the stromal collagen and cause corneal thinning.

20. Describe the pathology of Mooren's ulcer.

The histopathology of Mooren's ulcer suggests an immune process. The involved limbal cornea consisted of three zones.

  i. The superficial stroma is vascularized and infiltrated with plasma cells and lymphocytes. In this region, there is destruction of the collagen matrix. Epithelium and Bowman's layer are absent.
 ii. The midstroma shows hyperactivity of fibroblasts with disorganization of the collagen lamellae.
iii. The deep stroma is essentially intact but contains a heavy macrophage infiltrate. Descemet's membrane and the endothelium are spared.

Heavy neutrophil infiltration, as well as dissolution of the superficial stroma are present at the leading edge of the ulcer. These neutrophils show evidence of degranulation. The adjacent conjunctiva shows epithelial hyperplasia and a subconjunctival lymphocytic and plasma cell infiltration. Frank vasculitis is not present, and numerous eosinophils may present in the nearby involved conjunctiva during the course of healing.

21. Describe the pathophysiology of Mooren's ulcer.

The precise pathophysiological mechanism of Mooren's ulceration remains unknown, but there is much evidence to suggest that it is an autoimmune process, with both cell-mediated and humoral components.

On pathological examination plasma cells, neutrophils, mast cells and eosinophils have been found in the involved areas. High levels of proteolytic enzymes are found in the affected conjunctiva. Numerous activated neutrophils are found in the involved areas and these neutrophils are proposed to be the source of the proteases and collagenases that degrade the corneal stroma.

22. How cornea is immune privileged?

Anatomical and molecular barriers

  i. Blood–retinal barriers and lack of lymphatics
 ii. Paucity of antigen presenting Langerhans cells
iii. Dendritic cells and macrophages are absent
 iv. MHC class II-proteins are absent, express only low levels of MHC class I molecules.

a. Eye-derived immune tolerance (ACAID)

  i. ACAID is Anterior Chamber Associated Immune Deviation
 ii. ACAID acts by identifying any antigens in anterior chamber with the help of dendritic cells, enters venous system via trabecular meshwork bypassing lymphatics and destroyed in spleen by regulatory T cells by a complex process.

   b. Immune suppressive intraocular microenvironment

     i. FAS ligand on endothelial cells cause apoptosis of natural killer cells

     ii. Membrane bound and soluble proteins like TGF-β, thrombospon-din, MSH-α regulate macrophages, and dendritic cells.

23. How limbus is different from rest of cornea?

     i. Closer to conjunctiva, sclera, and episclera

     ii. Derives its blood supply and lymphatics from limbal capillary vessels that extend 0.5 mm into clear cornea

     iii. Source (reservoir) of immunocompetent cells like macrophages, Langerhan's cells, lymphocytes, and plasma cells

     iv. Circulating immune complexes can lodge in the limbal vessels

     v. Contains five times higher levels of C1 than central cornea which stimulates chemotaxis of neutrophils

     vi. Large concentration of IgM directed against IgG (RA factor) is greater in this site.

24. What are the investigations done to diagnose a case of Mooren's ulcer?

Mooren's ulcer is a diagnosis of exclusion.

Infectious etiologies should be excluded by appropriate smears and cultures.

This investigation may include a complete blood count with evaluation of the differential count, platelet count—baseline investigations done before starting immunosuppressive therapy.

     i. Erythrocyte sedimentation rate—marker of systemic inflammatory activity

     ii. Rheumatoid factor—to rule out rheumatoid-associated PUK

     iii. Complement fixation, antinuclear antibodies (ANA)—to rule out SLE

     iv. Antineutrophil cytoplasmic antibody (ANCA)—to rule out Wegener's granulomatosis

     v. Circulating immune complexes, liver function tests

     vi. VDRL and fluorescent treponemal antibody absorption (FTA-ABS) tests—syphilis

     vii. Blood urea nitrogen and creatinine

     viii. Serum protein electrophoresis

     ix. Urinalysis

     x. Chest roentgenogram

     xi. Additional testing is done as indicated by the review of systems and physical examination.

25. Describe the stepwise management of Mooren's ulcer.

The overall goals of therapy are to arrest the destructive process and to promote healing and re-epithelialization of the corneal surface. Most experts agree on a stepwise approach to the management of Mooren's ulcer, which is outlined as follows:

i. **Topical steroids**

Controlling inflammation by topical 1% prednisolone acetate in an hourly basis and tapering it over time, depending on the clinical response. This has to be supplemented with cycloplegic agents and anti-inflammatory drugs to reduce pain and inflammation

ii. **Conjunctival resection**

iii. **Systemic steroids and immunosuppressives**

Prednisolone (1 mg/kg body wt) after assessing systemic factors like diabetes mellitus, tuberculosis, and other immunosuppressive diseases

iv. **Additional surgical procedure (tectonic grafting)**

v. **Rehabilitation.**

26. What is the aim in treating peripheral ulcerative keratitis?

The aim of treatment in cases of peripheral ulcerative keratitis is to control the underlying inflammatory process, to promote healing of the ulcer and to avoid or prevent progression and complications.

27. Describe about medical management in peripheral ulcerative keratitis?

I. Local treatment

i. Antibiotics: to prevent secondary infection

ii. Cycloplegics: to alleviate pain

iii. Lubricants

iv. Collagenase inhibitors: tetracycline ointment

v. Antiglaucoma medications

vi. NSAIDS are contraindicated as they are

II. Systemic treatment

i. Systemic steroids

ii. Immunosuppressants

iii. Systemic collagenase inhibitors: Tetracycline 250 mg QID or Doxycycline 100 mg OD

28. Describe about surgical management in peripheral ulcerative keratitis.

i. Glue-assisted bandage contact lens

ii. Amniotic membrane grafts

iii. Patch grafts

iv. Superficial keratectomy

    v. Penetrating keratoplasty after full immunosuppression

   vi. Conjunctival resection

29. What parameters should be monitored in patients with chronic systemic steroid therapy?

     i. Patients should be monitored at 3 monthly intervals

    ii. Monitor weight

   iii. Blood pressure

   iv. Blood glucose

    v. Lipid profile

   vi. Bone scans annually

  vii. Supplements: calcium and vitamin D supplements should be given.

30. When is conjunctival resection advocated?

If the ulcer progresses despite the steroid regimen, conjunctival resection should be performed.

31. What is the rationale for performing conjunctival resection?

The rationale of this procedure is that the conjunctiva adjacent to the ulcer contains inflammatory cells that may be producing antibodies against the cornea and cytokines which amplify the inflammation and recruit additional inflammatory cell.

32. How is conjunctival resection performed?

Under topical and subconjunctival anesthesia, this consists of conjunctival excision to bare sclera extending at least 2 o'clock hours to either side of the peripheral ulcer, and approximately 4 mm posterior to the corneoscleral limbus and parallel to the ulcer. The overhanging lip of ulcerating cornea may also be removed. Postoperatively, a firm pressure dressing should be used.

33. What are other surgical procedures advocated at the second step?

Cryotherapy of limbal conjunctiva, conjunctival excision with thermocoagulation, keratoepithelioplasty, application of isobutyl cyanoacrylate.

34. What is keratoepithelioplasty?

In this procedure, donor corneal lenticules are sutured onto the scleral bed after conjunctival excision.

35. What is the rationale of keratoepithelioplasty?

It is postulated that the lenticules form a biological barrier between host cornea and the conjunctiva and the immune components it may carry.

36. When is systemic immunosuppression indicated?

The cases of bilateral or progressive Mooren's ulcer that fail the preceding therapeutic attempts will require systemic cytotoxic chemotherapy to bring a halt to the progressive corneal destruction.

37. What are the immunosuppressives and biologicals used in peripheral ulcerative keratitis?

   i. The commonly used agents include cyclophosphamide (2 mg/kg/day), azathioprine (2 mg/kg/body weight/day), and methotrexate (7.5–15 mg once weekly)

  ii. Milder disease: Antimetabolites (methotrexate, azathioprine, mycophenolate mofetil)

     a. Calcineurin inhibitors (cyclosporine A, tacrolimus)

 iii. Wegner's granulomatosis, rheumatoid arthritis, and sclerokeratitis

     a. First line: Cyclophosphamide

     b. Second line: Methotrexate and azathioprine

  iv. Rapidly progressive corneal melting, or one eyed pt with rapidly deteriorating second eye:

     a. Alkylating agents/antimetabolites + biologic response modifiers (Infliximab, Rituximab)

   v. Rapidly progressive systemic vasculitis: Rituximab infusions + antimetabolites/alkylating agents and systemic corticosteroids.

38. When is superficial lamellar keratectomy done and how is it useful?

It is done when all the steps of management fails. It arrests the inflammatory process and allows healing of stroma. After healing, corneal grafting can be done on a later date.

39. When is PKP done in cases of Mooren's ulcer?

An initial tectonic graft is done in the peripheral cornea to strengthen the peripheral cornea. In case the central cornea is involved, a large graft can be performed.

40. How is PKP done in these patients?

In these patients, a 13 mm tectonic corneal graft is first sutured in place of interrupted 10–0 nylon or prolene sutures with the recipient bite extending into the sclera so that the suture will not pull through the thin host cornea and then a 7.5 or 8.0 mm therapeutic graft is placed.

41. What are the common complications of PKP?

Associated cystoid macular edema and glaucoma may cause defective vision in patients undergoing PKP.

2.10. BAND-SHAPED KERATOPATHY

1. **What are the normal age-related changes of cornea?**
    i.   Flattening in the vertical meridian, leading to increased astigmatism (against the rule)
    ii. Decrease in thickness of cornea
    iii. Increase in the thickness of Descemet's membrane
    iv. Arcus senilis
    v.   Decrease in the endothelial cell count and decrease in luster.

2. **What is band-shaped keratopathy?**
    Deposits of calcium and hydroxyapatite in the basement membrane of epithelium, Bowman's, and superficial stroma, usually in the interpalpebral area is called as band-shaped keratopathy (also known as band keratopathy).

3. **What are the causes of band keratopathy?**
    i.   **Chronic ocular disease**
         – Chronic non-granulomatous uveitis—juvenile rheumatoid arthritis
         – Prolonged glaucoma (absolute)
         – Longstanding corneal edema
         – Phthisis bulbi
         – Spheroidal degeneration Norrie's disease—interstitial keratitis
    ii. **Hypercalcemia**
         – Hyperparathyroidism—primary and tertiary
         – Vitamin D excess
         – Milk alkali syndrome
         – Sarcoidosis
    iii. **Normocalcemia**—with elevated serum phosphorus
    iv. **Hereditary with or without other anomalies**
    v.   **Idiopathic**
    vi. **Chronic exposure to mercury**
         – Vapors
         – Eye drops due to the preservative phenyl-mercuric nitrate/acetate occurs only after months or years of usage. Can be central or peripheral
    vii. **Hereditary**
    viii. **Silicon oil instillation in aphakic eye.**

4. **What is the pathogenesis of band-shaped keratopathy?**
    Deposits often begin in the periphery and extend to involve the visual axis, thus occupying the interpalpebral area. The deposits are central in cases of chronic ocular inflammation.

Precipitation of calcium salts are due to:

i. Increase in Ca and P levels
ii. Increase in pH due to uveitis, evaporation of tears, and loss of Ca.
iii. Concentration by evaporation and thus dry eye is a predisposing factor.

Whole process is compounded by lack of blood vessels, hence preventing the buffering ability of blood serum to inhibit variations in tissue pH.

Small holes are noticed throughout representing areas in which corneal nerves penetrate Bowman's layer giving a "Swiss cheese appearance."

5. **What are the histopathologic findings in a case of band keratopathy?**
    i. Basophilic staining of the basement membrane of the epithelium
    ii. Calcium deposits in the Bowman's and anterior stroma, which coalesce resulting in fragmentation and destruction of Bowman's membrane
    iii. The deposits are initially gray and flat. But with progression they become white and elevate the epithelium
    iv. The calcium is deposited intracellularly in systemic hypercalcemia
    v. Fibrous pannus separates the Bowman's and epithelium.

6. **What are the signs and symptoms of band keratopathy?**

    Early stages—asymptomatic

    Late stages:

    i. *Decrease in visual acuity due to*
       Decrease in transparency
       Band across the papillary area

    ii. *Irritation and foreign body sensation* when the deposits either break or elevate the epithelium
        – Tearing and photophobia
        – Calcium may flake off

7. **What are the differential diagnoses of band keratopathy?**
    i. Calcareous degeneration of cornea is a similar process that involves all layers of cornea
    ii. Phthisis bulbi
    iii. Intraocular neoplasm
    iv. Extensive trauma.

8. **What are the indications of treatment?**
    i. When visual acuity is decreased
    ii. Mechanical irritation of lids
    iii. Epithelial breakdown.

9. **What are the methods of treatment?**

Treat the cause of the disease, if known. In addition, the following may be done:

Method – I

i. 4% cocaine applied over the cornea. Cocaine facilitates the removal of epithelium

ii. EDTA (Ethylene diamine tetra-acetic acid) is dropped from a 1.5 cm syringe well, and allowed to stand for a minute

iii. Cornea is then scraped with kimura spatula or scalpel blade until the band is removed

Method – II

i. EDTA is placed on a small strip of cellulose sponge

ii. Diamond bud is used to polish off the cornea

If there is no EDTA just anesthetize the cornea and scrape with blade until all gritty feeling material is removed.

Patching in the form of soft contact lenses and collagen shields along with cycloplegics and mild antibiotic are used until re-epithelialization.

Excimer laser phototherapeutic keratectomy can be tried only on smoother lesions.

2.11. ADHERENT LEUKOMA

1. **What are the types of corneal opacities?**

    i. Nebular (Nebula) corneal opacity is slight opacification of cornea allowing the details of iris and pupil to be seen through corneal opacity

    ii. Macular (Macula) corneal opacity: It is more dense than nebular corneal opacity, through it details of iris and pupil cannot be seen but margins can be seen

    iii. Leukomatous (Leukoma) corneal opacity: It is very dense, white totally opaque obscuring view of iris and pupil totally.

2. **What is adherent leukoma?**

    It is a leukomatous opacity in which the iris tissue is incarcerated within the layer of cornea.

3. **What are causes of adherent leukoma?**

    i. Perforated corneal ulcer

    ii. Penetrating injury

    iii. Operating wound.

4. **What is the mechanism of development of an adherent leukoma?**

    In a cornea which is structurally weak, due to either acute infection or old scar with thinning, the following events might take place

    Sudden exertion while sneezing and coughing
    ↓
    Acute rise of IOP
    ↓
    Weak floor of ulcer is unable to support their pressure
    ↓
    Perforated ulcer
    ↓
    Thereby sudden escape of aqueous
    ↓
    Sudden fall in IOP
    ↓
    Iris lens diaphragm moves forwards and comes in contact with the back of the cornea

5. **What are signs and symptoms of adherent leukoma?**

    Symptoms: Visual acuity is decreased if the adherent leukoma affects the central visual axis. In case of peripheral lesions, there may be a chance of *astigmatism.*

Signs:

  i. Corneal surface is flat, leukomatous and has decreased corneal sensation
 ii. There may be brown pigments dispersed from the iris on the back of the cornea
iii. The depth of the anterior chamber is irregular
 iv. The pupil is irregular in shape and drawn toward the adhesion
  v. The intraocular pressure may be raised.

6. What are the other complications associated with adherent leukoma?

    i. Perforation
   ii. Pseudocornea formation
  iii. Staphyloma formation
   iv. Ectatic cicatrix
    v. Atheromatus ulcer
   vi. Endophthalmitis
  vii. Panophthalmitis
 viii. Expulsive hemorrhage
   ix. Phthisis bulbi.

7. What are the advantages of perforation in a case of corneal ulcer?

  i. Pain is reduced due to lowering of IOP and egress of hypopyon
 ii. Rapid healing of the ulcer.

8. What are the reasons of phthisis bulbi?

  i. Large perforation may cause extrusion of the contents of the eyeball leading to shrinkage
 ii. Repeated corneal ulcer perforations may be sealed by exudates which may leak leading to fistula formation.

9. How do you do tattooing?

   i. After removing the epithelium, a piece of blotting paper of the same size as the opacity, soaked in fresh 2% platinum chloride solution, is kept over the opacity
  ii. On removing this filter paper, few drops of fresh 2% hydrazine hydrate solution are applied over the area which in turn becomes black
 iii. Eye is washed with saline
  iv. A drop of parolein is instilled and a pad and bandage applied
   v. The epithelium grows over the black colored deposit of platinum.

10. What is the treatment of choice for adherent leukoma?

   i. Optical iridectomy
  ii. Penetrating keratoplasty
 iii. Tattooing and synechotomy.

11. What is treatment for anterior staphyloma?

    i. Staphylectomy

    ii. Enucleation and prosthesis fitting.

12. What is the treatment for corneal fistula?

    i. Cyanoacrylate glue application

    ii. Bandage contact lens

    iii. Penetrating keratoplasty.

13. What is treatment of choice for panophthalmitis?

Evisceration and prosthesis

	Anterior synechia	Leukoma	Adherent leukoma	Anterior staphyloma
▪ **Definition**	Adhesion between iris and cornea	Dense white opacity of cornea	Adhesion between iris and leukoma	Adhesion between iris and ectatic leukoma
▪ **Etiology**	▪ Perforated corneal ulcer ▪ Iridocyclitis ▪ Closed angle glaucoma	▪ Healed corneal ulcer ▪ Healed keratitis ▪ Penetrating injury ▪ FB ▪ Corneal dystrophy	▪ Perforated corneal ulcer ▪ Penetrating injury ▪ Operating wound	▪ Perforated corneal ulcer ▪ Penetrating injury ▪ Operating wound
▪ **Visual acuity**	Normal	Impaired	Impaired	Impaired
▪ **Corneal surface**	Flat	Flat	Flat	Ectatic
▪ **Pigments**	Nil	Fine yellowish brown lines in the epithelium,	Brown pigment from iris are present	Brown pigment from iris are present
▪ **Anterior chamber**	Normal or shallow	Normal	Irregular or shallow	Absent or very shallow
▪ **Pupil**	Normal	Normal	Drawn toward adhesion	Not seen
▪ **Corneal sensation**	Normal	Impaired	Impaired	Impaired
▪ **Intraocular tension**	Normal or raised (Closed angle glaucoma)	Normal	Normal or raised (Secondary glaucoma)	Raised

2.12. BOWEN'S DISEASE

1. **What are the old terms to describe Bowen's disease?**
    i. Intraepithelial epithelioma
    ii. Bowenoid epithelioma.

2. **What are the new terms?**
    i. Ocular surface squamous neoplasia (OSSN)
    ii. Conjunctival intraepithelial neoplasia (CIN)
    iii. Corneal intraepithelial neoplasia.

3. **What is the common site of involvement?**
    Interpalpebral fissure, mostly at limbus.

4. **How does Bowen's disease present?**
    Typically, a patient presents with an isolated, slightly elevated, erythematous lesion with well-demarcated borders that fail to heal. Lesion has appearance of a second degree burn, does not bleed or itch and is devoid of hairs.

5. **What are the clinical forms of Bowen's disease?**
    i. Gelatinous
    ii. Papilliform
    iii. Leukoplakic
    iv. Nodular
    v. Diffuse.

6. **Which form masquerades as chronic conjunctivitis?**
    Diffuse form.

7. **What are the risk factors?**
    i. Exposure to sunlight
    ii. Human papilloma virus
    iii. Chronic inflammatory diseases—benign mucous membrane pemphigoid, chronic blepharoconjunctivitis
    iv. Ocular surface injury
    v. Exposure to chemicals—trifluridine, arsenic, petroleum products, cigarette smoking
    vi. HIV
    vii. Solar keratosis.

8. **What is limbal transition zone/stem cell theory?**
    Cells in limbal area have highly proliferating and long living property. Any alteration in this area causes abnormal maturation of conjunctival and corneal epithelial cells leading to OSSN.

9. **How do you differentiate squamous dysplasia from carcinoma *in situ*?**

   Squamous dysplasia: Atypical cells involve only part of epithelium
   Carcinoma in situ: Atypia involves throughout epithelium, not involving the basement membrane.

10. **What is the histopathological hallmark of Bowen's disease?**

    Histopathological hallmark of Bowen's disease is lack of penetration of cancerous cells into the dermis.

11. **How does squamous cell carcinoma present?**

    Average age of presentation of squamous cell carcinoma between 68 and 73 years, but primary squamous cell carcinoma in younger patients may be seen in those who are immunosuppressed.

    They may present as:
    i. Painless plaque/nodules with variable degree of scale, crust, and ulceration.
    ii. Papillomatous growths/cutaneous horns/cysts along the lid margins.

12. **What are various histopathological types of OSSN?**
    i. Dysplastic *lesions*
    ii. Carcinoma *in situ*
    iii. Squamous cell carcinoma
    iv. Spindle cell variant
    v. Mucoepidermoid carcinoma
    vi. Adenoid squamous carcinoma.

13. **Describe spindle cell variant.**

    It exhibits spindle-shaped cells that may be difficult to distinguish from fibroblasts. Positive immunohistochemical staining for cytokeratin confirms epithelial nature.

14. **Describe mucoepidermoid carcinoma.**

    It is a variant of conjunctival squamous cell carcinoma that in addition to squamous cells shows mucous secreting cells (stain positively with special stains for mucopolysaccharides such as muciramine, alcian blue, and colloidal iron).

15. **Describe adenoid squamous cell carcinoma.**

    It is an aggressive variant with extracellular hyaluronic acid but no intracellular mucin and invades eyeball. Metastasis to distant sites is common.

16. **From where does corneal OSSN arise?**

    It is controversial. Some investigators suggest that corneal epithelium may undergo dysplastic and cancerous changes, whereas others believe that origin is in limbus.

17. When do you suspect intraocular invasion?

It is often heralded by the onset of low-grade inflammation and secondary glaucoma. It is common in older patients.

18. What are the common sites of metastasis?

   i. Preauricular, submandibular, cervical lymph nodes
   ii. Parotid
   iii. Lungs
   iv. Bones
   v. Distant organs.

19. What is exfoliative cytology?

Using a platinum spatula, brush, and cotton wool tip, cells are obtained from conjunctival surface, followed by Papanicolaou and Giemsa stains.

20. What are advantages and disadvantages of exfoliative cytology?

Advantages

   i. Nature of lesion—benign or malignant
   ii. Sampling from multiple sites
   iii. DNA of cells can also be obtained.

Disadvantage

Superficial nature of sample, sometimes containing only keratinized cells.

21. What is impression cytology?

It is a method of obtaining cells from conjunctival lesions in which filter paper such as cellulose acetate, millipore filter, or biopore membrane are placed over ocular surface to sample superficial cells and then stained by Papanicolaou smear.

22. What is the treatment?

Localized lesion: Excision with autologous conjunctival or limbal transplantation or amniotic membrane graft (Mohs micrographic technique)

Diffuse

   i. Topical mitomycin 0.02% twice a day for 15 days followed by a relapsing period

5-FU

   ii. Interferon (alternative or adjunct to surgery)
   iii. Very large tumors—enucleation
   iv. Orbital involvement—exenteration.

23. What are the other treatment modalities available?

   i. Cryotherapy
   ii. Brachytherapy.

24. What is the mechanism of cryotherapy?

It obliterates microcirculation by lowering temperature within tissues resulting in ischemic necrosis of tumor cells.

25. What are the side effects of cryotherapy?

    i. Iritis

    ii. Increase or decrease in intraocular pressure

    iii. Inflammation

    iv. Edema and corneal scarring

    v. Sector iris atrophy

    vi. Ablation of peripheral retina

    vii. Ectropion

    viii. Superficial corneal vascularization

26. What are the commonly used radioactive materials in brachytherapy?

    i. Strontium 90

    ii. Ruthenium 106

    iii. Gamma radiation.

27. What are the complications of brachytherapy?

    i. Conjunctivitis

    ii. Dry eye

    iii. Scleral ulceration

    iv. Corneal perforation

    v. Cataract.

2.13. KERATOCONUS

1. **Name a few corneal ectatic conditions.**

   Keratoconus, keratoglobus, pellucid marginal degeneration, Terrien's marginal degeneration.

2. **What are the signs of keratoconus?**

   i. **External signs**
      Munson's sign
      Rizzuti phenomenon

   ii. **Slit-lamp findings**
      Stromal thinning
      Posterior stress lines (Vogt's striae)
      Iron ring (Fleischer's ring)
      Scarring—epithelial or subepithelial

   iii. **Retroillumination signs**
      Scissoring on retinoscopy
      Oil droplet sign ("Charleaux")

   iv. **Photokeratoscopy signs**
      Compression of mires inferotemporally
      ("egg-shaped" mires)
      Compression of mires inferiorly or centrally

   v. **Videokeratography signs**
      – Curvature map
        Localized increased surface power > 47D
        Inferior superior dioptric asymmetry > 1.4D
        Relative skewing of the steepest radial axes above and below the horizontal meridian
      – Elevation map
        Maximum elevation difference in posterior float > 50 μ
      – Pachymetry map
        Thinnest < 480 μ.

3. **Which gender is commonly affected by keratoconus?**

   Keratoconus has been seen a bit more commonly in males than in females.

4. **What are the biochemical alternations seen in corneas with keratoconus?**

   Various abnormalities suggested include:

   i. Decreased levels of glucose-6-phosphate dehydrogenase (G6PD)
   ii. Relative decrease in hydroxylation of lysine and glycosylation of hydroxylysine

    iii. Decrease in total collagen and a relative increase in structural glycoprotein

    iv. In patients with keratoconus, keratan sulfate is decreased and its structure is modified

    v. The ratio of dermatan sulfate to keratan sulfate is increased in keratoconus

    vi. Decrease in matrix metalloproteinase (MMP) inhibitors leading on to increased collagenolytic activity

    vii. There is a decreased level of α1 proteinase inhibitor, tissue inhibitor of metalloproteinase (TIMP)-1 and α2 macroglobin levels in keratoconus cornea

    viii. The loss of anterior stromal keratinocytes is due to apoptotic cell death

    ix. Keratinocytes have fourfold increased expression of interleukin-1 (IL-1) receptors. Interleukin-1 is released from epithelial and endothelial cells and IL-1 can cause loss of keratinocytes through apoptosis and loss of corneal stroma over a period of time.

5. What is Munson's sign?

Munson's sign is a V-shaped conformation of the lower lid produced by the ectatic cornea in down gaze.

6. What is Rizzuti's sign?

Conical reflection on the nasal cornea when a penlight is shown from the temporal side.

7. What are Vogt's striae?

Vogt's striae are fine vertical lines in the deep stroma and Descemet's membrane that parallel the axis of the cone and disappear transiently on gentle digital pressure.

8. What are Fleischer's rings?

The Fleischer ring is a yellow-brown to olive-green ring of pigment, which may or may not completely surround the base of the cone. The deposition occurs at the level of basal epithelium. Locating this ring initially may be made easier by using a cobalt filter and carefully focusing on the superior half of the corneal epithelium. Once located, the ring should be viewed in white light to assess its extent.

9. What is the clinical significance of Fleischer's ring?

It delineates the extent of the base of the cone of the keratoconus, which helps to mark the recipient during the penetrating keratoplasty.

10. What is acute hydrops?

The acute hydrops is caused by breaks in Descemet's membrane with stromal imbibition of aqueous through these breaks. The edema may persist for weeks or months, usually diminishing gradually, with relief of pain and resolution of the redness and corneal edema ultimately being replaced by scarring.

11. How is acute hydrops treated?

Acute hydrops is not an ophthalmic emergency and is treated conservatively with topical hypertonic agents, patching or soft contact lens and mild cycloplegics. The edema usually resolves within a few months.

12. What is the visual prognosis following healing of acute hydrops?

Acute hydrops usually heals by scarring. The scarring can flatten the cornea and decrease the astigmatism. The flattened cornea can be fitted with a contact lens easier.

13. Describe scissoring reflex on retinoscopy.

Scissoring reflex is appreciated well with dilated pupil. The central part of the cone is hypermetropic with regards to its periphery which is myopic. The scissoring reflex is produced due to presence of two conjugate foci in pupillary axis and high astigmatism.

During retinoscopy when the neutralization point is approached, the central zone produces a hypermetropic reflex which moves with the streak and the peripheral zone produces a myopic reflex which moves against the streak which produces the appearance of scissoring reflex.

14. Describe oil droplet sign.

It is seen with a dilated fundus examination. It is an annular dark shadow separating the bright reflex of the central and peripheral areas. It occurs due to complete internal reflection of the light.

15. What is swirl staining of cornea?

Swirl staining may occur in patients who have never worn contact lenses because basal epithelial cells drop out and the epithelium slides from the periphery as the cornea regenerates. Thus, a hurricane, vortex, or swirl stain may occur.

16. What is forme fruste keratoconus?

Forme fruste keratoconus or subclinical keratoconus is a clinical entity in which there is no frank clinical sign of keratoconus. However, the cornea is at risk of developing keratoconus at a later stage and can be diagnosed only by videokeratography. Cornea is considered suspicious when:

 i. The central keratometry is more than 47.0D
 ii. There is presence of an oblique astigmatism of >1.5D
 iii. Superior–inferior curvature disparity of >1.4D on videokeratography
 iv. The Massachusetts Eye and Ear Infirmary Keratoconus classification is currently used to detect cases of forme fruste keratoconus and variable grades of clinical keratoconus.

17. What are the systemic disorders associated with keratoconus?

    i. Crouzon's syndrome
   ii. Down's syndrome
  iii. Laurence–Moon–Bardet–Biedl syndrome
   iv. Marfan's syndrome
    v. Nail–patella syndrome
   vi. Neurofibromatosis
  vii. Osteogenesis imperfecta
 viii. Pseudoxanthoma elasticum
   ix. Turner's syndrome
    x. Xeroderma pigmentosa.

18. What are the ocular associations of keratoconus?

Can be classified into corneal disorders and noncorneal disorders.

Corneal disorders	Noncorneal disorders
Atopic keratoconjunctivitis	Retinitis pigmentosa
Axenfeld's anomaly	Vernal conjunctivitis
Corneal amyloidosis	Congenital cataracts
Essential iris atrophy	Leber's congenital amaurosis
Fuchs' corneal dystrophy	Gyrate atrophy
Microcornea	Posterior lenticonus
Lattice dystrophy	Aniridia

19. Why is keratoconus commonly associated with Leber's congenital amaurosis and Down's syndrome?

These two disorders are associated with increased incidence of eye rubbing. This is due to increased incidence of blepharitis in Down's syndrome and oculodigital sign in Leber's congenital amaurosis. Recent study by Elder suggests that the association might be due to genetic factors rather than eye rubbing.

20. What is the role of contact lens wear in causing keratoconus?

Contact lenses are suggested as a source of mechanical trauma to the cornea. It is extremely difficult to determine which came first, the contact lens wear or the keratoconus. It is possible that mechanical rubbing and hard contact lens wear can act as environmental factors that enhance the progression of the disorder in genetically predisposed individuals.

21. Describe the three types of cones seen in keratoconus.

    A. Nipple cone—small in size (< 5 mm)
       i. Steep curvature
      ii. Apical center usually lies central or paracentral
     iii. Easiest to fit with contact lens

    B. Oval cone—larger (5–6 mm) ellipsoid displaced inferotemporally

    C. Globus cone—larger (> 6 mm) may involve more than 75% of the cornea

      i. Most difficult to fit with contact lenses.

22. What is posterior keratoconus?

It's a congenital corneal anomaly unrelated to keratoconus which is characterized by protrusion of posterior corneal surface into the stroma and is usually sporadic, unilateral, and nonprogressive.

23. What are Rabinowitz's criteria for diagnosis of keratoconus?

    i. Keratometry value > 47.2D

    ii. Steepening of inferior cornea compared with the superior cornea of > 1.2D

    iii. Skewing of the radial axis of astigmatism by greater than 21D

    iv. Difference in central power of more than 1D between the fellow eye.

24. Describe the histopathology of corneas in keratoconus.

Thinning of corneal stroma, breaks in Bowman's layer, and deposition of iron in the basal layer of the corneal epithelium comprise a triad of the classic histopathologic features found in keratoconus.

    i. **Epithelium**—degeneration of basal cells
      – Breaks accompanied by downgrowth of epithelium into Bowman's layer
      – Accumulation of ferritin particles within and between basal epithelial cells

    ii. **Bowman's layer**—breaks filled with eruptions of underlying stromal collagen
      – Reticular scarring

    iii. **Stroma**—compactions and loss of arrangement of fibrils in the anterior stroma
      – Decrease in number of collagen lamellae

    iv. **Descemet's membrane**—rarely affected except in cases with acute hydrops

    v. **Endothelium**—usually normal.

25. Classify keratoconus based on keratometry.

i. Mild	< 45D in both meridians
ii. Moderate	45–52D in both meridians
iii. Advanced	> 52D in both meridians
iv. Severe	> 62D in both meridians.

26. **How is a case of keratoconus managed?**
    i. Glasses
    ii. Contact lenses
    iii. Collagen cross-linking
    iv. Intracorneal rings
    v. Deep anterior lamellar keratoplasty (DALK)
    vi. Penetrating keratoplasty (PKP).

27. **What are the various types of contact lenses used in the management of keratoconus?**
    i. Rigid gas permeable contact lens
    ii. Tricurve flex lens for nipple cone
    iii. Soper lens system
    iv. McGuire lens system
    v. Rose K design
    vi. Nicone design
    vii. Bausch and Lomb C series
    viii. Double posterior curve lenses
       - One central curve to fit the corneal apex
       - Another flatter curve peripheral to the central apical zone to fit the mid corneal periphery
    ix. Piggy back lenses—gas permeable firm lens is fitted upon a soft lens or flex lens system of a hard lens fitted in to the groove of a soft lens. Hard lens with a soft peripheral skirt.

28. **What is "three-point touch" technique of contact lens fitting?**
    The lens lightly touches the peak of the cone, then a very low vault over the edges of the cone, and lastly a thin band of touching near the edge of the lens. The name "three-point touch" refers to the edge-peak-edge pattern of the lens touching the cornea. The lens is kept as small as is optically possible. Since the lens will center itself over the peak of the cone, an off-center cone needs a bigger lens than a centered cone.

29. **What is the fluorescein pattern of a well-fit lens in a keratoconus patient?**
    i. Slight central bearing
    ii. Intermediate pooling of tears
    iii. Peripheral bearing or touch over some portion of the lens circumference and perhaps slight peripheral lift at the steepest site of the cone.

30. **What are SoftPerm lens?**
    The SoftPerm lens is a hybrid lens with a rigid, gas-permeable center surrounded by a soft, hydrophilic skirt. This lens may be indicated for patients with displaced corneal apexes or for patients who cannot tolerate

rigid lenses. However, in advanced keratoconus, in which a lens of larger diameter is useful, the lack of steep base curves in the SoftPerm lens (its steepest base curve is 6.5 mm) limits performance. In addition, the lens material has a low DK value (rigid lens, 14 DK; soft portion, 5.5 DK).

31. What is Soper lens system?

The objective of the Soper lens system is based on sagittal depth. The principle is that a constant base curve with an increased diameter results in increased sagittal depth and a steeper lens. The lenses included in the fitting set are categorized as mild (7.5 mm diameter, 6.0 mm optic zone diameter), moderate (8.5 mm diameter, 7.0 mm optic zone diameter), and advanced (9.5 mm diameter, 8.0 mm optic zone diameter). The initial trial lens is selected on the basis of degree of advancement of the cone. The more advanced the cone, the larger the diameter of the recommended lens; the smaller and more centrally located the apex, the smaller the diameter of the lens.

32. What is thermokeratoplasty?

Thermokeratoplasty is corneal flattening by heat application, which may regularize the corneal surface. It is often used to flatten the cornea at the time of keratoplasty to make trephining easier.

33. What is epikeratoplasty?

A corneal lenticule is sewn over the keratoconus area, flattening the cone, reducing the myopic astigmatism, and improving contact lens fit. It is preferred in conditions like Down's syndrome because of its noninvasive nature and decreased potential for corneal graft rejection.

34. What is excimer laser phototherapeutic keratectomy?

It is useful in management of patients with keratoconus who have nodular subepithelial corneal scars who are contact lens intolerant.

35. Why is prognosis of PKP good in cases of keratoconus?

   i. Absence of vascularization in the lesion
   ii. Keratoconus is a noninflammatory ectatic condition.

36. What is collagen cross-linkage?

Corneal collagen cross-linking using riboflavin is a noninvasive procedure which strengthens the weak corneal structure in keratoconus.

This technique works by increasing collagen cross-linking, which are the natural "anchors" within the cornea. Riboflavin eye drops are applied to the cornea, which is then activated by a ultraviolet (UVA) light. This increases the amount of collagen cross-linking in the cornea and strengthens the cornea. The technique uses riboflavin to create new bonds between the adjacent collagen molecules so that the cornea is about one-and-a-half times thicker and less malleable.

37. Explain the mechanism of action of collagen cross-linkage.

Application of riboflavin on the cornea along with penetration for approximately 200 μm and irradiation of the riboflavin molecules through UVA leads to loss of the internal chemical balance of the riboflavin molecules, producing oxygen free radicals. The riboflavin molecule becomes unstable and stabilizes only when it is linked to two collagen fibrils. A cross bridge is created between the collagen fibrils (i.e. cross-linking) to produce a general strengthening of the cornea.

38. What are the indications for C3R?

i. **Refractive indications**
   - Progressive keratoconus:
     • If two topography maps measured at an interval of 6 months or more show the following
       o Increase in k max by 1 diopter
       o Increase in astigmatism by 1 diopter
       o Decrease in pachymetry by 30 microns
       o Marked change in the topographic pattern to crab claw or increase in the hot spot
   - Keratoconus in young patients with borderline pachymetry at first visit
   - Pellucid marginal degeneration
   - Post refractive surgery ectasia

ii. **Nonrefractive indications**
   - Infective keratitis
   - Pseudophakic bullous keratopathy
   - Scleral C3R in glaucoma.

39. What are the contraindications for C3R?

i. Age less than 10 years
ii. Pachymetry less than 350 microns
iii. Corneal endothelial count less than 2400 cells/mm^2
iv. Presence of significant corneal opacity
v. Active VKC
vi. Corneal epithelial healing disorders
vii. Any other active disease of the eye
viii. Pregnancy.

40. Which are the modifications of C3R?

i. **Hypotonic C3R:**
   This uses 0.1% riboflavin (made using water for injection instead of high molecular weight dextran T500 which is used to prepare the isotonic 0.1% riboflavin drops)

   Indication: Thin corneas requiring C3R (350–400 microns)

Principle: Hypotonic drops when applied to the epithelium debrided cornea it leads to transient water retention and hence increase in the corneal thickness to approximately 350 microns. This decreases the endothelial damage from the UV light.

ii. **Transepithelial C3R/epi-on technique**:

C3R performed without debriding the epithelium is termed as epi-on C3R.

Advantages:
- Less painful
- Faster healing
- Reduces chances of corneal infections
- Can be performed in thinner corneas

Disadvantages:
- Less effective than the standard epi-off treatment
- Longer duration

iii. **Accelerated C3R**:

The UVA power is increased to 30 mW/cm^2 and duration is reduced to 3 minutes, hence keeping the total energy received by the tissue almost the same as in the standard technique.

Advantage:

Shorter duration and so better patient compliance is achieved

Disadvantage:

Still experimental and less effective than the standard technique.

41. Compare and contrast the clinical features of keratoconus, keratoglobus, Terrien's, and Pellucid marginal degeneration?

	Keratoconus	Keratoglobus	Terrien's	Pellucid
Age group	Progress during adolescence	Presents at birth	Presents at fourth to fifth decade	Presents between second and third decade
Appearance	Progressive thinning of central/para-central cornea	Globular deformation of entire cornea	Begins superiorly and spreads circumferentially	Causes inferior thinning of cornea
Vascularization	Absent	Absent	Forms pannus	Absent
Familial inheritance	Most cases are sporadic	Dominant inheritance with incomplete penetrance	Sporadic	Sporadic
Laterality	Bilateral, usually asymmetrical	Bilateral, usually asymmetrical	Unilateral or asymmetrically bilateral	Bilateral
Prognosis after PKP	Very favorable prognosis	Poor prognosis	Good prognosis after lamellar keratoplasty	Moderate

42. Which are surgical options for keratoconus treatment?

  i. Deep anterior lamellar keratoplasty (DALK)—replaces only the stroma upto Descemet's membrane.
  Advantages—reduced chances for immune rejection since the endothelial layer is preserved.
  Disadvantage—technically difficult procedure.
  Visual quality may be inferior to PK because of interface irregularities and astigmatism.
  ii. Intracorneal ring segment insertion
  iii. Penetrating keratoplasty—in the presence of Descemet's scarring DALK cannot be done. A penetrating keratoplasty is the only choice for visual rehabilitation.

43. What are intracorneal rings?

Intracorneal ring segments are PMMA/silicon semicircular rings which are inserted in mid-peripheral stroma, which helps to reduce high refractive error and provides better fitting of cornea.

44. How do intracorneal rings Intacs act?

Insertion of a ring of particular thickness in the mid-peripheral stroma will increase the thickness and corneal arc diameter. This will act like a hammock rod to cause central flattening. Two half-ring segments are inserted on either side of the cone.

45. What are the types of intrastromal corneal ring segments (ICRSs)?

There are four types of ICRS available, namely,

  i. INTACS
  ii. Ferrara rings
  iii. Bisantis segments
  iv. Myoring.

46. What are the indications and contraindications of ICRSs?

Indications:
  i. Keratoconus
  ii. Pellucid marginal degeneration
  iii. Post refractive surgery ectasia
  iv. Myopia (−1 to −3.0 D)
  v. Contact lens intolerance in keratoconus patients

Contraindications:
  i. Age < 21 years
  ii. Corneal scar involving the central optical zone
  iii. Pachymetry less than 450 microns at the site of insertion
  iv. Associated corneal dystrophy
  v. Collagen vascular diseases
  vi. Pregnancy and nursing women.

47. **What are the causes of prominent corneal nerves?**

Ocular causes:
   i. Keratoconus
   ii. Fuchs' dystrophy
   iii. Congenital glaucoma

Systemic causes:
   i. Leprosy
   ii. Neurofibromatosis
   iii. Multiple endocrine neoplasia.

2.14. STROMAL DYSTROPHIES

1. **What is the meaning of word dystrophy?**

   The word dystrophy is derived from the Greek word, *dys* = wrong, difficult; *trophe* = nourishment.

2. **Define corneal dystrophy.**

   Corneal dystrophies are a group of inherited corneal diseases that are typically bilateral, symmetrical, and slowly progressive and without relationship to environmental or systemic factors, causing loss of clarity of one or more layers of cornea.

3. **Define corneal degenerations.**

   Corneal degenerations may occur from physiological changes occurring from aging, or may follow an environmental insult such as exposure to ultraviolet light or secondary to a prior corneal disorder.

4. **What are the differences between corneal dystrophy and degenerations?**

	Dystrophy	Degenerations
1	Bilateral and symmetric	Unilateral or bilateral
2	Hereditary	Sporadic
3	Appears early in life	Occurs late in life and are considered as aging changes
4	Noninflammatory	Inflammatory
5	Avascular and located centrally	Often eccentric and peripheral and are related to vascularity
6	Usually painless except in recurrent epithelial erosions	Mostly associated with pain
7	Systemic associations are rare	Local and systemic conditions are common association

5. **Classify corneal dystrophies.**

   Classification according to the layers of cornea involved (anatomic) is most often used. Other classifications are based on genetic pattern, severity, histopathologic features, or biochemical characteristics.

Layer	Descriptive term
Epithelium	1. Epithelial basement membrane dystrophy (EBMD) (Map-dot-fingerprint, Cogan's microcystic) 2. Messman's (Juvenile epithelial) dystrophy
Bowman's layer	1. CDB I & II Reis–Bucklers dystrophy (Corneal dystrophy of Bowman's layer, type I)

(Continued)

(Continued)

Layer	Descriptive term
	Thiel–Behnke dystrophy (Corneal dystrophy of Bowman's layer, type II)

Stroma	1. Granular dystrophy
	   Type I
	   Type II
	2. Lattice dystrophy
	   Type I (Biber-Haab-Dimmer)
	   Type II (Meretoja syndrome)
	   Type III
	3. Avellino corneal dystrophy (combined granular-lattice)
	4. Macular dystrophy
	   Type I
	   Type II
	5. Gelatinous drop-like dystrophy (primary familial amyloidosis)
	6. Schnyder crystalline corneal dystrophy
	7. Fleck dystrophy
	8. Central cloudy dystrophy of Francois
	9. Congenital hereditary stromal dystrophy

Endothelium	1. Posterior polymorphous dystrophy (PPMD) 2. Fuchs' hereditary endothelial dystrophy 3. Congenital hereditary endothelial dystrophy (CHED I & II)

6. What is the age of presentation of the corneal dystrophies?

Most dystrophies become clinically apparent by second decade of life. There are some that may present in the first few years of life like epithelial basement membrane dystrophy and others like Fuchs' dystrophy, which may not become symptomatic until very late in life.

7. What is the mechanism of decreased vision in dystrophies?

i. Intraocular light scattering in the initial stages

ii. Disruption of geometric image caused by the corneal deposits and by the anterior corneal surface

iii. Recurrent corneal erosions and resultant subepithelial scarring

iv. Opacities causing obstruction to light

v. By affecting normal endothelial function as in CHED, Fuchs' dystrophy, etc.

8. What are the types of dystrophies affecting vision?

i. Macular dystrophy

ii. Lattice dystrophy

iii. Central crystalline

iv. Congenital hereditary endothelial dystrophy

v. Fuchs' dystrophy

9. **What are the types of dystrophies not affecting vision?**

   i. Granular
   ii. Fleck dystrophy.

10. **What are the modes of inheritance of corneal dystrophies?**

   Most of them are inherited as autosomal dominant except
   i. Macular (autosomal recessive)
   ii. Congenital hereditary endothelial dystrophy (type II)
   iii. Posterior polymorphous (rarely autosomal recessive)
   iv. Type III lattice (recessive).

11. **What is the frequency of recurrence of stromal dystrophy in a graft?**

   Among the stromal dystrophies frequency of regraft is highest in lattice dystrophy, followed by granular dystrophy, and then macular dystrophy. Of all the dystrophies the recurrence is very high for gelatinous drop-like dystrophy.

12. **Why is Avellino corneal dystrophy named so?**

   It was originally described in a small number of families who traced their roots to a place Avellino, in Italy. It is a combination of lattice and granular dystrophies.

13. **How is granular dystrophy inherited?**

   An autosomal dominant transmission with variable expression. Linked to chromosome 5q31, along with lattice, Avellino, and Reis-Bucklers dystrophy.

14. **What are the features of granular dystrophy?**

   i. Bilaterally symmetric and affects the central cornea
   ii. Glare and photophobia due to light scatter by the opacities
   iii. Vision remains normal in till around 40 years. In an affected patient, a diffuse, and irregular, ground-glass haze may appear in the superficial stroma
   iv. It is characterized by the discrete, white dense; round to oval granular opacities lie in the relatively clear stroma and form a variety of patterns, including arcuate chains and straight lines. *The intervening and peripheral areas of cornea are clear*
   v. They are characterized by focal extracellular aggregates of eosinophilic material occupying all levels of the stroma
   vi. A mutation in the BIGH3 gene localized to chromosome 5q31 is responsible for granular corneal dystrophy.

15. **What are the differential diagnoses of granular dystrophy?**

   Paraproteinemia A in a patient with leukemia can produce dense crystalline deposits in the cornea. Serum protein electrophoresis will show an M component spike in the patient with paraproteinemic keratopathy.

16. Classify lattice dystrophies.

Type	Predominant corneal location	Inheritance	Age of onset	Amyloid protein
Type I	Central, full thickness	Autosomal dominant	First–second decade	AA
Type II (coexisting systemic amyloidosis)	Peripheral radial pattern	Autosomal dominant	Third decade	Gelsolin
Type III	Peripheral radial pattern	Autosomal recessive	Sixth decade	AP

17. What are the characteristic features of lattice-I dystrophy?

The characteristic translucent lattice lines vary from a few small comma-shaped flecks to a dense network of large irregular ropy cords that contain white dots. The white dots and lattice lines consist of amyloid. In the corneal stroma they form fusiform deposits that push aside the collagen lamellae. Lattice dystrophy results from abnormal keratocyte synthesis.

18. What are the slit-lamp findings in lattice-II dystrophy?

Coarse translucent stromal lattice lines radiating centrally from the limbus sparing the central and intervening cornea.

19. What are the systemic features of lattice-II dystrophy?

i. Slowly progressive cranial and peripheral neuropathy
ii. Skin changes such as lichen amyloidosis, cutis laxa, blepharochalasis, protruding lips, and mask facies, and, variably ventricular hypertrophy and polycythemia vera.

20. What are features of lattice-III dystrophy?

i. Inherited as an autosomal recessive trait and has a late adult onset
ii. The disorder occurs unilaterally or bilaterally
iii. Usually, visual acuity is not greatly affected
iv. The lattice lines are thick and ropy and extend from limbus to limbus
v. Variably sized amyloid deposits accumulate beneath Bowman's layer and in the anterior stroma.

21. What are the components of amyloid?

Their chemical composition is unknown, but pre-albumin, transthyretin AP protein, and gelsolin (actin-modulating plasma protein, an amyloidogenic protein), are all associated with the amyloid deposits.

22. **Define Avellino dystrophy.**

Concurrent granular and lattice dystrophies in the same cornea.

23. **What are the clinical features of combined granular-lattice dystrophy?**

Exhibits an autosomal dominant inheritance pattern and appears in the first decade of life.

Granular	Lattice
The granular lesions resemble the sharply demarcated, round, focal deposits of isolated granular dystrophy, but they occur early in life and may be accompanied by a diffuse haze between the granules. The granular deposits are clustered in the anterior stroma	Whiter, and more polygonal or speculated occur later in life, and lack the classic glass-red refractile appearance in retroillumination. The lattice deposits appear in middle to posterior stroma

24. **What are the characteristic features of gelatinous drop-like dystrophy?**

   i. Gelatinous drop-like dystrophy is a rare, bilaterally symmetric, primary familial corneal amyloidosis.
   ii. Inherited as an autosomal recessive mapped to chromosome 1p.
   iii. The disorder manifests early in life in the first decade.
   iv. Presenting symptoms include photophobia, lacrimation, foreign body sensation, and progressive deteriorating vision.
   v. It is characterized by multiple, subepithelial, gelatinous excrescences that give the corneal surface a mulberry appearance.
   vi. The deposits appear opaque on direct illumination and translucent in retroillumination. In advanced case, they are accompanied by neovascularization.

25. **What are the characteristics of macular dystrophy?**

   i. It is an autosomal recessive disease
   ii. It involves both the central and peripheral cornea, and also all the layers of cornea
   iii. It is a heterogeneous disorder, on the basis of the type of an abnormal proteoglycan present
   iv. This condition requires penetrating keratoplasty earlier than other stromal dystrophies
   v. Recurrence after graft is less common when compared to lattice and granular dystrophy. The cornea is thinner than normal.

26. Classify macular dystrophy.

Based on the immune histochemical studies macular dystrophy are classified into two types as:

Type I	Type II
Most common. The antigenic keratin sulfate are absent from both serum and cornea	Antigenic keratin sulfate is both present in serum and cornea
Deficiency of sulfotransferase enzyme (an enzyme that catalyze the sulfation of kerato amino-glycans) leads to precipitation of less soluble keratin chains in the extracellular matrix causing loss of transparency	Dermatan sulfate proteoglycan molecule is shorter than that of normal individuals resulting in abnormal packing of collagen fibers

27. What is the substance that forms the stromal opacity in macular dystrophy?

The stromal opacities correspond to the deposition of abnormal keratin sulfate proteoglycans.

28. What are the clinical features of central crystalline dystrophy?

i. It is a bilateral disorder with autosomal dominant inheritance.
ii. It is characterized by deposition of subepithelial corneal crystals that appear early in life.
iii. Local disorder of corneal lipid metabolism. Pathologically, the opacities are accumulations of unesterified and esterified cholesterol and phospholipids.
iv. The crystals are generally deposited in an arcuate or circular pattern in the anterior, paracentral stroma). When they are relatively dense, they give the cornea a bull's eye appearance and may reduce vision.
v. Oil Red O stains the globular neutral fats red whereas the Schultz method stains cholesterol crystals blue-green.

29. What is the Weiss classification of central crystalline dystrophy (Schnyder's crystalline dystrophy)?

Weiss has recommended that this dystrophy be reclassified into two major clinical types:

i. With superficial stromal cholesterol crystals
ii. With diffuse full-thickness stromal haze alone.

30. What is Schnyder's dystrophy sine (without) crystals?

It is a rare dystrophy with diffuse stromal haze only are called Schnyder's dystrophy sine (without) crystals.

31. What are associated systemic conditions of central crystalline dystrophy?

Central crystalline dystrophy can be associated with hyperlipidemia, thyroid abnormalities, and genu valgum.

32. Describe Bietti's crystalline dystrophy.
   i. Bietti's crystalline dystrophy is autosomal recessive disorder.
   ii. It is characterized by marginal depositions of numerous, small crystals in the anterior peripheral corneal stroma and in the paracentral and peripapillary retina.
   iii. Visual acuity is retained throughout its course but pigmentary changes occur at the fovea and in the retinal periphery which produce poor dark adaption and paracentral scotomata.
   iv. The demonstration of crystals resembling cholesterol and other lipids suggest a systemic abnormality of lipid metabolism.

33. What are the features of fleck dystrophy?
   i. Uncommon nonprogressive stromal dystrophy begins very early in life and may be congenital. It shows extreme asymmetry.
   ii. Affected keratocytes contain two abnormal substances: excess glycosaminoglycan, which stain with Alcian blue and colloidal iron and lipids demonstrated by Sudan Black and Oil Red O.
   iii. Discrete flat gray-white dandruff-like opacities appear throughout the stroma to its periphery. Symptoms are minimal and vision is usually not reduced.

34. What are the features of central cloudy dystrophy of Francois?

Bilateral, symmetrical, and slowly progressive stromal dystrophy. Autosomal dominant inheritance. Extracellular deposition of mucopolysaccharide and lipid-like material has been described.

Clinically opacity is densest centrally and posteriorly and fades both anteriorly and peripherally. Opacities consist of multiple nebulous, polygonal, gray areas separated by crack-like intervening clear zones. Vision is usually not reduced.

35. Write short notes on congenital hereditary stromal dystrophy?
   i. Autosomal dominant disorder and consists of bilaterally symmetric central anterior stromal, flaky feathery opacities that are present at birth.
   ii. Congenital hereditary stromal dystrophy is nonprogressive but is often accompanied by searching nystagmus and esotropia.
   iii. Histopathologically, the stroma consists of alternating layers of tightly packed and loosely packed collagen fibrils about 15 nm in diameter.

iv. The treatment of choice is penetrating keratoplasty, although amblyopia usually limits visually acuity to 20/200.

36. How to differentiate CHSD and CHED?

CHSD	CHED
Nonprogressive condition Normal corneal thickness and absence of both epithelial edema and thickening of Descemet's membrane	Progressive in autosomal recessive condition Increased corneal thickness to about two to three times and diffuse gray-blue ground-glass appearance which is the pathological hallmark of disease

37. What are the various methods of diagnosing corneal dystrophies?

   i. Transmission electron microscopy—accurate method
  ii. Immunohistochemistry—identifies composition of deposits in dystrophic corneas
 iii. Molecular genetics—using common DNA determinants.

38. Name the substances that are found in various stromal dystrophies.

It can be remembered using the acronym.

Marilyn   — Macular
Monroe   — Mucopolysaccharides
Always   — Alcian blue
Gets   — Granular
Her   — Hyaline lipoprotein
Man   — Masson's trichrome stain
L   — Lattice
A   — Amyloid
City   — Congo red

Dystrophy	Material	Stain
Macular	Mucology	Alcian blue
Granular	Hyaline	Mucin
Lattice	Amyline	Congo red

39. What are the stains that are used in stromal dystrophies?

Stain for amyloid in lattice dystrophy:

   i. Pink to orange by Congo red.
  ii. Alternating red and green color when viewed through a rotating polarizing filter.
 iii. Yellowish green color against black background through two rotating filters.
  iv. Periodic Acid Schiff's and Masson's trichrome staining can also be used.

Stain for granular dystrophy (Hyaline lipoprotein):
Masson's trichrome staining gives bright red color.

Stain for macular dystrophy (Glycosoaminoglycans or mucopol-ysaccharides):
Blue color on staining with Alcian blue, cuprolinic blue, and colloidal iron.

40. How to treat a case of a stromal dystrophy?

  i. Observation and best corrected refractive correction by spectacles. Since most of the patients are asymptomatic during their initial stages of presentation it is better to observe
  ii. Treatment of symptoms of erosion:
      Lubricants
 iii. Excimer laser phototherapeutic keratectomy (PTK):
      Used to treat the superficial lesions
      It can also be used to treat recurrence of granular dystrophy in a penetrating keratoplasty because the recurrences are almost always superficial
  iv. Superficial keratectomy:
      Dense superficial juvenile variety can be treated by superficial keratectomy or lamellar keratoplasty, an advantage because multiple recurrences can be treated by multiple grafts
   v. Lamellar keratoplasty:
      For diseases involving the superficial stroma
  vi. Deep lamellar keratoplasty
 vii. Penetrating keratoplasty
      Indications: When dense opacities and subepithelial connective tissue reduce visual function to unacceptable levels. But recurrence is common affecting within 5 years.
      Macular dystrophy requires penetrating keratoplasty earlier than other stromal dystrophies.
      Recurrence after graft is less common in macular dystrophy when compared to lattice and granular dystrophy.

41. What is the differential diagnosis of congenital corneal opacity?

Acronym for differential diagnosis of neonatal cloudy cornea—STUMPED

S Sclerocornea
T Tears in Descemet's membrane
    Infantile glaucoma—most common cause
    Birth trauma
U Ulcer: Herpes simplex viral keratitis, bacterial, neurotrophic
M Metabolic disorders: Rare—mucopolysaccharidosis, mucolipidosis, tyrosinosis

P   Posterior corneal defect: Posterior keratoconus, Peter's anomaly—most common cause staphyloma

E   Endothelial dystrophy: Congenital hereditary endothelial dystrophy, posterior polymorphous dystrophy, congenital hereditary stromal dystrophy

D   Dermoid.

42. **What are the conditions that cause recurrent corneal epithelial erosions?**

Primary epithelial dystrophies	Map-dot-fingerprint basement membrane, Franceschetti's recurrent epithelial, epithelial rosette. Meesmann's epithelial
Stromal and endothelial	Reis-Bucklers, gelatinous drop-like, lattice
Dystrophies	Fuchs' endothelial
Systemic diseases	Epidermolysis bullosa

43. **How do you manage recurrent corneal erosions?**
    i. Lubricating eye drops and ointments
    ii. Epithelial debridement
    iii. Bandage contact lenses
    iv. Anterior stromal puncture to increase adhesions
    v. Excimer laser PTK.

2.15. FUCHS' ENDOTHELIAL DYSTROPHY

1. **What is Fuchs' dystrophy?**

   Fuchs' dystrophy (combined dystrophy) is defined as a bilateral, non-inflammatory progressive loss of endothelium that results in reduction of vision; the key features being guttae, folds in Descemet's membrane, stromal edema and microcystic epithelial edema.

2. **Describe the epidemiology of Fuchs' dystrophy.**
   i. Autosomal dominant, occasionally sporadic.
   ii. Female preponderance (4:1).
   iii. Elderly; onset of symptoms > 50 years.
   iv. Increased incidence of POAG (reason unclear).

3. **Describe the pathogenesis of Fuchs' dystrophy.**
   i. The primary cause of the dysfunctional endothelial cells is unknown.
   ii. Corneal swelling is thought to result from the loss of Na-K ATPase pump sites within the endothelium and an increase in permeability.
   iii. The deposition of aberrant collagen fibrils and basement membrane with thickening of Descemet's membrane is a result of endothelial cell transformation to fibroblast like cells.

4. **Describe the various hypotheses regarding the pathogenesis of Fuchs' dystrophy.**
   i. Believed to be due to an embryonic defect in the terminal induction or differentiation of neural crest cells resulting in abnormal morphology of the Descemet's membrane.
   ii. Hormonal influences are suspected as the phenotypic expression is more severe in women.
   iii. Endothelial inflammation secondary to trauma, toxins or infection results in endothelial cell pleomorphism, and a thickened abnormal Descemet's membrane.

5. **What are the symptoms of Fuchs' dystrophy?**
   i. Initially asymptomatic.
   ii. Decrease in vision (related to edema).
   iii. Pain due to ruptured epithelial bullae.
   iv. Symptoms are worse upon awakening.
   v. Painful episodes subside once subepithelial fibrosis occurs.

6. **Why are symptoms worse upon awakening?**

   The decrease in vision and glare in Fuchs' dystrophy are primarily due to varying degree of epithelial and stromal edema. Decreased evaporation of the tears during sleep decreases their osmolarity, leading to increased edema and decreased visual acuity upon awakening.

7. **Describe the clinical stages of Fuchs' dystrophy.**

   Stage: 1
   i. Asymptomatic
   ii. Central cornel guttae
   iii. Pigments on posterior corneal surface
   iv. Gray and thickened appearance of Descemet's membrane
   v. In more advanced cases, endothelium has a "beaten-bronze" appearance due to the associated melanin deposition.

   Stage: 2
   i. Painless decrease in vision and glare, severe on awakening
   ii. Stromal edema (ground-glass appearance)
   iii. Microcystic epithelial edema (occurs when stromal thickness has been increased by about 30%).

   Stage: 3
   i. Episodes of pain
   ii. Formation of epithelial and subepithelial bullae, which rupture.

   Stage: 4
   i. Visual acuity may be reduced to hand movements
   ii. Free of painful attacks
   iii. Appearance of subepithelial scar tissue.

8. **What are the differential diagnoses of Fuchs' dystrophy?**
   i. Posterior polymorphous dystrophy
   ii. Congenital hereditary epithelial dystrophy
   iii. Aphakic/pseudophakic bullous keratopathy
   iv. Chandler's syndrome
   v. Interstitial keratitis
   vi. Trauma
   vii. Intraocular inflammation.

9. **How is a diagnosis of Fuchs' dystrophy made?**
   i. Slit-lamp findings of guttae, stromal edema, epithelial bullae
   ii. Increased central corneal thickness on pachymetry
   iii. Specular microscopy.

10. **What are the features of Fuchs' dystrophy seen on specular microscopy?**
    i. Pleomorphism (increased variability in cell shape)
    ii. Polymegathism (increased variation in individual cell areas)
    iii. Decreased endothelial cell count
    iv. Guttae are seen as small dark areas with central bright spot in mild disease
    v. Later, severely disorganized endothelial mosaic is seen.

11. **What are the histopathological changes in Fuchs' dystrophy?**

Epithelium

i. Initially, intracellular edema in the basal cells
ii. Later, interepithelial and subepithelial pockets of fluids develop
iii. Map-dot and fingerprint scarring.

Bowman's membrane

i. Usually intact
ii. Subepithelial fibrosis, thick in advanced disease.

Stroma

i. Moderate thickening and edema.

Descemet's membrane

i. Diffusely thickened since deposition of collagen basement membrane-like material.
ii. Anterior banded layer—relatively normal.
iii. Posterior non-banded layer—thinned and irregular.
iv. Followed by a thick banded layer similar to the anterior banded zone and composing the guttae.

Endothelium

i. Lower cell density
ii. Enlarged cells
iii. Thinning of cells over Descemet's warts
iv. Fibroblast-like metaplasia in end stage.

12. **Why does rupture of bullae cause pain?**

Rupture of epithelial bullae exposes the underlying nerve ending and hence causes pain.

13. **Describe the medical management of Fuchs' dystrophy.**

i. Hyperosmotic eyed rops and ointment reduces the epithelial edema and improves both comfort and vision.
   – 5% NaCl drops 4–8 times/day.
   – 5% NaCl ointment at night.
ii. A hairdryer held at arm's length may help "dry-out" the corneal surface.
iii. Lowering of IOP is useful in some cases.
iv. Bandage contact lens is used to alleviate discomfort from bullae formation and rupture.

14. **Describe the surgical management of Fuchs' dystrophy.**

Indicated when diminished visual acuity impairs normal activities. If there is no corneal opacity due to subepithelial fibrosis, then DSAEK (Descemet's stripping automated endothelial keratoplasty) is done. A recent modification called DMEK (descemet membrane endothelial keratoplasty) is also being performed.

15. **What are all the surgical measures for Fuchs' dystrophy done for relief of pain?**

   i. Anterior stromal puncture

  ii. Bowman's membrane cauterization

 iii. Conjunctival hooding

 iv. Amniotic membrane transplantation.

2.16. ENDOTHELIAL DISORDERS AND BULLOUS KERATOPATHY

1. **Classify endothelial diseases.**

   i. **Primary endothelial diseases**
   Endothelial dystrophy:
   - Fuchs' endothelial dystrophy
   - Posterior polymorphous dystrophy
   - Congenial hereditary endothelial dystrophy
   - Iridocorneal endothelial syndrome.

   ii. **Secondary endothelial diseases**
   - Mechanical trauma to the endothelium
     - Intraocular foreign body
     - Corneal trauma
     - Cataract surgery
       o Preexisting endothelial disease
       o Surgical trauma
       o Intraoperative mechanical trauma
       o Postoperative trauma
       o Vitreous touch
       o IOL
   - Nonmechanical damage to the endothelium
     - Inflammation
     - Increased IOP
     - Contact lens (hypoxia).

2. **What is CHED?**

   Congenital hereditary endothelial dystrophy (CHED) is a dystrophy in which there is bilateral corneal edema. The corneal appearance varies from a blue-gray, ground-glass appearance to total opacification.

   Types: CHED 1
   CHED 2

3. **What are the features of CHED 1?**

   Autosomal dominant inheritance with the gene locus on 20p11.2–q11.2. It is less severe developing in the first and second year of life.
   Symptoms: Progressive defective vision is present. Nystagmus is absent.

4. **What are the features of CHED 2?**

   Autosomal recessive inheritance with the gene locus on 20p13. Present at birth. Relatively nonprogressive.

Symptoms of discomfort are less prominent despite profound epithelial and stromal edema. Nystagmus is common.

5. What is pathogenesis of CHED?

The association of enlarged stromal collagen fibrils suggests some primary development abnormality of both keratocyte and endothelium quantifying this disorder as an example of mesenchymal dysgenesis.

6. Is there an association between CHED and glaucoma?

A combination of congenital glaucoma and CHED may occur and should be suspected when persistent and total corneal opacification fails to resolve after normalization of IOP.

7. How do you differentiate between CHED and congenital glaucoma?

Sl No	Congenital glaucoma	CHED
1.	Photophobia present	No photophobia
2.	Tearing and redness	Eye white
3.	Megalocornea	Normal-sized cornea
4.	Epithelial edema	More of a thick cornea

8. What are corneal guttae?

Seen as a primary condition in middle age and old age. Reveals a typical beaten metal appearance of the Descemet's membrane. These warts like excrescences are abnormal elaboration of basement membrane and fibrillar collagen by distressed or dystrophied endothelial cells.

9. What are Hassall–Henle bodies?

Guttae located in the periphery of the cornea may be seen in patients as they get older. It is of no clinical signification.

10. What is posterior polymorphous dystrophy (PPMD)?

It is a rare, slowly progressive autosomal dominant or recessive dystrophy that presents early in life. It has been mapped to chromosome 20q11.

Pathogenesis: The most distinctive microscopic finding is the appearance of abnormal, multilayered endothelial cells that look and behave like epithelial cells or fibroblast.

These cells show:

   i. Microvilli
  ii. Stain positive for keratin
 iii. Show rapid and easy growth in culture
 iv. Have intercellular desmosomes
  v. Manifest proliferative tendencies

A diffuse abnormality of the Descemet's membrane (DM) is common including thickening and multilaminated appearance and polymorphous alteration.

11. What are PPMD's clinical manifestations?

The posterior corneal surface shows

  i. Isolated grouped vesicles
 ii. Geographic-shaped discrete gray lesions
iii. Broad bands with scalloped edges.

12. Association of PPMD.

   i. Iris membranes
  ii. Peripheral anterior synechiae
 iii. Ectropion uveae
  iv. Corectopia
   v. Polycoria
  vi. Glaucoma
 vii. Reminiscent of iridocorneal endothelial syndrome
viii. Alport's disease

13. What are the investigations to detect PPMD?

  i. Specular microscopy shows typical vesicles and bands
 ii. Confocal microscopy reveals alteration in Descemet's membrane.

14. Management of PPMD.

  i. Most patients are asymptomatic
 ii. Mild corneal edema can be managed as with early Fuchs' dystrophy
iii. Stromal micropuncture to induce subthelial pannus can be done to manage localized swelling
 iv. In severe disease glaucoma must be managed and corneal transplant may be required.

15. What is iridocorneal endothelial syndrome?

It is typically unilateral occurring in middle-aged women. It is a spectrum of disorders characterized by varying degrees of corneal edema, glaucoma, and iris abnormalities. It consists of the following three disorders with considerable overlap in presentation.

  i. Progressive iris atrophy
 ii. Iris nevus (Cogan-Reese) syndrome
iii. Chandler's syndrome.

16. What is the pathogenesis of ICE syndrome?

The primary abnormality lies in the endothelial cell which takes on the ultrastructural characteristics of epithelial cells. The abnormal endothelial cells proliferate and migrate across the angle and onto the surface of the iris, "proliferative endotheliopathy."

Glaucoma may be due to synechial angle closure secondary to contraction of the abnormal tissue. Herpes simplex virus DNA has been identified in some ICE syndrome corneal specimens.

17. **What are the specific features?**

Progressive iris atrophy: Characterized by severe iris changes such as holes, corectopia, etc.

The iris nevus (Cogan–Reese) syndrome: characterized by either a diffuse nevus which covers the anterior iris or iris nodules. Iris atrophy is absent in 50% of the cases although corectopia may be severe.

Chandler's syndrome:
  i. Characterized by hammered silver corneal endothelial abnormalities.
  ii. Presence of corneal edema.
  iii. Stromal atrophy is absent in 60% of cases.
  iv. Corectopia is mild to moderate.
  v. Glaucoma is usually less severe than in the other two syndromes.

18. **Treatment of iridocorneal endothelial (ICE) syndrome.**

Management of glaucoma:
  i. Medical treatment is usually ineffective
  ii. Trabeculectomy is frequently unsuccessful
  iii. Artificial filtering shunts is usually required
  iv. Penetrating keratoplasty for the corneal component.

2.17. KERATOPLASTY

1. **What is keratoplasty?**

   It is a surgical procedure wherein the abnormal recipient corneal tissue is replaced by donor corneal tissue either full thickness or partial thickness.

2. **Why is corneal transplant more successful than the other transplants?**

   Cornea is relatively immune privileged.

   Three factors are:
   - i. Absence of blood vessels
   - ii. Absence of lymphatics
   - iii. Anterior chamber associated immune deviation (ACAID).

3. **Indications for keratoplasty.**
   - i. **Optical:**
     - Pseudophakic bullous keratopathy
     - Keratoconus
     - Corneal scars
     - Fuchs' dystrophy
   - ii. **Tectonic:**
     - Stromal thinning
     - Descemetocele
     - Ectatic disorders
   - iii. **Therapeutic:**
     - Removal of infected corneal tissue refractory to maximal medical therapy.

4. **Common indications for keratoplasty in our country.**
   - i. Corneal scar: healed infectious keratitis or traumatic scar
   - ii. Acute infectious keratitis
   - iii. Regrafting
   - iv. Aphakic and pseudophakic bullous keratopathy
   - v. Corneal dystrophy especially macular corneal dystrophy
   - vi. Keratoconus.

5. **Common indications for keratoplasty in the West.**
   - i. Aphakic or pseudophakic bullous keratopathy
   - ii. Fuchs' dystrophy
   - iii. Keratoconus
   - iv. Corneal scar
   - v. Dystrophies.

6. **What are the types of keratoplasty?**
   - i. Full thickness or penetrating keratoplasty
   - ii. Partial thickness or lamellar keratoplasty.

7. **What are the types of lamellar keratoplasty?**

    i. **Anterior:**
        - Anterior lamellar keratoplasty
        - Deep anterior lamellar keratoplasty (DALK).

    ii. **Posterior:**
        - Posterior lamellar keratoplasty (PLK)
        - Deep lamellar endothelial keratoplasty (DLEK)
        - Descemet's stripping endothelial keratoplasty (DSEK)
        - Descemet's stripping automated endothelial keratoplasty (DSAEK)
        - Descemet's membrane endothelial keratoplasty (DMEK).

8. **What are the conditions having excellent prognosis with kerato-plasty?**

    i.   Keratoconus
    ii. Central avascular corneal scars
    iii. Granular dystrophy
    iv. Macular dystrophy
    v.   Pseudophakic bullous keratopathy.

9. **What are the conditions having worst prognosis with keratoplasty?**

    i.   Stevens–Johnson syndrome
    ii. Ocular cicatricial pemphigoid
    iii. Severe chemical burns
    iv. Dry eye of any etiology like collagen vascular disorders.

10. **What are the contraindications for donor's selection?**

    i.   Death due to an unknown cause
    ii.   Rabies
    iii. Certain infectious diseases of CNS like Jacob-Creutzfeldt, subacute sclerosing panencephalitis (SSPE), and progressive multifocal leuko encephalopathy
    iv.   HIV
    v.   Septicemia
    vi.   Systemic infections like syphilis, viral hepatitis B and C
    vii. Leukemia and disseminated lymphoma
    viii. Intraocular tumors.

11. **What is the importance of graft size and how much is it?**

    Usually donor cornea should be oversized by 0.5 mm from recipient cornea. In keratoconus same size can be used.
    Graft size is about 7.5–8.5 mm.

12. **What are the disadvantages of larger graft?**

    Larger graft may cause:
    i. Increased intraocular pressure

ii. Rejection
iii. Anterior synechiae
iv. Vascularization.

13. What are the disadvantages of smaller graft?

Smaller graft would give rise to astigmatism due to subsequent tissue tension.

14. Why should graft in keratoconus be same size?

Using same diameter trephines for both donor and host tissues helps by decreasing postoperative myopia.

15. What are the methods of anterior chamber entry in PKP?

  i. **Trephine:**
   Advantages:
   – Sharp vertical edges
   – Quick
   – Uniform entry in all 360°.
   Disadvantage:
     Not controlled and so chance of damage to intraocular structures.
  ii. **Blade:**
   Advantage:
     Controlled entry.
   Disadvantage:
     May not be uniform.

16. Where are the cardinal sutures placed in PKP?

The first suture is placed at 12 o'clock. The second suture is the most important suture and is placed at 6 o'clock position. The third and fourth sutures are put at 3 o'clock and 9 o'clock position, respectively. At the end of four cardinal sutures, a trapezoid should be formed.

17. What are the indications for interrupted sutures?

  i. Corneas of uneven thickness.
  ii. Corneas with localized areas of inflammation.
  iii. Vascularized, inflamed or thinned corneas where uneven wound healing is expected.
  iv. Corneas in which bites on the recipient side is very close to the sclera.
  v. Pediatric keratoplasties.

18. What are the advantages of interrupted sutures?

  i. Technically less difficult.
  ii. Permits elective removal in case of children and uneven wound healing.
  iii. Individual suture bites can be adjusted.
  iv. Selective sutures can be removed in case of infection.

19. What are the disadvantages of interrupted sutures?

Stimulates more inflammation and vascularization because of more knots.

20. When can continuous sutures be used?

In absence of inflammation, vascularization or thinning, continuous sutures can be used.

21. What are the advantages of continuous sutures?

    i. They allow more even distribution of tension around the wound.
    ii. Wound healing is more uniform.
    iii. Incites less inflammation because of less knots.
    iv. If double continuous is done, the second running suture can be placed in a manner that counteracts the torque induced by the first.

22. What are the disadvantages of continuous sutures?

Sectoral loosening or cheese wiring compromises the entire closure of the cornea.

23. What are torque and antitorque sutures?

When continuous sutures are radially arranged perpendicular to the limbus they are bound to induce some torque while tightening and so they are known as torque sutures.

When the sutures are typically placed 30–40° to the donor-recipient interface in the direction of suture advancement, they are known as antitorque sutures.

24. What are combined sutures?

When both types of suturing: continuous and intermittent are used to secure the graft it is called combined suture.

25. What is the advantage of combined sutures?

They have advantage of both. Interrupted sutures can be removed as early as 4 weeks later. Continuous suture can remain *in situ* to protect against wound dehiscence.

26. What are the guidelines for suture removal?

    i. Interrupted sutures can be removed before 6–12 months.
    ii. Combined interrupted sutures in steep meridian at 3 months.
    iii. Continuous sutures can be removed after 1 year.
    iv. Always remove suture by pulling on the recipient's side.
    v. Only loose sutures should be removed. Tight sutures may need to be cut or replaced.

27. What is lamellar keratoplasty?

Selective replacement of diseased recipient tissue wherein the partial thickness donor graft is placed in recipient corneal bed. This is prepared by lamellar dissection of abnormal corneal tissue, the donor graft being of similar size, and thickness as the removed pathological host cornea.

28. What are the advantages of anterior lamellar over penetrating keratoplasty?

    i. Extraocular procedure and hence devoid of intraocular complications like hyphema, endophthalmitis, etc.

    ii. Large graft can be placed.

    iii. Less chances of rejection.

    iv. Nonviable tissue (tissue with low endothelial count) can be used.

    v. Less stringent donor selection.

    vi. Faster recovery.

    vii. Better wound strength.

29. What are the disadvantages of lamellar keratoplasty?

    i. Procedure is technically more demanding.

    ii. Visual acuity can be impaired due to uneven dissection of recipient or donor corneal tissue and interface scarring.

    iii. Particulate debris trapped in lamellar interface.

    iv. Mechanical folds in the posterior layer over the visual axis due to flattening of this layer especially in keratoconus.

    v. Vascularization and opacification at the interface.

30. What are the indications for lamellar keratoplasty?

    i. **Anterior:**
- Localized superficial corneal scar
- Keratoconus
- Corneal and conjunctival tumors.

    ii. **Posterior:**
- Fuchs' dystrophy without corneal scarring
- Pseudophakic bullous keratopathy without scarring.

31. When do you prefer anterior lamellar keratoplasty and why?

Anterior keratoplasties are useful in treating:

    i. Keratoconus

    ii. Scars from refractive surgery or trauma

    iii. Stromal scarring from bacterial or viral infections

Healthy recipient endothelium is preserved thus decreasing graft rejection and prolonged graft survival.

32. When do you prefer posterior lamellar keratoplasty and why?

Posterior keratoplasties are used primarily for endothelial diseases like:

    i. Fuchs' endothelial dystrophy

    ii. Aphakic or pseudophakic bullous keratopathy.

Advantages of posterior lamellar keratoplasty are:

i. Posterior grafts do not require corneal surface incisions and suture so induced astigmatism is reduced and tectonic stability is greater.
ii. Quicker visual rehabilitation.
iii. Theoretically lesser chance of stromal rejection.
iv. No suture related complications as no sutures.
v. Strong wound.

33. What are the disadvantages of posterior lamellar keratoplasty (DSAEK/DMEK)?

i. Requires very high quality donor tissue.
ii. Requires costly instruments like microkeratome, artificial anterior chamber.
iii. Higher chance of primary graft failure.
iv. Higher chance of resurgeries like rebubbling.
v. Cannot be performed if there is a significant anterior stroma opacity.

34. What are inlay and onlay lamellar keratoplasties?

Inlay: Partial thickness of recipient cornea is removed by lamellar dissection and replaced by partial thickness of donor cornea.

Onlay: Partial thickness donor cornea is placed over a de-epithelized recipient cornea in which either a small peripheral keratectomy or lamellar dissection has been done (e.g. epikeratoplasty).

35. What are the techniques of deep anterior lamellar keratoplasty (DALK)?

DALK involves replacing the entire stroma barring the Descemet's membrane (DM). This can be achieved by:

i. Dissecting with balanced salt solution, ocular viscoelastic device
ii. Big bubble technique of Anwar where bubble is used to blow the Descemet's membrane off the rest of the cornea
iii. Melles' technique where a series of dissecting blades do a deep dissection to the cornea almost down to Descemet's membrane.

36. What is the difference between DLEK and DSEK?

In DLEK, manual lamellar dissection with corneal depth of 75–85% is done in the recipient. In DSEK, no lamellar dissection is necessary. Instead the DM is stripped off the central 8 mm of the cornea using a reverse Sinskey's hook followed by placement of the folded donor disk via sclero corneal tunnel.

37. What is the difference between DSEK and DSAEK?

DSEK: Donor dissection is done using a manual artificial anterior chamber.
DSAEK: Donor dissection is done using a microkeratome.

38. What is femtosecond DSEK?

In this the donor tissue is precut with laser. Rest of the steps continue like normal DSEK.

39 How is DSEK superior to DLEK?

DSEK:

i. Obviates complex recipient trephination and dissection techniques. Better visual outcome.

ii. Less potential for trauma to the anterior chamber and lens.

iii. Ability to perform corneal refractive surgery later on to correct refractive errors.

40. What is the advantage of DMEK?

The visual rehabilitation is superior to DSAEK, since only the Descemet's membrane and endothelium is transplanted without any stroma. However, it is technically difficult and there is a higher chance of graft dislocation.

41. What are the complications of keratoplasty?

Intraoperative complications:

i. Improper trephination: If smaller size trephine used for donor button instead of recipient button, complications of smaller graft like increased IOP may be seen.

ii. Damage to donor button during trephination.

iii. Incomplete trephination in recipient cornea-retained Descemet's membrane.

iv. Iris or lens damage.

v. Anterior chamber hemorrhage.

vi. Torn posterior capsule during combined keratoplasty with cataract surgery.

vii. Expulsive choroidal hemorrhage.

Postoperative complications:

i. Wound leaks and wound displacement

ii. Persistent epithelial defects

iii. Filamentary keratitis

iv. Suture-related complications:
- Suture exposure
- Suture-related infection
- Suture-related immune infiltrate

v. Elevated intraocular pressure

vi. Postoperative inflammation

vii. Anterior synechiae

viii. Pupillary block

   ix. Choroidal detachment or hemorrhage

   x. Fixed dilated pupil

   xi. Postoperative infection: Endophthalmitis rates post-PKP: 0.2–0.7%

   xii. Primary donor failure.

42. How is the donor tissue evaluated?

   i. Slit-lamp appearance for lusture, presence or absence of folds

   ii. Specular microscopy data

   iii. Death to preservation time

   iv. Tissue storage time

   v. Serology—hepatitis B and HIV.

43. What is the recommended lower limit for age of donors?

Donor corneas less than 1 year of age is not used, as these corneas are extremely flaccid and can result in high corneal astigmatism and myopia.

44. What is the recommended upper limit for age of donor?

The upper limit recommended by eye bank association of America is 70 years, but as long as the cornea is healthy, donor age does not matter.

45. What is the difference between graft rejection and failure?

Graft rejection is an immunologically mediated reversible loss of graft transparency in a graft which remained clear for at least 10–14 days following PKP.

Graft failure is irreversible loss of graft corneal transparency. It can be primary failure or late donor failure or end result of multiple rejection episodes.

46. Mention the most common types of rejection.

   i. Endothelial

   ii. Subepithelial

   iii. Epithelial

   iv. Stromal (in decreasing frequency).

47. What are the risk factors for rejection? Or Who are the high-risk patients?

Host factors:

   i. Corneal stromal vascularization

   ii. Regrafts: two or more higher chances

   iii. Coexisting conditions like uveitis, herpes simplex keratitis, atopic dermatitis, and eczema

   iv. Active ocular inflammation at the time of surgery

   v. Age: young patient.

Technical factors:

   i. Larger graft

   ii. Eccentric graft

   iii. Therapeutic keratoplasty

iv. Suture removal

v. Loose sutures arching vascularization.

48. What is the Khodadoust line?

Linear arrangement of endothelial precipitates composed of inflammatory cells which originate at vascularized end of peripheral donor cornea or at junction of anterior synechiae with endothelium and moves toward center of cornea. It is seen in endothelial type of rejection.

49. What are the conclusions of Collaborative Corneal Transplant Study (CCTS)?

i. Donor-recipient tissue HLA typing has no significant long-term effect on success of transplantation.

ii. ABO compatibility is more useful.

iii. In high-risk patients, high dose topical long-term steroids, good patient compliance, and close follow up gives successful corneal transplant.

50. What are the symptoms and signs of graft rejection?

Symptoms precede the signs.

Symptoms: Decreased vision

Photophobia and glare

Signs: Circumcorneal congestion

Keratic precipitates

Localized corneal edema

Generalized corneal edema

51. What are the types of graft failure?

i. *Primary graft failure:* The graft is irreversibly edematous, right from the immediate postoperative period. The causes are:

– Poor donor tissue

– Traumatic surgery destroying endothelium.

ii. *Secondary graft failure:* Causes are:

– Irreversible rejection

– Infection

– Trauma.

52. How do you treat endothelial rejection?

i. Topical 1% prednisolone acetate eye drops: Titrate according to the response

ii. Subconjunctival injection of 0.5 mg dexamethasone

iii. Oral prednisolone acetate 1 mg/kg body weight

iv. Intravenous methyl prednisolone acetate

v. If it is still irreversible, then to plan for a regraft

53. How do you treat graft failure?

Regraft.

3.1. UVEITIS—HISTORY AND CLINICAL FEATURES

1. **Why is uvea named so?**

   "Uvea" is derived from the Greek word "*uva*" meaning grape. When the sclera is removed, the center of the eyeball appears like a grape and hence the name.

2. **What does iris mean?**

   Iris is derived from a Greek word meaning rainbow/halo.

3. **Why do the iris and ciliary body often get involved together?**

   The presence of the major arterial circle causes the involvement of both the iris and ciliary body in pathological conditions. The blood supply to the choroid is essentially segmental and hence the lesions are also isolated.

4. **What is the importance of age in uveitis?**

   i. Children
      - Juvenile rheumatoid arthritis
      - Toxocariasis

   ii. Young adults
      - Behcet's disease
      - HLA-B27 associated uveitis
      - Fuchs' uveitis
      - Sarcoidosis
      - Herpes simplex
      - Toxoplasmosis

   iii. Middle age
      - Reiter's disease
      - Ankylosing spondylitis
      - Vogt–Koyanagi–Harada syndrome
      - White dot syndromes
      - Toxoplasmosis

iv. Elderly individuals
- Vogt–Koyanagi–Harada syndrome
- Herpes zoster ophthalmicus
- Tuberculosis
- Leprosy

5. **What is the importance of gender in uveitis?**

i. Males
- Ankylosing spondylitis
- Reiter's disease
- Behcet's disease
- Sympathetic ophthalmia
ii. Females
- Rheumatoid arthritis
- Juvenile rheumatoid arthritis

6. **What is the importance of race in uveitis?**

i. Caucasians–Ankylosing spondylitis
ii. Blacks–Sarcoidosis
iii. Orientals–Vogt–Koyanagi–Harada syndrome
iv. Orientals–Behcet's disease
v. Filipinos-Coccidioidomycosis

7. **Definitions.**

i. **Anterior uveitis:**
It is subdivided into:
- *Iritis:* Inflammation involving iris only.
- *Iridocyclitis:* Inflammation involving iris and anterior part of ciliary body (the pars plana).
ii. **Intermediate uveitis:** Predominant involvement of pars plana and extreme periphery of retina.
iii. **Posterior uveitis:** Inflammation beyond the posterior border of vitreous base.
iv. **Panuveitis:** Involvement of the entire uveal tract.
v. **Retinochoroiditis:** Primary involvement of retina with associated involvement of choroid.
vi. **Chorioretinitis:** Primary involvement of choroid with associated involvement of retina.
vii. **Vitritis:** Presence of cells in the vitreous secondary to inflammation of uvea, retina, optic nerve, and blood vessels.
viii. **Diffuse choroiditis:** Generalized inflammation of the choroid.
ix. **Disseminated choroiditis:** Two or more scattered foci of inflammation in the choroid, retina or both.

   x. **Exogenous infection:** Infection occurring as a result of external injury to uvea, operative trauma or any other event leading to invasion of microorganisms from outside.

   xi. **Endogenous infection:** Infection occurring as a result of microorganisms or their products released from a different site within the body.

   xii. **Secondary infection:** Infection of uveal tract due to spread from other ocular tissue.

8. How do you classify uveitis?

International Uveitis Study Group (IUSG) Classification

i. *Anatomical classification*

Term	Primary site of inflammation	Includes
Anterior uveitis	Anterior chamber	Iritis Iridocyclitis Anterior cyclitis
Intermediate uveitis	Vitreous	Pars planitis Posterior cyclitis Hyalitis
Posterior uveitis	Retina/Choroid	Choroiditis Chorioretinitis Retinochoroiditis Retinitis Neuroretinitis
Panuveitis	AC/Vitreous/Retina/Choroid	

ii. *Clinical classification*
- **Infectious:**
  - Bacterial
  - Viral
  - Fungal
  - Parasitic
- **Noninfectious:**
  - Known systemic association
  - No known systemic association
  - Masquerade:
    - Neoplastic
    - Non-neoplastic

Anatomical Classification

Tessler's Classification

i. Sclerouveitis
ii. Keratouveitis

iii. Anterior uveitis
iv. Iritis
v. Iridocyclitis
vi. Intermediate uveitis
vii. Cyclitis, vitritis
viii. Pars planitis
ix. Posterior uveitis
x. Retinitis
xi. Choroiditis

Pathological Classification

i. Granulomatous and non-granulomatous
ii. Suppurative and exudative

Etiological Classification

Infectious

i. **Exogenous:** *Staphylococcus, Pseudomonas, Propionibacterium acnes.*
Secondary—iridocyclitis associated with herpetic keratitis, iridocyclitis
associated with anterior and posterior scleritis.

ii. **Endogenous:**

Bacterial	TB
	Syphilis
	Gonorrhea
Viral	Herpes simplex
	CMV
	Measles
	Influenza
Fungal	Histoplasmosis
	Coccidioidomycosis
	Candidiasis
Parasitic	Toxoplasmosis
	Toxocariasis
	Onchocerciasis
	Pneumocystis carinii

Hypersensitivity/autoimmune

i. Lens-induced—autoimmune reaction to lens protein
ii. Sympathetic ophthalmia—autoimmunity to uveal pigment
iii. VKH-suspected autoimmune origin
iv. Behcet's

Toxic

i. Systemic toxins—onchocercal uveitis
ii. Endo-ocular uveitis—atrophic uveitis in degenerating eyes
iii. Iridocyclitis in RD due to unusual proteins reaching through retinal tear
iv. Chemical irritants—miotics and cytotoxic agents.

Associated with Systemic Conditions

i. Associated with arthritis
ii. Ankylosing spondylitis (AS)
iii. Rheumatoid arthritis (RA)
iv. Juvenile rheumatoid arthritis (JRA)
v. Psoriatic arthritis
vi. Associated with GIT disorders: Ulcerative colitis
vii. Associated with anergy: Sarcoidosis, leprosy, TB.

Associated with Neoplasms

i. Retinoblastoma, choroidal melanoma.

Idiopathic

i. Specific—Fuchs'
ii. Nonspecific—account for 25% of all uveitis.

Occurrence of Uveitis

i. Most common type of uveitis:
   Anterior uveitis is the most common type, followed by intermediate, posterior, and panuveitis.
ii. Commonest age group affected, i.e. 20–40 years.
iii. Common causes of uveitis in young adults:
   - Behcet's
   - Sarcoidosis
   - Fuchs' heterochromic iridocyclitis
   - Herpes simplex
   - Toxoplasmosis
iv. Causes of uveitis in middle ages
   - Reiter's
   - Ankylosing spondylitis
   - Vogt–Koyanagi–Harada (VKH) syndrome
   - White dot syndrome
   - Toxoplasmosis
v. Uveitic entities with sex predilection

Males	Females
Ankylosing spondylitis	RA
Reiter's syndrome	JRA
Behcet's	

vi. Racial influence on uveitis
   Caucasians   – Ankylosing spondylitis, Reiter's syndrome
   Black   – Sarcoidosis
   Orientals   – VKH, Behcet's
   Philipino   – Coccidioidomycosis
vii. Geographic influence on uveitis
   – "Histoplasmosis belt" of Ohio, Missouri and Mississippi—histoplasmosis
   – Japan and Mediterranean countries—Behcet's and VKH
   – San Jaoquin Valley of California—coccidioidomycosis
viii. Genetic/familial influence on uveitis
   – RA and Collagen disease
   – Syphilis
   – HIV and CMV
   – TB
   – Pars planitis

SUN (Standardization of Uveitis Nomenclature) Working Group "Activity of Uveitis" Terminology:
Inactive: Grade 0 cells in AC
Worsening activity: Two-step increase in level of inflammation
Improving activity: Two-step decrease in level of inflammation
Remission: Inactive disease for > 3 months after discontinuing all treatment for eye disease.

SUN Working Group "Descriptors in Uveitis":
Onset: Sudden/Insidious
Duration:
   Limited: < 3 months duration
   Persistent: > 3 months duration
Courses:
   Acute: sudden onset and limited duration
   Recurrent: repeated episodes separated by periods of inactivity without treatment 3 months duration
   Chronic: persistent uveitis with relapse in < 3 months after discontinuing treatment
   Remission: inactive disease for at least 3 months after discontinuing treatment.

9. **Name causes of acute and chronic posterior uveitis.**

   i. *Acute posterior uveitis* occurs in toxoplasmosis
   ii. *Chronic posterior uveitis* occurs in pars planitis and toxocariasis.

10. **Name causes of acute generalized uveitis.**

   i. Endophthalmitis
   ii. Sympathetic ophthalmia.

11. What are the causes of acute suppurative uveitis?

   i. Panophthalmitis

   ii. Endophthalmitis

   iii. Suppurative iridocyclitis.

12. Name causes of unilateral non-granulomatous uveitis.

   i. Fuchs'

   ii. Ankylosing spondylitis.

13. What are the causes of unilateral granulomatous uveitis?

   i. Viral

   ii. Lens induced.

14. What are the causes of bilateral granulomatous uveitis?

Infectious	*Noninfectious*
Tuberculosis	Sarcoidosis
Leprosy	Vogt–Koyanagi–Harada (VKH) syndrome
Syphilis	Sympathetic ophthalmia (SO)

15. What is Fuchs' heterochromic uveitis? What are the gonioscopic findings in Fuchs'? What are its sequelae?

Fuchs' uveitis is an unilateral idiopathic non-granulomatous anterior uveitis occurring in young adults. It is associated with heterochromia of the iris.

Gonioscopic finding in Fuchs'—fine filamentous vessels bridging angle.

Sequelae in Fuchs'   — cataract

                    — glaucoma

16. What are the causes of uveitis associated with vitritis?

   i. Pars planitis

   ii. Irvine–Gass syndrome

   iii. Active retinitis

   iv. Trauma.

17. What is the relevance of eliciting the following history in uveitis?

   i. Trauma/eye surgery—sympathetic ophthalmia

   ii. Vitiligo, alopecia, poliosis—Vogt-Koyanagi-Harada (VKH) syndrome

   iii. Rashes: Hyper/Hypopigmentation—leprosy

   iv. Low back pain/Joint pain—ankylosing spondylitis (AS), rheumatoid arthritis (RA), psoriatic arthritis

   v. Painful mouth ulcers—Behcet's syndrome

   vi. Dysentery, altered bowel habits—ulcerative colitis

   vii. Ringing in the ears, hearing loss, headache—VKH

   viii. Respiratory symptoms.

18. Why history of fever is important in uveitis?

    i. Tuberculosis

    ii. Syphilis

    iii. Leprosy

    iv. Leptospirosis

    v. Collagen vascular disorders

19. What are the systemic findings associated with uveitis?

Skin:

    i. Rash of secondary syphilis

    ii. Erythema nodosum, sarcoidosis, Behcet's

    iii. Psoriasis—plaques, arthritis

    iv. Keratoderma blennorrhagica, Reiter's syndrome

    v. Kaposi sarcoma

    vi. Leprosy

    vii. Vogt–Koyanagi–Harada syndrome

    viii. Sarcoidosis.

Hair:

    i. Alopecia: VKH, secondary syphilis

    ii. Poliosis: VKH.

Nails:

    i. Pitting

    ii. Psoriasis.

Dysentery

    i. Reiter's syndrome

Mouth ulcers

    i. Painful: Behcet's syndrome

    ii. Painless: Reiter's syndrome.

Arthritis

    i. RA

    ii. Juvenile RA

    iii. AS.

Gut involvement

    i. Ulcerative colitis

    ii. Crohn's disease.

Lungs

    i. TB

    ii. Sarcoidosis.

Urethritis/urethral ulcers

  i. VKH
 ii. Cytomegalovirus (CMV) infections
iii. Congenital toxoplasmosis
 iv. Syphilis.

CNS involvement

  i. VKH
 ii. CMV
iii. Behcet's
 iv. Congenital toxoplasmosis.

20. **Why do we ask for history of contact with pet animals/livestock?**

  i. Cat—toxocariasis, toxoplasmosis
 ii. Cattle—leptospirosis, cysticercosis, toxoplasmosis
iii. Pigs—cysticercosis, leptospirosis
 iv. Rat—leptospirosis.

21. **What is the mechanism of pain in uveitis?**

The pain is an acute spasmodic ciliary neuralgia superimposed on a dull ache. Since the iris is richly supplied with sensory nerves from the ophthalmic division of the fifth nerve, pain is very common. It is typically worse in the night. It is worse in the acute stage when there is tissue swelling hyperemia and release of high concentration of toxic materials.

22. **What are the symptoms in cyclitis/choroiditis?**

Cyclitis:

  i. Floaters
 ii. Redness due to ciliary congestion
iii. Tenderness over pars plana
 iv. Defective vision, in chronic cyclitis due to vitreous opacities.

Choroiditis:

  i. Asymptomatic, unless posterior pole is involved
 ii. Photopsia, due to irritation of rods and cones at the periphery of the lesion.
iii. Floaters—due to outpouring of exudate
 iv. Metamorphopsia due to irregular elevation in the retina. Initially a positive scotoma develops following which a negative scotoma develops. Hiatus or negative scotoma is sector shaped in severe lesions due to destruction of nerve fibers and blockage of retinal vessels causing damage to RPE in periphery.

23. What is the difference between photophobia and blepharospasm?

	Photophobia	Blepharospasm
Definition	Increased sensitivity/ abnormal intolerance to ambient light	Focal dystonia manifested by forceful, frequent involuntary eyelid closure
Etiology	Ocular: Blepharitis, Conjunctivitis, Keratitis, Dry Eye, Iridocyclitis, Vitritis, Optic Neuritis, Papilledema Non-ocular: Blepharospasm, Migraine, Traumatic Brain Injury	Benign Essential Blepharospasm (BEB)—B/L condition The exact cause of BEB is unknown and, by definition, it is not associated with another disease entity or syndrome. It is a diagnosis of exclusion
Pathophysiology	Afferent: Unmyelinated ciliary branches of ophthalmic nerve (V1)—branch of trigeminal nerve Center: Trigeminal Nucleus Caudalis (TNC) →Thalamus and Cortex (Nociceptive signals) Efferent: Facial nerve → Orbicularis oculi (blinking reflex)	Dysfunction in Basal Ganglia, Overacting Facial Nerve
Instillation of local anesthetic and on exposure to dark	Patient gets relieved of the symptom	Symptom persists
Treatment	Treat the cause	Periodic injection of a Botulinum Toxin A

24. Differentiate circumcorneal/ciliary and conjunctival congestion.

	Conjunctival	Circumcorneal
Site	In fornices	Circumcorneal
Color	Bright red	Pale red/violaceous
Type of discharge	Mucus	Serous
Branching of vessels	Dichotomous	Radially arranged around the cornea without branching
Origin	Posterior conjunctival vessels	Anterior ciliary vessels
Movement of vessels	Can be moved on moving conjunctiva	Cannot be moved
On pressure	Fill from fornix	Fill from limbus

25. What are the keratic precipitates? What is the importance of detecting them? What is their fate?

Keratic precipitates (KPs) comprise of lymphocytes, plasma cells, and phagocytes enmeshed in a network of fibrin. Mononuclear phagocytes are common in non-granulomatous KPs. Epithelial and giant cells are common in granulomatous KPs.

Significance of KPs:
  i. Gives clue to diagnosis
  ii. Evidence of inflammatory activity
  iii. It signifies involvement of ciliary body.

Fate of KPs:
  i. Hyalinization
  ii. May disappear after resolution of inflammation
  iii. May reduce in size
  iv. May become pigmented
  v. May get washed away during surgery.
Sometimes, if inflammation becomes chronic then non-granulomatous KPs may become larger and granulomatous.

26. Describe distribution of KPs.

von Arlt's triangle: A base down triangle on the inferior aspect of the corneal endothelium, where KPs aggregate due to convection currents of aqueous humor and gravity.
Ehrlich Tuck's line: Vertical line along the center of the endothelium
Central: Viral
Diffuse: Fuchs' heterochromic iridocyclitis
In the angle: Sarcoidosis.

27. What are the prerequisites for a keratic precipitate to occur?
  i. Defective nutrition of the corneal endothelium so that the cells become sticky and may desquamate in places
  ii. The convection currents in the anterior chamber (due to the difference of the temperature between the warm iris and the cool cornea)
  iii. Gravity.

28. Differentiate fresh/old and granulomatous/non-granulomatous KPs.

Fresh	Old
White	Pigmented
Round	Flat
Fully hydrated	Dehydrated
Smooth edges	Crenated edges

(Continued)

(Continued)

	Granulomatous	Non-granulomatous
Size	Large	Small to medium
Shape	Oval or Oblong	Usually circular
Color and Appearance	Yellow and greasy Mashed potato appearance	White—hydrated
Confluence	Often confluent	Usually non-confluent
Changes	Cause alteration of endothelium leading to prelucid halos May get pigmented	Pigmentation, dehydration, flattening

29. **What is flare? What is its significance? How is it examined and graded?**

The visualization of the path of the slit lamp when aimed obliquely across the anterior chamber (AC) is called flare.

Breakdown of blood–ocular barrier and damage to iris blood vessels cause proteins to leak into AC. This causes flare.

Flare in the absence of cells does not indicate active inflammation as damaged blood vessels leak for a long time after inflammation has resolved. Steroids are not indicated in the absence of cells.

Flare is examined at the slit lamp with maximum light intensity and magnification 1 mm long, 1 mm wide beam is directed at 45° to 60° to ocular surface.

Grading of flare:

Hogan's grading:

Faint—just detectable	=	1 +
Moderate—iris details clear	=	2 +
Marked—iris details hazy	=	3 +
Intense—fibrinous exudates	=	4 +

SUN Working Group Grading for AC flare:

Grade	Description
0	None
+1	Faint
+2	Moderate (Iris and lens details clear)
+3	Marked (Iris and lens details hazy)
+4	Intense (Fibrin/plasmoid aqueous)

30. **What are the types of AC reaction?**

Serous: Flare due to protein exudation.
Purulent: PMNs and necrotic debris causing hypopyon.
Fibrinous/plastic: Intense fibrinous exudates, hypopyon.
Sanguinoid: Inflammatory cells with RBCs, hypopyon.

31. What are the types of cells in AC? How are they graded?

i. Inflammatory cells (lymphocytes and PMN)
ii. Red blood cells (RBCs)
iii. Iris pigment cells
iv. Malignant cells, e.g. lymphoma.

Grading of cells

Hogan's grading:

None	=	0
5–10/field	=	1+
10–20/field	=	2+
20–50/field	=	3+
50/field	=	4+

SUN Working Group Grading of AC cells:

Grade	Cells in Fields
0	None
+0.5	1–5
+1	6–15
+2	16–25
+3	26–50
+4	>50

32. How is hypopyon formed in uveitis?

Hypopyon is a collection of leucocytes. Sufficient fibrin content in the anterior chamber causes cells to clump and settle down as hypopyon.

33. When is hyphema seen in uveitis?

i. Viral uveitis (especially zoster)
ii. Syphilis
iii. Ophthalmia nodosum
iv. Trauma
v. Masquerade syndrome.

34. What are the iris changes in uveitis?

i. Pattern change—iris crypts and furrows are obliterated
ii. Iris atrophy
iii. Heterochromia—Fuchs', viral
iv. Rubeosis
v. Synechiae
vi. Seclusio pupillae
vii. Occlusion pupillae
viii. Ectropion uveae
ix. Nodules—Koeppe's and Busaca's
x. Granulomas and lepra pearls.

35. What are the nodules seen in a case of uveitis? What are leprotic pearls?

There are two types of nodules seen in uveitis:

	Koeppe's	Busacca's
Location	At pupillary margin	Usually seen along collarette
Pathology	Ectodermal nodules	Mesodermal floccules
Color	Small usually white, but may be pigmented	Greenish white and larger than Koeppe's nodules
Conditions	Usually seen in granulomatous but may occur in non-granulomatous	Only in granulomatous never in non-granulomatous uveitis

Leprotic pearls:

They are iris nodules, pathognomic of leprosy and are situated between collarette and ciliary margin.

36. What is seclusio pupillae?

It is also called as annular or ring synechia. In this condition, the whole circle of the pupillary margin may become tied down to the lens capsule.

37. What is occlusio pupillae?

When the exudate becomes more extensive, it may cover the entire pupillary area, which then becomes filled by a film of opaque fibrous tissue and this condition is called as occlusio pupillae.

38. What is the differential diagnosis for iris nodules?

   i. Down's syndrome (Brushfield spots)
   ii. Epithelial invasion, serous cyst
   iii. Foreign body (retained)
   iv. Fungal endophthalmitis
   v. Iridocyclitis
   vi. Iris freckle
   vii. Iris nevus syndrome (Cogan-Reese)
   viii. Iris pigment epithelial cyst
   ix. Juvenile xanthogranuloma
   x. Leiomyoma
   xi. Malignant melanoma
   xii. Melanocytosis (ocular and oculodermal)
   xiii. Neurofibromatosis
   xiv. Retinoblastoma.

39. What are the pupil changes in uveitis?

In the acute stage: Miosis.
In the chronic stage: Posterior synechiae

Miosis is due to:
  i. Irritants causing muscle fibers to contract; sphincter effect overcomes dilator leading to constriction.
  ii. Vascularity allows unusual amounts of exudation, causing iris to become waterlogged and the pupil to become sluggish.
  iii. Radial nature of the vessels.

40. What are the various causes of complicated cataract?
  i. Uveitis
  ii. Trauma
  iii. Steroids (systemic steroids)
  iv. Chronic retinal detachment
  v. Radiation
  vi. RP
  vii. High myopia

40. Why is posterior subcapsular cataract more common in complicated cataract?
  i. Posterior capsule is thin and hence toxins can diffuse easily
  ii. Rate of metabolism is low

Since the metabolism is high in anterior lens capsule, toxins can be metabolized (easily washed away)

41. What are the characteristic features of complicated cataract?
  i. Bread crumb appearance
  ii. Polychromatic lusture

42. What are the vitreous changes in uveitis?
Vitreous changes:
  i. Opacities—fine, coarse, stingy snowball.
  ii. Posterior vitreous detachment (PVD).
  iii. Cellular precipitation posterior wall of vitreous, flare and cells, fluid in retrovitreal space.
  iv. Late shrinkage of vitreous may cause vitreal holes and retinal detachment (RD).
  v. Vitreous hemorrhage.

SUN Working Group Grading for vitreous cells:

Grade	No. of cells
0	None
+0.5	1–10
+1	10–20
+2	20–30
+3	30–100
+4	>100

43. What are the fundus changes in uveitis?

A. Optic disk:
   i. Papillitis (VKH)
   ii. Granuloma (Sarcoid)
   iii. Optic atrophy secondary to retinal damage
   iv. Disk hyperemia/edema.

B. Macula:
   i. Edema (pars planitis, birdshot chorioretinopathy)
   ii. Scar—toxoplasmosis.

C. Peripheral retina:
   i. Healed retinitis/choroiditis/retinochoroiditis
   ii. Retinal detachment
      – Serous (VKH)
      – Rhegmatogenous
      – Tractional
   iii. Vascular occlusion
   iv. Perivascular exudates
   v. Candle wax drippings, e.g. sarcoid
   vi. Sheathing, e.g. Eales' disease
   vii. Pars plana exudates—snow banking
   viii. Neovascularization
      – Peripheral—pars planitis
      – Macular—toxoplasmosis
      – Periphery and ONH sarcoidosis

44. What are the causes of defective vision in uveitis?

   i. Cornea:
      – Corneal edema
      – Keratic precipitates on endothelium

   ii. Anterior chamber:
      – Cells and flare

   iii. Pupil:
      – Miosis

   iv. Lens:
      – Complicated cataract

   v. Vitreous :
      – Vitreous cells
      – Vitreous hemorrhage

vi. Fundus:

Optic disc:

- Papillitis
- Papilledema
- Optic atrophy

vii. Macula:

- Edema
- Scar

viii. Peripheral retina:

- Retinitis/choroiditis/retinochoroiditis
- Retinal detachment
- Vascular occlusion

45. Differentiate choroiditis from retinitis.

Choroiditis	Retinitis
Yellow patch	White cloudy appearance
Distinct with defined borders	Indistinct borders
Involvement of vessels	Abundant vitreous cells
Vitreous minimal or absent	Sheathing of adjacent vessels
Subretinal hemorrhage	Surrounding retinal edema

46. What is the difference between active and healed choroiditis?

Active	Healed
Elevated lesion	Flat
Ill-defined margins	Distinct pigmented margins
Associated with vascular sheathing, hemorrhage and vitreous inflammation	No associated features

47. What are the intraocular pressure (IOP) changes that can occur in uveitis?

Low IOP:

i. Inflammation of ciliary body and failure to produce sufficient amount of aqueous
ii. Choroidal detachment
iii. Retinal detachment.

High IOP:

i. Trabeculitis
ii. Neovascular glaucoma (NVG)

iii. Clogging of trabecular meshwork by inflammatory debris
iv. Posner–Schlossman syndrome
v. Sclerosis of trabecular meshwork
vi. Peripheral anterior synechiae
vii. Iris bombe
viii. Steroid induced glaucoma.

48. What are the uveitic conditions associated with increased IOP?

i. Viral
ii. Toxoplasmosis
iii. Sarcoidosis
iv. Fuchs' heterochromic iridocyclitis
v. Posner–Schlossman syndrome
vi. Steroid-induced uveitis
vii. Lens-induced uveitis.

49. What are the characteristic features of Posner–Schlossman syndrome?

It is also known as hypertensive iridocyclitis crises. The features are:
i. Quiet eye
ii. Periodic raised intraocular pressure with flare and cells
iii. Reduced vision during these attacks and mimics angle closure glaucoma
iv. Treatment is by using atropine ointment.

50. What are the complications of iridocyclitis?

Corneal conditions:
i. Band keratopathy

Anterior chamber:
i. Posterior synechiae
ii. Iris bombe
iii. Seclusio pupillae
iv. Occlusio pupillae.
Secondary glaucoma (described above) .
Complicated cataract.
Cystoid macular edema.
Tractional RD.
Phthisis bulbi.

51. How does phthisis occur in uveitis?

Organization of vitreous forms a cyclitic membrane, contraction of which leads to a retinal detachment with base toward lens and apex toward optic disc. As the cyclitic membrane consolidates, the ciliary processes are drawn inwards, so that the ciliary body detaches leading to phthisis bulbi.

52. What are the causes of cystoids macular edema in uveitis?

    i. Acute severe iridocyclitis

   ii. Behcet's syndrome

  iii. Pars planitis

  iv. Endophthalmitis

   v. Birdshot chorioretinopathy.

53. What are the causes of macular chorioretinitis?

    i. Toxoplasmosis

   ii. Tuberculosis

  iii. Syphilis

  iv. Cytomegalovirus (CMV) retinitis

   v. Herpes simplex.

54. What are the causes of retinochoroiditis?

    i. Toxoplasmosis

   ii. Toxocara granuloma of retina/choroid

  iii. Septic (subacute bacterial endophthalmitis)

  iv. CMV retinitis

   v. Candida retinitis.

55. What are the causes of chorioretinitis?

    i. Tuberculosis

   ii. AMPPE

  iii. Geographical helical polypoidal choroidopathy

  iv. Birdshot choroidopathy

   v. Sympathetic ophthalmia

  vi. Presumed ocular histoplasmosis.

56. What is the characteristic description of active toxoplasmic retino-choroiditis?

"Headlight in fog" appearances.

57. What are the preoperative concerns while performing cataract surgery in an eye with uveitis?

    i. The eye should remain quiet for a minimum of 3 months before contemplating surgery under the cover of steroids.

   ii. In phacolytic and other lens-induced uveitis the above does not apply and cataract surgery could be done immediately.

58. What are the intraoperative steps to be taken while performing cataract surgery in a uveitic eye?

    i. Inadequate pupillary dilatation (to do sphincterotomy, iris hooks, sector iridectomy)

   ii. Complete cortical removal

iii. Minimal manipulation of iris

iv. To perform a prophylactic peripheral iridotomy

v. Perform capsulorhexis and facilitate in the bag intraocular lens placement

vi. To preferably use a heparin coated or an acrylic lens.

59. What are the indications of explanation of IOL's in a uveitic eye?

i. Propionibacterium gene endophthalmitis

ii. Persistent postoperative uveitis with haptic rubbing the iris due to "in sulcus" placement.

60. Name an uveitic entity in which intraocular placement of IOL is contraindicated. Why?

JIA (juvenile idiopathic arthritis) due to persistent severe uveitis causing cyclitic membrane leading to phthisis bulbi.

61. What are the uses of atropine in a case of uveitis?

i. It keeps the iris and ciliary body at rest

ii. It breaks the preexisting synechia and prevents new synechia from occurring

iii. It decreases hyperemia.

62. What is mydricaine?

It is a powerful mydriatic agent and is a combination of procaine, atropine, and adrenaline. 0.3 mL is given through the subconjunctival route.

3.2. SYMPATHETIC OPHTHALMIA

1. **Define sympathetic ophthalmia.**

   A specific bilateral inflammation of the entire uveal tract of unknown etiology, characterized clinically by insidious onset and progressive course
   with exacerbations and pathologically by a nodular or diffuse infiltration
   of the uveal tract with lymphocytes and epitheloid cells; almost univer-
   sally follows a perforating injury involving the uveal tissue.

   Exciting eye—injured eye developing the disease at a variable time after
   the injury.

   Sympathizing eye—the other eye which develops the disease synchro-
   nously or shortly afterwards.

2. **What are the predisposing causes for sympathetic ophthalmia?**
   i. *Perforating injuries—65%*
      – Perforating injury involving the uveal tissue and in the vast majority
        of cases rapid and reaction less wound healing is interfered by iris,
        ciliary body incarceration or foreign body retention.
      – Subacute inflammation in a soft shrunken eye in which delayed or
        incomplete wound healing is present.
      – Wounds in the ciliary region are most dangerous but not very
        common.
   ii. *Operative wounds—25%*
      – Incarceration of iris in the wound.
      – Iridectomy, iridencleisis.
   iii. *Non-perforating contusions* (subconjunctival scleral rupture)—10%
   iv. *Intraocular malignant melanomata*—rare
      – Complicated by perforation of the globe by invading tumor.
      – Necrotic tumors.

3. **Discuss the pathology of sympathetic ophthalmia.**
   i. Sympathetic ophthalmia is a clinicopathologic diagnosis and never a
      histological diagnosis alone.
   ii. Focal lymphocytic and plasma cell infiltration around large veins of
      choroid → coalesce to form multinucleated giant cells → formation
      of nodules of epitheloid cells with central giant cells surrounded by
      lymphocytes → infiltration of iris (posterior part) and diffuse infiltra-
      tion of choroid (especially outer layers).
   iii. Four characteristic histological findings in the sympathizing and
      exciting eye include:
      – Diffuse granulomatous uveal inflammation composed predomi-
        nantly of epitheloid cells and lymphocytes; eosinophil and plasma
        cells may be present—neutrophils are absent.
      – Sparing of choriocapillaries

– Epitheloid cells containing phagocytosed uveal pigment
– Dalen Fuchs' nodules:
  Collections of epitheloid cells between Bruch's membrane and the retinal pigment epithelium (RPE) with no involvement of the overlying neural retina and sparing of the underlying choriocapillaries.
  Some cells may come from transformation of the RPE.

4. **What are the clinical features of sympathetic ophthalmia?**

In sympathizing eye:
  i. Mild pain
  ii. Photophobia
  iii. Increased lacrimation
  iv. Blurring of vision
  v. Visual fatigue.

In exciting eye:
Decrease in vision and photophobia.

Signs in both eyes:
  i. Ciliary injection
  ii. Development of keratic precipitates on corneal endothelium
  iii. Partially dilated and poorly responsive pupil
  iv. Thickened iris
  v. Clouding of vitreous.

Posterior segment findings:
  i. Papillitis
  ii. Generalized retinal edema
  iii. Perivasculitis
  iv. Small yellow white exudate beneath RPE (Dalen-Fuchs' nodule)
  v. Areas of choroiditis
  vi. Exudative retinal detachment.

3.3. FUCHS' HETEROCHROMIC IRIDOCYCLITIS

1. **What are the signs and symptoms of Fuchs' heterochromic iridocyclitis?**

    Symptoms:
    - i. Decreased vision—due to cataract formation
    - ii. Floaters—due to vitreous opacities
    - iii. Discomfort—due to ciliary spasm
    - iv. Conjunctival injection
    - v. Asymptomatic
    - vi. Symptoms due to elevated IOP
    - vii. Change in iris color
    - viii. Hyphema
    - ix. Strabismus from juvenile cataract.

    Signs:
    Triad of:
    - i. Heterochromia
    - ii. Cataract
    - iii. Keratic precipitates.

    Heterochromia:
    - i. Iris pigments present in all three layers:
        - – Anterior border layer
        - – Stroma
        - – Posterior pigment epithelium
    - ii. There is atrophy of all the three layers.
    - iii. Atrophy of anterior border layer and stroma—**hypochromia** in many cases and **hyperchromia** in a few due to revealing of the posterior pigment epithelium.
    - iv. Blue irides—affected eye looks bluer or lighter than the other eye due to loss of orange brown pigment of the anterior border layer concentrated around the collarete. Rarely show hyperchromia.
    - v. Brown—usually affected eyes are hypochromic may appear normal also.
    - vi. Subtle heterochromia—best observed by naked unaided eye under natural day light or bright overhead light. Most sensitive method to identify heterochromia is to compare anterior segment photographs taken under standard conditions.
    - vii. May be congenital/acquired later in life.
    - viii. Bilateral cases—no heterochromia.

Iris characteristics:

i. Anterior border layer: depigmentation → lighter, translucent, whitish hazy appearance.
ii. Stroma—depigmentation and loss of volume → smooth iris surface → prominent radial vessels → visualization of the sphincter.
iii. Pigment epithelium affected: transillumination defects and abnormalities of the pupillary ruff.
iv. Iris nodules: rare, translucent near the pupillary margin.
v. Posterior synechiae is rare.
vi. Iris vessels:
  - Due to atrophy—normal iris vessels become conspicuous.
  - Radial and orderly dichotomous branching.
  - New vessels—fine, filamentous, sinuous, arborizing with anomalous branching pattern.
  - Seen on the surface of iris and anterior chamber angle.
  - Rarely may form fibrovascular membrane over trabecular meshwork—neovascular glaucoma occasional.
  - Incidence of rubeosis: 6–22%; more when iris fluorescein angiography is used.
  - May cause filiform hemorrhage arising as a fine stream of blood arising in or near the angle usually opposite to the site of puncture during paracentesis—**Amsler's sign**
  - Considered to be diagnostic and confirmatory test—but now its clinical utility is questioned.
  - Applanation tonometry and cataract surgery may cause bleeding.

Iridocyclitis:

Characteristic KPs –
  Stellate or round, whitish translucent with interspersed wispy filaments precipitated over the entire corneal endothelium diffusely.
Minimal anterior chamber cellular activity.

Cataract:

i. Posterior subcapsular cataracts
ii. Rapid advance to maturation.

Vitreous cells:

Individual cells, aggregates, stingy filaments, and occasional dense vitreous veils.

Glaucoma: 26–59%

Mechanism of glaucoma:
i. Rubeosis
ii. Peripheral anterior synechiae
iii. Lens-induced angle closure
iv. Recurrent spontaneous hyphema
v. Steroid response

3.4. VOGT–KOYANAGI–HARADA SYNDROME

1. **What is Vogt–Koyanagi–Harada (VKH) syndrome?**

   VKH syndrome or uveomeningitic syndrome is a systemic disorder involving many organ systems, including the eye, ear, integumentary, and nervous system.

2. **What are the clinical manifestations of VKH?**

   The American Uveitis Society adopted the criteria for the diagnosis of VKH syndrome in 1978 as follows:
   i. No history of ocular trauma or surgery.
   ii. At least three of four of the following signs:
      – Bilateral chronic iridocyclitis.
      – Posterior uveitis, including exudative retinal detachment, disk hyperemia or edema, and sunset glow fundus.
      – Neurologic signs of tinnitus, neck stiffness, cranial nerve or CNS problems or CSF pleocytosis.
      – Cutaneous findings of alopecia, poliosis, or vitiligo.

3. **What are the clinical manifestations of VKH?**

   Typical clinical manifestations of VKH syndrome:
   i. Bilateral panuveitis in association with multifocal serous retinal detachment.
   ii. Central nervous system manifestations—meningismus, headache, CSF pleocytosis
   iii. Auditory manifestations—hearing loss, tinnitus
   iv. Cutaneous manifestations—vitiligo, alopecia, poliosis.

   Most patients, present with severe bilateral uveitis associated with exudative retinal detachment and signs of meningismus.

4. **What are the differential diagnoses of VKH?**

   i. Idiopathic central serous choroidopathy
   ii. Nanophthalmos (axial length <19 mm)
   iii. Uveal effusion syndrome
   iv. Bilateral diffuse melanocytic hyperplasia
   v. Toxemia of pregnancy, renal disease
   vi. Posterior scleritis
   vii. Acute retinal necrosis syndrome
   viii. Primary B-cell intraocular lymphoma
   ix. Syphilis, tuberculosis, and sarcoidosis
   x. Sympathetic ophthalmia
   xi. Lupus choroidopathy.

5. **How will you investigate a case of VKH?**

   Fluorescein angiography (FA)

   i. Characteristic FA in acute stage of VKH demonstrates multiple punctate hyperfluorescent dots at the level of RPE.

   ii. These hyperfluorescent dots gradually enlarge and stain the subretinal fluid.

   iii. 70% of the patients have disc leakage.

   iv. In chronic stage, the angiogram shows multiple hyperfluorescent RPE window defects without progressive staining.

   v. Alternating hyper and hypofluorescence from RPE alteration causing "moth eaten" appearance can be found.

   Ultrasonography:

   Echographic manifestations of VKH are described by:

   i. Diffuse thickening of the posterior choroid with low to medium reflectivity.

   ii. Serous RD around posterior pole or inferiorly.

   iii. Vitreous opacities without PVD.

   iv. Posterior thickening of the sclera or episclera.

   Lumbar puncture:

   Lumbar puncture (LP) has not been used routinely in most recent studies. In a study by Ohno et al., more than 80% of the patients had CSF pleocytosis consisting mostly of lymphocytes. CSF pleocytosis occurs in 80% of the case within 1 week and resolves within 8 weeks.

   MRI discriminates the sclera from the choroid, which is not possible with computerized tomography and allows the detection of subclinical ocular and CNS disease. Choroidal thickening can be demonstrated even when the fundus and fluorescein angiogram appear normal.

3.5. BEHCET'S DISEASE

1. **Definition of Behcet's disease.**

   It is relapsing and remitting systemic vasculitis of unknown etiology characterized by oral and genital ulcers and ocular inflammation.
   With the triad of:
   i. Recurrent hypopyon—iritis
   ii. Oral ulceration
   iii. Genital ulceration.

2. **What is the etiology?**
   i. Viral agent—herpes simplex
   ii. Bacterial—streptococcal species
   iii. Genetic: HLA-B5   –   Ocular type
                       HLA-B12 –   Mucocutaneous
                       HLA-B27 –   Arthritic

3. **What is Behcet's Disease Research Committee Criteria?**

   Major Criteria:
   i. Oral aphthous ulceration
   ii. Skin lesions:
      – Erythema nodosum-like skin eruption
      – Subcutaneous thrombophlebitis
      – Cutaneous hypersensitivity
   iii. Ocular lesions
   iv. Recurrent hypopyon iritis or iridocyclitis
   v. Chorioretinitis
   vi. Genital aphthous ulceration.

   Minor Criteria:
   i. Arthritic symptoms and signs (arthralgia, swelling, redness in large joints).
   ii. Gastrointestinal lesions (appendicitis like pain, melena, diarrhea, and so on).
   iii. Epididymitis.
   iv. Vascular lesions (Obliterative vasculitis, occlusions, aneurysms).
   v. CNS involvement:
      – Brain stem syndrome
      – Meningoencephalomyelitic syndrome
      – Psychiatric symptoms.

4. **What are the anterior segment findings?**
   i. Iridocyclitis with hypopyon—19–31%.
   ii. Periorbital pain, redness, photophobia, and blurred vision.
   iii. Ciliary injection, fine KPs.

Hypopyon, does not coagulate—changes position with head movement

Attack lasts for 2–3 weeks and then subsides, recurrences are the rule with subsequent iris atrophy and posterior synechiae formation.

5. **What are the posterior segment findings?**

    i. Vitritis
    ii. Retinal vasculitis
    iii. Patchy perivascular sheathing and inflammatory exudates sur-rounding retinal hemorrhages
    iv. Retinal edema
    v. Severe vasculitis—thrombosis—ischemic retinal changes. BRVO/CRVO
    vi. Neovascularization—bleeding—fibrosis—RD (very rare)
    vii. Optic neuritis in acute phase
    viii. Progressive optic atrophy.

3.6. INVESTIGATIONS IN UVEITIS

1. **What are the indications for investigations in uveitis?**
   i. To arrive at a specific diagnosis.
   ii. To choose a correct therapeutic approach.
   iii. To rule out infection (steroids are used in majority of uveitic cases; they may exacerbate existing diseases like TB and toxoplasmosis).
   iv. To rule out tumors—because many tumors like leukemias and retinoblastomas masquerade as uveitis.
   v. To rule out presumed autoimmune disease.
   vi. To rule out associated systemic conditions, e.g. HLA-B27+ JRA may present as uveitis initially. HLA-B27 positivity forewarns the patient about the systemic nature of the disease and its prognosis.
   vii. To evaluate why vision has not improved nonresponders, poor responses, and early recurrences.
   viii. To assess the side effects of treatment, e.g. in Behcet's disease, immunosuppressants are used.
   ix. For academic and research purposes.

2. **Which uveitic entities do not need laboratory investigations for diagnosis?**
   i. Pars planitis
   ii. Fuchs' heterochromic iridocyclitis
   iii. Traumatic uveitis
   iv. Postoperative uveitis.

3. **Classify Investigations used in uveitis.**

   Laboratory
   i. Routine—TC, DC, ESR
   ii. Skin test
   iii. Serological test
   iv. Pathological test
   v. Special specimen examination, e.g. feces

   Non-laboratory
   i. Imaging techniques

4. **What are the hematological investigations done in uveitis? What is their significance? What is the normal value?**
   WBC (Total count):
   Normal count: 4,500–11,000 cells/muL

   Conditions where total count is raised:
   i. Exercise
   ii. Stress

iii. Infections

iv. Tissue necrosis (e.g. myocardial infarction, pulmonary infarction)

v. Chronic inflammatory disorder (e.g. vasculitis)

vi. Drugs (e.g. glucocorticoids, epinephrine, lithium)

Conditions where total count is decreased

i. Infections—viral (e.g. influenza, HIV, hepatitis)
   Bacterial (e.g. typhoid, TB)

ii. Nutritional—B_{12} and folate deficiency

iii. Autoimmune, e.g. SLE

5. **What are the clinical conditions which can cause raised neutrophils (neutrophilia)?**

   i. Inflammatory states

   ii. Nonspecific infections

   iii. Eclampsia

   iv. Hemolytic anemia

   v. Corticosteroids.

6. **What are the causes of decreased neutrophils (neutropenia)?**

   i. Congenital

   ii. Leukemia

   iii. Chemotherapy

   iv. Steroids

   v. Radiation

   vi. Vitamin B_{12}/Folate deficiency

   vii. Hemodialysis

   viii. Viral infections.

7. **What are the causes of raised eosinophils (eosinophilia)?**

   i. Parasitic infestation

   ii. Allergic disorders

   iii. Churg–Strauss syndrome

   iv. Cholesterol embolization

   v. Hodgkin's lymphoma

   vi. Addison's disease.

8. **What are the causes of decreased eosinophils (eosinopenia)?**

   i. Congenital

   ii. Leukemia

   iii. Chemotherapy

   iv. Steroids.

9. **What are the causes of raised basophils (basophilia)?**

   i. Stress

   ii. Inflammatory states

   iii. Leukemia.

10. What are the causes of decreased basophils (basopenia)?

   i. Urticaria
   ii. Agranulocytosis
   iii. Ovulation

11. What are the causes of increased lymphocytes (lymphocytosis)?

   i. Acute viral infections
   ii. Infectious mononucleosis
   iii. Acute pertussis
   iv. Protozoal—toxoplasmic infections
   v. Tuberculosis
   vi. Brucellosis
   vii. Chronic lymphocytic leukemia
   viii. Acute lymphocytic leukemia
   ix. Connective tissue disorders
   x. Thyrotoxicosis
   xi. Addison's disease
   xii. Splenomegaly with sequestration of granulocytes.

12. What are the causes of decreased lymphocytes (lymphocytopenia)?

   i. Common cold
   ii. Corticosteroids
   iii. HIV/viral/bacterial/fungal infections
   iv. Malnutrition
   v. Systemic lupus erythematosus
   vi. Stress
   vii. Prolonged physical exertion
   viii. Rheumatoid arthritis
   ix. Iatrogenic—radiation.

13. What are the causes of increased monocytes (monocytosis)?

   i. Infections—tuberculosis, syphilis, brucellosis, listeria, subacute bacterial endocarditis
   ii. Protozoal infections
   iii. Rickettsial infections
   iv. Myeloproliferative disorders
   v. Autoimmune diseases
   vi. Malignancies: Hodgkin's, leukemia
   vii. Sarcoid
   viii. Lipid storage diseases.

14. What are the causes of decreased monocytes (monocytopenia)?

   i. Immunosuppressed states
   ii. Bone marrow suppression
   iii. Radiation states

iv. Increased destruction: autoimmune states, carcinoma of hemato-poietic system

v. Hemodialysis.

15. What is erythrocyte sedimentation rate (ESR)?

Erythrocyte sedimentation rate or Biernacki reaction is defined as the rate at which erythrocytes precipitates in an hour.

16. What are the principles of ESR?

Erythrocyte sedimentation rate (ESR) is principally determined by the balance between pro-sedimentary factors and factors that resist sedimentation. The main pro-sedimentary factor is fibrinogen. The negative charge on the surface of RBCs called as potential is responsible for resisting the sedimentation of erythrocytes.

In inflammatory states, increase in fibrinogen causes the erythrocytes to stick to each other thereby causing "Rouleaux" formation and raised ESR.

17. What are the causes of raised ESR?

i. *Physiological:*
   - Pregnancy
   - Exercise
   - Menstruation

ii. Pathological:
   - Anemia
   - Endocarditis

iii. Renal disorders

iv. Osteomyelitis

v. Rheumatic fever

vi. Rheumatoid arthritis

vii. Thyroid disorder

viii. Tuberculosis

ix. Syphilis

x. HIV.

Causes of very high-raised ESR:

i. Giant cell arthritis

ii. Hyperfibrinogenemia

iii. Multiple myeloma

iv. Macroglobulinemia

v. Necrotizing vasculitis

vi. Polymyalgia rheumatica.

18. What are the drugs which can cause increased ESR?

i. Dextran

ii. Methyldopa

iii. Oral contraceptives
iv. Penicillamines
 v. Theophylline
vi. Vitamin A.

19. What are the causes of decreased ESR?

i. Congestive cardiac failure
ii. Hyperviscosity syndrome
iii. Hypofibrinogenemia
iv. Low plasma protein states
v. Polycythemia
vi. Sickle cell anemia
vii. Very high blood sugar levels
viii. Severe liver diseases
ix. Drugs—aspirin, cortisone, quinine.

20. What are the common methods to estimate ESR?

i. Westergren's method
ii. Wintrobe's method

21. What is tuberculin skin testing (TST)?

The Mantoux tuberculin test is the standard method of determining whether a person is infected with *Mycobacterium tuberculosis*. Reliable administration and reading of the TST requires standardization of procedures, training, supervision, and practice.

22. How is the TST administered?

The TST is performed by injecting 0.1 mL of tuberculin purified protein derivative (PPD) into the inner surface of the forearm. The injection should be made with a tuberculin syringe, with the needle bevel facing upward. The TST is an intradermal injection. When placed correctly, the injection should produce a pale elevation of the skin (a wheal) 6–10 mm in diameter.

23. How is the TST read?

The skin test reaction should be read between 48 and 72 hours after administration. A patient who does not return within 72 hours will need to be rescheduled for another skin test.

The reaction should be measured in millimeters of the induration (palpable, raised, hardened area, or swelling). The reader should not measure erythema (redness). The diameter of the indurated area should be measured across the forearm (perpendicular to the long axis).

24. How are TST reactions interpreted?

Skin test interpretation depends on two factors:
  i. Measurement in millimeters of the induration
  ii. Person's risk of being infected with TB and of progression to disease if infected.

25. What are false-positive reaction?

Some persons may react to the TST even though they are not infected with *Mycobacterium tuberculosis*. The causes of these false-positive reactions may include, but are not limited to, the following:
  i.   Infection with nontuberculosis mycobacteria
  ii. Previous BCG vaccination
  iii. Incorrect method of TST administration
  iv. Incorrect interpretation of reaction
  v.   Incorrect bottle of antigen used.

26. What are false-negative reactions?

Some persons may not react to the TST even though they are infected with *Mycobacterium tuberculosis*. The reasons for these false-negative reactions may include, but are not limited to, the following:
  i.   Cutaneous anergy (anergy is the inability to react to skin tests because of a weakened immune system).
  ii.   Recent TB infection (within 8–10 weeks of exposure).
  iii. Very old TB infection (many years).
  iv.   Very young age (less than 6 months old).
  v.   Recent live-virus vaccination (e.g. measles and small pox).
  vi.   Overwhelming TB disease.
  vii. Some viral illnesses (e.g. measles and small pox).
  viii. Incorrect method of TST administration.
  ix.   Incorrect interpretation of reaction.

27. Who can receive a TST?

Most persons can receive a TST. Tuberculin skin testing is contraindicated only for persons who have had a severe reaction (e.g. necrosis, blistering, anaphylactic shock, or ulcerations) to a previous TST. It is not contraindicated for any other persons, including infants, children, pregnant women, persons who are HIV infected, or persons who have been vaccinated with BCG.

28. How often can TST be repeated?

In general, there is no risk associated with repeated tuberculin skin test placements. If a person does not return within 48–72 hours for a tuberculin skin test reading, a second test can be placed as soon as possible. There is no contraindication to repeating the TST, unless a previous TST was associated with a severe reaction.

29. What is boosted reaction?

In some persons who are infected with *Mycobacterium tuberculosis*, the ability to react to tuberculin may wane over time. When given a TST, years after infection, these persons may have a false-negative reaction. However, the TST may stimulate the immune system, causing a positive, or boosted reaction to subsequent tests. Giving a second TST after an initial negative TST reaction is called two-step testing.

30. Why is two-step testing conducted?

Two-step testing is useful for the initial skin testing of adults who are going to be retested periodically, such as healthcare workers or nursing home residents. This two-step approach can reduce the likelihood that a boosted reaction to a subsequent TST will be misinterpreted as a recent infection.

31. Can TST be given to persons receiving vaccinations?

Vaccination with live viruses may interfere with TST reactions. For persons scheduled to receive a TST, testing should be done as follows:
i. Either on the same day as vaccination with live-virus vaccine or 4–6 weeks after the administration of live-virus vaccine.
ii. At least 1 month after smallpox vaccination.

32. Classification of the tuberculin skin test reaction.

Classification		
An induration of **5 or more millimeters** is considered positive in ■ HIV infected persons ■ A recent contact of a person with TB disease ■ Persons with fibrotic changes on chest radiograph consistent with prior TB ■ Patients with organ transplants ■ Persons who are immunosuppressed for other reasons (e.g. taking the equivalent of >15 mg/day of prednisone for 1 month or longer, taking TNF alpha antagonists	An induration of **10 or more millimeters** is considered positive in ■ Recent immigrants (<5 years) from high-prevalence countries ■ Injection drug users ■ Residents and employees of high-risk congregate settings ■ Mycobacteriology laboratory personnel ■ Persons with clinical conditions that place them at high-risk ■ Children <4 years of age ■ Infants, children, and adolescents exposed to adults in high-risk categories	An induration of **15 or more millimeters** is considered positive in any person, including persons with no known risk factors for TB. However, targeted skin testing programs should only be conducted among high-risk groups.

33. What is the role of chest X-ray in uveitis cases?

   i. To rule out active pulmonary TB
   ii. To look for sarcoidosis
   iii. To look for secondaries.

34. What is the basis of skin tests and what is the role of skin tests in uveitis?

The basis of all skin tests is delayed hypersensitivity type IV.

Uses of skin tests:

In diagnosis of
   i. Tuberculosis
   ii. Histoplasmosis
   iii. Coccidomycosis
   iv. To indicate anergy—sarcoidosis.
Pathergy test—Behcet's disease

35. What is Kveim test? How is it done?

   i. Kveim test—a skin test for sarcoidosis
   ii. Suspension of antigenic preparation of human sarcoid tissue prepared from spleen of sarcoidosis patients is injected intradermally
   iii. At the end of 6 weeks—a papule develops
   iv. Papule is biopsied for evidence of granuloma and giant cells
   v. Well-formed epithelial tubercles indicate a positive reaction
   vi. Sensitivity—positive in 80% patients of sarcoidosis.

Disadvantages:
   i. Requires standardization by testing in patients with sarcoidosis
   ii. It is usually negative in patients on steroid treatment.

36. How is Behçet's skin test done?

   i. The skin test for Behçet's disease is called Pathergy test
   ii. Intradermal injection of 0.1 mL of sterile saline solution
   iii. A pustule develops within 18–24 hours
   iv. Patient shows increased sensitivity to needle trauma
   v. *Disadvantage:* Only rarely positive in the absence of systemic activity.

37. What are the conditions associated with elevated antinuclear antibodies (ANA)?

   i. Systemic lupus erythematosus (SLE)
   ii. Juvenile rheumatoid arthritis (JRA)
   iii. Scleroderma
   iv. Hepatitis

v. Lymphoma

vi. Polyarteritis nodosa.

38. **List the conditions in uveitis which are associated with HLA.**

   i. HLA-B27 – Acute anterior uveitis, Reiter's syndrome
   ii. HLA-B51 – Japanese with Behçet's disease
   iii. HLA-DR4 – VKH
   iv. HLA-B7 – Macular histoplasmosis
   v. HLA-A29 – Birdshot chorioretinopathy
   vi. HLA-B8 – Sarcoidosis

39. **What is ELISA?**

   ELISA is enzyme-linked immunosorbent assay. It is very sensitive and specific.

40. **What are uses of ELISA in uveitis?**

   Used to detect antibodies of toxoplasma, toxocara, and herpes simples.

   Apart from blood, the test can also be done on aqueous and vitreous sample.

   Patients antibodies are bound to solid phase antigen and then incubated with enzyme tagged antibody. Measurement of enzyme activity provides measurement of specific antibody concentration.

41. **What are the serological tests for toxoplasmosis?**

   i. Toxoplasma dye test/Sabin–Feldman test
   ii. Hemagglutination test
   iii. Indirect fluorescent test
   iv. ELISA
   v. PCR.

42. **What serological tests for syphilis are commonly done in uveitis?**

   i. Non-treponemal test: VDRL
   ii. Treponemal test: FTA-ABS, TPHA.

43. **What is the role of VDRL and FTA-ABS in case of suspected syphilis?**

   i. FTA-ABS is done in syphilis because of its high sensitivity and specificity
   ii. VDRL is done to determine state of activity of disease and adequacy of treatment.

44. **What are the two new specific tests for syphilis?**

   MHA-TP, i.e. microhemagglutination assay for antibodies to *Treponema pallidum.*

   HATTS, i.e. hemagglutination treponemal test for syphilis as 90% positive for ANA fillies. IgG titer more confirmatory than IgM titer.

45. What is the importance of negative ANA?

Negative result is more important as it excludes the diagnosis.

46. When is ANA considered positive?

ANA is considered positive when titers are 1:10 or 1:20

47. Where is angiotensin-converting enzyme (ACE) produced?

By normal capillary endothelium cells and monocytes.

48. What is normal value of ACE?

Normal value

| Males | → | 12–55 | mmol/mL |
| Females | → | 11–29 | mmol/mL |

49. What conditions are associated with elevated ACE?

i. Increased in active sarcoidosis (falls to normal if there is systemic remission even if ocular inflammation is active; i.e. normal ACE does not rule out sarcoidosis)

ii. Also increased in untreated TB, leprosy, toxoplasmosis (thereby not specific for sarcoidosis).

50. What is human leukocyte antigen (HLA)?

Human leukocyte antigen (HLA) includes histocompatibility antigens present on the surfaces of most nucleated cells.

51. Where are genes for HLA antigens located?

HLA genes are located on short arm of chromosome 6.

Two classes are present

i. Class I—A, B, C

ii. Class II—D

52. What is the most important HLA in uveitis?

Most important is HLA-B27

HLA-B27: 58% of normal population

85% in ankylosing spondylitis

70–85% in Reiter's syndrome.

In patients with ankylosing spondylitis, HLA-B27 positivity implies 35% chance of developing acute uveitis, vis-a-vis 7% if negative.

53. What is the importance of serum calcium in uveitis?

Serum calcium—hypercalcemia occurs in 25% of patients with sarcoidosis but only rarely positive in isolated ocular sarcoidosis with systemic remission.

54. What is normal A:G ratio? Name conditions where it is reversed.

i. Normal A:G ratio is 1.5:1 to 2.5:1
ii. Decreased A:G ratio—conditions with elevated antibody concentration, e.g. chronic infections, SLE, RA, malignancy, collagen diseases
iii. Serum globulin is elevated in sarcoidosis.

55. What is significance of urine culture in cytomegalovirus (CMV) infection?

It is recovered from urine specimens from 100% patients with acute CMV infection.

56. What is PCR?

Polymerase chain reaction (PCR) works on the principle of amplification of a segment of DNA. It is used to identify infectious agents—bacteria, viruses, and parasites.

57. What are the uses of PCR in uveitis?

Currently used to detect viral DNA in eyes with ARN and to diagnosis ocular toxoplasmosis, TB.

58. What is the importance of serum lactate dehydrogenase (LDH) in uveitis?

Serum LDH is useful in the diagnosis of retinoblastoma, which can present as uveitis (masquerade syndrome).

59. Serum lysozyme—what is its importance in uveitis?

- Increased in TB, sarcoidosis, leprosy
- Normal levels 1–2 mg/dL

60. What is rheumatoid factor composed of?

i. 7S lgG
ii. 7S lgM
iii. 19S lgM.

61. What are the conditions in which rheumatoid factor is positive?

i. Rheumatoid arthritis
ii. Juvenile rheumatoid arthritis
iii. SLE
iv. Sjogren's syndrome
v. Scleroderma
vi. Infections, e.g. syphilis, infectious mononucleosis, hepatitis.

62. What are the conditions in which rheumatoid factor is negative?

i. JRA (pauciarticular variety)
ii. Seronegative spondyloarthropathies like psoriasis, ulcerative colitis, Crohn's disease, and Reiter's syndrome
iii. Ankylosing spondylitis.

63. What antibody testing methods are used in uveitis?

   i. ELISA

   ii. IFA

   iii. Complicated fixation test

   iv. Hemagglutination test.

64. How is anterior chamber (AC) paracentesis done?

It is done with a 26 gauge needle attached to 1 cc tuberculin syringe.

At the limbus a gutter is made with a blade; care taken to be parallel to plane of iris with bevel up.

It provides small amount of fluid (200–250 pg).

65. Who proposed AC paracentesis first?

Desmont.

66. What are the uses of AC tap?

   i. Detection of organisms by direct exam/culture

   ii. Microscopic study to rule out malignancy

   iii. Assessment of nonspecific biological enzyme, e.g. aqueous ACE

   iv. Immunological test for infection agent, e.g. ELISA to show herpes simplex in ARN

   v. Cell cytology.

67. How is cell cytology of aqueous sample done?

Small drop of aqueous is placed on the slide-fixed in absolute methanol for 10 minutes, air dried, stained with Giemsa for 1 hour, rinsed with 95% ethanol, and let to dry.

68. What are the therapeutic investigations done in uveitis?

   i. Vitrectomy

   ii. Trial of antituberculous treatment

   iii. Trial of steroids.

69. What are the cells found in AH in different condition?

Type of cells	Condition
Neutrophils	Bacterial infection
Eosinophils	Parasitic infection
Lymphocytes	Viral, fungal, autoimmune, and hypersensitivity uveitis
Macophages	Phacoanaphylactic/sympathetic ophthalmia
Tumor cells	Foreign body/masquerade syndrome

70. How is vitreous aspiration done?

   i. Done with 18–20 gauge needle

   ii. The aspirate is sent for cytology, antibodies, and culture.

71. Why is vitrectomy preferred over vitreous aspiration?

    i. Collection of more material

    ii. Apart from diagnostic use, it may also prove therapeutic, e.g. in pha-coanaphylactic uveitis

    iii. Less complications due to controlled traction on vitreous base

    iv. Avoids long-term hypotony

    v. Chorioretinal biopsy can also be taken with vitrectomy.

72. What are the indications and techniques for chorioretinal biopsy in uveitis?

The main indication is bilateral vision threatening disease not responding to treatment, in which etiology cannot be established.

Can be done by:

    i. Making scleral flap at site of lesion by microblade and Vannas scissors.

    ii. Can be also done endoretinally while doing vitrectomy with vitrectomy scissors and forceps.

73. What are the contraindications of chorioretinal biopsy?

Infections of retina and choroid.

74. What are the complications of chorioretinal biopsy?

    i. Choroidal hemorrhage

    ii. Retinal detachment

    iii. Infection

    iv. Proliferative vitreoretinopathy.

75. When is lacrimal gland biopsy done in uveitis?

Lacrimal gland biopsy is done in suspected sarcoidosis, but only if lacrimal glands are clinically enlarged or show increased uptake on gallium scan.

76. What are the indications for invasive procedures in uveitis?

    i. Uncontrolled uveitis

    ii. Endophthalmitis

    iii. Threatened vision

    iv. Doubtful malignancy

    v. Viral retinitis

    vi. Research tool.

77. How is feces examination useful in uveitis?

It is useful to diagnose the following organisms:

    i. *E. coli*

    ii. *E. histolytica*

    iii. *Ascariasis*

    iv. *Giardiasis* (can cause CME).

78. **What X-rays are taken in uveitis?**
    i. **X-ray chest:** TB, Sarcoidosis, histoplasmosis
       In TB—X-ray chest may show fibrocavitary lesions or miliary lesions.
       In sarcoidosis—findings can be divided into four stages.
       Stage 1: Bilateral lymphadenopathy and normal parenchyma.
       Stage 2: Bilateral lymphadenopathy and reticulonodular parenchymal infiltrates.
       Stage 3: Reticulonodular infiltrates alone.
       Stage 4: Progressive pulmonary fibrosis.
    ii. **X-ray sacroiliac joint:** in all young patients with acute unilateral iritis irrespective of presence or absence of low backache. This is because X-ray may be positive before patient is symptomatic in cases of ankylosing spondylitis.
    iii. **X-ray hands and feet:** Sarcoidosis
        CT/MRI brain is indicated in lymphoma.
    iv. **X-ray skull:** Cerebral calcifications in congenital toxoplasmosis, CMV.

79. **What is the importance of gallium scan?**
    i. Gallium is taken up by mitotically active liposomes of granulocytes.
    ii. Scanning is done 48 hours after intravenous injection of labeled gallium citrate.

80. **What is the importance of gallium scan in the diagnosis of sarcoidosis?**
    i. In acute systemic sarcoidosis, gallium scan of head, neck, and chest shows increased uptake.
    ii. This increased uptake + increased aqueous ACE—highly suggestive of sarcoidosis.

81. **In which condition is iris angiography done?**
    Fuchs' heterochromic iridocyclitis—new vessels—in the angle.

82. **What are the indications of FFA in uveitis?**
    i. Vogt–Koyanagi–Harada syndrome
    ii. Acute polypoidal multifocal PPE
    iii. Multiple evanescent white dot syndrome (MEWDS)
    iv. Serpiginous choroiditis.

83. **What are the major FFA findings in uveitis?**
    i. Cystoid macular edema
    ii. Sub retinal neovascular membrane
    iii. Disc leakage
    iv. Late staining of retinal vessels
    v. Neovascularization of retina
    vi. Retina vascular capillary drop out and reorganization
    vii. RPE perturbation.

84. **What are the uses of USG (ultrasonography) in uveitis?**
    i. To diagnosis masquerade syndromes like lymphoma, benign lymphoid hyperplasia, and diffuse melanoma.
    ii. To plan surgery in hazy media due to complicated cataract.
    iii. Vitreal disorders like hemorrhage, inflammation, pars planitis, retained lens fragments.
    iv. Optic disc edema and cupping.
    v. Macular edema and exudative detachment.
    vi. Choroidal thickening, uveal effusion, scieritis, Harada's disease, sympathetic ophthalmia hypotony.
    vii. To rule out Coat's disease and intraocular tumors.
    viii. Useful in VKH and toxocariasis.

85. **What is the importance of visual fields in uveitis?**
    i. Association with secondary glaucoma—glaucoma damage can be estimated
    ii. Behcet's syndrome
    iii. Uveitis syndromes are associated with neurologic disorders VF may be helpful in differentiating papillitis from juxtapapillary uveitis
    iv. Differentiating uveitis from heredodegenerative diseases, e.g. RP from bone spicule pigmentation seen in luetic uveitis
    v. In the early diagnosis and follow-up.

86. **What are the indications for lumbar puncture in uveitis?**
    i. VKH
    ii. Reticulum cell sarcoma
    iii. Intraocular lymphoma.

3.7. TREATMENT OF UVEITIS

1. **What are the aims of therapy?**
   i. To prevent vision threatening complications
   ii. To relieve the patient's discomfort
   iii. To treat the underlying cause if possible.

2. **What are the surgeries done in uveitis?**
   i. Cataract extraction
   ii. Pupillary reconstruction
   iii. Glaucoma surgery
   iv. Peeling of ERM
   v. Scleral buckling
   vi. Vitrectomy.

3. **What is the purpose of using mydriatics/cycloplegics?**
   i. Give comfort by relieving the spasm of ciliary body and sphincter of pupil.
   ii. Prevent the formation of posterior synechiae by using a short acting mydriatic to keep the pupil mobile.
   iii. Breakdown posterior synechiae.
   iv. Reduce exudation from the iris:
       1% atropine—most powerful and longest acting cycloplegic in severe acute inflammation. It is changed to a short acting agent, once inflammation subsides.

4. **Which short acting cycloplegics are used and what is their role?**
   Short acting cycloplegics are used as they keep the pupil mobile, which is the best mechanism to prevent synechiae formation.
   These agents include:
   i. Tropicamide 0.5%, 1.0%
   ii. Cyclopentolate 0.5%, 1.0%, 2.0%

   (*Note:* Side effect of cyclopentolate—chemoattractant for leukocytes and so it may prove bad for uveitis)

   When long acting cycloplegics are continued posterior synechiae occurs in dilated state thereby ill serving the very purpose of it.

5. **What are the preparations commonly used topically?**

i. Prednisolone acetate Suspension (Pred Forte)	0.12% and 1%
ii. Prednisolone sodium phosphate solution	0.12% and 1%
iii. Dexamethasone phosphate solution	0.1%
iv. Fluoromethalone	0.1% and 1%

Duration and frequency of application depends upon severity of inflammation.

Initially applied more frequently and tapered slowly over weeks as inflammation subsides.

Steroids should not be used topically more than 2–3 times/day without concomitant antibiotic drops applied once/twice daily.

Antibiotic-steroid combinations are usually used.

6. **What are the indications for periocular steroids?**
    i. Severe acute anterior uveitis, especially ankylosing spondylitis with severe fibrin membrane/hypopyon.
    ii. Adjunct to topical/systemic treatment in resistant cases of chronic anterior uveitis.
    iii. Intermediate uveitis.
    iv. Poor patient compliance.

7. **What are the advantages of periocular steroids over drops?**
    i. To achieve therapeutic concentration behind lens.
    ii. Drugs not capable of penetrating corneas are able to enter the eye by penetrating sclera.
    iii. Long lasting effect achieved when a depot preparation is used.

8. **What are the types of periocular preparations used?**
    i. Anterior sub-tenon—persistent severe anterior uveitis.
    ii. Posterior sub-tenon—intermediate uveitis, posterior uveitis.
    iii. Subconjunctival and retrobulbar injections.

9. **What are the types of periocular preparation used?**
    i. Triamcinolone acetonide 40 mg
    ii. Depo-medral (methylprednisolone acetate) 40 mg.

10. **What are complications of periocular steroids?**
    Topical complication + extraocular muscle fibrosis, scleromalacia, and conjunctival necrosis.

11. **Why is posterior sub-tenon (PST) injection given temporally and in what frequency?**
    Because it reaches macula when given temporally. It is given every 4–10 weeks. The injection site is close to insertion of inferior oblique, which corresponds to anatomical macula.

12. **What are indications for systemic treatment with oral steroids?**
    i. Intractable anterior uveitis (that has not responded to topical medications and anterior sub-Tenon's injections)
    ii. Intractable intermediate and posterior uveitis (that has not responded to PST).

13. What are contraindications to steroid treatment?

i. Inactive disease with chronic flare
ii. Very mild anterior uveitis
iii. Intermediate uveitis with normal vision
iv. Fuchs' uveitis
v. When antimicrobial treatment is more appropriate, e.g. candidiasis.

14. What are indications and dose of IV steroids?

i. IV pulse methylprednisolone 1 g over 1–2 hours can be employed in cases of severe inflammatory process that needs to be treated as rapidly as possible.
ii. IV methylprednisolone 1 g every day 3 days.

15. What are the indications for immunosuppressants?

i. Vision threatening intraocular inflammation
ii. Reversibility of the disease process
iii. No response to steroids
iv. Intolerable side effects of steroids.

16. Clinical conditions needing immunosuppressants according to IUSG.

i. Absolute   - Behcet's
             - Rheumatoid arthritis
             - Sympathetic ophthalmia
             - VKH
             - Serpiginous choroidopathy
ii. Relative - Intermediate uveitis in adults
             - Preretinal vasulitis
             - Chronic cycltis

17. What are the classes of immunosuppressives?

i. Antimetabolites   - Methotrexate
                      - Azathioprine
ii. Alkylating agents - Cyclophosphamide
iii. Antibiotics   - Cyclosporine
iv. Ergot alkaloid   - Bromocripine
v. Dapsone
vi. Colchicine   - Anti-inflammatory

18. What are indications and side effects of different immunosuppressants?

	Indications	Side effects
1. Cyclophosphamide	Behcet's RA SO	Marrow suppression Hemorrhagic cystitis Secondary malignancy
2. Chlorambucil	Behcet's SO	Marrow suppression Gonadal malignancy Secondary malignancy Hepatotoxicity
3. Methotrexate	SO Scleritis	Marrow suppression Ulcerative stomatitis Diarrhea
4. Azathioprine	Behçet's SLE Pemphigoid	Marrow suppression Secondary infection
5. Cyclosporine	Behçet's Birdshot chorioretinopathy Corneat graft rejection	Hepatotoxicity Nephrotoxicity Hyperuricemia
6. Bromocriptine	Adjunct to cyclosporine in anterior idiopathic uveitis	Nausea, vomiting Postural hypotension
7. Dapsone	Cicatricial pemphigoid	Hemolytic anemia Nausea
8. Colchicine	Behcet's	Nausea, vomiting Marrow suspension

19. What are indications for PKP in uveitis?

Corneal scarring caused by herpes simplex keratouveitis.

20. What are indications for vitrectomy?

    i. Diagnostic—endophthalmitis of suspected infective etiology

    ii. Therapeutic—progressive disease (hypotony) complications needing surgery, e.g. RD iris bombe with hypotony.

21. Ocular complications of steroids.

    i. Increased IOP

    ii. Decreased resistance to infection

    iii. Delayed healing of corneal/shear wounds

    iv. Mydriasis—may precipitate angle closure glaucoma

    v. Ptosis

    vi. Complicated cataract

    vii. Blurred vision

    viii. Enhances lytic action of collagenase

    ix. Paralysis of accommodation

x. Visual field changes
- Scotoma
- Constriction
    - Enlarged blind spot
    - Glaucoma field defect
xi. Problems with color vision
- Color vision defect
- Colored halos around lights
xii. Eyelids and conjunctiva
- Allergic reactions
- Persisted erythema
- Telangiectasia
- Depigmentation
- Poliosis
- Scarring
- Fat atrophy
- Skin atrophy
xiii. Cornea
- SPK
- Superficial corneal defects
xiv. Irritation
- Lacrimation
- Photophobia
- Ocular Pain
- Burning sensation
- Anterior uveitis
xv. Corneal/scleral thickness
- Increased—initial
- Decreased
xvi. Toxic amblyopia
xvii. Optic atrophy
xviii. May aggravate the following diseases:
- Scleromalacia perforans
- Corneal melting disease
- Behcet's disease
- Eales disease
- Presumptive ocular
xix. Retinal embolic phenomena

22. What are the systemic complications of steroids?

    i. Endocrine
- Adrenal insufficiency
- Cushing's syndrome
- Growth failure
- Menstrual disorders

    ii. Neuropsychiatric
- Pseudotumor cerebri
- Insomnia
- Mood swings
- Psychosis

    iii. Gastrointestinal
- Peptic ulcer
- Gastric hemorrhage
- Intestinal perforation
- Pancreatitis

    iv. Musculoskeletal
- Osteoporosis
- Vertebral compression fracture
- Aseptic necrosis of femur
- Myopathy

    v. Cardiovascular
- Hypertension
- Sodium and fluid retention

    vi. Metabolic
- Secondary diabetes mellitus
- Hyperosmotic ketoacidosis
- Centripetal obesity
- Hyperlipidemia

    vii. Dermatologic
- Acne
- Hirsutism
- Subcutaneous tissue atrophy

    viii. Immunologic
- Impaired inflammatory response
- Delayed tissue healing.

CHAPTER
4

Glaucoma

4.1. BASIC EXAMINATION OF GLAUCOMA AND TONOMETRY

1. **What are the methods of measurement of anterior chamber depth (ACD)?**
   i. Clinical method
      – Pen torch or eclipse technique
      – Split limbal technique
   ii. Subjective method
      – Qualitative: van Herick's method
      – Quantitative: Smith's method
   iii. Objective methods.

2. **What is pen torch shadow or eclipse technique?**
   It involves shining a pen torch temporal to the patient's eye and interpreting the light and shadow across the iris front surface.
   This may be done as follows:
      i. In this method, the patient is asked to look straight in primary gaze.
      ii. A pen torch is held parallel to iris plane.
      iii. The amount of iris that remains in shadow may then be interpreted as an indication of the depth of chamber.

   With a very narrow angle, the forward bulging iris leaves much of the nasal iris in shadow. A deep chamber with a wide angle allows reflection of light from most of the iris.

Grade 4	Good spread of light (open angle)	Fully illuminated
Grade 3	Partial shadow of distal iris	>2/3 illuminated
Grade 2	Increasing eclipse	1/3–2/3 illuminated
Grade 1	Large eclipse of distal iris due to forward bulging of iris (narrow angle)	<1/3 illuminated

3. **What is split limbal technique?**

van Herick's method can help measure nasal and temporal ACD, but for superior and inferior angles it gives no clue. Knowing superior angle depth is important as it is the narrowest and most likely to close.

    i. In split limbal technique, superior anterior chamber angle is illuminated with slit lamp but assessment is made with naked eye.

    ii. With the illumination in click position, a vertical slit should be placed at 12 o'clock.

    iii. Observe the arc of light falling on cornea and iris without the aid of slit lamp eyepiece

    iv. The angular separation seen at limbal corneal junction is an estimation of ACD in degrees.

Grade	Estimated angle
0	0°
1	10°
2	20°
3	30°
4	≥45°

4. **How do you do van Herick's method of assessment of ACD?**

It is a subjective method of estimation of ACD using a slit lamp by comparing the peripheral ACD with the peripheral corneal thickness.

PROCEDURE:

    i. The patient is positioned comfortably and looks straight toward the microscope.

    ii. The viewing system of slit lamp is parallel to visual axis and the illumination system is set at 60° temporal to the viewing system.

    iii. The angle is chosen as 60° so that the illuminating beam is approximately perpendicular to the limbus and as the angle is constant whenever the technique is used, this enables consistency of interpretation every time the patient is assessed.

    iv. The slit-lamp magnification should be set at 16× and slit length to maximum to allow an adequate depth of focus.

    v. An optical section of the cornea as thin as possible and as close to the temporal limbus as possible is viewed.

    vi. A comparison is made between the thickness of the peripheral cornea and the gap between the posterior surface of the cornea and the front of the iris where the beam first touches.

    vii. The ratio of these two measurements may be graded and interpreted.

    viii. Measurement at the nasal limbus can also be done.

van Herick estimate of angle width from ACD at the periphery:

Angle	Depth	Comment
Grade 4 angle	ACD = Corneal thickness	Wide open
Grade 3 angle	ACD = 1/4 to 1/2 corneal thickness	Incapable of closure
Grade 2 angle	ACD = 1/4 corneal thickness	Should be gonioscoped
Grade 1 angle	ACD <1/4 corneal thickness	Gonioscopy demonstrates dangerously narrow angle
Slit angle	ACD = Slit-like (extremely shallow)	
Closed angle	Absent peripheral anterior chamber	

5. What is Smith's method?

This was described by Smith in 1979. This technique differs from van Herick's in being quantitative.

The procedure is carried out as follows:

   i. The microscope is placed in the straight-ahead position in front of the patient. The illumination is placed at 60° temporally.
   ii. To examine the patient's right eye, the practitioner views through the right eyepiece and for the left eye through the left eyepiece.
   iii. A beam of 1–2 mm is orientated horizontally and focused on the cornea.
   iv. In this position, two horizontal streaks of light are seen: one on the anterior corneal surface and the other on the front surface of the crystalline lens.
   v. Altering the slit-height adjustment on the instrument is seen as a lengthening or shortening of the two horizontal reflexes.
   vi. Beginning with a short slit, the length is slowly increased to a point at which the ends of the corneal and lenticular reflections appear to meet.
   vii. The slit length at this point is then measured (it is assumed that the slit lamp is calibrated for slit length).
   viii. This length may be multiplied by a constant 1.34 to calculate ACD by Smith's method.
   ix. Eyes with ACD <2 mm should be dilated with caution.

Slit length (mm)	ACD (mm)
1.5	2.01
2.0	2.68
2.5	3.35
3.0	4.02
3.5	4.69

6. **What is adapted Smith's method?**

   i. It is used in those situations in which variable slit height is not possible.
   ii. In this case, the slit length is noted prior to measurement at a point where it corresponds to 2 mm. The instrument is then set up exactly as in the Smith method but with the initial angle of incidence at 80°.
   iii. By gradually closing the angle, the two reflected images on the cornea and lens appear to move closer and the angle at which they first touch is noted.
   iv. A corresponding value for the chamber depth for differing angles is then calculated.

7. **What are the objective methods?**

   i. Ultrasonography
   ii. AS-OCT, HD-OCT
   iii. Oculus Pentacam-Scheimpflug imaging
   iv. Pachometer slit-lamp attachment.

8. **What is the normal intraocular pressure (IOP)?**

   The normal IOP is between 10 mm Hg and 21 mm Hg.

9. **Why is 21 considered as upper limit?**

   IOP distribution in general population resembles a Gaussian curve but skewed toward right. Mean IOP is considered to be 15.5 ± 2.57 mm Hg. Two standard deviation above the mean is approximately 20.5 mm Hg as approximately 95% of the area under a Gaussian curve lies between the mean ± 2 SD. The concept of normal IOP limits is viewed as only a rough approximation.

10. **What are the two ways by which aqueous is secreted?**

    i. Active secretion by nonpigmentary ciliary epithelium—80%
    ii. Passive secretion by ultrafiltration and diffusion—20%.

11. **What are the factors that determine the level of IOP?**

    i. Rate of aqueous secretion
    ii. Resistance encountered in outflow channels
    iii. Level of episcleral venous pressure.

12. **What is normal episcleral venous pressure?**

    The normal range is 8–10 mm Hg.

13. **What are the causes of elevated episcleral venous pressure?**

    i. *Obstruction of venous drainage*
       - Thyroid eye disease
       - Pseudotumor

- Cavernous sinus thrombosis
- Jugular vein obstruction
- Superior vena cava obstruction
- Pulmonary venous obstruction
- Congestive heart failure
- Radiation.

ii. *Arteriovenous anomalies*

- Carotid-cavernous sinus fistula
- Sturge–Weber syndrome
- Dural fistula
- Venous varix
- Intraocular vascular shunts.

iii. *Idiopathic*

14. **What are the conditions that influence IOP?**
    i. Diurnal variation
    ii. Postural variation
    iii. Exertional influences
    iv. Lid and eye movement
    v. Intraocular conditions
    vi. Systemic conditions
    vii. Environmental conditions
    viii. General anesthesia
    ix. Food and drugs.

15. **How does the IOP vary diurnally?**

    The most common pattern is that the IOP is maximum in mid-morning and decreases as the day progresses to become minimum in the late evening or early morning. Some individuals show an elevation at nighttime. This diurnal variation is about 3–6 mm Hg in normal individuals and 10 mm Hg or more in a glaucomatous eye.

16. **What is this diurnal variation due to?**

    It is due to cyclic fluctuation of blood levels of adrenocortical steroids. Maximum IOP is reached 3–4 hours after the peak of plasma cortisol. The nighttime elevated IOP is due to the supine position along with the fluctuating cortisol levels.

17. **What are the types of diurnal variation curves?**

    There are four types of diurnal variation curves.

    They are:
    i. **Falling type**: maximal at 6–8 am followed by a continuous decline
    ii. **Rising type**: maximal at 4–6 pm
    iii. **Double variation type**: with two peaks 9–11 am and 6 pm
    iv. **Flat type** of curve.

18. **How does IOP vary with posture?**

The IOP rises (0.3–6 mm Hg) when the person is lying down. This may be because of increase in the episcleral venous pressure in the supine posture.

19. **How does IOP vary with exertion?**

Valsalva maneuvers increase IOP (by increasing episcleral venous pressure), while prolonged exercise decreases IOP (by metabolic acidosis and increased colloid osmotic pressure).

20. **How does IOP vary with lid and eye movement?**

Forcible eyelid closure raises IOP by 10–90 mm Hg. Repeated eyelid squeezing reduces IOP.
Widening of the lid fissure increases IOP by approximately 2 mm Hg. Conversely, with Bell's palsy, IOP is slightly reduced.

21. **How does IOP vary with intraocular conditions?**

Acute anterior uveitis causes a slight reduction in IOP because of decreased aqueous humor production. Rhegmatogenous retinal detachment also causes a reduction because of reduced aqueous humor production as well as shunting of aqueous humor from the posterior chamber through the vitreous and retinal hole into the subretinal space.
Inflammatory rise in IOP in anterior uveitis
Schwartz syndrome—rise in IOP in retinal detachment.

22. **How does IOP vary with systemic conditions?**

Systemic factors causing increased IOP:
   i. Systemic hypertension
   ii. Systemic hyperthermia
   iii. Adrenocorticotropic hormone and growth hormone stimulation
   iv. Hypothyroidism
   v. Diabetes
   vi. Obesity.

Systemic factors causing decreased IOP:
   i. Pregnancy
   ii. Hyperthyroidism
   iii. Myotonic dystrophy.

23. **How does IOP vary with environmental conditions?**

Exposure to cold decreases IOP (because of lowered episcleral venous pressure) while reduced gravity increases IOP.

24. How does IOP vary with food and drugs?

Agents increasing IOP:

  i. Caffeine
 ii. Corticosteroids
iii. Topical cycloplegics
 iv. Water (large volume of water consumption increases IOP: basis of water drinking test).

Agents decreasing IOP

General Anesthesia:

  i. Alcohol
 ii. Heroin and marijuana
iii. Tobacco smoking.

25. How does IOP vary with anesthetic agents?

In general, general anesthetic agents reduce IOP. However, trichloroethylene, ketamine, succinylcholine, and suxamethonium increase IOP.

26. Does heredity influence IOP?

IOP tends to be higher in individuals with enlarged cup-disk ratio and in relatives of patients with open-angle glaucoma.

27. What is tonography?

Tonography is a method used to measure the facility of aqueous outflow. The facility of outflow is called as the C value and it ranges from 0.22 to 0.30 µL/min/mm Hg.

28. How is tonography performed?

The clinician first takes the IOP measurement by using a Schiotz tonometer. The tonometer is placed on the cornea, acutely elevating the IOP. The rate at which the pressure declines with time is related to the ease with which the aqueous leaves the eye. The decline in IOP over time can be used to determine outflow facility.

Tonography technique:

  i. Patient in supine position
 ii. Topical anesthetic instilled
iii. IOP measured with two brief applications of electronic tonometer
 iv. 4 minute tracing of pressure at this position till a smooth tracing is obtained for full 4 minutes
  v. Slope is estimated by placing free hand line through middle of oscillations (readings at beginning and end noted)

vi. P0 and change in readings used to obtain C value from special tono-graphic tables.

$$F = C (P_0 - P_v)$$

F—aqueous outflow rate (microlitre/min), P0—IOP

C—coefficient of outflow facility, Pv—episcleral nervous pressure

29. What is the principle of digital tonometry?

Compressibility of ocular coats is estimated by sense of fluctuation perceived on palpation.

30. How is IOP measured digitally?

After asking the patient to look down, the sclera is palpated through the upper lid above the tarsal plate using the tip of two fingers. One finger is kept still and the other indents the globe lightly.

31. What are the types of tonometers?

   i. Indentation/impression tonometer:
  - Schiotz
  ii. Applanation tonometer
  - Goldmann, Mackay–Marg, Maklakov, pneumotonometer noncontact
 iii. Newer tonometers
  - Dynamic contour tonometer (DCT), ocular response analyzer (ORA).

32. What are the types of weights used in Schiotz tonometry?

A 5.5 g weight is permanently fixed to the plunger, which can be increased to 7.5 or 10 and 15 g by adding additional weights.

33. What are the advantages of Schiotz tonometry?

   i. Easy to use
  ii. Portable
 iii. Useful for screening
 iv. Cost-effective.

34. What are the disadvantages of Schiotz tonometry?

   i. **Ocular rigidity**: The more the scleral rigidity, the higher is the reading. Conversely, in conditions like high myopia, where the scleral rigidity is low, the IOP is underestimated.
  ii. **Corneal influences**: A steeper or thicker cornea causes a greater displacement of fluid during indentation tonometry, which leads to a falsely high tonometry reading.
 iii. **Blood volume alteration**: The variable expulsion of the intraocular blood during indentation tonometry may also influence IOP measurement.
 iv. **Moses effect**: The hole in the tonometer foot plate can be a source of error.

35. **What are the precautions to be taken before using Schiotz tonometry?**
    i. Touch the artificial cornea till the reading is at zero
    ii. Avoid pressure over the eyelids
    iii. Sterilize before using.

36. **What are the other types of indentation tonometers?**
    i. Herrington
    ii. Grants
    iii. Maurice.

37. **What are the types of applanation tonometers?**
    They are of two types:

Variable force	Variable area
i. Goldmann	i. Maklakov–Kalfa
ii. Perkins	ii. Applanometer
iii. Draeger	iii. Tonomat
iv. Mackay–Marg	iv. Halberg

38. **What is the principle of applanation tonometer?**
    It is based on Imbert–Fick law, which states that the pressure inside an ideal dry, thin-walled sphere equals the force necessary to flatten its surface divided by the area of the flattening.
    $$P = F/A$$

39. **What is the most common applanation tonometer used?**
    The one designed by Goldmann for use with Haag–Streit slit lamp.

40. **Volume of aqueous displaced during application using Goldmann application tonometer?**
    $0.5 \ \mu L$.

41. **How much of the anesthetized cornea does the circular plate flatten?**
    3.06 mm of corneal diameter is flattened, which is always constant. Hence, it is called constant area applanation tonometer.

42. **How is the pressure calculated?**
    When the area is made constant (3.06 mm) then 0.1 g reading corresponds to a pressure of 1 mm Hg.

43. **What is the rationale behind using a circular plate of a particular (3.06 mm) diameter?**
    At this diameter, the resistance of the cornea to flattening is counterbalanced by the capillary attraction of the tear film meniscus for the tonometer head.

44. Which dye is used and under what illumination?

Fluorescein dye (0.25%) is used and viewed under cobalt blue light.

45. What should be the angle between the source of illumination and microscope?

The angle should be approximately 60°.

46. What mark is the knob set before the procedure?

The knob is set at 1. If placed at zero, microvibrations are produced which can cause corneal erosions.

47. What is observed when viewed through the eyepiece?

The fluorescence of the stained tear facilitates visualization of the tear meniscus at the margin of the contact between cornea and bi-prism. A central blue circle, which is the flattened cornea, surrounded by two yellow semicircles which is the tear meniscus is seen.

48. What is the desired end point of an applanation tonometer?

The bi-prism which contacts the cornea produces two semicircles that should be equal in size and inner sides of the two should coincide.

49. What are the advantages of applanation tonometers over indentation tonometry?

   i. Reliable and accurate
  ii. Reproducible
 iii. Not influenced by scleral rigidity.

50. What are the disadvantages or source of errors of applanation tonometry?

   i. **Central corneal thickness:** Thicker corneas produce falsely higher reading while thinner corneas produce falsely lower readings. However, corneal thickening due to edema causes a falsely lower reading. An average error is 0.7 mm Hg per 10 microns of deviation from the mean of 520 microns.
  ii. **Semicircles**: Wider meniscus and improper vertical alignment cause falsely higher reading.
 iii. **Corneal astigmatism**: Since astigmatism produces an elliptical area of contact, there is an error in measurement. IOP is underestimated in cases of with the rule astigmatism and overestimated in cases of against the rule with approximately 1 mm Hg for every 4 D of astigmatism.
 iv. **Design**: It has a complex design and can be done only in sitting position.
  v. **Corneal irregularity**: It is not useful in case of corneal irregularity.
 vi. **Errors following corneal refractive surgery**: It will not be accurate following Lasik surgery.

51. How can errors due to astigmatism be minimized?

The tonometer prisms should be rotated so that the axis of the least corneal curvature is opposite the red line on the prism holder.

52. What are the methods of disinfection of tonometers?

The following chemicals can be used to sterilize the tip of applanation tonometers:

i. 3% hydrogen peroxide
ii. 70% isopropyl alcohol
iii. Diluted sodium hypochlorite solution (1:10)
iv. Heat-sterilized Schiotz tonometer.

53. What are the infections likely to be transmitted?

i. Adenovirus of epidemic keratoconjunctivitis (EKC)
ii. HSV—type 1
iii. HIV
iv. Hepatitis B.

54. How is IOP measured in conditions of corneal scarring?

The following tonometers can be used:

i. Noncontact tonometers
ii. Mackay–Marg
iii. Tonopen
iv. Pneumatic tonometers.

55. What are the advantages of tonopen?

i. Used in cases of corneal epithelial irregularities
ii. Measurement of IOP over bandage contact lens
iii. Useful in edematous and scarred corneas
iv. Useful in patients with nystagmus and head tremors
v. Used in operation theater
vi. Portable.

56. What is the principle of noncontact tonometers?

A puff of air creates constant force that deforms the central cornea. The time from an internal reference point to the moment of maximum light detection is measured and converted to IOP.

57. What are the disadvantages of noncontact tonometer (NCT)?

i. Tear film damage
ii. False-positives and false-negatives.

58. What are the newer modalities of IOP measurement?

i. Optical response analyzer
ii. Dynamic contact tonometer (Pascal)
iii. Rebound tonometer
iv. Proview phosphene tonometer.

59. What is the principle behind dynamic contact tonometer (DCT)?

Pressure applied to an enclosed fluid is transmitted undiminished to every part of closed system including walls of container. By applying DCT cornea is placed in a neutral shape so that pressure on interior surface equals pressure on exterior surface.

60. Advantages of DCT over Goldmann applanation tonometer.

   i. Pressure reading independent of corneal thickness
   ii. No mechanical calibration
   iii. No fluorescein staining
   iv. Direct display of pressure as numerical values

4.2. GONIOSCOPY

1. **What is gonioscopy?**

   It is a clinical technique that is used to examine structures in the anterior chamber angle and forms an important part of glaucoma evaluation.

2. **What is cycloscopy?**

   This is a technique of direct visualization of ciliary processes under special circumstances such as the presence of an iridectomy, wide iris retraction, aniridia, and some cases of aphakia. Main value is in conjunction with laser therapy to ciliary processes (transpupillary cyclophotocoagulation).

3. **What is the principle of gonioscopy?**

   Under normal conditions, light reflected from the angle structures is incident at the tear–air interface at an oblique angle, and is internally reflected. All gonioscopy lenses eliminate the tear–air interface by placing a plastic or glass surface adjacent to the front surface of the eye.

4. **What are commonly used contact lenses for gonioscopy?**

   i. **Direct gonioscopy (Gonio lens):**
   - Koeppe
   - Barkan
   - Worst
   - Swan–Jacob
   - Richardson

   ii. **Indirect gonioscopy (Gonio prism):**
   - Goldmann
   - Zeiss
   - Posner
   - Sussman

5. **Describe direct gonioscopy.**

   This is performed with a hand-held binocular microscope, a fiberoptic illuminator or a pen light, and a direct gonioscopy lens. It is performed with the patient in a supine position (e.g., in an operating room for infants under anesthesia). With direct gonioscopy lenses, an erect view of the angle structures is obtained.

6. **Describe indirect gonioscopy.**

Instruments:

1. Goldmann single mirror	Mirror in this lens has a height of 12 mm and tilt of 62 degrees from the plano front surface. Central well has a diameter of 12 mm, posterior radius of curvature— 7.38 mm
2. Goldmann three mirror	**Has two mirrors for examination of the fundus and one for the anterior chamber angle.** **Equatorial mirror (inclined at 73°):** It is largest and oblong shape enables visualization from posterior pole to equator. **Peripheral mirror (67°):** Intermediate in size, square shape enables visualization from equator to ora serrata. **Gonioscopy mirror (59°):** Smallest and dome shape used to visualize extreme periphery and the angle.
3. Zeiss four mirror (can be used for indentation gonioscopy)	All four mirrors are tilted at 64 degrees. Original four mirror lens is mounted on a holding fork called unger or holder. Posners lens has permanently attached holder rod. Sussmans lens is held directly. Patient's own tears are useful as fluid bridge.
4. Ritch trabeculoplasty	Two mirrors are titled at 59 degrees. Two are titled at 62 degrees; convex lens is present over one mirror of each set.
5. Trabeculens	Has a 30 D convex lens in a hollow funnel, with four mirrors at 62 degrees angles. It can be used as a diagnostic gonioprism, as well as for laser trabeculoplasty and iridotomy.

Techniques:

The cornea is anesthetized and with the patient positioned at the slit lamp, topical anesthetic is instilled, and the gonioprism is gently placed against the cornea with or without a fluid bridge (depending on type). Slit beam is narrowed, carefully avoiding direct illumination of the pupil. A corneal wedge is formed, to identify Schwalbe's line.

Visualization into a narrow angle can be enhanced by manipulating the Goldmann gonioprism, by asking the patient to look in the direction of the mirror being used.

7. **Comparison of direct and indirect gonioscopy.**

Sl No	Advantages	Disadvantages
Indirect		
1.	Equipment easily available	Orientation is confusing initially
2.	Quicker procedure	Difficult in narrow angles

(Continued)

(*Continued*)

SI No	Advantages	Disadvantages
3.	Compression can be done	
4.	Slit lamp provides good illumination and magnification	
Direct		
1.	Binocular comparison	Special equipment
2.	Simple orientation	Time consuming
3.	Can see over convex iris	Expensive
4.	Ideal for surgical intervention	
5.	Supine position comparable to normal anatomy	

8. **What is compression gonioscopy?**

This is also called as indentation gonioscopy. By varying the amount of pressure applied to the cornea by a Zeiss contact lens the physician can observe the effects, since this will cause the aqueous humor to be forced into the angle. This is used to differentiate appositional versus synechial angle closure. Compression gonioscopy can be performed by Zeiss Posner or Sussman lenses.

9. **Describe normal structures of the angle seen in gonioscopy.**

Starting at the root of the iris and progressing anteriorly toward the cornea, the following structures can be identified by gonioscopy (from behind forward):

i. **Ciliary body band**: This is a gray or dark brown band and is the portion of ciliary body that is visible in the anterior chamber as a result of the iris insertion into the ciliary body.

ii. **Scleral spur**: This is usually seen as a prominent white line between the ciliary body band and functional trabecular mesh work. This is the posterior lip of the scleral sulcus.

iii. **Trabecular meshwork**: This is seen as a pigmented band just anterior to the scleral spur. It has an anterior and posterior part. The posterior part is the primary site of aqueous outflow.

iv. **Schwalbe's line**: This is the junction between the angle structures and the cornea. It marks the transition between corneal endothelium and trabecular cells. It also marks termination of Descemet's membrane.

10. **Mention the clinical uses of gonioscopy.**

i. **Diagnostic:**

   – Differentiate between open-angle and angle-closure glaucoma
   – Early detection of narrow angles

- Helps in diagnosing secondary glaucomas like trauma (angle recession), neovascular (new vessels in the angle), pseudoexfoliative (deposition of pseudoexfoliation (PXF) material), and pigmentary glaucoma
- Helps in identifying tumor, cysts, foreign bodies, or blood in the angle
- Assess K–F ring (Wilson's disease).
- Postoperative evaluation:
  - Ostium
  - Cyclodialysis
  - Iridotomy

ii. **Therapeutic:**
- Indentation gonioscopy can be used to break an attack of acute angle closure.
- Useful to do goniotomy and goniophotocoagulation.

11. **How do you differentiate iris processes and peripheral anterior synechiae (PAS)?**

Iris process	PAS
Lacy, fenestrated	Solid, not fenestrated
Underlying angle structures visible through spaces between strands	Preclude any view of underlying structures

Iris processes are present in one third of the normal eyes. Generally insert at the level of scleral spur more in number in the nasal angle.

12. **How do you differentiate between the normal blood vessel in angle and the pathological angle vessels?**

Normal blood vessel in angle	Pathological angle vessels
Broad	Fine
It will not cross the scleral spur	Crosses the scleral spur
Do not arborize	Branch, arborize in trabecular meshwork

13. **How do you differentiate between Sampaolesi's line and pigmented trabecular meshwork?**

Sampaolesi's line	Pigmented trabecular meshwork
Located anterior to the corneal wedge	Posterior to the corneal wedge
Salt and pepper appearance	Brown sugar
Dark and granular	Fine
Discontinuous	Continuous

14. **Mention the causes of trabecular meshwork pigmentation.**
    i. Pigmentary glaucoma/pigment dispersion syndrome
    ii. PXF
    iii. Pseudophakic pigment dispersion
    iv. Trauma
    v. Following YAG laser iridotomy
    vi. Following acute angle-closure glaucoma
    vii. Anterior uveitis
    viii. Iris melanoma
    ix. Epithelial cysts
    x. Nevus of Ota
    xi. Darkly pigmented iris.

15. **What are the causes of blood in the angle?**
    i. Posttraumatic
    ii. Postsurgical
    iii. Postlaser
    iv. Ghost cells recognized as candy stripe pattern

16. **What are the causes of blood in Schlemm canal?**
    i. **Due to increased episcleral venous pressure**
       – Carotid-cavernous fistula
       – Dural shunt
       – Sturge–Weber syndrome
       – Obstruction of superior vena cava
       – Ocular hypotony
       – Post gonioscopy
    ii. **Due to low IOP**
       – Hypotony following trabeculectomy

17. **What are the causes of peripheral anterior synechiae?**
    i. Primary angle-closure glaucoma (PACG)
    ii. Anterior uveitis
    iii. Iridocorneal endothelial (ICE) syndrome
    iv. Secondary glaucoma following intraocular surgery (like wound leak, etc.)
    v. Trauma.

18. **What are the findings one can expect in gonioscopy following trauma?**
    i. Angle recession
    ii. Trabecular tears
    iii. Iridodialysis
       Cyclodialysis
    iv. Foreign bodies
       PAS (late onset)

GONIOSCOPIC GRADING OF ANGLES STRUCTURE

Shaffer's grading system

S.No	Angle grade	Numeric grade	Degrees	Clinical interpretation	Structure visible
1.	Wide open angle	4	35–40 degrees	Closure impossible	Up to ciliary body
2.	Open	3	25–35 degrees	Closure impossible	Up to ciliary body
3.	Moderately narrow	2	20 degrees	Eventual closure possible. But unlikely	Trabecular meshwork (pigmented)
4.	Extremely narrow	1	10 degrees	Closure possible	Only Schwalbe line. May be anterior TM (non pigmented) seen
5.	Slit angle	S	<10 degrees	Portions appear closed	No angle structures seen. But no obvious iridocorneal contact
6.	Closed angle	0	—	Closure complete	Iridocorneal contact

In grade 0—indentation gonioscopy with Zeiss goniolens is necessary to differentiate appositional from synechial angle closure.

1. **Define occludable angle.**

   This is a condition in which pigmented trabecular meshwork is not visible (Shaffer grade 1 or 0) without indentation or manipulation in at least three quadrants.

2. **Scheie's gonioscopic classification.**

S.No	Grade	Structure visible
1.	Wide open	All structure visible
2.	Grade 1 narrow	Hard to see the root of iris
3.	Grade 2 narrow	Ciliary body band obscured
4.	Grade 3 narrow	Posterior trabecular meshwork obscured
5.	Grade 4 narrow	Only Schwalbe's line visible

3. **Spaeth classification.**

   Takes four parameters into consideration.

   i. Site of iris root insertion

A	Anterior to TM (i.e. Schwalbe's line)
B	Behind Schwalbe's line (at the level of TM)
C	Centered at the level of scleral spur
D	Deep to scleral spur (i.e. anterior to CB)
E	Extremely deep inserted into CB

   ii. Width or geometric angle of iris insertion

   The angle between the intersection of imaginary tangents formed by peripheral third of iris and the inner wall of corneoscleral junction. It is graded as 10, 20, 30 degrees and 40 degrees.

   iii. Contour of peripheral iris near the angle

S	Steep or convex configuration
R	Regular or flat
Q	Queer—deeply concave

   iv. Intensity of trabecular meshwork pigmentation minimal or no pigment (Grade 0) to dense pigment deposition (Grade 4).

4.3. GLAUCOMA DIAGNOSTIC WITH VARIABLE CORNEAL COMPENSATION (GDx VCC)

1. **What are the key elements of the printout?**

   i. **The thickness map**

   Retinal nerve fiber layer (RNFL) thickness represented on color-coded map

   Thick RNFL—yellow, orange, red

   Thin RNFL—dark blue, light blue, and green.

   ii. **The deviation map**

   Location and magnitude of RNFL defects over the map.

   iii. **The TSNIT map**

   Displays RNFL thickness over the calculation circle (stands for temporal-superior-nasal-inferior-temporal)

   Normal TSNIT—map follows a double hump pattern, i.e.,

   Thick RNFL—superior, inferior

   Thin RNFL—nasal, temporal

   shows actual values along with shaded area representing normal range for that age.

   iv. **The parameters**

   - TSNIT average
   - Superior average
   - Inferior average
   - TSNIT standard deviation
   - Inter eye asymmetry.

2. **How is the measurement done? What area is measured and at how many points?**

   It is performed with an undilated pupil of at least 2 mm diameter. As the scanner has two mirrors that oscillate at 4000/sec, there is a high-pitched noise emitted.

   65,536 points are measured in a full 15 × 150 grid centered at the optic nerve head.

   The central ellipse denotes an area of 1.75 disk diameter in size.

   The reproducibility of images is 5–8 microns per measured pixel.

   Image quality check: A warning is given if image fails to meet criteria.

   The quality of image is affected by cataracts and poor media clarity.

3. **What are the abnormal patterns on the thickness map?**

   Abnormal patterns include:

   i. Diffuse loss of NFL, causing areas that should be yellow to fade to red

   ii. Focal defects are seen as concentrated dark areas (should be visible on fundus image as well)

   iii. Asymmetry between superior and inferior quadrants

   iv. Asymmetry between the two eyes

   v. Higher than normal nasal and temporal thickness (red and yellow where blue should be).

4. What is the sensitivity and specificity of GDx VCC?

   i. Sensitivity—96%

   ii. Specificity—93%

5. What are advantages of GDx VCC?

Advantages of GDx VCC:

   i. Easy to operate

   ii. Does not require pupillary dilatation

   iii. Good reproducibility

   iv. Does not require a reference plane

   v. Can detect glaucoma on the first exam

   vi. Early detection before standard visual field

   vii. Comparison with age-matched normative database

6. What are limitations of GDx VCC?

Limitations of GDx VCC:

   i. It does not provide optic nerve head analysis

   ii. Limited use in moderate/advanced glaucoma

   iii. Does not measure actual RNFL thickness (inferred value)

   iv. No clinical studies on detection of progression using this technology

   v. No database from the Indian population

   vi. Affected by anterior and posterior segment

Pathology such as:

   i. Ocular surface disorders

   ii. Macular pathology

   iii. Cataract and refractive surgery

   iv. Refractive errors (false-positive in myopes)

   v. Peripapillary atrophy (scleral birefringence interferes with RNFL measurement)

7. What is scanning laser polarimetry?

Scanning laser polarimetry is an imaging technology that is utilized to measure peripapillary RNFL thickness. It is based on the principle of birefringence. GDx is the trade name that uses this technology.

8. What is VCC?

VCC stands for variable corneal compensator, which has been created to account for the variable corneal birefringence in patients.

4.4. GLAUCOMA VISUAL FIELD DEFECTS

1. **What is visual field?**

   Traquair defined visual field as an island of vision in a sea of darkness. The island of vision is usually described as a three-dimensional graphic representation of differential light sensitivity at different positions of space.

2. **What is the extent of the normal visual field?**

Superior	: 60 degrees
Inferior	: 75 degrees
Nasally	: 60 degrees
Temporally	: 100–110 degrees

3. **What is blind spot?**

   This region corresponds to the optic nerve head, and because there are no photoreceptors in the area, it creates a deep depression within the boundaries of the normal visual field.

4. **What is kinetic perimetry?**

   Kinetic perimetry is one in which a target is moved from an area where it is not seen to an area where it is just seen, keeping size and intensity of the stimulus constant, e.g., Goldmann perimetry.

5. **What is static perimetry?**

   A stationary stimulus is presented at various locations with variable intensity, e.g., Humphrey's perimetry.

6. **What are the variables that can influence perimetry?**
   i. Alertness of the patient
   ii. Fixation must be constant and centered
   iii. Background luminance: should be maintained between 4 and 31 apostilbs
   iv. Brightness of the stimulus
   v. Patient refraction should be fully corrected
   vi. Pupil size should be constant (2–4 mm)
   vii. Increasing age is associated with a reduction in retinal threshold sensitivity
   viii. High cheekbones and sunken socket
   ix. Media clarity.

7. **What are the causes of generalized decrease in sensitivity of the visual field?**
   i. Glaucoma
   ii. Cataracts

   iii. Use of miotics

   iv. Gross uncorrected refractive errors

    v. Other media opacities.

8. What is an isopter?

A line on a visual field representation connecting points with the same threshold. It is usually done on a two-dimensional sheet of paper.

9. What is a scotoma?

Localized defect or depression in the visual field. An absolute defect persists even at the maximum stimulus, and a relative scotoma is seen in a weaker stimulus, but disappears on increasing the brightness of the stimulus.

10. What is a depression?

Depression is a decrease in expected retinal sensitivity.

11. What are the sequential progression of visual field defects in glaucoma?

     i. Generalized depression

    ii. Paracentral scotoma

   iii. Siedel's scotoma

   iv. Arcuate or Bjerrum scotoma

    v. Double arcuate or ring scotoma

   vi. Nasal step

  vii. Progressive contraction

 viii. Central island and temporal island with or without split fixation.

12. What are angioscotomas?

Angioscotomas are long branching scotomas above and below the blind spot, which are presumed to result from shadows created by the large retinal blood vessels.

13. What is Bjerrum's (arcuate's) area?

It is an arcuate area extending above and below the blind spot between 10 and 25 of fixation point.

14. What are the differential diagnosis for arcuate scotoma?

    i. **Chorioretinal lesions:**
   - Juxtapapillary choroiditis
   - Myopia with peripapillary atrophy
   - Panretinal photocoagulation.

   ii. **Optic nerve head lesions:**
   - Drusen
   - Retinal artery plaques
   - Chronic papilledema

  - Colobomas
  - Optic pit.

iii. **Anterior optic nerve head lesion:**
  - Electric shock
  - Retrobulbar neuritis
  - Cerebral arteritis
  - Ischemic optic neuropathy.

iv. **Posterior lesions of the visual pathway:**
  - Pituitary adenoma
  - Optochiasmatic arachnoiditis
  - Meningiomas of dorsum sella.

15. **What is paracentral scotoma?**

It is the earliest clinically significant field defect. It may appear either below or above the blind spot in Bjerrum area.

16. **What is Seidel's scotoma?**

When the disease progresses, paracentral scotoma joins with the blind-spot to form a sickle-shaped scotoma known as Seidel's scotoma.

17. **What is ring (or) double arcuate scotoma?**

It develops when the two arcuate scotomas join together at the horizontal raphe.

18. **What is Roenne's central nasal step?**

It is created when the two arcuate scotomas run in different arcs and meet to form a sharp right-angled defect at the horizontal meridian.

19. **What are the true baring and false baring of blindspots?**

When a small isopter is being studied, a patient with Seidel's scotoma may demonstrate a connection between the blindspot and nonseeing area outside the 25 degree radius. This is true baring of blind spot. A normal patient may exhibit false baring of blindspot, when the isopter is just outside blindspot.

20. **What is scotometry/campimetry?**

Estimation of defect of central fields by using tangent screen is termed as campimetry/scotometry.

21. **Which part of the visual field is tested using tangent screen?**

Central 300.

22. **What is the size of the tangent screen board?**

$1 m^2$ or $2 m^2$.

23. **At what distance should patient be seated?**

1 m or 2 m according to the tangent screen size.

24. What is the color and material of tangent screen?

The color of the screen is black felt.

25. What are the numbers of meridians that should be tested?

Eight meridians with one central fixation.

26. What is the size of the test object?

1–10 mm.

27. How many circles in a tangent screen?

There are 6 concentric circles from 50 to 300.

28. What is a wand?

It is a handle where the object is fixed. Spherical test objects are being mounted on the side of the wand near its tip.

29. What is a meridian?

The circles are divided into radial sections by diameter lines called meridians.

30. What is the color of the test objects used in tangent screen?

White, red, green, and blue.

31. Which is the color maximum used in checking visual fields?

White.

32. What is the specific use of colors used in tangent screen?

Red and blue are used for neuro cases, white is used for normal vision and glaucoma.

33. How to move the target in tangent screen?

   i. Normally it is from nonseeing to seeing area
   ii. When mapping the blind spot, it is from seeing to nonseeing area.

34. What are the types of manual perimeter?

   i. Goldmann's perimetry
   ii. Bjerrum's perimetry
   iii. Lister's perimetry.

35. What is Bjerrum's perimetry?

It is the quantitative test and subjective method of identifying central visual field defect.

36. What is blind spot?

It is the region of deep depression within the boundaries of the normal visual fields, corresponding to the optic nerve head that lies temporal to the fixation in the visual fields.

37. What is the location of the blind spot?

The center of the blind spot is 120–170 from the point of fixation on the temporal side and is situated 1.50 below the horizontal meridian.

38. What is the size of the blind spot?

The size of the blind spot is 7.5 mm in the vertical direction and 5.5 mm in the horizontal direction.

39. What are the classifications of scotoma?

According to the situation scotoma is divided into central, peripheral, paracentral, ring, absolute and relative, positive and negative scotoma.

40. What is central scotoma?

It includes the point of fixation. When it has a sufficient density, it interferes with or abolishes central vision altogether. For example, central scotoma caused by macular lesions.

41. What is paracentral scotoma?

It is situated to one side of the point of fixation.
For example, tobacco amblyopia.

42. What is ring/annular scotoma?

It encircles the point of fixation. For example, Retinitis pigmentosa.

43. What is peripheral scotoma?

It causes little disturbance of sight and may exist without the patients' knowledge, especially when situated away from the point of fixation.

44. What is a positive scotoma?

When the patient sees a black spot in his visual field.
For example, changes in eye media or retina.

45. What is negative scotoma?

When the scotoma exists as a defect in the visual field but is not perceived by the patient until the visual field of examination.

46. What is mobile scotoma?

If the opacities exist in the vitreous, the scotoma is mobile.
For example, Muscae volitantes

47. What is absolute scotoma?

It refers to the area of optic nerve head that is devoid of photoreceptors and is seen as vertically oval.
Perception of light is entirely lost over the absolute scotoma.

48. What is relative scotoma?

A scotoma in which there is a visual depression but not complete loss of light perception. For example, toxic amblyopia.

49. What is the importance of size of the test object?

The size of the scotoma depends on the size of the test object used. By using a large object it may be impossible to demonstrate a scotoma that is clearly demonstrable when a small test object is used.

50. Describe Bjerrum screen and its technique

   i. Bjerrum screen consists of a black felt screen measuring about 1 m² or 2 m² in size supported on a framework.

   ii. The patient should be seated at a distance of 1 or 2 m according to the size of the tangent screen.

   iii. The screen has a white object for fixation in its center around which are marked concentric circles from 50 to 300.

   iv. The patients fix it on the central dot with one eye occluded.

   v. A white target 1–10 mm diameter is brought from the periphery toward the center in various meridian.

   vi. Initially, the blind spot is charged which is normally located about 150 degrees temporal to the fixation point on a 1m tangent screen

51. How to perform the tangent screen examination?

   i. For a tangent screen examination, it is essential that the patient wears his/her glasses, if he/she has refractive error.

   ii. The examiner usually stands toward a side and keeps his/her eye on the patients' eye to ensure that the fixation is absolutely maintained.

   iii. The test object, the size of which correlated with the patient's visual acuity, is moved from the periphery toward the center.

   iv. The patients indicate when they see the test object, either by making a verbal response such as yes or by tapping the coin

   v. At all times, the fixation of the patient has to be checked

   vi. The easiest way is to map out the patient's blind spot first, which is smaller and closer to the fixation point.

   vii. Check the patient's response by rotating the test object, out of view, so that it is not visible to the patients at all.

   viii. Transfer the information from the felt screen to the chart carefully

   ix. Make sure to understand the proper degree of eccentricities and the meridian placements in the stitched chart and the recording diagram.

   x. Evaluate each scotoma for the depth with a small and a larger target.

52. How to calibrate the Bjerrum screen?

   i. Bjerrum screen is calibrated by means of a series of black thread sewn into the black cloth at intervals of 50 along the principal 300 meridian rotating from the fixation point.

   ii. These threads cannot be seen by the patients at 2 m, but it is visible to the examiner working at a close range.

   iii. Alternatively, Sinclair's rule may be used, which translates distance from the fixation point into the appropriate degree and also shows the different meridians.

53. What are the differences between neurological and glaucomatous field defects?

Neurological field defects	Glaucomatous field defects
i. It follows the vertical meridian	i. It follows horizontal meridian
ii. Absolute field defect	ii. Relative field defect, progress to absolute defect in late stage
iii. Field defects are mostly congruous.	iii. Field defects are incongruous.

54. What is standard automated perimetry (SAP)?

It is also called achromatic automated perimetry. With this procedure, threshold sensitivity measurements are usually performed at a number of test locations using white stimuli on a white background.

55. What is short wavelength automated perimetry (SWAP)?

This is also known as blue yellow perimetry. Standard perimeters are available that can project a blue stimulus onto a yellow background. Sensitivity to blue stimuli is believed to be mediated by small bi-stratified ganglion cells that typically have large receptive fields. This method is more sensitive to detect early stages of glaucoma.

56. What are the advantages and disadvantages of SWAP?

Advantages
i. Detects glaucoma early
ii. Can track progression.

Disadvantages
i. Tedious and time consuming
ii. More affected by refractive error and media opacities.

57. What is frequency doubling technology (FDT) perimetry?

The FDT perimeter was developed to measure contrast detection thresholds for frequency-doubled test targets. This test uses a low spatial frequency sinusoidal grating undergoing rapid phase reversal flicker. The instruments employ a 0.25 cycle per degree grating phase reversed at a rapid 25 Hz. It is believed that this stimuli employed in this test preferentially activate the M cells and are most sensitive in the detection of early glaucomatous loss.

58. What are the advantages and disadvantages of FDT perimetry?

Advantages
i. Portable
ii. Can be used in ambient illumination

iii. Relatively insensitive to refractive error
iv. Shorter learning curve
v. Faster than SAP.

Disadvantages

i. Affected by media opacity
ii. False-positives possible
iii. Ability to detect progression is questionable.

59. What is false-positivity?

When a patient responds at a time when no test stimulus is being presented, a false-positive response is recorded. False-positives more than 33% suggest an unreliable test.

60. What is false-negativity?

When a patient fails to respond to a stimulus presented in a location where a dimmer stimulus was previously seen, a false-negative response is recorded. False-positive more than 33% suggest an unreliable test.

61. What is threshold?

The differential light sensitivity at which a stimulus of a given size and duration of presentation is seen 50% of the time.

62. What is a decibel (dB)?

The measured light sensitivity is expressed in logarithmic units referred to as decibels. It is a 0.1 log unit. It is a relative term used both in static and kinetic perimetry. It refers to log units of attenuation of the maximum light intensity available in the perimeter. The standard staircase strategy used by automated perimeters employs an initial 4 dB step size that decreases to 2 dB on first reversal and continues until a second reversal occurs.

63. What are the testing strategies in automated perimetry?

i. Suprathreshold strategy	:	For screening purposes
ii. Threshold-related strategy	:	For moderate to severe defects
iii. Threshold strategy	:	Current standard for automated perimetry
iv. Efficient threshold strategies.	:	This is a shorter threshold testing typified by Swedish interactive thresholding algorithm (SITA) and takes only 50% of regular threshold strategy. Completes in shortest time, most practical to use, especially in large clinical settings.

64. What are the common programs for glaucoma testing using automated perimetry?

   i. Octopus 32   : Central 24 degree and 30 degree programs

  ii. Humphrey field   : 24-2 and 30-2 programs.
       analyzer (HFA).

These programs test the central field using a 6 degree grid. For patients with advanced visual field loss that threatens fixation, serial 10-2 should be used.

65. What are test programs of HFA?

   i. Central field test   : Central 30-2 test
                          Central 24-2 test
                          Central 10-2 test
                          Macula test

  ii. Peripheral field   : Peripheral 30/60-1
       test   Peripheral 30/60-2
                          Nasal step
                          Temporal crescent

 iii. Speciality test   : Neurological-20
                          Neurological-50
                          Central 10-12
                          Macular test

66. What is central 30-2 tests?

It is the most comprehensive from of visual field assessment of the central 30 degrees. It consists of 76 points at 6 degrees apart on either side of the vertical and horizontal axes. The inner most points are 3 degrees from the fixation point.

67. What is mean deviation?

It is the mean difference between the normative data for that age compared with that of collected data. It is more an indicator of the general depression.

68. What is pattern standard deviation?

It is a measure of variability between two different points within the field, i.e., it measures the difference between a given point and adjacent point. It determines localized field effect.

69. What is glaucoma Hemifield test (GHT)?

It compares the five clusters of points in the upper field (above the horizontal midline) with the five mirror images in the lower field. These clusters of points are specific to the detection of glaucoma outside normal limits.

70. **What are the indicators in automated perimetry that indicate glaucomatous progression?**

    i. Average fluctuations between two determinations of visual field will be more than 3 dB

    ii. Deepening of an existing scotoma is suggested by the reproducible depression of a point in an existing scotoma by >7 dB.

    iii. Enlargement of an existing scotoma is suggested by the reproducible depression of a point adjacent to an existing scotoma by >9 dB.

    iv. Development of a new scotoma is suggested by the reproducible depression of a previously normal point in the visual field by >11 dB, or of two adjacent, previously normal points by >5 dB.

71. **What are the criteria to grade glaucomatous field defects?**

Parameters	Early defects	Moderate defects	Severe defects
Mean deviation	<–6 dB	– 6 dB to –12 dB	>–12 dB
Corrected pattern standard deviation	Depressed to the P <5%	Depressed to the P <5%	Depressed to the P <5%
Pattern deviation plot			
1. Points depressed below P <5%	<18 (25%)	<37 (50%)	>37 (>50%)
2. Points depressed below P <1%	<10	<20	>20
Glaucoma hemifield test	Outside normal limits	Outside normal limits	Outside normal limits
Sensitivity in central 5 degrees	No point <15 dB	One hemifield may have point with sensitivity <15 dB	Both hemifields have points with sensitivity <15 dB

72. **What are Anderson's criteria?**

    i. GHT: Outside normal limits on at least two consecutive occasions.

    ii. Three or more nonedge points in a location typical of glaucoma all of which are depressed at P <5% and one of which is depressed at P <1% level on two consecutive occasions.

    iii. Corrected pattern standard deviation (CPSD) (it takes into account the short-term fluctuations, thereby highlighting the localized defects. It accounts for intraobserver variations), at P <5% level.

73. **What are the features of tangent screen?**

    i. It may be used at 1 or 2 m

    ii. It should have a uniform illumination of 7 foot candles

    iii. It should be large enough to allow testing of the full 30° of central field.

74. **What are the features of Goldmann perimetry?**

    i. It is a type of bowl perimetry
    ii. The maximum stimulus should be 1000 apostilbs
    iii. The background illumination should be 31.5 apostilbs
    iv. A threshold target is initially identified. Careful investigation of the 5°, 10°, and 15° isopters is necessary to detect early glaucoma.

75. **What are the other psychophysical tests useful in glaucoma?**

    i. High pass resolution perimetry
    ii. Motion detection perimetry
    iii. Electroretinography (ERG)
    iv. Pattern ERG
    v. Multifocal visual evoked potential.

4.5. ULTRASOUND BIOMICROSCOPY AND ANTERIOR SEGMENT OPTICAL COHERENCE TOMOGRAPHY (AS-OCT) IN GLAUCOMA

1. **What is UBM?**

   The ultrasound biomicroscope (UBM) is a high-frequency ultra-sound machine with 50–100 MHz transducers. It is used to image ocular structures anterior to the pars plana region of the eye in living patients.

2. **Give characteristics of the UBM image.**

   It produces cross-sectional images of anterior segment structures providing

   i. Lateral resolution of 50 μ
   ii. Axial resolution of 25 μ
   iii. Depth of penetration of approximately 4–5 mm
   iv. Field of view is 5 × 5 mm
   v. Vertical image lines 256
   vi. Scan rate is 8 frames/second

3. **What are qualitative uses of UBM?**

   i. **Glaucoma**
      – **Angle-closure glaucoma**
        Angle-closure can occur in four anatomic sites, the iris (pupillary block), the ciliary body (plateau iris), the lens (phakomorphic glaucoma), and behind the iris by a combination of various forces (malignant glaucoma and other posterior pushing glaucoma types). Differentiating these sites is the key to provide effective treatment. UBM is extremely useful in achieving this goal.
        • **Angle occludability**
          Darkroom provocative testing can be done generating objective results using UBM.
        • **Pupillary block**
          Unbalanced relative pressure gradient between anterior and posterior chamber results in anterior iris bowing, angle narrow-ing, and acute or chronic angle closure, seen on UBM.
        • **Plateau iris**
          Indentation UBM shows double-hump sign (as seen on inden-tation gonioscopy).

- **Malignant glaucoma**
  UBM clearly shows that all anterior segment structures are displaced and pressed tightly against the cornea with or without fluid in the supraciliary space.
- **Other causes of angle closure**
  Iridociliary tumor, enlargement of ciliary body due to inflammation or tumor infiltration, air or gas bubble after intraocular surgery, can be diagnosed on UBM. Can be used in pigment dispersion and pigmentary glaucoma and helps in visualization of the posterior bowing of the iris.
  - **Open-angle glaucoma**
    The only type of open-angle glaucoma showing typical finding on UBM is pigment dispersion syndrome. UBM shows widely open angle, posterior bowing of the peripheral iris, and increased iridolenticular contact.

ii. **Ocular trauma**
  - **Detection of foreign body**
    Wood and concrete: Shadowing artifact
    Metal and glass: Cosmetic artifact
    Detection of location of intraocular lens for research purposes
  - **Angle recession**
    UBM shows the separation between the longitudinal and circular ciliary muscles
  - **Cyclodialysis**
    Cyclodialysis cleft confirmed on UBM as an echolucent streak between the sclera and ciliary body, just posterior to the scleral spur.
  - Anterior Segment Tumors.

4. **What are quantitative uses of UBM in biometry of anterior chamber?**
   Quantitative uses in biometry of anterior chamber
   Determination of:
   i. Corneal thickness
   ii. ACD
   iii. Posterior chamber depth
   iv. IOL thickness
   v. Scleral thickness.

5. **Advantages and disadvantages of UBM**
   Advantages
   i. Quick
   ii. Convenient
   iii. Minimally invasive investigative tool

iv. Imaging of the anterior segment structures is possible even in eyes with corneal edema or corneal opacification that precludes gonio-scopic assessment.

Disadvantages

i. Bulky instrumentation

ii. Limited penetration into the eye

iii. Requires immersion technique.

6. How does OCT work?

OCT employs low coherence interferometry to obtain in vivo cross-sectional image of ocular tissues—using light instead of sound (unlike UBM), a beam is shore on structures of the eye and reflections returning from the structures are analyzed to produce real-time images.

7. What is the wavelength used?

i. For anterior segment: Longer wavelength (1310 nm)

ii. For posterior segment: Shorter wavelength (830 nm).

8. What are the advantages of OCT?

i. Noncontact

ii. Rapid

iii. Provides real-time cross-sectional view of the angle structures

iv. Less observer dependent

v. Used to diagnose or confirm appositional angle closure

vi. Used to evaluate effects of laser peripheral iridotomy (PI).

9. What are the disadvantages of OCT?

i. Poor ability to show details of the ciliary body and posterior surface of the iris.

ii. Cyclodialysis clefts and ciliary body tumors cannot be detected.

iii. Difficult to visualize the superior angle quadrant.

4.6. ANGLE-CLOSURE GLAUCOMA

1. **Classify angle-closure disease.**

   Many different classifications are cited for angle-closure disease

   Primary:

   i. **With pupillary block**
   - Primary angle closure (PAG; acute/subacute/chronic)—(old classi-fication wrt severity of symptoms)

   ii. **Without pupillary block**
   - Plateau iris syndrome
   - Plateau iris configuration

   Secondary:

   i. **With pupillary block**
   - Miotic induced
   - Swollen lens
   - Mobile lens syndromes (ectopia lentis/microspherophakia)

   ii. **Without pupillary block**
   - Synechiae to lens/vitreous/PCIOL
   - Anterior "PULLING" mechanisms (iris is pulled forward by some membrane)
     • Neovascular glaucoma
     • ICE syndromes
     • Post PKP
     • Aniridia
   - Posterior "PUSHING" mechanisms (iris is pushed forward by some posterior segment pathology with anterior rotation of the ciliary body)
     • Ciliary block glaucoma
     • Cysts of iris/ciliary body
     • Nanophthalmos
     • Intraocular tumors
     • Intravitreal air (pneumoretinopexy)
     • Suprachoroidal hemorrhage
       ○ Classic (based on clinical symptoms): Acute, subacute, chronic, latent
       ○ Classification based on level of obstruction to aqueous flow
       ○ Iris (pupil block/nonpupil block)
       ○ Ciliary body (plateau iris, cysts)
       ○ Lens (phakomorphic, phacotopic, anterior subluxation)
       ○ Posterior segment (malignant, silicone oil induced, Vitreous haemorrhage)

2. **What is the classification of PAC disease on the basis of natural history?**

  i. **PAC suspect:**
    - Greater than 180° of iridotrabecular contact
    - Absence of PAS
    - Normal IOP, disk, and visual fields.

  ii. **Primary angle closure**
    - Greater than 180° of iridotrabecular contact
    - Either elevated IOP and/or PAS
    - Normal disk and fields.

  iii. **Primary angle-closure glaucoma**
    - Greater than 180° of iridotrabecular contact
    - Elevated IOP plus optic nerve and visual field damage.

3. **What are the predisposing factors for angle-closure glaucoma?**

  The predisposing factors for ACG include:

  i. **Anatomical factors**
    - Eyes with small axial length (hypermetropia, nanophthalmos)
    - Smaller corneal diameter
    - Decreased corneal height
    - Shallow anterior chamber
    - Plateau iris configuration
    - Anteriorly placed iris lens diaphragm
    - Thicker and more curved lens (e.g., microspherophakia)
    - More anterior insertion of the iris into the ciliary body.

  ii. **Physiological factors**
    - Mid dilated pupil (emotional stress)
    - Dim illumination
    - Near work (accommodation)
    - Prone position.

  iii. **Demographic factors**
    - Increasing age
    - Family history
    - Gender: More common in females
    - Race: Indians, Eskimos, and other Asian groups.

  iv. **Psychosomatic factors**
    - Type-I personality.

4. **What are the two forms of iridotrabecular contact?**

  i. Appositional
  ii. Synechial.

5. **How does the risk of PACG increase with age?**
   i. Continuing growth of the lens thickness
   ii. More anterior position of the lens
   iii. Pupil becomes increasingly miotic.

6. **Why is the mid dilated pupil a significant cause of increased pupillary block?**
   i. Posterior vector of force of the iris sphincter muscle reaches its maximum during the mid-dilated time.
   ii. Peripheral iris is under less tension and is more easily pushed forward into contact with the trabecular meshwork.
   iii. Dilation also causes thickening and bunching of the peripheral iris. With full dilation, there is no contact between the lens and iris and hence there is no pupillary block.

7. **What is plateau iris syndrome?**
   The plateau iris syndrome is a form of PACG. It is less common than pupillary block and is observed most commonly in young adults. Plateau iris syndrome is caused by anatomically anterior position of the ciliary body with corresponding ciliary processes, which hold the peripheral iris in an anterior position overlying the trabecular meshwork. The iris is commonly located on the same plane as Schwalbe's line and a recess is present in the peripheral angle.

8. **How do you diagnose plateau iris syndrome?**
   Patients with plateau iris syndrome are characteristically asymptomatic but can present with signs and symptoms of acute, intermittent, or chronic angle closure. They demonstrate deep axial anterior chambers but narrow peripheral anterior chambers when examined with a slit lamp.
   On gonioscopic examination, the iris is flat instead of convex with a corresponding narrow anterior chamber angle. If indentation gonioscopy is used, the trabecular meshwork is visible with a sine wave appearance of the rolled-up peripheral iris due to the iris hanging over the anterior ciliary processes.
   To definitively diagnose plateau iris syndrome, a peripheral iridotomy must be performed; an anterior chamber angle that remains occludable confirms plateau iris syndrome.
   UBM definitively reveals the characteristic "plateau" configuration of the peripheral iris, with anterior placement of the ciliary body.

9. **What is plateau iris configuration?**
   Plateau iris configuration occurs when the typical iris configuration is present but without angle closure.

10. **How is plateau iris syndrome treated?**
    Most cases of suspected plateau iris syndrome have at least some component of pupillary block and patients are treated with peripheral iridotomy.

When the diagnosis of plateau iris syndrome is confirmed in a symptomatic patient, argon laser iridoplasty may be used to shrink the peripheral iris and relieve the closed angle.

11. **What are the drugs capable of precipitating angle-closure glaucoma in susceptible eyes?**

Drugs causing angle-closure glaucoma through pupillary block mechanism:

i. **Adrenergic agonists**
   - Phenylephrine
   - Ephedrine

ii. **Noncatecholamine adrenergic agonists**
   - Naphazoline
   - Salbutamol

iii. **Anticholinergics**
   - Tropicamide
   - Ipratropium bromide
   - Promethazine
   - Botulinum toxin

iv. **Medications with anticholinergic side effects**
   - Imipramine (tricyclic antidepressants)
   - Fluoxetine (SSRI).

Drugs causing angle-closure glaucoma through nonpupillary block mechanism:

i. **Cholinergics**
   - Pilocarpine
   - Carbachol
   - Anticholinesterase

ii. **Sulfonylureas**
   - Chlorpropamide
   - Glicazide
   - Glimepiride
   - Tolbutamide

iii. **Sulfa-Based Antibiotics**
   - Trimethoprim-sulfamethoxazole
   - Sulfadizine
   - Dapsone

iv. **Other Sulfa-Based Drugs**
   - Topiramate
   - Sumatriptan
   - Sotalol

v. **Anti-Inflammatory**
- Mefenamic acid

vi. **Sulfa-Based Diuretics**
- Acetazolamide
- Furosemide
- Bumetanide
- Chlorothiazide
- Chlorthalidone
- Metolazone
- Indapamide

vii. **Rheumatological Drugs**
- Sulfasalazine
- Probenecid
- Celecoxib

viii. **Anticoagulants**
- Heparin.

12. **What is the mechanism by which drugs can cause angle-closure glaucoma?**

Drugs can cause either pupillary block or nonpupillary block angle-closure glaucoma.

Nonpupillary block mechanism:

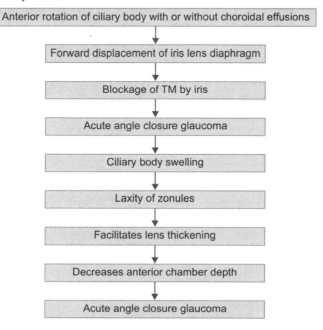

Anterior rotation of ciliary body with or without choroidal effusions

↓

Forward displacement of iris lens diaphragm

↓

Blockage of TM by iris

↓

Acute angle closure glaucoma

↓

Ciliary body swelling

↓

Laxity of zonules

↓

Facilitates lens thickening

↓

Decreases anterior chamber depth

↓

Acute angle closure glaucoma

13. **Why is the eye pain more in PACG than in POAG, even with the same IOP?**

The eye pain appears to be related more to the rapid rate of the rise in IOP than the actual pressure.

14. **What is the cause of defective vision in PACG initially?**

The blurred vision occurs first as a result of distortion of the corneal lamellae and later as a result of corneal epithelial edema.

15. **What is colored haloes due to?**

Haloes are due to corneal epithelial edema, which acts as a diffraction grating that breaks white light into its component colors.

16. **How does the colored haloes present?**

It presents with blue-green color in the center and yellow-red color in the periphery.

17. **What are the other conditions which can cause colored haloes?**

   i. Mucus on the cornea due to conjunctivitis
   ii. Incipient stage of cataract
   iii. Vitreous opacities
   iv. Snow blindness
   v. Tilt of IOL.

18. **What is Fincham test?**

Fincham or the stenopic test is a test used to distinguish between the haloes seen in incipient cataract and angle-closure glaucoma. A stenopic slit is placed in front of the eye and moved from one end of the pupillary aperture to the other. In glaucoma the halo remains intact while the halo in incipient cataract breaks into component colors.

19. **What is the incidence of developing angle closure in the fellow eye?**

About 50% within 5 years.

20. **Describe the clinical features of the various stages of angle-closure glaucoma.**

   i. **Prodromal stage:**
      – Presence of haloes
      – White eye
      – Intermittent attacks of mild pain
      – IOP may rise to 40–60 mm Hg

   ii. **Phase of constant instability:**
      – Intermittency is replaced by regularity
      – Increase in diurnal fluctuations

iii. **Acute congestive attack:**
- Circumcorneal congestion
- Corneal edema
- Pain and vomiting
- Shallow AC
- Pupil moderately dilated and vertically oval
- Very high IOP

iv. **Chronic closed-angle glaucoma:**
- Presence of PAS
- IOP remains high between attacks
- Decreased vision and fields

v. **Absolute glaucoma:**
- Vision is no PL
- Corneal sensation absent
- Dilated circum corneal vessels
- Atrophic iris and ectropion uvea
- Optic disk cupped
- Stony hard eye
- Scleral staphyloma.

21. **What are the differential diagnoses of acute angle-closure glaucoma?**

Evidence of compromised angle on gonioscopy or shallow anterior chamber:
i. Ciliary block glaucoma
ii. Neovascular glaucoma
iii. Iridocorneo endothelial (ECE) syndrome
iv. Plateau iris syndrome with angle closure
v. Secondary angle closure with pupillary block (phakomorphic glaucoma).

High-pressure open-angle glaucomas masquerading as acute angle closure:
i. Glaucomatocyclytic crisis
ii. Herpes simplex keratouveitis
iii. Herpes zoster ophthalmicus
iv. Pigmentary glaucoma
v. Exfoliative glaucoma
vi. Phako glaucoma.

22. **Why is the pupil in angle-closure glaucoma vertically mid dilated and nonreacting?**

It is due to iris sphincter ischemia and paresis due to high IOP.

23. **What is inverse glaucoma?**

In conditions like spherophakia, miotics increase the iris lens contact area due to slackening of the zonules (due to ciliary muscle contraction) leading to forward displacement of the lens, thus precipitating or aggravating the pupillary block.

24. **What are the gonioscopic findings in angle-closure glaucoma?**

In chronic angle closure, peripheral anterior synechiae is seen late in the course. In the subacute/acute congestive stages the angle shows an occludable configuration.

25. **How do you do gonioscopy in the presence of corneal edema?**

After application of one or two drops of anhydrous glycerin. Epithelial bullae are a relative contraindication for gonioscopy.

26. **What are the signs suggestive of previous attacks of angle closure?**
    i. Iris pigments on the back of cornea and endothelial loss
    ii. Peripheral anterior synechiae
    iii. Sectoral iris atrophy
    iv. Posterior synechiae
    v. Mid-dilated sluggishly reacting pupil
    vi. Glaukomflecken
    vii. Visual field loss
    viii. Diminished outflow facility
    ix. Optic nerve cupping.

27. **What are the various provocative tests used to diagnose angle-closure glaucoma?**

The various provocative tests include:
    i. Mydriatic test
    ii. Darkroom test
    iii. Prone test
    iv. Prone darkroom test
    v. Phenylephrine-pilocarpine test
    vi. Triple test.

Mydriatic test:

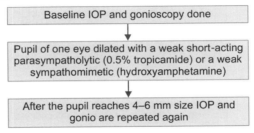

Baseline IOP and gonioscopy done

Pupil of one eye dilated with a weak short-acting parasympatholytic (0.5% tropicamide) or a weak sympathomimetic (hydroxyamphetamine)

After the pupil reaches 4–6 mm size IOP and gonio are repeated again

IOP rise >8 mm Hg or gonio showing angle showing closure test is considered positive. Some advocate an additional inclusion of tonography in the test, decrease of outflow facility by 30% is taken as positive.

Darkroom test:

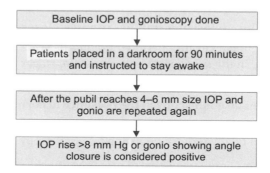

Prone test:

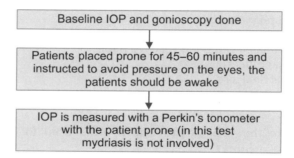

Darkroom prone test:

This test combines the features of darkroom test and prone test.

Phenylephrine-pilocarpine test:

This test uses 10% phenylepherine and 2% pilocarpine to produce a pupillary block by creating a mid dilated pupillary state.

Triple test:

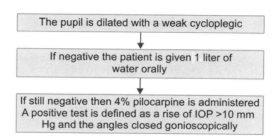

28. What are the optic nerve head changes seen in angle-closure glaucoma?

　i. In the acute stage the view is obscured by the corneal edema, but after the corneal edema clears out, the disk is seen to be congested with or without multiple hemorrhages. In chronic angle closure, the disk changes are similar to the changes seen in POAG.

　ii. In chronic congestive stage, the disk will be pale.

29. What are the field defects in angle closure glaucoma, during an attack?

There is generalized constriction of the fields.

30. Indications of trabeculectomy in angle closure glaucoma.

　i. Documented progression of ONH cupping inability to achieve target IOP despite laser procedures and maximal tolerable medical therapy.

　ii. Synechial angle closure (>270°).

31. What is the role of nonpenetrating glaucoma surgeries in angle closure glaucoma?

Angle closure glaucoma serves as a relative contraindication to non-penetrating glaucoma surgeries. Since the trabecular meshwork is very close to the root of iris, effective filtration may not occur.

32. What is Vogt's triad?

A triad of symptoms usually seen in postcongestive glaucoma or any treated case of angle closure glaucoma. It includes:

　i. Glaukomflecken

　ii. Patches of iris atrophy

　iii. Slightly dilated nonreacting pupil.

33. How do we manage the terminal stage of PACG?

The terminal stage of PACG, i.e., absolute glaucoma, is characterized by

　i. Painful blind eye

　ii. Ciliary congestion and caput medusa appearance of limbal vessels

　iii. Shallow AC

　iv. Atrophic iris

　v. Band keratopathy

　vi. Very high IOP (stony hard eyeball)

　vii. Optic atrophy.

Management

　i. Topical antiglaucoma medications

　ii. Topical steroids

　iii. Cycloplegics (preferably atropine).

If pain still persists

i. Cryophotocoagulation/cyclophotocoagulation

ii. Retrobulbar alcohol injection

iii. Evisceration/enucleation.

34. How is retrobulbar alcohol given (technique)?

Initially about 2–3 mL of lignocaine is injected in the retrobulbar region. The needle is then held in place while the syringe is replaced with a 1 mL syringe containing 95–100% alcohol (some prefer to use 50% alcohol). The alcohol is then injected into the retrobulbar space. This is effective for 3–6 months.

35. What do you anticipate following a retrobulbar alcohol injection?

i. Transient ptosis

ii. Eyelid swelling

iii. Ocular movement restriction

iv. Anesthesia (periocular)

v. Necrosis of ocular tissue.

36. What is combined mechanism glaucoma?

An eye with normal IOP and narrow angles, with otherwise normal anatomy is said to be defined as "anatomically narrow angles." A person like this may present with signs of angle closure such as increased IOP, PAS, iris atrophy, glaucomflecken. Such symptoms are likely to be diagnosed as PAC/PACG, and treated with an iridotomy. Diagnosis of combined mechanism (or POAG with anatomically narrow angles) is typically made in such a patient who experienced an acute attack of angle closure that was treated with a peripheral iridotomy. Iridotomy addresses the narrow angle component, and the ensuing treatment is aimed at the open-angle component of the patient's glaucoma.

37. What are the newer imaging technologies useful in diagnosis of angle closure?

i. UBM

ii. Anterior segment OCT.

38. Causes of increased IOP postlaser iridotomy?

i. Inflammation

ii. Steroid response

iii. PI not patent

iv. Plateau iris.

4.7. PRIMARY OPEN-ANGLE GLAUCOMA

1. **Define glaucoma?**

   Glaucoma is a multifactorial chronic progressive optic neuropathy with characteristic optic nerve head changes and corresponding visual field defects with an IOP detrimental to that optic nerve head.

2. **Electrolyte difference between human plasma and aqueous humor?**

Electrolyte	In aqueous (nM/ kgH$_2$O)	In plasma (nM/ kgH$_2$O)
Sodium	163	176
Chloride	126	117
Bicarbonate	22	26
pH	7.21	7.40
Ascorbate	0.92	0.06

   i. Aqueous humor is slightly hypertonic and acidic when compared to plasma.
   ii. It has marked excess of ascorbate and marked deficit of protein which are considered as its most striking features.
   iii. Other reported constituents:
      - Sodium hyaluronate
      - Amino acids
      - Norepinephrine
      - Coagulation components
      - Tissue plasminogen activator
      - Latent collagenase activity.

3. **What is the mechanism of aqueous humor outflow?**

   Aqueous humor leaves the eye through conventional and unconventional pathway.

   Conventional pathway or trabecular outflow pathway:

   Contributes to approx 70% to 95% of outflow.

   Aqueous humor formed by ciliary processes passes from posterior chamber to anterior chamber through pupil and exits via trabecular meshwork and Schlemm canal into episcleral and conjuctival veins through direct and indirect intrascleral channels.

Unconventional pathway:

Contributes to 5% to 30% of outflow.

  i. Uveoscleral outflow:

Aqueous humor passes through root of iris and interstitial spaces of ciliary muscle to reach suprachoroidal space. From there it passes to episcleral veins via scleral pores surrounding ciliary blood vessels and nerves, vessels of optic nerve membrane, or directly through collagen substance of sclera.

 ii. Uveovortex outflow:

Tracer studies in primates have also demonstrated aqueous outflow through vessels of iris, ciliary muscle, and anterior choroid to eventually reach vortex veins. However role of net fluid movement is clinically insignificant.

4. **What are the risk factors for POAG?**
     i. High IOP
    ii. Advanced age
   iii. Family history of glaucoma
    iv. Race (African and Latin ancestry)
     v. Myopia
    vi. Thinner corneas (CCT<555 microns)
   vii. Systemic diseases: diabetes mellitus, diastolic perfusion pressure <55 mm Hg.

5. **What percentage of risk is associated in family history?**
     i. First-degree relatives are at increased risk
    ii. Siblings are at 4 times increased risk
   iii. Offsprings are at twice the risk of normal population.

6. **What is the prevalence of POAG?**

   1–2% in persons older than 40.

7. **What is ONH?**
     i. ONH extends from retinal surface to the myelinated portion of the nerve posterior to lamina
    ii. Extends to 3 mm behind the sclera where the myelination starts.

8. **What are the types of axoplasmic flow and which one will be affected in glaucoma?**
     i. Orthograde foow (retina to LGB)
    ii. Retrograde flow (LGB to retina affected in glaucoma).

9. **What is phasing?**

The measurement of IOP at various times of day and night to record diurnal variation is known as phasing. This is being done since POAG patients manifest greater diurnal variation (≥ 6 mm Hg).

10. **What is the cause of diurnal variations/fluctuation?**

Fluctuation in aqueous humor production causes mean diurnal IOP measurement variation. The rate of aqueous formation falls to low levels during sleep and increases during the day, most likely in response to circulating catecholamines.

11. **What is the usefulness of diurnal variation measurement?**

   i. For diagnosing glaucoma
   ii. Explaining progressive damage despite apparent good pressure control
   iii. Evaluating the efficacy of therapy
   iv. Distinguishing NTG from POAG.

12. **What is the pathogenesis of glaucoma damage in POAG patients?**

The optic nerve damage from glaucoma is multifactorial and may involve genetic susceptibility factors, mechanical forces, ischemia, loss of neurotrophic factors, and neurotoxicity.

   i. Jaeger's schemic theory secondary to raised IOP which causes impaired perfusion of optic nerve.
   ii. Muller's mechanical theory of raised pressure gradient causing direct compression and axonal death
   iii. Susceptibility of ganglion cells
   iv. Loss of architecture of the connective tissue structures within the ONH.

13. **What are the genes associated with POAG?**

MYOC : Myocillin gene (1q21-23)
WDR36 gene (5q22)
OPTN optineurin gene (10p)
NTF4 gene (19q13.3)
Glaucoma has polygenic or multifactorial transmission

14. **What is the normal rate of loss of ganglion cells per year?**

5000 ganglion cells are lost every year in normal individuals by apoptosis.

15. **How do ganglion cells die?**

They die by a process called as apoptosis (preprogrammed genetic mode for individual cellular suicide).

16. What are the types of ganglion cells and which cell is susceptible for glaucomatous damage?

P cells   -   M cells
Ratio   -   8:1
P cells   -   Motion perception, scotopic information
M cells -   Acuity and color data
"M cells" loss in early glaucoma.

17. What are the studies done in POAG patients to define systemic risk factors?

i. Beaver Dam eye study
ii. Baltimore eye study
iii. Blue mountains eye study.

18. What is the importance of performing gonioscopy every year in open-angle glaucoma patients?

With advancing age, angle closure component may develop because of increasing thickness of lens which may warrant peripheral iridotomy to prevent pupillary block.

19. Define target pressure.

The IOP range below which risk of disease progression is sufficiently low so as to minimize the risk of any further vision loss during the lifetime of the patient by reducing the rate of ganglion cell loss to that of normal physiologic levels.

It depends on the IOP at the time of presentation, severity of damage, extent of damage, and rapidity of progression of visual field deterioration.

20. How is the target IOP set?

Individualized for each patient based on IOP at which damage has occurred, rate of progression, life expectancy/age.

Middle to high teens (mm Hg)—minimal damage (early NRR thinning without visual field loss)

Low to middle teens—moderate damage (cupping to the disk margin in one quadrant with early field loss)

High single digits—advanced damage (extensive cupping and field loss).

21. How does normal tension glaucoma (NTG) differ from POAG?

i. Mean IOP will always be less than 21 mm Hg on diurnal testing while optic nerve head damage and glaucomatous field loss are present.
ii. The cup is often shallow with pallor.
iii. Disk hemorrhages are more frequent.
iv. History of migraine, peripheral vasospasm, or chronic blood loss may be reported. Visual field changes are reported to be denser, steeper, and more closer to fixation.

22. **What are the sites of maximum resistance to outflow in POAG patients?**

    i. Juxtacanalicular part of trabecular meshwork offers maximum resistance to outflow.
    ii. Schlemm's canal.

23. **What are the reasons for this maximum resistance?**

    i. Altered corticosteroid metabolism
    ii. Dysfunctional adrenergic control
    iii. Abnormal immunologic process
    iv. Oxidative damage.

24. **What is the other reason besides trabecular outflow resistance for elevated IOP in patients with POAG?**

    Obstruction of collector channels by deposition of glycosaminoglycans.

25. **What are the histopathological findings in the anterior chamber angles of POAG patients?**

    i. Increase in extracellular matrix (ECM) in the juxtacanalicular region
    ii. Decreased number of pores in Schelmm's canal endothelium
    iii. ↑ amount of TGF-β in the aqueous humor
    iv. Alteration in trabecular beams in the form of fragmentation of collagen
    v. Thickened basement membrane
    vi. Fused trabecular beams
    vii Narrow intertrabecular spaces
    viii. Narrow collector channels
    ix. Decreased number of giant vacuoles.

26. **What is unique of vascular supply of ONH?**

    i. PCA and their branches have segmented distribution in choroid ONH (watershed zones)
    ii. Autoregulation
    iii. Blood flow in ONH is stable until IOP is > diastolic BP.

27. **What is the size of ONH?**

Vertical	1.88 mm
Horizontal	1.77 mm

28. **What are the optic nerve head changes in glaucoma?**

    i. **Papillary changes (actual changes in the optic disk)**
       – Vertical enlargement of cup
       – Asymmetric cupping (>0.2 difference in CD ratio)
       – Focal notching/polar notching
       – Concentric enlargement of cup

  – Deepening of cup—laminar dot sign
  – Saucerization
  – Disk with sharpened edge/rim.

ii. ***Peripapillary changes:***

  – Nerve fiber bundle defects: types:
    • Localized
    • Wedge shaped
    • Slit shaped
    • Diffuse loss
    • Mixed pattern
    • Reversal of pattern
  – Peripapillary choroidal atrophy:
    • Alpha zone
    • Beta zone
  – Disk hemorrhage: mostly inferotemporal quadrant

iii. ***Vascular changes:***

  – Baring of circumlinear vessels
  – Bayoneting sign
  – Collaterals between two veins at disk
  – Nasalization of vessels
  – Attenuation of retinal vessels.

29. What are the parapapillary changes in glaucoma?

The normal optic nerve head may be surrounded by zones that vary in width, circumference, and pigmentation. There are two zones—alpha and beta. Zone alpha is characterized by irregular hypopigmentation and by thinning of the overlying chorioretinal layers. Zone beta is located closer to the optic disk border and is usually more distinctive because of the visible sclera.

30. What is baring of circumlinear vessels?

Vessels that pass circumferentially across the temporal aspect of the cup have been called as circumlinear vessels. If they pass the exposed depths of the cup, they are bared. Baring of the circumlinear vessels is seen because, as the cup recedes, it exposes the vessel.

31. What is nasalization?

As the cup enlarges, the retinal vessels are displaced nasally. This can be an indicator for the progression of glaucoma.

32. What is the significance of disk hemorrhage?

It is a sign of active disease and they occur more frequently in NTG and precede visual field defects by several months. They occur most commonly inferotemporally and are flame shaped.

33. What is saucerization of the optic disk?

Occasionally, the glaucomatous damage to the optic disk produces a shallower background bowing of the disk rather than excavation. This is called saucerization.

34. What is the best method of evaluating the optic disk changes in glaucoma?

The best method is slit lamp combined with a 60, 78, or 90 D lenses.

35. What is the best method of documenting the optic disk changes in glaucoma?

Stereophotographic documentation of optic nerve head.

36. Why does increased cupping occur?

It is due to:
   i. Backward bowing of the lamina cribrosa
  ii. Elongation of the laminar beams
 iii. Loss of the ganglion cell axons in the rim of neural tissue.

37. Where does the increase in cupping start?

Large physiological cups are round in shape while vertical elongation occurs in glaucoma. The process frequently starts segmentally often in the lower temporal quadrant. This often causes an early appearance of an upper arcuate scotoma.

38. What are the types of pattern of glaucomatous cupping?

   i. Unipolar enlargement of cup
  ii. Bipolar enlargement of cup
 iii. Concentric enlargement of cup
  iv. Nasal cupping—rarely
   v. Cupping in reverse disk.

39. What are the differential diagnoses of glaucomatous cupping?

   i. Physiological:
     – Large physiological cup
     – Optic disk in high myopes
  ii. Pathological:
     – Congenital/hereditary:
       • Coloboma of ONH
       • Morning glory syndrome
       • Congenital pit
       • Tilted disk syndrome
       • Leber hereditary optic neuropathy

- Acquired :
  - Arteritic AION
  - Non arteritic AION
  - Compressive optic neuropathy
  - Methanol toxicity—toxic optic neuropathy
  - Shock optic neuropathy
  - Dominant optic atrophy
  - Posterior ischemic optic neuropathy
  - Cupping as sequelae to optic neuritis.

40. What is bean pot sign/cupping?

Bean pot cupping is a sign of advanced glaucomatous cupping where there is total cupping clinically seen as white disk with loss of all neural rim tissue and bending of all vessels at margins of disk.

Cross section of bean pot cup reveals extreme posterior displacement of lamina cribrosa and undermining of disk margins.

41. What is the main site of glaucomatous optic nerve damage?

Lamina cribrosa.

42. What are the changes in lamina cribrosa in glaucoma?

   i. Compression of lamina cribrosa plates
   ii. Posterior bowing
   iii. Collapse
   iv. Increase in lamina pore size occurs due to stretching of collagenous beams or by rupture of smaller beams
   v. Decrease structural support and blockage of axonal transport

43. What is the shape of the normal neuroretinal rim (NRR)?

The NRR is broadest in the inferior disk, then the superior disk, then the nasal disk, and thinnest in the temporal disk. (ISNT rule).

44. What is the shape of the normal cup disk ratio?

Because of the vertically oval optic disk and the horizontally oval optic cup, cup disk ratios are usually larger horizontally than vertically in normal eyes.

45. Why are the superior and inferior poles of optic disk affected first in glaucoma?

The superior and inferior poles have larger laminar pores and hence, the axon bundles traversing have less support by glial tissue. Thus they are more prone to damage.

46. Can cupping be reversed?

Reversal of cupping can happen in children and young patients following lowering of IOP, probably because the sclera is more elastic.

47. What is laminar dot sign?

Exposure of underlying lamina cribrosa caused by the deepening of cup and loss of extraneural connective tissue is recognized by the gray fenestra of the lamina which has been referred to as laminar dot sign.

48. How much ganglion cell loss should be there before visual field defects become manifest on white on white perimetry?

40% of ganglion cell loss occurs before visual field loss becomes apparent on white on white perimetry.

49. Why temporal and central fields are preserved?

i. Lamina septae are closely packed and thick along the horizontal meridian
ii. Resistant to mechanical deformation

50. What are the theories of glaucoma?

i. Multifactorial theory
ii. Muller's Mechanical Theory: Elevated IOP causes direct compression and death of neurons
iii. Von Jaeger's Vascular Theory: Decreased optic nerve head perfusion causes disturbance in autoregulation of ONH, leading to atrophy of neural elements, which pulls the optic nerve head posteriorlye Schnabel's Cavernous atrophy.

51. What is the role of glutamate in glaucoma?

i. Glutamate is normally present in retina, helps in verbal communication between cells
ii. Excessive glutamate is neurotoxic
iii. Elevated IOP renders neurons more permeable to glutamate
⟶ Activates NMDA receptors ⟶ Intracellular calcium influx ⟶ Activation of nitric oxide pathway ⟶ Apoptosis.

52. What are the modalities to detect preperimetric glaucoma?

i. Optical coherence tomography (OCT)
ii. GDx-VCC nerve fiber layer (NFL) analyzer
iii. Frequency doubling perimetry (FDP)
iv. Short wavelength automated perimetry (SWAP)
v. Heidelberg retinal tomography (HRT).

53. What is the role of corneal thickness in POAG?

The Goldmann's applanation tonometer is accurate only for a central corneal thickness measuring 520 µ. Thin corneas have falsely low measured IOP because force required to applanate is less. Thick corneas have falsely high reading.

54. What is the differential diagnosis of POAG?

   i. Pseudoexfoliative glaucoma
   ii. Pigmentary glaucoma
   iii. Elevated episcleral venous pressure
   iv. Postinflammatory glaucoma
   v. Steroid-induced glaucoma
   vi. Arteritic and nonarteritic anterior ischemic optic neuropathy (AAION and NAAION).

55. What is SLT?

It is selective laser trabeculoplasty wherein double frequency Nd:YAG 532 nm is used selectively to target melanin cells in trabecular meshwork.

56. Why miotics are ineffective in angle recession glaucoma?

Due to trabecular scarring, the miotics are ineffective while prostaglandin analogues are the drug of choice.

57. What are the types of disk damage in glaucoma?

   i. Type I (focal ischemic)
   ii. Type II (myopic glaucomatous)
   iii. Type III (senile sclerotic)
   iv. Type IV (concentrically enlarging)
   v. Mixed.

58. What is the concept of corneal hysteresis?

It measures the elasticity and the biomechanical properties of cornea hence IOP is measured more accurately by ORA.

59. When will you suspect an intracranial lesion in a patient with visual field defects?

   i. Pallor more than cupping
   ii. Asymmetric dyschromatopsia
   iii. Fields respecting vertical meridian
   iv. Contralateral ONH normal.

60. Nonglaucomatous conditions mimicking POAG?

   i. Chiasmal compression
   ii. AION
   iii. Toxic optic neuropathies
   iv. Hypotension (shock optic neuropathy).

61. How do you approach the diagnosis and treatment of open-angle glaucoma?

   i. Identify the risk factors
   ii. Careful optic nerve evaluation and documentation
   iii. Confirm visual field loss with automated perimetry

    iv. Reserve advanced imaging techniques for selected patients

    v. Differentiate ocular hypertension from POAG (may need follow-up for certain period)

    vi. Educate the patient regarding glaucoma and side effects of therapy

    vii. Institute therapy—single medication with less side effects and adequate follow-up

    viii. Ensure compliance each time

    ix. Switch over therapy to better drugs before addition

    x. Think of filtering surgery—if maximal tolerable medical therapy fails or in a noncompliant patient.

62. What are the problems associated with myopia and glaucoma?

    i. Faulty measurement of IOP due to decreased scleral rigidity

    ii. Increased chances of POAG due to
- Increasing ovality of the disk due to stretching or tractional vectors not evenly distributed across the myopic optic disk

    iii. Altered scleral rigidity and deformation of the posterior scleral structures can act as contributory factors.

63. What are the most common imaging techniques used for the diagnosis and evaluation of glaucoma?

They are:

    i. Heidelberg retina tomography (HRT) or confocal scanning laser ophthalmoscope (CSLO)

    ii. Optical coherence tomography (OCT)

    iii. Scanning laser polarimetry (also called as GDX).

64. What is HRT or CSLO?

It obtains three-dimensional images of the optic disk by acquiring high-resolution images, by using a 670 μ diode laser.

65. What are components of the HRT report?

    i. Patient demographic data

    ii. Topographic image (on the left upper corner of the printout)

    iii. Reflectance image (right upper corner)

    iv. Retinal surface height variation graph

    v. Vertical and horizontal interactive analysis

    vi. Stereometric analysis

    vii. Moorfields regression analysis

    viii. Glaucoma probability score.

66. What are the advantages and disadvantages of HRT?

Advantages:

    i. Rapid

    ii. Simple

    iii. No need for pupillary dilatation.

Disadvantages:

  i. Not useful for RNFL or macula

  ii. Operator dependent and hence high interobserver variability

  iii. Tends to overestimate rim area in small optic nerves.

67. What are the two types of OCT useful in glaucoma?

  i. Time domain

  ii. Spectral domain (Fourier domain).

68. Advantage of time domain OCT

  i. Possibility of evaluation of optic nerve head topography and RNFL thickness using a single instrument

  ii. Automatic demarcation of the optic nerve borders.

69. Why is spectral domain OCT superior to time domain OCT?

They utilize Fourier transform light to measure the back scattering of light without moving the reference arm which enables the measurements to be more precise.

70. Advantages of SD-OCT

  i. Faster

  ii. Higher resolution

  iii. Reduced motion artifacts

  iv. Real-time image quality information which can be compared to a normative database.

71. Disadvantages of SD-OCT

  i. Expensive

  ii. Quality of images poor in small pupil or media opacities

  iii. Image quality degrades in the deeper regions of the sample.

72. What are the recent developments in OCT technology?

  i. Adaptive optics

  ii. Swept source OCT.

4.8. NEOVASCULAR GLAUCOMA

1. **What are the other terminologies for neovascular glaucoma (NVG)?**
   i. Hemorrhagic glaucoma
   ii. Thrombotic glaucoma
   iii. Rubeotic glaucoma
   iv. Congestive glaucoma
   v. 100th day glaucoma.

2. **Who coined the term "neovascular glaucoma?"**
   Weiss et al.

3. **Describe the first sign of NVG.**
   i. Clinically new vessel tufts at pupillary margin.
   ii. By using investigative modalities, the first sign is increased permeability of the blood vessels at the pupillary margin as detected by fluorescein angiography on fluorophotometry.

4. **Why does ectropion uveae occur?**
   Radial traction due to contraction of the fibrovascular membrane in the angle and the iris pulls the posterior layer of the iris around the pupillary margin onto the anterior iris surface.

5. **Etiology of neovascular glaucoma.**
   i. **Ocular vascular diseases:**
      - Diabetic retinopathy
      - Ischemic CRVO
      - CRAO
      - BRVO
      - BRAO
      - Leber's miliary aneurysm
      - Sickle cell retinopathy
      - Coats' disease
      - Eales' disease
      - Retinopathy of prematurity
      - Persistent fetal vasculature.
   ii. **Ocular inflammation:**
      - Chronic uveitis
      - Chronic retinal detachment
      - Sympathetic ophthalmia
      - Endophthalmitis
      - Syphilitic retinitis
      - VKH
      - Leber's congenital amaurosis.

iii. **Neoplasms:**
  - Malignant melanoma
  - Retinoblastoma
  - Optic nerve glioma with venous stasis retinopathy
  - Metastatic carcinoma
  - Retinaocular cell sarcoma.

iv. **Systemic diseases:**
  - Diabetes mellitus
  - Sickle cell disease
  - SLE.

v. **Extraocular vascular disorders:**
  - Carotid artery obstruction
  - Congestive heart failure
  - Giant cell arthritis
  - Carotid cavernous fistula
  - Takayasu (pulseless) disease.

vi. **Miscellaneous:**
  - ROP
  - PHPV
  - Eales' disease
  - Coats' disease
  - RRD with PVR
  - Retinoschisis.

vii. **Precipitating ocular surgical causes:**
  - RD surgery
  - Cataract extraction
  - Vitrectomy
  - Radiation
  - Nd:YAG capsulotomy.

6. **Difference between new vessels and normal iris vessels.**

Features	New vessels	Normal vessels
Location	Pupillary margin, angles	Iris stroma
Arrangement	Irregular	Regular
Appearance	Thin	Tortuous
Course	Arborizing	Radial
Character	Fenestrated	Nonfenestrated
Scleral spur	Crosses	Does not cross
Fluorescein	Leakage	No leakage
Histology	Endothelial tube	Has all three coats
Blood–aqueous barrier	Poor	Intact

7. **Theories of neovasculogenesis**
   i. **Retinal hypoxia**: Vascular endothelial cells of blood vessels in retina release proangiogenic factors like FGF, VEGF, TGF-α, TNF α, angiogenin which incites a cascade leading to activation, proliferation, migration of endothelial cells—new vessel formation (e.g., PDR, ischemic CRVO).
   ii. **Angiogenesis factors**: "Tumor angiogenesis factor" released by tumors into the aqueous and vitreous, increases vasoproliferative activity.
   iii. **Chronic dilatation of ocular vessels**: Hypoxia of iris causes dilatation of its vasculature which is a stimulus for new vessel formation
   iv. **Vasoinhibitory factors from vitreous and lens**: Loss of these factors such as in pars plana vitrectomy and pars plana lensectomy increases rubeosis.

8. **What are the most commonly encountered proangiogenesis factors?**
   VEGF, FGF, TNF-α, IGF, IL-6, PDGF, TGF-β, angiogurin.

9. **What are the clinicopathological stages of NVG?**
   i. **Prerubeosis stage**: Patients may have arteriolar/capillary nonperfusion or optic disk neovascularization or retinal neovascularization. FFA shows leaking iris vessels and extensive retinal capillary closure. Vitreous fluorophotometry detects increased fluorescein appearance in the vitreous.
   ii. **Preglaucoma stage**: Also called rubeosis stage. IOP is normal. Slit lamp examination reveals dilated tufts of preexisting capillaries and new vessels over iris, especially at peripupillary area. NVA may also be present.
   iii. **Open-angle glaucoma stage**: Rubeosis more florid with anterior chamber (AC) reaction, high IOP, and open angles on gonioscopy. Angles are covered by translucent fibrovascular membrane extending to posterior iris.
   iv. **Angle closure glaucoma stage**: Raised IOP with florid NVI/NVA, ectropion uveae, and contracture of membrane in angles causing peripheral anterior synechiae which will lead to eventual total synechial angle closure.
   v. **Burnt-out stage.**

10. **What is Wands classification of the stages of NVG?**
    i. Stage 1: Vessels at the pupillary margin
    ii. Stage 2: Vessels up to collarette
    iii. Stage 3: Vessels up to angle
    iv. Stage 4: Vessels cross-scleral spur.

11. **What are the types of glaucoma occurring in NVG?**

Open-angle (pretrabecular type) and secondary angle closure glaucoma.

12. **Histopathological feature of open-angle glaucoma stage?**

The new vessels appear first as endothelial buds from capillaries of the minor arterial circle. The buds then become vascular tufts. The new vessels have thin walls with irregular endothelia and pericytes. A clinically invisible fibrous membrane develops along the vessels which then covers the angle and iris, obstructing trabecular meshwork.

13. **What is the cause of angle closure?**

Contraction of myofibroblasts present in fibrovascular membrane causes PAS and flattening of iris surface.

14. **Where do the new vessels arise from?**

They arise from microvasculature (capillaries, venules) of the vascular endothelial cell.

15. **In ischemic CRVO when does NVG occur?**

Usually between 3 and 5 months (100 days glaucoma) but anywhere from 2 months to 2 years (17–80%).

16. **What are the risk factors in diabetes that cause NVG?**

In an eye with diabetic retinopathy:
  i. Cataract extraction and vitrectomy
  ii. Cataract extraction with PCIOL implantation (increases anterior segment inflammation and disrupts blood retinal barrier).
  iii. Chronic RD
      (Lens and vitreous provide vasoconstrictive factors and serve as a diffusion barrier for angiogenic factors)
  iv. Longer duration of diabetes, associated hypertension, hypercholesterolemia.
  v. In extracapsular cataract extraction with capsule rupture, or loss of zonular support with exposure of vitreous.

17. **Name some occlusive vascular diseases causing NVI/NVG.**

  i. Carotid artery ligation
  ii. ICA obstruction, giant cell arteritis, Takayasu's disease.

18. **What are the differential diagnosis of NVG?**

  i. **Acute congestive stage of PACG** (does not have rubeosis of iris and angles, no fibrovascular membrane over iris and angles, no ectropion uveae).
  ii. **Uveitic glaucoma** (Keratic precipitates on endothelium, aqueous flare and cells; may have posterior synechiae, complicated cataract, band-shaped keratopathy in chronic cases; acute attack due to pupillary block).

iii. **Fuch's heterochromic iridocyclitis** (Eye is white and quiet, stellate KPs present, new vessels seen at angle but NVI and NVG rare, open-angle glaucoma may be present due to trabecular sclerosis).

iv. **ICE syndromes** (Corneal decompensation, corectopia, pseudopolycoria, iris atrophy).

v. **Old trauma** (Recession of angle, pigment clumps in trabecular meshwork; no NVI)

vi. **Lens-induced glaucoma**

19. **How is Fuch's heterochromic iridocyclitis different from NVG?**

Fuch's heterochromic iridocyclitis has the following features:

i. Eye is white and quiet

ii. New vessels seen at angle but new vessels on iris (NVI) and NVG rare (filiform vessels)

iii. Spontaneous hyphemas common

iv. Open-angle glaucoma may be present due to trabecular sclerosis.

v. Stellate KPs present

vi. Iris heterochromia present.

20. **What are the late complications of NVG?**

i. Painful bullous keratopathy (due to corneal decompensation or due to high IOP)

ii. Complete synechial angle closure (due to extensive synechial angle closure or due to the fibrovascular membrane contraction)

iii. Intractable glaucoma.

21. **Name other conditions in which fluorescein leaks from the pupillary margin.**

i. Exfoliation syndrome (at the site of pupillary ruff defects)

ii. Fuch's heterochromic iridocyclitis.

22. **Why does fluorescein leak?**

i. In NVI, gap junctions between the endothelial cells and fenestrations within basement membrane are present allowing leakage.

23. **Drugs contraindicated in NVG.**

i. Miotics—may increase inflammation and pain

ii. Epinephrine

iii. Prostaglandins (relative contraindication as membrane prevents uveoscleral outflow, may cause mild anterior uveitis).

24. **What is the role of atropine in treatment of neovascular glaucoma?**

i. causes pain relief by releaving ciliary spasm

ii. reduces inflammation

iii. increases uveoscleral outflow.

25. Treatment of choice in NVG.

Panretinal photocoagulation.

26. Mechanism of PRP influencing NVG.

Causes destruction of RPE and photoreceptor cells in posterior segment → Reduces oxygen requirement of posterior segment → Stimulus for release of angiogenesis factors reduced → Decreased proangiogenesis factors → Decreased anterior segment neovascularization.

27. Indications of prophylactic PRP.

   i. In diabetic retinopathy with peripupillary fluorescein leakage undergoing lensectomy or vitrectomy.
   ii. Ischemic CRVO with risk factors for developing NVI or NVA (extensive retinal hemorrhage or ischemia) where frequent ophthalmologic follow-up is not possible.
   iii. Proliferative diabetic retinopathy.

28. LASER treatment options in NVG.

   i. **Anterior segment**

   Goniophotocoagulation: is inadequate treatment for neovascular glaucoma by itself, it may be useful adjunct to panretinal photocoagulation in certain situations.
   Argon laser
   Eliminates vessels at the angle as they cross scleral spur by direct photocoagulation
   Exposure time: 0.2 sec
   Spot size: 50–100 μm
   Power 150–500 MW sufficient to blanch and constrict vessels.

   ii. **Posterior segment**

   – **Panretinal photocoagulation:**
   Parameters: Blue-green-argon laser
   Spot size: 500 μm
   Exposure time: 0.1 sec
   Power: 300 mW clear media; 500 mW—lenticular sclerosis
   End point: Moderate intense white burns
   Interburn distance—one half burn width apart
   Placement: 2 DD above, temporal and below center of macula
   500 mm from the nasal margin of disk extending to or beyond equator
   Number: 1800–2200 burns in 2–3 divided sittings over 3–6 week period.

- **Cyclophotocoagulation:**

  - **Trans-scleral contact cyclophotocoagulation techniques**

	1064 nm Nd:YAG	810 nm Diode
Power	5–6 J	1.5–2.5 W
Exposure time	0.5–0.7 sec	1–2 sec
Applications	30–40	16–18
Distance from limbus	0.5–1 mm	12 mm
Spot size	0.9 mm	100–400 microns

  - **Trans-scleral noncontact cyclophotocoagulation techniques**

	1064 nm Nd:YAG	810 nm Diode
Power	4–8 J	1200–1500 mW
Distance from limbus	1–2 mm	0.5–1 mm
Exposure time	20 ms	1 sec
Spot size	0.9 mm	100–400 microns
Depth of focus	3.6 mm beyond surface	3.6 mm beyond surface
Applications	30–40	100–400 microns

- **Transpupillary**: Argon laser
  - Exposure time: 0.1–0.2 sec
  - Spot size: 50–100 μm
  - Power: 700–1500 mW
  - White discoloration and brown concave burn
  - 180° treated

- **Intraocular:**
  - **Transpupillary visualization:** Argon laser
    - Exposure time: 0.1–0.2 sec
    - Power: 1000 mW
    - 3–5 per quadrant
    - White reaction with shallow tissue disruption
  - **Endoscopic visualization:** Argon laser
    - Illumination: 20 G probe (670 nm aiming beam)
    - Power of illumination: 1.2 Watt
    - 3.2 mm at/inside limbus
    - Power: 300 mW
    - 7–8 clock hours treated
    - Whitening and shrinkage of ciliary epithelium

29. Glaucoma surgical procedures in NVG

Filtering surgery: Trab with 5-FU (50 mg/mL-5 min) or MMC (0.2–0.4 mg/mL-2 min)
   i. **Modified trabeculectomy** with intraocular bipolar cautery of peripheral iris and ciliary processes
   ii. Trabeculectomy after intravitreal/intracameral injection bevacizumab 1.25 mg in 0.05 mL
   iii. **Drainage devices** or valves

Cyclodestructive procedure (cyclophotocoagulation/cyclocryotherapy).

30. How will you manage a case of NVG?

The main therapeutic goals will be to treat the underlying cause of neovascularization and prevent its further progression, to control the IOP and to provide symptomatic relief.

If the IOP is less than 40 mm Hg, the patient can be started on a combination of aqueous suppressants like topical β-blockers like timolol maleate 0.5% eyedrops bid, α_2 adrenergic agonists like 0.2% brimonidine tartrate eyedrops tds, or carbonic anhydrase inhibitors like dorzolamide hydrochloride 2% eyedrops tds.
   i. If the IOP is above 40 mm Hg, for initial control of IOP start the patient on 100 mL of 20% intravenous mannitol in a dose of 2 g/kg body weight over a period of 20–30 min after ruling out systemic hypotension or cardiac disease.
   ii. In the absence of history of sulfa allergy, nausea, and vomiting, tab. acetazolamide 250 mg bd or hyperosmotic agents like 50% oral glycerol at 1–1.5 g/kg body weight can be advised after ruling out diabetes mellitus. For symptomatic pain relief, atropine eye ointment 1% and topical prednisolone acetate 1% qid can be instilled.
   iii. Once epithelial edema subsides gonioscopic examination and fundus examination will be performed. If synechial angle closure does not extend for more than 270° and the patient has definite posterior segment ischemic pathology like PDR or ischemic CRVO, the patient can be advised for PRP in 3–4 sittings.
   iv. Once rubeosis regresses, glaucoma filtering surgery like trabeculectomy using wound modulators like 5-FU (50 mg/mL-5L min) or MMC (0.2–0.4 mg/mL-2 min) or a glaucoma drainage device like Ahmed valve will be done.
   v. If IOP is still not controlled, with hazy media, the patient can undergo panretinal cryotherapy with a cyclodestructive procedure like cyclocryotherapy or transscleral Nd:YAG cyclophotocoagulation.
   vi. If the IOP is still not controlled and the patient has severe pain in the blind eye, the patient can be advised retrobulbar alcohol injection for pain relief or enucleation after thorough and extensive counseling.

31. **Indication for transscleral panretinal cryoablation with cryotherapy**

Hazy media

32. **What is express shunt?**

3 mm long stainless steel tube with diameter of 400 μ having a 50 μ diameter lumen, implanted through limbus.

33. **Indication for cyclodestructive procedures in NVG?**

NVG with pain and poor visual potential with uncontrollable rubeosis and glaucoma.

34. **Newer treatments for NVG?**

   i. Anti-VEGF antibodies, e.g., bevacizumab
   ii. Alpha-interferon therapy
   iii. Troxerutin
   iv. Gene transfer of PEDF gene.

35. **Probe sizes.**

   i. Retinal cryotherapy: 2.5 mm (–70°C)
   ii. Cyclocryotherapy: 3.5 mm (–60 to –80°C).

36. **Define rubeosis iridis.**

Rubeosis iridis refers to new vessels on the surface of the iris regardless of the state of the angle or the presence of glaucoma.

37. **What is the role of bevacizumab (avastin) in neovascular glaucoma?**

In neovascular glaucoma, intravitreal bevacizumab (1.25 mg/0.05 mL) (avastin) can be administered through the pars plana route, 24–78 hours preceding surgery, with near total regression of iris neovascularization within 48 hours and some IOP lowering, an effect lasting for some weeks. Intracameral bevacizumab is also advocated by few experts for decreasing NVI prior to filtering surgery.

The rapid regression of new vessels allows both panretinal photocoagulation and glaucoma surgery with reduced risk of bleeding.

4.9. PIGMENTARY GLAUCOMA

1. **What is the typical profile of a patient presenting with pigmentary glaucoma (PG)?**

   Young (3rd decade), myopic, male, white race.

2. **Mention the chromosome related to pigment dispersion syndrome (PDS)?**

   Chromosome 7q and 18q

3. **What are the ocular findings in PG?**

   i. **Cornea:**
      - Krukenberg spindle
      - Increased corneal diameter
      - Corneal endothelial pleomorphism and polymegathism.

   ii. **Iris:**
      - Iris transillumination defects: seen in mid-periphery (in contrast to PXF glaucoma, where it is seen at the pupillary margins)
      - Pigment granules
      - Heterochromia
      - Anisocoria
      - Concave iris configuration
      - Posterior insertion into the sclera
      - Floppier iris stroma.

   iii. **Deep anterior chamber**

   iv. **Lens:**

   Pigment deposits on zonules, posterior lens surface (Zentmayer's ring or Scheie's line).

4. **What is the characteristic gonioscopic finding in PG?**

   i. The angle is wide open.
   ii. Dense, homogeneous dark brown pigment in the full circumference of the trabecular meshwork and pigmented Schwalbe's line is present.
   iii. The pigment can cover the entire width of the angle from the ciliary face to the peripheral cornea; a pigment line anterior to Schwalbe's line often referred to as Sampaolesi's line is seen.

5. **What are the differential diagnosis of pigmentation at the angles?**

   i. Aging
   ii. Pigmentary glaucoma
   iii. PXF glaucoma

    iv. Posttrauma

    v. Postintraocular surgery

    vi. Postlaser iridotomy

    vii. Uveitic glaucoma

    viii. Previous attack of angle closure glaucoma

    ix. Ocular melanosis

    x. IOL placement in sulcus.

6. What are the associated possible fundus findings in PG?

    i. Retinal detachments (6%–7%)

    ii. Lattice degenerations

    iii. RPE dystrophy.

7. What are the theories of mechanism of PG?

    i. **Inherited defect:**

       – Focal atrophy/hypopigmentation of iris pigment epithelium

       – Delay in melanogenesis

       – Hypertrophy of dilator muscle

       – Hypovascularity of the iris

    ii. **Mechanical theory (Campbell's theory):** Rubbing of lens zonules against mid peripheral iris due to iris concavity which release the pigments.

    iii. Anderson, et al. postulate that pigment production and mutant melanosomal protein genes may contribute to pigmentary glaucoma.

8. What is the mechanism of IOP rise in PG?

Two phenomena:

    i. Pigment release and

    ii. Diminished outflow facility.

9. What is reverse pupillary block?

An abnormally great iris–lens contact will prevent equilibration of aqueous between the two chambers, anterior and posterior. Therefore, the iris will assume an even more pronounced concave profile and the rubbing against the zonules will be facilitated. This has been named as "reverse pupillary block". Accommodation and exercise will also increase lens concavity and create a reverse block. The reverse block is relieved by a YAG laser iridotomy. The iris profile then loses its concavity to assume a planar configuration.

10. Histopathology of angle structures in PG.

Demonstrates pigment and debris in the trabecular meshwork cells. With advanced disease, the trabecular cell degenerates and wanders from their beams, allowing sclerosis and eventual fusion of the trabecular meshwork.

11. What are the differential diagnoses of PG?

i. PXF glaucoma (PXF material on endothelium, anterior lens capsule angles)
ii. Chronic uveitis (keratic precipitates on endothelium, aqueous flare and cells; may have posterior synechiae, complicated cataract, band-shaped keratopathy in chronic cases; acute attack due to pupillary block).
iii. Angle recession glaucoma
iv. Ocular melanosis
v. Trauma
vi. Herpes zoster
vii. Siderosis
viii. Hemosiderosin
ix. Pigmented intraocular tumors
x. Previous surgery (including laser surgery)
xi. Cysts of iris and ciliary body.

12. What are the differences between PXF and pigmentary glaucoma?

Feature	Pseudoexfoliative glaucoma	Pigmentary glaucoma
Profile	5th decade and older	3rd decade
Severity	Increases with age	Decreases/disappears in later life
Gender	Equal	Males (2:1)
Types of glaucoma	Open angle and angle closure	Open-angle glaucoma
Clinical features	Cornea: PXF, pigments on endothelium, guttatae	Krukenberg spindle
	Iris: Iris transillumination defects (peripupillary), moth-eaten appearance	Iris transillumination defects (mid-periphery), heterochromia, reverse pupillary block
	Pupil: PXF, poor mydriasis	Anisocoria
	Lens: Cataract, phakodonesis,	May be normal
	Zonular distribution of PXF	
Gonioscopy	Sampaolesi line	Increased trabecular pigmentation
Coarse pigmentation fine dense pigmentation obscuring angle structures		
Progression	40% with PXF develop glaucoma	35% with PDS develop glaucoma
Management	Surgical in most cases	Medical in most cases
Extraocular involvement	Systemic findings present—amyloid like material (CNS, CVS, kidney, liver)	No systemic association

13. **What is the treatment of PG?**

Medical:

i. Pilocarpine 1% eyedrops (miosis restricting pupillary movement and pigment release, direct effect on aqueous outflow)

ii. Carbonic anhydrase inhibitor—dorzolamide 2% eyedrops tds,

iii. Beta blockers—timolol maleate 0.5% eyedrops bd

iv. Pilocarpine is poorly tolerated by these young patients and also chances of higher incidence of retinal detachment.

Laser:

Nd:YAG laser iridotomy (Relieves the posterior bowing of iris in pigmentary glaucoma) to cure reverse pupillary block

i. Power: 4–8 mJ

ii. 1–3 pulses per burst.

Argon laser trabeculoplasty:

i. Power: 200–600 mW increased till blanch/bubble is seen. Low energy settings should be used due to heavy pigmentation

ii. Spot size: 50 μm

iii. Duration: 0.1 sec

iv. 50 burns over 180°

v. Burn site: Junction of anterior 1/3rd and posterior 2/3rd of trabecular meshwork.

Selective laser trabeculoplasty:

i. Frequency-doubled Q switched Nd:YAG laser (532 nm)

ii. Pulse duration: 3 ns

iii. Energy: 0.3–1.7 mJ

iv. Spot size: 400 μm

v. 50 adjacent laser spots over 180°

Surgery:

i. **Filtering surgery**—modified trabeculectomy with 5-FU (50 mg/mL-5 min) or MMC (0.2–0.4 mg/mL-2 min)

ii. **Drainage devices** or valves.

4.10. PSEUDOEXFOLIATION GLAUCOMA

1. **What is true exfoliation of lens capsule?**

   It is a delamination of anterior capsule. There is separation of superficial layers of lens capsule from the deeper layers to form a scroll-like margin, which occasionally float in the anterior chamber as thin, clear membranes. It was first described in glassblowers, hence it is called glassblower's cataract.

2. **What is the risk factor associated with capsular delamination?**

   Extended exposure to infrared radiation (prophylactic measure—use of protective goggles).

3. **What are the differential diagnoses of capsular delamination?**
   - i. Trauma
   - ii. Intraocular inflammation
   - iii. Idiopathically with advanced age.

4. **What is PXF?**

   PXF is a gray white fibrillogranular ECM material composed of a protein core (10–12 fibrils) surrounded by glycosaminoglycans. It is a sticky "Christmas tree" type of protein, aggregating a large number of elastic tissue and basement membrane proteins.

5. **What is glaucoma capsulare?**

   Occurrence of glaucoma in an eye with PXF syndrome is called glaucoma capsulare.

6. **What is the origin of PXF?**

   It is thought to be produced by abnormal basement membranes of aging epithelial cells in the trabeculum, equatorial lens capsule, iris, ciliary body, conjunctiva, and then deposited on the anterior lens capsule, zonules, ciliary body, iris, trabeculum, anterior vitreous phase, and conjunctiva.

7. **What are the epidemiological factors of significance?**
   - i. ↑Age →↑PXF
   - ii. Mostly bilateral but unilateral cases are also present
   - iii. More common between 60 and 70 years
   - iv. Mostly seen in Scandinavian, Japanese, Australian population.

8. **What is the incidence of glaucoma in patients with PXF syndrome?**

   Glaucoma is found to occur in 40% of patients with PXF.

9. **List the clinical features of PXF.**

   i. **Corneal changes**
      - PXF material deposited on the back of cornea
      - Associated with corneal guttata
      - Associated with spheroidal degeneration
      - Decrease in the endothelial density, polymegathism, and endothelial decompensation.

   ii. **Anterior chamber angle**
      - Increased trabecular meshwork pigmentation (uneven and coarse)
      - Sampaolesi's line: deposition of pigment at Schwalbe's line, not pathognomic of PXF.

   iii. **Iris changes**
      - Material deposited on iris tissue (anterior stroma)
      - Peripupillary iris transillumination defects (moth-eaten appearance).

   iv. **Pupil**
      - PXF material deposited on pupillary margin
      - Poor mydriasis (secondary to atrophy of muscle cells)
      - Sphincter atrophy.

   v. **Lenticular changes**

      PXF on anterior lens capsule has three distinct zones:
      - Translucent, central disk with occasional curled edges (absent in 20% of cases).
      - Central clear zone → corresponds to contact with moving iris
      - Peripheral granular zone → radial striations (most consistent).

   vi. **Zonules and ciliary body changes**
      - PXF may be detected earliest in the ciliary body or zonules
      - Involvement of zonules

      Subluxation or phakodonesis

10. **What is the mechanism by which PXF causes zonular weakness?**

    i. PXF material erupts through the basement membrane and invades the zonules creating areas of weakness (esp. in its origin—nonpigmented ciliary epithelium and insertion—pre-equatorial region of lens).

    ii. Proteolytic enzymes within the PXF material may facilitate zonular disintegration.

11. What is target sign in PXF glaucoma?

Deposits on the anterior capsule, in a manner resembling a target. This is a classic sign. The "target" appearance is caused by the iris clearing a circular area on the surface of the capsule due to movement of the iris. These deposits are normally only visible if the pupil is dilated.

12. What are the findings in iris fluorescein angiography in case of PXF syndrome?

   i. Hypoperfusion
  ii. Peripupillary leakage.

13. What are the specular microscopy findings in PXF syndrome?

   i. Decreased cell density of corneal endothelium
  ii. Altered size of endothelial cells
 iii. Altered shape of endothelial cells.

14. Describe the clinical classification of PXF based on morphologic alterations of anterior lens capsule.

   i. Preclinical stage (clinically invisible)
  ii. Suspected PXF (precapsular layer)
 iii. Mini-PXF (focal defect starts superonasally)
 iv. Classic PXF.

15. What are the differences in gonioscopic findings in PXF and pigmentary glaucoma?

PXF glaucoma	Pigmentary glaucoma
↓	↓
i. Uniform pigmentation in trabecular meshwork	i. More thicker pigmentation in an irregular manner
ii. Pigmentation does not extend beyond Schwalbe's line.	ii. Pigmentation extends anterior to Schwalbe's line occluding view of angle structures.

16. What are the intraocular complications of PXF syndrome?

   i. **Trabecular meshwork**
      – Open-angle glaucoma
      – Angle-closure glaucoma
      – Acute pressure rise

  ii. **Lens or zonules**
      – Phakodonesis
      – Subluxation/dislocation
      – Nuclear cataract
      – Zonular dialysis

iii. **Iris**
- Posterior synechiae
- Uveitis due to impaired blood–aqueous barrier
- Sphincter muscle degeneration
- Melanin dispersion
- Poor mydriasis

iv. **Cornea**
- Early endothelial decompensation

v. **Retina**
- CRVO
- Retinal detachment

17. **How does PXF syndrome cause vein occlusion?**

There is narrowing of the vessel lumen due to deposition of PXF material produced by the vascular endothelial cells. This in turn leads to occlusion of the veins causing CRVO.

18. **How does open-angle glaucoma in PXF differ from primary open-angle glaucoma?**

i. Greater diurnal fluctuation of IOP in PXF glaucoma.

ii. IOP in PXFglaucoma tends to run higher and more difficult to control

iii. Glaucomatous neuroretinal rim damage tends to be more diffuse in PXF cases (sectoral preference → primary open-angle glaucoma)

iv. PXF cases show ↑ tendency for glaucomatous optic atrophy.

19. **What are the ways in which PXF causes glaucoma?**

PXF causes open-angle and angle-closure glaucoma.

i. **Open-angle glaucoma is caused by the following mechanisms:**
- Blockage of trabecular meshwork by PXF material by
  - Active PXF material production within the trabecular meshwork, Schlemm's canal, and collector channels
  - Passive PXF material deposition in intertrabecular spaces
  Progressive accumulation → Swelling of juxtacanalicular meshwork
  ↓

  Gradual narrowing of Schlemm's canal
- Blockage of meshwork by liberated iris pigment
- Trabecular cell dysfunction
- Associated open-angle glaucoma.

ii. **PXF causes angle closure by the following mechanisms:**
- Zonular weakness → anterior movement of lens
- Lens thickening from cataract formation
- Increased adhesiveness of the iris to the lens due to PXF material, sphincter muscle degeneration, and uveitis.

20. **Why do a high percentage of PXF cases have occludable angles?**

Presence of shallower central and peripheral ACDs due to:
   i. Zonular weakness and forward movement of lens iris diaphragm
   ii. Lens thickening from cataract formation.

21. **What is the pathogenesis of PXF?**
   i. **Microfibril theory**: Elastic microfibril hypothesis which states that it's a type of elastosis with elastic microfibrils being secreted abnormally by local ocular cells.
   ii. **Basement membrane theory**: PXF may be a basement membrane proteoglycan
   iii. **Glycosaminoglycan theory**: Abnormal metabolism of glycosaminoglycans in the iris

22. **What are the ocular and systemic sites of PXF deposition?**

Ocular
   i. Lens capsule epithelium and zonules
   ii. Iris epithelium
   iii. Vascular endothelium
   iv. Corneal endothelium
   v. Schlemm's canal endothelium
   vi. Conjunctiva
   vii. Extraocular muscles
   viii. Orbital septa
   ix. Anterior hyaloid face of the vitreous
   x. Posterior ciliary arteries
   xi. Vortex veins
   xii. Central retinal vessels.

Systemic
   i. Lungs
   ii. Heart
   iii. Liver
   iv. Kidneys
   v. Skin
   vi. Gallbladder
   vii. Cerebral meninges.

23. **What are the differential diagnoses of PXF?**
   i. Uveitis
   ii. Capsular delamination
   iii. Primary amyloidosis
   iv. Pigment dispersion syndrome and pigmentary glaucoma
   v. Melanosis and melanoma.

24. What are the important points to be kept in mind while medically managing PXF glaucoma?

   i. Tends to respond less well with medical therapy than POAG

  ii. Treat aggressively with frequent follow-up

 iii. Higher diurnal variation of IOP in PXF to be kept in mind while deciding the target pressure for an individual

 iv. Consider argon laser trabeculoplasty/selective laser trabeculoplasty which has a higher success rate in PXF glaucoma than in POAG but shorter duration of effectiveness.

25. What is trabecular aspiration?

Surgical modality to remove intertrabecular and pretrabecular debris.

26. What are the important findings to be looked for during preoperative evaluation in PXF syndrome patients undergoing cataract surgery?

   i. Corneal endothelial compromise

  ii. Evidence of zonular dialysis → phakodonesis

Asymmetric ACD

UBM to confirm the extent of zonular dialysis

 iii. Poor pupillary dilatation

 iv. Posterior synechiae

  v. Lens subluxation.

27. What are the special features to be adopted in PXF cases undergoing cataract surgery to maximize postoperative outcome?

   i. Use corneal endothelium-friendly viscoelastics (chondroitin sulfate)

  ii. Expand the pupil

     – Kuglen hooks

     – Iris hooks

     – Minisphincterotomies

     – Sector iridectomy

 iii. Use of heparin surface-modified intraocular lens (to minimize postoperative iritis that is common in PXF cases postoperatively)

 iv. Capsular tension ring to manage zonular dialysis and stabilize the bag.

28. Which gene is associated with exfoliation syndrome?

A polymorphism in exon 1 of the LOXL1 gene.

4.11. UVEITIC GLAUCOMA

1. **What are the mechanisms of uveitic glaucoma?**

    i. **Open-angle mechanisms**
        - Clogging of trabecular meshwork and Schlemm's canal by inflammatory cells
        - Trabecular meshwork endothelial cell dysfunction
        - Edema of the trabecular meshwork
        - Prostaglandin-mediated breakdown of the blood–aqueous barrier
        - Steroid-induced glaucoma.

    ii. **Closed angle mechanism**

    Broadly classified as pupillary block and nonpupillary block mechanisms
        - **Pupillary block**
          • Inflammatory cells, fibrin, and debris collect in the angle
          • The peripheral iris adheres to the trabecular meshwork which leads to the formation of peripheral anterior synechiae
          • Anterior segment inflammation causes posterior synechiae formation
        - **Nonpupillary block**
          • The ciliary body edema can cause the anterolateral rotation of the ciliary body about its attachment to the scleral spur, which relaxes the lens zonules and causes the forward movement of a rounder lens.
          • The anterior face of the ciliary body and peripheral iris is then brought into contact with the trabecular meshwork, causing angle closure.
          Chronic inflammation may be associated with angle neovascularization, which causes synechiae to develop.

2. **Describe the development of glaucoma in an acquired immune deficiency syndrome (AIDS) patient.**

    i.   Bilateral acute angle-closure glaucoma has been reported in these patients which is due to choroidal effusion with anterior rotation of the ciliary body
    ii. B-scan echography is helpful in establishing the diagnosis by demonstrating diffuse choroidal thickening with ciliochoroidal effusion
    iii. These cases do not respond to miotics or iridotomy
    iv. Treatment with aqueous suppressants, cycloplegics, and topical steroids is reported to achieve complete resolution of the angle closure.

3. **What is Posner–Schlossman syndrome?**

    It is otherwise called as glaucomatocyclitic crisis. It is characterized by:

    i.   Recurrent attacks of mild anterior uveitis with marked elevation of IOP.
    ii. Virtually always unilateral
    iii. White eye with minimal congestion
    iv. Open-angle with occasional debris and characteristic absence of synechiae.
    v.   Apraclonidine is especially useful.

4. **Describe the management of uveitic glaucoma.**

    There are two components:

    CONTROL OF INFLAMMATION:

    Topical administration of corticosteroids is preferred for anterior segment and commonly used steroids include 1.0% prednisolone acetate or 0.1% dexamethasone. The drops are titrated depending on the response. When the response is insufficient, periocular injections (e.g., dexamethasone phosphate, prednisolone succinate, triamcinolone acetate, or methylprednisolone acetate) or a systemic corticosteroid (e.g., prednisone) may be required.

    Children with uveitis may have unique dosing requirements and drug-associated risks such as growth retardation with systemic corticosteroids.

    Nonsteroidal anti-inflammatory agents

    When the use of corticosteroids is contraindicated or inadequate, other anti-inflammatory drugs may be helpful.

    Prostaglandin synthetase inhibitors such as aspirin, imidazole, indoxyl, indomethacin, and dipyridamole have been effective.

    In severe cases, **immunosuppressive agents** such as methotrexate, azathioprine, or chlorambucil are used. These patients must be monitored closely for hematologic reactions.

    Newer cyclooxygenase inhibitors like → flurbiprofen, ketorolac, suprofen and diclofenac may provide useful anti-inflammatory effects without the risk of steroid-induced IOP elevation.

    Mydriatic cycloplegics → atropine (1%), homatropine (1–5%), or cyclopentolate (0.5–1%) is used to avoid posterior synechiae and to relieve the discomfort of ciliary muscle spasm.

    CONTROL OF GLAUCOMA

    Medical management

    i.   Topical β-blocker, α2-agonist, and carbonic anhydrase inhibitor are the first-line antiglaucoma drugs in uveitic glaucoma.
    ii. An oral carbonic anhydrase inhibitor may be added, and a hyperosmotic agent is used for a short-term emergency measure.

  iii. In eyes with acute fibrinous anterior uveitis and impending pupillary block with or without peripheral anterior synechiae, it may be reasonable to consider use of intracameral tissue plasminogen activator (6.25–12.5 µg).

  iv. Miotics and prostaglandins are contraindicated in the inflamed eye.

Surgical management

  i. Intraocular surgery should be avoided in active inflammation, eye should be quiescent for a minimum of 3 months before surgery.

  ii. When medical therapy is inadequate, surgery may be required.

  iii. Laser iridotomy is safer than an incisional iridectomy but fails usually due to iris inflammation, fibrin exudates, or late neovascularization.

  iv. Filtering surgery with heavy steroid therapy is indicated in open-angle cases that are uncontrolled with medical therapy. Additional use of subconjunctival 5-fluorouracil (5-FU) significantly improves the success rate in these cases.

  v. Laser trabeculoplasty is not effective in eyes with uveitis and open-angle glaucoma and it may cause an additional, significant rise in IOP and is generally contraindicated in these cases.

  vi. Surgical iridectomy during cataract surgery in uveitic cases can be performed to prevent postoperative angle closure due to pupillary block

  vii. Cyclodestructive surgery like transscleral Nd:YAG cyclophotocoagulation can be done in aphakic and pseudophakic eyes with limited visual potential.

  viii. Filtering devices like Ahmed valve may be placed when the inflammation is under control, but steroid cover is important to reduce inflammatory exudates from blocking the lumen during early post operative period.

4.12. STEROID-INDUCED GLAUCOMA

1. **Define steroid-induced glaucoma.**

   Corticosteriod-induced glaucoma is a secondary glaucoma of the open angle type caused by prolonged use of topical, periocular, intravitreal, inhaled, or systemic corticosteroids.

   i. 25% of general population develop increase in IOP after 4 weeks of QID topical steroids.

   ii. 5% of the population are super responders—they develop >10–15 mm Hg rise in IOP within 2 weeks.

   iii. Approximately 15% of super responders developing glaucoma require filtering surgery.

   iv. There is no racial or sexual predilection for steroid-induced glaucoma.

2. **What is steroid responsiveness?**

   The normal population can be divided into three groups on the basis of IOP response to a 6 week course of topical betamethasone

   i. High—marked elevation of IOP >30 mm Hg

   ii. Moderate—moderated elevation of IOP 22–30 mm Hg

   iii. Nonresponders—no change in IOP.

3. **What is the mechanism of steroid-induced glaucoma?**

   Steroids decrease aqueous outflow by the following mechanisms:

   i. Corticosteroids stabilize the lysosomal membranes and this inhibits the release of hydrolases. Glycosoaminoglycans cannot get depolymerized and retain water which leads to narrowing of the trabecular openings.

   ii. Endothelial cells using the trabecular meshwork act as phagocytes of debris; corticosteroids suppress their activity.

   iii. In POAG, an abnormal accumulation of dehydrocortisols leads to increased IOP.

   iv. Corticosteroids inhibit the synthesis of Prostaglandin whose normal function is to lower IOP.

   v. Glucocorticoids alter the trabecular meshwork cell morphology by causing an increase in nuclear size and DNA content

4. **Who are the people at risk of developing steroid-induced glaucoma?**

   i. Prolonged use of steroid drops for conditions like vernal conjunctivitis, uveitis, chronic blepharitis.

   ii. Long-term systemic steroid use in conditions like SLE, rheumatoid arthritis.

   iii. Use of steroid drops in patients with strong family history of glaucoma.

    iv. 50% of patients with progressive AMD or diffuse macular edema treated with intravitreal injection of 25 mg of triamcinolone acetonide

    v. Sub-Tenon depot triamcinolone in treatment of patients with pars planitis.

    vi. Diabetic patients

    vii. High myopes

    viii. Postrefractive surgeries

    ix. Asthmatics using inhaled and/or oral steroids.

5. Example of a systemic condition causing steroid-induced glaucoma.

Excessive secretion of endogenous corticosteroids associated with adrenal hyperplasia or adenoma can cause steroid-induced glaucoma.

6. Clinical picture of steroid-induced glaucoma in adults.

    i. Resembles chronic open-angle glaucoma with an open, normal appearing angle and absence of symptoms

    ii. May have acute presentation and IOP rises have been observed within hours after steroid administration

    iii. May mimic low-tension glaucoma when IOP increase has damaged the optic nerve head

7. Clinical picture of steroid-induced glaucoma in children.

    i. Children in general have lower incidence of positive steroid responses than adults.

    ii. Infants treated with steroids develop a condition resembling congenital glaucoma.

    iii. Increase in IOP has been reported in infants using steroid for
        1. Nasal and inhalational steroids.
        2. Eyedrops after strabismus surgery.

8. Diagnosis of steroid-induced glaucoma.

Diagnosis requires a high index of suspicion and questioning of patients specifically about steroid eyedrops, ointments, and pills.

9. Mention a few alternative drugs which have a lesser tendency to cause glaucoma.

    i. Medrysone

    ii. Loteprednol etabonate

These drugs have a lesser tendency to raise IOP.

10. Are there any genetic influences in the causation of steroid-induced glaucoma?

Myocilin gene as well as optineurin gene is upregulated in steroid-induced glaucoma.

11. Prevention of steroid-induced glaucoma.

Patient selection

    i. Good history and systemic conditions

    ii. Avoid steroids when safer drugs are available

    iii. Use least amount of steroid necessary

    iv. Establish baseline IOP before initiating therapy

    v. Monitor IOP for duration of steroid therapy

Drug selection—choose a drug that can achieve desired response by safest route in lowest concentration and with fewest potential side effects

    i. Topical drops are often associated with raised IOP

    ii. Periocular injection of long acting steroid—most dangerous

    iii. Systemic steroids—least likely to induce glaucoma

12. Mention a few words about the relative pressure effects of anti-inflammatory drugs.

    i. Corticosteroids—pressure-inducing effect is proportional to its anti-inflammatory potency. Hence betamethasone, dexamethasone, and prednisolone have increased tendency to induce glaucoma.

    ii. Nonadrenal steroids—closely related to progesterone with less pressure-inducing effects. For example, medrysone is used for treatment of extraocular disorders but has poor corneal penetration. Fluorometholone (0.1%) is more effective than medrysone.

    iii. NSAIDs
       – Act as COX inhibitors
       – May be effective in anterior segment inflammation
       – Act by reducing breakdown of blood–aqueous barrier
       – Do not cause increase in IOP
       – For example—oxyphenbutazone, flurbiprofen, diclofenac
       – Other drugs in this class are suprofen and ketorolac.

13. Management of steroid-induced glaucoma.

    i. The first step is to discontinue the drug—IOP returns to normal in a few weeks or replace with a milder anti-inflammatory drug

    ii. Excision of depot steroid if present

    iii. Antiglaucoma drugs can be used to control IOP

    iv. If unsuccessful filtering surgery should be considered after confirming progression in glaucomatous damages

    v. Patients with steroid-induced glaucoma respond poorly to argon laser trabeculoplasty.

4.13. LENS-INDUCED GLAUCOMA

1. **What is lens-induced glaucoma?**

   Lens-induced glaucoma is a group of secondary glaucoma that shares the lens as a common pathogenic cause.

2. **How will you classify lens-induced glaucoma?**

Open angle	Closed angle
Phakolytic glaucoma	Phakomorphic glaucoma
Lens particle glaucoma	Ectopia lentis
Phakoanaphylaxis glaucoma	

3. **What is the mode of presentation in phakolytic glaucoma?**

   Elderly patients with history of poor vision and sudden, rapid onset of pain and redness.

4. **What are the clinical features of phakolytic glaucoma?**
   - i. Conjunctiva: Hyperemia
   - ii. Cornea: Microcystic corneal edema
   - iii. Anterior chamber: Deep
     Prominent cell and flare reaction
     No keratic precipitates
     White flocculent material floating in the anterior chamber with or without pseudohypopyon
   - iv. Iridocorneal angle: Open
   - v. Lens: Mature, hypermature/morgagnian cataract
     1. Wrinkling of anterior lens capsule
   - vi. IOP: High, >35 mm Hg.

5. **Mechanism of phakolytic glaucoma.**

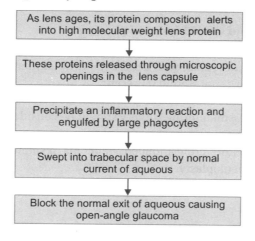

As lens ages, its protein composition alerts into high molecular weight lens protein

↓

These proteins released through microscopic openings in the lens capsule

↓

Precipitate an inflammatory reaction and engulfed by large phagocytes

↓

Swept into trabecular space by normal current of aqueous

↓

Block the normal exit of aqueous causing open-angle glaucoma

6. **How will you treat phakolytic glaucoma?**

The ultimate treatment is lens removal after control of IOP.

Medical: Reduction of IOP by:

β-blockers

Apraclonidine

Carbonic anhydrase inhibitor

Osmotic agents

Surgical: Cataract extraction.

7. **What are the precipitating events for lens particle glaucoma?**

   i. Remnants of cortical or epinuclear material after cataract surgery

   ii. Nd:YAG laser posterior capsulotomy.

8. **Describe the clinical features of lens particle glaucoma.**

i.	Cornea	: Microcystic corneal edema
ii.	Anterior chamber	: Free cortical material in the anterior chamber Dense flare and cells
iii.	Pupil	: Posterior and peripheral anterior synechiae
iv.	IOP	: Elevated.

9. **What is the treatment for lens particle glaucoma?**

Medical : Aqueous suppressants (decrease aqueous production)

Topical steroids (reduce inflammation)

Cycloplegics (inhibit posterior synechiae)

Surgical : Removal of lens debris

10. **Define phakoanaphylactic glaucoma.**

It is a rare entity in which patients become sensitized to their own lens protein following surgery or penetrating trauma resulting in granulomatous inflammation.

11. **Name two criteria to suspect phakoanaphylactic glaucoma.**

   i. Polymorphonuclear leukocytes must be present within the aqueous or vitreous

   ii. Circulating lens protein or particle content of aqueous must be insufficient to explain glaucoma.

12. **What is the clinical feature of phakoanaphylatic glaucoma?**

Anterior chamber : Moderate reaction

KPs present both on the corneal endothelium and anterior lens surface

Low-grade vitritis

Synechial formation

Residual lens material in the anterior chamber

13. **What is phakomorphic glaucoma?**

Secondary angle-closure glaucoma due to lens intumescence is called phakomorphic glaucoma.

14. **What is the differential diagnosis for phakomorphic glaucoma?**

Primary angle-closure glaucoma.

15. **How to differentiate phakomorphic glaucoma from PACG?**

Phakomorphic glaucoma	PACG
Rapid swelling of lens	Normal lens growth
Occurs in senile cataract, traumatic cataract	Occur in hypermetropic individual
Asymmetric central shallowing of AC	BE—shallow AC
Unilateral mature intumescent cataract	Normal lens

16. **Describe pathogenesis of phakomorphic glaucoma.**

Lens becomes intumescent (rapid development of cataract/traumatic cataract)

↓

Swollen lens obliterate the drainage (forcing root of iris against cornea)

↓

Result in angle-closure glaucoma.

17. **Treatment for phakomorphic glaucoma.**

i. The definitive treatment is surgery after controlling IOP.
ii. Reduction of IOP by:
    – Beta blockers, alpha adrenergic agonist, topical or systemic carbonic anhydrase
    – Topical steroids—surgical
        • YAG PI
        • Lens extraction.

18. **What is ectopia lentis?**

Displacement of the lens from its normal anatomic position.

19. **How does ectopia lentis cause secondary glaucoma?**

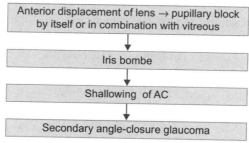

20. What are the causes of ectopia lentis?

Without systemic associations

  i. Familial ectopia lentis
  ii. Ectopia lentis et pupillae
  iii. Aniridia.

With systemic associations

   i. Marfan syndrome
  ii. Homocystinuria
  iii. Weill–Marchesani syndrome
  iv. Hyperlysinemia
   v. Sulfite oxidase deficiency
  vi. Stickler syndrome
  vii. Ehlers–Danlos syndrome.

21. What is the treatment of choice?

Laser iridotomy since it is PACG with pupillary block.

22. Medical management of ectopia lentis.

   i. Cyclopegics and mydriatics
  ii. Cycloplegics act by flattening the lens and pull it posteriorly and break pupillary block
  iii. Miotics—should be avoided since it may exaggerate pupillary block and make the glaucoma worse.

23. Surgical treatment of ectopia lentis.

   i. Lens removal is not indicated unless lens is in the AC or there is evidence of lens-induced uveitis.
  ii. Pars plana lensectomy is preferable if posterior lens displacement is present.

4.14. MEDICAL MANAGEMENT OF GLAUCOMA

1. **What is the goal of therapy in glaucoma?**

   To achieve a target IOP which will arrest or prevent optic nerve head damage and progression of field defects.

2. **What is target pressure?**

   The target pressure is estimated for each patient based on:
   i. Initial IOP,
   ii. Degree of existing damage,
   iii. Potential side effects, complications, and cost.

   Then it is continually reassessed and reset based on the clinical course. AAO guidelines suggest:
   - For mild damage (optic disk cupping but no visual field loss), the initial target pressure should be 20–30% below baseline.
   - For patients with advanced damage, the target pressure range may be a reduction of 40% or more from baseline.
   - For patients with NTG, a 30% reduction is recommended.

3. **What are the advantages of medical therapy of glaucoma?**

   i. Serious side effects are rare,
   ii. Most patients are easily controlled.

4. **What are the disadvantages of medical therapy?**

   i. Less effective than surgery to lower the IOP
   ii. Prolonged use may interfere with the success of future surgery, if necessary
   iii. Medical therapy tends to esclate with time
   iv. Nuisance factor and side effects may interfere with quality of life
   v. Costly
   vi. Effects tend to wean away with time
   vii. Difficulty in compliance.

5. **Classify drugs used in glaucoma.**

   i. **Cholinergic drugs**
      - **Parasympathomimetics**: Pilocarpine, carbachol
      - **Anticholinesterases**: Echothiophate iodide, phospholine iodide, physostigmine and demecarium.

   ii. **Adrenergic agents**
      - *Sympathomimetics:*

      Nonselective: Epinephrine, dipivefrine
      Selective (α-agonists): Clonidine, apraclonidine, brimonidine

– *Adrenergic blocking agents:*

Nonselective: Timolol, levobunolol, metipranolol, carteolol

Selective (β_1 antagonists): Betaxolol

iii. **Carbonic anhydrase inhibitors:**

Oral: Acetazolamide, methazolamide

Topical: Dorzalomide, brinzolamide

iv. **Hyperosmotic agents:**

Oral: Glycerol, isosorbide

Intravenous: Mannitol, urea

v. **Prostaglandins:**

Latanoprost, bimatoprost, travoprost, unoprostone

vi. **Neuroprotective agents:**

– NMDA receptor antagonists
– Calcium channel blockers
– NO synthetase inhibitors
– Antioxidants
– Vasodilators.

6. **What is the mechanism of action of pilocarpine?**

It is a directly acting parasympathomimetic.

In PACG: Pilocarpine constricts the pupil and pulls the peripheral iris from the trabecular meshwork, thereby relieving the pupillary block and in short-term management to prepare the eye for iridotomy

In POAG: Pilocarpine acts by causing contraction of the longitudinal ciliary muscle, which pulls the scleral spur to tighten the trabecular meshwork, thereby increasing aqueous outflow. It also increases the intertrabecular pore size.

7. **What are the contraindications to the use of pilocarpine?**

i. Neovascular glaucoma
ii. Uveitic glaucoma
iii. Phakolytic glaucoma.

8. **What are the adverse effects of pilocarpine?**

Functional side effects:

i. Browache (due to ciliary body spasm)
ii. Decreased vision in low illumination due to miosis
iii. Induced myopia (due to ciliary body contraction)
iv. Lacrimation due to punctal stenosis.

Anatomical side effects:

i. Conjunctival congestion
ii. Corneal epithelial staining
iii. Increased inflammation
iv. Cataract
v. Iris pigment cysts
vi. Retinal holes and detachment
vii. Increased vascular permeability formation of posterior synechiae and postoperative inflammation secondary angle-closure glaucoma on chronic use.

9. **What are the types of adrenergic receptors?**

   $\alpha_1, \alpha_2, \beta_1, \beta_2$

10. **Where are they located?**

    α_1 : Arterioles, dilator pupillae
    α_2 : Ciliary epithelium
    β_1 : Heart
    β_2 : Bronchi, ciliary epithelium.

11. **Which is the only cardioselective β-blocker?**

    Betaxolol.

12. **What are the contraindications for β-blockers?**

    i. Congestive cardiac failure
    ii. Second- or third-degree heart block
    iii. Bradycardia
    iv. Asthma
    v. COPD.

13. **What are the β-blockers used as antiglaucoma medication?**

i. Timolol	0.5% bd, 0.25%
ii. Betaxolol	0.5% bd
iii. Levobunolol	0.5% bd
iv. Carteolol	1%, 2%
v. Metipranolol	0.1%, 0.3% bd

14. **What is the mechanism of action of β-blocker?**

    Topical β-blockers inhibit cyclic adenosine monophosphate (cAMP) production in ciliary epithelium, thereby decreasing aqueous production (20–50%) and hence reducing the IOP (20–30%).

15. **Which is the ideal time to use timolol?**

    Timolol reduces aqueous production more, while taken in the morning. There is an IOP spike in the early morning due to increasing catecholamines during waking and hence this can be blunted.

16. **How is β-blockers classified?**
    i. Nonselective : Timolol
                       Carteolol
                       Levobunolol
                       Metipranolol
    ii. Selective   : Betaxolol

17. **What are the types of decrease in efficacy associated with timolol application?**
    i. Short-term escape—increase in the receptors
    ii. Long-term drift
    This decrease in efficacy may be due to the response of beta receptors to constant exposure to an antagonist.

18. **What are the different formulations of timolol?**
    i. Timolol maleate and in gel formulation
    ii. Timolol hemihydrate
    iii. Timolol potassium sorbate.

19. **What are the ocular side effects of α-blockers?**
    i. Allergy
    ii. Punctate epithelial erosions
    iii. Decreased tear secretion
    iv. Decreased corneal sensation.

20. **What are the systemic side effects?**
    CVS: Bradycardia, hypotension, heart failure
    RS: Bronchospasm, aggravating asthma, emphysema, bronchitis
    CNS: Sleep disorders, depression, forgetfulness, rarely hallucinations.

21. **What are the ways to decrease systemic absorption of topically administered drug?**
    i. Lacrimal occlusion following instillation
    ii. Closing the eyes for 3 minutes

22. **Which antiglaucoma drug is contraindicated in children?**
    Alpha-2 agonists are contraindicated in children because they cross blood–brain barrier (bradycardia, hypotension, apnea, and CNS depression).

23. **What are the advantages of gel-forming solution?**
    i. Stays longer
    ii. Better corneal penetration
    iii. Day long IOP control
    iv. Improves compliance
    v. Once daily dosing.

24. What is 0.5% levobunolol equivalent to?

0.5% timolol (but produces blepharoconjunctivitis more frequently)

25. What is the advantage of betaxolol?

It is the only cardioselective β-blocker. It has minimal respiratory side effects. It is also neuroprotective (topical betoxolol seems to increase the retinal blood flow).

26. What are the dosages in which brimonidine is available?

   i. 0.2% brimonidine tartate
  ii. 0.15% brimonidine purite
 iii. 0.1% brimonidine purite.

27. What is the action of highly selective α₂ adrenergic agonist (brimonidine)?

   i. Decreases aqueous formation
  ii. Increases uveoscleral outflow
 iii. Neuroprotection.

28. What are the drugs with neuroprotective effect?

Betaxolol, Brimonidine.

29. What is the mechanism of action of sympathomimetics?

They decrease aqueous production by the net inhibition of adenylate cyclase and the reduction of intracellular cAMP.

30. What are the side effects of epinephrine and dipivefrine?

Ocular:

   i. Black deposits (adrenochrome deposits in conjunctiva and cornea)
  ii. CME
 iii. Pupillary dilatation and hence contraindicated in angle-closure glaucoma.

Systemic:

   i. Tachycardia
  ii. Extrasystoles
 iii. Systemic hypertension
 iv. Palpitation.

31. What is dipivefrine?

Dipivefrine is a derivative prodrug of epinephrine.

32. Why is clonidine not used widely?

   i. Narrow therapeutic index
  ii. Causes systemic hypotension—worsening blood flow to the optic nerve head

iii. Causes sedation

iv. High incidence of cardiovascular side effects.

33. How does apraclonidine work?

Apraclonidine reduces IOP by:
  i. Reduced aqueous production
 ii. Improved trabecular outflow
iii. Reduced episcleral venous pressure.

34. What is the advantage of apraclonidine over clonidine?

Apraclonidine achieves substantial IOP reduction of clonidine without causing the centrally mediated side effects of systemic hypotension and drowsiness.

35. What are the antiglaucoma drugs with neuroprotective role?

 i. Brimonidine
ii. Betaxolol.

36. What are the side effects of α agonists (brimonidine)?

  i. Allergic blepharoconjunctivitis
 ii. Dry mouth
iii. Anterior uveitis
 iv. Somnolence
  v. Should be avoided in children and infants because of the increased risk of somnolence, hypotension, seizures, apnea, and serious derangements of neurotransmitters in the CNS.

37. What is apraclonidine?

Apraclonidine is a paraamino derivative of clonidine and it is a potent α_2 adrenergic agonist. Clonidine is believed to reduce aqueous humor production, which may be caused by constriction of afferent vessels in the ciliary processes.

38. What is the indication of 1% apraclonidine?

It has the advantage over clonidine in that it has minimal blood–brain barrier penetration and rapidly brings down the IOP in cases with short-term IOP elevations, such as following laser iridotomies.

39. What are the systemic side effects of α_2-agonists?

CVS: Bradycardia, vasovagal attack, palpitation, postural hypotension
GIT: Abdominal pain, nausea, vomiting, diarrhea.

40. What is the mechanism of action of carbonic acid inhibitors (CAI)?

They cause lowering of IOP by decreasing aqueous humor production, by inhibition of carbonic anhydrase II isoenzyme in ciliary epithelium.

41. What are the forms in which CAI are available?

Oral: Acetazolamide, methazolamide
Topical: Dorzolamide and brinzolamide

42. What is the dosage of oral CAI?

Acetazolamide, 250 mg tablets, over 6 hours or 500 mg sustained release capsules twice a day.

43. What are the side effects of CAI?

  i. **Ocular:**

  Transient myopic shift.

 ii. **Systemic:**

    – **Electrolyte imbalance:**
- Metabolic acidosis
- Potassium and chloride depletion
- Uric acid retention.

    – **Gastrointestinal disturbances:**
- Abdominal discomfort
- Metallic taste
- Nausea
- Diarrhea
- Anorexia.

    – **Genitourinary disturbances:**
- Nocturia
- Urolithiasis associated with dysurea
- Impotence.

    – **Central nervous system disturbances:**
- Drowsiness, headache, fatigue, paresthesias, and tingling sensations
- Irritability
- Vertigo
- Insomnia.

    – **Blood dyscrasias:**
- Agranulocytosis
- Neutropenia
- Aplastic anemia

    – **Dermatological side effects:**
- Exfoliative dermatitis
- Hair loss
- Pruritus
- Stevens–Johnson syndrome.

44. What are the topical CAI available?

2% dorzolamide hydrochloride eyedrops used three times a day and 1% brinzolamide used twice a day.

45. What are the side effects of topical CAI eyedrops?

i. **Ocular:**
- Ocular burning
- Stinging and discomfort
- Hypersensitivity reactions like periorbital dermatitis
- Superficial punctate keratitis.

ii. **Systemic:**
- Thrombocytopenia.

46. When should the CAI be avoided?

Renal transplant patients, renal failure patients, and those patients with known allergy to sulfa drugs and patients with chronic liver disease.

47. What is the mechanism of action of prostaglandins?

They cause increased uveoscleral outflow by three possible mechanisms, namely:
i. Widen the spaces in the uveoscleral route by degradation of collagen
ii. The relaxation of the ciliary muscle
iii. Remodeling the ECM of the ciliary muscle
    In addition , it also has a
iv. Mild neuroprotective effect.

48. What are the indications for prostaglandins?

i. All glaucoma as a first-line medication
ii. High chance for compliance since once a day dose.

49. What are the contraindications for prostaglandins?

i. Hypersensitivity
ii. Contact lens wear
iii. Relative contraindication in inflammatory glaucoma
iv. Stopped before cataract surgery.

50. What are the various prostaglandins available?

i. Latanoprost (0.005%)
ii. Travoprost (0.004%)
iii. Unoprostone (0.12%)
iv. Bimatoprost (0.03%).

51. What are the side effects of prostaglandins?

i. Increased pigmentation of eyelid skin
ii. Fat atrophy

  iii. Fornix shortening
  iv. Alterations in eyelid cilia, like hypertrichosis and increased pigmentation
  v. Conjunctival hyperemia
  vi. Reactivation of dendritic keratitis
  vii. Increased iris pigmentation due to upregulation of tyrosinase activity in melanocytes
  viii. Uveitis
  ix. Cystoid macular edema
  x. There is no systemic side effects.

52. Effects of prostaglandins on pregnancy.

First trimester—termination of pregnancy
Third trimester—premature labor.

53. Why is prostaglandin analogues used at bedtime?

Because they have a peak effect 10–14 hours after administration, bedtime application is recommended:
  i. To maximize efficacy
  ii. Decrease patient symptoms related to vascular dilatation.

54. What are the benefits of prostaglandins?

  i. Single dosing schedule
  ii. 30–35% reduction in IOP
  iii. Flat IOP curve
  iv. Nil systemic side effects.

55. What is the specific advantage of travoprost?

It has a good effect over the diurnal variation of IOP. BAK-free formulations are also available.

56. What is the mechanism of action of hyperosmotic agents?

  i. Increase the osmolarity of plasma and thereby water from the eye (mainly from the vitreous) moves to the hyperosmotic plasma. This movement of water reduces vitreous volume and causes lowering of IOP.
  ii. CNS action decreases the aqueous production.

57. What are the indications for hyperosmotics?

  i. Any form of acute glaucoma
  ii. To prepare the patient for surgery
  iii. Malignant glaucoma.

58. What is the contraindication for hyperosmotics?

  i. Anuria
  ii. Severe dehydration

iii. Severe cardiac decompensation

iv. Pulmonary edema.

59. What are the side effects of hyperosmotic agents?

i. **Ocular:**
   - Rebound of IOP
   - Intraocular hemorrhage.

ii. **Systemic:**
   - **GIT:**
     - Nausea
     - Vomiting
     - Abdominal cramps
     - Diarrhea
   - **CNS:** Hyperosmolarity and electrolyte imbalance causes:
     - Thirst
     - Chills
     - Fever
     - Confusion
     - Disorientation

iii. **Genitourinary system:**
   - Diuresis
   - Electrolyte imbalance
   - Dehydration
   - Hypovolemia.

iv. **Cardiovascular system:**
   - Angina
   - Pulmonary edema
   - Congestive cardiac failure.

v. **Others:**
   - Hyperglycemia
   - Hypersensitivity.

60. What is the most common instruction given to patients after IV mannitol?

Not to get up immediately after the injection, since it may lead to hypotension and, rarely, even coning of the brain.

61. What is the dosage of hyperosmotic agents?

Glycerol 50%	oral route	1–1.5 g/kg
Isosorbide 45%	oral route	1–2 g/kg
Mannitol 20%	IV	1–2 g/kg

62. What is the advantage of isosorbide over glycerol?

It can be safely given to diabetics unlike glycerol.

63. Why is mannitol the drug of choice for IV use?

    i. Less irritating to blood vessels

    ii. Can be used in diabetic patients

    iii. Can be used in renal failure patients.

64. What are the disadvantages of mannitol?

    i. Large volume

    ii. Dehydration

    iii. Diuresis.

65. What are the advantages of urea?

    i. Less cellular hydration

    ii. No caloric value

    iii. Penetrates eye readily.

66. What are the disadvantages of urea?

    i. Unstable

    ii. Thrombophelibitis and sloughing of skin at injection site, if extravasation occurs.

67. Onset of action and peak action of hyperosmotic agents

    i. mannitol—onset of action 15–30 minutes, peak action 30–60 minutes

    ii. glycerol—onset of action 10–30 minutes peak action 45–120 minutes

    iii. isosorbide—same as glycerol.

68. What is the percentage reduction of IOP in each class of drugs?

i. Prostaglandin analogs	: 25–32%	
ii. β-blockers	: 20–30%	
iii. Adrenergic agonists	: 15–20%	
iv. Parasympathomimetics	: 15–20%	
v. Carbonic anhydrase inhibitors	: 15–20%	

69. What are the disadvantages of using two or more drugs separately?

    i. Nonadherence to treatment

    ii. Poor compliance

    iii. Difficult scheduling

    iv. Washout effect

    v. Preservative toxicity

    vi. Cost.

70. **What are the parameters which need to be addressed when going in for fixed combination (FC)?**

   i. Need
   ii. Is IOP lowering effect superior?
   iii. Pharmacologically complementing mechanism of action
   iv. Similar dosing schedule.

71. **What are advantages of timolol 0.5% + dorzolamide 2% combination?**

   i. Reduces IOP more than either drug alone
   ii. Produces maximal or near maximal efficacy
   iii. Additive in their effect in spite of being aqueous suppressants
   iv. No electrolyte imbalance.

72. **What is the advantage of timolol and prostaglandin combination?**

   Prostaglandin   Increase uveoscleral outflow
   Timolol   Decrease aqueous inflow
   13–37% IOP reduction.

73. **Why should we not combine prostaglandins with pilocarpine?**

   Pilocarpine: Contracts ciliary muscle
                     Decrease uveoscleral outflow
                     Increase trabecular outflow
   Prostaglandins: Relaxes ciliary muscle
                     Increase uveoscleral outflow

74. **What is the fixed combination of prostaglandins?**

   Prostaglandins with timolol.

75. **What are the advantages of fixed combination?**

   i. Simple dosing and easy scheduling
   ii. More patient adherence
   iii. Maintains IOP at a lower level
   iv. Less preservative toxicity
   v. Less systemic toxicity
   vi. Economical.

76. **What are the disadvantages of fixed combination?**

   i. – Formulation of both drugs in single bottle → time of action. For example, for timolol, dosing first thing in the morning is preferred in order to effectively blunt an early morning pressure rise while minimizing the risk of systemic hypotension during sleep, when aqueous production is diminished. But prostaglandin analogs reach the peak effect 10–14 hours after administration. Hence bedtime application is recommended to maximize efficacy and decrease patient symptoms related to vascular dilatation. Therefore, when both these drugs are combined, dosage becomes an issue.

– Alters the individual potency of medication.

ii. Without confirming the efficacy of individual components, unnecessary exposure to drugs which will not be beneficial.

77. What are the choices of drugs in uveitic glaucoma?

Monotherapy or combination of any of these drugs timolol,brimonidine or dorzolamide.

78. What are prostamides?

Prostamides are COX-2 derived oxidation products of the endocannabinoids/endovanniloid anandamide.

79. What is maximal medical therapy?

The use of three drugs over a period of 3 months.

80. When to quit and move on to surgery?

i. Inability to maintain target IOP,

ii. Progressive glaucomatous damage on maximum medical therapy

iii. Intolerance

iv. Poor compliance.

81. What are neuroprotective drugs?

These drugs are thought to protect the optic nerve and include:

i. Memantine

ii. Nitric oxide synthetase inhibitors

iii. Peptides

iv. Cannabinoids

v. Calcium channel blockers

vi. Immunomodulation.

82. Which antiglaucoma medications are contraindicated in uveitis?

Miotics and prostaglandin analogs are contraindicated because they increase blood–aqueous barrier breakdown, thereby increasing inflammation.

83. What are prostamides closely related to?

PGF2 alpha is related to bimatoprost.

4.15. NEWER DRUGS IN GLAUCOMA

1. **Classify new ocular hypotensive agents.**
   i. Natural products: Cannabinoids
   ii. Activators of ECM hydrolysis: Matrix metalloproteinases (MMPs)
   iii. Cytoskeleton modulator: Ethacrynic acid
   iv. Protein kinase inhibitors
   v. Compounds that increase cGMP

2. **What are cannabinoids?**

   Mechanism of action:
   i. Vasodilatation of the efferent vessels in the anterior uvea
   ii. Modification of the surface membrane glycoprotein residues on the ciliary epithelium
   iii. Increased facility of outflow.

   Side effects:
   Tachycardia, hypotension, euphoria, and hyperemia of the conjunctiva. Pulmonary fibrosis and impaired neurologic behavior.

   Disadvantages:
   Systemic hypotension, which may be associated with reduced perfusion of the optic nerve head. These side effects of the cannabinoids thus far tested in humans seriously limit their usefulness in the treatment of glaucoma.

3. **What are the activators of ECM hydrolysis group?**

   Mechanism of action:
   An excessive accumulation of ECM material in the TM of glaucomatous eyes likely contributes to decreased aqueous outflow. Therefore, therapeutic manipulations that eliminate the excessive ECM should theoretically improve outflow facility and consequently lower IOP.

   Current drug under study from this group:
   i. Matrix metalloproteinases
      Activation of these enzymes reduces the excessive accumulation of ECM molecules, such as proteoglycans, collagens, fibronectins, and laminin, in the glaucomatous eye and in turn decreases hydrodynamic resistance of the outflow pathway.

      Disadvantages:
      MMPs, being proteins of large molecular mass, are not practical as medical treatment.

ii. Inducers of matrix metalloproteinases

Tert-butylhydroquinone, can upregulate MMP-3 expression in the TM cells and increase aqueous outflow facility in glaucoma and nonglaucoma eyes.

iii. Activator of glycosaminoglycan degradation compounds:

Products that catalyze the hydrolysis of glycosaminoglycans (GAGs) stimulate the degradation of ECM in the TM and increase the outflow. GAG-degrading enzymes, hyaluronidase and chondroitinase, consistently increase outflow facility and decrease IOP in study models. Similar to MMPs, these GAG-degrading enzymes are not practical for clinical use. AL-3037A (sodium ferri ethylenediamine tetraacetate), a small molecule with a chelated ferric ion, accelerates the ascorbate mediated hydrolysis of GAGs and enhances outflow facility by 15–20%. Future studies may discover other small molecules that stimulate the production or activation of these enzymes, which are more suitable as clinically useful therapeutic agents.

4. **What are protein kinase inhibitors?**

Mechanism of action: Exact mechanism of action is not fully understood. They likely increase aqueous outflow by affecting cytoskeleton of the TM or Schlemm's canal endothelial cells.

Current drug under study from this group:
i. Broad spectrum kinase inhibitors—H-7
ii. Inhibitors of protein kinase C—GF109203X
iii. Rho-associated coiled coil-forming kinase (ROCK) inhibitors—Y-27632 and H-1152.

Advantages:

Topically active and have great IOP-lowering efficacy.

Disadvantages:

Since kinases are involved in many cellular functions in most tissues, vigilance is needed for the potential local and systemic side effects of prolonged use of these compounds.

5. **What are cytoskeleton acting agents?**

Mechanism of action:

Compounds that disrupt the cytoskeleton (microfilaments, microtubules, intermediate filaments) can affect the cell shape, contractility, and motility, and these changes may be sufficient to alter the local geometry of the outflow pathway and consequently aqueous outflow.

Current drug under study from this group:
  i. Ethacrynic acid
 ii. Latrunculin B
iii. Swinholide A

Disadvantages:
  i. Poor corneal penetration
 ii. Corneal toxicity
iii. Trabecular meshwork toxicity.

These side effects have limited its clinical utility as a glaucoma therapeutic agent.

6. **What are compounds that increase cyclic GMP?**

Mechanism of action:

Cyclic GMP affects both aqueous production and outflow.

Activation of cyclic GMP-dependent protein kinases, which, by phosphorylation, leads to functional changes of various proteins, e.g., an inhibition of Na-K ATPase, leads to decrease in aqueous production.

Current drug under study from this group:
  i. Cyclic GMP analogs:
     Cell permeable analogs of cyclic GMP
 ii. Nitric oxide donors:
     Nitroglycerin, isosorbide dinitrate, sodium nitrite, hydralazine, minoxidil, sodium nitroprusside.
iii. Natriuretic peptides:
     Atrial natriuretic peptide (ANP)
     Brain-derived natriuretic peptide (BNP)
     C-type natriuretic peptide (CNP).
     Intracellular cyclic GMP levels can also be increased by the activation of guanylyl cyclases. Nitric oxide (NO) and compounds that release NO by hydrolysis (NO donors) are activators of the soluble guanylyl cyclases. Natriuretic peptides are activators of the membrane-bound guanylyl cyclases. Both NO donors and natriuretic peptides are effective IOP-lowering compounds.
     Disadvantages: Since they are peptides, cornea penetration and degradation by peptidases can be prohibitive hurdles for their clinical usefulness.
 iv. Compounds that increase natriuretic peptides:
     Candoxatril natriuretic peptides are degraded partly by a neutral endopeptidase NEP 24.11. Thus, inhibition of this enzyme increases tissue concentration of natriuretic peptides. Oral administration of candoxatril, a prodrug that is metabolized to an NEP 24.11 inhibitor, increases atrial natriuretic peptide (ANP) level and significantly lowers IOP by 2–3 mm Hg.

7. **Neuroprotection:**

Rationale for using neuroprotection:

It has been hypothesized that intraretinal or intravitreal glutamate levels that are neurotoxic to ganglion cells play a role in glaucoma and hence drugs which work against these agents can help in glaucoma management. They are also supposed to enhance the vascular supply and decrease proapoptotic factors.

Methods for neuroprotection

i. **Pharmacologic**
   - Glutamate receptor antagonists
     NMDA receptors: Memantine
     AMPA/kainate antagonists
   - Calcium channel blocker
     Nimodipine
   - β2-adrenergic agonists like brimonidine
   - Neurotrophic factors
     Neurotrophin 3
   - Nitric oxide synthase inhibitors
     Aminoguanidine
   - Reactive oxygen species scavengers
   - Apoptosis inhibitors
     Cytochrome C release inhibitors
     Caspase inhibitors

ii. **Immune modulation**

   Focal activation of the immune system in the optic nerve or retina as a way of preserving retinal ganglion cells and their functions. (Activated T lymphocytes primed to optic nerve constituents, e.g., myelin basic protein, would home to sites of injury and release factors that are neuroprotective.)

iii. **Preconditioning**

   Concept: An injury insufficient to cause irreversible damage often may result in increased resistance to future injury. This type of neuroprotection is difficult to translate directly into clinical use, as it requires a series of injuries insufficient to kill retinal ganglion cells and it may not be tolerated by the patient.

Neurorepair and regeneration

Neurorepair is the name given to the production and differentiation of new neurons. Regeneration is the name given to the extension of axons to their appropriate targets. Neurorepair focuses on the use of stem cells (embryonic stem cells, adult stem cells or more differentiated neural progenitor cells) to repopulate and repair damaged neuronal tissues.

8. **Neuroprotectors.**

   i. **Memantine**

   It is an N-methyl-D-aspartate (NMDA) receptor antagonist.

   Mechanism of action:

   The NMDA receptor is an ion channel that is activated by glutamate, allowing extracellular calcium to enter the cell. In normal physiologic conditions, the NMDA receptor has an important role in neurophysiologic processes, such as memory. However, excessive activation of the NMDA signaling cascade leads to "excitotoxicity" wherein intracellular calcium overloads neurons and causes cell death through apoptosis. Memantine blocks the excessive glutamate stimulation of the NMDA receptor of the regional ganglion cell and protects it from calcium mediated apoptosis.

   Uses: To treat CNS disorders like—Parkinson, Alzheimer's disease. Currently being studied as a neuroprotective agent in glaucoma.

   ii. **Nitric oxide synthase inhibitors**

   Aminoguanidine:

   Mechanism of action:

   Nitric oxide is a gaseous second messenger molecule. It has both physiologic and pathologic functions in blood flow, immune response and neuronal communication.

   The expression of nitric oxide is regulated by three different forms of nitric oxide synthase (NOS)—endothelial NOS (eNOS), neuronal NOS (nNOS) and inducible NOS (iNOS).

   Role of nitric oxide in the eye:

   Aqueous humor dynamics, maintaining a clear cornea, ocular blood flow, retinal function and optic nerve function. Excessive nitric oxide generated by iNOS in optic nerve astrocytes and microglia is associated with optic nerve damage. Aminoguanidine by inhibiting inducible nitric oxide (iNOS) synthase was shown to prevent retinal ganglion cell loss.

   iii. **Calcium channel blockers**

   Nimodipine

   Mechanism of action:

   Produce vasodilatation by inhibiting the entrance of calcium ions into vascular smooth muscle cells. Hence may protect the optic nerve head by improving vascular perfusion.

   They have also been shown to have ocular hypotensive activity.

   Current status: The level of evidence at this time, as well as the systemic side effects of calcium channel blockers, does not support the use of this class of drugs for the routine management of glaucoma.

iv. **Neurotrophic factors**

Neurotrophins are peptides that have an important role in the development and maintenance of various neuronal populations. Brain-derived neurotrophic factor, neurotrophin 3, and nerve growth factor have differential effects on the cell survival promotion, differentiation, or demise. The role for these biologically active peptides and their receptors in relation to the survival and death of ganglion cells is under study.

v. **Apoptosis inhibitors**

Caspases are a family of proteases that execute the dismantling and demolition of cells undergoing apoptosis. Caspases 8 and 9 have been shown to be activated in experimental glaucoma. Suppression of apoptosis using caspase inhibitors is an approach that has been explored with modest success.

9. **Other agents.**

i. **Tetrahydrocortisol**: A metabolite of cortisol, shown to lower the dexamethasone-induced ocular hypertension.

ii. **Mifepristone**: A specific glucocorticoid receptor antagonist lowers IOP, possibly by blocking the glucocorticoid receptor-mediated effects in ocular tissues.

iii. **Spironolactone**: A synthetic steroidal aldosterone antagonist with potassium-sparing diuretic-antihypertensive activity produced significant IOP reduction in glaucoma patients, which persisted 2 weeks after termination of the treatment.

iv. **Antazoline**: An antihistamine of the ethylene diamine class, shown to lower the IOP following topical administration apparently by decreasing aqueous production. Angiotensin-converting enzyme inhibitor: In a topical formulation has been shown to lower the IOP in dogs and humans with ocular hypertension or open-angle glaucoma.

v. **Organic nitrates**: Intravenous nitroglycerin or oral isosorbide dinitrate has been reported to lower IOP in glaucoma and nonglaucoma patients.

vi. **Melatonin**: A hormone produced by the pineal gland, was shown to lower the IOP in normal subjects. Demeclocycline, tetracycline, and other tetracycline derivatives: lower the IOP in rabbits, which appears to be related to reduce aqueous humor production. Acepromazine, an analog of chlorpromazine that is used as a tranquilizer in veterinary medicine, had no effect on IOP when given topically to normotensive rabbits, but reduced the pressure for at least 32 hours in rabbits with chronic IOP elevation produced by argon laser applications to the trabecular meshwork.

vii. **Alternative medicine**:

Ginkgo biloba extract (GBE): Leaf extracts of the ginkgo tree have many neuroprotective properties applicable to the treatment of non-IOP–dependent risk factors for glaucomatous damage. GBE exerts significant protective effects against free radical damage and lipid peroxidation. It preserves mitochondrial metabolism and ATP production. It partially prevents morphologic changes and indices of oxidative damage associated with mitochondrial aging. It can scavenge nitric oxide and possibly inhibit its production. It can reduce glutamate-induced elevation of calcium concentrations and can reduce oxidative metabolism in resting and calcium-loaded neurons and inhibits apoptosis. GBE has been reported to be neuroprotective for retinal ganglion cells in a rat model of chronic glaucoma.

4.16. LASERS IN GLAUCOMA

1. **What are the applications of laser in glaucoma?**
    i. **Therapeutic**
        – **To treat internal block:**
           Iridotomy (both argon and Nd:YAG and diode)
        – **To treat outflow obstruction:**
           Trabeculoplasty (argon)
           Trabeculopuncture (argon)
           Gonioplasty/iridoplasty (argon)
        – **Miscellaneous uses:**
           Cyclophotocoagulation (Nd:YAG)
           Cyclodialysis (Nd:YAG)
           Pupilloplasty (argon)
           Sphincterotomy (both)
           To rupture cysts of iris and ciliary body (both):
           Goniophotocoagulation (argon)
           Laser suturolysis
           Anterior hyaloidotomy
    ii. **Diagnostic**
        – Confocal scanning laser ophthalmoscope (optic nerve head evaluation)
        – Laser retinal Doppler flowmetry (optic nerve head perfusions).

2. **Mention commonly used lasers and their wavelengths.**

Laser	Wavelength (in nm)
Excimer	193
Argon blue-green	488–514
Nd:YAG	1064
Diode	810
CO_2	10600

3. **What are the principles used in lasers to treat glaucoma?**
    i. **Photodisruption:**
        When ultrashort pulses of laser are targeted at tissue, the latter is reduced to a form of matter called 'plasma'. This generates fluid forces (both hemodynamic waves and acoustic pulses) which propagate in all directions. This propagating force incises tissue. This forms the basis of Nd:YAG capsulotomies and iridotomies.
    ii. **Photocoagulation:**
        Any chromophore including iris and trabecular meshwork absorbs laser light and converts to heat energy. This causes coagulation of

tissue. When collagen is warmed during this process, it contracts and changes the microanatomy of tissues (trabeculoplasty). Likewise, the leaking blood vessels are sealed in neovascular glaucoma.

4. **What are the indications of laser iridotomy?**
   i. Acute angle-closure glaucoma
   ii. Prodromal stage of angle-closure glaucoma
   iii. Chronic angle-closure glaucoma
   iv. Aphakic or pseudophakic pupillary block
   v. Malignant glaucoma
   vi. Prophylactic laser iridotomy in fellow eye of angle closure
   vii. Nanophthalmos
   viii. Traumatic secondary angle closure
   ix. Microspherophakia
   x. Pigment dispersion syndrome
   xi. To penetrate nonfunctioning peripheral iridectomy
   xii. Combined mechanism glaucoma
   xiii. Alteration in angle structure due to lens like phakomorphic glaucoma.

5. **What are the contraindications of laser peripheral iridotomy?**
   i. Corneal edema
   ii. Corneal opacification
   iii. Flat anterior chamber
   iv. A completely sealed angle resulting in angle closure
   v. Primary synechial closure of the angle
   vi. Uveitis
   vii. Neovascular glaucoma
   viii. ICE syndrome.

6. **What is the mechanism by which argon produces peripheral iridotomy?**
Argon laser requires uptake of light energy by the pigment (thermal effect) and coagulates tissues. However, it requires more energy for iridotomy and is associated with more late closures compared to Nd:YAG laser.

7. **What are the conditions where argon laser is preferred over Nd: YAG in producing peripheral iridotomy?**
   i. Brown irides (it is used in sequential contribution with Nd:YAG)
   ii. Patients on chronic anticoagulant therapies (as Nd: YAG works on disruption and not on coagulation)
   iii. Angle-closure stage of neovascular glaucoma
   iv. Patients with blood dyscrasias like hemophilia

8. **What is the mechanism by which Nd:YAG laser produces a peripheral iridotomy?**

Nd:YAG works on the principle of photodisruption and is effective on all iris colors. Laser wavelength is near infrared range (1064 nm). It is always preferred over argon laser.

9. **Describe the technique of Nd:YAG PI.**

    i. **Preoperative preparation:**

        Cornea should be clear Pilocarpine 2%—3 times (5 minutes apart), is used to constrict the pupil. (The iris is stretched fully and at it's thinnest and easily penetrable.)

        Brimonidine or apraclonidine 0.2%— Half hour before procedure.

    ii. **Role of using a contact lens**: The lens provides firm control over eyeball and reduces saccades and extraneous eye movements that interfere with accurate superimposition of burns. The lens assists in

        – keeping the lids separated,
        – smoothens out cornea,
        – provide peripheral magnified view,
        – reduces unneccesary spread of damage by reducing axial expansion of plasma,
        – increases the power density of the spot. The Abraham lens which is used, consists of a fundus lens with a +55D planoconvex lens with a D button placed on its anterior surface. The button provides magnification without loss of depth of focus.

    iii. **The gonioscopy solution**: Absorbs excess heat delivered to the cornea, thus decreasing the incidence of corneal burns.

    iv. **Site**: Iridotomy spot may be placed in the upper nasal iris to avoid diplopia and macular burns. The laser is targeted at the crypts to ensure easy penetration. The red helium neon laser aiming beam is brought to focus when the multiple beams are brought into a single spot aimed through center of the contact lens.

        Energy: 3–10 mJ

        1–3 pulses per shot

        PI size should be 300–500 μ

    v. **Immediate post treatment:** Prednisolone acetate 1% is used every 2 hours for 1 day and then tapered over a week. The IOP is checked regularly at 1 hour, 1 day, 1 week, and 4 weeks. Gonioscopy is done at 1 week and dilation at 2 weeks. IOP status of the overlying corneal endothelium, anterior chamber reaction and iridotomy patency are evaluated. Gonioscopy is always performed to be sure that pupillary block has been relieved and to determine the extent of PAS. Smallest size iris opening that is acceptable following laser iridotomy is 60 µ or greater. More importantly, one must be able to see the lens capsule through the iridotomy to document relief of pupillary block by gonioscopy. Failing this, repeat treatment is indicated.

10. What are the signs of iridotomy penetration?

   i. Sudden gush of aqueous
  ii. Retroillumination shows a patent PI
 iii. Deepening of AC
 iv. Plomb of iris pigments
  v. Visualisation of anterior lens capsule.

11. What are the various techniques used in argon laser PI?

Hump, drumhead, and chipping are the techniques advocated for producing peripheral iridotomy with continuous wave argon laser.

Hump technique: Involves creating a localized elevation of iris with large-diameter low-energy burns and then penetrating the hump with a small intense burn.

Drumhead technique: Involves placing a large-diameter low-energy burn around the intended treatment site to put the iris on stretch and the area is penetrated with small high-energy burns.

Chipping technique: Especially useful in dark brown iris where standard settings may produce black char in iris stroma, making it difficult to penetrate the tissue. This is circumvented by using multiple short duration burns. This is called the chipping technique.

12. Common complications of laser peripheral iridotomy.

     i. Corneal burn
    ii. Uveitis
   iii. Elevated IOP
   iv. Hemorrhage
    v. Pigment dissemination and iris atrophy
   vi. Lens injury
  vii. Posterior synechia
 viii. Retinal damage
   ix. Corectopia
    x. Monocular diplopia
   xi. Malignant glaucoma
  xii. Glare

13. Difference between surgical iridectomy and laser iridotomy.

	Surgical iridectomy	Laser iridotomy
Margins	Clean cut, triangular	Ragged, irregular
Site	Near limbal incision site (mostly 12 o'clock)	Any clock hour on the iris surface
Closure	Not possible	Possible
Surrounding iris tissue	Not altered	May be associated with pigment dispersions

14. What are the indications for argon laser trabeculoplasty?

    i. Primary open-angle glaucoma
    ii. Exfoliative glaucoma
    iii. Pigmentary glaucoma
    iv. Glaucoma in pseudophakia
    v. Combined mechanism glaucoma
    vi. NTG
    vii. Noncompliance with medications
    viii. Inadequate medical control.

15. What are the contraindications for argon laser trabeculoplasty?

    i. Inflammatory glaucoma
    ii. ICE syndrome
    iii. Neovascular glaucoma
    iv. Synechial angle closure
    v. Developmental glaucoma

16. Describe the technique of argon laser trabeculoplasty.

    i. Preoperatively: Pilocarpine is used to constrict the pupil. 0.5% apraclonidine and topical xylocaine are instilled.
    ii. Contact lens: Ritch trabeculoplasty/Goldmann 3 mirror can be used.
    iii. Site: Equally spaced burns are applied to anterior half of trabecular meshwork at the junction of pigmented functional and nonfunctional trabecular meshwork.
    iv. Laser parameters: 180–360° of angle treated with argon blue green of 800–1200 mW; 0.1 sec exposure, 50 μmm spot size, 24 shots per quadrant.
    v. End point: Blanching of trabecular meshwork or appearance of an air bubble.

17. What is the mechanism of action of argon laser trabeculoplasty?

Explained by two theories:

Mechanical theory: Collagen shrinkage is produced at site of burns. There is stretching of trabecular meshwork between the burns which opens the meshwork pores and allows aqueous to flow better. Laser burns attract phagocytes that clean up the debris within the meshwork and allow aqueous to flow better.

Biological theory: It causes activation of macrophages to ingest and clear the debris thereby increasing the outflow facility.

18. **What are the complications of argon laser trabeculoplasty?**
    i. Pressure rise
    ii. Visual loss
    iii. Peripheral anterior synechiae
    iv. Uveitis
    v. Hyphema
    vi. Increased incidence of Tenon's cyst following trabeculectomy.

19. **What is the percentage decrease in IOP following argon laser trabec-uloplasty in POAG?**

    Average reduction is about 30%. About 50% of eyes remain well controlled after 5 years of treatment.

20. **What is the effect on success of trabeculectomy following ALT versus an eyes in which no laser was done previously?**

    The risk of encapsulated blebs following filtration surgery is up to 3 times more in eyes previously treated by ALT.

21. **What are the indications for selective laser trabeculoplasty?**
    i. Open-angle glaucoma
    ii. Failed argon laser trabeculoplasty
    iii. PXF glaucoma
    iv. Pigmentary glaucoma
    v. Juvenile glaucoma
    vi. Inflammatory glaucoma
    vii. Poorly compliant patient
    viii. End stage treatment.

22. **What are the contraindications for selective laser trabeculoplasty?**
    i. Angle closure glaucoma
    ii. Uveitic glaucoma
    iii. Angle recession glaucoma
    iv. Developmental glaucoma
    v. Neovascular glaucoma (NVG).

23. **What is the mechanism of action of selective laser trabeculoplasty?**

    Selective laser trabeculoplasty therapy targets the pigmented melanin containing cells (yellow) in the trabecular meshwork preventing thermal transfer to the surrounding tissue.

A cellular and biochemical model has been proposed.
Macrophages are recruited to the laser treatment zones which stimulate release of cytokines. These cytokines upregulate synthetic MMP, which increase the porosity of endothelial layers of trabecular meshwork and Schlemm's canal and increases aqueous outflow.

24. **What are the laser parameters used in selective laser trabeculoplasty?**

    Frequency doubled Q switched Nd:YAG laser is used.
    532 nm, pulse duration 3 ms
    Spot size 400 μ
    Energy 0.2–1.7 mW, 50–100 adjacent laser spots are applied.

25. **What are the future trends in laser trabeculoplasty?**

    Micropulse laser trabeculoplasty (MLT) using a 810 nm diode laser
    Titanium Sapphire LTP (SOLX 790) using 790 nm; 5-10 microseconds.

26. **What is laser iridoplasty?**

    It is also called gonioplasty and is a technique to deepen the angle. It is an iris flattening procedure done in:
    Plateau iris
    Nanophthalmos
    POAG in anatomically narrow angle.
    Adjunct to laser trabeculoplasty
    After Nd;YAG iridotomy where IOP is still not controlled

27. **What are the settings used for laser iridoplasty?**

    Settings—500 microns
    —200–400 mW power
    —0.2–0.5 second
    —20–24 spots over 360°
    —1mm away from iris root

28. **What is the role of lasers in cyclodestructive procedures?**

    Involves cyclophotocoagulation – A thermal method of destroying part of ciliary body.
    Approaches can be

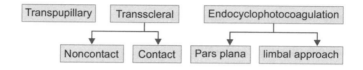

Transpupillary procedures are unpredictable and give disappointing results.

Transscleral route is the preferred modality.

In noncontact: There is slit lamp delivery of laser energy through air.

Contact method: Involves fiberoptic probe delivery directly to ocular surface.

Endocyclophotocoagulation: Involves use of intraocular laser probe to treat ciliary processes. Two options are available.

Pars plana route: Particularly useful in neovascular glaucoma in diabetic patients in whom vitrectomy is also needed.

Limbal route: Procedure is carried out through limbal incision. Useful in phakic, pseudophakic, and aphakic patients. It can be combined with cataract extraction.

29. **How is laser useful in malignant glaucoma?**

Laser hyaloidectomy/hyaloidotomy or vitreolysis is done. In malignant glaucoma anterior hyaloid acts as a barrier to fluid movement into anterior chamber. Laser (by Nd:YAG) is used to photodisrupt the anterior hyaloid face and relieve ciliovitreal compression.

Laser parameters: 100–200 µm
Spot size 1–11 mm

30. **What is laser suturolysis?**

Technique by which scleral flap sutures applied for closing flap in trabeculectomy can be lysed or cut using lasers.

31. **Describe the technique of laser suturolysis.**

Lasers used : Solid Nd:YAG laser or argon green
Timing   : Within 3–15 days to 2 months or more after use of mitomycin c after trabeculectomy
Indications : When the target IOP is not reached.
Lenses used : Zeiss gonioprism or Hoskins laser suturolysis lens
Duration   : 0.02–0.15 seconds
Spot size   : 50–100 nm
Power   : 200–1000 mW

Gentle pressure over conjunctiva makes sutures more visible.

32. **What are the complications of laser suturolysis?**

i. Conjunctival burns
ii. Flat anterior chamber
iii. Conjunctival flap leak
iv. Hypotonous maculopathy
v. Iris incarceration, hyphema
vi. Blebitis, endophthalmitis.

33. Describe technique of digital pressure.

Constant and firm digital compression is applied over inferior aspect of globe through the patient's lower lid while the eye is upturned. Duration of each compression should not last for more than 10 seconds.

34. What is goniophotocoagulation?

Used to ablate vessels which cross scleral spur.
Argon laser of 150–500 mW
100 μ spot size is used for 0.2 sec for this procedure.

35. What are the indications for transscleral cyclophotocoagulation?

   i. In refractory glaucoma when IOP is uncontrolled despite maximum tolerated medical treatment and failed filtration or high risk of failure of the same like in aphakic, pseudophakic, or neovascular glaucomas.
  ii. Glaucoma associated with inflammation
 iii. Eyes with previous failed filtering procedure or following penetrating keratoplasty.

36. Describe diode laser transscleral cyclophotocoagulation.

Anesthesia: Administer local anesthetic. Supplement with retro or peribulbar injections. Can be done in supine position or sitting at the slit lamp.

Energy levels of 0.5–2.75 J for 32 applications distributed over 360° of the ciliary body

Treatment quadrants: Over a 270° area involving inferior, nasal, and superior quadrants (16–18 applications reduces complications). Temporal quadrant is spared to allow for some ciliary production of aqueous humor. the 3 and 9 o'clock meridians are avoided to prevent damage to the long posterior ciliary arteries.

Treatment parameters:

Pigmentation	Starting power	Starting duration
Dark	1500 mW	2000 ms
Light	1750 mW	2000 ms

Pops may be heard during treatment indicating tissue disruption but they are not a prerequisite for effective treatment.

The G probe tip (gaasterland made) and eye surface is kept moist by methylcellulose or artificial tears.

Postoperative care: The eye is patched for 4–6 hours. Topical cycloplegics BD or more, topical steroids QID is given and tapered as inflammation subsides. All preoperative glaucoma medications except miotics are to be continued. Monitor patients at 1, 3, 6 weeks after treatment.

37. What are the complications of diode cyclophotocoagulation?

Commonly:

   i. Pain
   ii. Inflammation
   iii. Reduced visual acuity due to cystoid macular edema
   iv. Hypotony

Uncommon complications:

   i. Hypopyon
   ii. Corneal epithelial defect
   iii. Scleral thinning
   iv. Graft failure
   v. Malignant glaucoma
   vi. Suprachoroidal hemorrhage
   vii. Hyphema
   viii. Sympathetic ophthalmitis
   ix. Phthisis bulbi

4.17. TRABECULECTOMY

1. **What are the definitions of anatomical limbus?**

   The anterior limit of limbus is formed by a line joining the end of the Bowman's membrane and the end of Descemet's membrane (Schwalbe's line). The posterior limit is a curved line marking the transition between regularly arranged corneal collagen fibres to haphazardly arranged scleral collagen fibres.

2. **What are the definitions of the surgical limbus?**

   It is an annular band, 2 mm wide with the posterior limit overlying the scleral spur. It is divided into a
   i. Anterior bue zone (between Bowman's membrane and Schwalbe's line)
   ii. Posterior white zone (between Schwalbe's line and scleral spur)

3. **What are the types of filtering surgeries?**

   Filtering surgeries are of three types:
   i. Full thickness
   ii. Partial thickness
   iii. Nonpenetrating

   Full thickness (Example):
   i. Sclerectomy
   ii. Trephination
   iii. Thermal sclerostomy (Scheie's procedure)
   iv. Laser sclerostomy (ab externo/interno)
   v. Iridencleisis
   vi. Goniopuncture

   Partial thickness:
   i. Trabeculectomy

   Nonpenetrating:
   i. Viscocanalostomy
   ii. Canaloplasty
   iii. Deep sclerectomy

4. **What are "full thickness" operations?**

   These are filtering operations without a sclera flap. Entire thickness of the wall from the corneoscleral surface to the anterior chamber is removed.

5. **What is a "partial thickness" operation?**

   An operation with a partial thickness flap of sclera overlying the opening between the anterior chamber and the subconjunctival space, e.g., trabeculectomy.

6. **What is the advantage of partial thickness flap over full thickness?**
   i. Uniform control of IOP
   ii. Decrease risk of postoperative hypotony thus decrease risk of hypotonous maculopathy
   iii. Decreased risk of postoperative complication like hyphema, iris prolapse, shallow anterior chamber
   iv. Decreased risk of postoperative infection, endophthalmitis.

7. **Is the term trabeculectomy a misnomer?**
   Yes, because the block of tissue removed does not need to include trabecular meshwork to be successful. The procedure involves a peripheral posterior keratectomy more than removal of trabecular meshwork.

8. **What is the principle?**
   Trabeculectomy works mainly because of filtration. The basic mechanism is by creating a fistula at the limbus, which allows aqueous humor to drain from the anterior chamber, around the edges of the sclera flap and into the subconjunctival space from where it leaves by transconjunctival filtration or by absorption into the lymphatics and vessels of subconjunctival tissue.

9. **What are the indications for trabeculectomy in primary open-angle glaucoma?**
   Failed maximal tolerated medical therapy and failed laser surgery or poor candidates of laser with any of the following:
   i. Progressive glaucomatous optic nerve head damage
   ii. Progressive glaucomatous field loss
   iii. Anticipated optic nerve head damage or as a result of excessive IOP
   iv. Anticipated visual field damage
   v. Lack of compliance with anticipated progressive glaucomatous damage.

10. **What are the features of a good filtering bleb?**
    The blebs which are associated with good IOP control are:
    i. Avascular and transparent
    ii. Numerous microcysts in the epithelium
    iii. Either low and diffuse or more circumscribed and elevated.

11. **What are the signs of a failing bleb?**
    The signs of a failing bleb are:
    i. Reduced bleb height
    ii. Increased bleb wall thickness
    iii. Vascularization of the bleb
    iv. Loss of transparency
    iv. Loss of conjunctival microcysts
    v. Raised IOP.

12. What are the types of blebs following trabeculectomy?

There are 4 types:

   i. **Type 1 bleb**: Thin and polycystic appearance due to transconjunctival flow of aqueous. It is associated with good filtration.

  ii. **Type 2 bleb**: Flat, thin, and diffuse with a relatively avascular appearance, associated with good filtration. Conjunctival microcysts are usually visible with high magnification.

 iii. **Type 3 bleb**: Flat, not associated with microcystic spaces, contains engorged blood vessels on its surface. This bleb does not filter and hence the IOP is elevated.

 iv. **Type 4 bleb/encapsulated bleb/Tenon's cyst**: Localized, highly elevated, dome-shaped, cyst-like cavity of hypertrophied Tenon's capsule with engorged surface blood vessels. This bleb does not filter and hence the IOP is elevated.

  v. **Risk factors for Tenon's cyst:**
- Young individuals
- Previous conjunctival surgery
- Secondary glaucoma
- Laser trabeculoplasty
- Topical sympathomimetic therapy
- Tenon cyst in the fellow eye

13. What is the preoperative care?

   i. If IOP is very high then it is reduced to a safe level

  ii. Treat any ocular inflammation (reduced chances of establishing a lasting bleb)

 iii. Discontinue epinephrine/anticholinesterase to reduce vascular congestion and reduce intraoperative bleedings

 iv. Discontinue aqueous suppressant timolol (2 weeks prior) and carbonic anhydrase inhibitors (1–2 days prior) to prevent ocular hypotony and establish a filtering bleb

  v. Avoid gentamicin, which can irritate conjunctiva and produce congestion of eyes

 vi. Constrict pupil with pilocarpine 1% 3 times, 1 hour before the operation. It prevents iris prolapse

 vii. If aspirin had been used, it is discontinued for 5 days before surgery

viii. If eyes have new vessels, preoperative panretinal laser photocoagulation should be done first to induce regression of vessels and improve prognosis.

14. What are the steps of trabeculectomy?

   i. Anesthesia: under retrobulbar/peribulbar/subtenons/general anaesthesia (avoid massage in case of advanced glaucoma, can lead to snuff out phenomenon)

ii. A bridle suture is inserted 2 mm anterior to the limbus

iii. A conjunctival flap is fashioned superonasally. The flap may be based either at the limbus or at the fornix

iv. A triangle or rectangle based at the limbus is outlined on the sclera measuring 3 mm radially and 4 mm circumferentially by a wet field cautery. One may make a square/triangular flap. With a sharp pointed knife, incisions are made along the cautery marks through 2/3rd of the sclera thickness starting as anteriorly as possible behind the reflected flap.

v. One of the corners of the flap is held up with toolkit colibri forceps and dissection is started. A natural tissue plane will become apparent at about 1/3rd of scleral thickness. The dissection is done in an anti-direction in the same plane keeping the blade flat until the color turns from white to gray

vi. The dissection is continued until clear cornea has been reached

vii. Paracentesis is done at this stage

viii. The fistula is begun by entering the anterior chamber with a knife just behind the hinge of scleral flap

ix. This deep block is excised using Kelly Descemet's membrane punch

x. Internal ostium should be 1.5×2 mm

xi. A peripheral iridectomy is performed to prevent blockage of the internal ostium by the peripheral iris

xii. The superficial sclera flap is sutured with interrupted 10-0 nylon so that it is apposed lightly to the underlying bed

xiii. If necessary, AC can be reformed by injecting BSS through the paracentesis with a Rycroft cannula.

xiv. The conjunctival flap is sutured with 8-0 vicryl

xv. At the completion of surgery, one drop of 1% atropine eyedrop is instilled and a mixture of betamethasone and gentamicin (0.8 mL gentamycin, 0.3 mL betamethasone) is injected inferiorly under the conjunctiva

15. What are the structures removed in trabeculectomy?

From outside to inside:

i. Block of scleral tissue

ii. Schlemm's canal

iii. Trabecular meshwork

iv. Schwalbe's line

v. Block of peripheral cornea

vi. Iris.

(Tenon's removal is optional. Some surgeons prefer to remove it, as it is source for fibroblasts.)

16. **What are the advantages of fornix-based flap?**
    i. Easier to create
    ii. Good surgical exposure
    iii. Easier to identify surgical landmarks
    iv. Avoids postconjunctival scarring.

17. **What are the disadvantages of fornix-based flap?**
    i. Harder to excise Tenon's tissue
    ii. Spontaneous aqueous leak at limbus in early postoperative period
    iii. Caution when doing argon laser lysis of sclera flap sutures subconjunctival 5-FU injections and digital pressure in the early postoperative period
    iv. Late postoperative IOP not as low as limbus-based flap

18. **What are the advantages of limbus-based flap?**
    i. Easier to excise Tenon's tissue
    ii. Argon laser lysis of sclera flap sutures, subconjunctival 5-FU injections, and digital pressure can be done with more safety in the early postoperative period
    iii. Late postoperative IOP lower

19. **What are the disadvantages of limbus-based flap?**
    i. Anterior dissection of the conjunctival flap is difficult as incision in conjunctiva is made posterior to the fornix
    ii. Poor surgical exposure
    iii. More conjunctival manipulation

20. **Which are more preferred limbus/fornix-based flaps?**
    Studies comparing fornix-based or limbus-based trabeculectomies have demonstrated equivalent success in IOP control both with and without antimetabolites.

21. **What is the problem with sclerostomy at 12 o'clock?**
    Bleeding from perforating branch of an anterior ciliary vessel that passes through the sclera to enter the cilliary body 2–4 mm from the limbus.

22. **What are the preferred sites of sclerostomy for limbus- and fornix-based flap?**
    Limbus based—superotemporal quadrant as conjunctival incision can be made farther back in the fornix.
    Fornix based—superonasal quadrant is adequate.

23. **What is the purpose of a corneal incision?**
    Provides an entry for fluid into the AC at any stage of the operation.

24. What needles can one use for the corneal incision?

A dull needle. Because the top of a sharp needle will get caught in the corneal stroma.

25. What is the disadvantage of bridle suture under the superior rectus tendon?

Subconjunctival hemorrhage may occur.

26. What are the reasons for doing an iridectomy with trabeculectomy?

i. To prevent iris incarceration in the sclerostomy with blockage of aqueous outflow if it shallows postoperatively.

ii. To prevent pupillary block if posterior synechiae or a pupillary membrane develops secondary to postoperative intraocular inflammation.

27. What should be the size of iridectomy?

It should be basal and wider than the opening in the anterior chamber so that iris tissue does not block the opening.

28. When should the sclera flap be sutured more tightly?

i. Eyes with PACG and those with a history of malignant glaucoma

ii. Aphakic/highly myopic eyes prone to choroidal hemorrhage

iii. Nanophthalmic eye and eyes with elevated episcleral venous pressure prone to suprachoroidal infusion and flat anterior chamber.

29. Why should a tenonectomy be done?

i. Improves visibility of the nylon sutures in the postoperative period.

ii. Partially determines the effectiveness of suture lysis, which determines the final postoperative pressure.

30. What should be used to reform the AC?

Usually done with balanced salt solution
Healon (sodium hyaluronate) can maintain ACD prevent choroidal effusion or suprachoroidal hemorrhage, decrease the rate of postoperative hyphaema, and delay scarring of the bleb. However, IOP may be higher in the early postoperative period.

31. Why is hemostasis essential in trabeculectomy surgery?

Because blood in the anterior chamber under the conjunctival flap can produce scarring of the bleb and cause failure of filtration.

32. How can it be prevented?

i. The internal sclerostomy is made as far anteriorly as possible.

ii. Ensure effective hemostasis by proper cautery during the operation, over cautery should not be done as scleral flap will be thin.

33. What should be the postoperative evaluation of the eye?

    i. Extent of height of the bleb

    ii. Presence/absence of microcysts

    iii. Presence/absence of aqueous leak

    iv. Visibility of sclera flap sutures through overlaying conjunctival flap

    v. IOP

    vi. Clarity of cornea

    vii. AC depth

    viii. AC inflammation

    ix. Hyphema

    x. Choroidal detachment/suprachoroidal hemorrhage

    xi. Optic disk and macular appearance.

34. What is the role of atropine 1% scopolamine 0.25% postoperative?

By paralyzing the ciliary muscles they:

    i. Tighten the zonular lens – iris diaphragm – maximally deepening the anterior chamber

    ii. Maintain blood–aqueous barrier

    iii. Relief from ciliary spasm

    iv. Dilate the pupil

    v. Prevent the formation of posterior synechiae.

35. What are the factors contributing to poor prognosis in filtering surgery?

    i. Age < 40 years

    ii. Previous failed filter

    iii. Aphakia/pseudophakia

    iv. Neovascular glaucoma

    v. Active uveitis

    vi. Congenital glaucoma

    vii. Congenital disease, e.g., Stevens–Johnson, ocular pemphigoid.

    viii. Previous penetrating keratoplasty

    ix. Previous scleral buckle for retinal reattachment

    x. Previous topical medications

    xi. Chronic conjunctival inflammation

    xii. Previous conjunctival surgery.

36. What is the most common problem after trabeculectomy?

Shallowing of the AC postoperatively.

37. What are the main causes of a shallow AC for trabeculectomy?

Shallow AC can be associated with:

    i. **Hypotony:**

      – Wound leak

      – Excessive filtration

      – Serous choroidal detachment.

ii. **Raised IOP:**
  – Malignant glaucoma
  – Incomplete peripheral iridectomy with pupillary block
  – Delayed suprachoroidal hemorrhage.

38. What are the characteristics and treatment of wound leak?

Characteristics:
  i. Soft eye
  ii. Poor bleb
  iii. Positive Seidel's test.

Treatment:
  i. Immediate pressure dressing
  ii. Simmons scleral shell tamponade
  iii. Therapeutic soft contact lenses
  iv. Cyanoacrylate tissue adhesive covered with collagen shield.

If the defect is large, suturing of the defect, construction of new conjunctival flap created posterior to original flap or a conjunctival autograft can be considered.

39. What are the characteristics and treatment of excessive filtration?

Characteristics:
  i. Very low IOP
  ii. A good bleb
  iii. A negative Seidel's test
  iv. Choroidal detachment may be present.

Treatment:
  i. First step is firm patching
  ii. Simmons scleral shell
  iii. Therapeutic soft contact lenses
  iv. Aqueous suppressants (to promote spontaneous healing by temporarily reducing aqueous flow through the fistula)
  v. Atropine (to prevent pupillary block)
  vi. Steroids.

Surgical: Reformation of the anterior chamber with air, sodium hyaluronate or SF6 and drainage of choroidal detachment if they are very deep. Scleral flap and conjunctiva are resutured.

40. What are the characteristic features, cause, and treatment of ciliary block glaucoma?

Features:
  i. Hard eye
  ii. No bleb
  iii. Negative Seidel's test.

Cause:
– Blockage of aqueous flow at the secreting portion of the ciliary body, so that aqueous is forced backward into the vitreous

Treatment:
  i. Strong topical mydriatics
 ii. If this fails, osmotic agents – IV mannitol
iii. If osmotic agent fails, the anterior hyaloid phase is disrupted through a patent iridectomy with an Nd:YAG laser.
 iv. Needling of aqueous pockets in vitreous
  v. Removal of aqueous pockets from vitreous through sclerostomy and formation of anterior chamber by air through paracentesis.
 vi. If laser therapy fails, an anterior vitrectomy via the pars plana should be performed with a vitreous cutter and the entrapped fluid removed.

41. What are the complications of postoperative shallowing of the AC?
  i. Peripheral anterior synechiae
 ii. Corneal endothelial damage
iii. Cataract.

42. What are the causes of failure of filtration?
  i. **Intraocular factors:**
     – Obstruction of fistula by clot, iris, ciliary body, lens, vitreous
     – Bleb failure
     – Poor surgical techniques which prevent exit of aqueous from the anterior chamber
 ii. **Extraocular factors:**
     – Subconjunctival fibrosis
     – Individual racial and genetic factors.

43. What is the most common cause for bleb failure?
Subconjunctival fibrosis.

44. What is the management of failure of filtration?
Two causes for failure of filtration:
  i. Obstruction of fistula by iris/ciliary body/lens or vitreous
 ii. Failing filtering bleb

If there is obstruction:
  i. Low energy argon laser therapy can be done surrounding the obstruction
 ii. Internal bleb revision

If failing bleb:
  i. Increase the steroids to hourly dosing
 ii. Digital pressure

iii. Argon laser suturolysin: 50 µ spot size, 0.02–0.1 sec, 250–1000 mW power.

iv. If fibrin or clot is obstructing, intracameral tissue plasminogen activator (6–12.5 µg)

v. Restart antiglaucoma medications

vi. Repeat filtering procedure with antimetabolites or drainage implants.

45. How can the success rate of trabeculectomy be improved?

Preoperative techniques:

i. Treat surface infections

ii. Discontinue use of pilocarpine, aqueous suppresants, carbonic anhydrase inhibitor and aspirin.

iii. Decreased use of preservatives like BAK.

Intraoperative techniques:

i. Constriction of pupil

ii. Prevent conjunctival button hole or scleral flap disinsertion

iii. Internal ostium should be 1.5 × 2 mm. Iridectomy should be larger than this ostium to prevent blockage

iv. Tight wound closure.

Postoperative techniques:

By the use of antimetabolities which inhibit the wound healing.
Antimetabolites used are:

i. Corticosteroids

ii. 5-fluorouracil

iii. Mitomycin C

iv. Suramin

v. Beta radiation (strontium)

vi. Tissue plasminogen activator

vii. Gamma interferon

viii. Calcium ionophores.

46. What are the complications of antimetabolites?

Complications are more with MMC than 5-FU.

Most important complications are:

i. Early or late hypotony

ii. Bleb leak

iii. Bleb-related infection.

Others are:

Lids:

i. Punctal occlusion (more with 5-FU)

ii. Cicatricial ectropion.

Conjunctiva:

  i. Wound and suture track leaks

  ii. Disintegration of vicryl sutures.

Cornea:

  i. Erosion

  ii. Ulcer.

Endothelial toxicity is common with mitomycin and epithelial toxicity is common with 5-FU

  i. Pupillary block

  ii. Cataracts

  iii. Hypotonous maculopathy

  iv. Choroidal hemorrhage

  v. Malignant glaucoma.

47. **What are the advantages of argon laser suture lysis?**

  i. Scleral flap can be closed tightly intraoperatively

  ii. Decreases hypotony

  iii. Decreases choroidal separation

  iv. Decreases suprachoroidal hemorrhage

  v. Decreases the hospital stay.

48. **What are the instruments used for laser suture lysis?**

  i. Hoskins suture lysis lens

  ii. Edge of four mirror gonio prism

  iii. High magnification mandlekorn lens or blumenthal lens.

49. **What is the role of aqueous humor in wound modulation?**

It decreases stimulation of fibroblasts as aqueous humor contains lots of factors to inhibit active inflammation. The bleb is formed permanently without fibrosis.

50. **What is the role of postoperative digital pressure?**

  i. Encourages flow of fluid through the sclerostomy

  ii. Expands the filtering bleb

  iii. Prevents anatomic obstructions to filtration from becoming unalterable.

51. **When should digital pressure be applied?**

Rather than waiting for a bleb to fail, if the IOP rises above 12 mm Hg or if the target pressure is not achieved, digital pressure should be applied.

52. **What are the problems due to digital pressure?**

  i. Small subconjunctival hemorrhages

  ii. Hyphema.

iii. Rupture of a filtering wound

iv. Dehiscence of an incisional wound.

53. What are the complications of trabeculectomy?

   i. Intraoperative

  ii. Early postoperative

 iii. Late postoperative.

Intraoperative

     i. Conjunctival buttonhole/perforation

    ii. Amputation of sclera flap

   iii. Flap related—thick, thin, irregular, and buttonholing

   iv. Hemorrhage

    v. Damage of lens

   vi. Vitreous loss

  vii. Choroidal effusion

 viii. Cyclodialysis cleft

   ix. Malignant glaucoma

Early postoperative

     i. Hypotony and flat AC:
  - Conjunctival defect
  - Excessive filtration
  - Serous choroidal detachment

    ii. Hypotony and formed AC:
  - Hypotony maculopathy

   iii. Raised IOP and flat AC:
  - Delayed suprachoroidal hemorrhage
  - Malignant glaucoma
  - Incomplete PI with pupillary block

   iv. Raised IOP with deep AC:
  - Obstruction of fistula
  - Failing bleb

    v. Uveitis

   vi. Hyphema

  vii. Dellen

 viii. Loss of central vision

   ix. Ocular decompression retinopathy

Late postoperative

     i. Bleb infection/endophthalmitis

    ii. Cataract

   iii. Dissection of filtering bleb into cornea

   iv. Leaking filtering bleb

    v. Cyst of Tenon's capsule
   vi. Hyphema
  vii. Pupillary membrane
 viii. Corneal edema
   ix. Failure of filtration
    x. Malignant glaucoma
   xi. Upper eyelid retraction
  xii. Scleral staphyloma
 xiii. Sympathetic ophthalmia.

54. What are the methods for repairing a conjunctival buttonhole?

    i. Small pinpoint leaks can be sealed with cyanoacrylate glues or fibrin glues.
   ii. Direct microsurgical repair
  iii. Wing suture technique
  iv. Glaucoma (Simmond) shell technique
   v. Purse string suture.

55. What care should be taken during trabeculectomy surgery in aphakic/highly myopic eyes?

Such eyes are hypotonous and can develop intra/suprachoroidal hemorrhage.

56. How can a leaking filtering bleb be detected?

Many can be detected with 0.25% fluorescein; subtle leaks are seen with 2% fluorescein.

57. How is a leaking bleb managed?

    i. If the leak is minimal, chamber is of good depth, bleb is pale and elevated, then conservative treatment is done.
   ii. Aqueous flow with blockers and carbonic anhydrase inhibitors
  iii. Topical antibiotic – gentamicin which irritates the conjunctiva and facilitates healing of the conjunctival defect
  iv. Patching of the eye to lid movement
   v. If associated with flat AC, glaucoma shells
  vi. If not effective, then surgical repair is done.

58. What is the earliest evidence of a bleb infection?

Mild conjunctival hyperemia around the filtering bleb is the first sign. If treatment is delayed, there is a risk of endophthalmitis.

59. What is the treatment of bleb infection?

    i. Initial treatment is empirical
   ii. Topical antibiotics frequently
  iii. Topical steroids 12–24 hours after starting antibiotics

60. **What are the common organisms involved in bleb related endophthalmitis?**
    i. *Haemophilus influenzae*
    ii. *Staphyloccocus*
    iii. *Streptococcus.*

61. **What is the treatment of Tenon's cyst?**
    i. Usually resolve spontaneously within 2–4 months
    ii. However medical therapy may be needed to control IOP during this time.

62. **How are corneal dellen formed and what is the treatment?**
    Localized disruption of the precorneal tear film → corneal dehydration causes stromal thinning and dellen formation
    i. Usually occur in the horizontal plane within the lid fissure.
    ii. Treatment—artifical tears and patching
       If ineffective, steroid drops are decreased.

63. **Why is trabeculectomy more successful in older patients?**
    i. Atrophic Tenon's capsule
    ii. Decreased capacity for fibroblastic proliferation.

64. **What are the indicators for combined glaucoma and cataract surgery?**
    May be considered in patients with visually significant cataracts and:
    i. Inadequate control of IOP
    ii. Medication intolerance/poor compliance
    iii. Advanced glaucoma
    iv. Eyes requiring epinephrine compound
    v. Marginally functioning filter.

65. **What are the advantages of combined cataract surgery?**
    i. Earlier visual rehabilitation owing to cataract extraction
    ii. Reduces risk of early postoperative IOP spikes which is detrimental in eyes with severely excavated ONH
    iii. A one-time single intervention eliminates need for further surgery
    iv. Patient compliance is better.

66. **What are the disadvantages of combined approach?**
    i. Long-term IOP control seems questionable owing to loss of bleb function from enhanced episcleral scarring.
    ii. Increased incidence of postoperative complications hyphema, uveitis, shallow chambers, hypotony.

67. What are the advantages of 2 stage procedure over combined procedure?

More decrease in IOP as plain trabeculectomy decreases IOP by 41%. Lesser risk of postoperative complication like hyphema, inflammation, hypotony, and shallow anterior chamber.

68. What are the antimetabolites used routinely?

MMC and 5-FU.
Dosage: MMC: 0.2–0.5 mg/mL for 1–5 min
5-FU: 30 mg/mL for 5 min, subconjunctival dose is 5 mg.

69. What are the indications for adjuvant antimetabolite therapy?

High risk factors:

i. Neovascular glaucoma
ii. Previous failed trabeculectomy or artificial filtering devices
iii. Certain secondary glaucomas (e.g., inflammatory, posttraumatic angle recession, ICE syndrome).

Intermediate risk factors:

i. Patients on topical antiglaucoma medications (sympathomimetics) for 3 years
ii. Previous conjunctival surgery
iii. Previous cataract surgery

Low risk factors:

i. Black patients
ii. Patients under age of 40 years

70. Mechanism of action of 5-FU.

It inhibits DNA synthesis and is active on the 'S' phase of the cell cycle. Fibroblastic proliferation is inhibited, but fibroblastic attachment and migration are unaffected.

71. Mechanism of action of MMC.

It is an alkylating agent which selectively inhibits DNA replication, mitosis and protein synthesis. The drug inhibits proliferation of fibroblasts, suppresses vascular ingrowth, and is much more potent than 5-FU.

72. Where are the antimetabolites placed?

They are placed in the sub-Tenon's space, as the most common cause for failure is subconjunctival fibrosis.

73. Why is previous long-term use of medications associated with failure of trabeculectomy?

i. Increased fibroblastic proliferation in conjunctiva
ii. Reduced goblet cells
iii. Infiltration of conjunctiva with inflammatory cells.

74. What are the advantages of releasable sutures and laser suturolysis?

   i. Can leave eye with firm pressure

   ii. Can protect eye against low pressure and complications associated with low pressure

   iii. Can titrate eye pressure postoperatively.

75. Name full thickness surgeries

   i. Thermal sclerotomy (scheie procedure)

   ii. Sclerectomy- anterior lip sclerectomy and posterior lip sclerectomy

   iii. Trephination

   iv. Iridenclesis.

4.18. MODULATION OF WOUND HEALING IN GLAUCOMA FILTERING SURGERY

1. **What are the pharmacological techniques that interfere with wound healing to maintain success of trabeculectomy?**
   i. The preoperative and postoperative administration of glucocorticosteroids to control inflammation and thereby scarring
   ii. The local intraoperative and postoperative administration of antineoplastic agents such as mitomycin C and 5-fluorouracil to reduce fibroblast proliferation
   iii. The use of agents to interfere with the synthesis of normal collagen such as b-aminopropionitrile and penicillamine.

2. **What is the role of corticosteroids in glaucoma filtering surgeries?**
   i. They control inflammation and immune response at multiple points.
   ii. Anti-inflammatory mechanisms of corticosteroids include constriction of blood vessels, stabilization of lysosomes, inhibition of degranulation, impairment of leucocyte chemotaxis, reduction of lymphocyte proliferation, suppression of fibroplasia, inhibition of phospholipase A2 production, which subsequently prevents cyclooxygenase and lipoxygenase from producing prostaglandins, prostacyclins, thromboxanes, and leukotrienes.

3. **What is the role of NSAIDs in glaucoma filtering surgeries?**
   i. NSAIDS are heterogeneous group of agents that inhibit the enzyme cyclooxygenase from converting arachidonic acid into prostaglandins and thromboxanes.
   ii. They have been demonstrated to inhibit proliferation of human Tenon fibroblasts in culture.

4. **What is the role of mitomycin C in glaucoma filtering surgeries?**
   i. Mitomycin C is an alkylating agent isolated from the fermentation filtrate of *Streptomyces caespitosus.*
   ii. It inhibits DNA dependent RNA synthesis and binds to cellular DNA sites on cell membranes, forming free radicals and chelating metal ions.
   iii. Like 5-FU, mitomycin inhibits fibroblast proliferation, but unlike 5-FU, it affects cells in all phases.

5. **Describe the methods of administration of mitomycin C.**
   i. After outlining and partially dissecting the scleral flap to ensure integrity of the scleral tissues, the conjunctiva is inspected to rule out the presence of any tears or button holes.

ii. Mitomycin C dilution: The drug is available in a vial as purple color powder at a concentration of 2 mg/mL. It is further reconstituted with 5 mL distilled water or normal saline to make 0.4 mg/mL or in 10 mL to make 0.2 mg/mL. When reconstituted to concentration of 0.2 mg/mL, it is stable for 1 hr at room temperature.

iii. An amputated tip of 4.5 mm × 4.5 mm sized methylcellulose sponge soaked in a 0.2–0.5 mg/mL solution of MMC is then placed between the conjunctiva/tenon's capsule and episclera for 1–5 minutes.

iv. During this time, the edges of the conjunctival flap are pulled over the sponge so that the tissue edges are not exposed to the drug.

v. The area is then rinsed with copious amounts of balanced salt solution.

vi. A relatively tight scleral flap is prudent to reduce the likelihood of prolonged postoperative hypotony.

6. **What are the side effects of MMC?**

Irritation

i. Lacrimation
ii. Hyperemia
iii. Photophobia
iv. Ocular pain.

Eyelids and conjunctiva

i. Allergic or irritative reactions
ii. Erythema
iii. Conjunctivitis
iv. Avascularity
v. Hyperemia
vi. Blepharitis
vii. Granuloma
viii. Symblepharon.

Cornea

i. Corneal melting
ii. Edema
iii. Erosion
iv. Crystalline epithelial deposits
v. Endothelial decompensation
vi. Punctate keratitis
vii. Delayed wound healing
viii. Perforation
ix. Recurrence of herpes simplex.

Sclera

  i. Scleral melting (necrotizing scleritis)
 ii. Delayed wound healing
iii. Avascularity
 iv. Erosion
  v. Perforation
 vi. Calcium deposits.

Uvea

  i. Iridocyclitis
 ii. Hyperemia
iii. Hypopigmentation of iris.

Glaucoma

Punctal occlusion

Hypotony

7. **What is the role of 5-fluorouracil in glaucoma filtering surgeries?**

   i. 5-fluorouracil is a pyrimidine analog.
  ii. It is a folic acid antagonist.
 iii. It is active on the 'S' phase (synthesis phase) of the cell cycle
  iv. Mechanism of action is to prevent the reduction of folic acid to tetrahydrofolic acid by noncompetitive enzyme inhibition. This results in inhibition of DNA and RNA synthesis and eventual cell death.
   v. Inhibition of fibroblast proliferation has been regarded as the primary mechanism by which 5-FU enhances and maintains bleb function.

8. **Describe the methods of administration of 5-FU.**

   It can be given as subconjunctival injections or as an intraoperative application.

   i. **Subconjunctival injection of 5-FU**
      – Subconjunctival injection of 5-FU may be administered in an undiluted concentration (50 mg/mL), although many prefer to dilute it to 10 mg/mL.

   ii. **Dilution**
      – Five milligrams of the agent is drawn into a tuberculin syringe, after which the tuberculin needle is replaced with a 0.5 inch 30 gauge needle.
      – After administration of a topical anesthetic, at least 2 cotton-tipped applicators soaked in 4% topical lidocaine are used to swab and further anesthetize the tissues at the proposed injection site.
      – The injection is then given 90°–180° from the trabeculectomy site.

iii. **Dosage**
  - Twice daily for 1 week and once daily for the second week for a total of 21 injections (105 mg).

9. **What are the side effects of subconjunctival or intradermal 5-FU?**

Irritation
  i. Lacrimation
  ii. Ocular pain
  iii. Edema
  iv. Burning sensation

Eyelids or conjunctiva
  i. Cicatricial ectropion
  ii. Allergic reactions
  iii. Erythema
  iv. Hyperpigmentation
  v. Keratinization
  vi. Utricaria
  vii. Subconjunctival hemorrhages
  viii. Periorbital edema.

Cornea
  i. Superficial punctate keratitis
  ii. Ulceration
  iii. Scarring stromal
  iv. Keratinized plaques
  v. Delayed wound healing
  vi. Endothelial damage.

10. **How to choose an agent: 5-FU versus MMC?**
  i. Currently intraoperative 5-FU with supplementary postoperative 5% FU injections are used in most primary filtering surgeries.
  ii. 5% FU is also used in selected higher risk case, particularly those with MMC complications in a previous surgery or those at risk for hypotonous maculopathy.
  iii. MMC is used in most high-risk cases including aphakic or pseudo-phakic eyes, eyes with previous filtration failure surgery, eyes with a history of anterior segment neovascularization, and eyes with uveitis.
  iv. MMC is also used in selected cases of primary filtering surgery (e.g., when trabeculectomy with 5-FU has failed in the fellow eye).

11. **What is the latest advancement in glaucoma filtering surgery?**
  Photodynamic therapy with diffuse blue light coupled with a photosensitizing agent to kill fibroblasts may be another way to control the surface area of treatment and modulate healing. It will be important to determine

the effect of these agents on the overlying epithelium, because differentiated stable epithelium may have a suppressive effect on fibroblasts in the wound.

12. **What are the indications for antimetabolites in glaucoma filtering surgery?**

    i. **Patient factors:**
       - Young patients
       - Previous failed trabeculectomy
       - Previous conjunctival surgery (e.g., pterygium surgery)

    ii. **Ocular factors:**
       - Secondary glaucomas (neovascular, uveitic, traumatic, and pseudophakic glaucoma
       - Congenital/pediatric glaucoma.

13. **What are the measures to be taken to prevent antimetabolite toxicity?**

    i. Thorough irrigation after the prescribed time of applications
    ii. Water tight wound closure
    iii. Careful dissection to prevent button hole formation.

14. **What is the role of Ologen in glaucoma filtering surgeries?**

    i. Composed of 3-D collagen-glycosaminoglycan copolymers (Ologen)
    ii. Source: Porcine collagen
    iii. Mechanism of action:
       - Provides a scaffold for fibroblasts to grow randomly
       - Absorbs the aqueous and functions like a reservoir
       - Provides pressure on the sclera flap to create controlled drainage of aqueous
       - Gets biodegraded by 90–180 days.
    iv. Advantages:
       - Limits postoperative hypotony by the tamponading effect
       - Does not produce thin avascular blebs which are at risk for bleb infection and endophthalmitis
       - No special handling and disposal precautions
       - Not teratogenic like MMC.
    v. Disadvantage: LASER suture lysis is difficult when sutures are covered by the implant and not clearly visible

4.19. GLAUCOMA DRAINAGE DEVICES

1. **Define glaucoma drainage devices (GDD) (aqueous shunt devices).**

   Consists of an alloplastic tube leading to a large equatorial reservoir that drains aqueous humor from the anterior chamber.

2. **Define setons.**

   Setons are solid stents or wicks, using the principle of surface-tension flow for fluid to exit the anterior chamber, while structurally intended to maintain a patent drainage fistula.

3. **Define shunts.**

   Hollow tubular structure that allows bidirectional flow. (Open-tubed devices have been synthesized to serve as *shunts*, secured translimbally to allow flow subconjunctivally (e.g., Molteno or Baerveldt implants)).

4. **Define valves.**

   Allows unidirectional flow which needs an activating pressure to open it. For example, krupin or ahmed valve

5. **What are the common features of all GDDs?**

   i. Manufacturing drainage tube and explant portions of the devices from materials to which fibroblasts cannot firmly adhere.
   ii. Equatorial placement of explant portion of the device.
   iii. Similar diameter of all drainage tubes.
   iv. Ridge along edge of the explant plate where drainage tube inserts ensures.

   | Physical separation of enveloping capsule from posterior tube orifice | Directs the flow onto explant's upper surface |

   ↓
   Preventing occlusion.

6. **What is the principle of GDD?**

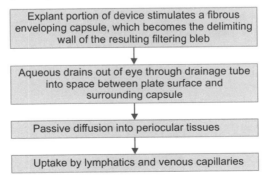

7. What are the factors that decide hydraulic conductivity of GDD?

Drainage capacity of bleb is directly proportional to surface area of capsule around explants. Resistance of capsule to flow is directly proportional to its thickness.

8. What are the indications of GDD?

All refractory glaucomas like:

    i. Uveitic glaucoma
    ii. Neovascular glaucoma
    iii. Congenital glaucoma
    iv. Refractory juvenile glaucoma
    v. Multiple failed trabeculectomy
    vi. Extensive conjunctival scarring
    vii. Post-PKP
    viii. Aniridia
    ix. Posttraumatic glaucoma.

Failed primary glaucomas

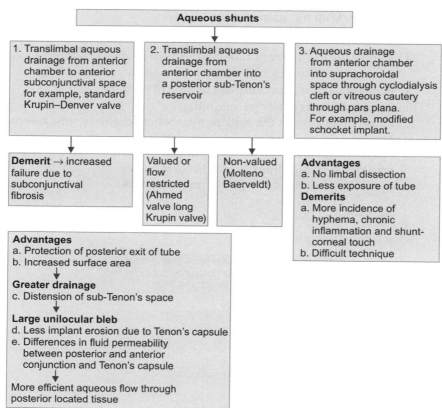

9. **Describe Molteno implant.**

   i. First implant with a nonvalved device
   ii. Material—polypropylene
   iii. Consists of a circular plate with a drainage tube
   iv. Outer diameter of drainage tube—0.63 mm
   v. Inner diameter of drainage tube—0.3 mm
   vi. Types—single plate, double plate and triple plate.

10. **Describe Baerveldt implant.**

   i. Nonvalved
   ii. Material—silicone

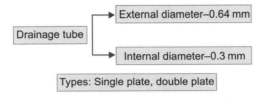

11. **Advantages of Baerveldt GDD.**

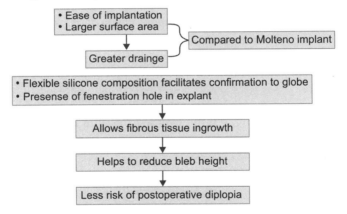

12. **What is the mechanism of action of Ahmed glaucoma valve?**

   i. Oval-shaped polypropylene plate 184 mm^2 (double plate – 364 mm^2) surface area is connected to a silicone drainage tube via 2 layers of silicone elastomer membrane that functions as a one way valve by Venturi effect (Bernoulli's principle)
   ii. Goal of keeping IOP between 8 mm Hg and 10 mm Hg
   iii. Venturi design (Bernoulli's principle).

The tension on the silicone membranes is designed to only allow outflow when the IOP is above 8–10 mm Hg. When the initial pressure in the anterior chamber is high, the valve fully opens. As the pressure is reduced, the membrane opening automatically reduces in size, diminishing the flow.

13. **Describe the optimed glaucoma pressure regulator.**

Silicone tube attached to a polymethyl methacrylate matrix of conductive resistors that regulate the flow of aqueous through capillary action.

14. **Preoperative evaluation in a case of glaucoma drainage devices.**
    i. Potential for useful vision is a must
    ii. Preoperative IOP
    iii. Upper lid position
    iv. Scleral exposure
    v. Tear film stability
    vi. Blepharitis (risk of late postoperative infection)
    vii. Corneal clarity– especially peripheral cornea
        For intraoperative
        Confirmation of tube location
    viii. Eyes with PCIOL
        – Shallow AC
        – Post PKP eyes
        – Endothelial cell function

        (All the above-mentioned risk factors are the indications for
          glaucoma drainage device with pars plana tube insertion
                          into vitreous cavity)

    ix. Presence of vitreous strands in anterior chamber → may occlude the tube tip.
    x. Cataract—for concurrent cataract surgery and glaucoma drainage device
    xi. Gonioscopy
        Assess PAS → areas to be avoided for tube insertion (peripheral anterior synechiae)
        Neovascularization of angle
        Preoperative treat to halt the

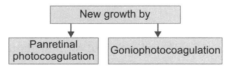

15. **What are the drugs to be stopped preoperatively?**
    i. Pilocarpine or echothiophate
        (To reduce postoperative inflammation)
        Continue all other glaucoma drugs till surgery
    ii. Warfarin.

16. **Types of surgical techniques for GDD implantation.**

i. **Limbal-based conjunctival flap**	**Fornix-based conjunctival flap**
Two layer closure securing Tenon's capsule and conjunctiva with separate running layers of absorbable sutures	If tissue coverage over the device is adequate ↓ Suturing only at lateral corners of flap

ii. **One stage installation**
  - One stage complete surgical installation with immediate function, done with devices that have flow restrictors or valves

iii. **Two stage installation**
  - Temporary ligature of tube on nonvalved devise for 2–3 weeks
  - Time for development of capsule and acceptable resistance to outflow.

17. **What are the types of temporary ligature sutures?**
  i. Rip cord—intraluminal occluding sutures left beneath the conjunctiva for pulling (4-0 chromic catgut).
  ii. Absorbable 8-0 polyglactin or 10-0 prolene tied around the tube (Released by argon laser suturolysis)
  iii. 5-0 nylon tied to side of tube and to an adjacent occluding structure like a spacer which is removed after 2–3 weeks.

18. **What is the cause of hypotony in both single and double stage techniques?**

Due to leakage around the surface of the tube, where it penetrates the eye wall.

19. **What is the difference between glaucoma drainage device bleb and trabeculectomy bleb?**

Features of GDD bleb:
  i. More posterior filtering bleb
  ii. More consistently organized surrounding capsule which is distinct and separable from overlying Tenon's capsule
  iii. Absence of conjunctival microcysts as seen in trabeculectomy.

20. **What is the preferred positioning of GDD?**
  i. Superotemporal quadrant
  ii. Centered at the equator and equally spaced between adjacent rectus muscles
  iii. Anterior edge of explant
     ↓
     8–10 mm posterior to corneoscleral junction
  iv. Explant plates are sutured to episclera
     ↓
     Complication encountered
     ↓
     Perforation of sclera.

21. **How to manage/identify perforation of sclera?**
  i. Identification → Gush of vitreous gel is seen
  ii. Management → Apply cryotherapy to the area
     Under direct observation by indirect ophthalmoscope.

22. **When do you suture the explant to the avascular insertion of superior rectus (instead of episclera)?**

    i. Staphyloma
    ii. Quiescent scleritis.

23. **What are the complications in superonasal placement of GDD?**

    i. Vertical strabismus—Pseudo-Brown's syndrome
    ii. Impact on optic nerve.

24. **What are the instances where the GDD can migrate?**

    i. Inadequate suturing
       ↓
       Posterior migration of explant
       ↓
       Extrusion of tube from anterior chamber
    ii. Postoperative hypotony
        ↓
        Drainage tube migrates anteriorly and impacts on cornea, lens or iris.

25. **Where do you place the 2nd plate in an explant with 2 plates?**

    The second plate and its interconnecting tube placed either above or below superior rectus muscle and attached by suturing in a similar manner to the first plate.

26. **How to install the drainage tube?**

Anterior chamber installation	Pars plana installation
▪ Tube shortened to the appropriate length with a sharp level to facilitate passage through a 23 gauge needle tract Tip → Beveled up surface ▪ Site of insertion ↓ Posterior edge of blue limbus ▪ Preparation of site of insertion ↓ Use wet field cautery ▪ 1.5–2 mm of tube should extend through the endothelium parallel to the plane of iris (prevents migration)	▪ Indications a. Aphakia and PCIOL eyes b. Post PKP eyes c. Eyes with shallow anterior chamber d. Decreased endothelial cell function ▪ Tip → Beveled down ▪ Needle tract oriented perpendicularly to scleral surface, 3–4 mm posterior to limbus ▪ Verify tube tip by direct visualization that it is free of vitreous ▪ Precautions: 1. Complete pars plana vitrectomy ↓ 2. Clearance of vitreous base in the quadrant of tube insertion

27. **What are the advantages of installation of drainage tube through 21 or 23 gauge needle tract compared to the traditional sclerectomy?**

    i. Ensures tight fit
    ii. Prevents aqueous leak around the tube.

28. **What are the advantages of scleral patch graft?**

    a. Covering the portion of tube exposed to lid contact (usually 3–5 mm of tube)

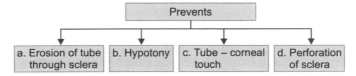

29. **How is the technique of scleral patch graft performed?**

    Full thickness scleral patch graft taken according to the size required.
    ↓
    Nonoccluding mattress suture is usually placed over the tube near its insertion.

30. **What is the complication of scleral patch graft?**

    i. Abrupt elevation of limbal conjunctiva
       ↓
       Corneal dellen formation
    ii. Scleral melt.

31. **What is the role of intracameral hyaluronic acid (Healon)?**

    Reforming the anterior chamber with intracameral hyaluronic acid at the end of the procedure through a paracentesis entry helps in:

    i. Decreasing postoperative hypotony and flat anterior chamber
    ii. Intraoperative evaluation of tube position
    iii. Slows the process of aqueous drainage in the immediate postoperative period.

32. **Compare valved and nonvalved GDD.**

    i. Advantage of valved → Simple one step procedure
    ii. Advantages regarding clinical safety and efficacy not clear over a short-term/long-term follow-up, appear to be equal.

33. **What is the principle behind sizing of nonvalved devices?**

    i. Larger devices → Younger, healthier eyes
    ii. Smaller devices → Older, sicker eyes.

34. How do you implant a modified Schocket device?

Bent 18 gauge needle is inserted into a sharp buckle capsule incision

↓

Segment of side perforated tubing fed into needle bore of 18 gauge needle and pulled into buckle capsule. (Segmented side perforated tubing later becomes intracapsular portion.)

↓

A tube segment placed between buckle capsule and anterior chamber

↓

Tight closure of buckle capsule incision

↓

Anchoring suture of 10° prolene is placed to prevent tube from slipping.

35. What is the level of IOP reduction as compared to trabeculectomy?

Percentage of IOP reduction achieved in GDD is less compared to trabeculectomy.

36. What are the contraindicated postoperative medications?

Increases vascularization of bleb capsule
  i. Miotics
 ii. Alpha agonists.

37. Complications of aqueous shunt surgery.

Intraoperative

  i. Hyphema: Injury to iris root with tube insertion
 ii. Lens damage: Improper tube length or direction
iii. Lens or corneal endothelial damage: Needle tip trauma
 iv. Scleral perforation and retinal tear; needle injury while suturing plate to globe
  v. Hypotony: Sclerotomy site too wide for tube, incomplete tube occlusion.

Early postoperative

  i. IOP elevation before occluding suture absorbs: Risk for nerves with advanced damage
 ii. Dellen: Elevated conjunctiva over patch graft causing poor tear lubrication
iii. Hypotony: Excessive aqueous run off with flat anterior chamber and choroidal effusion
 iv. Intraocular inflammation: Marked in eyes with chronic uveitis
  v. Suprachoroidal hemorrhage: Postoperative hypotony and high pre-operative IOP
 vi. Transient diplopia: Edema within the orbit and rectus muscles
vii. Endophthalmitis: Direct intraoperative contamination
viii. Aqueous misdirection: Initial postoperative hypotony and choroidal swelling.

Late postoperative

    i. Cataract progression: With or without direct mechanical injury, prolonged hypotony

    ii. Chorioretinal folds: Prolonged hypotony

    iii. Chronic iritis: History of uveitis or neovascularization

    iv. Corneal edema and graft failure; with or without cornea touch

    v. Persistent elevated IOP after tube open; thick fibrous capsule

    vi. Hypotony maculopathy: Excessive aqueous fluid runoff

    vii. Inadequate IOP control with properly functioning Baerveldt glaucoma drainage device: Hypertensive phase

    viii. Motility disturbance, strabismus, diplopia: Bleb displacement of globe, muscle fibrosis

    ix. Patch graft melting: Tube or plate erosion associated with poor lid closure, dry eye

    x. Retinal detachment: Scleral perforation, underlying disease such as diabetic retinopathy

    xi. Tube occlusion; blood, fibrin, iris, or vitreous

    xii. Tube migration: Poor fixation of plate to sclera

    xiii. Endophthalmitis: Associated with tube exposure.

38. How do you manage erosion of tube?

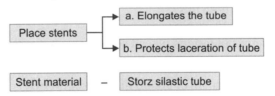

39. What are the phases of GDD surgery postoperatively?

Hypertensive phase   Hypotensive phase

Transient ↑IOP

in immediate postoperative.

40. What are the recent advances in GDD?

    i. Istent

    ii. Hydrus Schlemm's canal scaffold ivantis insertion

    iii. Cypass (suprachoroidal microstents)

    iv. Trabectome (internal trabeculotomy).

41. What is an Ex-PRESS shunt?

The Ex-PRESS shunt, consisting of a small stainless steel tube (equivalent to a 26-gauge needle) with a barbed end to anchor it in the trabecular tissue, through which it is placed on a stent and secured without suture.

4.20. CYCLODESTRUCTIVE PROCEDURES

1. **Classify cyclodestructive procedures.**

   Based on the destructive energy source
   - i. Diathermy
   - ii. β-irradiation
   - iii. Electrolysis
   - iv. Cryotherapy
   - v. Laser photocoagulation
   - vi. Therapeutic ultrasound
   - vii. Microwave cyclodestruction.

   Based on the route by which the energy reaches the ciliary process
   - i. Transscleral
   - ii. Transpupillary
   - iii. Intraocular.

2. **Describe the technique of penetrating cyclodiathermy.**

   Penetration of sclera (with or without preparation of conjunctival flap)
   Site: 2.5 mm to 5 m from corneolimbal junction
         1–1.5 mm electrode is used
         Current – 40–45 mA
         Duration – 10–20 second
   One or two rows of lesions placed several mm apart for approximately 180°.

3. **What is the mechanism of action in cyclodiathermy?**
   - i. Cell death within the ciliary body
   - ii. More posteriorly placed lesions create a draining fistula in the area of pars plana.

4. **What are the demerits of diathermy?**
   - i. Low success rate
   - ii. Hypotony
   - iii. Phthisical eye.

5. **What is the newer diathermy?**

   One pole diathermy unit.

6. **Describe the mechanism of action of cyclocryotherapy.**

   Ability of ciliary process to produce aqueous humor is destroyed by two mechanisms:
   - i. Intracellular ice crystal formation
   - ii. Ischemic necrosis.

7. **What is the additional effect of cyclocryotherapy other than IOP?**

It also causes destruction of corneal nerves and thus causes relief of pain.

8. **Describe the technique of cyclocryotherapy.**

Instruments
   i. Nitrous oxide or carbon dioxide gas cryosurgical units
   ii. Cryoprobe tips ranging from 1.5 to 4 mm. Commonly 2.5 mm is suggested for cyclocryotherapy.

Cryoprobe placement
   i. Placement of the anterior edge of probe, firmly on the sclera, 1 mm from corneolimbal junction temporally, inferiorly and nasally and 1 mm superiorly.

Number of cryoapplications
   i. 2–3 quadrants → 3–4 applications per quadrant
   ii. Rule of thumb → Treat less than 180° or 6 applications in each treatment session.

Freezing technique
   i. Temperature—60–80°C
   ii. Duration—60 seconds

Postoperative management
   i. Systemic analgesics
   ii. Topical corticosteroids—frequently
   iii. Cycloplegics
   iv. Preoperative glaucoma medications except miotics.

9. **What is the minimum time interval between repeated cyclotherapy?**

1 month.

10. **What is the additional measure taken for proper cryoprobe placement over ciliary process in cases of distorted anatomic land marks, e.g., buphthalmos?**

Transillumination (for delineating the pars plicata).

11. **List the complications of cyclocryotherapy.**
   i. Transient rise of IOP
   ii. Uveitis
   iii. Pain
   iv. Hyphema
   v. Hypotony and sometimes phthisis–Best avoided by treating a limited area each time
   vi. Choroidal detachment

    vii. Intravitreal neovascularization causing vitreous hemorrhage.
   viii. Anterior segment ischemia
     ix. Lens subluxation
      x. Sympathetic ophthalmia.

12. **List the indications for cyclocryotherapy/transscleral photocoagulation.**

      i. Relief for refractory ocular pain secondary to ↑IOP in blind eyes
     ii. Repeated failure of other glaucoma surgeries
   iii. Glaucoma following PKP
    iv. Chronic open-angle glaucoma in aphakia
     v. Congenital glaucoma
    vi. High-risk cases in which medical and other glaucoma surgical procedures have failed or not felt to be feasible
   vii. Patient who requires urgent IOP reduction but who is too sick to undergo incisional surgery.

13. **Describe the mechanism of action of transscleral cyclophotocoagulation.**

      i. *Reduced aqueous production*: Due to damage of pars plicata due to direct destruction of ciliary epithelium and reduced vascular perfusion.
     ii. *Increased aqueous outflow*: Due to increased pars plana or transscleral outflow.

14. **What are the types of lasers used in transcleral cyclophotocoagulation?**

      i. Nd:YAG lasers (yttrium-aluminum-garnet): 1064 nm
     ii. Semiconductor diode lasers: 750–810 nm
   iii. Krypton lasers

15. **What is the advantage of diode laser over Nd:YAG laser in cyclophotocoagulation?**

      i. The energy needed to produce comparable lesions is less with the diode laser than that required with the Nd:YAG laser.
     ii. Primarily because of the smaller size and greater durability of diode lasers, transscleral diode cyclophotocoagulation is currently most commonly performed cyclodestructive procedure.
   iii. Transcleral diode cyclophotocoagulation has the advantage of being quick and easy to perform.

16. **What are the advantages of semi-conductor diode lasers?**

      i. Greater absorption by uveal melanin
     ii. Solid state construction with compact size (portable)
   iii. Low maintenance requirements.

17. What are the types of cryoprobes?

Diameter   *Indications*

1 mm   — ICCE

2 mm   — Retinal cryotherapy

2.5–4 mm   — Cyclocryotherapy

> 4 mm   — Hammerhead probe –

Treatment of malignant melanoma.

18. Describe the preoperative preparation of the patient in laser cycloablation.

i. Retrobulbar anesthesia usually preferred over peribulbar.

ii. Contralateral eye patched to prevent entry of stray laser light.

19. What is the role of contact lens in Nd:YAG noncontact thermal mode?

i. Maintains lid separation

ii. Compress and blanch the conjunctiva. Allows more energy to reach ciliary body

iii. Provide measurement from the limbus (applying laser 0.5–1.5 mm behind limbus is optimum)

iv. Reduces laser back scatter at the air–tissue interface

v. Higher incidence of phthisis is observed when laser is applied with contact lens.

20. What is the protocol commonly followed for noncontact transscleral cyclophotocoagulation (Nd:YAG)?

i. 30–40 evenly spaced lesions for 360°.

ii. Approximately 8 applications per quadrant.

iii. Spare the 3 and 9 o'clock positions from laser applications due to long posterior ciliary vessels underneath.

21. What is the minimum time interval before retreatment in transscleral laser cyclophotocoagulation?

i. 1 month

ii. 2/3rd of cases do not require retreatments.

22. In which condition is a contact Nd:YAG transscleral cyclophotocoagulation indicated over a noncontact laser.

i. Pediatric patients with refractory glaucoma.

23. Describe complication of transscleral cyclophotocoagulation?

i. Conjunctival hyperemia

ii. Uveitis

iii. Malignant glaucoma

iv. Sympathetic ophthalmia

v. Ocular hypotony.

24. What are the measures taken to prevent full thickness sclerostomies?

i. Use of well-rounded, polished tips.

ii. Prior to treatment inspect the probes to make sure they are free of mucus and other debris.

iii. Constantly keep the eyeball moist.

25. What are the factors that influence the variability of tissue response in contact delivery systems?

i. Probe pressure

ii. Probe diameter

iii. Time of probe contact.

26. What is the prerequisite for transpupillary cyclophotocoagulation?

i. A sufficient number of ciliary processes (at least a quarter) must be visualized gonioscopically.

27. Describe the technique of transpupillary cyclophotocoagulation?

i. Argon laser

ii. Spot size – 100–200 μ

iii. Duration – 0.1–0.2 sec

iv. Energy level – 700–1000 mW

v. Desired effect – Produce a white discoloration as well as a brown concave burn with pigment dispersion or gas bubbles

vi. All the visible portions of ciliary processes are treated

vii. 3–5 applications for each process

viii. All visible processes treated up to a total of 180°.

28. What are the factors that decide the outcome of transpupillary cyclophotocoagulation?

i. Number of ciliary processes that can be visualized and treated

ii. Intensity of laser burns to each process

iii. Angle at which ciliary processes are visualised gonioscopically.

29. What are different types of intraocular photocoagulation?

i. With transpupillary visualization

ii. With endoscopic visualization (argon or diode laser)

30. Describe the technique of therapeutic ultrasound?

i. Immersion applicator or contact ultrasound (contains a distensible rubber membrane that can be inflated)

ii. 6–7 exposures of ultrasound delivered at an intensity level of 10 kW/cm^2 for 5 seconds each to scleral sites near the limbus.

31. **What is transscleral microwave cyclodestruction?**

   Direct application of high-frequency electromagnetic radiation over conjunctiva causes heat-induced damage to the ciliary body and causes a decreased production of aqueous humor.

32. **Describe the mechanism of action by which an ultrasound works in decrease IOP.**

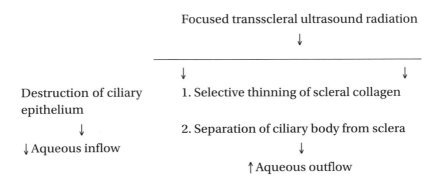

4.21. IMPORTANT GLAUCOMA STUDIES

1. **What are the important landmark studies in glaucoma?**
   i. Ocular Hypertension Treatment Study (OHTS)
   ii. Collaborative Initial Glaucoma Treatment Study (CIGTS)
   iii. Early Manifest Glaucoma Trial (EMGT)
   iv. Advanced Glaucoma Intervention Study (AGIS)
   v. Tube vs Trabeculectomy study (TvT).

2. **What are the findings of Ocular Hypertension Treatment Study (OHTS)?**

   Treating abnormally elevated IOP especially in high-risk individuals with topical medications delays or prevents the onset of glaucomatous damage.

3. **What are the findings of Collaborative Initial Glaucoma Treatment Study (CIGTS)? (Drugs vs Surgery)**
   i. To consider surgery first in patients with moderate or advanced disease
   ii. African–American patients and diabetics, however, do not do well with initial surgery
   iii. Filtering surgery is easier before eyedrops are used
   iv. Surgery reduces IOP spikes
   v. Major surgical complications were few.

4. **What are the findings of Early Manifest Glaucoma Trial (EMGT)?**
   i. Pressure lowering is beneficial in glaucoma treatment in all clinical situations
   ii. Every 1 mm of Hg of IOP reduction was associated with a risk of reduction of 10–13%.
   iii. Disease progression in patients can be variable
   iv. Mean IOP, not fluctuation, is what matters (in contrast to CIGTS).

5. **What are the results of Collaborative Normal Tension Glaucoma Study (CNTG)?**
   i. Glaucoma progression was slower in the treated group
   ii. Patients who had filtering surgery were more likely than the other patient groups to develop cataracts.

6. **What are the results of Advanced Glaucoma Intervention Study (AGIS)?**
   i. Lower mean IOP results in a reduced risk of visual field progression.
   ii. Patients were randomized to receive ALT – Trabeculectomy – Trabeculectomy (ATT) or Trabeculectomy – ALT – Trabeculectomy (TAT)
   iii. African–American patients were better off with ALT first (ATT).

7. **What are the results of tube vs trabeculectomy study (TvT)?**

   i. Tubes were as useful as trabeculectomy even in early cases
   ii. Shunts (tubes) had a higher long-term success rate and lower complications
   iii. Trabeculectomy had quicker pressure control.

CHAPTER
5

Lens and Cataract

1. **What is the size of the adult human lens?**

    It measures 9 mm equatorially and 5 mm anteroposteriorly. It weighs approximately 255 mg.

2. **What are the changes in the eye during accommodation?**
    - i. Contraction of the ciliary muscle
    - ii. Decrease in ciliary ring diameter
    - iii. Decrease in zonular tension
    - iv. More spherical shape of the lens
    - v. Decrease in lens equatorial diameter
    - vi. Increased axial lens thickness
    - vii. Steepening of the central anterior lens curvature
    - viii. Increased lens dioptric power.

3. **What is the level of amplitude of accommodation?**
    - i. Adolescents have 12–16 D of accommodation
    - ii. Adults at 40 have 4–8 D
    - iii. After 50, accommodation reduces to 2 D.

4. **What is lenticonus?**
    - i. It is a congenital, localized cone-shape deformation of the anterior or posterior lens surface.
    - ii. Anterior lenticonus is uncommon, bilateral, and associated with Alport's syndrome.
    - iii. Posterior lenticonus is more common, unilateral, and axial.

5. **What are the types of lens coloboma?**
    - i. *Primary coloboma:* Isolated wedge-shaped defect or indentation
    - ii. *Secondary coloboma:* Defect or indentation of the lens periphery caused by the lack of ciliary body or zonular development.

6. **How do you treat presbyopia during cataract surgery?**
    i. Monovision
    ii. Multifocal intraocular lens
    iii. Accommodating intraocular lens.

7. **What is Mittendorf's dot?**
    It is a remnant of the posterior pupillary membrane of the tunica vasculosa lentis and is located inferonasal to the posterior pole of the lens.

8. **What are the common causes of microspherophakia?**
    i. Weill–Marchesani syndrome
    ii. Marfan's syndrome
    iii. Peter's anomaly
    iv. Alport's syndrome
    v. Lowe syndrome.

9. **What are the common causes of cataracts in children?**
    i. **Bilateral cataracts:**
        – Idiopathic
        – Hereditary cataracts
        – Maternal infections like rubella, CMV, varicella, and syphilis
        – Ocular anomalies like aniridia and anterior segment dysgenesis syndrome.

    ii. **Unilateral cataracts:**
        – Idiopathic
        – Trauma
        – Persistent fetal vasculature
        – Posterior pole tumors.

10. **What are the conditions which can cause poorer visual result following cataract surgery in children?**
    i. Unilateral cataracts carry a poorer prognosis than bilateral cataracts
    ii. Patients with nystagmus
    iii. If adequate visual rehabilitation or treatment of amblyopia is not carried out.

11. **What are the causes of ectopia lentis?**
    i. Marfan's syndrome
    ii. Homocystinuria
    iii. Aniridia
    iv. Congenital glaucoma
    v. Trauma
    vi. Ehlers–Danlos syndrome
    vii. Sulfite oxidase deficiency

   viii. Hyperlysinemia

    ix. Ectopia lentis at papillae.

12. What are the features of Marfan's syndrome?

Systemic:

    i. Arachnodactyly

   ii. Long arm span

  iii. Chest deformities

  iv. Mitral valve prolapse

   v. Dilated aortic root

  vi. High arched palate.

Ocular:

    i. Axial myopia

   ii. Hypoplasia of dilator pupillae (difficulty in dilatation)

  iii. Superotemporal subluxation of lens

  iv. Pupillary block glaucoma

   v. Retinal detachment.

13. How is the lens status in various syndromes?

    i. *Marfan's syndrome:* Superotemporal subluxation with the presence of zonules

   ii. *Homocystinuria:* Llens subluxation inferiorly with absent zonules

  iii. *Weill–Marchesani:* Llens subluxation inferiorly along with microspherophakia.

14. What are the drugs which can cause cataracts?

    i. Corticosteroids

   ii. Phenothiazines and other antipsychotics

  iii. Topical miotics

  iv. Amiodarone

   v. Statins.

15. What is Vossius ring?

The imprinting of the pupillary ruff onto the anterior surface of the lens due to blunt trauma is termed as Vossius ring.

16. What are the characteristic types of cataract in specific situations?

    i. Trauma: Rosette cataract

   ii. Infrared rays (Glassblowers cataract): Exfoliative cataract

  iii. Chalcosis: Sunflower cataract

  iv. Diabetes: Snow-flake cataract

   v. Myotonic dystrophy: Polychromatic crystals in a Christmas tree pattern.

17. What are the experimental medical agents tried for reversal of cataracts?

 i. Aldose reductase inhibitors
 ii. Aspirin
 iii. Glutathione-raising agents.

18. What are the indications for cataract surgery?

 i. Reduced visual function due to cataract
 ii. Lens-induced disease such as phacolysis, phacoanaphylaxis, phacomorphic angle closure
 iii. Second eye cataract surgery to improve stereopsis and reduce anisometropia
 iv. Cataract limiting assessment or treatment of posterior segment disease
 v. Refractive lens extraction (clear lens) particularly in high ametropia.

19. What are the common types of cataract?

 i. Cortical cataracts: characterized by spokes, water clefts, and vacuoles due to osmotic imbalances in lens epithelial cells.
 ii. Nuclear cataract: result from accumulation of protein aggregates becoming more harder with time
 iii. Posterior subcapsular cataract: associated with diabetes, steroid use, and ocular inflammation.

20. What are the tests by which postoperative acuity can be estimated in the presence of a dense cataract?

 i. Laser interferometry
 ii. Potential acuity meter.

21. What are the tests to assess macular function in the presence of cataract?

 i. Maddox rod test
 ii. Photostress recovery time: normal is less than 50 seconds
 iii. Blue-light endoscopy
 iv. Purkinje's entoptic phenomenon
 v. ERG and
 vi. VEP.

22. What are cohesive viscoelastics?

They are high molecular weight agents with high surface tensions and high pseudoplasticity. They tend to be easily aspirated from the eye. Examples include Healon, Amvisc, Healon GV.

23. What are dispersive viscoelastics?

They are substances with low molecular weight and good coating abilities. They tend to be removed less rapidly. Examples include Viscoat and Vitrax.

24. **What are the advantages of peribulbar anesthesia as compared to retrobulbar anesthesia?**
    i. Lower risk of optic nerve damage
    ii. Lower risk of systemic neurological effects.

25. **What are the disadvantages of peribulbar anesthesia?**
    i. Need more anesthetic
    ii. More chemosis and congestion
    iii. May need more number of injections.

26. **What are the complications of retrobulbar and peribulbar anesthesia?**
    i. Retrobulbar hemorrhage
    ii. Globe penetration
    iii. Optic nerve damage
    iv. Extraocular muscle damage
    v. Neurological damage due to intrathecal penetration of drugs
    vi. Death.

27. **What are the different pump designs in phacoemulsification machines?**
    i. Peristaltic
    ii. Diaphragm
    iii. Venturi.

28. **What are the various techniques of nucleus fragmentation in phacoemulsification?**
    i. Divide and conquer
    ii. Stop and chop
    iii. Direct chop.

29. **What are the steps which can be taken to modify astigmatism following phacoemulsification?**
    i. Toric intraocular lenses
    ii. Limbal relaxing incisions
    iii. Astigmatic keratotomy.

30. **How do you treat astigmatism in cataract surgery?**
    i. Astigmatism <1 D—limbal relaxing incisions.
    ii. Astigmatism 1–3 D—toric IOL or LRIs, although toric IOLs are regarded to give more reliable results.
    iii. Astigmatism >3 D—a combination of toric IOL, LRIs (or corneal relaxing incisions) and/or strategic cataract incision placement.

31. What is SRK formula?

It was developed by Sanders, Retzlaff, and Kraff and is useful for calculating the required IOL power. IOL power $P = A - (2.5L) - 0.9K$, where "A" is the constant specific to the lens implant, "L" is the axial length and "K" is the average keratometry reading.

32. What are the various formulae used in IOL power calculation?

i. 1st generation:
- SRK
- Binkhorst
ii. 2nd generation:
- SRK II
- Hoffer
iii. 3rd generation:
- SRK-T
- Hoffer Q
- Holladay 1
iv. 4th generation:
- Holladay 2
- Haigis
- Olsen.

33. What are the commonly used IOL power calculation formulae?

i. Hoffer Q
ii. SRK/T
iii. Holladay 1, Holladay 2
iv. Haigis (especially for post-Lasik patients).

34. What are the ways to calculate IOL power in a patient who has undergone corneal refractive surgery?

i. Refractive surgery technique
   K = Pre-refractive surgery average K value + (change in refraction at corneal plane)
ii. Contact lens technique (when no pretreatment data exists)
iii. Special formulae such as Haigis formula.

35. How do you correct astigmatism during cataract surgery?

i. Incision placement: at the steepest meridian
ii. Limbal relaxing incisions
iii. Toric intraocular lenses
iv. Bio-optics (cataract followed by PRK).

36. What are the signs of posterior capsular rent?

    i. Deepening of AC
    ii. Difficulty in rotating the nuclear material that could previously rotate
    iii. Distorting pupil
    iv. Sudden appearance of red reflex
    v. Loss of followability of lens material and phaco efficacy during Phaco or I/A
    vi. Visible vitreous strands to the instrument's tip
    vii. Posterior or lateral movement of nucleus
    viii. Unusual movement or stress lines in capsular bag (capsular starring)
    ix. Frank descent of nuclear material into the vitreous
    x. If the lens does not center in the usual manner
    xi. If folded IOL becomes entangled with the capsular bag
    xii. Difficulty in aspiration of residual cortex.

37. What are the steps during which posterior capsular rent can happen?

    i. Anterior capsulorhexis
    ii. Hydrodissection
    iii. Cortex aspiration
    iv. Nucleotomy
    v. IOL implantation.

38. What are the steps to be taken in a case of intraoperative posterior capsular tear?

    i. Stop infusion of irrigating fluid
    ii. Avoid anterior chamber collapse by refilling viscoelastics
    iii. Mechanical anterior vitrectomy to take care of vitreous in the anterior chamber or in the wound
    iv Attempt retrieval of fragments only if they are accessible
    v. If a significant amount of cortex or nucleus falls into the vitreous, then pars plana vitrectomy is performed
    vi. The IOL is placed in the bag in the event of a small well-defined tear. In case of a big tear, but with an associated intact peripheral capsular rim, then the lens can be placed in the ciliary sulcus
    vii. Plan a peripheral iridectomy after IOL implantation
    viii. The incision is closed in a watertight manner
    ix. In the postoperative period, frequent use of topical steroidal drops and topical NSAIDs may be used.

39. What are the conditions which can cause shallow anterior chamber following cataract surgery?

    i. Conditions associated with increased intraocular pressure:
      – Pupillary block glaucoma

- Suprachoroidal hemorrhage
- Malignant glaucoma (ciliary block glaucoma)

ii. Conditions associated with decreased intraocular pressure
   - Leaking incision
   - Choroidal detachment.

40. How do you manage a case of aphakia?

i. Optical
   - Spectacles
   - Contact lens

ii. Surgical
   - Eyes with poor capsular support
     • Epikeratophakia
     • Iris supported IOL-iris claw lens, iris sutured PCIOL
     • Angle supported IOL
     • Scleral supported IOL
     • Capsule supported IOL
   - Eyes with good capsular support
     • In the bag placement
     • Simple sulcus placement
     • Membrane optic capture placement
     • Capsule membrane suture fixation of IOL.

41. What are the causes of glaucoma after cataract surgery?

The causes can be classified into:

i. Secondary open-angle glaucoma
   - Early causes (first postoperative week)
     • Retained viscoelastic
     • Big air bubble in AC
     • Aphakia with vitreous block
     • Damage to the angle structures intra-operatively
     • Distortion of angle due to improper suturing technique in ECCE
     • Preexisting chronic open angle glaucoma
     • Idiopathic
   - Intermediate causes (1 week to 2 months postop)
     • Preexisting chronic open angle glaucoma
     • Hyphema
     • Retained lens fragments or cortical matter in AC clogging the TM
     • Vitreous in AC
     • Post-operative inflammation
     • Steroid-induced glaucoma
     • Ghost cell glaucoma

- Late (> 2 months postop)
  - Preexisting chronic open angle glaucoma
  - Ghost cell glaucoma
  - Pressure on the angle structures by ACIOL
  - Pigment dispersion syndrome
  - Chronic inflammation
  - Uveitis Glaucoma Hyphema syndrome (UGH syndrome)
  - Pseudophakic NVG
  - Late occurring hemorrhages
  - Post ND YAG capsulotomy
  - Proliferation of iris melanocytes across TM
ii. Secondary angle-closure glaucoma
  - With pupillary block
    - Anterior hyaloid causing pupillary block
    - Optic capture
    - Hyphema blocking the pupil
    - Posterior synechiae following inflammation
    - Fibrinous aqueous
    - Silicon oil
  - Without pupillary block
    - Preexisting angle closure glaucoma
    - Inflammation/Hyphema
    - Prolonged AC shallowing
    - Iris incarceration in incision
    - IOL haptics
    - NVG
    - Epithelial/fibrous ingrowth
      Aqueous misdirection (malignant glaucoma).

42. What are the types of multifocal intraocular lenses?
  i. Diffractive: Incoming light is diffracted by an interference grid producing separate focal points simultaneously
  ii. Refractive: Optic composed of concentric rings of different power
  iii. Combined refractive and aphorized diffractive
  iv. Sector-shaped refractive.

43. What are the disadvantages of multifocal IOLs?
  i. Full correction may not be obtained
  ii. Night glare and haloes
  iii. Dysphotopsia
  iv. Decreased contrast sensitivity.

44. **What are the accommodating intraocular lenses?**

   These lenses have single optic and utilize a forward–backward axial movement of IOL in response to ciliary muscle contraction (e.g., Crystalens).

45. **What are the special steps taken for small pupil in cataract surgery?**
   i. Optimize mydriasis
      - Stop miotics in advance
      - Use topical NSAID along with mydriatics
   ii. Highly cohesive viscoelastics: used to dilate the pupil
   iii. Posterior synechiolysis
   iv. Iris hooks and pupil expanders.

46. **What are the special steps taken for zonule weakness/dehiscence?**
   i. Make the main incision opposite to the area of zonular weakness
   ii. Initiate the capsulorhexis toward the weak zonules using the intact zonules for counter traction
   iii. Use iris hooks
   iv. Careful hydrodissection and hydrodelineation
   v. Sufficient phaco power to avoid pushing the nucleus
   vi. Use capsular tension ring to stabilize the bag. If zonular loss is marked use Cionni ring and fix to sclera
   vii. Insert the leading haptic into the bag toward the area of zonular weakness and gently direct the trailing haptic into the bag with McPherson forceps.

47. **What are the special steps taken for brunescent cataract?**
   i. Larger capsulorhexis
   ii. Bottle height low to reduce irrigation volume
   iii. Move phaco tip slowly when sculpting
   iv. Use enough power to avoid pushing the lens
   v. Use burst mode of pulse mode to avoid chatter
   vi. Adequate viscoelastics, preferably a soft shell technique.

48. **What are the special steps taken for white cataract?**
   i. Use of Trypan blue 0.06%
   ii. Use smaller capsulorhexis since it may extend to periphery
   iii. Use higher density viscoelastic.

49. **What is soft shell technique?**
   i. Inject dispersive viscoelastic adjacent to the endothelium (Viscoat)
   ii. Then expand the AC below using cohesive viscoelastic, thus spreading the dispersive agent against the endothelium.

50. What are the potential risk factors for the development of posterior capsular opacification (PCO)?

  i. Younger age at surgery
  ii. Intraocular inflammation
  iii. Round-edged intraocular lenses are more prone to develop PCO than square edged IOLs
  iv. Smaller capsulorhexis
  v. Residual cortical material and anterior capsular opacity
  vi. Presence of intraocular silicon oil
  vii. PMMA IOLs are more likely to develop PCO than acrylic IOLs.

51. What are the signs of expulsive suprachoroidal hemorrhage?

  i. Sudden increase of intraocular pressure
  ii. Darkening of the red reflex
  iii. Wound gape
  iv. Expulsion of the lens, vitreous, and bright red blood
  v. Severe pain.

52. What are the risk factors for expulsive hemorrhage?

  i. Uncontrolled glaucoma
  ii. Arterial hypertension
  iii. Patients on anticoagulant therapy
  iv. Bleeding diathesis
  v. Prolonged hypotony.

53. How will you manage expulsive hemorrhage?

  i. Attempt to close the wound as quickly as possible
  ii. Posterior sclerotomies (5–7 mm posterior to the limbus).

CHAPTER
6

Retina

6.1. DIFFERENTIAL DIAGNOSIS OF RETINAL FINDINGS

1. **Retinal neovascularization**
    i. Diabetes
    ii. Retinal vein occlusion
    iii. Hypertension
    iv. Sickle cell retinopathy
    v. Ocular ischemic syndrome
    vi. Retinopathy of prematurity (ROP)
    vii. Familial exudative vitreoretinopathy
    viii. Norrie's disease
    ix. Eales' disease
    x. Inflammation: vasculitis, posterior uveitis
    xi. Hyperviscosity syndrome
    xii. Radiation retinopathy
    xiii. Talc emboli.

2. **Intraretinal hemorrhage**
    i. Diabetes
    ii. Retinal vein occlusion
    iii. Hypertension
    iv. Hyperviscosity syndrome
    v. Anemia
    vi. Ocular ischemic syndrome
    vii. Subretinal neovascularization (SRNV)
    viii. Associated with infections, e.g. HIV microangiopathy, Roth's spots
    ix. Valsalva retinopathy
    x. Eales' disease
    xi. Sickle cell retinopathy.

3. **Subretinal choroidal neovascularization**
   i. Age-related macular degeneration (ARMD)
   ii. Postinflammatory
   iii. Presumed ocular histoplasmosis syndrome (POHS)
   iv. Myopic degeneration
   v. Trauma
   vi. Dystrophies (Sorsby's, Best's, etc.)
   vii. Optic nerve drusen
   viii. Angioid streaks.

4. **Retinal telangiectasia**
   i. Diabetes
   ii. Hypertension
   iii. Previous retinal vein occlusion
   iv. Sickle cell retinopathy
   v. Idiopathic juxtafoveal telangiectasia
   vi. Radiation retinopathy
   vii. Coats' disease
   viii. Incontinentia pigmenti.

5. **Retinal vascular tortuosity**
   i. Polycythemia
   ii. Leukemia
   iii. Retinal vein occlusion
   iv. Dysproteinemia
   v. Sickle cell disease
   vi. Familial dysproteinemia
   vii. Mucopolysaccharidosis
   viii. Fabry's disease
   ix. Hyperviscosity syndrome
   x. Eales' disease
   xi. Racemose angioma
   xii. Epiretinal membrane.

6. **Retinal deposits**
   i. Exudates
      – Diabetes
      – Hypertension
      – Retinal vein occlusion
      – Vascular tumors
      – Coats' disease
   ii. Drusen
      – ARMD
      – Basal laminar drusen
      – Sorsby' fundus dystrophy

iii. Crystals	– Juxtafoveal telangiectasia
	– Tamoxifen
	– Bietti's crystalline retinopathy
	– Canthaxanthin toxicity
iv. White dots	– Multiple evanescent white dot syndrome (MEWDS)
	– Birdshot chorioretinopathy
	– Hereditary fundus albipunctatus
v. Flecks	– Stargardts
	– Fundus flavimaculatus
	– Hereditary fundus albipunctatus
vi. Yellow lesions	– Best macular dystrophy
	– Pattern dystrophy
	– ARMD
	– Harada's disease
	– Metastasis

7. **Cherry-red spots in the macula**
   i. Central retinal artery occlusion (CRAO)
   ii. Sphingolipidoses (Tay–Sachs, Gaucher, and Niemann–Pick)
   iii. Quinine toxicity
   iv. Traumatic retinal edema
   v. Ocular ischemic syndrome
   vi. Macular hole with surrounding retinal detachment.

8. **Macular edema**
   i. Diabetes mellitus
   ii. Retinal vein occlusion
   iii. Pseudophakic (Irvine–Gass)
   iv. SRNV
   v. Uveitis/scleritis
   vi. Hypertension
   vii. Choroidal ischemia
   viii. Retinitis pigmentosa
   ix. Vascular tumor
   x. Nicotinic acid toxicity.

9. **Macular star**
   i. Hypertension
   ii. Retinal vein occlusion
   iii. Papilledema
   iv. Inflammation: Choroiditis, posterior scleritis, vasculitis, neuroretinitis, toxoplasmosis, chronic infection, e.g., syphilis.

10. **Macular atrophy**
    i. ARMD
    ii. Pathological myopia
    iii. Stargardt's disease
    iv. Cone dystrophy
    v. Dominant retinal dystrophies
    vi. Best's vitelliform dystrophy
    vii. X-linked retinoschisis
    viii. Chloroquine toxicity
    ix. After pigment epithelial detachment
    x. Solar retinopathy.

11. **Bulls' eye maculopathy**
    i. Macular, cone or cone/rod dystrophies
    ii. Drug toxicity—chloroquine
    iii. Batten's disease
    iv. Benign concentric annular macular dystrophy
    v. Bardet—Biedl syndrome.

12. **Angioid streaks**
    i. Pseudoxanthoma elasticum
    ii. Paget's disease
    iii. Hemoglobinopathies
    iv. Ehlers–Danlos syndrome.

13. **Choroidal folds**
    i. Hypermetropia
    ii. Hypotony
    iii. Papilledema
    iv. Retrobular mass lesions
    v. Thyroid eye disease
    vi. Posterior scleritis
    vii. Scleral buckle
    viii. Choroidal tumors
    ix. Choroidal neovascularization.

14. **Roth spots (hemorrhage with white center)**
    i. Bacterial endocarditis
    ii. Leukemia
    iii. Severe anemia
    iv. Sickle cell disease
    v. Collagen vascular disease
    vi. Diabetes mellitus
    vii. Multiple myeloma
    viii. HIV retinopathy.

15. **Drugs causing toxic maculopathies**
    i. Aminoglycosides
    ii. Canthaxanthin
    iii. Chloroquine and hydroxy chloroquine
    iv. Chlorpromazine
    v. Quinine
    vi. Niacin
    vii. Interferon–alpha
    viii. Tamoxifen
    ix. Sildenafil (Viagra).

6.2. FUNDUS FLUORESCEIN ANGIOGRAPHY (FFA)

1. **What is luminescence, fluorescence, and phosphorescence?**

    i. Luminescence is the emission of light from any source other than high temperature. This occurs when there is absorption of electro-magnetic radiation, the electrons are elevated to higher energy states and then the energy is reemitted by spontaneous decay of the electrons to lower energy levels. When this decay occurs in visible spectrum, it is called luminescence.

    ii. Fluorescence is luminescence that is maintained only by continuous excitation, thus emission stops when excitation stops.

    iii. Phosphorescence is luminescence where the emission continues long after the excitation has stopped.

2. **What are the dyes used in ocular angiography?**

    i. Fluorescein sodium

    ii. Indocyanine green.

3. **Describe the chemical properties of fluorescein.**

    i. Orange-red crystalline hydrocarbon, related to phenolphthalein, resulting from the interaction of phthalic acid anhydride and resorcinol.

    ii. The chemical name is resorcinophthalein sodium, $C_{20}H_{10}Na_2O_5$

    iii. It has low molecular weight (376 daltons) and high solubility in water allows rapid diffusion.

4. **Describe the biophysical properties of fluorescein.**

    i. Maximum fluorescence at pH 7.4

    ii. Up to 80% protein bound (mainly albumin)

    iii. Only the remaining 20% is available for fluorescence

    iv. Rapid diffusion through intra- and extracellular spaces

    v. Elimination rapidly through liver and kidney in 24–36 hours

5. **Describe the absorption and emission peaks of fluorescein.**

    Sodium fluorescein gets excited by a light energy between 465 nm and 490 nm which is a blue spectrum and will fluoresce at a wavelength of 520 nm and 530 nm which is green yellow.

6. **What are the other uses of fluorescein in ophthalmology?**

    i. Applanation tonometry

    ii. To identify corneal epithelial defects

    iii. Contact lens fitting

    iv. Seidel's test

    v. Fluorescein dye disappearance test

vi. Ear film breakup time testing

vii. For nasolacrimal duct obstruction evaluation

viii. Fluorophotometry.

7. **What is the common bacterial contaminant of fluorescein solution?**

   Pseudomonas aeruginosa.

8. **What is fluorescein angiography?**

   It is a fundal photography performed in rapid sequence following intra-venous injection of fluorescein dye.

   It provides three main information:

   i. The flow characteristics in the blood vessels as the dye reaches and circulates through the retina.

   ii. It records fine details of the pigment epithelium and retinal circulation that may not otherwise be visible

   iii. It gives a clear picture of the retinal vessels and assessment of their functional integrity.

9. **Describe the history of FFA.**

   i. Ehrlich introduced fluorescein into investigative ophthalmology in 1882.

   ii. Chao and Flocks gave earliest description of FFA in 1958.

   iii. Novotony and Alvis introduced this into clinical use in 1961.

10. **Describe the principle of FFA.**

    Inner and outer blood–retinal barrier are the key to understand FFA. Both barriers control movement of fluid, ions, and electrolytes from intravascular to extravascular space in retina.

    i. *Inner blood–retinal barrier*

       – At the level of retinal capillary endothelium and basement membrane

       – Prevents all leaks of fluorescein and albumin-bound fluorescein

       – Thus, a clear picture of retinal blood vessels is seen in a normal angiogram.

    ii. *Outer blood–retinal barrier*

       – Composed of intact retinal pigment epithelium (RPE) which is impermeable to fluorescein

       – RPE acts as an optical barrier to fluorescein and masks choroidal circulation.

11. **What are the requirements to perform a FFA?**

    i. Fundus camera with two camera backs, timer, filters, and barrier.

    ii. 35 mm black and white film

    iii. 35 mm color film

    iv. 23 gauge scalp vein needle

   v. 5 mL syringe with 1.5 inch needle

  vi. 5 mL of 10% fluorescein solution

 vii. Tourniquet

viii. Emergency tray with medicines to counter anaphylaxis.

12. **Describe the filters used in FFA.**

   i. *A blue excitation filter* through which white light passes from the camera. The emerging blue light excites the fluorescein molecules in the retinal and choroidal circulations, which then emit light of a longer wavelength (yellow-green).

  ii. *A yellow-green barrier filter* then blocks any reflected blue light from the eye allowing only yellow-green light to pass through unimpaired to be recorded.

13. **What is the dosage of fluorescein used for FFA?**

Solutions containing 500–1,000 mg of fluorescein available in vials of

   i. 5 mL of 10% fluorescein (most commonly used)

  ii. 10 mL of 5% fluorescein

 iii. 3 mL of 25% fluorescein (preferred in opaque media).

14. **Describe the technique employed in FFA.**

A good quality angiogram requires adequate pupillary dilatation and a clear media.

   i. The patient is seated in front of the fundus camera

  ii. Fluorescein, usually 5 mL of a 10% solution is drawn up into a syringe.

 iii. A red-free image is captured

 iv. Fluorescein is injected intravenously over a few seconds.

  v. Images are taken at approximately 1 second intervals, 5–25 seconds after injection.

 vi. After the transit phase has been photographed in one eye, control pictures are taken of the opposite eye.

vii. If appropriate, late photographs may also be taken after 10 minutes and, occasionally, 20 minutes if leakage is anticipated.

15. **List some of the *main indications* for fluorescein angiography.**

Fluorescein angiography is used mainly for the study of abnormal ocular vasculature. The following are the main indications for fluorescein angiography:

   i. **Diabetic retinopathy**
  - Detecting any significant macular edema which is not clinically obvious.
  - Locating the area of edema for laser treatment.
  - Differentiating ischemic from exudative diabetic maculopathy.

- Differentiating between IRMA and new blood vessels if clinical differentiation is difficult.
- In the presence of dense asteroid hyalosis to detect occult NVE and NVD.

ii. **Retinal vein occlusion**
- Determining the integrity of the foveal capillary bed and the extent of macular edema following branch retinal vein occlusion
- Differentiating collaterals from neovascularization
- To determine capillary nonperfusion areas.

iii. **Age-related macular degeneration**
- Locate the subretinal neovascularization and determine its suitability for laser treatment.

iv. **Other indications**
- Locating subretinal neovascular membrane in various conditions (*high myopia, angioid streaks, choroidal rupture, and chorioretinitis*)
- Locating abnormal blood vessels (*e.g. idiopathic retinal telangiectasia*)
- Looking for breakdown of RPE tight junctions (*central serous retinal retinopathy*) or the blood–retinal barrier (*cystoid macular edema*)
- Help with diagnosis of retinal conditions (*e.g. Stargardt's disease gives a characteristic dark choroid*).

16. What are the contraindications of FFA?
  i. Renal failure
 ii. Juvenile asthmatics
iii. Recent cardiac illness
 iv. Previous adverse reactions
  v. Pregnancy (not proven; better to avoid).

Caution required in:
  i. Elderly patients
 ii. Blood dyscrasia
iii. Impaired lymphatic system.

17. What are the phases described in an angiogram?
  i. Choroidal (prearterial)
 ii. Arterial
iii. Arteriovenous (capillary)
 iv. Venous
  v. Late (elimination).

18. Describe the phases of a normal fluorescein angiography.
Normally 10–15 seconds elapse between dye injection and arrival of dye in the short ciliary arteries (arm to retina time). Choroidal circulation

precedes retinal circulation by 1 second. Transit of dye through the retinal circulation takes approximately 15–20 seconds.

  i. **Choroidal phase**

  Choroidal filling via the short ciliary arteries results in initial patchy filling of lobules, very quickly followed by a diffuse (blush) as dye leaks out of the choroidocapillaris. Cilioretinal vessels and prelaminar optic disk capillaries fill during this phase.

  ii. **Arterial phase**

  The central retinal artery fills about 1 second later than choroidal filling.

  iii. **Capillary phase**

  The capillaries quickly fill following the arterial phase. The perifoveal capillary network is particularly prominent as the underlying choroidal circulation is masked by luteal pigment in the retina and melanin pigment in the RPE. (At the center of this capillary ring is the foveal avascular zone (500 mm in diameter).)

  iv. **Venous phase**

  Early filling of the veins is from tributaries joining their margins, resulting in a tramline effect (laminar flow). Later, the whole diameter of the veins is filled.

  v. **Late phase**

  After 10–15 minutes little dye remains within the blood circulation. Dye which has left the blood to ocular structures is particularly visible during this phase.

19. What do you mean by laminar flow?

It happens in the venous phase of FFA. It is due to the following reasons

  i. Fluorescein from venules enter the veins along their walls.
  ii. Vascular flow is faster in the center of the lumen than on the sides, fluorescein seems to stick the sides creating the laminar pattern.
  iii. The dark central lamina is nonfluorescent blood that comes from the periphery which takes longer time to fluoresce because of its more distant location.
  iv. As the fluorescent filling increases in veins laminae eventually enlarge and meet resulting in complete fluoresce of retinal veins.

20. In which conditions does the arm to retina time increased in FFA?

  i. Carotid artery occlusion
  ii. Takayasu arteritis
  iii. Ocular ischemic syndrome
  iv. Conditions associated with reduced cardiac output.

21. What is A–V transit time?

i. It is the time from the appearance of dye in the retinal arteries to complete filling of the retinal veins.

ii. Normal—10–12 seconds.

22. Why does the fovea appear dark on FFA?

i. Absence of blood vessels in the foveal avascular zone.

ii. Blockage of background choroidal fluorescence due to increased density of xanthophyll at the fovea.

iii. Blockage of background choroidal fluorescence by the RPE cells at the fovea, which are larger and contain more melanin than elsewhere.

23. What is the normal size of foveal avascular zone?

Average is 650 microns.

Greater than 1,000 microns suggests ischemia.

24. What are the side effects of FFA?

They are transient and do not require treatment.

i. Staining of skin, sclera, tears, saliva, and urine (lasting 24–36 hours)

ii. Flushy sensation, tingling of lips, metallic taste.

25. What are the adverse reactions of FFA?

These require medical intervention.

Mild

i. Nausea and vomiting

ii. Vasovagal responses—dizziness, light-headedness.

Moderate

i. Urticaria

ii. Syncope

iii. Phlebitis

iv. Local tissue necrosis and nerve palsies (due to extravasation).

Severe

i. Respiratory—laryngeal edema, bronchospasm, anaphylaxis

ii. Neurologic—tonic clonic seizures

iii. Cardiac—arrest, death.

26. Methods to reduce the side effects of FFA.

i. Nil per oral

ii. Slow injection of the drug

iii. Reduced dosage of the drug

iv. Antiemetics.

27. **What are the abnormal fluorescein patterns?**

   i. **Hypofluorescence**

     Reduction or absence of normal fluorescence. It is any normally dark area on the positive print of any angiogram.

     It is seen in major two patterns:

     – Blocked fluorescence

     – Vascular filling defects.

   ii. **Hyperfluorescence**

     Appearance of areas that are more fluorescent which may be due to enhanced visualization of a normal density of fluorescein in the fundus or an absolute increase in the fluorescein content of the tissues.

     It is seen in several major patterns:

     – Window defect

     – Pooling of dye

     – Leakage

     – Staining of tissue.

   iii. **Pseudo fluorescence in FFA**

     – Normal occurrence in every angiogram.

     – Occurs late in angiogram.

     – Fluorescein material are activated within aqueous/vitreous and fluorescence reflected from fundus structures like optic disk.

     Pseudofluorescence is artefact of reflected fluorescein activated elsewhere in eye other than apparent fluorescence of structures due to inadequate barrier filters.

28. **What are true and false fluorescence?**

   i. Late fluorescence of optic disk: combination of true and pseudofluorescence

   ii. Dye bound to plasma protein penetrates vessel wall poorly hence only free dye enters aqueous

   iii. Dye in anterior segment is low, hence pseudofluorescence is also low.

   iv. Fluorescence of myelinated nerve fiber in late films is due to activated dye in aqueous/vitreous emitting fluorescence lately. This is called false fluorescence due to overlap of exciter and barrier filter.

29. **Describe the causes of hypofluorescence.**

   It can be because of blocked fluorescence or vascular filling defects

   i. **Blocked fluorescence**

     – *Pigments*

      RPE hypertrophy

      Melanin, xanthophyll at macula

Hemoglobin
- *Exudates*
- *Edema and transudates*
  diskiform degeneration
  Central serous retinopathy
  Detachment
- *Hemorrhage,* e.g. choroidal, retinal, subhyaloid

ii. **Vascular filling defects**

- Vascular occlusions of retinal, artery, vein, and capillary bed
- Choriocapillaries—nonperfusion, choroidal sclerosis.

30. How to differentiate blocked fluorescence and vascular filling defects?

Blocked fluorescence is most easily differentiated from hypofluorescence due to hypoperfusion by evaluating the ophthalmoscopic view where a lesion is usually visible that corresponds to the area of blocked fluorescence. If no corresponding area is visible clinically, then it is likely an area of vascular filling defect and not blocked fluorescence.

31. Describe the causes of hyperfluorescence.

i. **Preinjection phase**

Autofluorescence
Pseudofluorescence.

ii. **Increased transmission (window defect)**

- Atrophic pigment—drusen, RPE atrophy, albino epithelial window defect
- Leak
- Pooling (in space)
    - New vessels
    - Retinal
    - Subretinal—choroidal neovascular membrane (CNVM), central serous retinopathy (CSR)
- Staining (in tissue)
    - Retinal, e.g. soft exudate
    - Subretinal, e.g. drusen, scar tissue.

iii. **Abnormal vessels**

- Neovascularization
- Occlusions
- Micro- and macroaneurysms
- Telangiectasia, e.g. Coats' angiomatosis
- Shunts and collaterals subretinal
- Neovascular membrane tumors
- Retinal—retinoblastoma
- Subretinal—malignant melanoma, choridal hemangioma.

32. What is autofluorescence and pseudofluorescence?

i. *Autofluorescence* occurs when certain structures in the eye naturally fluoresce.
   - Optic nerve head drusen
   - Scar tissue
   - Astrocytic hamartoma
   - Cataractous lens.

ii. *Pseudofluorescence* is a false fluorescence indicating an inefficient filter system.
   - Old filters
   - Brand new filters
   - High humidity
   - Exposure to light.

33. What is leakage?

Leakage refers to the gradual, marked increase in fluorescence throughout the angiogram when:

i. Fluorescein molecules seep through the pigment epithelium into the subretinal space or neurosensory retina

ii. Out of retinal blood vessels into the retinal interstitium or

iii. From retinal neovascularization into the vitreous.

The borders of hyperfluorescence become increasingly blurred, and the greatest intensity of hyperfluorescence is appreciated in the late phases of the study, when the only significant fluorescein dye remaining in the eye is extravascular.

Examples include:

i. Choroidal neovascularization

ii. Microaneurysms

iii. Telangiectatic caplillaries in diabetic macular edema or

iv. Neovascularization of the disk.

34. Describe staining.

Staining refers to a pattern of hyperfluorescence where the fluorescence gradually increases in intensity through transit views and persists in late views, but its borders remain fixed throughout the angiogram process. Staining results from fluorescein entry into solid tissue or similar material that retains the fluorescein such as

i. Scar

ii. Drusen

iii. Optic nerve tissue or sclera.

35. Describe pooling.

Pooling refers to accumulation of fluorescein in a fluid filled space in the retina or choroid. The margins of the space trapping the fluorescein are usually distinct, as seen in an RPE detachment in central serous chorioretinopathy.

36. Explain transmission defect or window defect.

It refers to a view of the normal choroidal fluorescence through a defect in the pigment or loss of pigment in the RPE. In this pattern hyperfluorescence occurs early, corresponding to filling of the choroidal circulation, and reaches its greatest intensity with the peak of choroidal filling. The fluorescence does not increase in size or shape and usually fades in the late phases of the angiogram.

37. What are the angiographic findings in diabetic retinopathy?

   i. *Indications of FFA in DR*
     - Clinically significant macular edema
     - Macular ischemia
     - Fellow eye of high risk/severe PDR (asymmetric DR)
     - Suspected severe NPDR/PDR—to differentiate IRMA and NVE
     - Asteroid hyalosis
     - Featureless retina
     - To differentiate diabetic papillopathy from AION and NVD.

   ii. *Salient findings*
     The two most important phases of FFA in a diabetic eye are the mid-arteriovenous phase and the late venous phase.

     - *AV Phase*
       • The most important observations are capillary nonperfusion (CNP) areas outside the arcades and foveal avascular zone.
       • Foveal avascular zone changes in DR
         ○ Irregularity of FAZ margins
         ○ Capillary budding into FAZ
         ○ Pruning of the vessels
         ○ Widening of intercapillary spaces in perifoveal capillary bed
         ○ Enlargement of FAZ (normal diameter is 500 μ)
       • Leaking microaneurysms—many more than clinically evident are seen, and can be differentiated from dot hemorrhages
       • IRMA and new vessels are seen at the borders of CNP areas. The former leak minimally and the latter profusely.

     - *Late Phase:* Emphasizes leakage.

- *Mild non-proliferative diabetic retinopathy (NPDR)*
  - Microaneurysms—hyperfluorescent dots that may leak in later phases.
  - Superficial and deep retinal hemorrhages causing blocked choroidal fluorescence.
- *Severe NPDR:*
  - All features as in mild NPDR.
  - CNP areas—seen as areas of hypofluorescence and usually outlined by dilated capillaries unlike hypofluorescence caused by hemorrhages.
  - IRMAs—are segmental and irregular dilatation of capillary channels lying within CNP areas.
  - Venous abnormalities—such as dilatation, beading, looping, and reduplication.
  - Soft exudates cause blockage of choroidal fluorescence like retinal hemorrhages.
- *Proliferative diabetic retinopathy*
  - Neovascularization of disk (NVD) or neovascularization elsewhere (NVE) on retinal surface or elevated into vitreous—these leak the dye profusely which increases in later phase.
  - Preretinal (subhyaloid) hemorrhages are well outlined and these block both retinal and choroidal fluorescence.
- *Focal diabetic maculopathy:*
  - Focal leaks from microaneurysms in macular area.
  - Hard exudates cause blocked choroidal fluorescence.
- *Diffuse diabetic maculopathy (cystoid).*
  - Dilated retinal capillaries are seen leaking diffusely in the macular area.
  - Typical petalloid or honeycomb pattern of CME, may be seen in late phases.
  - Hard exudates typically are not seen.

38. **Describe the characteristic features of FFA in other common retinal pathologies.**
    i. **Cystoid macular edema**
       - Petalloid pattern of staining of cysts in macula
       - Disk may leak or stain
       - Leak into vitreous in late phases
    ii. Central **serous retinopathy**
       - 95% have one or more typical leakage points
       - Arteriovenous phase shows the leakage point

- In late phases
  - It spreads in all directions, i.e. ink-blot type of leakage
  - It first ascends forming smoke stack and then spreads like a mushroom or umbrella (7–20%)
- Scar will show hyperfluorescence with hypofluorescent patches
- Optic pit shows hyperfluorescence.

iii. **Macular hole**

- Pseudohole shows no abnormal fluorescence except for traction-induced retinal vascular leakage
- Outer lamellar hole—variable degree of window defect
- Inner lamellar hole—no transmitted fluorescence or minimal window defect
- Full thickness hole—granular hyperfluorescent window defects in arteriovenous phase. Surrounding elevation produces blockage of choroidal fluorescence which increase the contrast.

iv. **Branch retinal vein occlusion (BRVO)**

- Early arteriovenous phase shows delayed filling of involved vein
- Hemorrhages and cotton- wool spots produce blocked fluorescence
- NVD, NVE, capillary nonperfusion areas are seen
- Macular edema (perifoveal capillary leakage) and macular ischemia (broken FAZ)

v. **Central retinal vein occlusion (CRVO)**

- Delayed central venous filling and emptying
- Engorged and tortuous retinal veins
- NVD, NVE, capillary nonperfusion areas are seen
- Blocked fluorescence
- New vessels (early leakage) and collaterals (no leakage)

vi. **Anterior ischemic optic neuropathy (AION)**

- Early arteriovenous phase—hypofluorescence of the disk
- Mid-arteriovenous phase—patient capillaries leak and show edema
- Hypofluorescent areas remain as such due to capillary nonperfusion.

vii. **Subretinal neovascular membrane (SRNVM)**

- Early arteriovenous phase shows lacy irregular nodular hyperfluorescence
- Late phase shows leakage and pooling
- A lacy network of new vessels suggest a "classic" lesion, whereas diffuse leakage suggests an "occult lesion."

39. Describe indocyanine green (ICG) angiography.

Indocyanine green angiography is of particular value in delineating the choroidal circulation and can be a useful adjunct to FA in the investigation of macular disease in certain circumstances. About 98% of the ICG molecules bind to serum protein reducing the passage of ICG through the fenestrations of the choriocapillaries, which are impermeable to the larger protein molecules.

Indications:

   i. Exudative age-related macular degeneration
      - Occult CNV
      - CNV associated with PED
      - Recurrent CNV adjacent to laser scars
      - Identification of feeder vessels
  ii. Polypoidal choroidal vasculopathy
 iii. Chronic central serous retinopathy
  iv. Lacquer cracks and angioid streaks
   v. VKH
  vi. White dot syndromes
 vii. Choroidal melanoma.

40. Describe anterior segment angiography.

Abnormal blood vessels in the conjunctiva, cornea, and iris may be identified with fluorescein angiography.

Mainly iris angiography is done to diagnose

   i. Iris neovascularization
  ii. Iris tumors.

Findings:

   i. Normal iris vessels follow a fairly straight pattern from the iris root to the pupillary border with anastomotic connection between the vessels near the iris root and those of the collarete.
  ii. Rubeosis leak of fluorescein dye is extensive and occurs early in the angiography.

41. What is the principle of ICG angiography?:

ICG is a water soluble, tricarbocyanine anion dye with a molecular weight of 774.96 Da.

It absorbs near-infrared region of light with maximum absorption at 790 nm with a maximum emission at 835 nm.

Above 98% is bound to globulin, such as A1 – lipoprotein with negligible extra hepatic removal. High molecular weight in combination with high percentage bound to plasma protein reduces the amount of dye that exits through fenestration in choroidal vessels. Hence, it is suitable for studying the choroidal vascular network. Since it has a longer wavelength, it penetrates more and hence useful to study choroidal vessels.

42. **Why is CME stellate in the macular area as opposed to the honey-comb appearance of cystoid edema outside the macula?**

   i. The fovea contains only the following four layers of the retina—the ILM, the outer plexiform layer, the outer nuclear layer, and the rods and cones. No intermediate layers exist between the ILM and the outer plexiform layer in the fovea.

   ii. The outer plexiform layer is oblique in the foveal region, but outside the macular region, it is perpendicular.

43. **What are the other peculiarities in the macular region?**

   i. It is thinner.

   ii. The pigment epithelial cells are more columnar and have a greater concentration of melanin and lipofuscin granules than in the remainder of the fundus.

   iii. Xanthophyll is present.

   iv. Absence of retinal vessels for 400–500 mm in diameter.

44. **Why is the macular region black in FFA?**

   i. Absence of vessels

   ii. Differences in pigmentation.

6.3. ULTRASONOGRAPHY (USG)

1. What is an ultrasound?

Ultrasound is an acoustic wave that consists of oscillation of particles with a frequency greater than 20,000 Hz and hence inaudible.

2. What is the audible range?

20–20,000 Hz.

3. What is the frequency of diagnostic ophthalmic USG?

8–20 MHz.

4. What is an A-scan?

A—amplitude.
A-scan is one-dimensional acoustic display in which echoes are represented as vertical spikes. The spacing of spikes depends on the time it takes for the sound to reach an interface and the height indicates the strength of the returning echoes (i.e. amplitude).

5. What is B-scan?

B-Brightness.
B-scan produces two-dimensional acoustic sections. This requires focused beam with the frequency of 10 MHz. The echo is represented by a dot and the strength of the echo is depicted by brightness of the dot.

6. What is standardized echography?

Combined use of standardized A-scan and contact B-scan is called standardized echography.

7. What is M-mode?

M-mode (also called time motion (TM)) systems will examine temporal variations in tissue dimension, thus providing data concerning accommodation and vascular pulsations in tumors.

8. What are the basic probe orientations?

   i. Transverse
  ii. Longitudinal
 iii. Axial.

9. What are the indications for echography?

   i. Ocular media

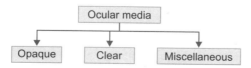

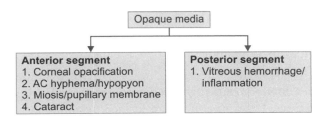

ii. Clear media

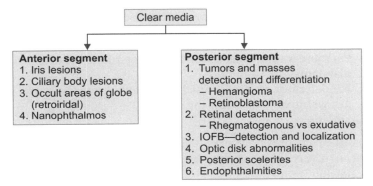

iii. **Miscellaneous**

- **Biometry:**
  - Axial eye length
  - AC depth
  - Lens thickness
  - Tumor measurement
- **Orbital indications:**
  - Pseudotumor
  - Thyroid myopathy
  - Orbital tumors.

10. **How does asteroid hyalosis show up in USG?**

   i. **B-scan**
   - Bright point like echo which is either diffuse or focal.
   - Clear area of vitreous between the posterior boundary of the opacities and the posterior hyaloid.

   ii. **A-scan**
   - Medium to high reflective spikes.

11. **How does vitreous hemorrhage (VH) show up in USG?**

   Aim:

   To establish the density and location of the hemorrhage and the cause of an unexplained hemorrhage.

Mild VH:

B-scan: Dots and short lines

A-scan: Chain of low amplitude spikes.

More dense hemorrhage

More opacities on B-scan and higher reflectivity on A-scan.

If blood organizes, larger interfaces are formed, resulting in membranous surfaces on B-scan and higher reflectivity on A-scan.

Because of gravity, blood may layer inferiorly, resulting in highly reflective pseudomembranes that may be confused with RD.

12. **How is USG useful in intraocular foreign body (IOFB)?**
    i. For more precise localization and to determine the extent of intraocular damage.
    ii. For determining, if a FB which is located next to the scleral wall, lies just within or just outside the globe.

Metallic FB

A-scan → Very high reflective spikes

B-scan → Very bright signal that persists at low sensitivity and marked shadowing (gain lowest).
    i. Standardized echography can monitor the response of FB to pulsed magnet, to determine if it can be removed magnetically.
    ii. Spherical FB (gun pellets/bullets)
        Reduplication/multiple signals due to reverberation of sound
        A-scan: Series of spikes of decreasing amplitude
        B-scan: Multiple short bright echoes in decreasing brightness
    iii. Glass FB: Produces extremely high reflection signal, only if the sound wave is perpendicular to the surface. If non-perpendicular, sound is reflected away from probe and hence, can be missed.

13. **How is USG useful in endophthalmitis?**
    i. **A-scan:** Chain of low amplitude spikes from vitreous cavity.
    ii. **B-scan:**
        – Diffuse low intensity vitreous echoes
        – Diffuse thickening of RCS complex
        – Serous/tractional RD may be seen.

14. **What is the normal RCS complex thickness?**
    1 – 1.5 mm

15. **What are the conditions with increased RCS thickness?**
    May be diffuse or focal
    i. Choroidal edema (high reflective)
        – Uveitis
        – Endophthalmitis

- Macular edema
- Vascular congestion
- Hypotony

ii. Inflammatory infiltration (low reflective)

- VKH syndrome
- Sympathetic ophthalmia
- Lymphoid hyperplasia of uvea

iii. Choroidal tumors

- Primary
- Metastatic

iv. Nanophthalmos.

16. How does PVD look in USG?

i. It can be focal or extensive and may be completely separated or remain attached to disk or at other sites (like NVE/tears/impact sites in trauma/arcades).

ii. B-scan—smooth, thick membranous with fluid undulating after movements.

iii. Scan—low (normal eye) to high (as in dense hemorrhage) reflectivity with marked horizontal and vertical spike after movements.

17. How does retinal detachment (RD) look in USG?

i. B-scan—bright, continuous folded membrane with more tethered restricted after movement—total RD is attached usually at disk and ora.

ii. A-scan—100% tall single spike at tissue sensitivity.

iii. Less than 100% spike is seen if retina is atrophic, severely folded or disrupted.

iv. Very mobile RD is seen if it is bullous.

v. Hemorrhagic RD produces echoes in the subretinal space.

vi. Configuration of RD should be determined which vary from very shallow, flat, and smooth membrane to a bullous folded and funnel-shaped membrane. The funnel shape may be open/closed and may be concave, triangular, or T-shaped.

vii. Long-standing RD may develop cyst with cholesterol crystals that produce bright echoes and RD may echolucent.

viii. Tractional RD

- Tent like if there is point adherence
- Table top RD.

18. USG findings in nanophthalmos.

i. Short axial length (14–20.5 mm)

ii. Shallow AC

iii. Diffuse RCS thickening (>2 mm)

iv. Normal-sized lens.

19. USG in choroidal melanoma.

i. Collar button or mushroom shaped-appearance
ii. Regular structure with low to medium reflectivity
iii. Marked sound attenuation on A-scan
iv. High vascularity indicated by marked spontaneous motion
v. Choroidal excavation which is seen in the base of the mass where the low reflective tumor replaces the normally high reflective choroidal layer
vi. Hemorrhage into globe and serous RD also seen.
vii. Extrascleral extension detected by well-circumscribed area of homogenicity that is situated mostly adjacent to lesion.
viii. Treated tumors—more irregular in structure, more highly reflective, and decreases in elevation.

20. USG in retinoblastoma.

A-scan—extremely high reflectivity
B-scan:

i. Large bright mass at high sensitivity
ii. At low sensitivity shows multiple bright echoes corresponding to calcium deposits
iii. Shadowing of sclera and orbit
iv. Diffuse tumor may not have calcification.

21. USG in choroidal hemangioma.

i. Solid, regularly structured, highly reflective.
ii. Internal vascularity—less pronounced than in melanoma.
iii. Lesions—mildly to moderately elevated with a dome-shaped configuration and are normally located posteriorly.

22. How will you different between thyroid myopathy and pseudotumor?

In thyroid myopathy, tendons are spared, with enlargement of muscle belly, whereas in pseudotumor, there will be diffuse enlargement of muscles (involving tendons) seen. Typical beer belly pattern is seen in thyroid-related myopathy.

23. What are the limitations of orbital ultrasonography?

i. Tumors located at the orbital apex are difficult to recognize because of the attenuation of sound and confluence of optic nerve and muscles that are inseparable ultrasonically.
ii. Tumors < 2 mm are not seen.
iii. Tumors originating/extending along the bony wall of the orbit do not present a reflecting surface perpendicular to the ultrasonic beam, and consequently do not produce distinct echoes (e.g. meningioma, osteoma, pseudotumor).
iv. Floor fractures, surgical defects of the orbital wall, as well as hyperostosis of bone, are not reliably detectable.

6.4. DIABETIC RETINOPATHY (DR)

1. **What are the characteristic features of retinal arteries?**

    Retinal arteries are end arteries.

2. **What are the various anatomical layers of retinal artery?**

    i. *Intima:* The innermost layer is composed of a single layer of endothelium.

    ii. *Internal elastic lamina:* Separates the intima from the media.

    iii. *Media:* It consists mainly of smooth muscle

    iv. *Adventitia:* It is the outermost and is composed of loose connective tissue.

3. **What are the outer and inner blood–retinal barriers?**

    i. *Outer blood–retinal barrier:* consists of basal lamina of the Bruch and zonal occludens between the retinal pigment epithelium (RPE).

    ii. *Inner blood–retinal barrier:* the endothelial cells of the capillaries linked by the tight junctions form the inner blood–retinal barrier,

4. **How do the RPE and the photoreceptors derive their nutrition?**

    RPE and layer of rods and cones are avascular and derive their nourishment from the choroidal circulation.

5. **What are the characteristics of retinal capillaries?**

    i. They supply the inner two thirds of the retina while the outer third is supplied by choriocapillaries.

    ii. There are two capillary networks—the inner (located in the ganglion cell layer) and the outer (in the inner nuclear layer).

6. **Why is proliferative diabetic retinopathy (PDR) more prevalent in insulin dependent diabetes mellitus (IDDM) than in NIDDM?**

    PDR is the result of prolonged, very high average blood glucose levels and such levels are seen more in patients with IDDM.

7. **What are the risk factors for developing DR in patients with DM?**

    i. Longer duration of the disease

    ii. Metabolic control—worsening of retinopathy occurs with poor control of hyperglycemia.

8. **What are the systemic factors which have an adverse effect on DR?**

    i. Duration of diabetes

    ii. Poor metabolic control of diabetes

    iii. Pregnancy

    iv. Hypertension

    v. Nephropathy

    vi. Anemia

    vii. Hyperlipidemia.

9. **What are the ocular conditions which decrease the progression of DR?**
   i. Chorioretinal scarring
   ii. Retinitis pigmentosa
   iii. High myopia
   iv. Optic atrophy
   (It is due to decreased retinal metabolic demand.).

10. **What are the causes of vision loss in diabetes?**
   i. **Anterior segment pathology**
      - Cornea—superficial punctuate keratitis, neurotrophic keratitis
      - Fluctuating refractive error
      - Cataract (snowflakes cataract, rapidly progressing)
   ii. **Posterior segment pathology**
      - Diabetic macular edema
      - Vitreous hemorrhage
      - Tractional and combined mechanism RD
      - Ischemic maculopathy
      - Vitreomacular traction
      - Laser or surgery-induced complications
      - Intravitreal injection-related complication
      - Neovascular glaucoma
      - Diabetic papillopathy
      - Non-arteritic anterior ischemic optic neuropathy
      - Wolfram's syndrome (type 1 diabetes, optic atrophy, hearing defect).

11. **What are the ocular manifestations of diabetes?**
   i. **Orbit**
      - Orbital cellulitis
      - Orbital mucormycosis
   ii. **Lid and adnexa**
      More susceptible for
      - Wart
      - Recurrent hordeolum
      - Blepharitis
      - Xanthelesma
   iii. **Conjunctiva**
      - Microaneurysm of bulbar conjunctiva
      - Dilatation
      - Tortuosity of vessels
   iv. **Cornea**
      - Reduced corneal sensitivity
      - Superficial punctate keratitis
      - Recurrent erosions

- Neurotrophic keratitis
- Tear film abnormality, reduced TBUT causing dry eye diseases
- Endothelial cell changes

v. **Iris**

- Rubeosis iridis
- Iris depigmentation
- Iris atrophy

vi. **Pupil**

- Miotic pupil
- Rigid pupil responding poorly to mydriatics

vii. **Lens**

Cataract—snowflakes and posterior subcapsular

viii. **Change in refractive error**

Hyperglycemia causes increased refractive index of lens and thus myopic shift where as hypoglycemia causes decreased refractive index of lens and thus inducing hyperopic shift.

ix. **Transient paralysis of accommodation**

x. **Extraocular movement**

Third, fourth, sixth nerve palsy

xi. **Retina**

Diabetic retinopathy and its sequelae like

- Vitreous hemorrhage
- Macular edema
- Isschemic maculopathy
- Tractional retinal detachment
- Combined mechanism RD

xii. **Optic disk**

- Diabetic papillopathy
- Non-arteritic ischemic optic neuropathy
- Wolfram syndrome: Optic atrophy, diabetes mellitus type 1 and hearing defect

xiii. **Glaucoma**

- More susceptible for development of POAG and its progression
- NVG Secondary to proliferative diabetic retinopathy.

12. **Explain the pathogenesis of diabetic microangiopathy.**

Diabetic microangiopathy occurs at the level of capillaries and comprise of:

i. **Capillaropathy**

- Degeneration and loss of pericytes
- Proliferation of endothelial cells
- Thickening of basement membrane and occlusion.

ii. **Hematological changes**

- Deformation of erythrocytes and rouleaux formation
- Changes in RBC leading to defective oxygen transport
- Increased plasma viscosity
- Increased stickiness and aggregation of platelets.

These changes result in microvascular occlusion and leakage.

13. **Mention the retinal vascular changes in DR.**

   i. *Capillaries:*
   - Occlusion
   - Dilatation
   - Microaneurysms
   - Abnormal permeability.

   ii. *Arterioles:*
   - Narrowing of terminal arterioles
   - Occlusion
   - Sheathing.

   iii. *Veins:*
   - Tortuosity
   - Looping
   - Beading
   - Sausage like segmentation.

14. **What are the functions of basement membrane?**

   i. Structural integrity to blood vessels
   ii. Filtration barrier for molecules of various sizes and charges
   iii. Regulate cell proliferation and differentiation.

15. **What is the ratio of endothelium cells to pericytes?**

   Normal endothelial cell: pericyte ratio is 1:1 and there is loss of intramural pericytes in DM.

16. **What are the causes of breakdown of blood–retinal barrier?**

   i. Opening of tight junction between adjacent endothelial cell processes
   ii. Fenestration of the endothelial cell cytoplasm (normally—absent)
   iii. Increased in foldings of plasma membrane at the basal surface of RPE cells
   iv. Increased transport by endocytic vessels.

17. **How does microvascular leakage occur?**

   Loss of pericyte results in distention of capillary walls which leads to breakdown in blood–retinal barrier and leakage of plasma.

18. **What is the cause of endothelial cell damage in DR?**

   It is due to increased sorbitol level in endothelial cells.

19. **What are the causes of RBC changes in DR?**

    It is due to increased growth hormone.

20. **What is the cause of increased platelet stickiness in DR?**

    Due to increased factor VIII.

21. **What are the features of non-proliferative diabetic retinopathy (NPDR)?**

    i. Retinal microvascular changes are limited to the confines of the retina and do not extend beyond the internal limiting membrane.
    ii. Findings include microaneurysms, areas of capillary nonperfusion, dot and blot retinal hemorrhages, and vascular abnormalities.

22. **What are the causes of defective vision in diabetic retinopathy?**

    i. **Retinal causes:**
       - Macular edema
       - Macular ischemia
       - Tractional retinal detachment involving macula
       - Rhegmatogenous retinal detachment involving macula (secondary to contraction of FVP causing retinal break)
       - Combined rhegmatogenous and tractional retinal detachment involving macula
       - Macular distortion secondary to contraction of fibrovascular proliferation
       - RPE atrophy and subretinal fibrosis (in long-standing DME)
       - Epiretinal membrane
       - Circinate retinopathy
       - Massive lipid exudation in lipaemia retinalis.
    ii. **Nonretinal causes:**
       - Neovascular glaucoma
       - Erythroclastic (RBC-induced) glaucoma
       - Ghost cell glaucoma
       - Snowflake cataract
       - Vitreous hemorrhage
       - Dense premacular subhyaloid hemorrhage
       - Diabetic papillopathy.

23. **Of these, what is the most important cause of defective vision?**

    Macular edema.

24. **What are the characteristic features of macula?**

    It is an area bounded by temporal arcades, 4 mm temporal, 0.8 mm inferior to the optic disk.
    It is 5 mm in diameter/3.5 disk diameter/18 degrees of visual angle
    Histologically, it has more than one layer of ganglion cells and has xanthophyll pigments.

25. What are the characteristic features of fovea?

It is an area of depression inside macula

It is 1.5 mm in diameter/1 disk diameter/5 degrees of visual angle

Histologically it has 6–8 layers of ganglion cells, tall RPE cells and a thick internal limiting membrane.

26. What are the characteristic features of foveola?

It is the central floor of fovea

It is 0.35 mm in diameter/0.2 disk diameter/0.54 minutes of visual angle

It is the thinnest part of retina. It has no ganglion cells or rods. It has only cones (150,000/mm²).

27. How will you classify diabetic retinopathy?

    i. Mild NPDR: At least one microaneurysm

    ii. Moderate NPDR:

       – Intraretinal hemorrhage or microaneurysm <ETDRS standard photograph 2A

       – Cotton wool spots, venous beading, and IRMA

   iii. Severe NPDR: 4:2:1 rule

   iv. Very severe NPDR: At least two of the criteria for severe NPDR

    v. High risk PDR

       – NVD >1/2 disk area

       – NVD plus vitreous or preretinal hemorrhage

       – NVE >1/2 disk area plus preretinal or vitreous hemorrhage

   vi. Advanced PDR: Tractional retinal detachment

28. Where will you find microaneurysms?

Between superior and temporal vascular arcades and within center of the circinate (wreath).

29. What is the size of the microaneurysm?

Minimum size of the microaneurysm should be 20 μ to be seen by DO.

30. What are microaneurysms?

They are localized saccular outpouchings of the capillary wall, often caused by pericyte loss. They are continuous with the blood vessels. They appear as red round intraretinal lesions of 30–120 μ in size and are located in the inner nuclear layer of the retina. However, clinically they are indistinguishable from dot hemorrhages. Fluorescein angiogram reveals hyperfluorescence. They are saccular outpouchings of the capillary wall probably arising at the weak points due to loss of pericytes.

31. What are hard exudates and where are they located?

They are caused by chronic localized retinal edema and appear at the junction of the normal and edematous retina. They are composed of lipoproteins and lipid-filled macrophages and are located mainly in the outer plexiform layer of the retina. FFA shows hypofluorescence.

32. **How do you differentiate drusen and hard exudates?**

   Drusen:

   i. Oval or round

   ii. Whitish or yellowish in color

   iii. Punched out areas of choroid or pigment epithelial atrophy

   Hard exudates:

   i. Waxy yellow lesions with distinct margin

   ii. Other features of DR-like microaneurysms and hemorrhages will be present.

33. **Why are the retinal superficial hemorrhages flame shaped?**

   These hemorrhages occur at the nerve fiber layer and they are flame shaped since they follow the architecture of the nerve fiber layer. They arise from superficial precapillary arterioles.

34. **Why are the inner retinal hemorrhages dot shaped?**

   This is because the inner retinal structures are perpendicular to the retinal surface.

35. **What are cotton wool spots?**

   Cotton wool spots are due to the ischemic infarction of the nerve fiber layer. Because of the ischemia, interruption of axoplasmic flow happens and buildup of transported material within axons occurs.

36. **What are causes of cotton wool spots?**

   They are:

   i. *Systemic diseases*

   - Diabetes
   - Hypertension
   - Collagen vascular diseases

   ii. *Vascular*

   - CRVO
   - BRVO

   iii. *Infections*

   - HIV retinopathy
   - Toxoplasmosis

   iv. *Hematological*

   - Leukemias
   - Anemia
   - Hypercoagulable states

v. *Others*
- Radiation retinopathy
- Purtchers retinopathy
- Interferon therapy.

37. Describe IRMA.

Intraretinal microvascular abnormality (IRMA) is frequently seen adjacent to capillary closure and they resemble focal areas of flat retinal neovascularization clinically. These are arteriovenous shunts that run from arterioles to venules. IRMA indicates severe NPDR and may herald the onset of the preproliferative stage of diabetic retinopathy (PPDR).

38. What is the difference between retinal collaterals, shunts, and neovascularization?

Collaterals: These are vessels which develop within the framework of the existing retinal vascular network. Collaterals originate from the retinal capillary bed, joining obstructed to non-obstructed adjacent vessels, or bypassing obstructions in a single vessel; i.e. veins are linked to veins, arteries linked to arteries, and less frequently, arteries are joined to veins. Flow these channels are generally slow. For example, branched retinal artery occlusion, retinal vein occlusion, sickle cell hemoglobinopathies, Leber's multiple military aneurysms

Shunts: These are arteriovenous communications, congenital, or developmental, in which blood passes directly from artery to vein without going through the normal capillary bed. Flow in these vessels is usually rapid. These vessels do not leak on FFA except large vascular malformations. For example, retinal angioma, Takayasu disease, Coats' disease

Neovascularization: These are new vessels originating and contiguous with the preexisting retinal vascular bed. They are located either within or adjacent to ischemic areas. These vessels usually leak on FFA. For example, proliferative diabetic retinopathy, CRVO, Coats' disease, Eales' disease, etc.

39. Why retinal edema commonly occurs at macula?
 i. High metabolic activity
 ii. Extremely high concentration of cells
 iii. Central avascular zone creates a watershed arrangement between the retinal and choroidal circulation, thus reducing the absorption of fluid.
 iv. Thickness and loose binding of inner connection fibers in Henle's layer
 v. Radial arrangement of Henle's layer
 vi. Lack of inner layers at the fovea.

40. Explain the pathological changes of diabetic maculopathy.

They are classified into:

i. **Intraretinal**
   - Macular edema
   - Macular ischemia

ii. **Preretinal**
   - Thickened posterior hyaloid
   - Thickened preretinal membrane
   - Macular traction
   - Macular ectopia.

41. What is normal foveal thickness?

According to ETDRS definition

i. Foveal thickness (212 ± 20 µm)—mean thickness in the central 1,000-µm diameter area

ii. Central foveal thickness (182 ± 23 µm)—mean thickness at the point of intersection of six radial scans.

42. What are the reasons for focal and diffuse macular edema?

This is the most common cause of visual impairment in the diabetic patients.

Focal edema: Due to localized leakage from microaneurysm leading to hard exudates ring formation and retinal thickening.

Diffuse edema (> 2 DD size): Due to generalized leakage from decompensated capillaries throughout the posterior pole.

43. What is clinical significant macular edema (CSME)?

i. Retinal thickening at or within 500 µ of the center of macula

ii. Hard exudates at or within 500 µ of the center of macula with adjacent retinal thickening

iii. Retinal thickening of 1 disk diameter (DD) or larger, any part of which is within 1 DD of the center of the fovea.

44. How does macular ischemia look clinically?

i. Signs are variable: Multiple cotton wool spots and attenuated arterioles may be seen.

ii. Macula may look relatively normal despite reduced visual acuity.

45. What are the FFA characteristics of macular ischemia?

i. Focal capillary dropout

ii. Enlargement of foveal avascular zone (FAZ)

iii. Occlusion of arterioles of the macula.

46. How do you manage clinically significant diabetic macular edema?

   i. Maximize medical control of blood glucose and blood pressure.

   ii. If it is a noncentric DMO, but meeting criteria of CCSMO with modified ETDS macular laser.

      Spot size: 100 µ

      Time: 0.1 second

      Space: 1 spot size apart

   iii. Center involving DMO >400 microns is treated with intravitreal injections of Ranibizumab (supported by NICE trial). Given monthly till vision is stable for 3 months. If the patient is pregnant or does not want the injection, then laser can be given.

   iv. To consider intravitreal fluocinolone acetonide for longstanding nonresponsive diabetic macular edema.

   v. *Surgery:*

      In cases with posterior hyaloid traction, pars plana vitrectomy and detachment of posterior hyaloid may be useful for treating DME.

47. Protocol for DME management

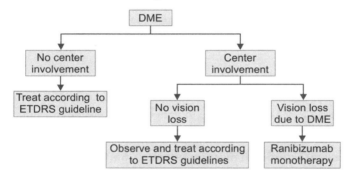

48. What are the characteristic features of preproliferative diabetic retinopathy?

   i. **Clinical features:**

     – Presence of cotton wool spots

     – Presence of IRMA

     – Venous beading

     – Narrowing of vessels

     – Dark blot hemorrhages.

   ii. **Fluorescein angiogram features:**

     – Extension of papillary nonperfusion areas.

49. What is the 4:2:1 rule?

ETDRS investigators developed the 4:2:1 rule to help clinicians identify patients at greater risk of progression.

    i. Diffuse intraretinal hemorrhages and microaneurysms in **4** quadrants

    ii. Venous beading in **2** quadrants

    iii. IRMAs in **1** quadrant.

50. What is the incidence of proliferative diabetic retinopathy in diabetic population?

5–10%. Type I patients are typically at risk.

51. What is the cause of neovascularization?

    i. Liberation of vasoformative angiogenic growth factors (VEGF, placental growth factor, pigment epithelial factor) elaborated by the hypoxic retina in an attempt to revascularize hypoxic areas are thought to produce neovascularization.

    ii. Inhibition of endogenous inhibitors like endostatin and angiostatin.

52. What is the common site for neovascularization?

It is mainly along major temporal arcade at the posterior pole and over the disk, arising most frequently from veins. Predilection of neovascularization over the disk to bleed is due to absence of internal limiting membrane and hence NVD is more dangerous than NVE.

53. What is high risk PDR?

High risk PDR was defined in the diabetic retinopathy study (DRS) as any one of the following:

    i. Mild NVD with vitreous hemorrhage

    ii. Moderate to severe NVD with or without vitreous hemorrhage ($\geq$ DRS standard 10A, showing one-fourth to one-third disk area of NVD).

    iii. Moderate NVE (one-half disk area) with vitreous hemorrhage.

54. What is the appearance of vitreous hemorrhage on ophthalmoscopic examination?

Black in color.

55. What are the various stages in the development of PDR?

    i. Fine new vessels with minimal fibrous tissue cross and extend beyond the ILM.

    ii. New vessels increase in size and extent with an increased fibrous component.

    iii. New vessels regress, leaving residual fibrovascular proliferation along the posterior hyaloid.

56. What is the most common type of RD that occurs in diabetes?

    i. Tractional RD

    ii. Combined RD and rhegmatogenous RD also occur.

57. What are the current indications for pars plana vitrectomy in PDR?

   i. Dense, non-clearing vitreous hemorrhage (VH).

   ii. Tractional retinal detachment involving or threatening macula

   iii. Combined tractional and rhegmatogenous retinal detachment

   iv. Diffuse diabetic macular edema associated with posterior hyaloid traction

   v. Significant recurrent vitreous hemorrhage despite maximal PRP.

58. What are the complications of PDR?

   i. Persistent VH

   ii. Tractional RD

   iii. Development of opaque membranes on posterior surface of detached hyaloid

   iv. Rubeosis iridis and NVG.

59. What are the landmark studies in DR?

   i. *Epidemiological studies:*

       – Wisconsin Epidemiology Study of DR (WESDR)

         In type I diabetics, retinopathy was seen in 13% of those with less than a 5-year duration of DM and in 90% of those with a duration of 10–15 years.

         In type II, in people not taking insulin, the corresponding rates are 24% and 53%.

   ii. *Studies which measured the efficacy of photocoagulation:*

       – DRS—proved the use of photocoagulation in the treatment

       – ETDRS—gave data regarding when to do photocoagulation.

   iii. *Study which measured the efficacy of vitrectomy:*

       – DRVS—proved the advantage of early vitrectomy in VH complicating PDR.

   iv. *Studies which measured the efficacy of metabolic control:*

       – DCCT—intensive glycemic control reduces DR and other microvascular complications of diabetes.

       – UKPDS—United Kingdom Prospective Diabetes Study.

       – Action to control cardiovascular risk in diabetes (ACCORD): Very intensive control of diabetes (HbA1C less than 6%) caused increased rate of death.

   v. *Studies measuring the efficacy of intravitreal injections:*

       – Diabetic retinopathy clinical research (DRCR) network: It showed that Ranibizumab was superior to laser or triamcinolone in diabetic macular edema.

       – READ 2 and RESTORE: Found that Ranibizumab was visually superior to laser alone in diabetic macular edema.

       – RISE and RIDE, and RESOLVE: showed Ranibizumab was superior to sham, for the treatment of diabetic macular edema.

60. What are the differential diagnosis for NPDR?

   i. CRVO
   ii. BRVO
   iii. Ocular ischemic syndrome
   iv. Hypertensive retinopathy
   v. Leukemia
   vi. Anemia
   vii. HIV microangiopathy.

61. What are the differential diagnosis for PDR?

   i. Vascular obstruction
   ii. Sickle cell retinopathy
   iii. Ocular ischemic syndrome
   iv. Sarcoidosis
   v. Eales' disease
   vi. Tuberculosis
   vii. Embolization from intravenous drug use.

62. What are the differential diagnosis for diabetic macular edema?

   i. CRVO or BRVO
   ii. Postoperative CME
   iii. Neovascular ARMD
   iv. Uveitic cystoid macular edema
   v. Epiretinal membrane
   vi. Vitreomacular traction
   vii. Hypotonous maculopathy.

63. What was the main study objective of diabetic retinopathy study (DRS)?

   If photocoagulation reduced the risk of severe visual loss in proliferative diabetic retinopathy.

64. What were the major methodology aspects of DRS?

   i. Randomization
   ii. One eye of each patient was assigned randomly to PHC (argon or xenon) and other eye for follow up. Eye on treatment was randomly assigned to argon or xenon arc.

65. What was the inference of DRS?

   i. Photocoagulation reduced risk of severe visual loss by 50% or more
   ii. Modest risks of decrease in visual acuity and constriction of visual fields (more for xenon)
   iii. Treatment benefit outweighs risks for eyes with high risk PDR.

66. What were the main study questions of early treatment diabetic retinopathy study (ETDRS)?

   i. Is photocoagulation effective in treating diabetic macular edema?

   ii. Is photocoagulation effective for treating diabetic retinopathy?

  iii. Is aspirin effective for preventing progression of diabetic retinopathy?

67. What were the results of ETDRS?

    i. *Aspirin use results:*

      – Aspirin use did not alter progression of diabetic retinopathy but reduced risk of cardiovascular morbidity and mortality.

   ii. *Early scatter photocoagulation results:*

      – Early scatter photocoagulation resulted in a small reduction in the risk of severe visual loss.

      – Early scatter photocoagulation is not indicated for eyes with mild to moderate diabetic retinopathy.

      – Early scatter photocoagulation may be most effective in patients with type 2 diabetes.

  iii. *Macular edema results:*

      – Focal photocoagulation for DME decreased risk of moderate visual loss, reduced retinal thickening and increased the chance of moderate visual gain.

68. What was the main study question of diabetic retinopathy vitrectomy study (DRVS)?

To evaluate the natural course and effect of surgical intervention on severe PDR and its complications.

69. What were the clinical recommendations?

    i. Early vitrectomy is advantageous for severe vitreous hemorrhage causing significant decrease in vision especially in type I diabetics.

   ii. Greater urgency for early surgery in uncontrolled fibrovascular proliferation or when proliferation has been treated partially by scatter photocoagulation.

  iii. Eyes with traction detachment not involving the fovea and producing visual loss do not need surgery until there is detachment of fovea, provided proliferation process is not severe.

70. What were the main study questions of diabetes control and complication trial (DCCT)?

    i. **Primary prevention study:** Will intensive control of blood glucose slow development and subsequent progression of diabetic retinopathy?

   ii. **Secondary prevention study:** Will intensive control of blood glucose slow progression of diabetic retinopathy?

71. What were the main study outcomes of DCCT?

    i. Intensive control reduced the risk of developing retinopathy and also slowed the progression of retinopathy.

ii. Intensive control also reduced the risk of clinical neuropathy and albuminuria.

72. **What were the study questions of United Kingdom Prospective Diabetes Study (UKPDS)?**

Will intensive control of blood glucose and intensive control of blood pressure reduce the risk of microvascular complications of DR?

73. **What were the main study outcomes of UKPDS?**

Intensive control of diabetes and blood pressure slowed the progression of diabetic retinopathy and reduced the risk of other microvascular complications of DR.

74. **What are the recent newer protocols in DRCR.net?**

    i. **PROTOCOL T**

    To determine relative efficacy and safety of intravitreous aflibercept, bevacizumab, ranibizumab in the treatment of diabetic macular edema.

    Conclusion:
    When the initial visual acuity loss was mild and there were no apparent differences, at worse levels of initial visual acuity aflibercept was more effective at improving the vision.

    ii. **PROTOCOL S**

    Panretinal photocoagulation vs intravitreous ranibizumab for PDR.

    Conclusion:
    Among eyes with PDR, treatment with ranibizumab resulted in visual acuity that was not inferior to PRP at 2 years.
    Although longer-term follow-up is need, ranibizumab may be a reasonable treatment alternative for patients with PDR.

    iii. **PROTOCOL I**

    Intravitreal ranibizumab for diabetic macular edema with prompt vs deferred laser treatment.

    Conclusion:
    5-year result suggest focal or grid laser treatment at initiation of intravitreal ranibuzumab is no better than deferring laser treatment for >24 weeks in eye with center involving DME with visual impairment.
    More than half of eyes in which laser treatment deferred may avoid laser for at least 5 years. Such eyes may require more injections to achieve these results.

6.5. LASERS IN DIABETIC RETINOPATHY

1. **What does the word LASER stand for and what is its basic principle?**

   LASER stands for **L**ight **A**mplification by **S**timulated **E**mission of **R**adiation.

   Principle: Electrons in lasing medium are excited to higher energy level, which then decay to a lower energy state with the release of a photon, which may be spontaneous or stimulated emission. This photon is then to target the tissue of interest.

2. **What are the types of laser tissue interaction?**

   i. Photocoagulation—absorption of light by pigments causes 10–20°C rise in temperature leading to protein denaturation/coagulation. For example, PRP for high-risk PDR.

   ii. Photoablation—high energy ultraviolet rays are used to break covalent bonds. For example, Excimer laser for refractive surgery.

   iii. Photodisruption—high energy pulsed laser strips electrons from molecules which form plasma. This expands causing a mechanical shock wave displacing tissue. For example, Nd-YAG laser capsulotomy.

   iv. Photoactivation—conversion of a chemical from one form to another using light. For example, Photodynamic therapy using verteporfin.

3. **What are the types of laser tissue interaction in the eye?**

   i. *Photochemical effects:*
      - Photoradiation (dye laser)
      - Photoablation (excimer lasers)

   ii. *Thermal effects:* Photocoagulation (argon, krypton laser)

   iii. *Ionizing effect:* Photodisruption (Nd:YAG laser).

4. **How does laser work?**

   The lasing material is placed in a resonant cavity, which has a mirror at each end. When a photon encounters an excited electron and stimulated emission occurs, the light emitted travels to and fro in the cavity and reinforces itself, producing coherent, monochromatic, and collimated light.

5. **What are the different types of lasers used?**

   i. **Based on types of laser media, lasers are classified as:**
      - **Solid-state lasers**
        - Ruby laser
        - Nd:YAG laser

- **Gas lasers**
  - Argon laser
  - Krypton laser
  - CO_2 laser
- **Liquid lasers**

  Dye laser (not much popular)
- **Semiconductor lasers**

  Diode lasers

ii. **Based on types of output modes:**

- **Continuous wave:** Coherent, monochromatic, and collimated light are produced continuously, e.g. argon lasers.
- **Pulsed mode**
  - **Mode locked:** Pulses in Q-switched mode are separated from each other by a specific time interval and all the wavelenghts are in phase.
  - **Q-switched mode:** Single, brief, and very high power pulsed, e.g. Nd:YAG, CO_2.
  - **Rerunning mode:** The pulses are not separated by specific time interval and the wavelengths are not in place.

6. What does solid-state laser use?

Solid-state lasers are ruby laser, Nd:YAG laser. The active element in ruby laser is chromium ion incorporated in sapphire crystal. In the Nd:YAG, the yttrium-aluminum-garnet is doped with neodymium ions.

7. What does gas laser use?

The gas lasers have an ionized rare gas as their active medium. For example argon and krypton lasers are ion lasers.

8. What does tunable dye laser mean?

It is a fluorescent organic compound dissolved in liquid solvent which, when optically pumped by laser/flash lamp laser, can emit laser radiation over a wide range of wavelength. The output wavelength can be changed over the possible lasing band by varying the tuning element.

9. What is phototherapy?

Necrosis of tumor/neovascularization using locally/systematically administered photosensitizer.

10. Mechanism by which phototherapy works?

Photochemically sensitized target tissue, when exposed to laser of proper wavelength, releases singlet oxygen. This damages the lesion by lipid per-oxidation. For example photodynamic therapy—verteporfin.

11. Few important lasers and their properties?

Laser type	Wavelength (nm)	Active medium	Primary damage mechanism	Applications
1. Argon	488–514	Gas	Photothermal Photochemical	Trabeculoplasty Iridotomy Iridoplasty PRP/PDT Laser Suturolysis Sclerotomy
2. CO_2	10,600 (Far IR)	Gas	Photothermal	▪ Oculoplastic surgery ▪ Laser Phacolysis ▪ Sclerostomy
3. Excimer	193 (UV)	Gas (Ar/F)	Photochemical	LASIK LASEK PRK/PTK Trabeculoplasty Sclerostomy
4. Nd:YAG	532 (green) 1064 (near IR)	Solid neodymium ion in yttrium aluminum **garnet** matrix	Photo disruption Photothermal	Capsulotomy Iridotomy Trabeculoplasty Phakolysis Sclerostomy PRP Cyclophotocoagulation Oculoplastic Surgery
5. Diode	(620–895) Red and IR	Solid **gallium** aluminum	Photothermal	PRP Iridotomy Iridoplasty Sclerostomy Suturolysis Trabeculoplasty Cyclophotocoagulation
6. Dye	310–1200 (UV-visible IR)	Fluorescent dye	Photothermal Photochemical	PKP PDT Iridotomy Sclerostomy Suturolysis

12. What are the lenses used in laser photocoagulation?

Negative power plano-concave lens	High plus power lens
Upright image	Real and inverted image
Superior image of small retinal area (focal laser)	Loss of fine resolution with wide field of view (PRP)
Same spot size as that selected	Magnifies the spot size selected
Hruby lens	Goldmann lens Rodenstock panfundoscope Mainster lenses PRP 165, focal/grid Volk lenses—superquad 160, area centralis

Lenses used for panretinal photocoagulation

Lens	Image magnification	Laser spot magnification	Field of view
Goldmann 3 mirror	0.93x	1.08x	140°
Mainster PRP 165	0.68x	1.96x	165–180°
Volk superquad	0.50x	2.00x	160–165°
Volk quadraspheric	0.51x	1.97x	120–144°

Lenses used in focal/grid laser photocoagulation

Lens	Image magnification	Laser spot magnification	Field of view
Mainster focal/grid	0.96x	1.05x	90–121°
Mainster high mag	1.25x	0.8x	75–88°
Volk area centralis	1.06x	0.94x	70–84°

13. How can you increase the burn intensity?

$$\text{Burn intensity} = \frac{(\text{Burn duration}) \times (\text{Power setting})}{\text{Spot size}}$$

So intensity can be increased by:
- ↑ duration
- ↑ power
- ↑ spot size.

14. How does Nd:YAG laser work?

It uses a trivalent neodymium ion, which is excited in YAG matrix by an external exciting source (flash lamp/other laser diode).

15. What is the special property of Nd:YAG?

Nd ion laser works at 1064 nm (near infrared) and can be used as a continuous wave laser. Because of longer wavelength, it would penetrate tissue which would otherwise scatter shorter wavelength.

16. How can it frequency doubled?

Bypassing through KTP crystal (potassium titanium phosphate). The emitted wavelength is 532 nm.

17. What is the use of frequency doubling?

At this wavelength, it is well absorbed by hemoglobin and RPE and hardly any by xanthophyll. This property makes it excellent for use in retina and vitreous disorders.

18. What is Q-switching?

Q-switching causes giant pulse formation.

In this technique a laser can be made to produce a pulsed output beam. Because the pulse duration is so short, the total power delivered per pulse is not very high but the peak power per pulse is very high.

19. What are the uses of Q-switched Nd:YAG laser?

i. Capsulotomy
ii. Iridotomy
    Hyaloidotomy—release of loculated preretinal blood into vitreous cavity.

20. What are the properties of laser light?

i. *Coherence:* The photons are in phase with each other in time and space.
ii. *Collimation:* Light amplification of photons produced in parallel beam.
iii. *Monochromatic:* Photons are emitted in a single wavelength.
iv. *High intensity.*

21. What is the difference between photocoagulation and photoablation?

Photocoagulation: Process, by which light energy is converted into heat energy, resulting in coagulation of tissue proteins and producing a burn.
Photoablation: High energy photons are able to break the intramolecular bonds of the corneal surface tissue enabling a fine layer to be removed with each pulse without thermal damage to remaining cornea.

22. What are the fundus pigments?

i. Melanin—in RPE and choroids
ii. Xanthophyll—in macula (ganglion cells)
iii. Hemoglobin—in blood vessels.

23. What is the absorption spectrum of pigments in the retina?

Pigments in the retina	Absorbs	Reflects
Melanin	All wavelength	
Xanthophyll	Blue	Yellow and red
Hemoglobin	Blue, green, and yellow	Red

24. **What are the various parameters used in laser photocoagulation?**
    i. Spot size—ranges 50 μ–1,000 μ
    ii. Exposure time—0.01–5 seconds
    iii. Power—0–3000 mW.

25. **What is the relationship between spot size and energy requirements in laser?**
    To decrease energy, spot size is increased except in xenon arc where a decrease of energy is caused by decreasing spot size.

26. **When do we use different time duration laser burns?**
    Shorter duration burns (0.05 seconds) are more comfortable
    Longer burns (0.1—0.2 seconds) are more effective and less likely to rupture Bruch's membrane.

27. **What are the factors, which determine the effectiveness of any photocoagulation?**
    i. Penetration of light through ocular media.
    ii. Amount of light absorbed by the pigment and converted to heat.

28. **What are the indications of photocoagulation in eye?**
    i. Diabetic retinopathy
    ii. Retinal vascular abnormalities
       – BRVO (grid, sector)
       – ICRVO with NVG
    iii. Subretinal neovascularization
    iv. Retinal break
    v. Vascular tumors
    vi. Iridectomy
    vii. Trabeculoplasty
    viii. Vasculitis
    ix. Coloboma
    x. Optic nerve pit.

29. **What are the indications of laser photocoagulation in diabetic retinopathy?**
    i. Clinically significant macular edema.
    ii. Paramacular edema.
    iii. Proliferative diabetic retinopathy:
       – High risk PDR
       – Early PDR
         • Patients with poor compliance
         • During pregnancy
         • Patients with systemic diseases

- Pending cataract surgery
- Rubeosis
- Severe/very severe NPDR (irregular follow-up).

30. What are the laser types used in the treatment of macular edema?

  i. Direct/focal
 ii. Grid for diffuse leakage
iii. For circinate leakage, treat within the circinate.

31. DRCR.net Focal/Grid Photocoagulation (modified-ETDRS) Technique?

Features	Focal	Grid
Wavelength	Green-Yellow	Green-Yellow
Area	Direct treatment of all leaking microaneurysms in areas of retinal thickening 500–3,000 μ from center of macula	Areas of edema not associated with microaneurysms. ■ 500–3,000 μ superior, and inferior to macula and 500–3,500 μ temporally ■ No burns within 500 μ from disk or over the maculopapillary bundle
Spot size	50 μ	50 μ
Burn duration	0.05–0.1s	0.05–0.1s
Power	100–400 Mw	100–400 Mw
Intensity	Grade 3 burn evident beneath all microaneurysms	Bare visible (light gray) 2 visible burn width apart

32. What is the intensity of photocoagulation burns?

  i. Grade I (light)   Faint retinal blanching
 ii. Grade II (mild)   Hazy translucent retinal burn
iii. Grade III (moderate)   Opaque gray/dirty white
iv. Grade IV (heavy)   Dense chalky white

33. What are the disadvantages of green laser?

  i. Attenuated by nuclear sclerosis
 ii. Cannot do immediately after FFA, since residual vitreous fluorescein provides troublesome fluorescence with green illumination
iii. Absorbed by luteal pigments in the foveal region and hence yellow laser is preferable.

34. How does laser work in clinically significant macular edema (CSME)?

  i. Direct closure of leaking vascular microaneurysms due to laser-induced endovascular thrombosis and heat-induced contraction at the vessel wall. It acts by increasing filtration by RPE

ii. Thermally damaged RPE alters outer retinal–blood barrier thereby favoring fluid movement from retina to choroid

iii. Photoreceptor destruction increases inner retinal oxygenation, which results in vasoconstriction decreased blood flow and therefore decreased vascular leakage

iv. RPE damage causes retinal capillary and venule endothelial proliferation, which restores inner blood–retinal barrier.

v. Decreases the amount of retinal leakage by decreasing total surface area of leaking retinal vessels.

35. **What are the side effects of focal photocoagulation?**
    i. Paracentral scotoma
    ii. Transient increased edema/decreased vision
    iii. Choroidal neovascularization
    iv. Subretinal fibrosis
    v. Photocoagulation scar expansion
    vi. Inadverdent foveal burn.

36. **How long should we wait for macular edema to resolve following laser before deciding on retreatment?**

    Up to 4 months.

37. **What is the minimal level of visual acuity to give focal treatment in macular edema?**

    Focal treatment has to be given even if vision is 6/6 or better if the edema is clinically significant.

38. **What are the indicators of poor prognosis in CSME for laser photocoagulation?**
    i. Extensive macular capillary nonperfusion (ischemic maculopathy)
    ii. Diffuse disease
    iii. Cystoid macular edema (long)
    iv. Lamellar macular hole
    v. Foveal hard exudates plaque.

39. **What are the indications for PRP?**
    i. High risk PDR
    ii. Others:
       – Rubeosis with/without NVG
       – PDR developing in pregnancy
       – Early PDR or severe NPDR with increased risk for progression (poor compliance, fulminant course in fellow eye, uncontrolled systemic diseases like hypertension, nephropathy, anemia, etc.)
       – Widespread retinal ischemia/capillary drop outs on FFA of >10 DD area.

40. **What is the mechanism of action of panretinal photocoagulation (PRP)?**

    i. Conversion of hypoxic areas to anoxic areas
    ii. Greater perfusion from the choroidal circulation by achieving a closer approximation of the inner layer of the retina with choriocapillaries.
    iii. Destruction of badly perfused capillaries and grossly hypoxic retina thus diverting available blood to a healthier retina.
    iv. Destruction of leaking blood vessels which create abnormal hemodynamic situation in the diabetic retina thereby normalizing the vascular supply of the macular region.

41. **What are the parameters of PRP?**

    Blue green argon/Fd Nd:YAG lasers

Spot size:	200–500 μ
Exposure time:	0.1–0.2 seconds
Power:	200–500 mW
End point:	Moderately intense white burns
Inter burn distance:	One burn width apart
Placement:	2 DD above, temporal, and below center of macula.

    500 μ from nasal margin of the optic disk and extends to or beyond the equator.

    To avoid direct treatment of:

    i. Major retinal vessels
    ii. Macula
    iii. Papillomacular area
    iv. Area of gliosis
    v. Retinal hemorrhage
    vi. Chorioretinal scars.

42. **What are the approximate number of burns required for completing PRP?**

    1,800–2,200 burns in 2–3 divided sittings over 3–6 weeks period.
    Multiple sessions decrease the risk of:

    i. Macular edema
    ii. Exudative RD
    iii. Choroidal detachment
    iv. Angle closure glaucoma.

43. **What are the indications of additional laser treatment after initial PRP?**

    For recurrent or persisting neovascularization.

44. What is the placement or number for additional burns in PRP?

   i. In between prior treatment scars

  ii. Anterior to previous scars

 iii. Posterior pole—2 DD away from the macula

Number at least 500–700.

45. What are the complications of PRP?

Functional complications:

   i. Decreased night vision

  ii. Decreased color vision

 iii. Decreased peripheral vision

 iv. Loss of 1 or 2 lines of visual acuity

  v. Glare, photopsia.

Anatomical complications:

i. *Anterior segment:*

  – Cornea burns

     • Erosion

     • SPK'S

  – Shallowing of AC

  – Iris

     • Iritis

     • Atrophy

     • Damage to sphincter

     • Posterior synechiae

  – Lens

     • Lens opacities

ii. *Posterior segment:*

  – Foveal burn

  – Occlusion of vein/artery

  – Retinal hemorrhage

  – Choroidal hemorrhage—due to rupture of Bruch's membrane/choroidal detachment

  – Macular edema following extensive PRP

  – Macular pucker

  – Contraction of fibrous tissue leading to tractional RD

  – CNVM

  – Subretinal fibrosis

  – Scar expansion.

46. What are the causes of pain during PRP?

   i. Inadequate anesthesia

  ii. High power or long duration burns

   iii. Large number burns

   iv. Focussed on the choroid rather than the retina

   v. Treatment over the long posterior ciliary nerves on the horizontal meridian

   vi. Peripheral treatment.

47. What are the differences between choroiditis pigmentation marks and old laser marks?

	Choroiditis pigmentation	Old laser marks
i.	Irregular	Regular with equal spacing
ii.	Pigmentation is peripheral	Pigmentation is in the center
iii.	Anywhere	Spare the macular regions and immediately surrounding the disk

48. What is the goal of PRP?

   i. To cause regression of existing neovascular tissue

   ii. To prevent new vessel formation.

49. Why is PRP done inferiorly first?

So that if a hemorrhage occurs only the superior retina is left to be lasered which is easier.

50. What is the wavelength of argon laser?

Argon blue green emits both blue (488 nm) and green (514 nm).

51. What are the advantages of argon laser?

   i. Coherent radiation—more efficient delivery

   ii. High monochromacity

   iii. Very small spot size.

52. What are the disadvantages of argon laser?

   i. Absorption by cataract lens

   ii. Poor penetration through vitreous hemorrhage

   iii. Uptake by macular xanthophyll (blue green)—cannot be used for treatment around macula

   iv. High intraocular scattering leads to less precise retinal focusing.

53. What is the wavelength of krypton red?

Krypton red—647 nm.

54. What are the advantages of krypton?

   i. Useful in treatment of lesions within foveal avascular zone and papillomacular bundle (as not absorbed by xanthophylls).

   ii. Better penetration through nuclear sclerotic cataracts (decreased absorption by lens) and through moderate vitreous hemorrhage (decreased absorption by hemoglobin) because of decreased intraocular scattering.

55. What are the disadvantages of krypton laser?

Red light must have melanin for its absorption

  i. Less effective for treating vascular abnormalities because of poor absorption by hemoglobin

  ii. Less effective for pale fundus

  iii. Increased pain and hemorrhage due to deeper choroid penetration.

56. What are the modes of delivery of lasers?

  i. Slit lamp

  ii. Indirect ophthalmoscopy

  iii. Endolaser.

57. What are the various lenses used?

  i. All-purpose fundus contact lens.

    – Goldmann contact lens

    – Karickhoff lens

  ii. Contact lens for macular photocoagulation

    – Volk super macula

    – Mainstar high magnification   } Real inverted

    – Volk area centralis

    – Mainstar standard lens

  iii. For peripheral photocoagulation

    – Rodenstock panfundoscopic

    – Volk trans equator   } Inverted real magnified

    – Mainster widefield

    – Mainster ultrafield

  iv. Noncontact lenses

    – 60 D

    – 78 D

    – 90 D.

58. What are the indications of laser PHC through indirect ophthalmoscopy delivery?

  i. PRP in patients with hazy media, patients unable to sit, early anterior segment postoperative period

  ii. Retinopathy of prematurity

  iii. Peripheral proliferative lesions as in pars planitis, Eales', sickle cell retinopathy, Coats' disease

  iv. Peripheral retinal breaks

  v. Retinal PHC following pneumatic retinopexy

  vi. Retinal and choroidal tumors: Choroidal malignant melanoma, retinoblastoma.

59. What are the advantages of laser PHC through indirect ophthalmoscope delivery?

Treatment of patients with:

   i. Hazy media

  ii. Poorly dilated pupils

 iii. In presence of intraocular gas bubbles

 iv. For patients unable to sit at a slit lamp

  v. For peripheral lesions.

60. Which is more responsive to treatment, flat, or elevated new vessels?

   i. Flat vessels

  ii. Because absorption of laser energy by elevated lesions is less.

61. Which is more likely to bleed, NVD, or NVE? Why?

NVD. Because of the absence of internal limiting membrane over the disk.

62. What is to be done when bleeding occurs during photocoagulation?

   i. Bleeding can be stopped by increasing the pressure of the contact lens on the globe.

  ii. By increasing the laser energy and hitting the bleeding point repeatedly.

63. What are the relative indications for retrobulbar anesthesia in photocoagulation procedures?

   i. Significant ocular pain

  ii. Significant eye movement

 iii. Treatment near the foveal center to avoid incidental foveal burns.

64. What are the indications of anterior retinal cryotherapy?

   i. Progressive proliferative diseases (NVD, NVE, or NVI) despite full PRP

  ii. When media opacities (cataract, VH) preclude PRP.

65. What are the diameters of various cryoprobes used in ophthalmology?

Endocryopexy—1 mm

ICCE—1.5 mm

Retina—2–2.5 mm.

66. What are the recent advances in laser photocoagulation?

   i. Pattern Scanning Laser—PASCAL® (Topcon Inc.)

     – Laser—double frequency Nd-YAG 532 nm laser and 577 nm Yellow Laser

     – Uses a microprocessor-driven scanner that produces a variety of scalable patterns, viewable on a computer screen and selected by the physician. Allows the operator to apply multiple spots almost simultaneously, with a single foot pedal depression, multiple laser burns in a rapid predetermined sequence in the form of a pattern array produced by a scanner.

- Advantages
  - Faster 56 spots in 0.6 seconds—reduces treatment duration
  - Lesser pain and better patient comfort
  - Perfect spacing of spots—no accidental confluence/overlapping
  - End point management system—reduction of fluence decreases collateral damage to surrounding tissue compared with conventional laser.
- Disadvantages
  - The efficacy of PASCAL laser, however, appears to be diminished compared to conventional laser therapy when the same number of laser spots were delivered.

ii. Micropulse laser—IRIDEX 577 nm

- Using a micropulse mode, laser energy is delivered with a train of repetitive short pulses (typically 100–300 microseconds "on" and 1,700–1,900 microseconds "off") within an "envelope" whose width is typically 200–300 milliseconds.
- Mechanism of action—stimulate the RPE and have a beneficial effect on its activation.
- Advantages—the length of pulses shorter than the thermal relaxation time of the target tissue and allows tissues to cool before the next pulse to limit damage to adjacent areas thereby minimize scarring.
- Uses—macular edema, central serous chorioretinopathy (CSCR), CNVM.

iii. Navigated Lase—NAVILAS

- Combines color fundus photography, FA, and IR imaging with a target locked frequency-doubled solid-state laser (wavelength 532 nm).
- Features:
  - Computer-based treatment planning—superimposed FFA and live retinal images for targeting
  - Safety/eye-tracking feature—minimize inadvertent laser treatment
  - Accuracy
  - Multimodal integration—FA, OCT, ICG
  - Patient comfort
  - Treatment ease
  - Documentation.

6.6. HYPERTENSIVE (HTN) RETINOPATHY

1. **What are the different classifications of HTN retinopathy?**

   There are two main classifications:

   i. Keith–Wagener–Barker classification
   ii. Scheie's classification

2. **What is the Keith–Wagener–Barker classification?**

   It is divided into four groups:

   Group 1—minimal constriction of the arterioles with some tortuosity

   Group 2—abnormalities in Group 1 with definite focal narrowing and arteriovenous nicking

   Group 3—group 1 and 2 abnormalities and hemorrhages, exudates, cotton wool spots

   Group 4—above findings along with optic disk edema.

3. **What is Scheie's classification?**

   Scheie classified changes of hypertension and arteriosclerosis separately. Scheie's classification of hypertensive retinopathy:

   Stage 0—no visible retinal vascular abnormalities
   Stage 1—diffuse arteriolar narrowing
   Stage 2—arteriolar narrowing with areas of focal arteriolar constriction.
   Stage 3—diffuse and focal arteriolar narrowing with retinal hemorrhages
   Stage 4—all above findings with retinal edema, hard exudates, and optic disk edema.

   Scheie's classification of arteriolosclerosis:
   Stage 0—normal
   Stage 1—broadening of arteriolar light reflex
   Stage 2—light reflex changes and arteriovenous crossing changes
   Stage 3—copper wiring of arterioles
   Stage 4—silver wiring of arterioles.

4. **What is Salus's sign?**

   Deflection of vein as it crosses the arteriole.

5. **What is Gunn's sign?**

   Tapering of veins on either side of arteriovenous (AV) crossing.

6. **What is Bonnet's sign?**

   Banking of veins distal to arteriovenous (AV) crossings.

7. **What is the cause of arteriolar light reflex?**

   It is the light reflected from the convex surface of normal arteriolar wall.

8. **What is copper wiring?**

   When the light reflex from the vessel wall takes on a reddish brown hue due to increase in arteriolosclerosis it is called copper wiring.

9. **What is silver wiring?**

   When there is severe arteriolosclerosis and no blood is seen inside the vessel wall it is called silver wiring.

10. **What is the reason for arteriolar narrowing?**

    When there is rise in blood pressure, it excites the pliable and non-sclerotic retinal vessels to increase their vascular tone by autoregulation.

11. **What is a cotton wool spot?**

    It is an area of focal ischemic infarct of the nerve fiber layer as a result of axon disruption.

12. **What are flame-shaped hemorrhages?**

    These are the hemorrhages present in nerve fiber layer from superficial precapillary arterioles and hence assuming the architecture of nerve fiber layer.

13. **What are the differential diagnoses of flame-shaped hemorrhages?**

    They are:
    i. HTN retinopathy
    ii. Diabetic retinopathy
    iii. CRVO
    iv. BRVO
    v. Ocular ischemic syndrome
    vi. Eales' disease
    vii. Hemoglobinopathies.

14. **What are hard exudates?**

    They are caused by chronic retinal edema. They develop at the junction of the normal and edematous retina and are composed of lipoprotein and lipid rich macrophages located within the outer plexiform layer.

15. **What are the differential diagnoses of hard exudates?**

    They are:
    i. Diabetic retinopathy
    ii. HTN retinopathy
    iii. BRVO
    iv. CRVO
    v. Coats' disease
    vi. Retinal artery macroaneurysm
    vii. Radiation retinopathy
    viii. Eales' disease.

16. **What is macular star?**

It is the deposition of hard exudates in a star-shaped pattern around the fovea. This is due to chronic macular edema in hypertensive retinopathy.

17. **What are the differential diagnoses of macular star?**

They are:
- i. HTN retinopathy
- ii. Neuroretinitis
- iii. Papilledema
- iv. CRVO
- v. BRVO.

18. **What is the hallmark of accelerated hypertension?**

Optic disk swelling.

19. **How is hypertensive eye disease divided on the basis of ocular tissue involved?**

It is divided into:
- i. HTN retinopathy
- ii. HTN choroidopathy
- iii. HTN optic neuropathy.

20. **What are different phases of HTN retinopathy?**

It is divided into:
- i. Vasoconstrictive phase
- ii. Exudative phase
- iii. Sclerotic phase.

21. **What are the changes in vasoconstrictive phase?**

Fundus changes:
- i. Diffuse arteriolar narrowing
- ii. Focal arteriolar narrowing
- iii. Reduction of arteriole to venule ratio (Normal—2:3).

22. **What are the changes in exudative phase?**

Fundus changes:
- i. Flame-shaped hemorrhages
- ii. Cotton wool spots
- iii. Hard exudates.

23. **What is the finding in sclerotic phase?**

Fundus changes:
- i. Sclerosis of vessel wall (copper wiring and silver wiring)
- ii. Arteriovenous crossing changes (Salus's sign, Bonnet's sign, Gunn's sign).

24. What are the complications of HTN retinopathy?

They are:
- i. Macroaneurysms
- ii. Central retinal artery or vein occlusion
- iii. Branch retinal artery or vein occlusion
- iv. Epiretinal membrane formation
- v. Macular edema
- vi. Retinal neovascularization
- vii. Vitreous hemorrhage.

25. What is HTN arteriolosclerosis?

It is progressive increase in the elastic and muscular component in the walls of the arterioles.

26. What is onion skin appearance of the vessel wall?

In long-standing hypertension elastic tissue forms multiple concentric layers. Muscular layer is replaced by collagen fibers and the intima is replaced by hyaline thickening. These give the appearance of onion skin.

27. What are the risk factors for HTN choroidopathy?

It is commonly seen in acute HTN and young patients. Risk factors are:
- i. Toxemia of pregnancy
- ii. Malignant HTN
- iii. Renal disease
- iv. Pheochromocytoma
- v. Acquired diseases of connective tissue.

28. What are the fundus changes in HTN choroidopathy?

Fundus changes are:
- i. Elsching's spots and Siegrist's streaks
- ii. Serous retinal detachments
- iii. Macular star
- iv. RPE depigmentation
- v. Subretinal exudates
- vi. Choroidal sclerosis.

29. What are Elschnig's spots?

They are small black spots surrounded by yellow halos representing RPE infarct due to focal occlusion of choriocapillaries.

30. What are Siegrist's streaks?

They are flecks arranged linearly along the choroidal vessels; indicative of fibrinoid necrosis.

31. How is choroidal circulation different from retinal circulation?

Choroidal circulation has got following peculiarities:

   i. Profuse sympathetic nerve supply

  ii. No autoregulation of blood flow

 iii. No blood–ocular barrier.

Hence, increased blood pressure is directly transferred to choroidal choriocapillaries which initially constrict but further increase in blood pressure overcomes the compensatory tone, resulting in damage to the muscle layer and endothelium.

32. What is HTN optic neuropathy?

It is characterized by:

   i. Swelling of the optic nerve head (ONH)

  ii. Blurring of the disk margins

 iii. Hemorrhages over the ONH

 iv. Ischemia and pallor of the disk

33. What are the differential diagnosis of HTN optic neuropathy?

They are:

   i. CRVO

  ii. AION

 iii. Radiation retinopathy

 iv. Diabetic papillopathy

  v. Neuroretinitis.

34. What is malignant hypertension?

Diastolic blood pressure of >120 mm Hg

It is characterized by fibrinoid necrosis of the arterioles. Choroidopathy and optic neuropathy are more common but retinopathy also occurs in malignant hypertension.

35. What are ocular manifestations in pregnancy-induced HTN (PIH)?

They are divided as:

Conjunctiva—

   i. Capillary tortuosity

  ii. Conjunctival hemorrhages

 iii. Ischemic necrosis of conjunctiva

Hypertensive retinopathy changes

Choroid—serous detachments

Optic nerve—disk edema and rarely optic atrophy.

36. How do you manage PIH?

The fundus findings that occur generally return to normal in response to appropriate medical management or upon spontaneous or elective delivery. The role of ophthalmologist is limited.

37. What is the management of HTN retinopathy?

Control of the hypertension is the key step. An ophthalmologist mainly plays a supportive role to a primary care physician in the diagnosis and management of systemic hypertension with prompt referral.

6.7. CENTRAL RETINAL VEIN OCCLUSION (CRVO)

1. **What are the main types of CRVO?**
   i. *Ischemic* (nonperfused/ hemorrhagic/complete (ICRVO))
   ii. *Nonischemic* (perfused/partial/incomplete (NICRVO)).

2. **What is indeterminate CRVO?**
   A CRVO is categorized as indeterminate when there is sufficient intra-retinal hemorrhage to prevent angiographic determination of perfusion status.

3. **Which type of CRVO is more prevalent in younger age group?**
   Nonischemic CRVO.

4. **Which type of CRVO more prevalent in older age group?**
   Ischemic CRVO.

5. **Which type of CRVO is known to recur in the same eye again?**
   Nonischemic CRVO.

6. **What is the crucial period for the development of neovascularization after the ischemic insult?**
   First 7 months. (The risk period may span up to 2 years.)

7. **What percentage of patients with neovascularization develops NVG?**
   33% of patients with iris neovascularization develop NVG.

8. **What is the need for distinction between two types of CRVO?**
   i. Prediction of the risk of subsequent ocular neovascularization.
   ii. Identification of patients who will have poor visual prognosis.
   iii. Determination of the likelihood of spontaneous visual improvement.
   iv. Decision as to appropriate follow-up interval.

9. **Mention the causes for CRVO.**
   i. *Systemic vascular disease:*
   - Hypertension (artery compresses the vein)
   - Thrombosis of the central retinal vein
   - Diabetes
   - Hyperlipidemia
   - Hematological alterations like hyperviscosity syndrome, blood dyscrasias
   - Leukemia

ii. *Ocular disease:*
   - Primary open angle glaucoma
   - Ischemic optic neuropathy
   - Events compressing the proximal part of the optic nerve like retrobulbar hemorrhage, orbital pseudotumor, optic nerve tumors

iii. *Inflammatory/autoimmune vasculitis:*
   - Systemic lupus erythematosus
   - Behcet's disease
   - Sarcoidosis

iv. *Infectious vasculitis:*
   - HIV
   - Syphilis
   - Herpes zoster

v. *Medications:*
   - Oral contraceptives
   - Diuretics
   - Hepatitis B vaccine

vi. *Others:*
   - After retrobulbar block, dehydration, pregnancy.

10. **Where is the common site of occlusion in nonischemic CRVO?**
   6 mm behind lamina cribrosa.

11. **What is the common site of occlusion in ischemic CRVO?**
   At the region of lamina cribrosa or immediately posterior it.

12. **How do we check for raised central retinal vein pressure?**
   Digital ophthalmodynamometry.

13. **How is this done?**
   In normal eyes, the central retinal vein spontaneously pulses or can be made to wink or collapse with minimal ocular pressure through the eyelids. In CRVO, the vein and artery link together, or in extreme cases, the artery is more easily compressed than the vein

14. **Why does ischemic CRVO present with a more malignant picture?**
   In ischemic CRVO, the site of occlusion is closer to the disk, i.e. it is at lamina cribrosa or immediately posterior to it, where only a few collaterals are present to drain the blood. So there is a marked increase in venous pressure with a more malignant picture at presentation. Nonischemic CRVO has occlusion more proximally with plenty of collaterals to drain the blood.

15. How does glaucoma cause CRVO?

    i. The pressure in CRV at optic disk depends upon the IOP, the former being always higher than the latter to maintain blood flow. A rise of IOP would produce retinal venous stasis and sluggish venous outflow—one of the factors in Virchow's triad for thrombus formation

    ii. The central retinal artery and veins are subjected to compression from mechanical stretching of lamina cribrosa, while passing through rigid sieve like openings especially in POAG

    iii. Nasalization and compression of vessels.

16. How does CRVO cause glaucoma?

    i. Neovascular glaucoma (open-angle and closed-angle types).

    ii. In the management of macular edema in CRVO, intravitreal steroid may cause steroid-induced glaucoma.

17. What are the risk factors for the conversion of nonischemic CRVO to ischemic CRVO?

    i. *Ocular risk factors:*

        – Nonischemic CRVO with V/A at presentation of <6/60

        – Presence of 5–9 disk areas of nonperfusion on angiography

    ii. *Systemic risk factors:*

        – Elderly individuals (>60 years)

        – Associated cardiovascular disease

        – Blood dyscrasias

        – Nocturnal hypotension.

18. What are the pathological changes in CRVO?

    i. Hemorrhagic infarction of inner layer of retina

    ii. Neovascularization of disk, retina, iris, angle

    iii. Thickening of retina, reactive gliosis

    iv. Intraretinal edema.

19. What is the most common cause of visual loss in CRVO?

Macular edema.

20. Why do patients of CRVO complain of defective vision in the early morning?

The fall in the blood pressure during sleep (nocturnal hypotension) alters the perfusion pressure and so the venous circulation is further slowed down, converting partial thrombosis to complete thrombosis.

21. Why do patients with CRVO have amaurosis fugax?

The thrombosis formation in central retinal vein completely cuts off the retinal vascular blood flow resulting in transient obscuration of vision with field defects. However, due to the sudden rise in the blood pressure at the arterial end of the retinal vascular blood flow, the freshly formed thrombus is pushed out of the site of block and relieves the ischemia, resulting in the return of vision and field normality.

22. **Which type of CRVO is usually asymptomatic?**

Nonischemic CRVO.

23. **Which type of CRVO presents with amaurosis fugax?**

Nonischemic CRVO.

24. **Which type of CRVO presents with sudden loss of vision?**

Ischemic CRVO.

25. **What is the commonest field defect in CRVO?**

Central scotoma.

26. **What are the clinical tests used in the evaluation of CRVO?**

Clinical tests can be classified into two categories:

Morphological
i. Ophthalmoscopy
ii. FFA

Functional
i. Visual acuity
ii. RAPD
iii. Visual fields
iv. ERG

27. **Differentiate between nonischemic and ischemic CRVO.**

Features	Nonischemic CRVO	Ischemic CRVO
1. V/A	Better than 6/60	Worse than 6/60(3/60-HM)
2. Anterior segment	Normal RAPD++	RAPD+/– NVI, NVA +/– NVG features
3. Fundus	Less retinal hemorrhage at posterior pole Cotton wool spot +	Abundant and extensive retinal superficial hemorrhage Cotton-wool spot + + +
4. Field defects	50–75%	100%
5. ERG changes	+/–	+ + (decreased 'b'wave amplitude)
6. FFA changes	Few nonperfusion areas	Nonperfusion areas >10 DD
7. Course	Majority resolve completely (48%)	Majority do not resolve, leading to ocular morbidity

28. **What is the importance of relative afferent pupillary defect (RAPD) in the setting of CRVO?**

Uses:
i. Higher sensitivity at earliest stages
ii. It gives reliable information in spite of hazy media.
iii. It can detect conversion of nonischemic to ischemic CRVO.
iv. It is a noninvasive and inexpensive diagnostic tool.

Limitations:

i. To test for RAPD, it is essential to have a normal fellow eye and normal optic disk and pupil in both eyes. For example, not useful in pharmacologically miotic or mydriatic pupil, glaucomatous disk damage or optic neuropathy.

ii. The amount of RAPD is influenced by the size of the central scotoma because it is modified more by the number of retinal ganglion cell involved than by the area of the retina. For example, NICRVO with central large, dense, macular edema may show a RAPD.

29. What will be the fundus picture in ischemic CRVO?

i. Widespread retinal hemorrhages (Tomato ketchup fundus)
ii. Retinal venous engorgement and tortuosity
iii. Cotton-wool spots
iv. Macular edema
v. Optic disk edema.

30. What is the footprint of asymptomatic NICRVO?

Retinocapillary venous collaterals on optic disk.

31. What is the importance of ocular neovascularization in CRVO?

i. Ocular neovascularization is seen in 2/3 of ischemic CRVO.
ii. Ocular neovascularization if seen in nonischemic CRVO, should raise the suspicion of other associated conditions like
   – DM and other proliferative retinopathy
   – Carotid artery disease.

32. Which is the commonest site of neovascularization in ischemic CRVO?

Iris.

33. What is the importance of ischemic index in CRVO?

$$\text{Ischemic index} = \frac{\text{Nonperfusion area}}{\text{Total area of retina}}$$

The risk of developing neovascularization is directly proportional to the degree of ischemic index.

Ischemic index:

0–10%	— < 1% develop NVG
10–50%	— 7% develop NVG
> 50%	— 45% develop NVG.

34. What are the indications of FFA in CRVO?

FFA should be performed after the acute phase is over since the hemorrhages during the acute phase will not provide accurate information.

i. To look for any macular ischemia before treatment
ii. To evaluate the extent of capillary nonperfusion (CNP)

iii. In cases of nonischemic CRVO, follow-up changes can be identified such as conversion to ischemic type.

35. FFA findings in ischemic CRVO and nonischemic CRVO.

Ischemic CRVO:

i. Hypofluorescence due to retinal capillary nonperfusion, blockage from retinal hemorrhages
ii. Increased arteriovenous transit time
iii. Macular area shows pooling due to edema and nonperfusion areas suggestive of macular ischemia
iv. NVD and NVE show leakage
v. Vessel wall staining.

Nonischemic CRVO:

i. Delayed AV transit time
ii. Blockage by hemorrhages
iii. Nonperfusion areas are minimal
iv. Late leakage
v. FFA may become normal after NICRVO resolves.

36. How do you differentiate between ischemic CRVO and nonischemic CRVO by FFA?

Ischemic CRVO	>10 DD of CNP area
Nonischemic CRVO	<10 DD of CNP area

37. Is ERG useful in differentiating ICRVO from NICRVO?

i. Amplitude reduction of "b"wave has 80% sensitivity and specificity in differentiating ICRVO from NICRVO. It does not require normal fellow eye and can be done in patients with optic nerve and pupil abnormalities also. In ischemic CRVO
ii. "b" wave amplitude decreased to less than 60% of normal
iii. "b" wave amplitude reduced by 1 standard deviation or more, below the normal mean value.

38. What are the investigations to be done in patients with CRVO?

History:	Age
	Sex
	Occupation/lifestyle
	DM/HTN
Ocular:	Slit lamp examination
	Direct/indirect ophthalmoscopy
	Field charting
	FFA
	ERG

General:	BP, pulse rate
	Systemic examination
Specific investigations:	BP
	ECG
	Full blood count and ESR
	FBS and lipids
	Urine albumin and serum creatinine
	Plasma protein electrophoresis

Young patients have to be specifically screened for
Thrombophilia screening
Autoantibodies (anticardiolipin, lupus anticoagulant, ANA, DNA, ACE)
Homocysteine.

39. What is the DD for CRVO?
  i. D/D of papilledema
  ii. D/D of cotton wool spots.

40. How will you manage CRVO?
  i. Treat the associated cause like hypertension, diabetes, elevated cholesterol
  ii. Intravitreal triamcinolone acetonide for treating macular edema
  iii. Intravitreal anti-VEGF agents to reduce macular edema
  iv. Surgical decompression of CRVO via radial optic neurotomy which involves sectioning the posterior scleral ring and retinal vein cannulation with an infusion of tissue plasminogen activators have been reported.

41. What are the findings of central vein occlusion study group (CVOS)?
The CVOS findings were the following:
  i. Even though grid laser treatment in the macula reduced angiographic evidence of macular edema, it yielded no benefit in improved visual acuity.
  ii. The most important risk factor predictive of iris neovascularization in CRVO is poor visual acuity. Scatter PRP failed to decrease the incidence of iris neovascularization. CVOS recommended waiting for at least 2 o'clock hours of iris neovascularization to show on undialted gonioscopy before performing photocoagulation.

42. What is significant anterior segment neovascularization?
More than 2 o'clock hours neovascularization of iris (NVI) and/or angle (NVA).

43. When is PRP indicated in CRVO?
  i. Patient presenting with NVI or NVA
  ii. Patient presenting with NVD or NVE, even without NVA or NVI.

44. When is prophylactic PRP indicated in CRVO?

Patient with **ischemic CRVO** where regular follow-up is not possible.

45. Is grid photocoagulation useful in macular edema due to CRVO?

No.

46. Why is there no improvement of visual acuity after grid in CRVO as against that seen in BRVO or early stages of DME? (CVOS).

   i. Difference in the pathophysiology of the diseases.
   ii. CRVO usually results in the diffuse capillary leakage involving all the macular area, unlikely in BRVO or background DR.
   iii. In BRVO, macular edema may have more angiographically normal parafoveal capillaries.
   iv. Also in BRVO, collateral channels typically develop temporal to the macula crossing the horizontal raphe. This may permit a greater normalization of venous circulation in the recovery phase (as opposed to CVO, where collaterals channels develop at the optic nerve).
   v. In CRVO—macular edema involves the center of the fovea and additionally includes all four quadrants in the parafoveal region. May adversely affect the recuperative process in the macula.

47. What is the role of steroids in management of CRVO?

Decreases macular edema in nonischemic CRVO.
Treatment of CRVO in young is especially secondary to phlebitis.
Dexamethasone implants (OZURDEX) has been used and has shown to be of benefit in the GENEVA studies.

48. What are the other intravitreal injections which can be given?

   i. Cruise trial: found monthly intravitreal 0.5 mg, ranibizumab for 6 months is useful, especially when macular edema is present.
   ii. COPERNICUS and GALILEO trials: found monthly intravitreal 2 mg Aflibercept (VEGF Trap eye) to be useful.

49. What is the role of cyclocryotherapy?

Procedure:

   i. 180° of the ciliary body is treated at one time, employing six spots of freezing, 2.5 mm posterior to the limbus.
   ii. The 3.5 mm probe is allowed to reach –60° to –80°C and is left in place for 1 minute each.

50. What is anterior retinal cryotherapy (ARC)?

Indication in NVG: In cases in which the cornea, lens, and vitreous is hazy to allow adequate PRP.

Procedure:

i. A 2.5 mm retinal cryoprobe is used. The first row of application is performed 8 mm posterior to limbus, three spots between each rectus muscle.

ii. Second row of application is performed 11 mm behind the limbus, four spots between each rectus muscle.

iii. Probe is applied for approximately 10 seconds.

51. Complications of ARC.

i. Tractional and exudative RD

ii. Vitreous hemorrhage.

52. What is the visual outcome in patients with CRVO?

Depends on the vision on presentation

Nonischemic CRVO—final V/A is better than 6/60 in 50% patients.

Ischemic CRVO–final V/A is worse than 6/60 in 93%, worse than 3/60 in 10%.

53. Why is visual prognosis in young patients good?

i. Due to absence of significant retinal ischemia

ii. Young patients with healthy blood vessels may be able to tolerate brief periods of CRVO better than older individuals.

54. What is the differential diagnosis of CRVO?

i. Ocular ischemic syndrome

ii. Hyperviscosity retinopathy

iii. Diabetic retinopathy

iv. Papilledema.

6.8. CENTRAL RETINAL ARTERY OCCLUSION (CRAO)

1. **What does central retinal artery supply?**

   Central retinal artery is a branch of ophthalmic artery that enters the eye within the optic nerve and supplies the blood to the inner layers of the retina, extending from the inner aspect of the inner nuclear layer to the nerve fiber layer. Therefore, CRAO leads to damage predominantly to the inner layers of the retina.

2. **What are the causes of CRAO?**

   i. Atherosclerosis-related thrombosis
   ii. Carotid embolism
   iii. Giant cell arteritis
   iv. Cardiac embolism which may be calcific emboli or vegetations or thrombus or myxomatous material
   v. Periarteritis
   vi. Thrombophilic disorders
   vii. Sickling hemoglobinopathies
   viii. Retinal migraine.

3. **Where is the occlusion present in CRAO?**

   Occlusion is most commonly present at the level of lamina cribrosa (80%).

4. **What are the features of atherosclerosis?**

   Atherosclerosis is characterized by focal intimal thickening comprising cells of smooth muscle origin, connective tissue, and lipid containing foam cells.

5. **What are the risk factors of atherosclerosis-related thrombosis?**

   Risk factors are:
   i. Aging
   ii. Hypertension
   iii. Diabetes
   iv. Hyperhomocysteneimia
   v. Increased LDL cholesterol
   vi. Obesity
   vii. Smoking
   viii. Sedentary lifestyle.

6. **Where does carotid embolism originate from and what are the types of emboli?**

Carotid embolism mostly originates from an atheromatous plaque at the carotid bifurcation and less commonly from the aortic arch. The emboli may be of:

   i. Cholesterol *(Hollenhorst plaques):* appear as intermittent showers of minute, bright, refractile, golden to yellow-orange crystals. They rarely cause significant obstruction to the retinal arterioles and are frequently asymptomatic.
   ii. *Calcific emboli:* single, white nonscintillating and are often on or close to the disk. Calcific emboli are more dangerous than the others as they cause permanent occlusion of the central retinal artery or its branches.
   iii. *Fibrin-platelet emboli:* are dull, gray, multiple elongated particles that occasionally fill the entire lumen. They may cause retinal transient-ischemic attacks with resultant amaurosis fugax and occasionally complete obstruction.

7. **What is the incidence of CRAO?**
   i. 1 per 10,000 outpatients
   ii. Above the age of 60 years
   iii. Bilateral in 2–3% of cases—to rule out cardiac valvular diseases, giant cell arteries, and vascular inflammations.

8. **Describe the clinical features of CRAO.**
   Symptoms
   i. Sudden painless loss of vision.
   ii. In a few cases, visual loss is preceded by amaurosis fugax.
   iii. Visual acuity—counting fingers to PL+ve in 90% of cases.
      – In case of PL–ve—suspect associated ophthalmic artery occlusion or optic nerve damage.
   Signs
   i. RAPD—within seconds after CRAO.
      – will be present even when fundus appears normal during the early phases of CRAO.
   ii. Anterior segment is usually normal initially.
   iii. Rubeosis iridis at the time of obstruction is rare.
      – If present, suspect concomitant carotid artery obstruction.
      – Rubeosis iridis in CRAO develops at a mean of 4–5 weeks after obstruction, with a range of 1–15 weeks and seen in 18% of eyes.
   iv. Yellowish white opacification of superficial retina in the posterior pole except fovea. This loss of retinal transparency is due to ischemia of inner half of retina. This usually resolves in 4–6 weeks.
   v. Cherry-red spot in the foveal area due to extremely thin retina, allowing view of underlying retinal pigment epithelium and choroids.

     vi. In early stages, the retinal arteries are attenuated. The retinal veins are thin, dilated, or normal.

        In severe cases, segmentation or "box caring" of blood vessels in arteries and veins are seen.

    vii. In 20% of CRAO, Hollenhorst plaque–(glistening, yellow cholesterol embolous) that arises from atherosclerotic, deposits in the carotid artery.

   viii. NVD in 2–3%.

     ix. Late fundus picture:

       – Consecutive optic atrophy

       – Attenuated blood vessels to a relatively normal fundus picture

       – When present, pigmentary changes may indicate carotid or ophthalmic artery occlusion.

9. Mention the differential diagnosis of CRAO.

      i. Acute ophthalmic artery occlusion (usually no cherry-red spot)

     ii. Other causes of cherry-red spot like Tay-Sachs diseases, Neimann-Pick disease, some cone dystrophies, etc.

    iii. Berlin's edema

    iv. Anterior ischemic optic neuropathy

     v. Inadvertent intraretinal injection of gentamicin.

10. What is cherry-red spot?

Cherry-red spot at the macula is a clinical sign seen in the context of thickening and loss of transparency of the retina at the posterior pole. The fovea being the thinnest part of the retina and devoid of ganglion cells, retains relative transparency, due to which the color of the choroids shines through.

In case of lipid storage diseases, the lipids are stored in the ganglion cell layer of the retina, giving the retina a white appearance. As ganglion cells are absent at the foveola, this area retains relative transparency and contrasts with the surrounding retina.

11. What are the causes of cherry-red spot?

      i. CRAO

     ii. Sphingolipidoses like Gaucher's disease, Neimann–Pick disease, Tay–Sachs disease, Goldberg syndrome, Faber syndrome, gangliosidosis GM1-type 2, Sandoff's disease

    iii. Berlin edema/commotio retinae

    iv. Macular retinal hole with surrounding retinal detachment

     v. Quinine toxicity

    vi. Hollenhorst syndrome (chorioretinal artery infarction syndrome)

   vii. Cardiac myxomas

  viii. Severe hypertension

    ix. Temporal arteritis

     x. Myotonic dystrophy syndrome.

12. What are the systemic diseases associated with CRAO?

    i. Atheromatous vascular diseases

    ii. Diabetes mellitus

    iii. Hypertension

    iv. Cardiac valvular/occlusive disease

    v. Carotid occlusive disease

    vi. Compressive vascular disease

    vii. Blood dyscrasias

    viii. Embolic disease

    ix. Vasculitis

    x. Spasm following retrobulbar injection.

13. What are the ocular diseases associated with CRAO?

    i. Precapillary arterial loops

    ii. Optic disk drusen

    iii. Increased IOP

    iv. Toxoplasmosis

    v. Optic neuritis.

14. How do you treat a case of CRAO?

CRAO is an ophthalmic emergency. Treatment has to be instituted as soon as the diagnosis of CRAO is made even before work up of the case.

    i. **Bringing down the IOP**

       – Dislodges the embolus.

       – Produces retinal arterial dilation and increases retinal perfusion

         • Ocular massage with gonioscope preferred

         • Paracentesis of anterior chamber

         • IOP lowering drugs.

    ii. **Vasodilation**

        • Carbogen inhalation

        • Retrobulbar or systemic administration of vasodilators

        • Sublingual nitroglycerin.

    iii. **Fibrinolysis**

    Mode and Effects of Treatment

       – **Ocular massage**

         • Done digitally or by direct visualization of the artery by using a contact lens (Goldmann lens)

         • Compression of globe for approximate 10 seconds to obtain retinal arterial pulsation or flow cessation followed by 5 seconds of sudden release which is continued for approximately 20 minutes

         • Improvement of retinal blood flow is seen as reestablishment of continuous laminar flow and increase in width of blood column and disappearance of fragmented flow.

- **Anterior chamber paracentesis**
  - Causes sudden decrease in IOP. As a result the perfusion pressure behind the obstruction will push on an obstructing embolus.
    Technique: Performed at the slit lamp using topical anesthesia with a twenty-five gauge needle.
    Generally 0.1–0.2mL of aqueous is removed.
- **IOP lowering agents**

  Act in the same mechanism as AC paracentesis.
  - 500 mg of IV acetazolamide
  - 20% IV mannitol
  - Oral 50% glycerol.
- **Vasodilators**
  - Carbogen (95% of O_2 + 5% CO_2 mixture).
  - Inhalation of 100% O_2 in the presence of CRAO produces a normal pO_2 at the surface of the retina via diffusion from the choroids.
  - CO_2 is a vasodilator and can produce increased retinal blood flow.
    - In the absence of CO_2-O_2 mixture, rebreathing into a paper bag can be considered.
  - Retrobulbar or systemic papavarine or tolazoline.
  - Sublingual nitroglycerin.
- **Fibrinolytic agents**
  - Administered through supra orbital artery. This produces 100 times higher doses of fibrinolytic agent at the central retinal artery than IV administration due to retrograde flow into ophthalmic artery.
  - Injection of urokinase into the internal carotid artery through femoral artery catheterization has been tried.
  - Systemic thrombolysis using plasminogen has also shown improvement in CRAO patients.

Work up/Investigations

  i. A detailed history regarding hypertension, diabetes, cardiac diseases, and other systemic vascular diseases, e.g. giant cell arteritis.
 ii. Check pulse (to rule out atrial fibrillation) and BP
iii. ESR, FBS < glycosylated Hb < TC, DC, PT, and APTT.
   - In young patients (<50 years) consider lipid profile, ANA, RF, FTA- ABS, serum electrophoresis, Hb electrophoresis, and antiphospholipids antibodies.
 iv. Carotid artery evaluationdigital palpation/duplex USG
  v. ECG, echo
 vi. FFA and ERG.

15. What is the FFA picture in CRAO?

  i. Delay in arterial filling.
 ii. Prolonged A-V transit time.
iii. Complete lack of filling of arteries is unusual.
 iv. Choroidal vascular filling is usually normal in eyes with CRAO.
  v. If there is marked delay in choroidal filling in the presence of cherry-red spot—suspect ophthalmic artery occlusion or carotid artery occlusion.
 vi. Though the arterial narrowing and visual loss persists, the fluorescein angiogram can become normal after varying time following CRAO.

16. What is the ERG picture in CRAO?

  i. "b" wave diminution—due to inner retinal ischemia.
 ii. "a" wave is generally normal.

17. What are the causes of sudden visual loss?

  i. **Painless loss of vision:**

   – CRAO
   – Retinal detachment
   – Retrobulbar neuritis
   – Methyl alcohol poisoning
   – Vitreous hemorrhage

 ii. **Painful loss of vision:**

   – Acute congestive glaucoma
   – Optic neuritis
   – Traumatic avulsion of optic nerve
   – Meningeal carcinomatosis

6.9. RETINAL DETACHMENT (RD)

1. **What are the layers of retina?**

    From outer to inner:
    - i. Retinal pigment epithelium (RPE)
    - ii. Layers of rods and cones
    - iii. External limiting membrane
    - iv. Outer nuclear
    - v. Outer plexiform
    - vi. Inner nuclear
    - vii. Inner plexiform
    - viii. Ganglion cell layer
    - ix. Nerve fiber layer
    - x. Internal limiting membrane.

2. **Define macula.**

    It is an area of 4,500 μ in size between the temporal around where the ganglion cells are 2 or more in layers.

3. **Define fovea and foveola.**

    Fovea: is a depression in the inner retinal surface at the center of the macula with a diameter of 1.5 mm. Ophthalmoscopically, it gives rise to an oval light reflex because of the increased thickness of the retina and internal limiting membrane at its border.

    Foveola: forms the central floor of the fovea and has a diameter of 0.35 mm. It is the thinnest part of the retina, is devoid of ganglion cells and consists only of cones and their nuclei.

4. **What are the layers of Bruch's membrane?**
    - i. Basement membrane of RPE
    - ii. Inner loose collagenous zone
    - iii. Middle layer of elastic fibers
    - iv. Outer loose collagenous zone
    - v. Basement membrane of the endothelium of the choriocapillaries.

5. **What are the layers of choroid?**

    Four layers from without inwards:
    - i. Suprachoroidal lamina (lamina fusca).
    - ii. Stroma of choroids:
        - – Outer layer of choroidal vessels → (Haller's layer)
        - – Inner layer of choroidal vessels → (Sattler's layer)
    - iii. Choriocapillaries
    - iv. Bruch's membrane or lamina vitrae.

6. **What is the blood supply of choroid?**

   Posterior choroid up to the equator: Short posterior ciliary arteries. These arise as two trunks from the ophthalmic artery. Each trunk divides into 10–20 branches which pierce the sclera around the optic nerve and supply the choroid in a segmental manner.

   Anterior choroid: Recurrent ciliary arteries, long posterior ciliary artery, and anterior ciliary artery.

7. **What is the blood supply of retina?**

   Outer four layers (pigment epithelium, layer of rods and cones, external limiting membrane, and outer nuclear layer) get their nutrition from choriocapillaries.

   Inner six layer (outer plexiform layer, inner nuclear layer, inner plexiform layer, layer of ganglion cells, nerve fiber layer, and internal limiting membrane) get their blood supply from central retinal artery.

8. **What is vitreous base?**

   Vitreous base straddles ora serrata, extending 1.5–2 mm anteriorly and 1–3 mm posteriorly.

9. **What are the normal attachments of vitreous to retina?**
   - i. Around vitreous base
   - ii. Around the optic disk
   - iii. Around the fovea
   - iv. Around the peripheral blood vessels.

10. **What is the composition of vitreous?**

    99% water with volume of 4 cc. Liquid phase contains hyaluronic acid. Collagen types—II, IX, and XI.

11. **What are the landmarks of vortex vein?**

    Vortex ampulae are located just posterior to the equator in the 1, 5, 7, and 11 o'clock meridian.

12. **What are the landmarks of long posterior ciliary artery?**

    Yellow lines that start behind the equator and runs forward at 3 and 9 o'clock position with accompanying nerves.

13. **How does a normal retina remain attached?**
    - i. An interphotoreceptor matrix between the cells forms a "glue" that helps to maintain cellular apposition.
    - ii. RPE function as a cellular pump, to remove ions and water from the interphotoreceptor matrix providing a "suction force" that keeps the retina attached.
    - iii. Vitreous acts as a tamponade.

14. What is syneresis?

Contraction of gel, which separates its liquid from solid component.

15. What is synchysis?

Liquefaction of gel.

16. What is a retinal break?

A retinal break is a full thickness defect in the sensory retina connecting the vitreous cavity and the potential or actual subretinal space.
They can be tears or holes.

    i. **Tears:** are caused by dynamic vitreoretinal traction.

   ii. **Holes:** caused by chronic atrophy of sensory retina and are less dangerous than tears.

Operculated holes: When a piece of retina has been pulled away from the rest of the retina and when this piece of retina attached to the detached vitreous face floats internal and anterior to the hole, the piece of retina is called operculum and the hole, an operculated hole.

17. What are the factors responsible for break?

    i. Dynamic vitreoretinal traction

   ii. Underlying weakness on peripheral retina due to predisposing degeneration.

18. Name the most common site of breaks.

Upper temporal quadrant (60%).

19. What is primary and secondary break?

Primary   — break responsible for RD

Secondary   — break not responsible for RD.

20. What is retinal dialysis?

Retinal dialysis is the disinsertion of neurosensory retina from neuropigment epithelium of pars plana.

21. What is the most common and pathognomic site for dialysis in blunt trauma?

Upper nasal quadrant.

22. What is the most common site for non-trauma dialysis?

Inferior temporal quadrant.

23. What are giant tear and horseshoe tear?

Giant tear: A tear involving 90° or more of the circumference of the globe. They have vitreous gel attached to the anterior margin of the break. Common site—immediate post-oral retina.

Horseshoe tear: is a retinal tear which takes the shape of a horseshoe with the ends pointing toward the ora. The tongue of retina inside the horseshoe is called a flap. Horseshoe tear is always a sequelae of lattice degeneration. HST is formed when attempt to PVD at lattice edges tear off the retina creating Horseshoe-shaped tear.

24. **What are the peripheral retinal degenerations not associated with RD?**

    Benign peripheral retinal degenerations are:
    i. Peripheral cystoid degenerations
    ii. Snowflakes
    iii. Pavingstone degenerations
    iv. Honeycomb degenerations
    v. Drusen.

25. **Which are the peripheral retinal degenerations which predispose to RD?**
    i. Lattice degeneration
    ii. Snail track degeneration
    iii. Retinoschisis
    iv. White without pressure
    v. Diffuse chorioretinal atrophy.

26. **What is lattice degeneration?**

    Lattice degeneration is sharply demarcated, circumferentially oriented, spindle-shaped areas of retinal thinning. There is discontinuity of internal limiting membrane with variable atrophy of underlying sensory retina. It is present in 8% of normal population and 40% of patients with RD and commonly associated with myopia.

    Most common location: Between equator and posterior border of vitreous base, more in the superotemporal quadrant. Lattice may be complicated by retinal tears or atrophic holes. It should be treated prophylactically in those with past history of detachment in the fellow eye, family history of detachment, recently acquired horseshoe tears and aphakic patients.

27. **What is snail track degeneration?**

    These are sharply demarcated bands of tightly packed snowflakes which gives the peripheral retina a white frost like appearance. Round holes may be seen in the snail track and overlying vitreous liquefaction may be present. Snail track degeneration is a predisposing condition for RD.

28. What is retinoschisis?

Horizontal splitting of the peripheral sensory retina into two layers, namely an

i. Outer (choroidal layer)
ii. Inner (vitreous layer)

There are two main types:

- *Typical:*
  - Split is at the outer plexiform layer
  - Does not extend posterior to the equator
  - Outer layer is uniform
  - Less transparent inner layer.
- Reticular:
  - Split is at the nerve fiber layer
  - Extends posterior to the equator more often, may involve the fovea.
  - Outer layer is not homogenous and may have dark areas
  - Greater transparency of the inner layer.

Seen in 5% normal population above 20 years, and common among hypermetropes. This is a predisposing condition for RD.

29. What is white with pressure (WWP)?

Translucent gray appearance of retina induced by indenting it.

30. What is white without pressure?

It is a gray appearance of retina even without indenting it.

31. What is posterior vitreous detachment (PVD)?

It is a separation of cortical vitreous from the internal limiting membrane (ILM). It may be complete or incomplete. Acute PVD may cause retinal tears, rhegmatogenous retinal detachment, avulsion of blood vessel in the periphery and vitreous hemorrhage.

32. Why is there tessellation in the fundus?

i. Decreased pigmentation in the RPE
ii. Increased pigmentation in the choroid.

33. What is Weiss ring?

Weiss ring is a solitary floater consisting of the detached annular attachment of vitreous to the margin of the optic disk.

34. What are the standard color codes used in fundus drawings?

i. Detached retina	—*Blue*
ii. Attached retina	—*Red*
iii. Retinal veins	—*Blue*

iv.	Retinal breaks	—*Red with blue outlines*
v.	Flap of retinal tear	—*Blue*
vi.	Thinned retina	—*Red hatches outlined in blue*
vii.	Lattice degeneration	—*Blue hatches outlined in blue*
viii.	Retinal pigment	—*Black*
ix.	Exudates	—*Yellow*
x.	Vitreous opacities	—*Green*

35. What is retinal detachment (RD)?

Retinal detachment is defined as the separation of neurosensory retina (NSR) from the retinal pigment epithelium (RPE) with accumulation of fluid in the potential space between NSR and RPE.

36. What are the types of RD?

i. Rhegmatogenous
ii. Tractional
iii. Exudative
iv. Combined tractional and rhegmatogenous.

37. What is rhegmatogenous RD (RRD)?

Rhegma—break
RRD occurs secondary to a full thickness defect in the sensory retina which permits the fluid from synchytic (liquefied) vitreous to enter the subretinal space. There are two types of rhegmatogenous RD—primary and secondary.

Primary: retinal break has not been preceded by an antecedent condition (e.g. degenerations) and is usually preceded by PVD.

Secondary: retinal break has been preceded by an antecedent condition like lattice, etc.

38. What are the prerequisites for RRD?

i. Presence of retinal break
ii. Liquefied vitreous gel
iii. Traction over/at break keeping it open to allow fluid to pass in subretinal space.

39. What are the important causes of liquefaction of vitreous in early childhood which can predispose to RRD?

i. Trauma
ii. High myopia
iii. Inflammation (vitritis)
iv. Retinochoroidal coloboma
v. Genetic predisposition like Stickler's syndrome, Marfan's syndrome, Ehlers-Danlos, etc.

40. What are the symptoms of RRD?

i. *Flashes or photopsia:* due to vitreoretinal traction
ii. *Floaters:* due to microbleeding from retinal tear
iii. *Field defects:* due to spread of subretinal fluid (SRF) posterior to equator.

41. What are flashes due to?

The perception of flashes or photopsia is due to the production of phosphenes by pathophysiologic stimulation of retina. During PVD, as the vitreous separates from the retinal surface, the retina is disturbed mechanically stimulating a sensation of light. Ocular migraine is a differential diagnosis.

42. What is the significance of floaters?

i. Sudden appearance of one large floater near the visual axis is mostly due to PVD (Weiss ring).
ii. Appearance of numerous curvilinear opacities within the visual field indicates vitreous degeneration.
iii. Floaters due to vitreous hemorrhage is characterized by numerous tiny black dots, followed by cobwebs as the blood forms clots.

43. What is the significance of visual field?

The quadrant of visual field in which field defect first appears is useful in predicting the location of primary retinal break (which will be in opposite quadrant). Patients tend to be less aware of superior field defects and hence patients with inferior RD may not be symptomatically aware. High bullous detachments cause dense field defects, while flat detachments produce relative field defects.

44. What are the symptoms perceived by a patient with acute vitreous hemorrhage?

Shower of floaters/reddish smoke.

45. What are the signs of fresh signs of RRD?

i. Marcus Gunn pupil
ii. IOP lowers by about 5 mm Hg than the other eye
iii. Mild anterior uveitis
iv. Tobacco dusting in the vitreous
v. Retinal breaks
vi. Detached retina has a convex configuration and a slightly opaque and corrugated appearance with loss of underlying choroidal pattern.

46. Why is the intraocular pressure (IOP) decreased in certain RDs?

An eye with rhegmatogenous RD typically has decrease IOP and is due to the following factors:

    i. **Early transient pressure drop** may result from inflammation and reduced aqueous production.

    ii. **Prolonged hypotony** may be caused by posterior flow, presumably through a break in the RPE.

47. What is Schwartz syndrome?

RRD is typically associated with decreased IOP. Schwartz described a condition in which patient presents with unilateral intraocular pressure elevation, retinal detachment, and open anterior chamber angle.

48. Why is IOP raised in certain RD's?

Chronic low grade uveitis in RDs damage the trabecular meshwork

In long-standing RDs

Rubeosis iridis (NVI)

Increased IOP

49. What is "tobacco dusting"?

    i. Pathognomonic of RRD

    ii. Present in the anterior vitreous phase

    iii. The cells represent macrophages containing shed RPE.

50. What is the incidence of retinal detachment in myopes?

40% of all RDs occur in myopes.

51. What are the reasons for high myopes to have RRD?

    i. Increased stretch of the retina over the bigger eye ball

    ii. Incidence of lattice generation is higher

    iii. Incidence of PVD is higher

    iv. Macular hole

    v. Vitreous loss during cataract surgery

    vi. Diffuse chorioretinal atrophy.

52. Which are the systemic conditions associated with rhegmatogenous RD?

    i. Marfan's syndrome

    ii. Ehlers–Danlos syndrome

    iii. Stickler syndrome

    iv. Goldmann–Favre syndrome

    v. Homocystinuria.

53. Why is detached retina gray?

Retina is transparent normally and the normal color of retina is due to the underlying choriocapillaries showing through the transparent retina. However, in detachment, the following factors make the retina look gray.

 i. Detached retina is away from capillaries
 ii. Presence of subretinal fluid
 iii. Retinal edema.

54. Why is configuration of SRF important?

Because SRF spreads in gravitational fashion and its shape is governed by anatomic limits (ora and optic nerve), it can be used to locate primary break.

55. What are the factors promoting SRF into the break?

 i. Ocular movements
 ii. Gravity
 iii. Vitreous traction, at the edge of the break
 iv. PVD.

56. What is Lincoff's rule?

Lincoff's rules are a set of guidelines on finding the retinal break based on the configuration of the retinal detachment. SRF usually spreads in gravitational fashion and its shape is governed by anatomical limits and location of the primary retinal break. If the primary break is located superiorly, SRF first spreads inferiorly on the same side of the break and then spreads superiorly on the opposite side of the fundus.

 i. A shallow inferior RD in which SRF is slightly higher on the temporal side points to a primary break on that side.
 ii. A primary break at 6 o'clock will cause inferior RD with equal fluid levels.
 iii. In a bullous inferior RD, the primary break usually lies above the horizontal meridian.
 iv. If a primary break is in the upper nasal quadrant, the SRF will revolve around the optic disk and then rise on the temporal side until it is level with the primary break.
 v. A subtotal RD with a superior wedge of attached retina points to a 1° break located in the periphery nearest its highest borders.
 vi. When the SRF crosses the vertical midline above the primary break is near to 12 o'clock the lower edge of the RD corresponding to the side of the break.

57. How does a RD progress?

They can go through any of the following patterns:

 i. Usually most detachments progress to total detachments.
 ii. "Stable detachment" form demarcation lines and does not settle (commonly in inferior breaks).

   iii. Settling of retinal break spontaneously, (only superior retinal breaks) as RD settles inferiorly the site of original break flattens.

   iv. Rarely by scarring, spontaneous closure of retinal hole may occur resulting in reattachment.

58. What are late secondary changes in RD?

   i. Retinal thinning.
   ii. Proliferative vitreoretinopathy (PVR) changes
   iii. Subretinal demarcation line (3 months)
   iv. Intraretinal cyst formation (1 year)
   v. Pigmentation.

59. What are demarcation lines?

Demarcation line is formed due to pigment epithelial proliferation and migration at the boundary of the detached and attached retina and is a sign of the chronicity of the condition. It takes about 3 months for the demarcation lines to develop.

60. What is vitreoretinal traction?

It is the force exerted on the retina by structures originating in the vitreous.

Types:

   i. Dynamic—it is induced by rapid eye movement, where there is a centripetal force toward the vitreous cavity. Responsible for retinal tears and rhegmatogenous RD.

   ii. Static—independent of ocular movements and plays an important role in pathogenesis of tractional RD and proliferative vitreoretinopathy.

It may be:

   i. Tangential → epiretinal fibrovascular membranes
   ii. Anteroposterior traction → contraction of fibrovascular membranes
   iii. Bridging (trampoline) traction → contraction of fibrovascular membranes which stretch from one part of the posterior retina to another or between vascular arcades which tends to pull the two involved points together.

61. What is tractional retinal detachment (TRD)?

Tractional RD occurs when the neurosensory retina is pulled away from the RPE by contracting vitreoretinal membranes in the absence of a retinal break.

62. What are the conditions causing tractional RD?

   i. Diabetes
   ii. Trauma

iii. Vascular occlusions
iv. Cataract extraction with vitreous incarceration
v. Perforating or penetrating injury to the globe
vi. Sickle cell hemoglobinopathies
vii. Retrolental fibroplasia
viii. Persistent hyperplastic primary vitreous (PHPV)
ix. Pars planitis
x. Eales' disease
xi. *Toxoplasma* and *Toxocara* infections.

63. What is the pathogenesis of exudative RD?

Diseases of choroids and retina

Damages RPE

Allow passage of fluid (transudate) from choroids into subretinal space

64. What are the causes of exudative RD?

i. *Inflammatory:*	VKH
	Peripheral uveitis
	Excessive cryopexy
	Extensive photocoagulation
	Choroidal effusion
ii. *Systemic:*	Renal failure
	Hypertension
	Dysproteinemia and macroglobulinemia
iii. *RPE defect:*	RPE detachment
	CSR
iv. *SRNV:*	ARMD
	Presumed histoplasmosis
	Angioid streaks
	Choroidal rupture
v. *Tumors:*	Malignant melanoma
	Metastasis
	Retinoblastoma

65. How do you differentiate between the three types of RD?

Rhegmatogenous, tractional, and exudative.

Features	Rhegmatogenous	Exudative	Tractional
History	Photopsia visual field defects	Systemic factors such as malignant hypertension, eclampsia, and renal failure	Diabetes, penetrating trauma, sickle cell disease
Retinal break	Present	No break or coincidental	No primary break, May develop secondary break
Extent of detachment	Extends to ora early	Gravity dependent, extension to ora is variable	Frequently does not extend to ora
Retinal motility	Undulating bulla or folds	Smoothly elevated bullae, usually without folds	Taut retina, concave surface. Peaks to traction points
Retinal elevation and shape	Low to moderate; convex sometimes	Varies—may be extremely high convex concave	Elevated to level of focal traction
Evidence of chronicity	Demarcation lines, intraretinal macrocysts, atrophic retina	Usually none	Demarcation lines
Pigment in vitreous	Present in 70% of cases	Not present	Present in trauma cases
Vitreous changes	Frequently syneretic, posterior vitreous detachment, traction on flap of tear	Usually clear, except uveitis	Vitreoretinal traction
Subretinal fluid	Clear	May be turbid and shift rapidly to dependent location with changes in head position	Clear, no shift
Choroidal mass	None	May be present	None
Intraocular pressure	Frequently low	Varies	Usually normal
Transillumination	Normal	Blocked transillumination if pigmented choroidal mass is present	Normal
Examples of conditions causing detachment	Peripheral retinal degeneration, PVD, CMV retinitis, Stickler syndrome, Marfan's syndrome, Ehlers–Danlos syndrome	Uveitis, metastatic tumor, malignant melanoma, Coats' disease, Vogt–Koyanagi–Harada syndrome, Retinoblastoma	Proliferative diabetic retinopathy, retinopathy of prematurity, *Toxocara* sickle cell retinopathy, posttraumatic vitreous traction

66. What is the differential diagnosis of leukokoria?

  i. **Congenital:**
   - Norrie's disease
   - Incontinentia pigmenti
   - Autosomal dominant exudative vitreoretinopathy

  ii. **Developmental:**
   - Retinopathy of prematurity
   - Myelinated nerve fiber layer
   - Coloboma
   - Persistent hyperplastic primary vitreous (PHPV)
   - Congenital cataract

  iii. **Inflammatory:**
   - CMV retinitis
   - *Toxoplasma*
   - *Toxocara.*

  iv. **Tumor:**
   - Retinoblastoma

  v. **Vasculitis:**
   - Coats' disease

  vi. **Others:**
   - Retinal detachment
   - Vitreous hemorrhage.

67. What are the conditions exhibiting abnormal retinal embryogenesis?

  i. Retinal dysplasia
  ii. Norrie's disease
  iii. Fundus coloboma
  iv. Optic nerve pits
  v. Persistent fetal vasculature.

68. What are the diseases which simulate retinal detachment?

  i. Retinoschisis
  ii. Choroidal detachment
  iii. Vitreous hemorrhage
  iv. Endophthalmitis
  v. Melanoma of choroid with exudative detachment
  vi. Intraocular cysticercosis
  vii. Uveal effusion syndrome
  viii. Severe vitritis.

69. What are the complications of longstanding RD?

   i. Uveitis

   ii. Complicated cataract

  iii. Rubeosis iridis

   iv. Glaucoma

   v. Band keratopathy

   vi. Phthisis.

70. What are the types of traumatic RD?

   i. Tractional

   ii. Rhegmatogenous

  iii. Combined.

71. What is the pathogenesis of traumatic RD?

Penetrating trauma → Vitreous incarceration at the site of penetration injuries

        Vitreoretinal traction

        The weakest area is in the temporal periphery.

Blunt trauma → Compression of AP diameter of globe and simultaneous expansion at equatorial plane. It can cause retinal dialysis (frequent in the upper nasal quadrant) or can cause macular or equatorial holes.

        Causes

        Dialysis, tears (equatorial), macular holes.

72. How to differentiate between rhegmatogenous retinal detachment and retinoschisis?

Features	Rhegmatogenous retinal detachment	Retinoschisis
Symptoms	Photopsia and floaters are present	Photopsia and floaters are absent as no vitreoretinal traction
Visual field defect	Relative scotoma	Absolute scotoma
Detachment	Convex with undulated appearance with mobility	Convex, smooth, thin and immobile, localized
	Presence of tobacco dusting, demarcation, and intraretinal cysts	Absence of such findings
Laser photocoagulation	Does not create burn due to underlying SRF	Will create a burn
Associated refractive Error	Myopia	Hypermetropia
Location	Superiotemporal	Inferotemporal

73. **Differentiate between retinal detachment (RD) and choroidal detachment (CD) clinically.**

Features	RD	CD
Symptoms	Photopsia and floaters are present	Absent (no vitreoretinal traction)
Appearance	Convex, undulated, mobile on eye movements. Lighter in color	Brown, convex, smooth, bullous detachment which is relatively immobile. Darker in color
Macula	May be involved	Elevations do not extend to the posterior pole because they are limited by the firm adhesion between the suprochoroidal lamellae and sclera where the vortex veins enter the scleral canals
IOP	Normal/low	Very low
Periphery examinations	Scleral indentation required for periphery examination	Peripheral retina and ora serrata may be seen without scleral indentation
Anterior chamber	Normal depth	Shallow

74. **How do you classify proliferative vitreoretinopathy (PVR) changes associated with RD?**

Modified Retina Society Classification/Silicone Study Classification		
Grade	Name	Clinical sign
A	Minimal	Vitreous haze, vitreous pigment clumps
B	Moderate	Wrinkling of inner retinal surface, rolled edge of retinal break, retinal stiffness, tortuosity, ↓ motility of vitreous
CP 1–12 (clock hours)	Marked	Posterior to equator focal, diffuse or circumferential full thickness folds, subretinal strands
CA 1–12 (clock hours)	Marked	Anterior to equator focal, diffuse, circumferential full thickness folds, subretinal strands, anterior displacement, anterior condensed vitreous strands
D	Massive	Fixed retinal folds in four quadrants; D-1 wide funnel shape; D-2 narrow funnel shape; D-3 closed funnel (optic nerve head, not visible)

75. **What are the factors governing visual function following surgical reattachment?**

If the macula has been involved the prognosis is poorer. It is especially more poorer if

i. The time of involvement is more than 2 months
ii. Height of macular detachment and age >60 years negatively affect visual restoration.

76. **What is the principle of retinal detachment surgery?**
    i. Identify all the breaks (See the break)
    ii. Create a controlled injury to the retinal pigment epithelium and retina to produce a chorioretinal adhesion at the site of all retinal breaks (seal the break).
    iii. Employing an appropriate technique such as scleral buckling and/or intravitreal gas to approximate the retinal breaks to the underlying treated retinal pigment epithelium.

77. **What is an explant?**

    Buckling element (silicon) sutured directly onto the sclera to create a buckle height.

78. **What is an implant?**

    Buckling element placed within the sclera to create a buckle height.

79. **What are the types of buckles used?**
    i. Radial explant: placed at right angles to limbus
    ii. Sequential circumferential explants: placed circumferentially to limbus to create a sequential buckle
    iii. Encircling circumferential explants: 360° buckle
    iv. Soft silicon sponges for radial or circumferential buckling
    v. Hard silicon straps: used for 360° buckling
    vi. Hard silicon tyres.

80. **What are the indications for radial buckling?**
    i. Large U-shaped tears, particularly when "fish mouthing" is anticipated (especially if it is a single break)
    ii. Posterior retinal beaks.

81. **What are the indications for segmental circumferential buckling?**
    i. Multiple breaks located in one or two quadrants and varying distance from ora serrata
    ii. Anterior breaks
    iii. Wide breaks, dialysis, and giant tears.

82. **What are the indications for encircling buckle (360°)?**
    i. Break involving three or more quadrants
    ii. Extensive RD without detectable breaks particularly is eyes with hazy media
    iii. Lattice degeneration, snail track degeneration involving three or more quadrants
    iv. Along with vitrectomy.

83. **What are the preliminary examinations to be done before surgery?**
    i. Check all clinically important lesions to see if it is correctly indicated in drawing.

ii. Access retinal mobility by moving eye with squint hook. Good retinal motility indicates absence of significant PVR and hence carries a good prognosis.

iii. Try to appose the retinal break, to the RPE by indenting the sclera with squint hook; if this can be done with case, drainage of SRF may not be necessary.

iv. Assess the dimensions of retinal breaks, by comparing them with the diameter of optic nerve head (1.5 mm).

v. Assess whether the break is anterior or posterior to the equator.

84. What are the steps in scleral bucking surgery?

i. Preliminary examination
ii. 360° peritomy
iii. Traction (bridle) sutures around the recti
iv. Inspection of sclera
v. Localization of the break
vi. Cryotherapy
vii. Scleral buckling
viii. Drainage of SRF
ix. Intravitreal air or BSS injection
x. Closure of the peritomy.

85. What precautions should be taken during peritomy?

Care should be taken not to damage the plica semilunaris, tears in conjunctiva and muscle.

86. What is the purpose of bridle sutures?

i. To stabilize the globe
ii. To manipulate it into optimal position during surgery.

87. How do you take bridle sutures?

i. Insert a squint hook under rectus muscle
ii. Pass a reverse mounted needle with a 4-0 black silk suture under the muscle tendon
iii. Secure the suture by twisting it around the forceps and cut externally.

88. What are the complications associated with taking bridle suture?

i. Damage to vortex veins
   The inferior vortex veins are more anteriorly placed, and can be damaged by a posterior insertion of squint hook under inferior rectus. If vein is damaged, do not cauterize, wait for bleeding to stop
ii. Rupture of muscle belly due to excessive traction on the sutures
iii. Muscle disinsertion.

89. What is the purpose of examining sclera?

i. *To detect scleral thinning:*
It is characterized by gray color due to underlying choroids. Complications due to it are:
   - Penetration of the needle into choroid and retina while the scleral bite is taken.
   - Sutures may cut through the thin sclera after the sutures are tied.

ii. *To detect anamolous vortex veins:*
As it can be damaged during cryotherapy, scleral buckling, and SRF drainage.

90. What are the three modalities used for prophylaxis of retinal detachment?

i. Cryotherapy
ii. Laser photocoagulation
iii. Scleral buckling for large tears.

91. What are the principles in the prophylactic management of retinal breaks?

i. *Breaks needing treatment:* High myopia, Aphakic eyes, symptomatic tear, any break with SRF more than 1 DD, any break greater than 1 o'clock hour, family history of RD, systemic conditions like Marfans, Ehlers–Danlos

ii. *Breaks needing only observation:* Asymptomatic holes, asymptomatic tears.

92. What is the principle of cryotherapy?

It is based on Joule Thompson effect, which states that when gas is allowed to pass through a narrow passage and under high pressure, it cools to a determined ($-70°$) temperature. Cryotherapy causes freezing of the intracellular and extracellular water to ice. This leads to tissue death and sterile with septic necrosis and an inflammatory reaction. Scarring will result in stronger than normal bond between the sensory retina, RPE and choroids. This permanently seals the break.

93. What are the indications for cryotherapy of retinal breaks? What is the temperature generated by cryoprobe and what is the probe size?

Indications:

i. Hazy ocular media
ii. Peripherally located tears near the ora
iii. Tears at the region of vortex veins and at the large ciliary vessels
iv. Small pupils

Temperature of probe: $-80°$

Probe size: Standard size of 2.5 mm.

94. What is the technique of cryotherapy?

i. Using indirect ophthalmoscope locate the break
ii. Indent the sclera gently with cryoprobe and bring the RPE as close as possible to the break
iii. Start freezing until sensory retina has returned "white"
iv. Repeat cryo until the entire break has been surrounded.
Cryoprobe position is changed only after complete thawing.

95. How is laser retinopexy done?

i. Laser source: Double frequency Nd:YAG, diode.
ii. Instruments: Slit lamp or indirect ophthalmoscope, Goldmann 3 mirror lens or wide angle fundoscopic lens.
iii. Spot size: 200–500 µ
iv. Duration: 0.1–0.2 seconds
v. Power: 150–400 mW
vi. Burn placement: ½ burn width apart for at least three rows. Lesion should be surrounded 360° or if closer to the ora, should be treated in U-shaped pattern around the posterior edge of the lesion.

96. What are the indications for subretinal fluid (SRF) drainage?

i. Difficulty in localization of retinal breaks in bullous detachments
ii. Longstanding RD as SRF is viscous
iii. Bullous RD
iv. Ganglion RD
v. Glaucomatous cyclitis
vi. Resurgeries.

97. What are the methods of SRF drainage?

i. Prang: Here digital pressure is applied till central retinal artery is occluded and choroidal vasculature is blanched. Then full thickness perforation is made with 27 gauge hypodermic needle to drain SRF. Air is injected to form the globe.
ii. Cut down: Radial sclerotomy is made beneath the area of deepest SRF. Mattress suture may be placed across the lips of the sclerotomy. Prolapsed choroidal knuckle is examined with +20 D lens for large choroidal vessels. After ruling this out, light cautery is applied to knuckle to avoid bleeding and knuckle is perforated with 25 gauge hypodermic needle.

98. What are the advantages of SRF drainage?

It provides immediate contact between sensory retina and RPE with flattening of the fovea. If this contact is delayed, the stickiness of RPE wears off and adequate adhesion may not occur, resulting in nonattachment of retina.

99. What are the precautions taken before drainage of SRF?

   i. Examine the fundus to make sure, SRF has not shifted

   ii. Avoid vortex vein

   iii. IOP should not be elevated (it may cause retinal incarceration).

100. How do you know that SRF drainage is completed?

By the presence of pigments.

101. What are the complications of SRF drainage?

   i. Choroidal hemorrhage

   ii. Ocular hypotony

   iii. Iatrogenic break

   iv. Retinal incarceration

   v. Vitreous prolapse

   vi. Damage to long posterior ciliary arteries and nerves

   vii. Endophthalmitis.

102. What are the indications for internal tamponade in scleral buckling?

   i. Superior break

   ii. Hypotony

   iii. Retinal folds

   iv. Fish mouthing

   v. Posterior breaks.

103. What are the causes of failed scleral buckling surgery?

   i. Improper positioning of buckle

   ii. Missed holes and iatrogenic inadvertent retinal perforations

   iii. Residual vitreous traction

   iv. PVR

   v. Infection and extrusion of buckle.

104. What are the complications of scleral buckling and retinal detachment surgery?

Immediate

   i. Failure to reattach retina

   ii. Iatrogenic break

   iii. CRAO

   iv. Anterior segment ischemia

   v. Excessive cryo resulting in exudative RD

Early

   i. Choroidal detachment

   ii. Vitritis

   iii. Bacterial endophthalmitis

   iv. Acute orbital cellulitis

Late
  i. Extraocular muscle (EOM) imbalance
  ii. Exposure of implant
  iii. Infection
  iv. Ptosis
  v. Maculopathy
  vi. Cataract
  vii. Proliferative vitreoretinopathy
  viii. Macular pucker.

105. Who are the best candidates for pneumatic retinopexy?
  i. A detachment caused by a single break, in superior 8 o'clock hours
  ii. The break should not be more than 1 o'clock hour.
  iii. Multiple breaks but in 1–2 o'clock hours of each other
  iv. Free of systemic disease (rheumatoid arthritis) (who can maintain position)
  v. Phakic patients
  vi. Total PVD

106. Which are the cases not suitable for pneumoretinopexy?
  i. Breaks larger than 1 o'clock hour or multiple breaks extending over more than 1 o'clock hour of retina
  ii. Breaks in the inferior part of the retina
  iii. Presence of PVR, grades C and D, since this surgery does not relieve vitreoretinal traction
  iv. Physical disability
  v. Severe uncontrolled glaucoma cloudy media.

107. How is this procedure done?
The eye to be treated is massaged well to reduce the IOP. Selected gas is drawn through a 0.22 μ millipore filter. Injection is given, 4 mm posterior to the limbus in the region of pars plana temporally. The 30 gauge needle is directed toward the center of the vitreous to ensure penetration of the pars plana epithelium and the anterior hyaloid face. With the injection side uppermost and the needle is vertical, the gas is injected moderately. To prevent leakage, from the injection site, the head is turned to the opposite side.

108. What are the principles of pneumoretinopexy?
Intraocular gases keep the retinal break closed by the following properties:
  i. Mechanical closure and thus RPE pump removes excessive SRF
  ii. Surface tension
  iii. Buoyancy.

109. What are the complications of pneumoretinopexy?

    i. Subretinal migration of gas
    ii. Gas entrapment at the injection site
    iii. Iatrogenic macular detachment
    iv. New retinal breaks
    v. Vitreous incarceration in the paracentesis site
    vi. Subconjunctival gas
    vii. Cataract and glaucoma
    viii. Fish-eggs formation.

110. What are the advantages and disadvantages of pneumatic retin-opexy with that of scleral buckling?

Advantages of pneumoretinopexy:
    i. Postoperative vision is better
    ii. Morbidity is less
    iii. Attachment results are similar
    iv. Incidence of cataract is less
    v. Economical

Disadvantages:
    i. Need for postoperative positioning
    ii. Needs closer monitoring.

111. What are the indications for vitrectomy in RD?

    i. PVR grade C2 or more
    ii. Giant retinal tear and dialysis
    iii. Posterior break
    iv. Associated with vitreous hemorrhage
    v. Combined RRD with TRD
    vi. Colobomatous detachment
    vii. Inadequate pupillary size
    viii. Associated cataract surgery
    ix. Associated intraocular foreign bodies.

112. What are the substances used as vitreous substitutes in RD surgery?

    i. **Intraocular Gases:**

Nonexpansile	*Expansile*
a. Air	a. SF6
b. SF6: Air mixture	b. C3F8
c. C3F8: Air mixture	

    ii. **Silicon Oil**
    iii. **Perfluorocarbon Liquids (PFCL)**

113. What are the characteristics of intraocular gases?

   i. *Air:* Average duration of action : 3 days
       Maximum size : Immediate
       Average expansion : No expansion
       Advantages : Low cost and universal availability
       Disadvantage : Shorter time of action.
  ii. *SF6:* Average duration of action : 2 days
       Maximum size : 36 hours
       Average expansion : Doubles
       Advantages : Smaller amount of gas required No need for reinjecting the gas in case a new break develops
       Disadvantages : Air travel contraindicated for a prolonged time
 iii. *C3F8:* Average duration of action: 38 days
       Maximum size : 3 days
       Average expansion : Quadruples
       Advantages and disadvantages : Similar to SF6

114. What are the common silicon oils used?
   i. Polydimethyl siloxane (PDMS)
  ii. Trifluoromethyl siloxane.

115. What is the mechanism of action of silicon oils?
Silicon oils provide retinal tamponade for a larger period more than the intraocular gases. Since it is heavier than water, it allows subretinal fluid to drain through peripheral retinal break. It can act as a mechanical instrument to cleave planes and also acts as an internal tamponade.

116. What are the indications for the use of silicon oil?
   i. Retinal detachment complicated by PVR changes
  ii. Traumatic RD
 iii. Giant retinal tears
 iv. Tractional and combined retinal detachments
  v. RD associated with choroidal colobomas
 vi. RD associated with infectious retinitis.

117. What are the complications of silicon oil?
   i. Silicon oil migration under the retina
  ii. Suprachoroidal silicon oil
 iii. Silicon oil keratopathy
 iv. Inverse hypopyon
  v. Glaucoma
 vi. Vitreous floaters.

118. What are the advantages of silicon oil over intraocular gases?

  i. Intraoperative advantages:
- Better intraoperative visualization
- Easier retinopexy
- Control of hemorrhage and effusion

  ii. Postoperative advantages:
- Longer lasting tamponade
- Posturing less critical
- Better immediate visual acuity
- Air travel not contraindicated.

119. What are perfluorocarbon liquids (PFCL)?

They are fully fluorinated synthetic analogs of hydrocarbons containing carbon-fluoride bonds.

120. What are the characteristic of PFCL that enables them to be used as a vitreous substitute?

  i. Optical clarity
  ii. Similar refractive index that of water
  iii. High density
  iv. Biologically inert
  v. High cohesive force.

121. What are the commonly used PFCL materials?

  i. Perfluor-n-octane
  ii. Perfluorotributylamine
  iii. Perfluorodecalin

122. What are the indications of PFCL?

  i. RD with PVR
  ii. RD with giant retinal tear
  iii. Traumatic RD
  iv. Lens/IOL dislocation into vitreous
  v. Management of suprachoroidal hemorrhage.

123. Who is the father of RD surgery?

Jules Gonin (1923) treated retinal break by ignipuncture.

124. Who invented scleral buckling?

Custodis.

125. Who invented vitrectomy?

Machemer in 1971.

6.10. ENDOPHTHALMITIS

1. **Define endophthalmitis.**

Endophthalmitis is an inflammation of the internal layers of the eye resulting from intraocular colonization of infection agents and manifesting with an exudation into vitreous cavity.

2. **Classify endophthalmitis.**

i. ***Based on route of entry:***
   – Exogenous: Pathogen is introduced from outside
     • Postoperative
     • Posttraumatic
   – Endogenous: Pathogen is introduced from ocular circulation

ii. ***Based on microorganisms:***
   – **Bacterial**
     • ***Gram-positive***
       ○ *Staphylococcus epidermidis*
       ○ *Staphylococcus aureus*
       ○ *Streptococcus pneumoniae*
       ○ *Streptococcus viridans*
       ○ *Peptostreptococci*
       ○ *Corynebacterium*
       ○ *Propionibacterium acnes*
       ○ *Actinomyces*
     • ***Gram-negative***
       ○ *Pseudomonas aeruginosa*
       ○ *Proteus mirabilis*
       ○ *Klebsiella*
       ○ *Haemophilus influenzae*
       ○ *Escherichia coli*
   – **Fungal**
     • *A*spergillus
     • Candida
     • Cephalosporium
     • Penicillium
     • P*aecilomyces*

iii. ***Based on duration:***

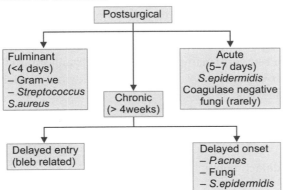

3. **What are the symptoms of endophthalmitis?**
   i. Decrease in vision (94% in EVS study)
   ii. Pain
   iii. Tearing
   iv. Photophobia
   v. Redness
   vi. Blepharospasm.

4. **What are the signs of endophthalmitis?**

i. Lids	Edema
ii. Conjunctiva	Chemosis, circumcorneal congestion
iii. Cornea	May be clear or
	Gross edema
	Limbal ring abscess
	Wound dehiscence
	Suture abscess
iv. Anterior chamber	Flare and cells
	Hypopyon
	Exudate
v. Iris	Posterior synechiae
vi. Pupil	Sluggish or absent pupillary reflexes
vii. Vitreous	Cells and exudates.

   Fundal glow
   Grading of media clarity (based on EVS)
   i. >20/40 (6/12) view of retina
   ii. 2° order retinal vessel visible
   iii. Some vessels visible but not second order
   iv. No vessels visible
   v. No red reflex.

5. **What are the differential diagnosis of endophthalmitis?**

Surgical	*Nonsurgical*
i. Fibrinous reactions	i. Retained IOFB
ii. Dislocated lens	ii. Pars planitis
iii. Chemical response	iii. Old vitreous hemorrhage
iv. Complicated surgery (manipulation)	iv. Toxoplasmosis/*Toxocara*
v. Microscopic hyphema	v. Necrotic retinoblastoma
vi. Phacoanaphylaxis	

6. **What is the role of USG in endophthalmitis?**
   To diagnose:
   i. Vitritis
   ii. Choroidal detachment

    iii. Retinal detachment

    iv. Dislocated lens/nucleus

    v. Radiolucent IOFB

    vi. Parasitic infestation.

7. What are the common organisms implicated in traumatic endophthalmitis?

    i. *Bacillus* species

    ii. Gram-negative species (*Pseudomonas*)

    iii. Fungi.

8. What are the common organisms implicated in endogenous endophthalmitis?

    i. *Candida*

    ii. *Neisseria*

    iii. *Bacillus.*

9. What are the common organisms implicated in postoperative endophthalmitis?

    i. *Pseudomonas*

    ii. *Nocardia*

    iii. *S. epidermidis*

    iv. *Haemophilus influenzae* (associated with bleb-related endophthalmitis).

10. Define "laboratory confirmed growth."

    i. At least semiconfluent growth on solid media.

    ii. Any growth on more than or equal to two media

    iii. Growth on one media supported by gram-positive stain.

11. What are the objectives in endophthalmitis treatment?

Primary

    i. Control/eradicate infection

    ii. Manage complication

    iii. Restoration of vision

Secondary

    i. Symptomatic relief

    ii. Prevent panophthalmitis

    iii. Maintain globe integrity.

12. What are the important determinants in outcome?

    i. Time duration between onset of infection and presentation

    ii. Virulence and load of organism

    iii. Pharmacokinetics and spectrum of drug activity.

13. **Modalities of treatment**

Medical   *Surgical*
  i. Antimicrobial   Vitrectomy
 ii. Anti-inflammatory
iii. Supportive

14. **What are the steps taken before intravitreal injection?**
   i. Informed consent
  ii. Check if vision is at least perception of light
 iii. Echography
 iv. To check for wound integrity
  v. Suture abscess
 vi. Lens status
vii. IOP.

15. **What are the materials for intravitreal injection?**
   i. Clean glass slides
  ii. Culture places
 iii. Tuberculin syringe
 iv. 26 gauge half inch, 23 gauge 1 inch needle
  v. Antimicrobial vials
 vi. Lid speculum, sterile cotton-tipped applicator
vii. Topical xylocaine hydrochloride 4%.

16. **What are the steps in intravitreal injection?**
   i. Informed consent
  ii. Paint periocular region with povidone iodine and wash cul-de-sac with solution of same
 iii. Apply topical xylocaine hydrochloride 4% adequately
 iv. Visualize injection site from limbus (3.0 mm if aphakic, 3.5 mm if pseudophakic, 4 mm if phakic)
  v. Stabilize globe and insert 26–30 gauge needle with bevel up toward anterior or midvitreous.
 vi. Inject drug drop by drop
vii. If multiple drugs are to be given, replace syringe but not needle
viii. Check IOP at end
 ix. Subcutaneous antibiotic is given and eye is patched.

17. **What are the advantages of vitrectomy?**
   i. Decrease infection and inflammatory load
  ii. Provides undiluted specimen for culture
 iii. Increases antimicrobial drug concentration within the eye
 iv. Enables rapid visual recovery by removing media opacities.

18. **What are the cardinal principles in vitrectomy?**
    i. Maximum cutting rate
    ii. Minimum suction
    iii. Do not attempt to induce PVD
    iv. Do not attempt to go close to retina.

19. **What are the indications for vitrectomy in infectious endophthalmitis?**
    i. Severe cases at manifestation defined as loss of red reflex, loss of light reflex, afferent pupillary defect and corneal ring infiltrate, etc.
    ii. All cases demonstrating gram-negative bacteria in microbiology
    iii. Cases where vitreous infection precludes retinal examination
    iv. Vitreous abscess
    v. Cases not responding to initial medical therapy.

20. **What are the causes of treatment failure?**
    i. Late presentation/delayed diagnosis
    ii. Highly virulent organism
    iii. Drug resistance
    iv. Inadequate drug concentration
    v. Complications (RD)
    vi. Poor visibility for pars plana vitrectomy
    vii. Faulty diagnosis
    viii. Failure to recognize a nidus of infection, e.g. dacryocystitis.

Endophthalmitis Vitrectomy Study (EVS)

21. **What was the main objective of the EVS?**
    To determine role of early pars plana vitrectomy (PPV) in comparison to intravitreal injection in patients with postoperative endophthalmitis and also identify the role of systemic antibiotic treatment in these cases.

22. **What were the outcome measures of this study?**
    Visual acuity and media clarity at the end of 3–9-month follow-up.

23. **Mention the inclusion and exclusion criteria for this study.**
    Inclusion criteria
    i. Bacterial endophthalmitis within 6 weeks of cataract surgery or secondary IOL implantation.
    ii. Visual acuity of PL or better, but worse than 20/50 with relatively clear cornea and anterior chamber view.

    Exclusion criteria
    i. History of (H/o) of other intraocular surgery
    ii. Presentation after 6 weeks
    iii. Fungal infection

   iv. Previous intraocular antibiotic

   v. Retinal and choroidal detachments

   vi. Drug sensitivity to lactams.

24. What were the drugs used in the study?

   i. *Intravitreal*

     – Vancomycin (1,000 µg in 0.1 mL)

     – Amikacin (400 µg in 0.1mL)

      (No intravitreal corticosteroids were used.).

   ii. *Systemic*

     – Ceftazidime (2 g, 8 hourly)

     – Amikacin (7–5 mg/kg BD)

      If allergic to lactams, oral ciprofloxacin 750 mg BD was used

   iii. *Subconjunctival*

     – Vancomycin   (25 mg/0.5 mL)

     – Ceftazidime   (100 mg/0.5 mL)

     – Dexamethasone   (6 mg/0.25 mL)

   iv. *Topical*

     – Vancomycin (50 mg/mL)   every 4 hours

     – Amikacin (20 mg/mL)   every 4 hours

25. What were the major conclusions of study?

   i. There was no difference in final visual acuity or media clarity with or without the use of systemic antibiotics.

   ii. In patients whose initial visual acuity was hand motions or better, there was no difference in visual outcome whether or not an immediate vitrectomy was performed.

   iii. In patients with only light perception vision, vitrectomy was much better than intravitreal injections alone.

26. What is sterile postoperative endophthalmitis?

This is caused by the following:

   i. Postoperative inflammation to retained lens matter

   ii. Residual chemicals

   iii. Toxicity of residual monomers on PMMA

   iv. Mechanical irritation of iris and ciliary body.

27. Most common organism in bleb-related endophthalmitis.

   i. *Streptococcus*

   ii. *Haemophilus influenzae.*

28. What is the mode of treatment in severe _P. acnes_ infection?

  i. Vitrectomy

  ii. Total capsulectomy

  iii. IOL explantation combined with intraocular and systemic antibiotics.

29. What are the organisms common in endogenous endophthalmitis?

Fungal	_Bacteria_
Candida	Bacillus cereus
Aspergillus	

30. What are the organisms common in posttraumatic endophthalmitis?

Bacterial	_Fungal_
S. epidermidis	Fusarium
Bacillus cereus	
In children	
Streptococcal species.	

31. How does treatment of endogenous endophthalmitis differ from other types?

  i. Both bacterial and fungal in the initial phase are treated with intensive intravenous therapy.

  ii. Only if infection is not responding to medical intravenous therapy then intravitreal is considered.

32. What drug is contraindicated in endogenous endophthalmitis?

Corticosteroids.

33. How to prepare the commonly recommended intravitreal drugs in postoperative endophthalmitis?

Antibacterial

  i. Vancomycin hydrochloride (1,000 µg in 0.1 mL)

   – The drug is available as a powder in strength of 500 µg.

   – Reconstitute this with 10 mL of sterile solution for injection or saline.

   – This gives a strength of 50 mg in 1 mL and hence 10 mg in 0.2 mL.

   – 0.2 mL of this drug is drawn into a tuberculin syringe and this is further diluted with 0.8 mL of sterile saline to give a strength of 10 mg in 1 mL and hence 1,000 µg (1 mg) in 0.1 mL.

  ii. Ceftazidime hydrochloride (2.25 mg in 0.1 mL)

   – The drug is available as a powder in a strength of 500 mg powder.

   – Reconstitute this with 2 mL of sterile saline solution for injection to give a strength of 250 mg in 1 mL (225 mg of active ingredient) and 25 mg (22.5 mg) in 0.1 mL.

- 0.1 mL of the drug is drawn into a tuberculin syringe and diluted further with 0.9 mL of sterile solution to give a strength of 25 mg (22.5 mg) in 1 mL and hence 2.25 mg in 0.1 mL.

iii. Cefazolin hydrochloride (2.25 mg in 0.1 mL)

Same as for ceftazidime.

iv. Amikacin sulfate (400 μg in 0.1 mL)

- The drug is available as a solution in a strength of 100 mg in 2 mL vial (50 mg in 1 mL) and 10 mg in 0.2 mL.
- 0.2 mL of the drug is drawn into a tuberculin syringe and diluted further with 2.3 mL of sterile solution to give a strength of 10 mg in 2.5 mL and hence 4000 μg in 0.1 mL.

v. Gentamicin sulfate (200 μg in 0.1 mL)

- The drug is available as a solution of 80 mg in 2 mL vial (40 mg in 1 mL) and 4 mg in 0.1 mL.
- 0.1 mL of the drug is drawn into a tuberculin syringe and diluted further with 1.9 mL of solution to give a strength of 4 mg in 2 mL (2 mg in 1mL) and hence 200 μg in 0.1 mL.

Antifungal

i. **Amphotericin B (5 μg in 0.1 mL)**

- The drug is available as a 50 mg powder vial.
- Reconstitute this with 10 mL of dextrose 5% to give a concentration of 5 mg per mL and 500 μg in 0.1 mL.
- Take 0.1 mL into a tuberculin syringe and dilute further with 9.9 mL of dextrose 5% to give a concentration of 500 μg in 10 mL and 50 μg per mL and 5 μg in 0.1 mL.

ii. **Voriconazole**

- One vial of voriconazole contains 1 mg of the drug in powder form.
- It is reconstituted with 1 cc normal saline.
- 0.1 mL of the drug solution now contains 0.1 mg or 100 micrograms of voriconazole which is the recommended dose for intravitreal injection.
- 0.1 mL of the drug is withdrawn and injected into the vitreous cavity.

Corticosteroids

Intravitreal dexamethasone (400 μg in 0.1 mL)

i. The drug is available as a solution in strength of 8 mg in 2 mL vial (4 mg in 1 mL) and hence 0.4 mg (400 μg) in 0.1 mL.

ii. 0.1 mL of the drug may be withdrawn directly into a tuberculin syringe without any further dilution.

34. What are the recommended doses of systemic antibiotics in endogenous endophthalmitis?

Chloramphenicol—1–1.5 mg IV 6 hourly   Ceftaxime—2 g IV 4 hourly
Cefuroxime—3 g IV 8 hourly   Moxalactam—2–4 g IV 6–8 hourly
Ampicillin—2–4 g IV 4 hourly   Ceftizoxime—2 g IV 6 hourly
Vancomycin—500 mg IV 6 hourly   Penicillin G—2 mU IV 2 hourly.
Gentamicin—8 mg/kg/day IV

Intravenous treatment should continue at least for a period of 10–14 days.

6.11. RETINITIS PIGMENTOSA

1. **Define retinitis pigmentosa.**

   Retinitis pigmentosa is a clinically and genetically heterogenous group of progressive hereditary disorders that diffusely and primarily affect photoreceptor and pigment epithelial function, and that are associated with progressive cell loss and eventually atrophy of several retinal layers.

2. **What are synonyms of RP?**
   i. Tapetoretinal degeneration
   ii. Primary pigmentary retinal degeneration
   iii. Pigmentary retinopathy
   iv. Rod-cone dystrophy
   v. Retinal dystrophy.

3. **What is the prevalence rate of RP?**
   Between 1/3000 and 1/5000.

4. **What is the earliest presentation of RP?**
   Nyctalopia (night blindness) and progressive visual field disturbances. By the age of 30 years more than 75% of the patients become symptomatic.

5. **What are the causes of nyctalopia (night blindness)?**
   i. *Congenital stationary night blindness*
      – Presenting with normal fundus—AD, AR, X-linked forms
      – Presenting with abnormal fundus—fundus albipunctatus, Oguchi's disease
   ii. *Progressive night blindness*
      – Retinitis pigmentosa
      – Choroidal diseases like choroideremia, gyrate dystrophy, diffuse choroidal atrophy
      – High myopia
      – Progressive glaucoma
      – Retinitis punctata albescens
      – Vitamin A deficiency
      – Liver cirrhosis (alcoholic)
      – Tapetoretinal degenerations
   iii. *Spurious night blindness*
      – Nuclear cataract
      – Postrefractive surgery.

6. **What is day blindness (hemeralopia)?**
   i. Posterior subcapsular cataract
   ii. Hereditary retinoschisis
   iii. Intraocular iron.

7. **What are the causes of central vision loss in RP?**
   i. Posterior subcapsular cataract
   ii. Cystoid macular edema
   iii. Cellophane maculopathy
   iv. Diffuse vascular leakage
   v. Macular preretinal fibrosis
   vi. RPE defects.

8. **What are the visual field defects in RP?**
   i. *Paracentral scotoma:* starts 20° from fixation
   ii. *Ring scotoma:* Outer edge of the ring expands rapidly to the periphery while the inner ring contracts toward fixation.
   iii. *Constricted tunnel field of vision (tubular vision).*

9. **What is the cause of ring like scotomas in the visual field?**
   The pigmentary changes extend both posteriorly and anteriorly giving rise to ring like scotoma in the visual field.

10. **What are the conditions which can cause tubular vision?**
   i. Retinitis pigmentosa
   ii. Glaucoma
   iii. High myopia
   iv. Aphakic glasses
   v. Extensive choroiditis
   vi. Extensive panretinal photocoagulation
   vii. Chronic atrophic papilledema
   viii. Hysteria and malingering
   ix. Alcohol poisoning.

11. **What are the diagnostic criteria for RP?**
   i. Bilateral involvement
   ii. Loss of peripheral vision and night vision
   iii. Rod dysfunction
      – Dark adaptation
      – ERG
   iv. Progressive loss in photoreceptor function.

12. **Which photoreceptors are involved?**
   Both cones and rods involved, but rod is predominantly involved.

13. **What is the mode of inheritance?**
   i. Autosomal recessive: 60%
   ii. Autosomal dominant: 10–25%
   iii. X-linked: 5–18%

14. **Discuss the prognosis of inheritance pattern of RP.**
   i. Best prognosis—AD
   ii. Worst prognosis—X-linked

15. What is the triad of RP?

    i. Arteriolar attenuation

   ii. Retinal bone spicule pigmentation

  iii. Waxy disk pallor.

16. What are the causes of retinal vessel attenuation?

The exact cause is unknown but it is thought to be a secondary change. It is thought to be the result of:

    i. Increased intravascular oxygen tension due to decreased oxygen consumption by degenerating outer retinal layers

   ii. Closer proximity of retinal vascular network to the choroidal circulations as a result of retinal thinning.

17. What are the differential diagnosis of retinal vessel narrowing?

     i. Arteriosclerosis

    ii. Hypertensive retinopathy

   iii. Coarctation of aorta

   iv. Hyperbaric oxygen therapy

    v. Apparent narrowing (hypermetropia, aphakia)

   vi. Inflammatory disorders like temporal arteritis, polyarteritis nodosa.

18. What is the cause of "bone spicule pigment deposits"?

Pigments getting released from the degenerating retinal pigment epithelium migrates into the inner retina and accumulates in the inner retina around the blood vessels, especially at the vessel branchings producing a perivascular cuffing and bone spicule pigment formation.

19. What are the conditions causing pigmentation in retina?

      i. Retinitis pigmentosa

     ii. Senile changes (degenerative pigmentation)

    iii. Inflammatory conditions like rubella, congenital syphilis (salt and pepper fundus), toxoplasmosis.

    iv. CMV retinitis

     v. Toxic: Chloroquine, phenothiazines, clofazamine

    vi. Iatrogenic: Photocoagulation, cryotherapy

   vii. Trauma

 viii. Spontaneously settled retinal detachment

    ix. Hereditary chorioretinal dystrophies like fundus flavimaculatus, pigmented paravenous chorioretinal atrophy

     x. Choroideremia

   xi. Peripheral retinal pigment degeneration.

20. What is the site of pigmentary deposition in the initial stages of RP?

It is found at the midperipheral, equatorial region of the fundus. This part of the retina is the one to develop first and according to the principle of abiotrophy undergoes degeneration first as well.

21. **What are the conditions which cause consecutive optic atrophy (waxy disk pallor)?**
    i. Retinitis pigmentosa
    ii. High myopia
    iii. Extensive photocoagulation
    iv. Diffuse chorioretinitis
    v. CRAO.

22. **What is the cause of waxy disk pallor in RP?**
    The waxy disk pallor is due to a thick preretinal membrane centered on the disk that extends over the retina in all quadrants. The preretinal membrane appears to originate from fibrous astroglial cells in the optic nerve. The reorganization of fibrous astrocytes into the thickened retinal membrane over the optic nerve could contribute to the appearance of waxy pallor of the optic disk.

23. **What are the classic fundus appearance in a case of RP?**
    i. Optic nerve changes
       - Variable waxy pallor disk
       - Consecutive optic atrophy
    ii. Vessel changes
       Arteriolar narrowing
    iii. General retinal changes
       - Pigment within the retina—generalized granularity or discrete
       - Pigment clumps or bone spicule appearing pigment deposits
       - A generalized mottling or moth-eaten pattern of the RPE
       - A refractile appearance to the retina
    iv. Macular changes
       Loss of foveal reflex
       Maculopathy (three types)
       - Atropic
       - Cellophane
       - CME
    v. Vitreous changes
       Stage 1: Fine colorless dust particles
       Stage 2: Posterior vitreous detachment
       Stage 3: Vitreous condensation
       Stage 4: Collapse.

24. **What are the changes in macula?**
    Three types of macular lesions
    i. Atrophy of the macular area with thinning of RPE and mottled transmission defects of fluorescein angiography
    ii. Cystic lesion or partial thickness holes within the macula with radial, inner retinal traction lines and/or various degrees of preretinal

membranes causing a "surface wrinkling phenomenon" (cellophane maculopathy)

iii. Cystoid macular edema and increased capillary permeability.

25. What are the vitreous particles seen in RP?

Fine melanin pigment granules, pigment granules, uveal melanocytes, retinal astrocytes, and macrophages like cells.

26. What are the associated ocular features?

i. Myopia
ii. Keratoconus
iii. Open-angle glaucoma
iv. Posterior subcapsular cataract
v. Optic disk drusen
vi. Microphthalmus.

27. What are the causes of cataract formation in RP?

It is possibly caused by pseudoinflammatory pigmental cells in the vitreous and is of the central posterior subcapsular variety. Ultrastructurally the cataracts of RP are not unique expect for focal epithelial degeneration, which may cause osmotic instability.

28. What is to be kept in mind when performing cataract surgery in retinitis pigmentosa?

i. Patients with retinitis pigmentosa and complicated cataract who undergo cataract surgery may suffer from capsular phimosis as a postoperative complication.
ii. Performing a larger rhexis and use of capsular tension ring (CTR) may be useful approaches to minimize the complication.

29. Discuss the theories of RP.

i. Vascular theory
   - Sclerosis of choroid and choriocapillaries
   - Sclerosis of retinal vessels
ii. Pigmentary theory
   - Changes in neuroepithelium and pigmentary epithelium
iii. Abiotrophy
iv. Premature seniling and death of cells of specified tissues—equatorial parts are affected first because it is the first to attain full development.

30. What are the variants of RP?

i. *Inverse RP or central RP:*
   Pigments are more seen centrally and the equatorial and peripheral retina may be spared.
ii. *Sectoral RP:*
   Pigmentary changes are confined to one quadrant. Visual function remains good for many years.

iii. *RP with exudative vasculopathy:*
It is bilateral and consists of vascular anomalies, serous RD and lipid deposits in retinal periphery.

iv. *Unilateral RP:*
These are patients with unilateral pigmentary degeneration.

v. *RP sine pigmento:*
Typical symptoms and the presence of signs except pigmentary deposition.

vi. *Retinitis punctata albescens:*
Fine white punctate lesions in the midperiphery at the level of pigment epithelium with symptoms of RP.

31. What are the tests of visual function done in patients with RP?

i. *Electroretinogram (ERG):*
 – Very useful to determine early loss of photoreceptor function
 – Prognostic information in some cases of RP
 – Useful in evaluating therapeutic modalities of retinal dystrophies

ii. *Dark adaptations and visual sensitivity:*
To measure visual sensitivity, a test light positioned on a given area of the retina is dimmed to a subthreshold level and is then made gradually brighter. The intensity at which it is perceived is defined as visual threshold and may be expressed in log units.

Dark adaptation involves the measurement of the absolute thresholds at given time intervals as the retina adapts to the dark. The Goldmann–Weekers adaptometer is the most commonly used.

iii. *Visual fields*

iv. *Fundus reflectometry:*
Useful technique for quantitative assessment of photopigment regeneration

v. *Contrast sensitivity:*
It is a more sensitive test of macular function

vi. *Electro-oculogram (EOG):*
The EOG is thought to measure the functions of both the photoreceptors and retinal pigment epithelium. Although EOG is abnormal in RP even in early stages, ERG is more preferred.

vii. *Visually evoked response*

viii. *Fluorescein angiography:*
It is useful in patients with exudative vasculopathy and cystoid macular edema.

ix. *Vitreous fluorophotometry:*
It is a method of evaluating the blood–retinal barrier by quantifying the leakage of fluorescein from retinal vessels into the posterior vitreous. It is useful to detect abnormality of the blood–retinal barrier. Patients with RP have a marked elevation of the dye concentration in the vitreous.

32. What is the significance of the various waves in ERG?

The a-wave is the initial cornea-negative deflection, it is hypothesized to arise from the photoreceptors.

The b-wave is the largest wave of the ERG and is a cornea-positive wave. There is general consensus that the b-wave reflects primarily the activity of depolarizing (on) bipolar cells and also from the Muller cells.

The c-wave is a cornea-positive wave on the ERG. It is generated from the retinal pigment epithelium mainly in response to rod photoreceptors.

33. How is ERG useful in RP?

 i. Patients with advanced RP have non-detectable rod and cone responses
 ii. In patients with early disease, a and b waves generated by the photo-receptors in response to white light under dark-adapted conditions are reduced in amplitude
 iii. In all genetic subtypes of RP, the pure rod responses have "b" wave amplitudes which are non-detectable or reduced with either pro-longed or normal implicit times.

34. What is non-detectable ERG?

Defined as less than 10 micro volts.

35. What are the conditions which can cause nonrecordable ERG?

 i. Leber's congenital amaurosis
 ii. Retinal aplasia
 iii. Retinitis pigmentosa
 iv. Total retinal detachment.

36. What are histopathological changes of RP?

 i. Rod and cone outer segments—shortened and disorganized (but inner segment remains (normal)
 ii. In the area of visual loss from RP, there is total loss and decrease in photoreceptor number
 iii. Pigmented cells invade the retina.
 • Typical RPE cells away from the RPE layer and macrophage like cells that contain melanin also found in retina.

37. What are the systemic associations with RP?

 i. *Usher's syndrome:*
 Congenital sensory neural deafness with RP
 ii. *Lawrence–Moon–Biedl syndrome:* components are
 – Retinal dystrophy
 – Mental retardation
 – Truncal obesity
 – Hypogonadism
 – Polydactyly

iii. *Cockayne syndrome:*
RP with infantile onset of growth failure, cutaneous photosensitivity to UV light, cachexia, dementia, cerebellar dysfunction, and joint contractures

iv. *Alstrom syndrome:*
Cone-rod dystrophy, interstitial nephropathy, progressive sensory neural deafness.

v. *RP with neurological disorders:*
These are lysosomal storage diseases with accumulation of insoluble autofluorescent lipopigments in a variety of tissues. They are characterized by symptoms of RP along with cerebellar degeneration and extrapyramidal signs. They are of the following types:

- Infantile form: Haltia–Santavuori syndrome
- Late infantile form: Jansky–Bielschowsky syndrome
- Juvenile form: Batten–Spielmeyer–Vogt syndrome
- Hallervorden–Spatz syndrome

vi. *Spinocerebellar degenerations (Pierre-Maries's hereditary cerebellar ataxia)*

vii. *Kearns–Sayre syndrome (mitochondrial myopathy)*
Pigmentary degeneration of the retina, external ophthalmoplegia, and complete heart block.

viii. *Refsum's syndrome (phytanic acid storage disease)*
RP with peripheral neuropathy, cranial neuropathy, cerebellar involvement, cardiomyopathy and sudden death.

ix. *Mucopolysaccharidosis: Sanfilippo's and Schie's syndrome*

x. *Abetalipoproteinemia Bassen-Kornzweig syndrome*
RP with infantile steatorrhea and failure to thrive.

38. What are the types of Usher's syndrome?

Type I: Congenital, bilateral sensorineural deafness, and no intelligible speech.
Type II: Nonprogressive moderate to profound congenital sensory neural hearing impairment and late manifestation of RP
Type III: Type I patients with ataxia.

39. Why is deafness associated with RP?

i. Common origin of RPE and the epithelium of organ of Corti
ii. The cilium of inner air and the cilium of the photoreceptors may fail to develop due to a defective gene in Usher syndrome.

40. How do you manage a case of RP?

i. Clinical evaluation and investigation
ii. Treatment of allied conditions
iii. Low vision aids
iv. Genetic counseling
v. Psychological and vocational counseling.

41. Discuss the treatment of RP.

  i. *Surgical procedures*
    – To increase retinal blood flow
    – Injections of vitamins and minerals, vasodilators, penicillamine, tissue therapy with placental extract, cortisone, transfer factor, muscle transplant.

 ii. *Topical therapy*
    Dimethyl sulfoxide

iii. *Injections*
    – Yeast RNA and subretinal injections to fetal retinal cells
    – Beneficial effects of 15,000 IU/day of vitamin A has been reported

 iv. *Light deprivation*
    Dark glasses during outdoor activities—CPF (corning photochromatic filter)

  v. *Optical aids*
    – *Mirrors and prisms* mounted on spectacles for peripheral field expansion
    – *Field expanders*
      • Drawbacks like distortion of depth perception
    – *Reverse Galilean telescopes*
      • Diminish central visual acuity to an unacceptably low level
    – *Low vision aid*
      • Magnifiers and closed circuit television
    – *Image intensifiers*
    – *High intensity lantern.*

42. What are the recent treatment modalities in RP?

   i. Argus II epiretinal prosthesis (bionic eye)
  ii. Retinal chip research
 iii. Stem cell
 iv. Gene therapy
  v. Analysis of leukocyte DNA
 vi. Hormone estrogen injection.

6.12. RETINOBLASTOMA (RB)

1. **What is the most common intraocular malignancy of childhood?**
   Retinoblastoma.

2. **What are the other common childhood malignancies?**
   i. Rhabdomyosarcoma
   ii. Neuroblastoma
   iii. Ewing's sarcoma
   iv. Wilms' tumor.

3. **What is the incidence of retinoblastoma?**
   1 in 17,000 live births in western countries.

4. **What are the modes of presentations?**
   i. Heritable—40%
   ii. Nonheritable—60%

5. **What is the pathogenesis?**
   RB1 tumor suppressor gene is located on long arm of chromosome 13 at region 14. It codes for RB nucleoprotein, which normally suppresses cell division. Any mutation in RB gene will cause retinoblastoma.

6. **What are the nonocular cancers common in heritable retinoblastoma?**
   i. Pinealoma
   ii. Osteosarcoma
   iii. Melanoma
   iv. Malignancies of brain, lungs.

7. **From where does it arise?**
   It arises from primitive retinal cells before differentiation.

8. **What is the common age of presentation?**
   First year of life in bilateral cases
   Second year of life in unilateral cases.

9. **Why is retinoblastoma seldom seen after 3 years of age?**
   Primitive retinal cells disappear within first few years of life.

10. **What are the patterns of tumor spread?**
    i. Endophytic (vitreous): Retina is not detached.
    ii. Exophytic (subretinal space): Retina is detached.
    iii. Optic nerve invasion
    iv. Diffuse infiltration of retina
    v. Metastasis.

11. **What is the histopathological hallmark of differentiated retinoblastoma?**

    Rosettes formation.

12. **Describe Flexner–Wintersteiner rosette.**

    It is an expression of retinal differentiation. Cells surround a central lumen lined by refractile structure. Refractile lining corresponds to external limiting membrane of retina. It is characterized by single row of columnar cells with eosinophilic cytoplasm and peripherally situated nuclei.

13. **Describe Homer–Wright rosette.**

    It consists of cells which form around a mass of neural fibers. No lumen is present.

14. **What are the differences between Flexner–Wintersteiner and Homer–Wright rosettes?**

Flexner–Wintersteiner rosette	Homer–Wright rosette
It consists of columnar cells around central lumen	It consists of cells around a mass of neural fibers. No lumen is present
Hyaluronidase is present	Hyaluronidase is absent
It is also seen in medulloepithelioma	It is also seen in neuroblastoma, medulloblastoma, medulloepithelioma

15. **What are fleurettes?**

    Cluster of tumor cells with long cytoplasmic processes project through a fenestrated membrane and resembles a bouquet of flowers. It represents photoreceptor differentiation.

16. **What are the presenting features of retinoblastoma?**

       i. Leukokoria—56% (white reflex in the pupillary area)
      ii. Strabismus—20%
     iii. Vitreous opacity
      iv. Pseudohypopyon
       v. Iris heterochromia
      vi. Spontaneous hyphema
     vii. Inflammation mimicking orbital cellulitis
    viii. Vitreous hemorrhage
      ix. Glaucoma
       x. Corneal edema
      xi. Proptosis.

17. **What is the differential diagnosis of leucocoria?**

       i. Persistent hyperplastic primary vitreous (PHPV)
      ii. Coats' disease
     iii. Toxocariasis
      iv. Retinopathy of prematurity (ROP)

  v. Coloboma of choroid
  vi. Cataract
  vii. Vitreous hemorrhage (VH)
  viii. Retinal detachment (RD)
  ix. Retinal dysplasia.

18. **What are the signs of regression in case of endophytic retinoblastoma?**
  i. Pigmented atrophic ring at the circumference of tumor
  ii. Translucency of tumor.

19. **What are the predictive factors of metastasis?**
  i. Orbital invasion
  ii. Optic nerve invasion
  iii. Massive choroidal invasion
  iv. Tumor volume >1 cm^3.

20. **What are the investigations useful in diagnosis of retinoblastoma?**
  i. X-ray skull
  ii. USG
  iii. MRI
  iv. Specular microscopy (seeding of tumor cells in the endothelium).

21. **What are the features of retinoblastoma in X-ray?**
  i. Expansion of optic canal
  ii. Diffuse or finely stippled calcification.

22. **How does USG help in cases of retinoblastoma?**
  i. Tumor dimension
  ii. Orbital shadowing
  iii. Calcification
  iv. Helpful in hazy media.

23. **How does CT help?**
  i. To determine the size, extraocular extent of tumor
  ii. Calcification
  iii. Optic nerve evaluation.

24. **How does retinoblastoma present in MRI?**
  i. Hyperintense in T1 weighted images
  ii. Hypointense in T2 weighted images.

25. **What are the investigations contraindicated in retinoblastoma?**
  i. FNAC and incisional biopsy are contraindicated. It may lead to tumor seeding into orbit
  ii. CT scan carries risk of secondary tumor formation.

26. **Describe the types of retinoblastoma based on USG.**
  i. Solid—early lesion
  ii. Cystic—advanced tumor cells floating in vitreous.

27. What are the inflammatory conditions that mimic retinoblastoma?

i. Toxocariasis
ii. Posterior uveitis
iii. Orbital cellulitis
iv. Congenital toxoplasmosis.

28. What are the neoplastic conditions that mimic RB?

i. Retinal astrocytic hamartoma
ii. Medulloepithelioma
iii. Leukemia
iv. Rhabdomyosarcoma.

29. Name a few diseases having intraocular calcification.

i. Retinoblastoma
ii. Toxoplasmosis
iii. Tuberculosis
iv. Cysticercosis
v. Syphilis
vi. *Toxocara* endophthalmitis
vii. Coats' disease.

30. What are the classification systems used in retinoblastoma?

i. Reese–Ellsworth classification
ii. International classification system.

31. What is international classification?

Group A (Very-low risk)	Small tumor <3 mm confined to retina; 3 mm from fovea, 1.5 mm from optic disk
Group B (Low risk)	Tumor >3 mm confined to retina in any location with clear SRF <6 mm from tumor margin
Group C (Moderate risk)	Localized vitreous subretinal seeding (>6 mm in total from tumor margin). If there is more than 1 site of subretinal/vitreous seeding, then total of these sites must <6 mm.
Group D (High risk)	Diffuse vitreous and/or subretinal seeding (>6 mm in total from tumor margin). If there is more than 1 site of sub-retinal/vitreous seeding, then total of these sites must >6 mm SRF >6 mm from tumor margin
Group E (Very-high risk)	No visual potential or any one of the following: 1. tumor in anterior segment 2. tumor in ciliary body 3. NVG 4. VH obscuring tumor of significant hyphema 5. phthisical or pre-phthisical 6. orbital cellulitis like presentation.

32. What are the various treatment modalities available for RB?

    i. Enucleation

    ii. Chemotherapy

    iii. Radiotherapy

    iv. Cryotherapy

    v. Transpupillary thermotherapy

    vi. Photocoagulation.

33. How do you plan to treat retinoblastoma?

    i. Unilateral nonheritable retinoblastoma:

    Group A: Photocoagulation and cryotherapy

    Group B: 3–4 cycles of chemotherapy. Solitary lesion can be treated using a radioactive plaque

    Group C: 6 cycles of chemotherapy

    Group D: Enucleation

    ii. Bilateral retinoblastoma: Symmetrical disease

    Group A: Photocoagulation and cryotherapy

    Group B to C: Same treatment like unilateral disease

    Group D: 6 cycles of three drug chemotherapy

    iii. Bilateral retinoblastoma: Asymmetrical disease.

    If the worst eye is in group E, then primary enucleation is recommended.

34. What are the precautions to be taken while enucleating retinoblasmic eye?

Special considerations for enucleation in retinoblastoma:

    i. Minimal manipulation

    ii. Avoid use of clamps, snares, or cautery

    iii. Avoid perforation of the eye

    iv. Harvest long (>15 mm) optic nerve stump

    v. Inspect the enucleated eye for macroscopic extraocular extension and optic nerve involvement

    vi. Harvest fresh tissue for genetic studies

    vii. Place a primary implant

    viii. Avoid biointegrated implant if postoperative radiotherapy is necessary

35. What is the role of chemotherapy in management of retinoblastoma?

    i. Chemo reduction of tumor in association with local therapy

    ii. To reduce the possibility of orbital recurrence

    iii. Suspected/documented metastasis.

36. What are the common chemotherapeutic agents used in management of retinoblastoma?

    i. Day 1—vincristine + etoposide + carboplatin

ii. Day 2—etoposide
Standard dose (3 weekly, 6 cycles):
Vincristine—1.5 mg/m^2 (0.05 mg/kg for children <36 months and maximum dose <2 mg)
Etoposide—150 mg/m^2 (5 mg/kg for children <36 months)
Carboplatin—560 mg/m^2 (18.6 mg/kg for children <36 months)
High dose (3 weekly, 6–12 cycles)
Vincristine—0.025 mg/kg
Etoposide—12 mg/kg
Carboplatin—28 mg/kg.

37. **What is periocular chemotherapy?**
Subtenon carboplatin had been tried. 2 mL of 10 mg/mL solution is injected.

38. **What are the side effects of periocular chemotherapy?**
Orbital myositis, optic atrophy.

39. **What are the indications of focal therapy?**
i. Small tumor <3 mm in diameter and height located in visually non crucial areas.
ii. As an adjuvant in large tumors/vitreous/subretinal seeding.

40. **What are the lasers used in the management of retinoblastoma?**
Xenon arc, argon laser. Focal consolidation is most often accomplished with transpupillary therapy.

41. **Where do you prefer cryoablation and laser photoablation?**
Laser photoablation is preferred for posteriorly located tumors and cryoablation for anteriorly located tumors because of the risk of optic nerve and macular damage. RD can occur in cryo scar.

42. **What is the indicator of satisfactory freezing during cryotherapy in retinoblastoma?**
Vitreous overlying tumor must be frozen.

43. **What is the aim of modern treatment?**
To save life as well as salvage vision.

44. **What are the absolute indications for enucleation?**
i. Tumor >50% of globe
ii. Orbital or optic nerve involvement
iii. Anterior segment involvement with or without neovascular glaucoma.

45. **What are the types of radiation therapy?**
i. External beam therapy
ii. Intensity modulated radiation therapy
iii. Brachytherapy.

46. What are the limitations of external beam radiotherapy?

    i. Increased risk of second independent primary malignancy, e.g. osteosarcoma

    ii. Radiation-related sequelae like midface hypoplasia, cataract, optic neuropathy, vasculopathy.

47. What are factors that influence the prognosis of retinoblastoma?

    i. Tumor size

    ii. Amount of vitreous/anterior chamber seeding

    iii. Presence/absence of choroidal invasion

    iv. Degree of tumor invasion of optic nerve or subarachnoid space.

48. Name the cryotherapy technique followed in treatment of retinoblastoma.

Triple freeze thaw technique.

49. What is the new gene therapy used in the treatment of retinoblastoma?

Targeted therapy uses adenoviral-mediated transfection of tumor cells with thymidine kinase renders tumor cells susceptible to systemically administered ganciclovir.

50. What is trilateral RB?

Bilateral retinoblastoma with pinealoblastoma.

51. Importance of genetic counseling in the management of retinoblastoma.

In patients with a positive family history, 40% of the siblings would be at risk of developing retinoblastoma and 40% of the offspring of the affected patient may develop retinoblastoma.

In patients with no family history of retinoblastoma, if the affected child has unilateral retinoblastoma, 1% of the siblings are at risk and 8% of the offspring may develop retinoblastoma.

In cases of bilateral retinoblastoma with no positive family history, 6% of the siblings and 40% of the offspring have a chance of developing retinoblastoma.

6.13. AGE-RELATED MACULAR DEGENERATION (ARMD)

1. **Definition of ARMD.**
   i. It is a spectrum of disease.
   ii. Associated with visual loss, RPE changes, drusens, geographical atrophy of the retina, SRNVM (subretinal neovascular membrane)
   iii. Usually in person aged above 50 years
   iv. Drusen alone without visual loss not considered as ARMD.

2. **Definition of early ARMD (according to the International Epidemiological Age-related Maculopathy Study Group).**
   i. Degenerative disorder in persons >50 years characterized by presence of any of the following:
   ii. Soft drusen >63 μm
   iii. Area of hyperpigmentation and/or hypopigmentation associated with drusen but excluding pigment surrounding small, hard drusen
   iv. VA is not a criterion for diagnosis.

3. **What are the risk factors for AMD?**
   i. Age—incidence, prevalence, and progression all increases with age.
   ii. Gender—female > male: 2:1 (Blue Mountains Eye Study)
   iii. Race—more in Whites
   iv. Ocular risk factor—hyperopia
   v. Family history—four times higher risk
   vi. Oxidative stress—accumulation of prooxidant melanin oligomers in RPE are responsible.
   vii. Systemic hypertension
   viii. Smoking—increases the risk
   ix. Light exposure—photooxidative damage mediated by reactive O_2 intermediates. Dietary and medication factor—very high doses of zinc, vitamin C, vitamin E, and β-carotene provide a modest protective effect on progression to advanced neovascular AMD.
   x. Genetic factors–1q 25—31 and 10q26 increases risk
   xi. Cataract surgery.

4. **What are the clinical features of ARMD?**
   i. Blurred Vision—dry ARMD: Asymptomatic or gradual loss of central vision; Wet ARMD: Rapid onset of vision loss
   ii. Difficulty in night vision
   iii. Decreased contrast sensitivity
   iv. Decrease saturation of colors
   v. Distorted vision (metamorphopsia)
   vi. Central scotomas
   vii. Slow recovery of visual function after exposure to bright light.

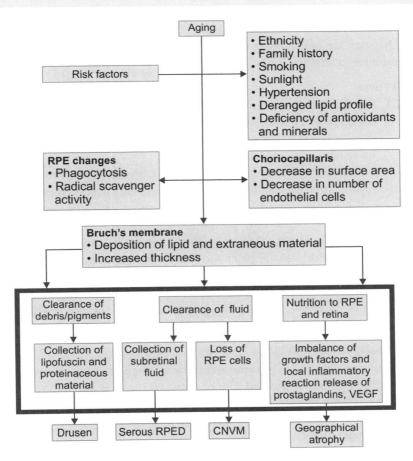

5. **What is the classification of AMD?**

AREDS (Age-Related Eye Disease Study) classification:

i. No AMD—category 1—control group—no or few small drusen <63 µ

ii. Early AMD—category 2—combination of multiple small drusen, few intermediate drusen (63–124 µ), or RPE abnormalities

iii. Intermediate AMD—category 3—extensive intermediate drusen, at least one large drusen (125 µ) or geographic atrophy not involving the center of the fovea

iv. Advanced AMD—category 4—characterized by one or more of the following in one eye:
   – Geographic atrophy of the RPE and choriocapillaries involving the center of fovea
   – Choroidal neovascularization (CNV)
   – Serous and/or hemorrhagic detachment of sensory retina or RPE
   – Retinal hard exudates
   – Subretinal and sub-RPE fibrovascular proliferation
   – diskiform scar.

6. What are drusens?

Drusens are aggregation of hyaline material located between Bruch's membrane and the RPE.

Types:

i. **Small, hard drusen:** Referred simply as drusen <63 µm

ii. **Large, soft drusen:** > 63 µm, ill-defined borders and vary in size and shape. They have a tendency toward confluence.

Three types (on basis of pathogenesis):

- Granular soft drusen: About 250 µm (2x vein width) with a yellow solid appearance, there confluence resulting in sinuous shapes.
- Soft serous drusen and drusenoid pigment epithelial detachments (PEDs): > 500 µm, may have pooled serous fluid, appearing blister like.
- Soft membranous drusen: Clinically between 63 and 175 µm (0.5–1.5 vein width), appear paler and shallower than the granular drusens.

iii. **Regressing drusens:** Drusens begin to regress when the overlying RPE fails. They become whiter and harder due to inspissation of contents. Hypo- and hyperpigmentation develops over the surface, margins become irregular and foci of calcification appear.

7. Classify CNV/SRNVM.

Histologically CNV is growth of abnormal, fragile new vessels between the Bruch's membrane and RPE or between the RPE and neurosensory retina. These vessels sprout from the choriocapillaries and proceed inwards through the defects in the Bruch's membrane.

i. **Topographic classification:**

- Extrafoveal (> 200 µm from foveal center)
- Juxtafoveal (1–199 µm from foveal center)
- Subfoveal—under the fovea.

ii. **Angiographic classification:**

- **Classic CNV**—reveals fairly discrete hyperfluorescence in early phase of angiogram that progressively intensifies throughout the transit phase, with intense late leakage of dye into the overlying neurosensory retinal detachment.
- **Occult CNV** is of two forms:
  - FVPED (Fibrovascular PED)—appears 1–2 minutes after dye injection. It appears as an irregular elevation of RPE with stippled leakage into overlying neurosensory detachment in early and late phase.
  - Late leakage of undetermined source: Regions of stippled or ill-defined leakage into overlying neurosensory detachment without a distinct source focus that can be identified in the early frames of angiogram.

8. **What is pigment epithelium detachment and how to identify PED in fluorescein angiography?**

Pigment epithelium detachment (PED): Appears as sharply demarcated, dome-shaped elevations of RPE. If filled with serous fluid they transilluminate. Four types of PED (on basis of angiographic pattern):

   i. **FVPED (Fibrovascular PED)**—appears 1–2 minutes after dye injection. It appears as an irregular elevation of RPE with stippled leakage into overlying neurosensory detachment in early and late phase.

   ii. **Serous PED**—uniform bright smooth and sharp hyperfluorescence with rapid homogenous filling that starts in early phase without leakage in late phase of angiogram. May or may not overlie CNVM.

   iii. **Drusenoid PED**—reveals hyperfluorescence in midphase which increases in late phase with faint hyperfluorescence of drusen and late staining. Does not have CNVM.

   iv. **Hemorrhagic PED**—dark sub-RPE blood, which blocks choroidal fluorescence on angiography.

9. **What is RPE rip/tear?**

Occurs as a complication in serous or fibrovacular PED at the border of attached and detached RPE due to stretching forces of the underlying fluid or from the contractile forces of the fibrovacular tissue. Clinically, it is seen as area of hypopigmentation with hyperpigmented wavy border on one side due to rolling in of the free edge of torn RPE.

10. **What is diskiform scar?**

It is the last stage in the evolution of neovascular AMD just as geographic atrophy as in dry AMD. Clinically apparent white to yellow subretinal scar with intervening areas of hyperpigmentation composed of fibrovascular complex is called diskiform scar.

11. **How do you differentiate dry ARMD and wet ARMD?**

Dry or nonexudative ARMD	Wet or exudative ARMD
More common	Less common
Atrophic and hypertrophic changes in the RPE underlying the central retina (macula) as well as deposits (drusen) on the RPE	Abnormal blood vessels called choroidal neovascular membranes develop under the retina
May progress to the exudative form of ARMD	Leak fluid and blood, and ultimately cause a blinding diskiform scar in and under the retina
Visual loss can occur particularly when geographic atrophy of the RPE develops in the fovea and causes a central scotoma	Causes severe visual loss as a result of leaky CNVMs

12. **What are the investigations for ARMD?**
    i. Fundus fluorescein angiography (FFA)
    ii. Indocyanine green (ICG) angiography
    iii. Optical coherence tomogram (OCT)
    iv. Multifocal electroretinography (MERG)
    i. **Fundus fluorescein angiography (FFA)**
      - *Classic CNV*—reveals fairly discrete hyperfluorescence in early phase of angiogram that progressively intensifies throughout the transit phase, with intense late leakage of dye into the overlying neurosensory retinal detachment.
      - *Occult CNV* is of two forms:
        • FVPED (fibrovascular PED)—appears 1–2 minutes after dye injection. It appears as an irregular elevation of RPE with stippled leakage into overlying neurosensory detachment in early and late phase.
        • Late leakage of undetermined source—regions of stippled or ill-defined leakage into overlying neurosensory detachment without a distinct source focus that can be identified in the early frames of angiogram.
    ii. **Indocyanine green (ICG) angiography**—can facilitate visualization of choroidal vasculature and CNVM through hemorrhage. ICG angiography can show CNVM as localized hot spots or as diffuse hyperfluorescent plaques.
    iii. **Optical coherence tomogram (OCT)**—high reflective thickened Bruch's/RPE complex that is characteristic of CNV in AMD. For monitoring the therapeutic response to photodynamic therapy (PDT) and anti-VEGF therapy.

13. **What are the differential diagnosis for CNVM?**
    i. Idiopathic polypoidal chorioidal vasculopathy (IPCV)
    ii. Myopia
    iii. Angioid streaks
    iv. Presumed ocular histoplasmosis syndrome.

14. **What are the treatment options available for ARMD?**
    i. **Early AMD**—no proven treatment
    ii. **Intermediate AMD**—the combination treatment of antioxidant, vitamins and minerals causes significant reduction in both the development of advanced AMD and vision loss.

Supplement	Dose (daily)
Vitamin C	500 mg
Vitamin E	400 IU
β-carotene	15 mg
Zinc oxide	80 mg
Cupric oxide	2 mg

iii. **Neovascular ARMD**
   - The VEGF inhibitors have become the first-line therapy for treating neovascular AMD.
     Ranibizumab (Lucentis)—dose: 0.3–0.5 mg in 0.03/0.05 mL every month intravitreally or as needed.
   - **Bevacizumab (Avastin)**—dosage between 1.25 and 2–5 mg monthly or as needed.
   - **Pegaptanib sodium (Macugen)**—dose: 0.3 mg injected every 6 weeks intravitreally.
   - **Cortisone**—triamcinolone in dosages of 4, 8, and 25 mg was used intravitreally, mainly as an adjunct to PDT. Side effects: Raised IOP and rapid cataract development.

Treatment according to location of CNVM:
   i. **Subfoveal CNV**—anti-VEGFs, verteporfin PDT, and thermal laser photocoagulation.
   ii. **Juxtafoveal CNV**—anti-VEGF is the primary therapy. PDT with verteporfin can also be used.
   iii. **Extrafoveal CNV**—anti-VEGFs, still a role for thermal laser treatment (as defined by the MPS).

Photodynamic therapy (PDT)
Mechanism of action: Initially, a drug (verteporfin) is administered. The drug gets concentrated in the immature endothelium of CNVM, and light-activation induces a photochemical reaction in the target area that causes immunologic and cellular damage, including endothelial damage of new vessels causing subsequent thrombosis and occlusion of the vasculature.

Procedure:
   i. Intravenous infusion of verteporfin (a benzoporphyrin derivative monoacid)—light-activated drug.
   ii. After 15 minutes the laser light (689 nm) is applied for 90 seconds.
      Avoid direct sunlight for about 2–5 days after treatment.
      Follow-up every 3 monthly.

Contraindicated in porphyria.

Transpupillary thermotherapy (TTT)
Modified infrared diode laser (810 nm) attached to the slit lamp is used. Used in treatment of subfoveal CNVM (classic, occult, or mixed).

15. **What are the newer modalities of treatments for ARMD?**
   i. **VEGF-trap**—regeneron-recombinant soluble VEGF receptor protein.
   ii. **Anecortave acetate**—15 mg every 6 monthly delivered by periocular posterior juxtascleral delivery.
   iii. **Small interfering RNA (siRNA)**—
      C and-5 therapy—it silences the gene that promote the overgrowth of blood vessels that lead to vision loss by shutting down the production of VEGF.

Sirna-027 therapy—modified siRNA that specifically targets VEGF receptor 1, a component of the angiogenic pathway found on endothelial cells.

16. **What surgical treatment options are available for ARMD?**
    i. **Macular translocation**—the aim of the surgery is to relocate the central neurosensory retina (fovea) away from the CNV, to an area of healthier RPE, Bruch's membrane, and choroid.
    ii. **Iris/retinal pigment epithelium transplantation**—fetal or mature RPE transplanted.
    iii. **Surgical removal**—failed to show a beneficial effect on vision in elderly patients with AMD.
    iv. **Retinal rotation**—extrafoveal RPE can maintain foveal function. Surgery has not been widely adopted.
    v. **Transplantation**—transplantation of the autologous RPE. It is performed in two different ways—the transplantation of a freshly harvested RPE suspension immediately after membrane removal and transplantation of a full thickness RPE-choroidal patch excised from the midperiphery of the retina and translocated subfoveally.

17. **What are the rehabilitation measures for ARMD patients?**
    i. Provision of low vision aids.
    ii. Visual handicap registration.
    iii. Training and coping strategies.
    iv. Statutory and voluntary support services in the community.

18. **Name the studies for ARMD.**
    i. **MARINA** (Minimally Classic/Occult Trial of the Anti-VEGF Antibody Ranibizumab in the treatment of Neovascular AMD)
    ii. **ANCHOR** (Anti-VEGF Antibody for the treatment of Predominantly Classic CNV in AMD)
    iii. **VISION** (VEGF Inhibition Study in Ocular Neovascularization)
    iv. **VIP** (Verteprofin in PDT)
    v. **TAP** (Treatment of Age-Related Macular Degeneration with Photodynamic therapy)
    vi. **PIER** (A Phase IIIb, Multicenter, Randomized, Double-Masked Degeneration with photodynamic therapy).

19. **What is MARINA trail?**
    i. Done for minimally classic and occult with no classic lesion
    ii. Divided into three groups—i. Sham injection. ii. Ranibizumab 0.3 mg every 4 weeks for 24 months. iii. Ranibizumab 0.5 every 4 weeks for 24 months.
    iii. After 2 years, mean visual acuity was better in Ranibizumab group versus placebo.

20. What is ANCHOR trail?

    i. This study was done for predominantly classic CNVM

   ii. Ranbizumab is superior to verteporfin in this condition

  iii. Divided into three groups:

      – Verteporfin PDT + Sham injection

      – Sham injection + Lucentis 0.3 mg every 4 weeks for 24 months

      – Sham + Verteporfin PDT + Lucentis 0.5 mg every 4 weeks for 24 months

  iv. Result—visual gain of 15 letters or more in:

    6% in group (i)

    36% in group (ii)

    40% in group (iii).

6.14. VITRECTOMY

Instrumentation:

1. **What are all the instruments used in vitrectomy?**
   i. The cutter
   ii. The intraocular illumination source
   iii. The infusion cannula
   iv. Accessory instruments like scissors, forceps, flute needle, endodiathermy, and endolaser delivery system.

2. **What is the number of oscillations in the guillotine blade?**
   i. Usually 1500 times/min
   ii. Latest—over 2500 times/min.

3. **What is the normal length of the infusion cannula? In which circumstances longer cannula is used?**
   Normal length is 4 mm. In special conditions like choroidal detachment or eyes with opaque media, 6 mm cannula is used.

4. **What are all the expanding agents? Why are they used?**
   i. Air
   ii. Sulfur hexafluoride which lasts for 10–14 days
   iii. Perfluoroethane which lasts for 30–35 days
   iv. Perfluoropropane which lasts for 55–65 days
   v. Expanding agents are used to achieve prolonged intraocular tamponade.

5. **Indications for vitrectomy.**
   i. **Anterior segment indications**
      – Glaucoma—ghost cell glaucoma due to vitreous hemorrhage
      – Cataract
        a. Lensectomy in eyes which need vitrectomy
        b. Dislocated lens fragments
      – Pupillary membranes
   ii. **Posterior segment indications**
      – **Indications for vitrectomy in diabetic retinopathy**
        • **Vitreous hemorrhage, especially if**
          o Longstanding
          o Bilateral
          o Disabling because of frequent recurrences
          o Retinal neovascularization is inactive
        • **Traction retinal detachment, especially if**
          o The macula is detached
          o It is of recent onset
        • **Combined traction/rhegmatogenous detachment**

- **Macular heterotopia of recent onset**
- **Macular epiretinal membranes**
- **Florid retinal neovascularization—(controversial)**

iii. **Other posterior segment indications**
   - Retinal detachment with proliferative vitreoretinopathy
   - Giant tears
   - Opaque media
   - Trauma
   - Macular pucker
   - Endophthalmitis
   - Uveitis
   - Acute retinal necrosis
   - Massive suprachoroidal hemorrhage
   - Macular hole
   - Retinopathy of prematurity
   - Sickle cell retinopathy
   - Dislocated intraocular lenses
   - Choroidal neovascular membrane
   - Diagnostic vitrectomy and retinal biopsy.

6. **What are the types of vitrectomy?**
   i. Open sky
   ii. Closed
      - Single port
      - Two port
      - Three port
      - Four port.

7. **What is the technique of three port pars plana vitrectomy?**
   i. A hand support is essential for intravitreal surgery. The surgeon rests both hands throughout the operation, avoiding fatigue and achieving fine control of the intravitreal manipulations.
   ii. Under aseptic precautions, plastic drape is pushed down into the space between the patient's head and the hand support, forming a trough to collect fluid that would otherwise spill onto the floor.
   iii. Small radial incisions through the conjunctiva and Tenon's capsule are made superonasally, superotemporally, and inferotemporally.
   iv. The sclerotomy incisions in the standard threeport vitrectomy technique are typically placed at the 10 and 2 o'clock positions at the same distance from the limbus as the infusion cannula.
   v. The entry incisions of size only to allow passage of instrument are parallel to the corneoscleral limbus and are 4 mm from it in phakic eyes and 3.5 mm in aphakic and pseudophakic eyes.

The first incision is for the infusion cannula, which is placed in the inferotemporal quadrant, just inferior to the lateral rectus.

A mattress suture which will secure the 4-mm diameter cannula infusion line is preplaced prior to entering the eye.

vi. After the infusion cannula is secured by its mattress suture, incisions are made in the superonasal and superotemporal quadrants for the vitrectomy instrument and the fiberoptics light pipe.

Before entering the eye, the surgeon must be certain that the instrument is functioning properly.

vii. If the pupil will not dilate, the iris must be retracted using pupillary stretching techniques or iris pins.

viii. **Vitrectomy**

The safest removal of vitreous is achieved using low suction (100–150 mm Hg) and a high cutting rate (400 cpm). This permits removal of small quantities of vitreous with each "bite" and reduces the risk of pulling on the vitreous base and of suddenly aspirating and cutting a detached retina.

After the vitreous has been removed and blood on the retinal surface has been aspirated, supplementary panretinal photocoagulation is given with the endolaser or with the laser indirect ophthalmoscope to diabetics who require it.

ix. Once the media have been cleared and the intraocular portion of the surgery has been completed, the cornea is covered to prevent foveal burns by the operating microscope. The scleral incisions are closed with 8-0 nylon sutures and the conjunctival incisions with 6-0 plain catgut.

The surgeon must carefully examine the peripheral retina for iatrogenic breaks.

8. **Mention the intraoperative complications of vitrectomy.**

     i. Cornea

Avoid corneal trauma especially in diabetic patients as they are vulnerable to recurrent erosion.

Do not perform corneal contact procedures such as tonometry, ERG, contact lens examinations.

Moisten cornea repeatedly throughout the procedure.

Endothelial damage during instrumentation and infusion; intraocular irrigating solutions are toxic to the corneal endothelium.

     ii. Cataract

Surgeon may inadvertently cause a break in the lens capsule with an instrument.

     iii. Choroidal hemorrhage

     iv. Choroidal detachment

v. Retina
- Iatrogenic tears, the worst operative complication of vitrectomy, have been reported to occur in approximately 20–25% of cases.
- One-third of all iatrogenic breaks are in the region of the sclerostomies, which must be carefully inspected by indirect ophthalmoscopy and scleral depression at the end of the procedure.
- If there is no vitreoretinal traction, cryotherapy of a peripheral tear with an intraocular gas tamponade will seal the tear.

9. **What are all the postoperative complications?**
    i. Cornea
    - Persistent stromal edema is twice as common in diabetics as in nondiabetics.
    - Formerly, as many as 15% of diabetic patients had significant postoperative corneal decompensation, and as many as 3% required a corneal transplant. More recent studies show a marked decrease in corneal complications.
    ii. Glaucoma
    - Neovascular glaucoma—11–26% of diabetic eyes go on to neovascular glaucoma.
    - Erythroclastic glaucoma
    - Chronic open-angle glaucoma the incidence of chronic open angle glaucoma after vitrectomy has been reported to be as high as 22% with most of the cases developing 5 or more years postoperatively.
    iii. Hypotony
    iv. Cataract
    Inadvertent touch by the vitrectomy instruments, toxicity of the intraocular irrigating solutions, and prolonged contact between the lens and long-lasting intraocular gases may all cause cataract.
    v. Vitreous hemorrhage
    vi. Anterior hyaloid fibrovascular proliferation
    vii. Retinal detachment
    Rhegmatogenous retinal detachment has been reported to occur in approximately 5–15% of cases.
    viii. Endophthalmitis
    ix. Sympathetic ophthalmia
    x. In association with vitrectomy, therefore, the placement or alteration of buckling material or manipulation of the extraocular muscles may produce:
    - Strabismus
    - Anterior segment necrosis
    - Postoperative infection
    xi. Extrusion of scleral buckling materials.

10. What are the factors contributing to neovascular glaucoma?
   i. Preoperative factors:
     – Neovascularization of the iris
     – Florid retinal neovascularization
     – Panretinal photocoagulation
     – Aphakia
   ii. Operative factors:
     – Removal of the lens
     – Failure to reattach the retina (50% cases).

11. What are the contraindications of vitrectomy?
   i. If the eye has no light perception
   ii. In the presence of suspected or active retinoblastoma
   iii. Active choroidal melanoma.

6.15. CENTRAL SEROUS CHORIORETINOPATHY (CSCR)

1. Define central serous chorioretinopathy.

It is a sporadic disorder of the outer blood–retinal barrier, characterized by a localized detachment of sensory retina at the macula secondary to focal RPE defect, usually affecting only one eye.

2. List out the risk factors that cause CSCR.

    i. Type A personality

    ii. Emotional stress

    iii. Untreated hypertension

    iv. Alcohol use

    v. Systemic lupus erythematosus

    vi. Organ transplantation

    vii. Gastroesophageal reflux

    viii. Cushing's disease

    ix. Pregnancy.

3. Age in which CSCR is common?

    i. Common among young or middle aged men, 30–50 years of age.

    ii. Men typically outnumber women with a ratio of at least 6:1.

    iii. In patients older than 50 years the ratio is changed to 2:1.

4. Classify CSCR.

CSCR are generally classified as:

    i. Typical CSCR

    ii. Atypical CSCR.

       Histologically CSCR (Spitnaz classification) has been classified as

       Type 1—detachment of sensory retina

       Type 2—RPE detachment

       Type 3—intermediate type—both sensory retina and RPE are elevated.

5. What are the clinical features of typical CSCR?

    i. Best corrected visual acuity of 6/60 or better

    ii. Macular detachment greater than 3 DD

    iii. Pin point ink blot, smoke stack leakage in FFA

    iv. Spontaneous resolution.

6. What are the common clinical features in CSCR?

At presentation:

    i. Unilateral blurred vision

    ii. Micropsia

    iii. metamorphopsia

    iv. Loss of color saturation.

Signs
  i. A round or oval detachment of the sensory retina is present at the macula.
 ii. Yellowish subretinal deposits forming a spot pattern.

7. **What are the FFA findings in CSCR?**
   i. Smoke stack:
      – Less common (10%)
      – Early phase—small hyperfluorescent spot due to leakage of dye through RPE
      – Late phase—fluorescein passes into the subretinal space and ascends vertically to the upper border of detachment, and then spreads laterally until the entire area is filled with dye
   ii. Ink blot:
      – Is more common
      – Early phase—shows hyperfluorescent spot
      – Late phase—spot gradually enlarges centrifugally until the area is filled with dye.

8. **What are the conditions during which management of CSCR becomes important?**
   Laser photocoagulation is carried out only when the following guidelines are met:
     i. Unresolving CSCR of 4 months or more duration.
    ii. If spontaneous recovery does not occur within a month in a patient with or without a history of recurrent CSCR in the same eye or if the other eye associated with visual loss due to previous episodes of CSCR.
   iii. For patients with occupational needs for binocular vision (pilot, surgeons).
    iv. In the acute stage, photocoagulation at the site of leakage can result in resolution of subretinal fluid in 3–4 weeks.

9. **What are the settings for laser therapy in CSCR?**
   Two or three moderate intensity burns are applied to the leakage sites to produce mild graying of the RPE.
   Spot size of 200 µ for 0.2 seconds and power of 80 MW titrated to 30 MW once the blanching signs are seen in RPE.

10. **What are all the differential diagnosis of CSCR?**
    i. Choroidal neovascular membrane
   ii. VKH
  iii. Optic disk pit
   iv. Posterior scleritis
    v. Rhegmatogenous retinal detachment.

6.16. ANGIOGENESIS

1. Name the angiogenic molecules.
   i. VEGF (vascular endothelial-growth factor)
   ii. Fibroblast growth factor
   iii. Integrins
   iv. Angioprotein
   v. Protein kinase C
   vi. Ephrins.

2. Name antiangiogenic factors.
   i. Pigment epithelial-derived factor
   ii. Matrix metalloproteinases
   iii. Angiostatin
   iv. Endostatin
   v. Thrombospondin
   vi. Steroids.

3. How many types of VEGF are present?
   i. VEGF-A
   ii. VEGF-B
   iii. VEGF-C
   iv. VEGF-D
   v. VEGF-E.

4. How many isoforms of VEGF-A are present?
   i. VEGF-206
   ii. VEGF-189
   iii. VEGF-165
   iv. VEGF-145
   v. VEGF-121.

5. Which is the main isoform of VEGF?
   VEGF A 165 is the predominantly expressed isoform. It is critical for both developmental and pathological neovascularization.

6. What is the role of other VEGF?
   i. VEGF B,C,D—play role in tumor angiogenesis and development of the lymphatic system
   ii. VEGF E—has similar angiogenic activity to VEGF A.

7. Where are the VEGF receptors found?
   i. Endothelial cells
   ii. Retinal epithelial cells
   iii. Bone marrow-derived epithelial cells.

8. **What are the factors upregulating VEGF?**

    i. Hypoxia
    ii. Hypoglycemia
    iii. β-estradiol
    iv. Epidermal growth factor
    v. Insulin-like growth factor
    vi. Pigment-derived growth factor
    vii. Fibroblast growth factor.

9. **What is the source of VEGF?**

    i. Muller cells
    ii. Endothelial cells of vessels.

10. **What are the properties of VEGF?**

    i. Stimulates angiogenesis
    ii. Increases vascular permeability
    iii. Proinflammatory action
    iv. Endothelial survival factor and fenestration factor
    v. Neuroprotective factor.

11. **What are the pathologic role of VEGF?**

    i. Neovascular AMD
    ii. Diabetic retinopathy
    iii. Retinal vein occlusion
    iv. Retinopathy of prematurity
    v. Corneal neovascularization
    vi. Iris neovascularization
    vii. Systemically, it has a role in cancer, psoriasis, rheumatoid arthritis.

6.17. INTRAVITREAL INJECTIONS

1. **What is the need for intravitreal injections?**
    i. Poor ocular penetration of systemically administered drugs especially posterior segment attributed to blood aqueous and retinal barrier.
    ii. Higher efficacy of local treatment due to desired dose at target site.
    iii. Reduced systemic toxicity.

2. **What are the common diseases treated by intravitreal injections?**
    i.   AMD
    ii. CSME/PDR
    iii. Retinal vein occlusions
    iv. Endophthalmitis
    v.   Uveitis
    vi. CME
    vii. CNVM secondary to multiple retinal diseases.

3. **What are the indications for intravitreal steroids?**
    i.   Diabetic macular edema—diffuse/refractory CME
    ii. Venous occlusions with macular edema
    iii. Uveitic macular edema
    iv. Pseudophakic macular edema
    v.   Adjunct to vitreoretinal surgery
    vi. Ocular hypotony
    vii. ARMD.

4. **Classify VEGF family. What are the isoforms of VEGF-A and its significance in management?**
    i.   VEGF-A, B, C, D, E, and PlGF
    ii.   VEGF-A isoforms 121, 145, 165, 189, and 206.
    iii. 121—dSoluble, unbound to extracellular matrix (ECM)
    iv.   165—intermediately soluble, binds somewhat to ECM-critical for developmental and pathologic retinal angiogenesis
    v.   189—sequestered to ECM
    vi.   Pegaptinib—binds only to VEGF-A 165 isoform
    vii. Bevacizumab—binds to all VEGF-A isoforms
    viii. Ranibizumab—binds with higher affinity to VEGF-A than bevacizumab
    ix.   Aflibercept—binds with maximum affinity to VEGF-A. Also with VEGF-B and PlGF.

5. **What is its mechanism of action?**
   i. Decrease expression of VEGF and VEGFR-2
   ii. Increase expression of decoy VEGFR-1
   iii. Decrease expression of ICAM-1.

6. **Complication of intravitreal steroids.**
   i. Ocular HTN
   ii. Progression of cataract
   iii. Inflammation
       – Sterile endophthalmitis-idiosyncratic reaction to vehicle or contaminant
       – Pseudo endophthalmitis-white crystals enter the AC and appear as hypopyon. Seen in aphakic or pseudophakic patients with PC rent.
       – Infectious endophthalmitis
   iv. RD
   v. Glaucoma
   vi. Local SCH.

7. **Indications for anti-VEGF.**
   i. Neovascular AMD
   ii. Diabetic retinopathy
   iii. Retinal vein occlusion with CME
   iv. Iris neovascularization—intracameral
   v. ROP
   vi. Corneal neovascularization—intracameral.

8. **Indications for anti-VEGF in DR.**
   i. Diffuse macular edema
       – Primary
       – Adjuvant with laser
       – Steroid responder
   ii. PDR
       – Post-PRP refractory PDR
       – Vitreous hemorrhage
       – Preoperative injection—2–3 days prior to surgery to reduce the vascularity and intraoperative bleeding
       – Neovascular glaucoma.

9. **Strategies in anti-VEGF therapy**
   i. Inhibition of VEGF production
   ii. Neutralisation of free VEGF
   iii. Blockage of VEGF receptors and intracellular signal transduction pathways
   iv. Inhibition of endothelial cellular response to VEGF.

10. Anti-VEGF agents

   i. Bevacizumab—Avastin
   ii. Ranibizumab—Lucentis
   iii. Pegaptanib—Macugen
   iv. VEGF trap—Eyelea
   v. Squalamine lactate—Evizon
   vi. Sirna 027
   vii. SU 5416

11. What is the half-life of various anti-VEGF?

   i. Lucentis—9 days
   ii. Macugen—10 days
   iii. Avastin—21 days.

12. Anti-VEGF comparison

Intravitreal drug	Bevacizumab	Ranibizumab	Triamcinolone	Aflibercept
Intravitreal dose	1.25 mg	0.3 FDA 0.5 (commonly used)	2 mg, 4 mg	2 mg
Strength in vial	25 mg/mL	0.5m/0.05 mL	40 mg/mL	2 mg/0.05 mL
Amount to be injected	0.05 mL	0.05 mL	0.1 mL	0.05 mL
To be repeated after	1 month	1 month	3–4 months	2 months
No. of injections/vial	30–40	1	Up to 10	1

13. Differences between Avastin and Lucentis

Avastin	Lucentis
▪ Full-length antibody ▪ Designed for IV administration ▪ T ½ 20 days ▪ Less frequent injection ▪ Less potent in binding ▪ Less penetration ▪ More uveitis—as larger foreign protein Comparatively Cheaper	▪ Fragment antigen binding ▪ Ocular administration ▪ T ½ 9 days ▪ Affinity matured—5–10 times more potent in binding to all isoforms ▪ Penetrates full thickness of retina Comparatively Costlier

14. Complication of anti-VEGF

   i. **Ocular:**
     – Endophthalmitis
     – IOP rise
     – Uveitis

- Vitreous hemorrhage
- RPE tear
- RRD (Rhegmatogenous retinal detachment)
- Cataract
- SCH (Subconjunctival hemorrhage)

ii. **Systemic:**
- Nonocular hemorrhage
- Death

iii. **Contraindication**
- Pregnancy
- Active ocular infection/inflammation.

15. **Guidelines for peri-injection management**
   i. Informed written consent for intravitreal therapy
   ii. Confirmation of the patient identity, eye, and the medication to be injected
   iii. Pupillary dilation
   iv. Topical anesthetic
   v. 10% povidone iodine—skin and periocular area
   vi. 5% Povidone iodine—conjunctival cul-de-sac
   vii. Sterile drape
   viii. Lid speculum—to isolate eye lashes.

16. **Preparation of the injection**
   i. Drugs dispensed in single dose vial
      - Ranibizumab and triamcinolone acetonide
      - Surface of the rubber cork is cleaned with alcohol swab
      - Drop of povidone iodine is placed for 2–3 minutes
   ii. Drugs dispensed in multidose vial—bevacizumab
      - Single dose sterile injections dispensed by pharmacy
      - One vial distributed among many patients by the ophthalmologist (4 mL vial containing 100 mg).

17. **Site of injection**
   i. Inferotemporal quadrant—preferred because of wide space, pars plana is wider here, if the patient has bells phenomenon then its advantageous.
      - Wide space to give injection
      - Pars plana is wider
      - Advantages especially in the presence of Bell's phenomena
   ii. 3.5 mm posterior to the limbus for a pseudophakic
   iii. 4 mm—phakic eye.

Age	Distance of injection from limbus
1–6 months	1.5 mm
6 months–1 year	2 mm
1–2 years	2.5 mm
2–6 years	3 mm
7 years onwards	4 mm phakic 3.5 mm pseudophakic 3 mm aphakic

18. **Needle size**
    i. Use a needle of 27-gauge or smaller with a length of 0.5–0.62 inches
    ii. Insert the needle at least 6 mm toward the center of the eye
    iii. Injections with crystalline TA are frequently applied with 27-gauge needles, while most liquid injections use 30-gauge needles.

19. **Anesthesia**
    i. Topical anesthetic drops
    ii. Lignocaine soaked cotton tipped swabs
    iii. Lignocaine gel
    iv. Subconjunctival injection of anesthetic agents.

20. **Procedure**
    i. Patient is asked to look away from site of injection (superonasally)
    ii. Mark the injection site using the caliper
    iii. The needle is inserted perpendicular through sclera with the tip aimed toward the center of the globe (to avoid any contact with the posterior lens)
    iv. Remove needle slowly and carefully
    v. A sterile cotton-tipped applicator is used to prevent reflux and to steady the eye
    vi. Once the needle is withdrawn any of following can happen
       - Liquid vitreous coming out
       - Spot of subconjunctival hemorrhage
       - Treatment—no special measured are required.

21. **The injection procedure**
    The angle of the incision through the sclera may be directed in an oblique, tunneled fashion, as rectangular radial incisions should not be performed since it may remain open, inducing vitreous or drug reflux under the conjunctiva, as well as severe chemosis and even hypotony in vitrectomized eyes.

22. Postinjection procedure

   i. Indirect ophthalmoscopy after any intravitreal injection

  ii. Normal disc perfusion as assessed by color of disc and venous pulsation

 iii. Vision should be grossly tested by show of fingers

 iv. Povidone iodine 5%—conj cul-de-sac

  v. Eye patched for 4 hours

 vi. Antibiotic eyedrops for 1–2 weeks.

23. Various drugs and their doses

Therapeutic agent	Absolute indications	Relative indications	Standard dosage
Triamcinolone Acetonide	Refractory CSME, refractory pseudophakic CME, CRVO, BRVO	—	2 mg in 0.05 mL/ 4 mg in 0.1 mL
Macugen (pegaptanib sodium)	CNVM -Wet AMD - Non-AMD	Refractory CSME, PDR, NVG, CRVO, BRVO	0.3 mg in 90 µL
Lucentis (ranibizumab)	CNVM -Wet AMD - Non-AMD	Refractory CSME, PDR, NVG, CRVO, BRVO	0.3 mg in 0.05 mL
Avastin (bevacizumab)	CNVM -Wet AMD - Non-AMD	Refractory CSME, PDR, NVG, CRVO, BRVO	1.25 mg in 0.05 mL

Drug	Indication	Dosage
Dexamethasone	Cystoids macular edema	400 microgram in 0.1 mL
Vancomycyin	Endophthalmitis	1 mg in 0.1 mL
Amikacin	Endophthalmitis	0.4 mg in 0.1 mL
Ceftazidime/cefazoline/ cefotaxim	Endophthalmitis	2.25 mg in 0.1 mL
Amphotericin B	Endophthalmitis	5 µg in 0.1 mL
Air	Pneumatic retinopexy	0.5–0.8cc
SF6 (100%)	Pneumatic retinopexy	0.5 mL
C3F8 (100%)	Pneumatic retinopexy	0.3 mL
Gancyclovir	CMV retinitis	2.5 mg in 0.05 mL
Avastin	ROP	0.675 mg in 0.03 mL

24. What are the studies in DR related to intravitreal injections?

Title	Purpose	Conclusion
RESOLVE 2005	Safety and efficacy of RBZ in DME involving foveal center	RBZ is effective in improving BCVA and is well tolerated in DME
RIDE AND RISE (2007)	Efficacy and safety of intravitreal RBZ in DME	RBZ rapidly and sustainably improved vision, reduced the risk of further vision loss, and improved macular edema in patients with DME with low rates of ocular and nonocular harm
BOLT 2007	Bevacizumab vs macular Laser therapy (MLT) in CSME	The study support the use of bevacizumab in patients with center involving CSME without advanced macular ischemia
DA VINCI 2008	VEGF Trap-Eye vs LASER in DME	VEGF Trap-Eye produced a statistically significant and clinically relevant improvement in BCVA compared with macular LASER in DME at 24 and 52 weeks
PROTOCOL I (2010)	Intravitreal ranibizumab for diabetic macular edema with prompt vs deferred laser treatment	5 years result suggest focal or grid laser treatment at initiation of intravitreal ranibuzumab is no better than deferring laser treatment for >24 weeks in eye with center involving DME with visual impairment
PROTOCOL S (2015)	Panretinal photocoagulation vs intravitreous ranibizumab for PDR	Among eyes with PDR, treatment with ranibizumab resulted in visual acuity that was not inferior to PRP at 2 years Although longer-term follow-up is needed, ranibizumab may be a reasonable treatment alternative for patients with PDR
PROTOCOL T (2016)	To determine relative efficacy and safety of intravitreous aflibercept, bevacizumab, ranibizumab in the treatment of diabetic macular edema	All three anti-VEGF groups showed VA improvement from baseline to 2 years with a decreased number of injections in year 2. Visual acuity outcomes were similar for eyes with better baseline VA. Among eyes with worse baseline VA, aflibercept had superior 2-year VA outcomes compared with bevacizumab, but superiority of aflibercept over ranibizumab, noted at 1 year, was no longer identified

Neuro-ophthalmology

7.1. NORMAL PUPIL

1. **Define pupil.**

   The pupil is an opening present in the center of the iris that controls the amount of light passing to the retina.

2. **What are the muscles involved in pupillary action and where are they derived from?**

   i. Sphincter
   ii. Dilator
   Both are derived from neuroectoderm.

3. **What is the normal shape and size of the pupil and how does it vary with age?**

   i. Normal pupil is approximately circular and usually placed slightly eccentrically towards the nasal side (inferonasal).
   ii. Average size (2.4–4 mm)
   iii. Larger in myopes
   iv. Smaller in hypermetropes
   v. Constantly smaller in very young and very aged because of decreasing sympathetic activity.
   vi. Largest in adolescence.

4. **What is the size of pupil when maximally dilated and maximally constricted?**

   Dilated pupil: 10 mm
   Constricted pupil: 1–1.5 mm.

5. **At what age does the pupillary light reaction start and what is the range at birth?**

   i. Premature baby has no pupillary light reaction until 3 weeks of gestational age.
   ii. Gradually increases up to 2 mm at birth.

6. **Trace the light reflex pathway.**

 i.

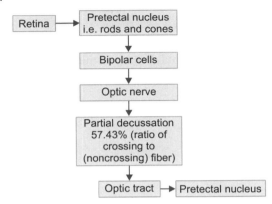

 ii. Intercalated neurons from the pretectal complex to parasympathetic motor pool

 (Edinger–Westphal of oculomotor nuclear complex)

   Parasympathetic outflow from Edinger–Westphal nucleus

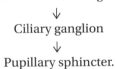

   Ciliary ganglion
   ↓
   Pupillary sphincter.

7. **How do you test the light reflex pathway?**

 i. **Direct response:**

  – The person testing should cover both eyes of the patient with palms of his hands or with two cards.

   One eye is then uncovered. Pupil should contract briskly and contraction should be maintained.

   Similar response should be noted in the other eye.

  – Patient should be asked to sit in a dimly lit room.

   Person testing should use a point light source or a pen torch.

   Patient should be asked to look into a distance approximately 6 meters (to avoid accommodation reflex).

   Light should be brought from temporal side focusing onto the nasal side.

 ii. **Indirect response:**

  – Criteria similar to that done in card test:

   It is obtained by uncovering one eye in such a way that it is not exposed to direct light while the other is alternately covered and exposed.

– Criteria are:
- Dim light
- Point light source
- Patient looking into distance
- Light should be brought from temporal side focusing onto the nasal side, so that it does not fall on the other eye and the reflex is observed in the unstimulated eye.

8. **Trace the near reflex pathway.**

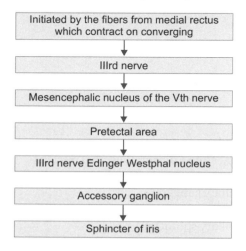

Initiated by the fibers from medial rectus which contract on converging

↓

IIIrd nerve

↓

Mesencephalic nucleus of the Vth nerve

↓

Pretectal area

↓

IIIrd nerve Edinger Westphal nucleus

↓

Accessory ganglion

↓

Sphincter of iris

9. **How do you test pupillary reactions for accommodation?**
   Normal light
   i. Ask the patient to look into the distance
   ii. Suddenly ask the patient to fixate to a close object at 6 inches from the patient's nose.

   Most accurately
   i. Patient is facing a wall between two windows and a small object is fixated for about half a minute 50 cm from his eye.
   ii. This is gradually moved towards his eyes as it approaches a distance of 40 cm, slight contraction should be noted, which becomes stronger when the distance is 20–15 cm.

10. **Describe other pupillary reactions.**
    i. **Hemianopic pupillary reaction of Wernicke's syndrome:** It is a crude method to estimate the function of nasal and temporal half of retina. Point pencil of light is used.
    ii. **Orbicularis (lid) reflex:** Is elicited by observing the pupillary contraction which occurs when a forcible attempt is made to close the lid while they are held apart by fingers or speculum.

iii. **Oculosensory reflex:** It is elicited by touching the cornea or the conjunctiva lightly with a cotton, and the pupil responds by dilating and then contracting. The reaction of the pupil will be sluggish, when light is thrown on the nonfunctioning part of retina.

11. How do you measure the size of the pupil?

Pupillometer.

12. Name some pupillometers.

   i. **Haabs:** It is a rough method of examination of the pupil size measurement by direct comparison of the aperture of the pupil with a series of circular disks of graduated sizes.
   ii. Similar method with ophthalmoscope is used in Morton's ophthalmoscope.
   iii. **Projection pupillometer:** Depends on the projection of the scale on the eye of the subject
       a. Priestley Smith's keratometer and pupillometer
       b. Bumke's
   iv. **Sanders:** It is a device attached to the corneal microscope of Zeiss. The light is reflected into the eye through a movable glass plate, which is graded in tint, in such a way that different parts transmit a different proportion of incident light. The degree of contraction can be accurately decided at different illumination and the least intensity at which the pupillary reaction starts can be noted.
   v. **Hemiakinesia meter:** This instrument is helpful in eliciting hemi-anopic pupillary response. This is possible because the illuminating system is duplicated. This provides for momentary stimulation of the peripheral retinal element, both in horizontal and oblique meridians.

13. What are the other methods of pupillometry?

   i. Photographic
   ii. Cinematographic
   iii. Electronic.

14. What is normal pupillary cycle time?

It is measured in slit lamp in dimly lit room.

A stopwatch is needed; time taken from the time the light is on to the constant contraction of pupil without any oscillation is noted. Normal 900 msec/cycle.

7.2. ABNORMAL PUPILS

1. **What are the characteristics of Marcus Gunn pupil?**
    Afferent pupillary defect
    Causes:
    i.   Optic neuropathy
    ii. Extensive retinal damage
    iii. Amaurotic pupil.

2. **What are the characteristics of Adie's tonic pupil?**
    i.   Idiopathic
    ii.   Female predilection
    iii. Dilated pupil with poor to absent light reaction
    iv.   Slow constriction to prolonged near effort and slow redilatation after near effort
    v.   Vermiform constriction of the iris sphincter on slit lamp examination
    vi.   Demonstrates cholinergic supersensitivity to weak (0.125%) pilocarpine solution
    vii. It may be associated with diminished deep tendon reflexes.

3. **What are the characteristics of Argyll Robertson pupil?**
    i.   Miotic, irregular pupils
    ii.   Light reflex absent
    iii. Accommodation reflex present
    iv.   *Etiology:* Neurosyphilis, diabetes mellitus, chronic alcoholism, multiple sclerosis, sarcoidosis
    v.   Site of lesion: Most likely in the region of sylvian aqueduct (dorsal midbrain).

4. **What are the characteristics of Hutchinson pupil?**
    i.   Seen in comatose patient
    ii.   Unilateral dilated poorly reactive pupil
    iii. *Etiology:* Due to expanding intracranial supratentorial mass that is causing downward displacement of hippocampal gyrus and uncal herniation compressing the third cranial nerve.

5. **What are the characteristics of Horner's pupil?**
    i.   Miosis
    ii.   Anhydrosis of the affected side of the face
    iii. Apparent enophthalmos due to narrow palpebral fissure
    iv.   Ptosis of the upper lid.

6. **What are the characteristics of Horner's syndrome?**
    i. Cocaine test
    ii. Paredrine test

    Causes of Horner's syndrome
    i. First-order neuron lesion
        – Cerebrovascular accident
        – Demyelinating disease
        – Neck trauma
        – Syringomyelia
        – Arnold–Chiari malformation
        – Neoplasm
    ii. Second order neuron lesion (preganglionic)
        – Chest lesions—Pancoast tumor, mediastinal mass, cervical rib
        – Neck lesions—trauma, thyroid lesion
        – Third order neuron lesion (postganglionic)
            • Migraine
            • Otitis media
            • Cavernous sinus lesion
            • Carotid–cavernous fistula.

7. **Can midbrain lesions have relative afferent pupillary defect (RAPD)?**
    Yes. Since the efferent fibers are present up to the Edinger–Westphal nucleus. Beyond Edinger–Westphal nucleus, there will be no RAPD. Optic nerve lesion causes same eye RAPD whereas optic tract lesions would produce fellow eye RAPD, since the nasal fibers have crossed over and nasal retina maintains eye and pupillary reactions.

7.3. OPTIC NERVE HEAD

1. **What are the dimensions of the optic nerve?**

   The optic nerve extends from the eye ball to the optic chiasma. It measures about 3.5–5.5 cm in length. The diameter ranges from 3 mm in orbit to 7 mm near the chiasma.

2. **Define optic nerve head (ONH).**
   i. It is the part of the optic nerve that extends from the retinal surface to the myelinated portion of the optic nerve just behind sclera
   ii. In reference to glaucoma, the ONH is defined as the distal portion of optic nerve that is directly susceptible to elevated IOP
   iii. The terms "disk" and "papilla" refers to the portion of the ONH that is clinically visible by ophthalmoscopy.

3. **What are the dimensions of ONH?**
   i. It is 1 mm long (anteroposterior)
   ii. Diameter—1.5 mm horizontally and 1.75 mm vertically
   iii. Mean area of disk—2.7 mm^2.

4. **Describe the parts of ONH.**
   i. Superficial nerve fiber layer—the prelaminar zone anterior to the level of Bruch's membrane (pars retinalis)
   ii. The prelaminar zone—level with the choroids (pars choroidalis)
   iii. The lamina cribrosa (pars sclerosis)
   iv. The retrolaminar portion, immediately behind the lamina.

5. **What is physiological cup?**
   i. Central depression of optic disk is known as physiological cup.
   ii. It is slightly pushed to the temporal side of the disk due to heaping of nasal fibers.
   iii. From the center of this depression, vessels emerge, usually hugging the nasal side.
   iv. Usually symmetrical in the two eyes.

6. **What are the dimensions of the physiological cup?**
   i. Median cup volume 0.28 mm^2
   ii. Median cup depth 0.63 mm^2
   iii. Mean cup area 0.72 mm^2.

7. **What is neuroretinal rim (NRR)?**
   i. The tissue outside the cup is termed the NRR and contains the retinal nerve axons as they enter the ONH
   ii. Rim area ranges from 0.8 to 4.66 mm^2
   iii. It is widest inferotemporally.

8. **What is the normal shape of cup?**

   i. Cup is 8% wider in the horizontal so that NRR is wider above and below.

   ii. Cup area correlates with disk area and hence is large in large disks and small in small disks.

9. **What is cup/disk ratio?**

   i. Ratio of the cup and disk width measured in the same meridian. Its median value is 0.3.

   ii. An asymmetry between both eyes of greater than 0.2 has been taken to signify enlargement and to be of diagnostic importance in glaucoma.

   iii. The vertical ratio is used as simple index of rim integrity in chronic glaucoma.

10. **Why is the ONH considered a major zone of transition?**

   i. Nerve fibers pass from an area of high tissue pressure within the eye to a zone of low pressure that correlates with intracranial pressure.

   ii. Transition from an area supplied by central retinal artery alone to an area supplied by other branches of ophthalmic artery.

   iii. The axons become myelinated immediately at the posterior end of ONH.

11. **What is scleral ring?**

   The layers of the retina abruptly cease before the optic nerve is reached. The pigment epithelium and the underlying choroid may not extend right up to the nerve, thus leaving a white scleral ring surrounding disk.

12. **What is conus?**

   i. If the scleral ring is accentuated it is termed as conus—a crescent-shaped configuration usually seen on the temporal side.

   ii. Large inferior conus is frequently associated with other abnormalities and approximately to a staphyloma.

13. **What is crescent?**

   The pigment epithelium may stop short some distance from the disk and the remaining space up to the margin of the optic nerve is covered by the choroid. It is usually crescent shaped and situated temporally (also known as choroidal ring).

14. **What is parapapillary chorioretinal atrophy?**

   A crescent-shaped region of chorioretinal atrophy at temporal margin of normal disks and may be exaggerated in chronic glaucoma or high myopia. There are 2 types of zone:

   i. Zone alpha

   ii. Zone beta.

15. **What are zone alpha and zone beta?**

   i. **Zone beta**
      - Inner zone
      - Exhibits chorioretinal atrophy with visibility of sclera and large choroidal blood vessels
      - Seen more frequently in patients with POAG
      - Contributes to absolute scotoma.

   ii. **Zone alpha**
      - More peripheral zone
      - Displays variable irregular hyper and hypopigmentation of RPE
      - Larger in patients with POAG, but frequency is similar in glaucoma and normal subjects
      - Contributes to relative scotoma.

16. **What is the site of emergence of retinal vessels?**

   The retinal vessels emerge on the medial side of the cup, slightly decentered superonasally.

17. **What is the significance of venous pulsation?**

   i. Absence of spontaneous venous pulsation is an early sign of papilledema.
   ii. 20% of normal population will not have spontaneous venous pulsation.
   iii. Pulsations cease when intracranial pressure exceeds 200 mm of water.

18. **What is the significance of retinal arterial pulsation?**

   Visible retinal arterial pulsations are rare and usually pathological implying for example
   i. Aortic incompetence
   ii. High intraocular pressure.

19. **What is microdisk and macrodisk?**

   i. Macrodisk, whose area lies greater than 2 standard deviations above the mean ($>4.09 \text{ mm}^2$)
      - Primary macrodisk: May be associated with optic nerve pit, morning glory syndrome
      - Secondary macrodisk: Seen with acquired globe enlargement such as high myopia and buphthalmos
   ii. Microdisk, whose area is less than 2 standard deviations below mean ($<1.29 \text{ mm}^2$).

20. **What is the relationship between size of optic disk and certain ONH diseases?**

   Small optic disks have a smaller number of optic nerve fibers and a smaller anatomical reserve.

    i. Nonarteritic ION is commoner in small ONH due to problems of vascular perfusion and of limited space

    ii. Same is true for ONH drusen

    iii. Pseudopapilledema is also encountered with smaller ONH, particularly in highly hypermetropic eyes.

21. Are there any racial differences in disk?

There is a racial difference in disk diameter. Blacks have larger disks and hence larger cups.

22. What is the meniscus of Kuhnt?

It refers to the central connective tissue that covers the non-myelinated fibers of the optic disk on the vitreous side.

23. What is the limiting tissue of Elschnig

    i. This is the border tissue or limiting tissue that separates the fibers of ONH from the retina and choroids.

    ii. It is essentially a derivative of the connective tissue of the choroids and sclera.

24. How many nerve fibers converge to form the disk?

There are approximately 1.2 million retinal nerve fibers.

25. Why is there a blind spot corresponding to the area of the ONH?

Because there are no rods or cones at the ONH, there is a physiological blind spot in the visual field.

26. What is the arrangement of retinal fibers at ONH?

    i. Those from the peripheral part of the retina lie deep in the retina but occupy the most peripheral part of optic disk; while fibers originating closer to ONH lie superficially and occupy a more deeper portion of the disk.

    ii. The arcuate nerve fibers occupy the supero- and inferotemporal portion of ONH and are most sensitive to glaucomatous damage accounting for early loss in corresponding region of visual field.

    iii. The papillomacular fibers spread over approximately one-third of distal optic nerve, primarily inferotemporally where axonal density is higher. They intermingle with extramacular fibers which might explain the retention of central visual field.

27. What do you mean by medullated nerve fibers at ONH?

Normally optic nerve fibers become medullated beyond lamina cribrosa. Occasionally myelin sheathing extends anterior to the lamina reaching a variable distance on the surface of the retina.

28. What is the composition of ONH?

Four types of cells:

   i. Ganglion cell axons
   ii. Astrocytes
   iii. Capillary associated cells
   iv. Fibroblasts.

29. What type of glial element is present at the disk?

   i. The prominent glial element is astrocyte.
   ii. It supports the bundles of nerve fibers.
   iii. Provides cohesiveness to the neural compartment by arranging themselves to form an interface with all mesodermal structures (like vitreous, choroids, sclera, etc.).
   iv. Also serves to moderate the conditions of neuronal functions. For example:
     – By absorbing extracellular potassium ions released by depolarizing axons
     – Storing glycogen for use during transient oligemia.

30. What is the vascular supply of ONH?

   i. Mainly posterior ciliary arterial circulations
   ii. Central retinal arterial circulations

31. Describe the vascular supply to the different parts of the ONH.

   i. Surface nerve fiber layer—supplied by capillaries derived from retinal arterioles.
   ii. Prelaminar region—supplied mainly from centripetal branches of peripapillary choroidal vessels.
   iii. Lamina cribrosa region—supplied by centripetal branches of the short posterior ciliary arteries. Some also delivered via the circle of Zinn–Haller, which encircles the prelaminar region and is fed via the short posterior ciliary arteries.
   iv. Retrolaminar region—supplied by centrifugal branches from central retinal artery and centripetal branches from pial plexus formed by branches of choroidal artery, circle of Zinn, central retinal artery and ophthalmic artery.

32. What is the venous drainage of ONH?

   i. Primarily via the central retinal venous system
   ii. Under conditions of chronic compression or CRVO, preexisting connections between superficial disk veins and choroidal veins— *Optociliary veins*, enlarge and shunt blood to choroids.

33. What are the features of microvascular bed of ONH?

   i. It resembles the retinal and CNS vessels anatomically
- Pericytes (mural cells) engulf the capillaries
- Nonfenestrated endothelium has tight junctions

  ii. The optic nerve vessels share with those of the retina and CNS the following physiological properties of
- Autoregulation
- Presence of blood–brain barrier.

34. What is the significance of autoregulation?

   i. Because of autoregulation the rate of blood flow in the optic nerve is not much affected by intraocular pressure.

  ii. In optic nerve the flow level is not affected by increase in BP because vascular tone is increased by autoregulation thus increasing the resistance to flow.

35. What is the main control of flow in optic nerve vessels?

Anterior to lamina cribrosa, autoregulation controls flow.

36. Why does fluorescein diffuse toward the center of the optic disk from its boundary during FFA?

The choroid is not separated from the ONH by a cellular layer that has tight junctions. Hence extracellular materials may diffuse into the extracellular space of the ONH.

37. How do you examine the ONH?

   i. Direct ophthalmoscope
- For disk examination
- Nerve fiber layer (NFL) through red free filter

  ii. Indirect ophthalmoscope
- Young children
- Uncooperative patients
- High myopes
- Substantial media opacities

 iii. Slit lamp using posterior pole lens such as Hruby lens, 60, 78, 90 diopter lens.

38. What is the location of ONH with respect to foveola?

The center of ONH is approximately 4 mm superonasal to the foveolar.

39. In what percentage of eyes is cilioretinal artery seen?

32%.

40. What is the difference between congenital and myopic crescents?

- Most temporal crescents are myopic and are acquired during life due to continuous growth process.

- True congenital crescents are present at birth and remain unchanged throughout life.

41. What are the congenital anomalies of ONH?

   i. Coloboma of ONH
- Results from a defective closure of fetal fistula
- It may be confined to the ONH or may include choroids, retina, iris and lens.
- Ophthalmoscopic appearance—the nerve is surrounded by peripapillary atrophy and shows extensive cupping and pallor.

   ii. Optic pit—usually located near the disk margin and often associated with serous detachment of the macula.

   iii. Situs inversus of the vessels: The right eye's ONH vascular pattern appears like that of the left eye.

   iv. Situs inversus of the disk: The scleral canal is directed nasally and the vessel divisions sweep nasally for a considerable distance before assuming their usual course.

   v. Bergmeister's papilla:
- A large stalk like vascularized tissue extending into the vitreous cavity from ONH.
- It is due to persistence of remnants of fetal vasculature extending from ONH to the lens.

42. What is corpora amylacea?

   i. They are small hyaline masses, of unknown pathologic significance and occurring more commonly with advancing age, derived from degenerate cells.

   ii. They are oval, highly refractile, either homogenous or showing concentric lamination and are enclosed in a definite capsule.

   iii. They occur normally in the optic nerve as in other parts of the CNS.

43. Why in papilledema does the disk swell easily but not the adjacent retina?

This is because in the prelaminar region loose glial tissue does not bind the axon bundle together as do the Muller cells of the retina.

44. What are the ocular signs of head injury?

   i. Torchlight signs: Subconjunctival hemorrhage (with no clear posterior demarcation)

   ii. Fundus signs:
- Papilledema
- Traumatic optic neuropathy (normal fundus with afferent pupillary defect)
- Purtscher's retinopathy

iii. Field signs
   – Homonymous hemianopia
iv. Pupillary signs:
   – Fixed dilated pupil due to
     • Transtentorial herniation (Hutchinson's pupil)
     • Traumatic IIIrd N palsy
     • Traumatic mydriasis
     • Orbital blowout fracture
   – Small pupil
     • Horner's syndrome
     • Pontine hemorrhage
v. Motor signs
   – Cranial nerve palsies
   – Internuclear ophthalmoplegia

7.4. OPTIC NEURITIS

1. **Define optic neuritis.**

   Literally means "Inflammation of the optic nerve" but it is defined as a demyelinating disorder of the optic nerve characterized by sudden monocular loss of vision, ipsilateral eye pain and dyschromatopsia.

2. **Classification of optic nerve inflammation.**

   Ophthalmoscopically
     i. Papillitis
    ii. Retrobulbar neuritis
   iii. Neuroretinitis.

   Etiologically
     i. Demyelinating
    ii. Parainfectious
   iii. Infectious.

   Structurally
     i. Perineuritis or peripheral optic neuritis
    ii. Inflammation of optic nerve substance.

3. **What are the causes of optic neuritis?**
     i. Etiology is numerous, most cases are idiopathic
    ii. 90% cases are demyelinating diseases of optic nerve
   iii. 20–40% cases develop signs and symptoms of multiple sclerosis (MS) in optic neuritis.

   – **Infectious diseases**
     • Bacterial—bacterial endocarditis, syphilis, meningitis, chronic mastoiditis (lateral sinus thrombosis), brucellosis, endogenous septic foci
     • Viral diseases poliomyelitis, acute lymphocyte meningitis, Coxsackie B virus encephalitis, recurrent polyneuritis, Guillain–Barré syndrome
     • Parasitic diseases sandfly fever, trypanosomiasis, neurocysticercosis.

   – **Ischemic diseases**
     • Atherosclerosis
     • Diabetes mellitus
     • Takayasu's disease
     • Carotid vascular insufficiency.

   – **Inflammatory diseases**
     • Collagen vascular diseases
     • Giant cell arteritis

4. **What are the triad of symptoms of optic neuritis?**

   i. Loss of vision
   ii. Ipsilateral eye pain and
   iii. Dyschromatopsia.

5. **What are the other symptoms of optic neuritis?**

   The associated visual symptoms are movement phosphenes, sound-induced phosphenes, and visual obscurations in bright light, and Uhthoff's symptom.

6. **What is the cause of pain in optic neuritis?**

   According to Whitnall's hypothesis, pain of optic nerve inflammation is caused by traction of the origins of the superior and medial recti on the optic nerve sheath at the orbital apex.

7. **Describe dyschromatopsia in optic neuritis.**

   Impaired color vision (dyschromatopsia) is always present in optic neuritis. In the absence of a macular lesion, color desaturation is a highly sensitive indicator of optic nerve disease. Color vision, a parvocellular-ganglion cell function, is abnormal in patients with acute and recovered optic neuritis. The localized loss of red and green perception to be the most sensitive test of interference with optic nerve function.

   Color vision defects are highly sensitive indicators of a previous attack of optic neuritis. Color vision defects can be detected clinically using Hardy–Rand–Ritter or Ishihara pseudoisochromatic plates. More sensitive testing can be achieved with the Farnsworth Munsell 100 Hue test.

   Typically the patient observes a reduced vividness of saturated colors. In color terminology saturation refers to the purity of color, and desaturation is the degree to which a color is mixed with white.

   Some patients who are shown a red target characterize the sensation as darker (i.e. red is shifted toward amber), whereas others say the color is bleached or lighter (i.e. red is shifted towards orange).

8. **Describe Uhthoff's phenomenon.**

   Uhthoff's symptom, episodic transient obscuration of vision with exertion, occurs in isolated optic neuritis and in MS.

   However, exertion is not the only provoking factor for Uhthoff's symptom.

   Typically, the patient has blurring of vision in the affected eye after 5–20 min of exposure to the provoking factor. Color desaturation may also occur. After resting or moving away from heat, vision recovers to its previous level within 5–60 min.

   In optic neuritis, Uhthoff's symptom correlates significantly with multifocal white matter lesions on brain MRI ($P < 025$).

Conversion to MS in patients followed for a mean of 3.5 year is significantly greater in patient with Uhthoff's symptom ($P < 01$).

Uhthoff's symptom also correlates with a higher incidence of recurrent optic neuritis.

Uhthoff's symptom in MS can be detected by Farnsworth Munsell 100 Hue testing and Octopus perimetry, as well as by fluctuations of VEP amplitudes and contrast sensitivity.

9. **What are the clinical signs of optic neuritis?**

   The clinical signs of optic neuritis are those of optic nerve disease. They include:

   i. Visual acuity (distance and near)—reduced
   ii. Dyschromatopsia
   iii. Contrast sensitivity—impaired
   iv. Stereoacuity—reduced
   v. Visual field—generalized depression, particularly pronounced centrally
   vi. Afferent pupillary defect
   vii. Optic disk(s)—hyperemia and acute swelling.

10. **What is the name of the chart used to test contrast sensitivity?**

    Pelli–Robson chart.

11. **How is stereoacuity checked?**

    Titmus polaroid 3 D vectograph stereoacuity test.

12. **What is Pulfrich effect?**

    Patients notice reduced brightness and difficulty in depth perception. Because optic nerve damage results in delayed transmission of impulses to the visual cortex, patients with unilateral or markedly asymmetric optic neuritis will experience the Pulfrich effect, a stereo illusion.

13. **What are the visual field defects in optic neuritis?**

    i. Involvement of the visual field during an attack of optic neuritis, as well as following recovery, can be extremely variable.
    ii. In acute optic neuritis, the cardinal field defect is a widespread depression of sensitivity, particularly pronounced centrally as a centrocecal scotoma.
    iii. When acuity is severely impaired perimetric field charting is unreliable and confrontation testing is recommended.
    iv. As vision improves multiisopter kinetic Goldmann perimetry or computer-assisted automated static perimetry using a Humphrey Field Analyzer or Octopus perimeter are sensitive techniques for serial testing.

v. A finding of generalized depression, paracentral scotomas, or scattered nerve fiber bundle–related defect(s) between 5° and 20° from fixation, may indicate sequelae of prior demyelinating optic neuropathy.

14. What are the optic disk finding in optic neuritis?

i. The appearance of the optic disk may be normal.

ii. Swollen (papillitis) in 23%, blurred or hyperemic in 18%, and blurred with peripapillary hemorrhages around the disk in 2%.

iii. Temporal pallor suggests a preceding attack of optic neuritis.

iv. In recovered optic neuritis, 6 months after the first attack, a normal disk can be present in 42% of eyes; temporal pallor present in 28%; and total disk pallor evident in 18%.

v. In MS in remission, optic pallor is present in 38% of cases.

15. What are the retinal findings in optic neuritis?

i. Two retinal signs are associated with optic neuritis and multiple sclerosis:

ii. Retinal venous sheathing due to periphlebitis retinae and

iii. Defects in the retinal nerve fiber layer.

16. What are the investigations in optic neuritis?

There is usually no need for investigative studies in a healthy adult presenting with typical acute, monosymptomatic, unilateral optic neuritis and an unremarkable medical history. However the following tests may be performed.

i. Complete blood counts

ii. ESR

iii. Rule out diabetes

iv. Rule out infectious disease etiology like
   – Tuberculosis—chest X-ray, Montoux (important as steroids will be used in treatment of optic neuritis)
   – Syphilis
   – HIV 1 and 2
   – Hepatitis B

v. Any other suspected infectious disease serology

vi. Rule out inflammatory disease conditions like
   – SLE, collagen vascular diseases—ANA, RA, ANCA, anti-double strand DNA
   – Giant cell arteritis—temporal artery biopsy.

17. What are the neuroimaging in optic neuritis?

CT, MRI, VEP, pattern electroretinogam.

18. What are the MRI finding in optic neuritis?

    i. Enhancing optic nerve on T1 contrast fat saturated
- Best seen on coronal images
- On axial images, may have tran-track' enhancement pattern simulating optic nerve sheath meningioma

   ii. On T2 with fat saturation (or STIR images)—mildly enlarged, hyperintense optic nerve

  iii. Acute and chronic MS lesions appear bright in T2 images.
- Lesions are round or ovoid in periventricular white matter, internal capsule and corpus callosum (perpendicular to vente rides, at callososeptal interface)
- They may also be linear with finger like appearance (Dawson's fingers) on sagittal or coronal scaring periventricular region.

19. What are the VEP finding in optic neuritis?

Prolongation of p_100 latency is seen optic neuritis.

20. What are the differential diagnosis of optic neuritis?

Unilateral optic neuritis

    i. Ischemic optic neuropathy
   ii. Rhinogenous optic neuritis
  iii. Syphilis
  iv. HIV-associated optic neuropathies
   v. Infectious optic neuropathy
  vi. Nonorganic factitious visual loss.

Simultaneous or sequential bilateral optic neuritis

When optic neuritis strikes both eyes, simultaneously or sequentially, the disorder must be distinguished from the following:

    i. Devic's disease
   ii. Immune-mediated optic neuropathy
  iii. Nutritional amblyopia
  iv. Jamaican optic neuropathy
   v. Leber's hereditary optic neuropathy and
  vi. Functional blindness.

21. What is Devic's disease?

Devic's disease (Neuromyelitis optica) is an inflammatory CNS-demyelinating disease that is considered to be a variant of MS. Affects both eyes simultaneously or sequentially in children, in young adults, and in the elderly and is accompanied by transverse myelitis within days or weeks.

Neuromyelitis optica has also been reported in association with SLE and pulmonary tuberculosis.

Familial cases of acute optic neuropathy and myelopathy may be linked to an inherited mutation in mitochondrial DNA (mtDNA), possibly a cytochromic oxidase subunit 2 mutation at nucleotide position 7706.

22. **Treatment trials of optic neuritis.**

Optic Neuritis Treatment Trial (ONTT) and Longitudinal Optic Neuritis Study (LONS).

Purpose

i. To assess the beneficial and adverse effects of corticosteroid treatment for optic neuritis.

ii. To determine the natural history of vision in patients who suffer optic neuritis.

iii. To identify risk factors for the development of multiple sclerosis in patients with optic neuritis.

The treatment phase of the study was called the Optic Neuritis Treatment Trial (ONTT), whereas the current long-term follow-up phase is called the Longitudinal Optic Neuritis Study (LONS).

Prior to the Optic Neuritis Treatment Trial (ONTT), well-established guidelines for treating optic neuritis did not exist. Although corticosteroids had been used to treat this disease, studies to demonstrate their effectiveness had not been satisfactory.

Patients were randomized to one of the three following treatment groups at 15 clinical centers:

i. Oral prednisone (1 mg/kg/day) for 14 days

ii. Intravenous methylprednisolone (250 mg every 6 hours) for 3 days, followed by oral prednisone (1 mg/kg/day) for 11 days.

iii. Oral placebo for 14 days.

Each regimen was followed by a short oral taper. The oral prednisone and placebo groups were double masked, whereas the intravenous methylprednisolone group was single masked.

The rate of visual recovery and the long-term visual outcome were both assessed by measures of visual acuity, contrast sensitivity, color vision and visual field at baseline, at seven follow-up visits during the first 6 months, and then yearly. A standardized neurologic examination with an assessment of multiple sclerosis status was made at baseline, after 6 months, and then yearly.

Patient eligibility

The major eligibility criteria for enrollment into the ONTT included the following:

i. Age range of 18–46 years
ii. Acute unilateral optic neuritis with visual symptoms for 8 days or less.
iii. A relative afferent pupillary defect and a visual field defect in the affected.
iv. No previous episodes of optic neuritis in the affected eye.
v. No previous corticosteroid treatment for optic neuritis or multiple sclerosis.
vi. No systemic disease other than multiple sclerosis that might be the cause of the optic neuritis.

Results

The study has defined the value of baseline ancillary testing, the typical course of visual recovery with and without corticosteroid treatment, the risks and benefits of corticosteroid treatment, and the 5-year risk of the development of multiple sclerosis after optic neuritis.

These results are briefly summarized below:

i. Routine blood tests, chest X-ray, brain MRI, and lumbar puncture are of limited value for diagnosing optic neuritis in a patient with typical features of optic neuritis.
ii. Brain MRI is a powerful predictor of the early risk of multiple sclerosis after optic neuritis.
iii. In optic neuritis patients with no brain MRI lesions, the following features of the optic neuritis are associated with a low 5-year risk of multiple sclerosis: lack of pain, optic disk edema (particularly if severe), peripapillary hemorrhage, retinal exudates and mild visual loss.
iv. Visual recovery begins rapidly (within 2 weeks) in most optic neuritis patients without any treatment, and then improvement continues for up to 1 year. Although most patients recover to 20/20 or near 20/20 acuity, many still have symptomatic deficits in vision.
v. The probability of a recurrence of optic neuritis in either eye within 5 years is 28%. Visual recovery after a second episode in the same eye is generally very good.
vi. Treatment with high dose, intravenous corticosteroids followed by oral corticosteroids accelerated visual recovery but provided no long-term benefit to vision.
vii. Treatment with standard-dose oral prednisone alone did not improve the visual outcome and was associated with an increased rate of new attacks of optic neuritis.

viii. Treatment with the intravenous followed by oral corticosteroid regimen provided a short-term reduction in the rate of development of multiple sclerosis, particularly in patients with brain MRI changes consistent with demyelination. However, by 3 years of follow-up, this treatment effect had subsided.

The treatments were generally well-tolerated, and side effects during the treatment period were mild.

23. What are the visual field defects noted in ONTT?

   i. Generalized visual field depression was present in 48.2% of eyes
   ii. Altitudinal or other nerve-fiber bundle-type defects were present in 20.1% of eyes
   iii. Central or centrocecal scotoma was present in 8.3% of eyes
   iv. Other defects were present in 23.4% of eyes.

7.5. PAPILLEDEMA

CLINICAL FEATURES AND CAUSES

1. **Definition of papilledema.**

   Bilateral passive hydrostatic, noninflammatory edema of the optic disk or nerve head due to raised intracranial pressure.

2. **What is the place of production and pathway of CSF?**

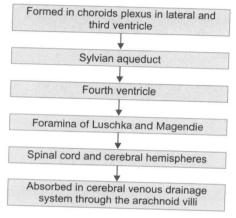

3. **What is normal CSF pressure?**

   Normal CSF pressure in adults = 80–200 mm H_2O
   Pressure >250 mm H_2O elevated.

4. **What is meant by the term "axoplasmic transport"?**

   i. Optic nerve axoplasmic transport, transports material (proteins and organelles) from the retinal ganglion cells to the entire axons and to its termination in the lateral geniculate body where some of the material is degraded and returned to the cell body via the retrograde transport system.

   ii. Orthograde axoplasmic transport (from eye to the brain) has a slow component (proteins and enzymes) that progress at 0.5–3.0 mm/day an intermediate component (mainly mitochondria) and a rapid component (subcellular organelles) that moves at 200–1,000 mm/day.

   iii. Retrograde axoplasmic transport of lysosomes and mitochondria (from the brain to the eye) also occurs at an intermediate rate.

5. **What is the relationship between IOP and papilledema?**

   Normally the IOP (14–20 mm Hg) is higher than the tissue pressure in the optic nerve (6–8 mm Hg). This pressure differential is the force driving the axoplasm in the region of the lamina cribrosa.

Hence, a fall in the IOP or an increase in the optic nerve tissue pressure following a rise in the CSF pressure will interfere in the axoplasmic flow, leading to stasis and accumulation of the axoplasm.

6. What are the theories of papilledema?

i. Inflammatory theory by Gowers and Leber—edematous inflammation was set up by toxic material associated with intracranial disease

ii. Vasomotor theories by Kornder—papilledema caused by venous stasis which was part of a generalized increase in systemic venous pressure due to an accentuated inhibitory action of vagus resulting from central stimulation of increased intracranial pressure

iii. Axoplasmic stasis theory by Hayreh.

The most accepted theory is Hayreh's theory of axoplasmic stasis.

7. What is Hayreh's theory of pathogenesis of papilledema?

i. Patency of the meningeal spaces surrounding the optic nerve and intracranial structures and transmission of increased CSF pressure, to the region posterior to the optic nerve sheath is the first step.

ii. There is free diffusion of substances from the CSF to the optic nerve and thereby increases the optic nerve tissue pressure in the setting of increased intracranial tension.

iii. Increased optic nerve tissue pressure causes alteration of pressure gradient across lamina cribrosa which causes blockage of axoplasmic flow from retinal ganglion cells to lateral geniculate body.

iv. Venous changes are secondary due to compression of fine vessels lying in the prelaminar region and in the surface layers by the swollen axons.

8. How frequent is the occurrence of papilledema in children?

i. Infants: Uncommon due to open fontanels

ii. Children age 2–10 years common due to increased infratentorial tumors.

9. What are the causes of papilledema?

i. **Space-occupying lesions**
- Neoplasms—infratentorial tumors (common)
- Abscess—temporal lobe
- Inflammatory mass
- Subarachnoid hemorrhage
- Infarction
- A–V malformations.

ii. **Focal or diffuse cerebral edema**
- Trauma
- Toxic
- Anoxia

  iii. **Reduction in size of cranial vault**
     Craniosynostosis
  iv. **Blockage of CSF flow**
     Noncommunicating hydrocephalus
   v. **Vitamin A toxicity**
  vi. **Reduction in CSF resorption**
     – Communicating hydrocephalus
     – Infectious meningitis
     – Elevated CSF proteins (meningitis)
     – Spinal cord tumor, Guillain–Barre syndrome (GBS)
 vii. **Increased CSF production**
viii. Idiopathic **intracranial hypertension (pseudotumor cerebri).**

10. Which tumors are more prone to develop papilledema and why?

Tumors of the midbrain, parietooccipital and cerebellum mostly cause papilledema

    Tumors → Infratentorial (more common)
           → Supratentorial

– Infratentorial tumors—produce papilledema by obstruction of the aqueduct or by compression of vein of galen or the posterior superior sagittal sinus.
– Supratentorial tumors—produce papilledema by deflection of the falx and pressure upon the great vein of Galen.

Others—intracranial masses—metastatic tumors, brain tumors.

11. Which intracranial tumor is least likely to cause papilledema?

– Medulla oblongata tumors
– Tumor of the anterior fossa

12. What are the common causes of papilledema in children?

Posterior fossa tumors—medulloblastoma.

13. What are the stages of papilledema?

   i. Early
  ii. Established
 iii. Chronic
 iv. Atrophic

(As suggested by Hughlings Jackson in 1871)

14. What are the clinical features of early papilledema?

   i. Visual symptoms are mild or absent
  ii. Optic disk shows hyperemia and blurring of superior and inferior margins and blurring of retinal nerve fiber layer
 iii. The physiological cup is normal.

15. **How does the edema progress?**

The edema (blurring of the optic nerve) starts at the superior and interior margins and extends around the nasal side and finally the temporal side (SINT).

16. **What are the pathological features of papilledema?**
    i. Signs of passive edema without evidence of inflammation
    ii. Edematous changes are located in front of the lamina cribrosa
    iii. Axoplasmic stasis is seen
    iv. Nerve fibers become swollen and varicose and ultimately degenerate
    v. Proliferation of neuralgia and mesoblastic tissue around the vessels becomes thickened.

17. **What are the clinical features of established papilledema?**
    i. Transient visual obscuration—5 seconds, rarely exceeds 30 seconds at irregular intervals
    ii. Visual acuity normal or decreased
    iii. Enlargement of blind spots
    iv. Gross elevation of the disk surface with blurred margins
    v. Obliteration of the cup
    vi. Venous pulsation absent
    vii. Microaneurysm formation and capillary dilatation on disk margin
    viii. Flame shaped hemorrhages, cotton-wool spots
    ix. Circumferential retinal folds (Paton's lines)
    x. Hard exudates on hemorrhages and macula (macular fan).

18. **Why do transient visual obscurations occur in papilledema?**

Transient visual obscurations of vision may occur in one or both eyes simultaneously with rapid recovery usually lasting seconds but sometimes lasting hours.

Patients may experience up to 20–30 attacks per day, with obscurations precipitated by change of posture or from the lying down to sitting or standing position.

The cause of these transient obscurations is related to transient compression or ischemia of the optic nerve.

Spasms of the ophthalmic artery/posterior cerebral artery, ciliary aqueduct obstruction by a tumor producing a ball valve effect causing transient ophthalmology.

19. **What is the usual duration of the transient obscuration of vision in papilledema and its precipitating factors?**
    i. 5 seconds. It rarely exceeds 30 seconds at irregular interval.

   ii. Precipitated by:
- Standing up from a sitting position
- Stooping
- Turning the head abruptly.

20. Name other conditions causing transient obscuration of vision.

   i. Amaurosis fugax
- usual duration 5–15 min
- Fundi may show emboli

   ii. Retinal migraine
- Duration 15–20 min
- Frequently accompanied or followed by headache

  iii. Acute glaucoma
- Several hours

  iv. Hemicrania
- 15–45 min

   v. Epileptic fits (partial)
- Few seconds.

21. In how many percentages of normal individuals can we see pulsations over the optic nerve head?

Absence of spontaneous venous pulsations—occurs when the intracranial pressure rises above 200 mm H_2O. This can be misleading if seen during the times of fluctuation of increased intracranial pressure when it may be below 200 mm H_2O. Absence of spontaneous venous pulsations may be a finding in 20% of normal population.

22. What is macular fan?

The nerve fibers in the macula are arranged in a radial fashion. Hence hard exudates and hemorrhages are arranged in a radial manner in the macula, which are more prominent on the nasal side of the fovea due to the vascular compromise in and around the disk.

23. What are the clinical features of chronic (vintage) papilledema?

Visual acuity is variable with constricted visual field. Optic disk changes are:

   i. Champagne-cork appearance with no exudates and hemorrhages
   ii. Central cup obliterated but peripapillary retinal edema absorbs
  iii. Small white opacities on the disk—corpora amylacea
  iv. Pigmentary changes in macula.

24. What are the clinical features of atrophic papilledema?

   i. Visual acuity is severely impaired with constriction of visual field
   ii. Optic disk grayish-white with indistinct margins as a result of gliosis

iii. Narrow retinal vessels due to sheathing of vessels, which are extension of gliosis

iv. Reduced disk elevation—flat disk.

25. What are the causes of optic atrophy in papilledema?

i. Increased intracranial pressure compromises the vascular supply (focal infarct, ischemia, axon damage) which cause nerve fiber atrophy. Decreased vascularity of the disk causes pale gray color leading to secondary optic atrophy

ii. Appearance depends on the fact that absorption of exudates causes organization and formation of fibrous tissue on the disk. This fibrous tissue obscures the lamina cribrosa and fills in atrophic cup, then extends over the edges which are thus ill-defined along vessels and perivascular sheath

iii. Number of vessels also decreases (Kestenbaum's sign).

26. What is the other staging system of papilledema?

Frisen's grading system

Stage 0

i. Mild nasal elevations of the nerve fiber layer

ii. A portion of major vessels may be obscured in upper pole

Stage 1: Very early papilledema

i. Obscuration of the nasal border of the disk

ii. No elevation

iii. Disruption of normal retinal nerve fiber layer

iv. Concentric or radial retino choroidal folds

Stage 2: Early papilledema

i. Obscuration of all the borders

ii. Elevation of nasal border

iii. Complete peripapillary halo

Stage 3: Moderate papilledema

i. Obscuration of all the borders

ii. Increased diameter of optic nerve head

iii. Obscuration of one or more segments of major blood vessels leaving the disk

iv. Peripapillary halo, irregular outer fringe with finger-like extensions

Stage 4: Marked papilledema

i. Elevation of the entire nerve head

ii. Obscuration of all the borders

iii. Peripapillary halo

iv. Total obscuration on the disk of a segment of major blood vessels

Stage 5: Severe papilledema
  i. Dome shaped protrusions representing anterior expansion of optic nerve head
  ii. Peripapillary halo
  iii. Total obscuration of a segment of major blood vessels
  iv. Obliteration of optic cup
  v. Obscuration of all the borders.

27. How does the blurring of disk margins appear in papilledema?

It usually appears first in the upper and lower margins. Usually at the upper nasal quadrant, spreading then round the nasal margin and appearing last at the temporal margin (SINT).

28. Why are the upper and lower quadrants affected first?

The distribution depends on the density of capillaries, with the papillo-macular bundle occupying the greater part of the outer aspect of the disk. The upper and lower quadrants are the most heavily crowded with nerve fibers.

29. Why is there an enlargement of blind spot?

It is due to separation of the retina around the disk by the edema.
  i. Due to compression, detachment and lateral displacement of the peripapillary retina and due to generalized decrease in sensitivity of the peripapillary retina. The outer layer of the neural retina may buckle, and rods and cones are displaced away from the end of the Bruch's membrane
  ii. ***Stiles–Crawford effect:*** This phenomenon proposes that the wrinkles and the folds in the peripapillary retina cause light to fall obliquely on the photoreceptors thus making the light a less effective stimulus.

30. List the differential diagnosis for enlargement of blind spot.
  i. Papilloedema
  ii. Papillitis
  iii. Glaucoma
  iv. Progressive myopia
  v. Coloboma of optic nerve
  vi. Inferior conus
  vii. Juxtapapillary choroiditis
  viii. High alcohol consumption
  ix. Drugs
    – Aldosterone
    – Betamethasone
    – Vitamin A
    – Prednisolone.

31. **What are the visual field defects common in cases of papilledema?**
    i. Enlargement of blind spots
    ii. Concentric contractions more common
    iii. Relative scotoma first to green and red
    iv. Complete blindness
    v. Homonymous hemianopia
    vi. Central and arcuate scotomas
    vii. Most commonly involves inferior nasal quadrant.

32. **What are the systemic features of increased intracranial pressure?**
    i. Headache—more severe in the morning, worsening progressively. Intensifies with head movement
    ii. Sudden nausea—projectile vomiting
    iii. Horizontal diplopia caused by stretching of the VI nerve over the petrous tip (false localizing sign). Sometimes IV nerve palsy
    iv. Loss of consciousness/generalized motor rigidity
    v. Bilaterally dilated pupil (rare).

33. **What are the causes of headache, loss of consciousness and generalized motor rigidity?**

    Headache: associated with increased intracranial pressure is due to stretching of the meninges while sharply localized pains can be due to involvement of sensory nerve at the base of the skull or localized involvement of the meningeal nerves.

    Loss of consciousness: occurs from compression of the cerebral cortex and the reduction of its blood supply.

    Generalized motor rigidity: Herniation of the hippocampal gyrus through the tentorium from increased intracranial pressure results in crowding of the temporal lobe into the incisura of each side.

    Tentorial herniation thus places pressure on the crura cerebri, resulting in generalized motor rigidity. Finally, direct pressure on the nerves and dorsal midbrain produces bilaterally dilated pupils that do not respond to light stimulation.

34. **How is the elevation of the disk seen on direct ophthalmoscopy?**

    First with a direct ophthalmoscope retinal vessels below the disk are focused and then the vessels above the disk are seen.

    A difference of 2–6 D may be found between the focus of the vessels on the top of the disk and those on the retina.

    A difference of 3 D is equivalent to approximately 1 mm difference of level at the fundus.

35. **Which refractive error may mimic papilledema?**

    Astigmatism and hypermetropia (pseudoneuritis): It is a condition usually occurring in hypermetropic eyes when the lamina is small and the nerve fibers are heaped up as they debouch upon the retina.

36. What are the earliest features of resolution in papilledema?

    i. Retinal venous dilatation and disk capillary dilatation regression

    ii. Disappearance of disk hyperemia.

37. What are the last abnormalities which usually resolve after treatment of papilledema?

    i. Blurring of disk margins

    ii. Abnormalities of the peripapillary retinal nerve fiber layer.

38. What are the poor prognostic factors for papilledema?

    i. Rapidity: The more rapid the onset, the greater the danger of permanent visual loss.

    ii. Duration of papilledema

    iii. Papilledema of more than 5 D, extensive retinal hemorrhages and exudates and macular scar

    iv. Early pallor of the disk and attenuated arterioles

    v. Gliosis of the disk

    vi. Obscurations of vision and presence of opticociliary shunts.

39. Mention the criteria for idiopathic intracranial hypertension?

(Modified from criteria established by WE Dandy)

    i. Signs and symptoms of increased intracranial pressure.

    ii. Absence of localizing findings on neurologic examination.

    iii. Absence of deformity, displacement and obstruction of ventricular system and otherwise normal neurodiagnostic studies except for increased cerebrospinal fluid pressure (>200 mm H_2O in nonobese patient and >250 mm H_2O in obese patient).

    iv. Awake and alert patient.

    v. No other cause of increased intracranial pressure present.

40. What are the diagnostic criteria of pseudotumor cerebri?

    i. Symptoms and signs solely attributable to increased intracranial pressure

    ii. Elevated CSF pressure

    iii. Normal CSF composition

    iv. Normal neuroimaging studies

    v. No other etiology of intracranial hypertension identified

    vi. Treated with diuretics and lumbar puncture.

41. What are the drugs that may produce a secondary pseudotumor cerebri?

    i. Nalidixic acid

    ii. Penicillin

    iii. Tetracycline

    iv. Minocycline

    v. Ciprofloxacin

    vi. Nitrofurantoin

42. Why are pupillary reactions normal in cases of early and established papilledema?

Because neuronal conduction is not dependant on axonal transport but rather on the myelin sheath.

43. What is the differential diagnosis of papilledema?

   i. Papillitis

   ii. Pseudopapilledema due to:

     – High hypermetropia

     – AION (nonarteritic)

     – Drusens of optic nerve

   iii. Optic neuritis

   iv. Tilted optic disk

   v. Hypoplastic disk

   vi. Myelinated nerve fiber.

44. How can one differentiate between pseudopapilledema and papilledema?

Pseudopapilledema—

   i. Swelling never more than 2 D

   ii. No venous engorgement, edema or exudates

   iii. Blind spot is not enlarged

   iv. FFA—no leaking.

45. How can one differentiate between optic neuritis (papillitis) and papilledema?

Optic neuritis

   i. Relative apparent pupillary defect

   ii. Moderate swelling; 2–3 D shelving gradually into the surrounding retina

   iii. Central scotoma with field loss of color discrimination

   iv. Visual symptoms are marked

   v. Acute depression of central vision

   vi. Usually uniocular

   vii. Associated vitreous opacities.

Papilledema

   i. Normal pupil

   ii. Severe swelling of the optic disc

   iii. Enlargement of the blind spot

   iv. Visual symptoms are minimal

   v. Usually bilateral

46. How can one differentiate crowded disk and tilted disk from papilledema?

   i. Peripapillary nerve fiber layer and retinal vessels that traverse it remain normal

   ii. Venous pulsations are usually present

iii. No vascular engorgement/hemorrhages
iv. No cotton-wool spots
v. An oval disk with one side displaced posteriorly, usually at the inferior margin and the other side elevated anteriorly, usually at the superior margin
vi. Oblique direction of retinal vessels
vii. High myopia/moderate oblique myopic astigmatism is usually present.

47. Differentiate between nonarteritic AION from papilledema.

i. Associated with hypertension–40%, diabetes mellitus–24%
ii. Visual acuity decreased >6/60
iii. Color vision defective
iv. Altitudinal field defects.

48. Differentiate between papilledema and optic disk drusen.

i. Drusen—common in children and young
ii. Familial and very slow growing
iii. Visual defects do not correspond to location of the drusen.
iv. Small optic nerve head
v. Calcified laminated globular aggregates on the disk.
vi. FFA is normal.

49. Differentiate between hypertensive retinopathy and papilledema.

Hypertensive retinopathy—is characterized by:

i. Less venous dilatation
ii. More marked arterial narrowing
iii. Abnormalities of arteriovenous crossings with
iv. Retinal hemorrhages and exudates more scattered than confined to the proximity of the disk.

50. Differentiate between optic neuritis, papilledema, ischemic neuropathy.

Features	Optic neuritis	Papilledema	Ischemic neuropathy
Symptoms			
Visual	Rapidly progressive loss of central vision	No visual loss +/– transient obscuration	Acute field defect (common altitudinal)
Others	Tender globe, pain on motion, orbit or browache	Headache, nausea, vomiting	None (headache in cranial arteritis)
Bilaterality	Rare	Always	Unilateral in acute stage. Second eye involved sub-sequently with picture of Foster–Kennedy syndrome

(Continued)

(*Continued*)

Features	Optic neuritis	Papilledema	Ischemic neuropathy
Signs			
Pupil	No anisocoria ↓ light reaction on side of neuritis	No anisocoria Normal reaction unless asymmetric atrophy	No anisocoria ↓ light reaction on side of disk infarct
Visual acuity	Decreased	Normal	Variable (Severe loss common in arteritis)
Fundus	Variable degrees of disk swelling with few flame hemorrhages, cells in vitreous	Variable degrees of disk swelling, hemorrhages, cystoids infarcts	Usually segmental disk edema with few flame hemorrhages
Visual prognosis	Vision usually returns to normal or functional levels	Good	Poor prognosis

51. What are the causes of unilateral optic disk edema?

Oculoorbital

   i. Papillitis

   ii. Drusen

  iii. Ischemic optic neuropathy

   iv. Central retinal venous occlusion

   v. Optic nerve glioma/meningioma

   vi. Ocular hypotony

Mixed intracranial

   i. Unilateral optic atrophy and true papilledema (Foster–Kennedy syndrome)

   ii. Pre-existing atrophy before development of increased ICP (pseudo-Foster–Kennedy syndrome)

  iii. Unilateral high myopia and true papilloedema

   iv. Cavernous sinus thrombosis

   v. Carotid-cavernous fistula

Pure intracranial

   i. Posterior fossa tumor

   ii. Pseudo tumor cerebri

  iii. Subarachnoid hemorrhage

   iv. Brain abscess

   v. Optochiasmatic arachnoiditis.

52. What are the causes of bilateral optic disk edema with normal visual function?

   i. Hypertensive retinopathy

   ii. Spinal cord tumors

   iii. Guillain–Barre syndrome

   iv. Hypoxemia and anemia

   v. Cyanotic congenital heart disease.

53. What is Foster–Kennedy syndrome?

This refers to specific clinical findings characteristically seen in frontal lobe/olfactory groove tumors especially meningioma. The syndrome is believed to occur subsequent to increased intracranial tension as a result of an asymmetrical frontal lobe mass which compresses the optic nerve on one side leading to atrophy while the other side demonstrates papilledema due to the increased ICT.

54. What are the features associated with Foster–Kennedy syndrome?

These include anosmia (if the olfactory nerve is affected), nausea, projectile vomiting (suggestive of increased ICT), emotional lability and memory loss (suggestive of frontal lobe lesions).

55. What is the treatment of Foster–Kennedy syndrome?

The treatment of the condition is symptomatic relief from the features of increased ICT, and treatment of the etiology (tumor) of the condition.

56. What is pseudo-Foster–Kennedy syndrome?

Pseudo-Foster–Kennedy syndrome is defined as preexisting optic atrophy in one eye, whereby the affected atrophied optic nerve cannot demonstrate changes of papilledema even in the presence of increased ICT. The other eye manifests with disk edema. There is no intracranial mass that can be deemed to be cause of an increase in the ICT in such cases.

INVESTIGATIONS

1. What is the investigation of choice in papilledema?

   i. MRI with or without contrast is the best investigation of choice

     – MRI angiography

     – MRI venography

       • To rule out arterial disease and venous obstruction (thrombosis)

       • Arnold–chiari malformations

       • To see structured lesions (mainly posterior fossa lesions)

       • To see hydrocephalus

   ii. Fascial resolution is better in MRI which provides three-dimensional image

   iii. Soft-tissue lesions are well appreciated.

2. **What is the role of CT scan in papilledema?**
   i. To rule out intracranial lesions that would produce increased intracranial pressure and rule out obstructive hydrocephalus.
      - Acute vascular causes—like subarachnoid, epidural, subdural, intracranial hemorrhages, acute infarctions
      - After head injury—cerebral edema
   ii. Patient with contraindication to MRI like pacemaker, metallic clip, metallic foreign body.

3. **What is the role of lumbar puncture (LP) in papilledema?**
   i. Diagnostic—to evaluate for intracranial hypertension by recording the opening pressure
   ii. To send CSF for microbial/infectious studies like—TLC, DC, glucose, protein, cytology, VDRL
   iii. Therapeutic—pseudotumor cerebri.

4. **What is the main hazardous disadvantage of LP?**
   It is usually contraindicated because of the danger of herniation of the brain into the foramen magnum which causes pressure on medulla leading to sudden death in cases with intracranial space occupying lesions with midline shift.

5. **What are the complications of lumbar puncture?**
   i. Poor compliance
   ii. Painful to the patient
   iii. Difficult in obese patients
   iv. May produce a remission of PTC by creating a permanent fistula through the dura mater
   v. Spinal epidermoid tumors
   vi. Infection.

6. **How does CT scan help in diagnostic of disk edema due to Graves disease?**
   It shows marked enlargement of extraocular muscle with compression of optic nerve leading to disk edema.

7. **What are the X-ray findings in papilledema in children and adults?**
   Adults
   i. Demineralization of subcortical bone leading to loss of "lamina dura" (white line) of sellar floor followed by thinning of dorsum sella and the posterior clinoid process.
   ii. In extreme cases the sella becomes very shallow and flattened with its floor and anterior wall demineralized and the posterior clinoid process and dorsum sella destroyed.

iii. Increased intracranial tension causes enlargement of the emissary veins in occipital region.

iv. Congenital cyst or chronic subdural hematoma may show localized thinning or bulge.

Children

i. Presents with sutural diastasis, i.e. sutural widening

ii. Increased convolutional markings with thining of the bone

iii. Any separation beyond 2 mm is suspicious of increased tension.

8. **What are the FFA findings in papilledema?**

Early phase

i. Disk capillary dilatation

ii. Dye leakage spots

iii. Microaneurysm over the disk.

Late phase

i. Leakage of dye beyond disk margin

ii. Pooling of dye around the disk as vertically oval pooling.

TREATMENT OF PAPILLEDEMA

1. **What is the medical and surgical treatment for benign intracranial hypertension?**

   i. Medical treatment
      - Acetazolamide 500 mg BD
      - Dehydrating agent—oral glycerol
      - Corticosteroids
      - Weight reduction

   ii. Surgical
      - Repeated LP
      - Decompression
      - Shunting procedure—lumboperitoneal shunt.

2. **How many times lumbar puncture can be done before subjecting the patient for decompression?**

   Multiple lumbar punctures can be done to relieve the increased intracranial tension. LP needle creates a sieve that allows sufficient regress egress of CSF, so that ICT is normalized.

3. **How long does it take for regression of papilledema following treatment?**

   Fully developed papilledema may disappear completely within hours, days or weeks depending on the way in which intracranial tension is lowered.

Brain tumor—papilledema can resolve 6–8 weeks after successful craniotomy to remove a brain tumor.

Peudotumor cerebri—resolution of papilledema within 2–3 weeks after lumboperitoneal shunts in idiopathic intracranial hypertension and several days after optic nerve sheath fenestration.

4. **During treatment of papilledema, how is therapeutic success determined?**
   i. Relief of headache
   ii. Diminished frequency of transient visual obscuration
   iii. Regression of papilledema
   iv. Stability or improvement of field defects
   v. Weight reduction.

5. **Indications of decompression.**
   i. Failure of medical treatment as evidenced by clinical signs
      – Marked degree of swelling (>5 D)
      – Great engorgement of veins
      – Presence of extensive hemorrhage
      – Early appearance of exudate spots
   ii. Progressive headaches unrelieved with medical treatment
   iii. Progressive optic neuropathy evidenced by early contraction of visual field.

6. **Which patient of pseudotumor cerebri should be treated? And how?**
   i. Those patients who develop
      – Signs of visual loss from chronic papilledema (optic neuropathy)
      – Intractable headaches
      – Persistent diplopia
   ii. Treatment
      – Repeated LP
      – Decompression
      – Shunting procedure

7. **How do you manage a case of pregnancy-induced hypertension (PIH) presenting with papilledema?**
   i. General—bed rest
   ii. Diet—only fluids
   iii. Sedative—phenobarbitone/diazepam
   iv. Control of BP
   v. Control edema—proteinurea/diuretic/frusemide, hypertonic glucose
   vi. Finally if patient does not respond to treatment, pregnancy has to be terminated.

8. **What are the operative disk decompression done to relieve papilledema?**

    i.   Subtemporal decompression
    ii. Suboccipital craniectomy
    iii. Direct fenestration of optic nerve sheath (ONSD) via medial or lateral orbitotomy.

9. **What is the procedure of ONSD?**

    The surgeon makes a window or multiple incisions in the normally bellowed anterior dural covering of the optic nerve sheath using either a lateral or a medial approach (the latter preferred).

10. **What are the features and treatment of fulminant IIH (idiopathic intracranial hypertension)?**

    i.   Features
         - Rapid onset of symptoms
         - Significant visual loss
         - Macular edema
         - Cerebral venous thrombosis and meningeal process should be considered
         - Malignant cause requires rapid treatment
    ii. Treatment
         - IV corticosteroids and insertion of lumbar drain used while waiting for definitive treatment.

11. **How do you manage a patient with PTC?**

    i.   No symptoms of papilledema
         - Periodic monthly review
         - If vision is normal for 3 months, then 2-monthly review
    ii. With transient obscuration of vision/signs of optic nerve dysfunction
         - T. acetazolamide–1 g daily depending on patient's tolerance
         - Re-examine the patient every 2–3 weeks for signs of compromise
    iii. With progressive optic neuropathy
         - T. acetazolamide–corticosteroid (80–100 mg/day)
    iv. Other treatment modalities
         - Repeated LP
         - Lumboperitoneal shunt
         - Optic nerve sheath decompression

12. **If the patient has visual symptoms only, what is the treatment of choice?**

    i.   Bilateral optic nerve sheath decompression.

13. **If the patient has headache only with no visual symptoms, what is the treatment of choice?**

    Lumboperitoneal shunt.

7.6. OPTIC ATROPHY

1. **Define optic atrophy.**

   Optic atrophy describes a group of clinical conditions which have abnormal pallor of the disk as a common physical sign. It is not a disease but a pathological end point of any disease that causes damage to the ganglion cells and axons with overall diminution of the optic nerve and visual acuity.

2. **What are the features of optic atrophy?**

   i. Loss of conducting function
   ii. Abnormal pallor of the disk
   iii. Proliferation of glial tissue
   iv. Reduction in number of capillaries
   v. Destruction of nerve fibers
   vi. Diminished volume of nerve fiber bundle
   vii. Increased excavation

3. **What are the clinical features of optic atrophy?**

   i. Reduced visual acuity
   ii. RAPD/APD
   iii. Defective color vision
   iv. Visual field loss central, paracentral, altitudinal scotomas

4. **What is the normal color of disk and why?**

   The disk is reddish pink in color with a mild pale physiological cup in the center.

   The normal color of the disk depends on following factors:

   i. *Composition of the optic disk*
      – Axons of retinal ganglion cells
      – Blood capillaries
      – Astrocytes
      – Connective tissue
   ii. *Relationship of these structures to each other*
   iii. *Behavior of light on falling on the disk*
   iv. *Vascularity of the disk.*

5. **What is the pathology of optic atrophy?**

   There are two main factors:
   i. Degeneration of optic nerve fibers
   ii. Proliferation of astrocytes and glial tissue

   The disease may be focal, multifocal or diffuse causing axonal interruption and their destruction by:
   i. Direct effect

   ii. Investing glial tissue

  iii. Decreasing capillary blood supply—gross shrinkage and atrophy of optic nerve.

6. What are the causes of pallor in optic atrophy?

Optic nerve degeneration causes:

   i. Reduced blood supply and disappearance of smaller vessels from view

  ii. Glial tissue formation occurs which is opaque

 iii. Loss of tissue causes visibility of opaque scleral lamina.

7. What is Kestenbaum capillary number?

Capillaries on normal disk were counted by Kestenbaum to be 10–12. In optic atrophy it was reduced to 6 or less.

8. What is Wallerian degeneration (ascending or antegrade optic atrophy)?

Primary lesion is in the optic nerve head, retina or choroid, which proceeds towards the brain. Visual axons are severed and their ascending segment disintegrates.

There is swelling and degeneration of terminal buttons of axons within the lateral geniculate body.

9. Which fibers are first to be affected in ascending optic atrophy?

Rate of degeneration is proportional to thickness of nerve fibers. Hence, larger axons degenerate faster than small caliber axons.

10. Causes of ascending optic atrophy?

    i. Retinitis pigmentosa

   ii. CRAO

  iii. Glaucoma

  iv. Papilledema

   v. Toxic amblyopia

  vi. Extensive panretinal photocoagulation.

11. How soon can ascending optic atrophy set in and completed?

The process can be identified within 24 hours and completed within 7 days.

12. What pathological process occurs in lateral geniculate body (LGB) in optic atrophy?

Transsynaptic changes occur in layer 1, 2, 3 and 5. Axons are reduced in size and not in number. Shrinkage and reduction of cytoplasm especially. Endoplasmic reticulum—reduced Nissl granule staining is seen.

13. **Examples of transsynaptic antegrade atrophy.**
    i. Glaucoma
    ii. After trauma
    iii. After enucleation.

14. **What is the earliest sign of optic atrophy?**
    Retinal nerve fiber layer changes are seen even before the onset of disk pallor or field defect. This defect can be slit like wedge shaped/diffuse loss.

15. **What is descending optic atrophy?**
    Refers to retrograde degeneration of axons. The primary lesion is in the brain or optic nerve. The atrophic process proceeds towards the eye leading to secondary effects on the optic disk and the retina.

16. **What is the time span of completion of descending optic atrophy?**
    Approximately 6–8 weeks. The time course of this descending degeneration is independent of the distance of the injury from the ganglion cell body.

17. **What are the histopathological hallmarks of optic atrophy?**
    i. Loss of myelin and axon fibers
    ii. Loss of the parallel architecture of the glial columns
    iii. Gliosis
    iv. Widening of the space separating the optic nerve and meninges
    v. Thickening of the pial septa of the nerve to occupy space lost by nerve fiber loss.

18. **Define primary optic atrophy (POA).**
    There is orderly degeneration of optic nerve fibers and is replaced by columns of glial tissue without any alteration in the architecture of the optic nerve head. This reflects a chronic process that has not been preceded by swelling or congestion of optic disk.

19. **Describe the features of primary optic atrophy.**
    i. Chalky white disk
    ii. Sharply defined margins
    iii. Lamina cribrosa is well seen
    iv. Surrounding retina and retinal vessels and periphery are normal
    v. Shallow, saucer shaped cup seen

20. **What are the common causes of primary optic atrophy?**
    i. *Retrobulbar neuritis*
    ii. *Compressive lesions of optic nerve, e.g.*
       – Pituitary tumors

    – Meningiomas

    – Gliomas

  iii. *Traumatic optic atrophy*

  iv. *Demyelinating diseases, e.g. tabes dorsalis, multiple scelrosis.*

21. What is secondary optic atrophy (SOA)?

It is characterized by marked degeneration of optic nerve fibers with excessive proliferation of glial tissue resulting in loss of entire architecture of optic nerve head.

It is preceded by swelling or congestion of the optic nerve head.

22. What are the causes of secondary optic atrophy?

  i. Papillitis

  ii. Papilledema.

23. Describe features of secondary optic atrophy.

    i. Gray or dirty gray pallor of the disk

    ii. Poorly defined margins

   iii. Physiological cup is obliterated and is filled with proliferating fibroglial tissue

   iv. Peripapillary sheathing and narrowing of arteries

    v. Veins are tortuous and sometimes narrowed

   vi. Hyaline bodies and drusens in and around the disk.

24. What is the most common cause of altitudinal pallor?

Acute ischemic optic neuropathy.

25. What is the most common cause of segmental optic atrophy?

Temporal pallor: This is due to degeneration of axial fibers of the retrobulbar optic nerve resulting in atrophy of papillomacular bundle.

26. What are the types of field defects occurring due to temporal pallor?

Centrocecal scotoma or central scotoma due to loss of papillomacular bundle.

27. How does wedge-shaped pallor occur?

Branch retinal artery occlusion leads to degeneration of infarcted ganglion cells causing atrophy of the corresponding wedge of the disk.

28. What is the most common cause of consecutive optic atrophy (COA)?

Central retinal artery occlusion. It is an ascending type of optic atrophy. Other causes are:

    i. Degenerative—RP, cerebromacular degeneration, myopia

    ii. Post-inflammatory—choroiditis, chorioretinitis

   iii. Extensive PRP

   iv. long-standing RD.

29. **What are the clinical features of consecutive optic atrophy?**
    i. Disk has a waxy pallor
    ii. Normal disk margin
    iii. Marked attenuation of arteries
    iv. Associated retinal pathology may be seen
    v. Normal physiologic cup.

30. **What is cavernous optic atrophy?**
    This is nothing but glaucomatous optic atrophy (Schnabel's). This is characterized by axonal degeneration without any proliferation of glial tissue resulting in formation of caverns with marked excavation of the optic disk. The caverns are filled with hyaluronic acid.

31. **What is the mechanism of ischemic optic atrophy?**
    Occurs when perfusion pressure of the ciliary system falls below the IOP.

32. **Causes of ischemic optic atrophy.**
    i. Systemic hypertension
    ii. Temporal arteritis
    iii. Atherosclerosis
    iv. Diabetes
    v. Collagen disorders

33. **When does optic atrophy manifests in CRAO?**
    2–3 weeks.

34. **Name some chemicals causing optic atrophy.**
    i. Arsenic
    ii. Lead
    iii. Benzene
    iv. Chromium
    v. Nitro- and dinitro-benzene.

35. **What are the drugs which can cause optic atrophy?**
    i. Quinine (total blindness in small doses in susceptible persons)
    ii. Ethambutol
    iii. Streptomycin
    iv. INH
    v. Chloroquine (Bull's eye maculopathy)
    vi. Oral contraceptives.

36. **What is the most common cause of toxic amblyopia?**
    Tobacco—in cigar and pipe smokers.

37. What is the pathogenesis and features of tobacco-induced optic atrophy?

Cyanide is the normal constituent of tobacco which is detoxified by sulfur metabolism to harmless thiocyanate. In tobacco users sulfur metabolism is deranged. There is degeneration of the axial portion of retrobulbar optic nerve due to demyelination. The resulting toxic degenerative neuritis leads to secondary fibrosis and gliosis within papillomacular bundle. It is associated with a deficiency of vitamin B12.

38. What is the treatment of tobacco amblyopia?

i. Abstention from tobacco and alcohol
ii. Injections of hydroxocobalamine 1000 µg intramuscularly. The dose should be repeated five times at intervals of 4 days.

39. Name some metabolic disorders causing optic atrophy.

i. Diabetes
ii. Thyroid ophthalmopathy
iii. Cystic fibrosis
iv. Nutritional amblyopia
v. Hypophosphatasia
vi. G-6-PD deficiency
vii. Mucopolysaccharidosis
viii. Acute intermittent porphyria—Menkes disease.

40. What is nutritional amblyopia?

It is due to atrophy of papillomacular nerve fibers caused by deficiency of vitamin B12, B6, B1, B2 and niacin.

Characterized by—

i. Progressive bilateral visual loss
ii. Centrocecal scotoma
iii. Temporal pallor.

41. What is the pathogenesis of tropical amblyopia?

Common in people eating cassava. Occurs due to reduced levels of serum cyanocobalamin and absence of sulfur containing amino acids.

42. What are the features of tropical amblyopia?

i. Bilateral blurred disk
ii. Temporal pallor
iii. General features like—ataxia, paresthesia of lower extremities, tinnitus, deafness, absence of deep tendon reflexes, posterior column sensory loss.

43. **Which variants of diabetes cause optic atrophy?**

   i. Juvenile diabetes mellitus
      - Autosomal recessive
      - Pronounced rod and less severe cone dystrophy (Wolfram syndrome)
   ii. DIDMOAD syndrome—diabetes mellitus, diabetes insipidus, optic atrophy, deafness.

44. **Specify the types of mucopolysaccharidosis causing optic atrophy.**

   i. Hurler's syndrome
   ii. Sanfilippo's syndrome.

45. **What is the mechanism of traumatic optic atrophy?**

   i. Tears in the nerve substance
   ii. Perforation of nerve by fractured bone spicules
   iii. Hemorrhage into nerve sheath
   iv. Contusion necrosis
   v. Avulsion of optic nerve.

46. **What is the most common site of injury leading to traumatic optic atrophy?**

   A blow to the lateral wall of the orbit.

47. **What is the time span after which the optic atrophic process manifest clinically first as temporal pallor in traumatic optic neuropathy?**

   2–4 weeks.

48. **What could be the pathophysiology of reversible loss of vision in traumatic optic neuropathy?**

   Compression of the intracanalicular portion of the optic nerve due to edema.

49. **What is the cause of intermittent visual claudication?**

   Takayasu disease—loss of vision may occur during exercise and improves at rest.

50. **What percent of foveal fibers must be present for normal visual acuity?**

   44% of foveal fibers.

51. **Name some hereditary causes of optic atrophy.**

   i. Congenital/infantile optic atrophy—recessive and dominant form
   ii. Leber's optic atrophy
   iii. Behr's optic atrophy

52. What are the differential diagnoses of optic atrophy?

   i. Coloboma of disk
  ii. Optic pit
 iii. Morning glory syndrome
  iv. Medullated nerve fibers
   v. Myopic disk
  vi. Optic disk hypoplasia
 vii. Drusens of the disk.

53. Name histopathological techniques to highlight demyelination of optic nerve.

   i. Special myelinophilic stains
     – Luxol fast blue
     – Weigert stain
  ii. Paraphenylenediamine—stains remnants of optic nerve myelin long after the degeneration/atrophy has occurred.
 iii. Demyelination is indicated in a hematoxylin and eosin tissue section by the more compact nature of the nerve parenchyma.

54. What is the specific color vision loss in optic nerve disorders?

Optic nerve disorders manifest a relative red-green deficiency.

55. How can color vision loss due to retinal and optic nerve pathology be differentiated?

Retinal diseases manifest a relative blue-yellow deficiency whereas optic nerve disorders show a relative red-green deficiency.

56. Name some causes of traction optic atrophy.

   i. Glaucoma
  ii. Post-papilledema
 iii. Sclerosed calcified arteries
  iv. Aneurysm of internal carotid artery
   v. Bony pressure at the optic foramen
  vi. Tumors of optic nerve sheath, pituitary, frontal temporal or sphenoidal lobes
 vii. Swelling of optic nerve which may get strangulated at the optic foramen
viii. Inflammatory adhesion in basal arachnoiditis.

57. What are the types of segmental or partial optic atrophy?

   i. Temporal pallor
  ii. Altitudinal pallor
 iii. Wedge-shaped pallor.

58. Classify optic atrophy.

Pathological

i. Ascending

ii. Descending

Ophthalmoscopical

i. POA

ii. SOA

iii. COA

Etiological

i. Consecutive

ii. post-inflammatory

iii. pressure/traction

iv. toxic

v. metabolic

vi. traumatic

vii. hereditary

viii. circulatory.

59. How is optic atrophy classified ophthalmoscopically?

i. Primary

ii. Secondary

iii. Consecutive

iv. Cavernous or glaucomatous

v. Segmental or partial.

60. How can methyl alcohol poisoning occur commonly?

Methanol (methyl alcohol) is found in cleaning materials, solvents, paints, varnishes, Sterno fuel, formaldehyde solutions, antifreeze, gasohol, "moonshine," Windshield washer fluid (30–40% methanol), and duplicating fluids. It is consumed as local liquor (wood alcohol).

61. What are the features of methyl alcohol poisoning?

i. Nonspecific symptoms such as headache, dizziness, nausea, lack of coordination, confusion, drowsiness

ii. Central nervous system (CNS) involvement in the form of unconsciousness, semiconsciousness, giddiness

iii. Visual symptoms are the predominant presenting features

iv. Shock may occur as a late event

v. Unconsciousness and death with sufficiently large doses.

62. How does methyl alcohol poisoning affect the optic nerve?

The symptoms of methanol poisoning are nonspecific except for the visual disturbances. Ocular changes consists of:

i. Retinal edema

    ii. Blurring of the disk margins
   iii. Hyperemia of the disks and
   iv. Optic atrophy as a late sequelae.

Metabolic acidosis is the most striking disturbance seen in methanol poisoning. It is probably due to the accumulation of formic acid and lactic acid.

Formic acid inhibits cytochrome oxidase in the fundus of the eye. Disruption of the axoplasm is due to impaired mitochondrial function and decreased ATP production. Swelling of axons in the optic disk and edema result in visual impairment.

The ocular changes correlate to the degree of acidosis. Retinal damage is due to the inhibition of retinal hexokinase by formaldehyde, an intermediate metabolite of methanol.

63. What is the treatment of methyl alcohol poisoning?

The essential therapy of methanol poisoning is adequate alkalinization and ethanol administration. Ethanol competes with methanol for the enzyme alcohol dehydrogenase in the liver, thereby preventing the accumulation of toxic metabolites of methanol in the body. The recommended dose of ethanol is 0.6 g/kg body weight (a loading dose) followed by an infusion of 66 mg/kg/hour in nondrinkers and 154 mg/kg/hour in chronic drinkers.

Dialysis is recommended in those patients who have visual disturbances, blood methanol of 50 mg% or more, ingestion of more than 60 mL of methanol and severe acidosis not corrected by sodium bicarbonate administration.

64. What are the features of excessive use of artificial sweeteners containing aspartame (NutraSweet)?

     i. Decreased vision—including blindness in one or both eyes
    ii. Blurring, "bright-flashes," tunnel vision, "black spots"
   iii. Double vision
    iv. Pain in one or both eyes
     v. Decreased tears
    vi. Difficulty in wearing contact lens
   vii. Unexplained retinal detachment and bleeding.

65. How do artificial sweetening agents affect the optic nerve?

Each of the components of aspartame—phenylalanine (50%); aspartic acid (40%); the methyl ester, are converted to methyl alcohol or methanol (10%) and further to formaldehyde which is toxic to the retina and optic nerves. Methanol causes swelling of the optic nerve and degeneration of ganglion cells in the retina.

66. Fundus portraits of different types of optic atrophy.

Primary	Secondary	Consecutive	Cavernous	Temporal
Disk	**Disk**	**Disk**	**Disk**	**Disk**
Chalky white in color	Gray dirty gray pallor	Waxy pallor of the disk	-Vertical pallor of cup-notching of NRR -Pallor of rim	Disk is pale on the temporal side
Sharply defined margins	Poorly defined margins	Normal disk margin	-Visibility of lamina pores–vlaminar dot sign -Backward bowing of lamina cribrosa	Clear disk margin
Lamina cribrosa well seen	Physiological cup obliterated and filled with fibroglial tissue obscuring view of lamina cribrosa	Normal physiological cup	-Bayoneting and nasalization of retinal vaessels -Splinter hemor -rhages at the disk margin -Saucerization of optic disk	
Vessels	**Vessels**	**Vessels**	**Vessels**	**Vessels**
Retinal vessels normal	Peripapillary sheathing of arteries and narrowing of arteries		Baring of cicumlinear vessels	
	Veins are tortuous and narrowed; occasionally sclerosed or hyaluronized	Marked attenuation of arteries	Peripapillary halo and atrophy	Vesels are normal
Surrounding retina normal	Hyaline bodies or drusen seen in and around the disk		Nerve fiber layer defect	

67. How is optic atrophy treated?

There is no real cure or treatment for optic atrophy. Therefore, it is important to have regular eye exams (especially if there is a family history of eye diseases), and to see an ophthalmologist immediately if any changes in vision are noted.

7.7. OPTIC DISK ANOMALIES

1. **What are congenital optic disk anomalies?**

   Definition: Unusual configuration of the disk(s) typically present since birth.

   Key features: Small, pale or unusual shaped disk may reflect mere curiosities or significant anomalies associated with visual field defects.

   Associated features: Abnormalities of the surrounding retina (e.g. in morning glory syndrome, anterior segment (e.g. in iris coloboma), face or brain occasionally may be seen.

   Congenital optic nerve head (ONH) anomalies are important because:
   - i. Relatively common
   - ii. Some may be mistaken for papilledema
   - iii. Some may give rise to visual field defects
   - iv. Some are associated with CNS malformation
   - v. Some may be associated with other ocular abnormalities.

2. **What are the features of congenital optic nerve head (ONH) anomalies?**

   Following are the general concepts useful in evaluating and managing children with congenital optic disk anomalies:
   - i. Children with bilateral optic disk anomaly generally present in infancy with poor vision and nystagmus; those with unilateral anomaly present during preschool years with sensory esotropia.
   - ii. CNS malformations are common in patients with malformed optic disks.

     Small optic disk is associated with malformations of cerebral hemisphere, pituitary infundibulum and midline intracranial structures (septum pellucidum, corpus callosum)

     Large optic disks of morning glory configuration are associated with the trans-sphenoidal form of basal encephalocele.

     Large optic disks of colobomatous configuration may be associated with systemic anomalies.

     MRI is advisable in infants with small optic disks (unilateral or bilateral) and in infants with large optic disks who have either neuro-developmental deficits or mid facial anomalies suggestive of basal encephalocele.
   - iii. Color vision is relatively preserved in an eye with a congenitally anomalous optic disk in contrast to the severe dyschromatopsia in acquired optic neuropathies.
   - iv. Any structural ocular abnormality that reduces visual acuity in infancy may lead to superimposed amblyopia. Occlusion therapy therefore should be tried in patients with unilateral optic disk anomalies and decreased vision.

3. **What are the features of optic nerve hypoplasia?**

The most common optic disk anomaly encountered in ophthalmologic practice.

Incidence has increased in recent times because of maternal alcohol and drug abuse.

Pathogenesis:

Primary failure of retinal ganglion cell differentiation at the 13 to 15 mm stage of embryonic life.

Ophthalmoscopic appearance:

  i. Abnormally small optic nerve head.
 ii. Gray in color and is often surrounded by a yellowish mottled peri-papillary halo, bordered by a ring of increased or decreased pigmentation (double-ring)
iii. Major retinal blood vessels are tortuous.
 iv. Histopathologically, subnormal number of optic nerve axons with normal mesodermal elements and glial supporting tissue.
  v. Double ring sign
     – Outer ring—normal junction between the sclera and lamina cribrosa.
     – Inner ring—abnormal extension of retina and RPE over the outer portion of lamina cribrosa.

Visual acuity

  i. Ranges from 6/6 to no PL
 ii. Localized visual field defects
iii. Generalized constriction of visual fields.

Systemic associations

  i. Superior segmental ONH—type 1 DM.
 ii. Growth hormone deficiency is most common.
iii. Neonatal hypoglycemia or seizures with ONH—congenital pan hypopituitarism.

Investigation

Magnetic resonance imaging (MRI) demonstrates thinning and attenuation of prechiasmatic intracranial optic nerve.

4. **What are excavated optic disk anomalies?**

  i. Morning glory disk anomaly
 ii. Optic disk coloboma
iii. Peripapillary staphyloma

5. **What are the features of morning glory disk anomaly?**

It is a congenital, funnel-shaped excavation of the posterior fundus that incorporates the optic disk.

Ophthalmoscopically

i. The disk is markedly enlarged, orange or pink in color, and it may appear to be recessed or elevated centrally within the confines of a funnel-shaped peripapillary excavation.

ii. A wide annulus of chorioretinal pigmentary disturbance surrounds the disk within the excavation.

iii. A white tuft of glial tissue overlies the central portion of the disk.

iv. Blood vessels appear increased in number and often arise from the disk periphery; have a straight course.

v. Macula may be incorporated in the excavation (macular capture).

Features

i. Morning glory anomaly is usually a unilateral condition.

ii. Visual acuity 6/60 to finger counting.

iii. Females > males.

iv. Rare in blacks.

v. Associated with transsphenoidal form of basal encephalocele.

vi. Patient with transsphenoidal encephalocele usually display a characteristic malformation complex consisting of midfacial anomalies, hypertelorism, widened bitemporal diameter, depressed nasal root and V-shaped fusion line involving the upper lip.

vii. A transsphenoidal encephalocele may appear clinically as a pulsatile posterior nasal mass or a "nasal polyp" high in the nose.

viii. Morning glory disk anomaly patients are at risk of acquired visual loss.

ix. In 30% serous retinal detachment starts in the peripapillary area and extends to the posterior pole.

6. What are the features of optic disk coloboma?

i. Coloboma means mutilated.

ii. Coloboma of the optic disk results from incomplete or abnormal coaptation of the proximal end of the embryonic fissure.

iii. In optic disk coloboma, a sharply defined, glistening white, bowl-shaped excavation occupies an enlarged optic disk.

iv. Excavation is decentered inferiorly, reflecting the position of the embryonic fissure.

v. Inferior neuroretinal rim is thin or absent while superior is spared.

vi. Iris and ciliary coloboma often co-exist.

vii. Axial scan show crater like excavation of the posterior globe at its junction with optic nerve.

viii. Visual acuity may be decreased.

ix. Optic disk coloboma may arise sporadically or inherited in an autosomal dominant fashion.

x. Eyes with isolated optic disk coloboma are prone to develop serous macular detachments.

7. **What are the features of peripapillary staphyloma?**

It is a rare, unilateral, deep fundus excavation which surrounds the disk.

Peripapillary staphyloma	Morning glory disk
Deep, cup-shaped excavation	Less deep, funnel-shaped excavation
Optic disk: Relatively normal and well defined	Optic disk: Grossly anomalous and poorly defined
Absence of glial and vascular anomalies	Central glial bouquet; anomalous vascular pattern

8. **How do you differentiate morning glory syndrome from optic disk coloboma?**

Ophthalmoscopic findings

Morning glory disk	Optic disk coloboma
1. Optic disk lies within the excavation	1. Excavation lies within the optic disk
2. Symmetrical defect	2. Asymmetrical defect
3. Central glial tuft	3. No central glial tuft
4. Severe peripapillary pigmentary disturbance	4. Minimal peripapillary pigmentary disturbance
5. Anomalous retinal vasculature	5. Normal retinal vasculature

Systemic and ocular findings

Morning glory disk	Optic disk coloboma
Females > males	No sex or racial predilection
Rarely familial	Often familial
Rarely bilateral	Often bilateral
No iris, ciliary body or retinal colobomas	Iris, ciliary and retinal colobomas common
Rarely associated multisystem genetic disorder	Often associated multisystem genetic disorder
Basal encephalocele common	Rare

9. **What are the features of megalopapilla?**

Features:

2 phenotypic variants

i. First is a common variant in which abnormally large optic disk (>2.1 mm in diameter)
   – Frequently bilateral with large cup-to-disk ratio where the cup is round or horizontally oval with no vertical notching differentiating it from a normal tension glaucoma.

ii. Second phenotypic variant, the normal optic cup is replaced by grossly anamolous noninferior excavation that obliterates the adjacent neuroretinal rim.

10. What are the features of optic pit?

    i. Round or oval, gray, white or yellowish depression in the optic disk.
    ii. Commonly involve the temporal optic disk but may be situated in any sector.
    iii. Temporally located pits are often accompanied by adjacent peripapillary pigment epithelial changes.
    iv. One or two cilioretinal arteries are seen to emerge from the bottom or margin of the pit in 50% cases.
    v. Typically unilateral; disk is larger than in the fellow eye.
    vi. Serous macular elevation develops in 25–75% cases.
    vii. Maculopathy become symptomatic in third to fourth decade of life.

11. What are the sources of fluid in an optic disk pit?

    i. Vitreous cavity via the pit
    ii. Subarachnoid space
    iii. Blood vessels at the base of pit
    iv. Orbital space surrounding the dura.

12. What are the features of congenital tilted disk syndrome?

Fairly common, nonhereditary, bilateral condition in which the superotem-poral optic disk is elevated and the inferonasal disk is posteriorly displaced, resulting in an oval–appearing disk, with its long axis obliquely oriented.

Accompanying features:

    i. Situs inversus of retinal vessels
    ii. Congenital inferonasal conus
    iii. Thinning of inferonasal RPE and choroid
    iv. Bitemporal hemianopia
    v. Affected patient may have myopic astigmatism
    vi. Disk is small, oval or d-shaped with axis oblique
    vii. Visual field defects involving the upper temporal quadrants may be present as a result of inferonasal fundus changes.

13. What are the features of Aicardi syndrome?

Cerebroretinal disorder of unknown etiology.

Clinical features:

    i. Infantile spasms
    ii. Agenesis of corpus callosum
    iii. A characteristic EEG pattern termed as "hypsarrhythmia"
    iv. A pathognomonic optic disk appearance consisting of multiple depigmented "chorioretinal lacunae" clustered around the disk
    v. Histopathologically these lacunae are well circumscribed, full thickness defects, limited to the RPE and the choroids
    vi. Other congenital optic disk anomaly may accompany the chorioretinal lacunae.

Ocular associations:

    i. Microphthalmos
    ii. Retrobulbar cyst
    iii. Pseudoglioma

　　iv. Retinal detachment, macular scars
　　 v. Cataract
　　vi. Pupillary membrane, etc.

Systemic associations:
　　 i. Vertebral malformations (fused vertebra, scoliosis, spina bifida)
　　 ii. Costal malformations (absent ribs, fused ribs or bifurcated ribs)
　　iii. CNS anomalies include:
Agenesis of corpus callosum, cortical migration anomalies and malformations.

14. **What are the features of optic disk drusen?**
　　　 i. Intrapapillary drusen are crystalloid, acellular refractile bodies that often appear in long-standing anomalously elevated disk.
　　　 ii. Incidence in general population is 0.3–2%.
　　　iii. Bilateral and familial "emerge" over time.
　　　iv. Patients with retinitis pigmentosa and angoid streak show increase incidence.
　　　 v. Thought to develop from stagnant axoplasm dammed up by a small disk, a tight cribriform plate, or a narrow scleral canal.
　　　vi. May be small or large; superficial or deep.
　　　vii. Produce field loss, sparing 10° of visual field.

Investigations
　　　 i. Fluorescein angiography: Drusen shows late staining with fluorescein (hyperfluorescence); whereas in papilledema the staining disk often shows feathery leakage into the adjacent nerve fiber layer.
　　　 ii. Autofluorescence: Drusen shows autofluorescence when viewed with 430 nm wavelength (blue) light source using a yellow filter.
　　　iii. CT scan: Drusen show mineralization.
　　　iv. Ultrasonography: Drusen reflect sound waves.

Differentiating drusen from early *papilledema* pose a diagnostic challenge.

Drusens have the following features:
　　　 i. Absent optic cup
　　　 ii. Disk has a pink/yellow color and margin has a "lumpy" appearance
　　　iii. Emerging vessels show anomalous premature branching
　　　iv. Autofluorescence.

15. **What are the features of myelinated nerve fibers?**
　　　 i. Myelination of the optic nerve begins in the fetus, approaching the optic chiasm by about 7 months of gestation.
　　　 ii. Myelination stops usually at lamina cribrosa at about 1 month of age, and is complete by about 10 months after birth.
　　　iii. In approximately 0.5% of population myelination continue past the optic disk and into the nerve fiber layer of the retina.
　　　iv. Characteristically, myelinated nerve fibers are white, and feathered at the edges and
　　　 v. Do not have any effect on visual fields but the blind spot may be enlarged.

7.8. ANTERIOR ISCHEMIC OPTIC NEUROPATHY

1. **Define anterior ischemic optic neuropathy.**

   Anterior ischemic optic neuropathy (AION)—defined as the segmental or generalized infarction within the prelaminar or laminar portion of the optic nerve. Caused by occlusion of the short posterior ciliary arteries.

2. **Give the clinical classification of anterior ischemic optic neuropathy.**

   i. Arteritic AION
   ii. Nonarteritic AION.

3. **What are the risk factors for nonarteritic anterior ischemic optic neuropathy?**

   Risk factors
   i. Nicotine smokers
   ii. Diabetes (diabetic papillopathy—common in juvenile diabetics)
   iii. Hypertensives and patients with migraine—long-standing HTN is thought to affect the autoregulation of blood flow to the optic nerve head
   iv. Hypercholesterolemia
   v. Cerebrovascular disease
   vi. Carotid artery disease
   vii. Acute severe blood loss
   viii. Uremia
   ix. Favism resulting in an acute hemolytic anemia
   x. Nocturnal hypotension
   xi. Elevated IOP
   xii. Uncomplicated cataract extraction
   xiii. Rarely associated with cavernous sinus thrombosis and radiation optic neuropathy.

4. **What is the pathogenesis of nonarteritic anterior ischemic optic neuropathy?**

   Nonarteritic anterior ischemic optic neuropathy is thought to be caused by vascular insufficiency. This hypothesis is supported by the following facts.

   Abrupt onset of visual loss which is typical of a vascular disease:
   i. Common in older patients with systemic vasculopathies
   ii. Closure of small blood vessels in histopathology specimens
   iii. Lack of evidence of inflammation.

   The prelaminar and laminar portions of the optic nerve is supplied by an elliptical arterial circle called Zinn's corona or Haller's circle formed by the anastomosis around the optic nerve between medial and lateral paroptic short posterior ciliary arteries. The ellipse is divided into superior and inferior parts by the entry points of the lateral and medial short posterior ciliary arteries, providing an attitudinal blood supply to the anterior optic nerve. Reduced perfusion pressure within the territory of the paraoptic branches of the short posterior ciliary arteries results in an altitudinal visual field loss.

Optic disks of patients with AION are usually small with little or no physiologic cupping. A small cup-to-disk ratio implies a small optic disk diameter and small scleral canal resulting in crowding of nerve fibers through a restricted space in the lamina cribrosa. The ischemia in AION causes axoplasmic flow stasis, which causes compression of the capillaries within this crowded disk resulting in further ischemia.

Hence the "disk at risk" is one with:
   i. Small physiologic cup.
   ii. Elevation of disk margins by a thick nerve fiber layer.
  iii. Anomalies of blood vessel branching.
   iv. Crowded and small optic nerve head.

Blood flow to the optic nerve head is directly proportional to the perfusion pressure and is inversely proportional to the vascular resistance in the blood vessels. Vascular resistance is influenced by the blood vessel wall changes, which are affected in disease states such as hypertension, diabetes mellitus, arteriosclerosis and vasospasm.

5. **What are the clinical features of nonarteritic anterior ischemic optic neuropathy?**
   i. Affects patients between 45–70 years of age.
   ii. Patients present with monocular sudden painless visual loss. 2/3rd of cases have a moderate to severe impairment and 1/3rd of cases are spared or have minimal visual impairment.
  iii. Diminished color perception. The degree of color vision loss is directly related to the amount of visual acuity loss (as opposed to patients with optic neuritis where color vision is significantly impaired despite minimal loss of visual acuity).
   iv. Visual field defects most often in the form of inferior altitudinal defects which spare fixation. Other field defects such as central scotomas, arcuate defects, quadrantic defects and generalized constriction may also occur.
   v. Relative afferent pupillary defect.
   vi. On ophthalmoscopic examination, there may be:
       – Focal or diffuse disk swelling
       – Disk may be pale or hyperemic and
       – May have splinter hemorrhages at the disk margin.

About 7% of cases have associated with hard exudates in a star pattern at the macula which may be misdiagnosed as neuroretinitis.

Focal hyperemic telangiectatic vessels may appear on the optic disk of an eye with NAION within day or weeks of onset of symptoms. This phenomenon is called luxury perfusion—a vascular autoregulatory response to ischemia.

Disk swelling resolves in 1–2 months with the development of optic atrophy but with no cupping and attenuated vessels.

6. **What are the investigations used in nonarteritic anterior ischemic optic neuropathy?**
    i. ESR
   ii. C-reactive protein
  iii. Serum lipids
   iv. Blood glucose
    v. Packed cell volume and
   vi. Fibrinogen levels.

7. **What is the treatment for nonarteritic anterior ischemic optic neuropathy?**

   No therapy is of significant benefit.

   Medical therapy
    i. Underlying systemic conditions should be treated.
   ii. Patients should discontinue smoking.
  iii. Antiplatelet agents and anticoagulants have been tried.
   iv. Steroids–its role is controversial.

   Surgical therapy
    i. Stellate ganglion block.
   ii. Optic nerve sheath decompression.

   The ischemic optic neuropathy decompression trial:
    i. It is a multicenter prospective study of nonarteritic anterior ischemic optic neuropathy.
   ii. The primary objective of this study was to assess the safety and efficacy of optic nerve sheath decompression (ONSD) versus careful observation of patient with NAION. The secondary objectives were documentation of the natural history of the disease, identification of risk factors and assessment of the contralateral eye risk as well as other nonocular vasoocclusive events.
  iii. The study found that 42.7% of patients on careful observation, at 6 months, showed an improvement in visual acuity by 3 lines or more while in 45% little or no change occurred.

iv. In the patients who underwent ONSD, only 32.6% of patient had an improved visual acuity of 3 lines or more while 43.5% experienced little or no change.

v. Hence, optic nerve sheath decompression ONSD did not appear to be effective in the management of nonarteritic anterior ischemic optic neuropathy.

vi. Optic nerve sheath decompression group also studied the role of aspirin in nonarteritic anterior ischemic optic neuropathy and concluded that its role in prevention of NAION is still unclear.

8. What are the causes of arteritic anterior ischemic optic neuropathy (AAION)?

   i. Giant cell arteritis or temporal arteritis (most common cause type of AAION)
   ii. Rheumotoid arthritis
   iii. HZV infection
   iv. Relapsing polychondritis
   v. Takayasu's arteritis
   vi. Behcet's disease
   vii. Polyarteritis nodosa
   viii. Systemic lupus erythematosis
   ix. Churg–Strauss angiitis.

9. What are the clinical features of AAION?

   i. Sudden monocular profound loss of vision which is preceded by transient visual obscurations and flashes of light
   ii. Bilateral involvement may occur
   iii. Periocular pain may or may not occur
   iv. Patients have pale swollen disks with splinter hemorrhages. The disks typically look chalky white. The disk edema resolves leaving behind a markedly cupped disk.

10. What are the ocular features of giant cell arteritis?

   i. Amaurosis fugax
   ii. CRAO
   iii. AION
   iv. Choroidal infarcts
   v. Cotton-wool spots
   vi. Anterior segment ischemia
   vii. Hypotony
   viii. Conjunctival and episcleral congestion
   ix. Corneal edema
   x. Extraocular muscle ischemia
   xi. Oculomotor nerve palsy
   xii. Ophthalmic artery occlusion
   xiii. Cortical blindness.

11. What are the systemic manifestations of giant cell arteritis (GCA)?

   i. Malaise

   ii. Weight loss, depression, fever

   iii. Polymyalgia rheumatica—stiffness and pain of proximal muscle groups in the morning and after exertion

   iv. Jaw claudication

   v. Headache

   vi. Palpable, nodular and nonpulsatile temporal artery

   vii. Anemia

   viii. Myocardial infarction

   ix. Stroke

   x. Renal failure

12. How do you diagnose arteritic anterior ischemic optic neuropathy (AAION)?

   i. ESR—normal in 20% of cases

    usually >50 mm/hr (by Westergren's method)

    age related normal for males is $age \dfrac{mm/hr}{2}$

    and for females is $age + \dfrac{10\ mm/hr}{2}$

   ii. C-reactive protein—raised

   iii. Fluorescein angiography—delayed or absent filling of the choroidal circulation

   iv. Alkaline phosphate level in serum—raised

   v. ANA—positive

   vi. Temporal artery biopsy

    – gives a definitive diagnosis

    – a 3 cm long specimen should be taken as skip lesions are evident.

Occult GCA: Ocular involvement without associated signs and symptoms but with raised ESR and temporal artery biopsy positive for GCA.

13. How do you treat arteritic anterior ischemic optic neuropathy (AAION)?

Systemic steroids is the main stay. The treatment protocol is as follows:

IV methyl prednisolone 1–2 g/day

          +   }   for 3 days

Tab prednisolone 80 mg/day

Then,

Tab prednisolone   60 mg × 3 days

                40 mg × 4 days

Taper by 5 mg/week till 10 mg/day

Maintenance dose of 10 mg/day for 12 months

Throughout the treatment the signs, symptoms and ESR is monitored.

7.9. OCULOMOTOR NERVE

1. **Enumerate the salient features in the embryology of 3rd nerve.**
   i. 3rd nerve develops in the cranial portion of the neural tube from the most medial row of neuroblasts, the somatic efferent column.
   ii. 3rd nerve nucleus becomes visible at the 8–9 mm stage.

2. **What are the functional components of third nerve?**
   i. Somatic efferent—fibers to extraocular muscles
   ii. General somatic afferent—carries proprioceptive impulses from these muscles
   iii. General visceral efferent—parasympathetic supply to eye.

3. **Describe the anatomy of third nerve nucleus.**
   Location: Midbrain at the level of superior colliculus.
   Dimension: Longitudinal column of large multipolar neurons, 10 mm in length, in the floor of cerebral aqueduct.
   Relations: Above it extends as far as the floor of the third ventricle. Below it is related to the nucleus of trochlear nerve.
   Blood supply: Nuclei and the fascicles are supplied by median group of arteries that arises from the bifurcation of basilar artery at the origin of superior cerebellar and posterior cerebral arteries.

4. **What are the components of third nerve nucleus?**
   i. Principal nucleus
   ii. Edinger–Westphal nucleus dorsal to the principal nucleus.

5. **What is Warwick's classification of principal nucleus?**

Nucleus	Muscle supplied
i. Dorsolateral	Inferior rectus
ii. Intermediate	Inferior oblique
iii. Ventro median	Medial rectus
iv. Paramedian	Superior rectus
v. Caudal central	Levator palpebrae superioris

6. **Which nucleus has a contralateral innervation and what is its significance in diagnosis?**
   Fibers from paramedian group nucleus are partly crossed and supply the contralateral superior rectus. Therefore, a nuclear third nerve palsy of one side causes a paresis of contralateral superior rectus.

7. **Which nucleus is unpaired and has a bilateral supply?**
   Both levator palpebrae superioris muscles are supplied by a single midline caudal subnucleus. Lesion that damages this region thus produces a bilateral symmetric ptosis.

Some lesions of the oculomotor nuclear complex may spare this region causing a fixed dilated pupil and ophthalmoparesis but no ptosis.

8. **Describe the anatomy of Edinger–Westphal (EW) nucleus.**
   i. The E–W nucleus is made up of small multipolar neurons.
   ii. It consists of two lateral components and a medial component united anteriorly.
   iii. Anterior part of median component and lateral components are parasympathetic.
   iv. Cranial half of this is concerned with light reflexes.
   v. Caudal half is concerned with accommodation reflex.
   vi. Posterior part of E–W nucleus is forked and previously was erroneously termed as convergence nucleus of perlia.

   The nucleus for the proprioreceptive fibers is situated in the trigeminal nerve nuclear complex. They reach the nucleus either through the communication to ophthalmic nerve in the cavernous sinus or through the connections between oculomotor nucleus and mesencephalic nucleus of trigeminal nerve.

9. **Describe the blood supply of third nerve.**
   i. In the subarachnoid space, the nerve receives vascular twigs from the posterior cerebral artery, superior cerebellar artery and the tentorial and dorsal meningeal branches of the meningohypophyseal trunk of the internal carotid artery.
   ii. In cavernous sinus, the tentorial, dorsal meningeal and inferior hypophyseal branches of the meningohypophyseal trunk supply the nerve along with branches from ophthalmic artery.

10. **Describe the topographic arrangement of fibers within the third nerve.**
    i. Within the subarachnoid space, pupillomotor fibers appear to be located superficially in the superior portion of the nerve. The fibers in this portion of the third nerve are arranged in a superior and inferior division.
    ii. Within the cavernous sinus and orbit, the pupillary fibers are located in the inferior division of the nerve. The position of the fibers going to the specific EOM is unknown.

11. **What are the muscles supplied by the third nerve?**
    i. The superior division innervates the
       – Superior rectus
       – Levator palpebrae superioris.
    ii. The inferior division innervates the
       – Inferior rectus
       – Medial rectus

 – Inferior oblique
 – Sphincter muscle of the iris (pupil)
 – Ciliary muscle (accommodation).

12. **What is ciliary ganglion?**

It is a peripheral parasympathetic pinhead size ganglion situated at the apex of the orbit, between the optic nerve medially and the lateral rectus laterally, in the central surgical space.

13. **What are the various roots of the ciliary ganglion?**

 i. Parasympathetic root is a branch from the nerve to inferior oblique, carrying preganglionic fibers from Edinger–Westphal nucleus.
 ii. Sympathetic root carries postganglionic fibers from the superior cervical sympathetic ganglion.
 iii. Sensory root is a twig from nasociliary nerve.

14. **What are types of third nerve palsies?**

 i. Congenital
 ii. Acquired.

15. **What are the causes of congenital third nerve palsies?**

 i. **Aplasia** or hypoplasia of the third nerve nucleus.
 ii. **Birth trauma:** It is due to the damage to the subarachnoid portion of the 3rd nerve, either at its exit from the brainstem or just before it enters the cavernous sinus.
 iii. *Syndromes associated with congenital 3rd nerve palsy:*
 – *Congenital adduction palsy with synergistic divergence:* Patients with this syndrome have congenital unilateral paralysis of adduction associated with simultaneous bilateral adduction on attempted gaze into the field of action of the paretic medial rectus muscle.
 – *Vertical retraction syndrome:* Main features are limitation of movement of the affected eye on elevation or depression associated with a retraction of the globe and narrowing of the palpebral fissure.
 – Oculomotor nerve paresis with cyclic spasms.

16. **What are the various levels at which third nerve can be affected in an acquired palsy?**

At the level of:

 i. Oculomotor nucleus
 ii. Oculomotor nerve fascicle
 iii. In the subarachnoid space
 iv. At or near the entrance to the cavernous sinus
 v. Within the cavernous sinus
 vi. Within the supraorbital fissure
 vii. Within the orbit
 viii. Uncertain or variable location.

17. **What are the causes of IIIrd nerve palsy?**

Any focally destructive lesion along the course of the third cranial nerve can cause oculomotor nerve palsy or dysfunction. Some of the most frequent causes include the following:

i. Nuclear portion
   - Infarction
   - Hemorrhage
   - Neoplasm
   - Abscess

ii. Fascicular midbrain portion
   - Infarction
   - Hemorrhage
   - Neoplasm
   - Abscess

iii. Fascicular subarachnoid portion
   - Aneurysm
   - Infectious meningitis—bacterial, fungal/parasitic, viral
   - Meningeal infiltrative
   - Carcinomatous/lymphomatous/leukemic infiltration, granulomatous inflammation (sarcoidosis, lymphomatoid granulomatosis, Wegener granulomatosis)

iv. Fascicular cavernous sinus portion
   - Tumor—pituitary adenoma, meningioma, craniopharyngioma, metastatic carcinoma
   - Vascular
   - Giant intracavernous aneurysm
   - Carotid artery—cavernous sinus fistula
   - Carotid dural branch—cavernous sinus fistula
   - Cavernous sinus thrombosis
   - Ischemia from microvascular disease in vasa nervosa
   - Inflammatory—Tolosa–Hunt syndrome (idiopathic or granulomatous inflammation).

v. Fascicular orbital portion
   - Inflammatory—orbital inflammatory pseudotumor, orbital myositis
   - Endocrine (thyroid orbitopathy)
   - Tumor (e.g. hemangioma, lymphangioma, meningioma).

18. **What is the most common cause of isolated IIIrd nerve palsy with pupillary involvement?**

Intracranial aneurysms

19. **What are the investigations for a IIIrd nerve palsy?**
    i. *Basic investigations*
       – Blood sugar
       – Blood pressure
       – Lipid profile
       – ESR—to rule out giant cell arteritis
    ii. *X-ray skull lateral view*—to rule out sellar lesions involving the cavernous sinus.
    iii. In complicated third nerve palsies where other neural structures are involved, have the patient undergo an MRI/MRA.
    iv. In isolated third nerve palsies with no pupillary involvement where the patient is over 50, MRI scanning, an ischemic vascular evaluation, and daily pupil evaluation is indicated.
    v. If the patient is under 50 and has a nonpupillary involved isolated third nerve palsy, intracranial angiography is indicated since ischemic vasculopathy is less likely to occur in this age group than is aneurysm. In majority of cases it can pick aneurysms >3 mm in size.
    vi. Cerebral *angiography*—angiography is the definitive test for berry aneurysm in all intracranial locations. If the adult patient of any age presents with a complete or incomplete isolated third nerve palsy with pupillary involvement, consider this to be a medical emergency and have the patient undergo intracranial angiography immediately (CT angiography or MR angiography). In these cases, the cause is likely subarachnoid aneurysm and the patient may die if the aneurysm ruptures.
    vii. Children under the age of 14 rarely have aneurysms; the majority of third nerve palsies in this age group are traumatic or congenital.
    viii. Lumbar puncture—the main purpose of lumbar puncture is to demonstrate the presence of blood in cerebrospinal fluid, an inflammatory reaction, neoplastic infiltration, or infection.
    ix. Cytologic examination of cerebrospinal fluid is used to diagnose meningeal carcinomatosis and lymphomatous or leukemic infiltration.

20. **How does aneurysms affect the IIIrd nerve and what is its most common site?**
    i. Aneurysms usually arise from the junction of internal carotid and posterior communicating arteries.
    ii. In its course towards the cavernous sinus, the IIIrd nerve travels lateral to the posterior communicating artery and may be injured by
       – Direct compression
       – Hemorrhage
       – Major rupture
       – During aneurysm surgery.

21. **Why are pupillary fibers spared in ischemic lesions and more commonly affected in compressive lesions?**

The pupillomotor fibers are arranged in outer layers of the IIIrd nerve and are therefore closer to the nutrient blood supply enveloping the nerve. So they are spared in 80% of ischemic lesions but being outer, are affected in 95% of compressive lesions.

22. **Why is IIIrd nerve more commonly affected in cavernous sinus lesions?**

The IIIrd nerve is firmly attached to the dura adjacent to the posterior clinoid process just posterior to the cavernous sinus, so is more vulnerable to

   i. Stretch
   ii. Contusion injuries
   iii. Frontal head trauma
   iv. Aneurysms
   v. Surgery in the perisellar region.

23. **What are the causes of painful IIIrd nerve palsy with pupil involvement?**

   i. Posteriorly draining, low flow carotid-cavernous fistula
   ii. Tumors
   iii. Compressive lesions—aneurysms of posterior cerebral and basilar vessels
   iv. Intrinsic lesions of the IIIrd nerve—schwannomas and cavernous angiomas

24. **How can you demonstrate whether fourth nerve is involved, in the situation of a third nerve palsy?**

The patient is asked to abduct the eye and then look down. If the fourth nerve is functioning the eye should intort.

25. **Localization of 3rd nerve lesions and clinical manifestations.**

Structure involved	Clinical manifestations
Lesions affecting OM nucleus:	
1. Oculomotor nucleus	Ipsilateral complete third palsy. Contralateral ptosis and superior rectus paresis
2. Oculomotor subnucleus	Isolated muscle palsy (inferior rectus)
3. Isolated levator subnucleus	Isolated bilateral ptosis
4. Paramedian mesencepalon	Plus minus syndrome (ipsilateral ptosis and contralateral eyelid retraction)

(Continued)

(*Continued*)

Structure involved	Clinical manifestations
Lesions affecting OM fascicles:	
1. Isolated fascicle	Partial or complete third nerve palsy with or without pupillary involvement
2. Fascicle and superior cerebellar peduncle	Ipsilateral 3rd nerve palsy with contralateral ataxia and tremor (Claude's syndrome)
3. Fascicle and cerebral peduncle	Ipsilateral 3rd nerve palsy with contra-lateral hemiparesis
4. Fascicle and red nucleus/ substantia nigra	Ipsilateral 3rd nerve palsy with contralateral choriform movements (Benedict's syndrome)

26. What are the features of nuclear IIIrd nerve palsy?

  i. Ptosis—always bilateral
  ii. Mydriasis and cycloplegia—always bilateral
  iii. Contralateral superior rectus paresis or bilateral superior rectus paresis
  iv. Incomplete involvement of different subnuclei
  v. Bilateral total IIIrd nerve palsy can happen without ptosis.

27. How does fascicular IIIrd nerve palsy present?

Damage to fascicular or subarachnoid portion of the IIIrd nerve presents as

  i. Isolated pupillary dilation with reduced light reaction
  ii. Ophthalmoplegia with or without pupillary involvement.

28. What are the factors responsible for IIIrd nerve palsy in hippocampal gyrus herniation?

  i. Direct compression of the IIIrd nerve
  ii. Mechanical stretching of IIIrd nerve
  iii. Shifting of basal arteries with herniating brainstem—posterior cerebral arteries drawn tightly across the dorsal surface of IIIrd nerves.

29. What is Hutchinson's pupil?

Dilation of one pupil when the other is contracted, resulting from compression of the third nerve due to:

  i. Meningeal hemorrhage at the base of the brain
  ii. Herniation of the uncus of the temporal lobe through the tentorial notch.

The effect is caused by pressure of the posterior cerebral artery on the superior surface of the oculomotor nerve where the pupillary fibers are concentrated.

30. What is sphenocavernous syndrome?

Characterized by paralysis or paresis of the IIIrd, IVth and VIth nerves within the cavernous sinus or the superior orbital fissure.

    i. Associated with involvement of the first division of the Vth nerve.

    ii. Optic nerve involvement can cause visual loss.

    iii. Oculosympathetic paresis may lead to proptosis and edema of eyelids and conjunctiva.

31. What is pseudo-orbital apex syndrome?

Large intracranial masses may expand to such a degree that they compress the intracranial optic nerve or cavernous portion of the IIIrd nerve and prevent adequate venous drainage from the orbit, resulting in pseudo-orbital apex syndrome.

32. Enumerate some common lesions causing sphenocavernous syndrome.

    i. Aneurysms

    ii. Meningiomas

    iii. Pituitary tumors

    iv. Craniopharyngiomas

    v. Nasopharyngeal tumors

    vi. Metastatic tumors

    vii. Infectious/inflammatory.

33. What are the common causes of pupil sparing IIIrd nerve palsy?

The most important cause is ischemia, due to:

    i. Diabetes

    ii. Hypertension

    iii. Atherosclerosis
  - Migraine
  - Systemic lupus erythematosus
  - Giant cell arteritis.

34. How can a pupil sparing isolated IIIrd nerve palsy be investigated?

Ischemia lab work-up

    i. Blood pressure

    ii. Complete blood count

    iii. ESR

    iv. Blood sugar, glycosylated Hb

    v. VDRL, FTA–ABS (TPHA).

35. How long does it take for pupil sparing palsy to recover?

Ischemic IIIrd nerve palsies resolve within 4–16 weeks without treatment and the resolution is almost complete.

36. What is aberrant regeneration of the IIIrd nerve or oculomotor synkinesis or misdirection syndrome?

Aberrant regeneration occurs as a consequence of complete IIIrd nerve palsy in which there is gross limitation of ocular movement amounting to virtual paralysis. The regenerating autonomic and voluntary nerve fibers grow along the wrong myelin tubes that contained functioning neurons before degeneration.

37. Why is aberrant degeneration seen commonly in IIIrd nerve palsy?

The IIIrd nerve supplies a number of different muscles. The regenerating sprouts from axons that previously innervated one muscle group may ultimately innervate a different muscle group with a different function.

38. What are the clinical presentations of aberrant regeneration of IIIrd nerve?

i. *Lid-gaze dyskinesis*
 – *Pseudo von Graefe sign:* Some of the nerve fibers to the interior rectus may end up innervating the elevator so that the lid retracts when the patient looks down.
 – *Inverse Duane's syndrome:* Some of the medial rectus fibers may end up supplying some of the innervation to the levator so that the lid retracts when the patient adducts his eye.

ii. *Pupil-gaze dyskinesis:*
 Pseudo-Argyll Robertson pupil: Some of the medial rectus fibers may end up innervating the pupillary sphincter muscle so that there is more pupil constriction during convergence than as a response to light.

39. What are the two forms of aberrant regeneration?

i. Primary: No preceding IIIrd nerve palsy
ii. Secondary aberrant regeneration: After IIIrd nerve palsy.

40. What are the syndromes associated with IIIrd nerve palsy?

i. **Benedict's syndrome**—involves the fasciculus as it passes through the red nucleus. It causes ipsilateral IIIrd nerve palsy and contralateral extrapyramidal signs.

Level of lesion: Red nucleus.

ii. **Weber's syndrome**—involves fasciculus as it passes through the cerebral peduncle. Causes ipsilateral third nerve palsy and contralateral hemiparesis.

iii. **Nothnagel's syndrome**—involves fasciculus at the level of superior cerebellar peduncle. Causes ipsilateral IIIrd nerve palsy and cerebellar ataxia.

iv. **Claude's syndrome**—combination of Benedict and Nothnagel syndrome.

v. **Uncal herniation syndrome**—a supratentorial space occupying mass ivcauses downward displacement and herniation of the uncus across tentorial edge compressing the IIIrd nerve. A dilated and fixed pupil (Hutchinson's pupil) in a patient with altered consciousness may be the presenting feature.

vi. **Orbital syndrome**—while crossing the superior orbital fissure any division of the IIIrd nerve may be affected causing paresis of structures innervated by them.

vii. **Cavernous sinus syndrome**—occurs in association with IV, V, VI nerves and oculosympathetic paralysis. IIIrd nerve cavernous palsy is usually partial and pupil sparing.

41. What is primary oculomotor nerve synkinesis?

Acquired oculomotor synkinesis may occur as a primary phenomenon, without a preexisting acute IIIrd nerve palsy. Common causes are slowly growing tumors of:

i. Cavernous sinus-meningioma, aneurysms, trigeminal schwannomas

ii. Subarachnoid space.

42. What are the indications of neurological imaging in IIIrd nerve palsy?

i. All children <10 years irrespective of pupillary findings

ii. Children >10 years with pupil involvement

iii. If pupil becomes dilated after 5–7 days of onset

iv. Multiple cranial nerves affected

v. No improvement is seen within 3 months

vi. Signs of aberrant degeneration of the nerve develop

vii. Other neurological signs.

43. How can IIIrd nerve palsy be managed?

Medical management

i. Medical management is watchful waiting, since there is no direct medical treatment that alters the course of the disease. Nearly all patients undergo spontaneous remission of the palsy, usually within 6–8 weeks.

ii. Treatment during the symptomatic interval is directed at alleviating symptoms, mainly pain and diplopia.

iii. Nonsteroidal anti-inflammatory drugs (NSAIDs) are the first-line treatment of choice for the pain. Diplopia is not a problem when ptosis occludes the involved eye.

iv. When diplopia is from large-angle divergence of the visual axes, patching one eye is the only practical short-term solution.

   v. When the angle of deviation is smaller, fusion in primary position often can be achieved using horizontal or vertical prism or both.

  vi. Since the condition is expected to resolve spontaneously within a few weeks, most physicians would prescribe the Fresnel prism.

Surgical management

   i. For practical purposes, surgical care of third cranial nerve palsy includes clipping, gluing, coiling or wrapping of the berry aneurysm by a neurosurgeon in the acute stage.

  ii. Patients who do not recover from third cranial nerve palsy after 6–12 months may become candidates for eye muscle resection or recession to treat persistent and stable-angle diplopia.

 iii. Some of these patients also may require some form of lid-lift surgery for persistent ptosis that restricts vision or is cosmetically unacceptable to the patient.

  iv. Neurosurgery: Third cranial nerve palsy due to berry aneurysm, with or without concomitant subarachnoid hemorrhage, requires neurosurgical management in most cases.

   v. Ophthalmology: The ophthalmologist provides symptomatic treatment for diplopia using
     – Occlusion
     – Prism
     – Eye muscle surgery
     – Lid-lift procedures for ptosis
     – Botulinum toxin into the lateral rectus muscle.

  vi. In treatment for nonresolving 3rd nerve palsy due to DM—first correct the squint before correcting the ptosis (otherwise there would be diplopia).

44. What are the indications of follow-up in IIIrd nerve palsy?

   i. Truly isolated palsy—which may be still evolving. Review within 2 weeks

  ii. Age >40 years

 iii. H/O diabetes or hypertension.

45. For how long is surgical intervention deferred in IIIrd nerve palsy?

   i. Strabismus and lid surgeries can be considered after six months. Most ischemic palsies have complete recovery by 3 months (maximum 6 months).

  ii. In complete traumatic palsies, recovery is usually not complete and surgical correction of squint is quite difficult.

46. What are the differential diagnosis of IIIrd nerve palsy?

   i. Neuromuscular disease—myasthenia

  ii. Orbital diseases—myositis

 iii. Cavernous sinus lesions

 iv. Chronic meningitis

  v. Midbrain pathology.

47. What are the differentiating features between concomitant/non-paralytic and nonconcomitant/paralytic squint?

Features	Paralytic squint	Nonparalytic squint
1. Onset	Usually sudden	Usually slow
2. Diplopia	Usually present	Usually absent
3. Ocular movements	Limited in the direction of paralysed muscle	Full
4. False projection	It is positive: the patient cannot correctly locate the object in space when seeing in the direction of the paralyzed muscle, in early stages	Negative
5. Head posture	Particular head posture depending on the muscle paralyzed, may be present	Normal
6. Nausea and vertigo	Present	Absent
7. Secondary deviation	More than primary deviation	Equal to primary deviation
8. Pathological sequelae in muscles	Present	Absent

7.10. FOURTH NERVE PALSY

1. **What are the peculiarities of the fourth nerve?**

   Trochlear nerve palsy is the most common cause of acquired vertical strabismus in the general population.

   i. It is the only cranial nerve to have a dorsal emergence.
   ii. It has all the fibers crossed.
   iii. It is the most slender cranial nerve.
   iv. It has the longest intracranial course of all the cranial nerves (75 mm).

2. **Where is the nucleus of the fourth nerve located?**

   It is situated in the midbrain at the level of the inferior colliculus anterolateral to cerebral aqueduct and dorsal to medial longitudinal bundle.

3. **What are the symptoms of fourth nerve palsy?**

   These are due to superior oblique palsy, which leads to:

   i. **Diplopia:** It can be vertical, some degree of horizontal and torsional. The last one is more pronounced on down gaze, i.e. in the field of action of superior oblique muscle.
   This in turn leads to symptoms like **asthenopia,** difficulty in walking down the stairs and difficulty in reading.
   ii. **Image tilting:** The image is tilted in the direction of affected side. This symptom is rare in congenital palsy.
   iii. **Anomalous head posture:** To prevent diplopia, the face is turned and head is tilted toward uninvolved side and the chin is depressed. This position places the eyes in a position where cooperation of affected muscle is not required.

4. **How does one test involvement of the fourth nerve?**

   Bielschowsky's head tilt test: It is employed to diagnose paretic superior oblique as well as vertical rectus muscle in hypertropia.

   The three steps are:

   Step 1: Identify the type of hypertropia (RHT or LHT).

   Step 2: Identify whether vertical deviation increases on dextroversion or levoversion.

   Step 3: Determine whether vertical deviation increases on tilting the head toward the right or left. If the hypertropia is due to weakness of one of the 8 vertically acting muscles, the paretic muscle is identified by answering these questions. Each step cuts possible number of muscles in half. After the last step only one muscle remains.

In a superior oblique paralysis, there is ipsilateral hypertropia, which increases on contralateral gaze and ipsilateral head tilt.

5. **How does one test involvement of the fourth nerve in the presence of 3rd nerve palsy?**

   i. In presence of 3rd nerve palsy, fourth nerve function is tested by asking the patient to depress the abducted eye and watching for intorsion.

   ii. Isolated fourth nerve palsy can occur in ishemic conditions, e.g. diabetes mellitus and herpes zoster.

6. **How does one test the torsional component of the fourth nerve?**

   i. Double Maddox rod test:
      - Done to quantify the torsional component of diplopia
      - >10° of torsion is suggestive of bilateral fourth nerve palsy

   ii. Landcaster's red green test

   iii. Ophthalmoscopic examination

   iv. Hess's charting.

7. **What are the differential diagnosis of vertical diplopia?**

   i. *Skew deviation:*
      - It is a vertical misalignment of visual axis
      - It may be transient, constant or alternating, concomitant or incomitant
      - Due to imbalance of supranuclear inputs
      - Associated with brainstem and cerebellar signs and symptoms
      - Not associated with torsional diplopia or cyclodeviation

   ii. *Myasthenia gravis:*
      - Can involve isolated superior oblique and mimic fourth nerve palsy
      - Shows diurnal variation
      - Can involve other extraocular muscles
      - Tensilon test positive
      - EMG and ACh receptor antibodies positive

   iii. *Thyroid ophthalmopathy:*
      - Other signs of hyperthyroidism are present
      - T_3, T_4 levels suggestive
      - In superior oblique palsy the hypertropia is worse on **down gaze,** while in thyroid ophthalmopathy it is worse in **up gaze.**

8. **What are the causes of superior oblique paresis?**

   i. Fourth nerve palsy

   ii. Traumatic (may be bilateral)

   iii. Vascular mononeuropathy

   iv. Diabetic

   v. Decompensated congenital paresis
  vi. Posterior fossa tumor (rare)
 vii. Cavernous sinus/superior orbital fissure syndromes
viii. Neurosurgical procedures
  ix. Herpes zoster
   x. Myasthenia gravis
  xi. Graves' myopathy (fibrotic inferior oblique, superior rectus)
 xii. Orbital inflammatory pseudotumor
xiii. Orbital injury to trochlea.

9. **What are the syndromes associated with fourth nerve palsy?**

   i. **Nuclear-fascicular syndrome:** Distinguishing nuclear from fascicular lesions is virtually impossible due to short course of fascicles within the midbrain.

    Common etiologies are:
    – Hemorrhage
    – Infarction
    – Demyelination
    – Trauma.

  ii. **Subarachnoid space syndrome:**
    Causes:
    – Trauma
    – Basal meningitis
    – Neoplasms like pinealomas and tentorial meningiomas and aneurysms.
     When bilateral-site-anterior medullary velum.
     Associated signs and symptoms of the condition are present.

 iii. **Cavernous sinus syndrome:** Associated with other cranial nerve palsies like third, sixth, fifth and ocular sympathetic paralysis.

 iv. **Orbital syndrome:** It occurs due to trauma, inflammation and tumors.
    Seen in association with other cranial nerve palsies, e.g. 3rd, 5th, 6th.
    Associated orbital signs are proptosis, chemosis and conjunctival injection.

  v. **Isolated fourth nerve palsy**
    Congenital:
    Diagnostic keys: large vertical fusion amplitude (10–15 prism diopters)
    FAT (family album tomography) scan.
    Acquired:
    In ischemic conditions, e.g. diabetes mellitus and in herpes zoster.

10. **Describe the management of superior oblique paresis.**

    Medical management:

    i. Primary aim is to **prevent diplopia** while waiting for spontaneous improvement

    ii. Occlusion of one eye with a patch or opaque contact lens can be done

    iii. Fresnel's prism can be used for vertical displacement

    iv. Treatment of diabetes and hypertension is done appropriately

    v. Evaluations at frequent intervals during waiting period

    vi. Role of botulinum toxin is controversial.

    With this treatment superior oblique function may:

    i. *Recover completely,* e.g. in cases of ischemia, closed injury, after relief of compression from tumor or aneurysm.

    ii. *Recover incompletely* leaving the patient with mild but persistent vertical diplopia, torsional diplopia or both.

    iii. *No recovery,* e.g. mesencephalic injury or transection of trochlear nerve.

    Chances of further improvement after 6 months are rare.

    Surgical management:

    i. About 50% of patients require re-surgery in future

    ii. The available options are:
    – Weaken the antagonist, i.e. weakening of ipsilateral inferior oblique
    – Weaken the yoke muscle, i.e. weakening of the contralateral inferior rectus
    – Weakening of ipsilateral superior rectus
    – Strengthening of superior oblique
    – More than one muscle surgery.

11. **What is Knapp's classification?**

    The choice of surgery is decided by **Knapp's classification.** It depends on magnitude of hypertropia in the diagnostic positions of gaze. There are 7 classes. For every class a specific surgery is recommended.

    i. **Class 1:**
    – Hypertropia is greatest in adduction and elevation.
    – Ipsilateral inferior oblique overaction is present. Treatment is inferior oblique myomectomy.

    ii. **Class 2:**
    – Hypertropia is greatest in adduction and depression.
    – Treatment is superior oblique tuck (8–12 mm) with recession of contralateral inferior rectus as second procedure.

    iii. **Class 3:**
    – Hypertropia is of equal magnitude in entire paralyzed field of gaze.

   – Treatment is ipsilateral inferior oblique myotomy.
   – But if hypertropia is more than 25 prism diopters, it is combined with superior oblique tuck.

iv. **Class 4:**
   – Hypertropia is more in entire paralyzed field of gaze and in down gaze also.
   – Contracture of ipsilateral superior rectus or contralateral inferior rectus.
   – Forced duction test is done.
   – Treatment is as in class 3 plus recession of ipsilateral superior rectus or contralateral inferior rectus.

v. **Class 5:**
   – Hypertropia is more in all down gazes.
   – Treatment is superior oblique tuck, recession of ipsilateral superior rectus or contralateral inferior rectus.

vi. **Class 6:**
   – Bilateral fourth nerve palsy.
   – Treatment is as in classes 1–5, but bilateral surgery.

vii. **Class 7:**
   – Classic superior oblique paralysis associated with restriction of elevation in adduction (pseudo Brown's syndrome)
   – Cause is direct trochlear trauma.

7.11. ABDUCENS NERVE PALSY

1. **Location of the nucleus.**

   Its nucleus is located in the pons in the floor of the fourth ventricle, at the level of the facial colliculi.

2. **What are the causes of 6th nerve palsy?**

   Nonlocalizing:
   - i. Increased intracranial pressure
   - ii. Intracranial hypotension
   - iii. Head trauma
   - iv. Lumbar puncture or spinal anesthesia
   - v. Vascular, hypertension
   - vi. Diabetes/microvascular
   - vii. Parainfectious processes (postviral; middle ear infections in children)
   - viii. Basal meningitis

   Localizing:
   - i. Pontine syndromes (infarction, demyelination, tumor); contralateral hemiplegia; ipsilateral facial palsy, ipsilateral horizontal gaze palsy (± ipsilateral internuclear ophthalmoplegia); ipsilateral facial analgesia.
   - ii. Cerebellopontine angle lesions (acoustic neuroma, meningioma): in combination with disorders of the eighth, seventh and ophthalmic trigeminal nerves (especially corneal hypoesthesia), nystagmus, and cerebellar signs. –
   - iii. Clivus lesions (nasopharyngeal carcinoma, clivus chordoma).
   - iv. Middle fossa disorders (tumor, inflammation of medial aspect of petrous): facial pain/numbness, ± facial palsy.
   - v. Cavernous sinus or superior orbital fissure (tumor, inflammation, aneurysm): in combination with disorders of the third, fourth, and ophthalmic trigeminal nerves (pain/numbness).
   - vi. Carotid-cavernous or dural arteriovenous fistula.

   Common causes of sixth nerve palsy:
   - i. Collier's sphenoidal palsy
   - ii. Superior orbital fissure syndrome
   - iii. Arteriosclerosis
   - iv. Hypertension
   - v. Diabetes
   - vi. Trauma and raised ICT.

3. **What are the clinical features of 6th nerve palsy?**

Symptoms:

Horizontal diplopia—uniocular, painless and increases on looking toward lateral side.

An abnormality of the abducens nerve is the most likely cause of strictly horizontal double vision, especially if it is worse at a distance than near, and worse on lateral gaze.

Signs
   i. Limitation of abduction
  ii. Esotropia in primary position
 iii. Uncrossed diplopia
  iv. Slight face turn toward side of diplopia.

All other ocular movements are normal.

In early cases, secondary deviation is greater than primary deviation (nonconcomitant).

Later due to contractures developing in the ipsilateral antagonist they become equal (concomitant).

Still later with the development of contractures in contralateral synergist (with secondary underaction of antagonist of contralateral synergist) the primary deviation increases.

Uncrossed horizontal diplopia
   i. Increases towards paralyzed side
  ii. Horizontal displacement of image
 iii. Vertical displacement also occurs due to increased effectiveness of obliques in adduction
  iv. Field of binocular vision constricted towards the affected side.

4. **What are the features seen on Hess charting?**
   i. Enlargement toward the direction of action of ipsilateral antagonist MR and opposite MR (contralateral synergist)
  ii. Contraction away from the direction of action of LR muscle of opposite eye (antagonist of contralateral synergist)
 iii. False projection outward toward the paralyzed side.

5. **What are the conditions that mimic the sixth nerve palsy?**
   i. Thyroid ophthalmopathy
  ii. Myasthenia gravis
 iii. Medial wall orbital blowout fracture
  iv. Duane's syndrome (type 1)
   v. Mobius syndrome

    vi. Spasm of the near reflex

   vii. Essential infantile esotropia

  viii. Divergence paralysis.

    ix. Post scleral buckling/squint surgery.

6. What are the syndromes associated with abducens nerve palsy?

    i. *Brainstem syndrome:*

       – Brainstem lesion affecting 6th nerve also affects 5th, 7th, 8th nerves.

       – Structures in the lower pons affected by a lesion of 6th nerve:

         • Oculomotor sympathetic central neuron: Ipsilateral horner's syndrome

         • Para pontine reticular fiber (PPRF): Ipsilateral horizontal conjugate gaze palsy

         • Medial longitudinal fascicle (MLF): Ipsilateral internuclear ophthalmoplegia

         • Pyramidal tract: contralateral hemiparesis.

       – *Millard–Gubler syndrome:*

       Due to the lesion in the ventral paramedian pons.

       Clinical features:

         • Ipsilateral 7th nerve paresis

         • Ipsilateral 6th nerve paresis

         • Contralateral hemiparesis.

       – *Raymond's syndrome:*

         • Ipsilateral 6th nerve paresis

         • Contralateral hemiparesis.

       – *Foville's syndrome:*

       Due to the lesion in the pontine tegmentum.

         • Horizontal conjugate gaze palsy.

         • Ipsilateral Horner's syndrome.

         • Ipsilateral 5,6,7 cranial nerve palsies.

         • Ipsilateral paralysis of the abduction.

    ii. **The subarachnoid space syndrome:**

       – Vascular: compression of the nerve by atherosclerosis and aneurysm of the anterior inferior cerebellar artery or posterior inferior cerebellar artery or the basillar artery.

       – Posterior fossa causes: Space-occupying lesion (SOL) above the tentorium, posterior fossa tumors, structural anomalies, head trauma.

Mechanism: All these causes leads to increased intracranial pressure (ICP) which leads to the downward displacement of the brainstem. This may cause stretching of the 6th nerve, which is tethered at its exit from the pons and in Dorello's canal. This gives rise to the "nonlocalizing" 6th nerve palsies of raised ICP.

- Other causes: Meningitis—often bilateral palsy.

   Basal tumors: like meningioma, chordoma and Schwannoma.

   After lumbar puncture—with or without raised ICP.

iii. **Petrous apex syndromes:**

Contact with the petrous pyramid makes the portion of the 6th nerve within the Dorello's canal susceptible to pathologic processes affecting the petrous bone.

- **Gradenigo's syndrome:**

   At the Dorello's canal the 6th nerve lies adjacent to mastoid air cells. So severe mastoiditis leading to inflammation of tip of the petrous bone causes inflammation of the 6th nerve. Mechanism is by the inflammatory involvement of the inferior petrosal sinus or pseudotumor cerebri leading to raised ICP with 6th nerve paresis.

   In addition the Gasserian ganglion and facial nerve are also nearby to the petrous apex leads to involvement of the 5th and 7th cranial nerves.

   Features:

   • Ipsilateral 6th nerve palsy
   • Ipsilateral decreased hearing
   • Ipsilateral facial pain in the distribution of the 5th nerve
   • Ipsilateral facial paralysis.

- **Petrous bone fracture:**

   Basal skull fractures following head trauma may involve the 5th, 6th, 7th and 8th cranial nerves.

   Associated findings—hemotympanum, Battle's sign, CSF otorrhea.

- **Pseudo-Gadenigo's syndrome:**

   Lesions other than inflammation can involve petrous apex and produce symptoms suggestive of Gradenigo's syndrome.

   Causes:

   • Tumors/aneurysms of the intrapetrosal segment of the internal carotid artery (ICA).
   • Nasopharyngeal carcinoma.
   • Cerebellopontine angle tumor like acoustic neuroma.

Mechanism:

The nasopharyngeal carcinoma extends through foramina at the base of the skull, spreading beneath the dura to damage the extra-dural portions of the 5th and 6th nerves.

The cerebellopontine angle tumor can cause:

- 5th, 6th, 7th and 8th cranial nerves paralysis
- Ataxia
- Papilledema.

- **Lateral sinus thrombosis or phlebitis:**
  Leads to involvement of the inferior petrosal sinus causing 6th nerve palsy.

iv. **The cavernous sinus syndrome:**

The nerve runs within the body of the sinus, in close relation to the ICA. Some oculosympathetic fibers within the cavernous sinus which leave the ICA and join briefly with 6th nerve before joining the ophthalmic division of 5th nerve.

This is responsible for the isolated 6th nerve palsy with ipsilateral Horner's syndrome.

Causes of the 6th nerve palsy in cavernous sinus lesion:

- Vascular: ICA aneurysm, direct carotid—cavernous fistula, dural carotid-cavernous fistula.
- Neoplastic: meningioma, metastasis, pituitary adenoma, Burkitt's lymphoma.
- Inflammatory: Granulomatous: TB, sarcoid.
  Nongranulomatous: Sphenoid sinus abscess.

v. **The orbital syndrome:**

The nerve enters the orbit through the superior orbital fissure within the annulus of Zinn. The nerve supplies the lateral rectus muscle only a few mm from the superior orbital fissure. For this reason, isolated 6th nerve within the orbit is rare.

Causes:

- Intraorbital tumor
- Orbital trauma
- Inflammatory pseudotumor
- Orbital cellulitis

vi. **Isolated 6th nerve palsy:**

- ***Benign transient isolated 6th nerve palsy:*** Occurs rarely. In children, it is caused most often by viral illness and recent vaccination. In adults, it is caused most often by vascular lesion like HT, DM, IHD.

  – *Chronic isolated 6th nerve palsy:* Some patients don't recover spontaneously and have no obvious lesion despite an extensive evaluation.

7. **How will you manage 6th nerve palsy?**

   i. Usually will recover spontaneously within 3–4 months, but sometimes recovery may take up to 1 year, in case of traumatic etiology.
   ii. If it does not recover then some serious pathology like tumor, aneurysm, stroke are often present. If the nerve palsy has not shown much improvement over 3–4 months, or if other cranial nerve involvement appears then further evaluation is needed.
   iii. Correction of the strabismus—should not be considered until 8–10 months have passed without improvement unless it is known that 6th nerve is no longer intact.
   iv. During this period one can do occlusion of one eye either by patching or by using opaque contact lens. Children <8 years should undergo alternate patching of the eyes to prevent amblyopia.
   v. Prisms can be used for the correction of diplopia.
   vi. Chemodenervation of the antagonist medial rectus muscle with botulinum toxin can be used. Strabismus surgery whenever required usually consists of either weakening of the ipsilateral medial rectus combined with strengthening of the ipsilateral lateral rectus or some type of transposition procedure.

8. **Which muscle is spared in retrobulbar block?**

   Superior oblique as the trochlear nerve lies outside the muscle cone.

7.12. MYASTHENIA GRAVIS

1. **What is myasthenia gravis (MG)?**

   Myasthenia gravis is an acquired autoimmune disorder of neuromuscular transmission.

2. **What is the literal meaning of myasthenia gravis?**

   From Greek *Mys* = muscle and *asthenia* = weakness and Latin *gravis* = heavy or weighty.

3. **What is the pathophysiology of myasthenia gravis?**

   Myasthenia gravis is an autoimmune disease in which antibodies are directed against postsynaptic acetylcholine receptors. There is a slight genetic predisposition: particular HLA types seem to be predisposed for MG (B8 and DR3 more specific for ocular myasthenia).

4. **What is the recent thought on the pathophysiology of myasthenia gravis?**

   It has recently been realized that a second category of gravis is due to auto-antibodies against the MuSK protein (muscle specific kinase), a tyrosine kinase receptor which is required for the formation of the neuromuscular junction. Antibodies against MuSK inhibit the signaling of MuSK normally induced by its nerve-derived ligand, agrin. The result is a decrease in patency of the neuromuscular junction, and the consequent symptoms of myasthenia.

5. **What is the source of antibody in myasthenia?**

   The antibodies are produced by plasma cells that have been derived from B cells. These plasma cells are activated by T helper cells. The thymus plays an important role in the development of T cells, which is why myasthenia gravis may be associated with thymoma.

6. **What is the role of the thymus gland in myasthenia gravis?**

   T helper cells which have been activated in the thymus probably stimulate the production of the acetylcholine receptor autoantibodies. Up to 65–70% myasthenics have thymic hyperplasia with 5–20% incidence of thymoma.

7. **Does the level of acetylcholine receptor antibody titer correlate with the severity of the disease?**

   No. The level of the acetylcholine receptor antibody titer does not correlate well with the severity of the disorder.

8. **What are the symptoms of myasthenia gravis?**

   Ocular symptoms:

   i. Drooping of upper lid
   ii. Diplopia.

Systemic symptoms:
  i. Weakness and fatigability of skeletal muscles
  ii. Mild generalized disease: facial and bulbar muscles affected
  iii. Severe generalized disease: impairment of respiration.

9. **Classify myasthenia gravis.**

   The most widely followed classification of myasthenia gravis is that of Osserman which is as follows:
   i. Ocular myasthenia
   ii. Generalized myasthenia:
       – Mild generalized myasthenia: Slow progression, no crisis, responds well to drugs.
       – Moderately severe generalized myasthenia. Severe skeletal or bulbar involvement but no crisis, response to drugs is less than satisfactory.
   iii. Acute fulminant myasthenia: Rapid progression of clinical symptoms with respiratory crisis, poor response to drugs, high incidence of thymoma and high mortality.
   iv. Late severe myasthenia: Symptoms same as in acute fulminating type. The difference is that the progression from class 1 to class 2 has occurred slowly, i.e. over two years.

10. **What are the commonly involved muscles in myasthenia?**

    Muscles that control eye and eyelid movement, facial expression, chewing, talking and swallowing are especially susceptible. The muscles that control breathing and neck and limb movements can also be affected. Often the physical examination is within normal limits.

11. **What is the reason for predilection for eye muscle?**

    There are several lines of thought:
    i. Slight weakness in a limb may be tolerated, but slight weakness in the extraocular muscles would lead to misalignment of the two eyes, even a small degree of which could lead to diplopia. Eyes may also be less able to adapt to variable weakness, because extraocular muscles use visual rather than proprioceptive (body position sensing) cues for fine-tuning.
    ii. Compared to extremity muscles, extraocular muscles are smaller, served by more nerve fibers, and are among the fastest contracting muscles in the body. This higher level of activity may predispose them to fatigue in MG.

12. **Which extraocular muscle is most commonly involved?**

    Medial recti are most commonly affected.
    Myasthenic ophthalmoparesis can mimic any pupil sparing ocular motility disorder.

13. Why is the pupil and ciliary muscle unaffected?

Myasthenia involves skeletal and not visceral musculature and therefore the pupil and ciliary muscle are unaffected.

14. How do you examine a case of suspected ocular myasthenia?

Muscle fatigability can be tested for many muscles. A thorough investigation includes:

i. Looking upward and sidewards for 30 seconds: ptosis and diplopia.
ii. "Peek sign": After complete initial apposition of the lid margins, they quickly (within 30 seconds) start to separate and the sclera starts to show.

15. What is ice pack test?

i. Cooling may improve neuromuscular transmission. In a patient with myasthenia gravis who has ptosis, placing ice (wrapped over a towel) over an eyelid will lead to cooling of the lid, which leads to improvement of the ptosis
ii. A positive test is clear resolution of the ptosis, with at least more than 2 mm of improvement
iii. The test is thought to be positive in about 80% of patients with ocular myasthenia.

16. What is lid fatigue test?

In this test, the patient is asked to keep looking up for several minutes and then observed for the appearance of worsening of ptosis.

17. What is sleep test?

Resolution of ptosis or ophthalmoparesis after 30-minute period of sleep, with reappearance of the sign 30 seconds to 5 minutes after awakening.

18. What is enhanced ptosis?

With bilateral ptosis, enhanced ptosis may be seen, where one upper eyelid becomes more ptotic when the other upper eyelid is manually elevated. This phenomenon is explained by Hering's law of equal innervation to yoke muscles.

19. What is Cogan's eye lid twitch?

When the patient looks down for at least 10–20 seconds and then makes an upward saccade back to primary gaze, a transient overshoot of the upper eyelid may be seen. This may be followed by nystagmoid twitches of the upper eyelid and then downward drifting of the eyelid to a normal or ptotic position. This is caused by rapid recovery on resting in down gaze and easy fatigability in up gaze of the myasthenic levator muscle.

20. What are the blood tests done to diagnose myasthenia gravis?

If the diagnosis is suspected, serology can be performed in a blood test to identify antibodies against the acetylcholine receptor.

21. What is repetitive nerve stimulation test?

i. Muscle fibers of patients with myasthenia gravis are easily fatigued. By repeatedly stimulating a muscle with electrical impulses, the fatigability of the muscle can be measured. This is called the repetitive nerve stimulation test.

ii. In single fiber electromyography, which is considered to be the most sensitive (although not the most specific) test for myasthenia, a thin needle electrode is inserted into a muscle to record the electric potentials of individual muscle fibers. By finding two muscle fibers belonging to the same motor unit and measuring the temporal variability in their firing patterns (i.e. their 'jitter'), the diagnosis can be made.

22. What is edrophonium test?

Edrophonium inhibits enzyme acetylcholinesterase (which destroys acetylcholine in the neuromuscular junction) thereby increasing the available acetylcholine.

Before test, ptosis, ocular motility eye alignment should be assessed.

Initially atropine sulfate (0.6 mg) is given.

Dose of edrophonium: 0.5–1.0 mg/kg.

In adults—1–2 mg test dose given watch for positive response. If there is no improvement remaining 8–9 mg given in increments of 0.1–0.2 cc waiting for 45–60 seconds between increments.

Onset of action: 30–60 seconds after IV injection.

Effect resolves within 5 minutes.

23. What is neostigmine test?

Neostigmine is a longer acting antiacetylcholinesterase that can also be used similarly.

Dose: 0.03 mg/kg or 1.0–1.5 mg intramuscularly, preceded by atropine 1 cc (0.6 mg) intramuscular (IM).

24. What is the role of atropine in edrophonium test?

It serves two purposes in the test—

i. First, it counters the muscarinic side effects of edrophonium, especially cardiac arrhythmias.

ii. Second, placebo responders may improve with this alone.

25. **What are the conditions which can give false positive responses in edrophonium test?**
    i. Intracranial mass lesions
    ii. Orbital apex syndrome from metastasis
    iii. Multiple sclerosis
    iv. Amyotrophic lateral sclerosis
    v. Lambert–Eaton syndrome
    vi. Guillain–Barre syndrome.

26. **What are the imaging tests done in myasthenia gravis?**
    i. Chest X-ray is frequently performed to diagnose:
       – Lambert–Eaton syndrome
       – Widening of the mediastinum suggestive of thymoma
    ii. Computed tomography (CT) or magnetic resonance imaging (MRI) are more sensitive ways to identify thymomas, and are generally done for this reason.

27. **How does the pulmonary function test help in monitoring of myasthenia gravis progression?**
    Spirometry (lung function testing) is done to assess respiratory function (FEV1) or the peak expiratory flow rate (PEFR) may be monitored at intervals in order not to miss a gradual worsening of muscular weakness.

28. **What is transient neonatal myasthenia?**
    In the long-term pregnancy does not affect myasthenia gravis. Up to 10% of infants with parents affected by the condition are born with transient (periodic) neonatal myasthenia (TNM) which generally produces feeding and respiratory difficulties. A child with TNM typically responds very well to acetylcholinesterase inhibitors. Immunosuppressive therapy should be maintained throughout pregnancy as this reduces the chance of neonatal muscle weakness, as well as controlling the mother's myasthenia.

29. **What are the myasthenic symptoms in children?**
    Three types of myasthenic symptoms in children can be distinguished:
    i. *Neonatal:* In 12% of the pregnancies with a mother with MG, she passes the antibodies to the infant through the placenta causing neonatal myasthenia gravis. The symptoms will start in the first two days and disappear within a few weeks after birth. With the mother it is not uncommon for the symptoms to even improve during pregnancy, but they might worsen after labor.
    ii. *Congenital:* Children of a healthy mother can, very rarely, develop myasthenic symptoms beginning at birth. This is called congenital myasthenic syndrome or CMS. CMS is not caused by an autoimmune

process, but due to synaptic malformation, which in turn is caused by genetic mutations. Thus, CMS is a hereditary disease. More than 11 different mutations have been identified and the inheritance pattern is typically autosomal recessive.

iii. *Juvenile:* Myasthenia occurring in childhood but after the peripartum period.

The congenital myasthenias cause muscle weakness and fatigability similar to those of MG. The symptoms of CMS usually begin within the first two years of life, although in a few forms, patients can develop their first symptoms as late as the seventh decade of life. A diagnosis of CMS is suggested by the following:

– Onset of symptoms in infancy or childhood
– Weakness which increases as muscles tire
– A decremental EMG response, on low frequency, of the compound muscle action potential (CMAP)
– No anti-AChR or MuSK antibodies
– No response to immunosuppressant therapy
– Family history of symptoms which resemble CMS.

30. **What are the various autoimmune diseases associated with myasthenia gravis?**

Myasthenia gravis is associated with various autoimmune diseases, including:

i. Thyroid diseases, including Hashimoto's thyroiditis and Graves' disease
ii. Diabetes mellitus type 1
iii. Rheumatoid arthritis
iv. Lupus and demyelinating CNS diseases.

Seropositive and "double-seronegative" patients often have thymoma or thymic hyperplasia. However, anti-MuSK positive patients do not have evidence of thymus pathology.

31. **What is the management of myathenia gravis?**

Symptomatic therapy

Acetylcholinesterase inhibitors: neostigmine and pyridostigmine can improve muscle function by slowing the natural enzyme cholinesterase that degrades acetylcholine in the motor end plate; the neurotransmitter is therefore around longer to stimulate its receptor. Usually one can start with a low dose, e.g. 3×20 mg pyridostigmine, and increase until the desired result is achieved. If taken 30 minutes before a meal, symptoms will be mild during eating. Side effects, like perspiration and diarrhea can be countered by adding atropine. Pyridostigmine is a short-lived drug with a half-life of about 4 hours.

Disease modifying therapy
i. *Medical*
   - Immunosuppressive drugs: Prednisone, cyclosporine, mycophenolate mofetil and azathioprine may be used.
   - Treatments with some immunosuppressives take weeks to months before effects are noticed.
ii. *Surgical*
   Thymectomy, the surgical removal of the thymus, is essential in cases of thymoma in view of the potential neoplastic effects of the tumor. It is usually indicated in all patients with myasthenia.

32. **What is the role of steroids in the treatment of myasthenia gravis?**
   Steroids are useful in inducing remission. However, because of the possible side effects, the treatment with steroids is reserved for severe cases.

33. **What are the drugs exacerbating the symptoms of myasthenia?**
   The adverse effects of many medications may provoke exacerbations; therefore, carefully obtaining a medication history is important. Some of the medications reported to cause exacerbations of myasthenia include the following:
   i. *Antibiotics*—macrolides, fluoroquinolones, aminoglycosides, tetracycline and chloroquine
   ii. *Antidysrrhythmic agents*—β-blockers, calcium channel blockers, quinidine, lidocaine, procainamide and trimethaphan
   iii. *Miscellaneous*—diphenylhydantoin, lithium, chlorpromazine, muscle relaxants, levothyroxine, adrenocorticotropic hormone (ACTH) and paradoxically, corticosteroids.

34. **What is cholinergic crisis?**
   i. One of the confusing factors in treating patients with MG is that insufficient medication (i.e. myasthenic crisis) and excessive medication (i.e. cholinergic crisis) can present in similar ways.
   ii. Cholinergic crisis results from an excess of cholinesterase inhibitors (i.e. neostigmine, pyridostigmine, physostigmine) and resembles organophosphate poisoning. In this case, excessive ACh stimulation of striated muscle at nicotinic junctions produces flaccid muscle paralysis that is clinically indistinguishable from weakness due to myasthenia.
   iii. Myasthenic crisis or cholinergic crisis may cause bronchospasm with wheezing, bronchorrhea, respiratory failure, diaphoresis and cyanosis.
   iv. Miosis and the SLUDGE syndrome (i.e. salivation, lacrimation, urinary incontinence, diarrhea, GI upset and hypermotility, emesis)

also may mark cholinergic crisis. However, these findings are not inevitably present.

v. Despite muscle weakness, deep tendon reflexes are preserved.

35. How is myasthenic crisis treated?

A myasthenic crisis occurs when the muscles that control breathing weaken to the point that ventilation is inadequate, creating a medical emergency and requiring a respirator for assisted ventilation. In patients whose respiratory muscles are weak, crises—which generally call for immediate medical attention—may be triggered by infection, fever, an adverse reaction to medication or emotional stress.

If the myasthenia is serious (myasthenic crisis), plasmapheresis can be used to remove the putative antibody from the circulation. Also, intravenous immunoglobulins (IVIG) can be used to bind the circulating antibodies. Both of these treatments have relatively short-lived benefits, typically measured in weeks.

36. What are the complications in a patient with myasthenia?

i. Respiratory crisis
ii. Pulmonary aspiration
iii. Permanent muscle weakness
iv. Side effects related to medication used and surgery related complications.

37. What are the other ancillary treatment modalities for reducing ocular disabilities in other myasthenia?

Ptosis—can be corrected with placement of crutches on eyeglasses ptosis tape to elevate eyelid droop.

Diplopia—can be addressed by occlusion with eye patching, frosted lens, occluding contact lens or by simply placing opaque tape over a portion of eyeglasses, plastic prisms (Fresnel prisms).

38. What are the differences between myasthenia gravis and myopathy?

Features	Myasthenia gravis	Myopathy
Ptosis	Asymmetrical	Symmetrical
Diplopia	Present	May or may not be present
Diurnal variation	Present	Absent
Fatigability	Present	Absent
Response to the stigmine	Positive	Negative
Clinical course	Variable characteristics	Slowly progressive
Other eye signs	Absent	Retinal pigment disturbance may be present
Age	Any age	Any age—under 20 suspect heart block

39. **Differential diagnosis of myasthenia gravis.**

Prominent ocular signs

  i. Mitochondrial myopathy: Progressive external ophthalmoplegia

  ii. Oculopharyngeal muscular dystrophy

  iii. Intracranial mass lesion

  iv. Senile ptosis

Bulbar dysfunction

  i. Motor neuron syndromes

  ii. Polymyositis

  iii. Thyroid disorders

  iv. Oculopharyngeal dystrophy

Generalized myasthenia gravis

  i. Lambert–Eaton syndrome (LES)

  ii. Botulism

  iii. Congenital myasthenic syndromes

  iv. Myopathies or muscular dystrophies.

7.13. NYSTAGMUS

1. **Define nystagmus.**

    It is defined as a regular, rhythmic, involuntary, repetitive, to-and-fro movement of the eye.

2. **Classification of nystagmus.**

    Based on physiology and pathology

    Physiological
    i. End gaze
    ii. Optokinetic
    iii. Vestibulo-ocular reflexes (VOR)

    Pathological
    i. Sensory deprivation (ocular)
    ii. Motor imbalance nystagmus
       – Congenital nystagmus
       – Spasmus nutans
       – Latent nystagmus
       – Ataxic nystagmus
       – Downbeat nystagmus
       – Upbeat nystagmus
       – Convergent refraction nystagmus
       – See-saw nystagmus of Maddox
       – Periodic alternating nystagmus

    Based on the type of nystagmus
    i. Pendular
    ii. Jerk

    Based on direction of movement
    i. Horizontal
    ii. Vertical
    iii. Rotatory

    Congenital/infantile
    i. Acquired
    ii. Toxic/drug/metabolic
    iii. Neurological
    iv. Functional/voluntary.

3. **What are the types of nystagmus?**

    There are different types depending upon:
    i. **Rate:** The number of to-and-fro movements in one second. It is described in hertz (Hz).
       – Slow (1–2 Hz)

- Medium (3–4 Hz)
- Fast (5 Hz or more)

ii. *Amplitude*
- Fine (<5)
- Moderate (5°–15°)
- Large (>15°)

iii. *Direction*
- Horizontal
- Vertical
- Rotational

iv. *Movement*
- Pendular
- Jerk.

4. **What is the anatomic basis of nystagmus?**

The goal of the eye movement control system is to maintain images of objects steady on the retina to preserve visual acuity. The slow eye movement systems that provide this stability of images are:

i. Visual fixation
ii. Vestibular system
iii. Optokinetic system
iv. Neural integrator
v. Smooth pursuit system
vi. Vergence eye movement system.

5. **What are the main points in history-taking in nystagmus?**

Following points should be asked in history

i. Present from birth or not
ii. Oscillopsia
iii. Vertigo
iv. Visual loss
v. Diplopia.

6. **What are the other movement disorders which can mimic a nystagmus?**

i. *Nystagmoid movements* are those which are not regular and rhythmic in nature.

ii. *Ocular bobbing:* Fast downward movement of both eyes followed by a slow drift back towards mid position. It is usually seen in patients with severe brainstem dysfunction.

iii. *Ocular dipping:* Slow downward movement of eyeball followed by delayed rapid upward movement and spontaneous roving horizontal eye movements.

  iv. ***Ping pong gaze:*** Slow roving horizontal conjugate movement from one extreme to the other occurring regularly or irregularly every few seconds. It is seen in acute diffused bilateral cerebral disease with intact brainstem.

  v. ***Ocular dysmetria:*** Seen in cerebral disease.

  vi. ***Ocular flutter:*** Brief, horizontal, bilateral ocular oscillation occurring intermittently when the patient looks straight or changes his gaze. Seen in certain cerebellar diseases.

  vii. ***Opsoclonus:*** Consists of large amplitude, involuntary, repetitive unpredictable conjugate chaotic saccades in horizontal, vertical and torsional planes. Causes include organophosphorus poisoning, Epstein-Barr virus infection and hypertension.

  viii. ***Superior oblique/myokymia:*** It consists of intermittent monocular torsional movement of one eyeball. Associated with torsional diplopia. It responds to carbamazepine. Causes midbrain tectal tumors.

7. What are the two components of jerk nystagmus and how is the direction defined?

The two components are slow component in one direction and a fast one in the opposite direction. The direction is defined by direction of the fast component as viewed by the patient.

8. What is Alexander's law?

It states that the amplitude of jerk nystagmus is largest in the gaze of the direction of its fast component.

9. What is null point?

It is the position of gaze in which the nystagmus is lessened or totally absent.

10. What are the causes of monocular nystagmus?

  i. Strabismus

  ii. Amblyopia

  iii. Internuclear ophthalmoplegia.

11. What are the features of congenital nystagmus (manifest)?

  i. Most common type (80%)

  ii. Presence from birth

  iii. Binocular

  iv. Horizontal and pendular

  v. Remains horizontal even in vertical gaze

  vi. Disappears at one position—null point

  vii. Decreases on convergence, eye closure

    viii. Absent during sleep
    ix. No oscillopsia, normal vision
    x. Particular head posture
    xi. Associated head oscillations may be there
    xii. Inversion of optokinetic nystagmus.

12. What are the features of pendular nystagmus?
    i. May have horizontal, vertical, torsional component
    ii. May be congenital or acquired
    iii. Associated with visual problems
    iv. Most common cause being demyelination of the neural circuit known as the myoclonic triangle (the dentato-rubro-olivary pathways—associated with visual loss oscillopsia, palatal myoclonus).

13. What are the features of gaze evoked nystagmus?
    i. Fast phase is towards the direction of gaze (up on looking up, down on looking down)
    ii. Amplitude may be greater towards the side of lesion
    iii. Drug-induced nystagmus tends to be minimal in down gaze.

14. What are the features of vestibular nystagmus?
    i. Seen in primary position
    ii. Purely horizontal or horizontal rotatory
    iii. Fast component opposite to the side of lesion
    iv. Suppressed by visual fixation, increased when fixation is removed
    v. Intensity increases in the direction of fast phase (**Alexander's law**)
    vi. Associated vertigo, tinnitus.

15. What are the features of downbeat nystagmus?
    i. Primary position nystagmus
    ii. Fast component downwards
    iii. Oscillopsia often present and may precede
    iv. Best elicited by looking down and out
    v. Craniocervical junction lesions, e.g. Arnold–Chiari malformations and certain drugs.

16. What are the features of upbeat nystagmus?
    i. Fast phase beats upward.
    ii. Lesion in the posterior fossa—either brainstem or cerebellar vermis or some drugs.

17. What are the features of seesaw nystagmus (of Maddox)?
    i. Primary position nystagmus worsens on down gaze.
    ii. One eye elevates as well as intorts while the other eye descends and extorts.
    iii. Site of lesion is parasellar, parachiasmal.

18. **What are the features of Bruns nystagmus?**

    i. A combination of large amplitude, low frequency horizontal nystagmus on looking to the ipsilateral side (due to cerebellar component) and small amplitude, high frequency nystagmus on looking contralaterally and in primary position (due to vestibular component)

    ii. Often seen in tumors of cerebellopontine angle.

19. **What are the features of optokinetic nystagmus?**

It is a normal nystagmus which results when a person gazes at a succession of objects moving past in one direction. For example, gazing from a fast moving train. The nystagmus is always in the direction opposite to the direction of movement of the object.

20. **What is the significance of eliciting optokinetic nystagmus?**

    i. To test presence of some vision (in malingering and children)

    ii. To test integrity of the horizontal and vertical gaze centers for saccadic and pursuit movements

    iii. To differentiate homonymous hemianopia of occipital cortical lesion from that of a lesion of optic radiation and adjacent opticomotor pathway (parietal lobe lesion). (In parietal lobe lesions, it will be lost due to disruption of the smooth pursuit pathways.).

21. **How will you detect the side of the parietal lobe lesion by demonstrating optokinetic nystagmus?**

Nystagmus will be absent or defective when the targets are moved toward the side of the lesion, i.e. away from hemianopia. This is called positive optokinetic nystagmus sign (OKN) and suggests a parietal lobe lesion, usually a neoplasm.

22. **What is latent nystagmus?**

It is a type of congenital jerk nystagmus that occurs during fixation when one eye is covered. This is frequently associated with strabismus.

23. **What is spasmus mutants?**

    i. It is a triad of nystagmus, head nodding and torticollis.

    ii. Onset is between 4 months and 1 year and lasts for 1–4 years.

    iii. Indicates serious neurological problem.

    iv. Has vertical and torsional components.

24. **How do you clinically differentiate congenital nystagmus from others?**

A good rule is that horizontal nystagmus which remains horizontal even on vertical gaze is always congenital nystagmus until proved otherwise.

25. **How do you induce caloric nystagmus?**

Cold or warm water is irrigated into the external auditory canal. With cold water, the fast phase will be in opposite direction while with warm water, the fast phase will be in the same direction. "**COWS**" (Cold Opposite Warm Same).

26. What should be the position of the patient to show caloric induced nystagmus?

Patient should be supine with the head bent forward by 30° so that the horizontal semicircular canals are almost horizontal in position.

27. What is the significance of demonstrating caloric nystagmus?

i. To test the integrity of vestibular-ocular system
ii. To induce eye movement in patients who are incapable of moving them in response to command—either because of their state of consciousness or because of their orientation.

28. What are the degrees of nystagmus?

i. 1st degree: Nystagmus only in the direction of fast component.
ii. 2nd degree: Nystagmus also in primary position gaze.
iii. 3rd degree: Nystagmus in addition to the above two gazes is also present in the direction of slow component.

29. What is the role of perinatal history in nystagmus?

History of intrauterine infection (rubella, *Toxoplasma*), maternal alcohol abuse or anticonvulsion drugs (optic nerve hypoplasia), neonatal asphyxia or neonatal seizures (cerebral damage) are very helpful in case of nystagmus.

30. What is the role of family history in nystagmus?

i. Most common X-linked
ii. Autosomal dominant is also likely but autosomal recessive is rare.

31. What are the treatment modalities in nystagmus?

i. **Optical aids**
   – Prisms—to shift gaze into the null point.
   – Soft contact lens—helps probably by stimulating trigeminal afferent—especially in congenital nystagmus.

ii. **Biofeedback**
   – Training mechanism to decrease nystagmus—visual and auditory

iii. **Medical modalities**
   Baclofen in acquired periodic alternating nystagmus
   Clonazepam, anticholinergic in downbeat nystagmus
   Menantine and gabapentene help in acquired pendular nystagmus

   Botulinum toxin
   Injected into the retrobulbar space or into the extraocular muscles in the better eye especially in pendular nystagmus. There may be

transient improvement in the visual acuity and oscillopsia. However, the side effects override the small and transient improvements.

iv. **Surgery**

This helps correct the head posture by shifting the null point from an eccentric location to a straight ahead position in visually disabling nystagmus.

- Kestenbaum–Anderson procedure

  By recession of horizontal muscles, the versions are blocked

- Faden operation

  Acts like a recession by creation of a more posterior attachment, first reducing the area of contact.

7.14. VISUAL FIELDS IN NEURO-OPHTHALMOLOGY

1.   What is the purpose of perimetry in neuro-ophthalmology?

  i.   To detect generalized or focal defects in the island of vision that may identify the location of pathology affecting the visual pathways.

  ii. To aid in differential diagnosis since different pathologies may produce different kinds of field defects.

  iii. To quantitate severity of defects in order to detect any progression, recovery or response to therapy.

  iv. To reveal hidden visual loss in patients who may be totally unaware of such defects.

2.   What are the types of visual field testing?

  i.   Confrontation

  ii. Amsler grid

  iii. Tangent screen

  iv. Goldmann perimetry

  v.   Static perimetry—octopus/humphrey visual analyzer

  vi. Newer tests—swap, high pass resolution, flicker, motion and displacement.

3.   What are the chiasmal anatomical variations?

  i.   Prefixed (10%) chiasm lies on the tuberculum sellae and pituitary tumor can compress posterior chiasm or optic tract.

  ii. Normally fixed (80%) chiasm lies on the diaphragm and projects backwards on to the dorsum sellae and pituitary tumor can compress the anterior chiasm.

  iii. Post fixed (10%) chiasm lies on the dorsum sellae , posterior to fossa and pituitary tumor compress the optic nerves.

4.   What are the field defects in lesions of the optic chiasma?

  i.   Bitemporal (heteronymous) hemianopia

  ii. Traquair's junctional scotoma

  iii. Incongruous contralateral homonymous hemianopia (very rare)

  iv. Posterior involvement affects crossing macular fibers—bitemporal hemiscotomas.

Compression of chiasma:

  i.   From below, e.g. pituitary adenoma—defects start superiorly and progress inferiorly in the temporal hemifields.

  ii. From above, e.g. craniopharyngioma, suprasellar meningioma—defects start inferiorly and progress superiorly in the temporal hemifields.

iii. Binasal hemianopia: rare. A rare neuro-ophthalmic cause is aneurysm of internal carotid artery producing compression of temporal fibers ipsilaterally and also contralaterally by displacing chiasma against opposite internal carotid artery.

5. **What is junctional scotoma?**

Inferonasal retinal fibers cross into the chiasm and cross anteriorly approximately 4 mm in the contralateral optic nerve (Wilbrand's knee) before turning back to join uncrossed inferotemporal temporal fibers in the optic tract.

Lesion in this region causes ipsilateral central scotoma and contralateral superotemporal defect. This is called junctional scotoma.

6. **What are the field defects in optic tract lesions?**

- Homonymous contralateral, incongruous hemianopia.

7. **What are the pupillary abnormalities in optic tract lesion?**

   i RAPD: On the opposite side of the lesion (eye with temporal field loss)
   ii. Behr's pupil: Anisocoria with larger pupil on the side of hemianopia
   iii. Wernicke's pupil: Light stimulation of a "blind" retina causes no pupillary reaction, while light projected on an "intact" retina produces normal pupillary constriction.

8. **What are the field defects in lesions of the lateral geniculate body?**

Such defects are generally rare.

   i. Incongruous homonymous hemianopia
   ii. Quadruple sectoranopia
      a. Homonymous hemianopia with sparing of a horizontal sector
      b. Occurs with infarction of anterior choroidal artery.
   iii. Relatively congruous, homonymous, horizontal sectoranopia
   iv. Only a horizontal sector involved
   v. Occurs with infarction of lateral choroidal artery.

9. **What are the characteristics of internal capsule lesion?**

Internal capsule lesion results in contralateral homonymous hemianopia with contralateral hemianaesthesia due to damage of thalamocortical fibers.

10. **What are the field defects in temporal lobe lesions?**

- Mid peripheral/peripheral contralateral homonymous superior quadrantanopia (pie in the sky).

11. What are the nonvisual manifestations of temporal lobe lesions?

   i. Seizures
   ii. Formed hallucinations.
   iii. If it affects uncinate gurus it is called uncinate fits characterized by an aura of unusual taste or smell.

12. What are the field defects in parietal lobe lesions?

   i. Contralateral inferior homonymous quadrantanopia (pie on the floor)
   ii. Homonymous hemianopia, denser inferiorly.

13. What are the nonvisual manifestations of parietal lobe lesions?

   i. Word blindness and visual agnosias
   ii. Numbness on contralateral side
   iii. Loss of tactile stimulation
   iv. Gerstmann syndrome (when dominant parietal lobe is affected) a combination of acalculia, agraphia, finger agnosia, and left-right confusion.

14. What is extinction phenomenon?

Seen in parietal lobe lesions. Patients with this phenomenon may not have a true visual field defect but may not perceive objects on one half of visual field when both sides are simultaneously stimulated.

15. What are the field defects in occipital lobe lesions?

   i. Exquisitely congruous contralateral, homonymous hemianopia
   ii. Macular 'sparing'
   iii. Macular 'splitting'
   iv. Central, macular homonymous hemianopia
   v. Temporal crescent sparing.

16. What are the reasons for macular sparing?

   i. Dual blood supply, from the terminal branches of middle cerebral artery and from the posterior cerebral artery.
   ii. Bilateral representation of macula.
   iii. Functional overlap of two sides of visual field.

17. What is cortical blindness?

It is seen in bilateral occipital lobe infarcts. Pupillary reflex are normal. Anton syndrome is denial of blindness and is classically associated with cortical blindness.

Homonymous Hemianopia

1. **What are the characteristics of optic tract hemianopia?**
   i. Reduction in ipsilateral visual acuity, defects with both bitemporal and hemianopic character
   ii. Incongruity
   iii. Associated bow-tie optic atrophy (from selective involvement of decussated axons)
   iv. A contralateral relative afferent pupillary defect.

2. **What are the causes of homonymous hemianopia?**
   Optic tract lesions—visual conduction system posterior to optic chiasma and anterior to lateral geniculate body.
   i. Saccular aneurysms of internal carotid artery.
   ii. Pituitary tumors—pituitary adenomas—chromophobe (the most common), basophil, acidophil, mixed, adenocarcinoma,
   iii. Metastases
   iv. Demyelinating diseases
   v. Trauma
   vi. Migraine.

   Temporoparietal lesions—temporal lobe lesions—pie in the sky and later pie on the floor if parietal lobe is involved.
   i. Vascular accidents thromboembolism, vasospasm, subdural hematoma, fracture skull
   ii. Tumors—meningioma, glioma, retinoblastoma, pinealoma, ependymoma, metastases
   iii. Demyelinating diseases—Schilder's disease, Krabbe's leukodystrophy, PMLE, migraine.

   Occipital lesions
   i. Vascular accidents thromboembolism, vasospasm, subdural hematoma, fracture skull, subclavian steal phenomenon
   ii. Vertebrobasilar insufficiency
   iii. Tumors—meningioma, glioma, retinoblastoma, pinealoma, ependymoma, metastases
   iv. Demyelinating diseases—Schilder's disease, Krabbe's leukodystrophy, PMLE, migraine
   v. Trauma
   vi. Poisons—digitalis, LSD, mescaline, opium, carbon monoxide
   vii. Migraine.

Bitemporal Hemianopia

1. **What are the causes of bitemporal heminopia?**

Chiasmal lesions
   i. Aneurysm of internal carotid artery, intrasellar, syphilitic, septic
   ii. Vascular—arteriosclerosis, arterial compression.
   iii. Chiasmal basal arachnoiditis, chiasmal neuritis—tuberculosis, syphilis, cysticercosis
   iv. Tumors—meningioma, glioma, retinoblastoma, pinealoma, ependymoma.

Pituitary lesions
   i. Hyper/hypo pituitarism
   ii. Pituitary tumors
   iii. Pituitary adenomas—chromophobe (the most common), basophil, acidophil, mixed, adenocarcinoma
   iv. Third ventricle enlargement
   v. Metastases.

Perisellar lesions
   i. Suprasellar tumors—craniopharyngioma, meningioma, frontal lobe tumors, ependymoma
   ii. Chordoma
   iii. Presellar tumors—meningioma of olfactory groove, neuroblastoma
   iv. Parasellar tumors—sphenoid bone meningioma, metastases, disseminated sclerosis.

Injury
Most common causes include:
   i. In children—craniopharyngioma and chiasmal glioma
   ii. In 20–40 years age—pituitary tumors
   iii. Above 40 years—meningioma, basal arachnoiditis, aneurysms.

2. **What are the clinical features of bitemporal hemianopia?**

   i. Monocular/binocular visual field defects that respect vertical meridian.
   ii. Asymmetry of field loss is the rule, such that one eye may show advanced deficits, including reduced acuity, whereas only relative temporal field depression is found in the contralateral field.
   iii. With few exceptions, these slow-growing tumors produce insidiously progressive visual deficits in the form of variations on a bitemporal theme.

iv. Most tumors are slow growing and so are the progress of visual symptoms.

v. Aneurysms may provoke sudden worsening or fluctuations in vision that mimic optic neuritis, at times with confounding improvement during corticosteroid therapy.

vi. Without temporal fields, objects beyond the point of binocular fixation fall on non-seeing nasal retina, so that a blind area exists, with extinction of objects beyond the fixation point.

vii. Suprasellar tumors of presumed prenatal origin, such as optic gliomas or craniopharyngiomas, may be associated with congenitally dysplastic optic disks.

3. What are the conditions that can mimic chiasmal field defects?

i. Tilted disks (inferior crescents, nasal fundus ectasia)

ii. Nasal sector retinitis pigmentosa

iii. Bilateral cecocentral scotomas

iv. Papilledema with greatly enlarged blind spots

v. Overhanging redundant upper lid tissue

vi. Dominant optic atrophy

vii. Ethambutol toxic optic neuropathy.

4. What is the treatment of visual field defects?

i. Visual field defects, particularly of the homonymous variety or those present in one-eyed patients, frequently pose unique problems of eye movement. Such patients typically experience difficulty in moving the eye very far into a large "blind" area.

ii. A prism with the base oriented toward the blind area and covering only the portion of the spectacle lens corresponding to the blind area can produce a favorable result. For example, a patient with sight in only the left eye and a left hemianopia would be helped in "seeing" objects in his left field with a base-out Fresnel prism applied to the temporal portion of the left lens.

iii. With a small eye movement from the primary position (no prism) to the left (into the prism), the visual field would be shifted by the amount of the eye movement plus the power of the prism. Thus, a small flick of the eye to the left would provide the subject with a large view of the visual scene normally lying in his "blind" area.

7.15. CAVERNOUS SINUS THROMBOSIS

1. Describe briefly anatomy of cavernous sinus.

i. The cavernous sinuses are irregularly shaped, trabeculated and consist of incompletely fused venous channels located at the base of the skull in the middle cranial fossa.

ii. They lie on either side of the sella turcica, are just lateral and superior to the sphenoid sinus and are immediately posterior to the optic chiasma.

iii. Each cavernous sinus is formed between layers of the dura mater, and multiple connections between the 2 sinuses exist.

iv. The cavernous sinuses receive venous blood from the facial veins (via the superior and inferior ophthalmic veins) as well as the sphenoid and middle cerebral veins. They, in turn, empty into the inferior petrosal sinuses, then into the internal jugular veins and the sigmoid sinuses via the superior petrosal sinuses.

v. There are no valves, however, in this complex web of veins, blood can flow in any direction depending on the prevailing pressure gradients.

vi. The internal carotid artery with its surrounding sympathetic plexus passes through the cavernous sinus.

vii. The third, fourth and sixth cranial nerves are attached to the lateral wall of the sinus.

viii. The ophthalmic and maxillary divisions of the fifth cranial nerve are embedded in the wall.

This intimate juxtaposition of veins, arteries, nerves, meninges and paranasal sinuses accounts for the characteristic etiology and presentation of cavernous sinus thrombosis.

2. What are the causes of cavernous sinus thrombosis?

Causes can be divided into:

Septic or infective:

i. Most cases of septic cavernous sinus thrombosis are due to an acute infection in an otherwise normal individual. However, patients with chronic sinusitis or diabetes mellitus may be at a slightly higher risk.

ii. The causative agent is generally *Staphylococcus aureus*, although *streptococci*, *pneumococci*, and fungi may be implicated in rare cases.

– Infection of the face

• Especially the middle 1/3rd,

• Causative organism: *Staphylococcus aureus*

• Bacteria → facial vein and pterygoid plexus → ophthalmic vein → cavernous sinus

- Sinusitis
  - it can be involving the sphenoid or the ethmoid sinuses
  - It can be
    - Acute: Caused by gram-positive organisms viz. *S. aureus*, pneumococci
    - Chronic: Caused by gram-negative organisms, coagulase negative staphylococci, fungi, e.g. *Aspergillus, Mucoraceae*
- Dental infections: (10%)
  - Common with maxillary teeth
  - Common pathogens involved in odontogenic septic cavernous sinus thrombosis are
    - Streptococci
    - *Fusobacteria*
    - *Bacteriodes*
- Otitis media:
  - Cavernous sinus thrombosis is rare complication
  - Seen in untreated, incompletely treated, incorrectly treated disease
- Orbital cellulitis:
  - Rare

Aseptic or noninfective:
  i. Polycythemia
  ii. Sickle cell disease or trait
  iii. Paroxysmal nocturnal hemoglobinuria
  iv. Arteriovenous malformations
  v. Trauma
  vi. Intracranial surgery
  vii. Vasculitis
  viii. Pregnancy
  ix. Oral contraceptive pills
  x. Congenital heart disease
  xi. Dehydration
  xii. Marasmus
  xiii. Compression or obstruction due to expanding mass (e.g. pituitary adenoma, meningioma) → sterile thrombosis
  part of the paraneoplastic hypercoagulability syndrome.

3. **What are the clinical features of cavernous sinus thrombosis?**
   History:
   i. Patients generally have sinusitis or a midface infection (most commonly a furuncle) for 5–10 days. In up to 25% of cases where a furuncle is the precipitant, it will have been manipulated in some fashion (e.g. squeezing, surgical incision).

ii. Headache, fever and malaise typically precede the development of ocular findings. As the infection tracks posteriorly, patients complain of orbital pain and fullness accompanied by periorbital edema and visual disturbances.

iii. In some patients, periorbital findings will not develop early on and the clinical picture is subtle.

iv. Without effective therapy, signs will appear in the contralateral eye by spreading through the communicating veins to the contralateral cavernous sinus. This is pathognomonic for cavernous sinus thrombosis. The patient rapidly develops mental status changes from CNS involvement and/or sepsis. Death will follow shortly thereafter.

Ocular and physical examination:

Other than the findings associated with the primary infection, the following signs are typical:

i. Initially, signs of venous congestion may present.
   - Chemosis
   - Eyelid edema
   - Periorbital edema

ii. Manifestations of increased retrobulbar pressure follow.
   - Exophthalmos
   - Ophthalmoplegia

iii. increased intraocular pressure (IOP)
   - Sluggish pupillary responses
   - Decreased visual acuity is common due to increased IOP and traction on the optic nerve and central retinal artery.

iv. Cranial nerve palsies are found regularly.
   - Isolated sixth nerve dysfunction may be noted before there are obvious orbital findings
   - Impaired extraocular movements.

v. Depressed corneal reflex is possible.

vi. Appearance of signs and symptoms in the contralateral eye is diagnostic of cavernous sinus thrombosis, although the process may remain confined to one eye.

vii. Meningeal signs may be noted, including nuchal rigidity, Kernig's and Brudzinski's signs.

viii. Systemic signs indicative of sepsis are late findings. They include chills, fever, shock, delirium and coma.

Ocular features depend on the origin of the infection.

i. Anterior infection (facial, dental, orbital) → acute presentation in the following order:
   - Deep seated pain around the eye
   - Increase temperature

- Orbital congestion
- Lacrimation
- Conjunctival edema
- Eyelid swelling
- Ptosis
- Proptosis
- Ophthalmoparesis

Such patients are usually toxic with +ve blood cultures.

ii. Sphenoid sinusitis/pharyngitis →
- Delayed presentation of signs
- Subacute or chronic
- Isolated abducens nerve paresis is the most consistent early neurologic sign

iii. Secondary to otitis media →
- Signs and symptoms are slow
- Protracted course.

Visual loss is common and causes are—ischemic oculopathy, ischemic optic neuropathy, neurotrophic keratopathy (corneal ulceration).

Aseptic: Signs and symptoms are similar to the septic type but without any laboratory or clinical evidence of infection.
- No fever, chills, leukocytosis, or signs and symptoms suggestive of meningitis
- Pain around and behind the eye
- Loss of corneal sensations, decreased facial sensations
- Ophthalmoparesis
- Proptosis, chemosis are less severe
- Sympathetic dysfunction
- Increased intraocular pressure
- Stasis retinopathy

Visual loss is usually uncommon regardless of the severity.

4.   What are the differential diagnosis of cavernous sinus thrombosis?

Differential diagnosis of cavernous sinus thrombosis	
Diagnosis	**Signs/symptoms**
Traumatic retrobulbar hemorrhage	▪ Accumulation of blood within the orbit ▪ History of trauma or surgery ▪ Bullous subconjunctival hemorrhage ▪ Pain, decreased vision, lid ecchymosis, increased IOP, proptosis
Orbital cellulitis	▪ Lid edema, erythema and tenderness ▪ Pain and fever but normal vision
Orbital fracture and ruptured globe	▪ History of trauma ▪ Periocular bruising, enophthalmos ▪ Pain, decreased vision, lid edema, restricted eye movements

(Continued)

(*Continued*)

Conjunctivitis	▪ Conjunctival follicles and/or papillae ▪ Red eye, decreased vision, lid edema, discharge ▪ Corneal neovascularization ▪ Itching and/or pain
Diagnosis	**Signs/symptoms**
Thyroid-related orbitopathy	▪ Lid retraction, lid lag, scleral show ▪ Foreign body sensation, decreased tearing ▪ Dyschromatopsia, diplopia, proptosis, decreased vision
Cavernous sinus thrombosis	▪ Altered level of consciousness ▪ Dilated and sluggish pupils; CN IIIrd, IVth, and/or VIth palsies ▪ Fever, nausea, vomiting ▪ Chemosis and lid edema, proptosis
Lacrimal gland neoplasia	▪ Temporal upper eyelid swelling ▪ Inferonasal globe displacement ▪ Tearing, pain, diplopia ▪ Palpable mass under superotemporal orbital rim
Orbital inflammation– idiopathic (orbital pseudotumor)	▪ Acute onset of orbital pain, headaches ▪ Binocular diplopia, decreased vision, proptosis, lid edema ▪ Induced hyperopia, decreased corneal sensation, increased IOP
Orbital vasculitis	▪ Systemic signs and symptoms (sinus, renal, pulmonary, skin) ▪ Fever, increased ESR (erythrocyte sedimentation rate)

5. **How do you investigate a case of cavernous sinus thrombosis?**

   i. Cavernous sinus thrombosis is a clinical diagnosis and lab studies are seldom specific.

   ii. Hematological investigation:
   - Most patients exhibit a polymorphonuclear leukocytosis, often marked with a shift towards immature forms.
   - Complete blood count is done to look for polycythemia as an etiologic factor.
   - Decreased platelet count would support thrombotic thrombocytopenic purpura; leukocytosis might be seen in sepsis. In addition, if heparin is used as treatment, platelet counts should be monitored for thrombocytopenia.
   - Blood cultures generally are positive for the offending organism.

   iii. Immunological tests:
   - Antiphospholipid and anticardiolipin antibodies should be obtained to evaluate for antiphospholipid syndrome.
   - Tests that may indicate hypercoagulable states include protein S, protein C, antithrombin IIIrd, lupus anticoagulant and leiden factor V mutation. These evaluations should not be made while the patient is on anticoagulant therapy.

    iv. Electrophoresis—sickle cell preparation or hemoglobin electrophoresis

    v. Cerebrospinal fluid examination—examination of the cerebrospinal fluid is consistent with either a parameningeal inflammation or Frank meningitis.

6. **What are the imaging studies done in cavernous sinus thrombosis?**

Computed tomography (CT) is the investigation of choice to confirm the diagnosis.

    i. On noncontrast study—thrombosis of the cavernous sinus can be appreciated as increased density.

    ii. Contrast scan reveal filling defects within the cavernous sinus. Empty delta sign appears on contrast scans as enhancement of the collateral veins in the superior sagittal sinus walls surrounding a non-enhanced thrombus in the sinus.

    iii. Negative CT cannot reliably rule out cavernous sinus thrombosis when the clinical suspicion is high.

    iv. Useful in ruling out other conditions such as neoplasm and in evaluating coexistent lesions such as subdural empyema. CT of the sinuses is useful in evaluating sinusitis; CT of the mastoids may be helpful in lateral sinus thrombosis.

Magnetic resonance imaging (MRI)

    i. Magnetic resonance imaging shows the pattern of an infarct that does not follow the distribution of an expected arterial occlusion. It may show absence of flow void in the normal venous channels.

    ii. Magnetic resonance venography (MRV) is an excellent method of visualizing the dural venous sinuses and larger cerebral veins.

    iii. Single-slice phase-contrast angiography (SSPCA) takes less than 30 seconds and provides rapid and reliable information.

    iv. If magnetic resonance studies are not diagnostic, conventional angiography should be considered.

Contrast studies

    i. Carotid arteriography is an invasive procedure and is therefore associated with a small risk.

    ii. Direct venography can be performed by passing a catheter from the jugular vein into the transverse sinus with injection outlining the venous sinuses.

7. **How do you treat a case of cavernous sinus thrombosis?**

Emergency department care:

    i. The mainstay of therapy is early and aggressive antibiotic administration. Although *S. aureus* is the usual cause, broad-spectrum coverage for gram-positive, gram-negative and anaerobic organisms should be instituted pending the outcome of cultures.

ii. Anticoagulation with heparin may be considered. The goal is to prevent further thrombosis and reduces the incidence of septic emboli. Heparin is contraindicated in the presence of intracerebral hemorrhage or other bleeding diathesis.

iii. Corticosteroids may help to reduce inflammation and edema and should be considered as an adjunctive therapy. When the course of cavernous sinus thrombosis leads to pituitary insufficiency, however, corticosteroids definitely are indicated to prevent adrenal crisis.

iv. Surgery on the cavernous sinus is technically difficult. The primary source of infection should be drained, if feasible (e.g. sphenoid sinusitis, facial abscess).

Medical treatment

Antibiotic therapy ideally is started after appropriate cultures but should not be delayed if there are difficulties in obtaining specimens. Antibiotics selected should be broad-spectrum, particularly active against *S. aureus*, and capable of achieving high levels in the cerebrospinal fluid.

Drug categories: i. Antibiotics ii. Anticoagulants iii. Corticosteroids.

– **Antibiotics**—empiric broad-spectrum coverage for gram-positive, gram-negative, and anaerobic organisms. Therapy must be comprehensive and should cover all likely pathogens in the context of the clinical setting.

The common antibiotics are:

- Oxacillin (2 g IV q4h)
- Ceftriaxone (2 g IV 112h)
- Metronidazole (500 mg IV q6h)

– **Anticoagulants**—unfractionated IV heparin and fractionated low molecular weight subcutaneous heparins are the 2 options in anticoagulation therapy.
  Dose: 80 mg/kg IV bolus; then 18 mg/kg IV infusion; titrate

– **Corticosteroids**—these agents have anti-inflammatory properties and cause profound and varied metabolic effects. In addition, these agents modify the body's immune response to diverse stimuli.

Complications of cavernous sinus thrombosis:

i. Meningitis
ii. Septic emboli
iii. Blindness
iv. Cranial nerve palsies
v. Sepsis and shock.

Prognosis

Septic cavernous sinus thrombosis:

   i. Mortality is up to 30%, with the majority of survivors suffering permanent sequelae and neurological deficit.
  ii. Full recovery is seen in <40%
 iii. Rarely Frohlich's syndrome has been reported.

Aseptic cavernous sinus thrombosis:

   i. Variable
  ii. Depends on the underlying cause
 iii. Extent and severity of neurologic dysfunction
  iv. Mortality rate is much low
   v. Damage to the cranial nerves → persistent pareses, trigeminal neuralgia
  vi. Permanent visual loss is rare but can occur.

7.16. CAROTICOCAVERNOUS FISTULAS

1. **Define caroticocavernous fistula.**

   It is an abnormal communications between the cavernous sinus and dural veins and the carotid arterial system.

2. **Classify caroticocavernous fistula.**

Cause	Velocity of blood flow	Anatomy
Traumatic	High flow	Direct and dural
Spontaneous	Low flow	Internal carotid and external carotid, or both.

   High flow: Carotid-cavernous fistulas, characterized by direct flow into the cavernous sinus from the intracavernous carotid artery.

   Causes: These usually are traumatic and most often diagnosed in young men.

   Low flow: Spontaneous shunts occur between the cavernous sinus and one or more meningeal branches of the internal carotid artery (usually the meningohypophyseal trunk), the external carotid artery, or both. These shunts have a low amount of arterial flow and almost always produce signs and symptoms spontaneously.

   Causes:
   - i. Spontaneously
   - ii. In the setting of atherosclerosis, hypertension,
   - iii. Collagen vascular disease,
   - iv. During or after childbirth,
   - v. Elderly, especially women.

3. **Describe dural shunts.**
   - i. Dural shunts between the arterial and venous systems have lower flow.
   - ii. They may produce symptoms in younger patients spontaneously or in older patients due to hypertension, diabetes, atherosclerosis or other vascular disorders.
   - iii. Anatomically, these shunts arise between the meningeal arterial branches and the dural veins.
   - iv. The meningohypophyseal trunk and the artery of the inferior cavernous sinus provide the arterial supply to most dural shunts.
   - v. Such shunts may be due to an expansion of congenital arteriovenous malformation, or due to spontaneous rupture of one of the thin-walled dural arteries that transverse the sinus.

4. What are the ocular manifestations of carotico-cavernous fistulas?

Ocular signs of carotico-cavernous fistulas are related to venous congestion and reduced arterial blood flow to the orbit. These abnormalities usually are unilateral, but can be bilateral or even contralateral to the fistula.

Conjunctiva: Chemosis of the conjunctiva and arterialization of the episcleral vessels occurs in most patients. Arterialization of episcleral veins is the hallmark of all carotico-cavernous fistulas or dural shunts

Glaucoma: Stasis of venous and arterial circulation within the eye and orbit may cause ocular ischemia and increased episcleral venous pressure may cause glaucoma.

Orbit

i. Exophthalmos is a common sign that occurs in almost all patients who have carotico-cavernous fistulas. rapid-flow fistulas may develop exophthalmus within hours or several days.

ii. The orbit can become "frozen," with no ocular motor function; usually, this is accompanied by conjunctival chemosis and hemorrhage. Vision may be reduced markedly as a result of optic nerve ischemia.

iii. "Pulsating exophthalmos" is uncommon in carotico-cavernous fistula. Usually, the orbit is rigid from hemorrhage and edema and incapable of "pulsation".

Bruits: Bruits associated with fistulas and dural shunts can be appreciated both subjectively and objectively. A bruit can be heard best when the examiner uses a "bell stethoscope" over the closed eye, over the superior orbital vein, or the temple. A subjective bruit (heard by the patient) almost always can be obtained from the history; however, an objective bruit heard over the orbit or temple by auscultation is relatively uncommon.

A bruit is not pathognomonic of carotico-cavernous fistula. It also can be heard in normal infants, in young children, and in severe anemia.

Optic nerve: Immediate or delayed visual loss occurs frequently in direct carotico-cavernous fistulas, due to optic nerve ischemia from apical orbital compression.

Long-standing fistulas can lead to loss of vision as a result of distention of the cavernous sinus or of retrobulbar ischemia.

Cranial nerve palsy

i. Diminished arterial flow to cranial nerves within the cavernous sinus may cause diplopia.

ii. The abducens nerve is affected most often as it lies in the cavernous sinus itself.

iii. Since the third and fourth nerves are encased in the superior internal dural wall of the sinus, they may be protected from changes caused by the fistula.

iv. Mechanical restriction from venous congestion and orbital edema also may contribute to limitation of eye movements.

Fundus picture

i. Ophthalmoscopic findings due to venous stasis and impaired retinal blood flow include retinal venous engorgement and dot and blot retinal hemorrhages.

ii. Central retinal vein occlusion may be observed in high-velocity carotico-cavernous fistulas with arterialized venous channels.

iii. High episcleral and intraocular pressures rarely results in damage to the optic nerve.

iv. In the unusual cases of central vein occlusion, neovascular glaucoma can occur.

5. **Investigations of choice in CCF?**

Digital subtraction angiography.

7.17. CAROTID ARTERY OCCLUSION

1. **What are the common modes of presentation of carotid artery occlusion to an ophthalmologist?**

    i. ***Transient*** ischemic ***attack.*** If the transient ischaemic attack involves the carotid system, the symptoms include hemiparesis, hemisensory loss, aphasia and transient monocular blindness (amaurosis fugax).

    ii. ***Purely*** ocular ***symptoms,*** such as
    - Paratransient ischemic attack or complete visual loss due to an artery obstruction
    - Decreased visual acuity
    - Pain resulting from the ocular ischemic syndrome.

    iii. Other patients are asymptomatic and any ocular findings consistent with carotid artery disease are incidental.

2. **What is amaurosis fugax?**

    Amaurosis fugax ("fleeting darkness or blindness"; ocular transient ischemic episode).

    i. Most common symptom of carotid artery disease.

    ii. This phenomenon may be defined as a painless unilateral, transient loss of vision that usually progresses from the periphery toward the center of the field.

    iii. Often, the visual deficit takes the pattern of a dark curtain descending from above or ascending from below.

    iv. Complete or subtotal blindness follows in seconds and lasts from 1 to 5 minutes (rarely longer).

    v. Vision returns to normal within 10–20 minutes, at times by reversal of the pattern of progression.

    vi. The return of vision can be sectorial or altitudinal and is occasionally described as a "curtain rising."

    vii. Generally, the vision returns to normal immediately after an attack. The frequency of these attacks varies from one or two attacks per month to 10 or 20 per day.

    viii. The retina—if observed during an amaurotic attack—may be normal or it may show obstruction (such as in central retinal artery obstruction).

    ix. It may exhibit migratory white retinal emboli (within the retinal arterioles and in association with disruption of the arterial circulation) or it may show cholesterol emboli moving through the arterial system.

    x. It is important to recognize amaurosis fugax as a transient ischemic attack because it is frequently caused by microembolization from an atheromatous ulcerative lesion in the ipsilateral extracranial carotid artery, at least in older patients.

xi. About a third of all patients with an untreated transient ischemic attack can be expected to have a stroke; this rate is about four times greater than that of an age-matched population.

3. **What are causes of amaurosis fugax?**
   i. Migraine
   ii. Hematology disorders
   iii. Ocular hypertension
   iv. Arterial hypotension
   v. Vasospasm
   vi. Temporal arteritis
   vii. Pseudotumor cerebri
   viii. Structural cardiac defects
   ix. Ophthalmic artery stenosis
   x. Ophthalmic artery aneurysms.

4. **What is ocular ischemic syndrome?**

   Ocular ischemic syndrome refers to the constellation of ophthalmic features that result from chronic hypoperfusion of the entire arterial supply to the eye, including the central retinal, posterior ciliary and anterior ciliary arteries.

   The occlusion is at the level of:
   i. The carotid artery
   ii. Proximal to the point where the central retinal and ciliary arteries branch from the ophthalmic artery.

5. **What is the clinical presentation of ocular ischemic syndrome?**
   i. Patient, typically more than 50 years old, is more likely to be male than female.
   ii. Patient reports having a loss of vision in one or both eyes over a period of weeks to months.
   iii. Ocular or periocular pain here may or may not be associated, it is found in approximately 40% of persons with ocular ischemic syndrome. Typically, the pain is described as a dull ache over the eye or brow.
   iv. Ischemia to the anterior segment structures, or ocular angina, is thought to be the cause of this pain in some cases.
   v. History of difficulty adjusting from bright light to relative darkness represents inability of ocular circulation to supply enough oxygen to sustain increases retinal circulation.
   vi. Similar complaints occur after exertion, change in posture and postprandial period.
   vii. Additionally, the patient may relate a history of transient focal neurologic deficits.

Ocular symptoms and signs of carotid artery occlusion

Symptoms
  i. Visual loss
 ii. Pain–"ocular angina" (40% case)
iii. Prolonged recovery after light exposure
 vi. Amaurosis fugax (10% cases)
  v. Associated with transient focal neurologic deficits.

Signs
    i. Spontaneous retinal arterial pulsations
   ii. Midperipheral retinal hemorrhage
  iii. Cholesterol emboli
   iv. Disk edema—AION
    v. Neovascularization of disk, retina, iris
   vi. Narrowed retinal arterioles
  vii. Dilated retinal veins
 viii. Arteriovenous communications.

Other peculiar presentations
  i. Ipsilateral Horner's syndrome
 ii. Carotid dissection
iii. Ischemic anterior uveitis
 iv. Neovascular glaucoma.

Systemic associations—most patients will have already been diagnosed with diabetes mellitus, hypertension, ischemic heart disease, cerebrovascular disease.

Differential diagnosis
  i. Diabetic retinopathy
 ii. Nonischemic CRVO

Diagnostic workup
Prompt noninvasive vascular workup is mandatory
  i. To confirm carotid vascular disease
 ii. Establish cause (atheroma, emboli, dissection, vasculitis, compression, etc.)
iii. Ocular and cerebral tolerance of carotid occlusion.

Investigations
  i. Carotid color doppler
 ii. Cerebral angiography and arteriography (gold standard)
iii. Digital subtraction angiography.
 iv. Ultrasonography
  v. MRI angiography

vi. Spiral CT angiography

vii. Fundus fluorescein angiography.

6. **What are the features of ocular ischemic syndrome on fluorescein angiogram?**

Characteristic fluorescein angiographic features reflect the chronic hypoperfusion of the retinal and choroidal circulations, as well as ischemic damage to the neurosensory retina and retinal vessels.

i. Prolonged arteriovenous transit time

ii. Prolonged arm-to-retina circulation times (over 20 seconds)

iii. Retinal vascular staining

iv. Retinal capillary nonperfusion

v. Delayed or patchy choroidal filling

vi. Macular edema.

7. **What are the other tests that can be done for diagnosing ocular ischemic syndrome?**

i. **Photopic stress test**

A marked difference in photopic stress recovery times between the two eyes is suggestive of macular disease, such as ocular ischemic syndrome; diseases of the optic nerve would be less affected.

ii. **Electroretinography**

Eyes with ocular ischemic syndrome show a decreased amplitude of both the a-and b-waves. The b-wave, which corresponds to the inner retinal layer, probably reflects the function of the bipolar and/or Müller cells, and it is diminished by compromised perfusion of the central retinal artery.

The a-wave correlates with photoreceptor function and is affected by choroidal ischemia.

iii. **Orbital color doppler imaging**

Central retinal and posterior ciliary artery peak systolic velocities markedly reduced.

iv. **Ophthalmodynamometry and oculoplethysmography**

The normal ophthalmic artery has a systolic pressure of approximately 100 mm Hg and a diastolic pressure of approximately 60 mm Hg.

In ocular ischemic syndrome, the systolic pressure is often less than 40 mm Hg, and the diastolic pressure may be less than 10 mm Hg. It is often useful to measure an unaffected contralateral eye for comparison.

v. **Carotid duplex (b-mode and doppler) scanning**

Although safe and inexpensive, has limitations, less reliable than carotid angiography in distinguishing between a completely occluded artery and one that is nearly occluded, used as screening techniques for atherosclerotic disease.

vi. **Carotid angiography (digital subtraction aortogram)**
Despite its expense and low but definite morbidity rate, carotid angiography remains the most reliable method of assessing atherosclerotic carotid disease, and it serves as the "gold standard" in the evaluation of all other tests of the carotid arteries.

8. **What is the treatment of ocular ischemic syndrome?**
Treatment directed primarily at
   i. Treating ocular neovascularization and neovascular glaucoma.
  ii. Restoring blood flow into the eye with surgery.

Treatment of ocular neovascularization
   i. Fundus fluorescein angiography to determine cause of NVD/NVE.
  ii. Retinal ablative procedures—PRP/anterior retinal cryoablation still remains the first modality of treatment.

Systemic antiplatelet therapy
   i. Aspirin
  ii. Ticlopidine
 iii. Pentoxifylline
  iv. Dipyridamole
   v. Clopidrogel

Indications for medical management
   i. Inoperable carotid disease
  ii. Nonstenotic carotid disease
 iii. Medical contraindication to surgery.

Surgical management: In most cases, carotid endarterectomy remains the treatment of choice for symptomatic patients with severe stenotic atherosclerotic disease of the internal carotid artery.

7.18. OPHTHALMOPLEGIA

1. **What are the types of ophthalmoplegia?**

    i. *Total ophthalmoplegia*—if all the extrinsic and intrinsic muscle of one or both eyes are paralyzed.

    ii. *External ophthalmoplegia*—if only the extrinsic muscle of one or both the eyes are paralyzed.

    iii. *Internal ophthalmoplegia*—if only the intrinsic muscles (sphincter pupillae and ciliary muscle) of one or both eyes are paralyzed.

    iv. *Painful ophthalmoplegia*—the syndrome of painful ophthalmoplegia consists of periorbital pain or hemicranial pain combined with ipsilateral ocular motor palsies, oculosympathetic paralysis, and sensory loss in the distribution of ophthalmic and occasionally maxillary division of trigeminal nerve. The etiology of painful ophthalmoplegia may be divided into those with the involvement of cavernous sinus/superior orbital fissure and those without the involvement of the same.

2. **Describe briefly anatomy of the superior orbital fissure.**

    Superior orbital fissure connects the middle cranial fossa with the orbit. It lies between the roof and lateral wall of the orbit and is a gap between greater wing and lesser wing of sphenoid, and is bounded by

    i. Body of sphenoid medially

    ii. Lesser wing of sphenoid above

    iii. Greater wing of sphenoid below

    iv. A part of frontal bone may complete the fissure laterally

    Subdivisions—a common tendinous ring (tendon of Zinn) encircles the optic foramen and middle of superior orbital fissure and gives origin to recti muscles of the eye ball. The central part of the fissure within the ring is called oculomotar foramen.

3. **What are the structures passing through the superior orbital fissure?**

    The various structures transmitted are:

    Above the common tendinous ring

    i. Trochlear nerve medially

    ii. Frontal nerve laterally

    iii. Superior ophthalmic vein

    iv. Rarely recurrent lacrimal artery.

    Through the oculomotor foramen

    i. Superior division of 3rd cranial nerve

    ii. Inferior division of the 3rd cranial nerve

    iii. Nasociliary nerve

iv. Sympathetic root of ciliary ganglion

v. Abducent nerve inferonasally.

Below the tendinous ring—inferior ophthalmic vein.

4. **What are the causes of parasellar syndrome producing painful ophthalmoplegia?**

    i. Trauma

   ii. Vascular

      – Intracavernous sinus carotid artery aneurysm

      – Posterior carotid artery aneurysm

      – Carotid artery fistula

      – Cavernous sinus thrombosis

  iii. Neoplasm

      – Primary intracranial neoplasm—pituitary adenoma, meningioma, sarcoma, craniopharyngioma, neurofibroma, Gasserian ganglion neuroma and epidermoid

      – Primary cranial tumor—chondroma, chordoma, giant cell tumor

      – Local metastasis—nasopharyngeal tumor, cylindroma, chordoma, squamous cell carcinoma

      – Distant metastasis—lymphoma, multiple myeloma

      – Inflammation

         • Bacterial—sinusitis, mucocele

         • viral—herpes zoster

         • fungal—mucormycosis

         • spirochetal—Treponema pallidum

         • *Mycobacterium*

         • unknown causes—sarcoidosis, Wegner's granulomatosis, Tolosa–Hunt syndrome.

5. **What are the causes of painful ophthalmoplegia with no involvement of the cavernous sinus/superior orbital fissure?**

    i. Orbital disease

      – Idiopathic orbital inflammation (pseudotumor)

      – Contigious sinusitis

      – Mucormycosis or other fungal infection

      – Metastatic tumor

      – Lymphoma/leukemia.

   ii. Diabetic ophthalmoplegia

      – Mononeuropathy

      – Multiple cranial nerve palsy

  iii. Posterior fossa aneurysm

      – Posterior communicating artery

      – Basilar artery

  iv. Cranial arteritis

   v. Migrainous ophthalmoplegia

  vi. Gradenigo's syndrome

 vii. Reader's syndrome

viii. Trauma.

6. **What are the ways in which trauma can produce ophthalmoplegia?**

Craniocerebral trauma may produce painful ophthalmoplegia in various ways namely

   i. Basilar skull fracture with ocular motor damage

  ii. Intracavernous carotid artery injury with subsequent aneurysm formation

 iii. Caroticocavernous fistula

 iv. Painful ophthalmoplegia may occur as an acute phenomenon or as delayed phenomenon.

   – **Acute painful ophthalmoplegia**

    • *Cranial nerve involvement*—immediate paralysis of IIIrd, IVth, VIth cranial nerves is a well known complication of closed head trauma.

    • *Orbit involvement*—the direct injury to the orbit can cause immediate impairment of ocular motility due to trauma to the ocular muscles, orbital hemorrhage and edema, or entrapment of the muscle or fasciae in the fracture site.

   – **Delayed painful ophthalmoplegia**

   This may be due to various reasons

    • Progression of the local edema after injury to the ocular motor nerve or to the orbit which tends to produce maximal impairment within few days after injury and manifestation itself as a worsening of the immediate impairment.

    • Progressive brainstem edema which becomes maximal within few days after the injury and is generally accompanied by other brainstem signs. This may be due to the injury to the blood vessels outside the brainstem rather than direct brainstem injury.

    • Sixth nerve and rarely fourth nerve paresis due to increased intracranial pressure without herniation, and third nerve paresis due to transtentorial herniation can all result from verity of mass lesions secondary to head injury.

    • Post-traumatic sphenoid mucocele can cause painful ophthalmoplegia usually after delay of months or years.

    • Sudden severe exophthalmos and painful ophthalmoplegia due to an orbital meningocele occurring one month after a frontal fracture has been reported.

7. What are the features of ophthalmoplegia due to intracavernous carotid artery aneurysm?

    i. Compromise about 3% of all intracranial aneurysm.

   ii. Most of these syndromes occur in middle aged individuals, without the history of incident head trauma.

  iii. The onset of signs and symptoms may be abrupt but may be slow and insidious.

  iv. Pain in and around the eye and face is the prominent symptom.

   v. The sixth nerve being the close relation of the internal carotid artery is affected first and in most cases third and fourth nerve are involved subsequently.

  vi. Trigeminal sensory loss is regarded as the classical manifestation of this disease.

 vii. Aneurysmal expansion can produce additional findings that vary with its directions.

    – Anterior expansion—can produce exophthalmos and ipsilateral and ipsilateral visual failure due to optic nerve compression.

    – Posterior expansion—may extend as far as petrous part of temporal bone and give rise to ipsilateral hearing loss.

    – Inferior expansion—into the sphenoid sinus with subsequent rupture explains the massive and sometimes fatal epistaxis suffered by the patients.

    – Medial erosion of the aneurysm into the sella turcica can produce signs and symptoms which mimic a pituitary tumor.

8. Why is pupil spared in intracavernous carotid artery aneurysm causing third cranial nerve paresis?

    i. The small pupil may be due to simultaneous involvement of the both the third nerve and the sympathetic fibers surrounding the internal carotid artery (ICA).

   ii. The absence of large pupil in the cavernous sinus lesion may sometimes reflect sparing of the inferior division of the third nerves.

9. Where do you ligate the carotid artery?

    i. Ligation of the carotid in the neck with or without intracranial clipping distal to the aneurysm

   ii. Occlusion of the carotid artery by the detachable balloon catheter.

10. What are the features of ophthalmoplegia due to carotico-cavernous fistula?

    i. This represents the direct communication between the intracavernous carotid artery and the surrounding cavernous sinus.

   ii. The large majority arises traumatically.

iii. Spontaneous fistula may develop. Causes:
   a. Pre-existing aneurysm.
   b. Angiodysplasias, such as Ehler-Danlos or pseudo-xanthoma elasticum.
iv. The clinical features usually develop immediately although there may be a delay. The degree of the external symptom depends on the amount of the anterior drainage of the shunted blood.

11. What are the clinical features of caroticocavernous fistula?

   i. *Conjunctiva:* There is arterialization of the bulbar conjunctiva often with marked proptosis and chemosis. Conjunctival prolapse with inversion of the fornix may occur.
   ii. *Cornea:* Exposure keratitis. And possible corneal anesthesia from the fifth nerve damage.
   iii. *Orbit:* Severe proptosis with limitation of the eyelid closure.
   iv. *Glaucoma* is usually due to increased episceleral venous pressure with open angles. Neovascular glaucoma may develop secondary to hypoxic retinopathy. Blood in the trabecular meshwork is the common finding on gonioscopy.
   v. *Bruit* may accompany these finding.
   vi. *Cranial nerves:* Any of the cranial nerves may be involved.
   vii. *Vision:* Visual loss may be due to
      – Traumatic optic neuropathy
      – Ocular steal phenomenon
      – Hypoxic retinopathy due to decreased ocular blood flow.

Management: The treatment of choice is balloon immobilization.

12. What are the features of ophthalmoplegia due to pituitary apoplexy?

   i. Pituitary tumors frequently invade the cavernous sinus and cause cavernous sinus syndrome
   ii. Pituitary apoplexy, which occurs as a result of infarction of the pituitary adenoma, which has outgrown its blood supply.
      – It can be precipitated by radiation therapy, trauma and pregnancy.
      – The condition is characterized by acute onset of headache, painful ophthalmoplegia, bilateral amaurosis, drowsiness or coma and subarachnoid hemorrhage.
      – Headache is usually of sudden onset, generalized or only retrobulbar.
      – Unilateral or bilateral ophthalmoplegia is due to involvement of IIIrd, IVth and VIth cranial nerve in the cavernous sinus.
      – The CSF shows xanthochromia, pleocytosis and elevated protein levels.
      – CT scan often shows infarction of the tumor with hemorrhage in and above enlarged sella.

Treatment

It is a life threatening condition and needs prompt treatment.
Corticosteroids are the mainstay of treatment.
If there no improvement, surgical transnasal decompression is done.

13. **What are the classical triad of pituitary apoplexy?**
    i. Headache
    ii. Diplopia
    iii. Subarachnoid hemorrhage

14. **What are the features of cavernous sinus meningiomas?**
    i. Manifest as slowly progressive, painless lesion occurring in older women, they may occasionally present as sudden painful ophthalmoplegia.
    ii. Presents with ptosis, diplopia and parasympathetic pupillary involvement.
    iii. The demonstration of primary aberrant regeneration of the third nerve without a preceding neuropathy is exceedingly suggestive meningioma.
    iv. Management includes observation, radiation, surgical therapy or combination of all the three. They are extremely radiosensitive.

15. **What are the features of nasopharyngeal tumors?**

Ophthalmic signs and symptoms	Otolaryngeal symptoms
1. Proptosis	1. Nasal congestion
2. Facial pain	2. Facial discomfort
3. Eye pain	3. Sinusitis
4. Visual loss	4. Facial swelling
5. Epiphora	5. Erythema
6. Globe displacement	6. Headache
7. Limitation of extraocular movements	7. Epistaxis
8. Diplopia	8. Nasal mass
9. Photophobia	9. Difficulty in chewing
10. Conjunctival chemosis	10. Facial numbness
11. Palpebral mass within the orbit	
12. Bony erosion	
13. Dacrocystitis	
14. Horner's syndrome	

16. **What are the features of Tolosa–Hunt syndrome?**
    This is a variant of acute inflammatory pseudotumor affecting the cavernous sinus or superior orbital fissure.

The diagnostic criteria are:

i. Steady boring retro orbital pain which may precede ophthalmoplegia.
ii. Second, third or fourth cranial palsy with or without Horner's syndrome.
iii. Symptoms lasting for days to weeks.
iv. Occasional spontaneous remission, although neurological defect may persist.
v. Recurrent attacks in the intervals of months to years.
vi. No evidence of disease outside cavernous sinus.

Pathology—orbital periostitis with granulomatous vasculitis in the cavernous sinus.

Investigations:

i. Hematological tests are nonspecific.
ii. CSF analysis is unremarkeble.
iii. Carotid angiography shows abnormalities in the configuration of intracavernous carotid artery in the form of irregular narrowing or constriction. These changes resolved with steroid therapy.
iv. Orbital venography shows occlusion of superior ophthalmic vein on the affected side. There may be partial or absent filling of cavernous sinus. Follow-up venography shows persistent filling defects, suggestive of fibrosis in the involved areas.

Treatment: Corticosteroids are the mainstay of the treatment.

7.19. MALINGERING

1. **What are the tests to detect malingering?**
   i. **Total binocular blindness**
      – **Observation**
        - Truly blind moves cautiously, bumps into things naturally; hysterics avoids objects, "seeing unconsciously," malingerer goes out of his or her way to bump into objects.
        - Patients who are truly blind in both eyes tend to look directly at the person with whom they are speaking, whereas patients with nonorganic blindness, particularly patients who are malingering, often look in some other direction.
        - Similarly, patients claiming complete or near complete blindness often wear sunglasses, even though they do not have photophobia, and external appearance of eyes is perfectly normal.
      – *Pupillary response*—earliest and single most important test.
        - Intact direct and consensual response excludes anterior visual pathway disease.
        - In patients with better than NPL, there is no consistent relationship between amount of visual loss and pupillary deficit.
      – *Menace reflex*—blinking to visual threat.
      – *Reflex tearing*—sudden strong illumination thrown into eyes difficult to suppress reflex tearing in a patient with good visual acuity.
      – *Signature*—truly blind patients have no difficulty in doing signature. While functionally blind patients sign their name with exaggerated illegibility.
      – Another way to detect nonorganic visual loss in a patient who claims to be unable to see shapes and objects in one or both eyes is to ask patient to touch the tips of index fingers of both hands together. If the patient claims loss of vision in one eye only, opposite eye is patched before test is performed.
        As physician knows, the ability to touch the fingers of both hands together is based not on vision but on proprioception. Thus patient with organic blindness can easily bring the tips of the fingers of two hands together, whereas patients with nonorganic blindness, particularly malingerer will not do so. As the patient's hand is held up in front of him, and he is asked to look at his hand, the malingerer tends to look to the right or left, anywhere but not at his hand.
      – *Optokinetic nystagmus* (**OKN**)—if patient claims no perception of light, light perception only, or perception of hand movements in one or both eyes. Rotating optokinetic drum or horizontally moving tape can be used to produce a horizontal jerk nystagmus that indicates intact vision of at least 3/60. It is important in this regard

that the images on the tape or drum be sufficiently large that the patient is not able to look around them. When testing a patient who claims complete loss of vision in one eye only, we begin test in rotating the drum or moving the tape in front of the patient while he/she has both eyes open. Once we elicit good OKN, cover the unaffected eye with palm of our hand or a hand held occluded. The patient with nonorganic loss of vision is one eye will continue to slow jerk nystagmus.

- *Mirror test*—a large mirror held in front of patient's face, and patient is asked to look directly ahead. Mirror is then rotated and twisted back and forth, causing image in mirror to move. Patients with vision better than NPL show nystagmoid movement of the eyes, because they cannot avoid following the moving mirror.
- *Visual-evoked potential (VEP)*—flash and pattern reversal stimuli correlation exists between check size and level of acuity. Although difficult, it is possible to consciously alter response to pattern reversal stimulation with convergence, meditation, intense concentration. P300 component of VEP is suggestive of conscious stimulation of the cerebral tissue even though the patient says that he does not view the pattern stimulus.

ii. **Total monocular blindness**
More common than binocular blindness, tends to occur with malingering. Can use any of the above tests with unaffected eye occluded.

- **Diplopia tests**
  - Suspected eye occluded while strong prism held with apex bisecting pupil of good eye. Patient admits monocular diplopia. As suspected eye uncovered, the entire prism is placed before good eye, producing binocular diplopia. If patient still reports diplopia, functional blindness is revealed.
  - Make patient walk up and down stairs with vertical prism over allegedly blind eye.
  - Prism dissociation tests

    Can be used to detect mild degrees of nonorganic monocular visual loss. In these tests patient is first asked if he or she has experienced double vision in addition to loss of vision in affected eye. If answer is negative, the patient is told that the examiner will test, the alignment of both eyes and that test should produce vertical double vision.

    A 4 prism diopter loose prism is then placed base down in front of unaffected eye at the same time that 0.5 prism diopter loose prism is simultaneously placed with base in any direction over the eye with decreased vision.

    In this way the patient does not become suspicious that examiner is paying specific attention to one or the other eye.

A 6/6 or larger letter projected at a distance, the patient is asked if he/she has double vision.

When patient admits diplopia, she/he is then asked whether the two letters are of equal quality or sharpness, and an assessment of visual acuity can be made.

- **Fixation tests**
  - 10 prism base out test
    - relies upon refixation movement to avoid diplopia
    - 10 D base out prism in front of normal eye produces shift of both eyes with refixation movement of the other eye.
  - Vertical bar (reading)
    A ruler is held 5 inches from nose in between eyes while patient reads at near. Overlap of visual fields allow a binocular person to read across the bar. If patient reads without interruption, functional blindness confirmed. Can also use prism in front of suspect eye, resulting in diplopia, which should interrupt reading.
- **Fogging tests**
  - With both eyes open on the phoropter, patient starts reading eye chart. Examiner progressively adds more plus to the good eye while patient keeps reading.
    Final line read is patient's visual acuity in suspected eye.
  - Crossed cylinder technique
    A variation of this test is the use of paired cylinders. A plus cylinder and minus cylinder of same power (usually from 2 to 6 diopters) are placed at parallel axes in front of the normal eye in a trial frame. The patient's normal correction is placed in front of the affected eye. The patient is asked to read with both eyes open, a line that previously has been read with the normal eye but not with the affected eye.
    As patient begins to read, the axis of one of the cylinders rotated through 10°–15°. The axes of two cylinders thus will no longer be parallel due to blurring of vision in normal eye.
    If patient continues to read the line or can read it again when asked to do so, he/she must be using affected eye.
  - Instill cycloplegic agent into unaffected eye while doing applanation tension, have patient read at near.
- **Color tests**
  - Red/green duochrome in projector, red/green glasses worn such that red lens covers suspected eye. Eye behind red lens sees letters on red and not on green side of chart. And eye behind the green lens sees only letters on the green side.

If patient reads the entire line, the suspected eye is being used.

- Red/green glasses and worth four dot test—patient should see appropriate number of dots.

- *Ishihara color testing*

  In this test, use of red and green filter in front of each eye, while subject views Ishihara's color plates. The numbers and lines on Ishihara plates are visible only through red filter while plates 1 and 36 are seen by all persons even if color blind, and are more distinctly seen through this filter. Even with visual acuity of 3/60, all color plates are can be seen through red filter.

  The test for detecting functionally impaired vision is performed as follows:

  After testing visual acuity of each eye, the patient is given the red and green goggles with red filter over the eye with alleged impaired vision. With sound eye, patient will not see plates through green filter. If the patient sees the plates, the visual acuity must be 3/60 or better. If there is no response the goggles should be switched so that the red filter will be over the sound eye, and if the patient does not respond even 1 and 36, then test should be done without any goggles to prove wrong answers.

- *Polaroid glasses and vectorgraphic slides*

  Polarizing lenses can be used in several ways to detect nonorganic visual loss in patients with decreased vision in one eye only.

  In American Optical Polarizing Test, the patient wears polarizing glasses, and the test object, a project-o-chart slide projects letters alternately so that one letter is seen by both eyes, the next by the left eye, the next by right eye and so on.

  Another test uses polarizing lens placed before a projector. The patient is asked to read the chart while wearing polarizing lenses, with one eye or the other being allowed to see the whole projected image at a time, with vertical polarizer in one eye and horizontal polarizer in the other eye.

- *Red Amsler grid test*

  Using red-green filters, red Amsler grid test is useful in cases with unilateral field loss when the professed visual field defect extends to within 10° of fixation. A paracentral scotoma must be demonstrated monocularly with Amsler grid. The patient is then asked to look at red Amsler grid on black background, using red filter in front of eye with scotoma and green filter in front of normal eye. The red on black can be seen only through red filter.

  A positive response indicates a credibility problem and proves functional visual loss.

- *Stereoscopic tests*
  Stereoacuity is directly proportional to Snellen's acuity. Test plates used are Titmus fly or Randot test.
  40 seconds of arc stereoacuity compatible with not worse than 20/20 or 6/6 Snellen's acuity OU.

  Relationship of Visual Acuity and Stereopsis

Visual acuity	Stereopsis
6/6	40 seconds
6/9	52 seconds
6/12	61 seconds
6/18	78 seconds
6/24	94 seconds
6/36	124 seconds
6/60	160 seconds

iii. **Diminished vision**
Simulation of visual acuity less than 6/6 is more difficult to detect. Binocular or monocular can use most of the tests above plus the following:
  - Doctor killing refraction (DKR) or toothpaste refraction
    Start with 6/5 line and express disbelief the patient could not see big letters on the 6/6 line then proceed up chart until patient reads.
  - Visual angle—varying test distance with eye chart, Landolt's C rings or Tumbling E block such that patient sees a smaller visual angle or demonstrates inconsistencies. For example, reading 6/6 letter at 10 feet is equivalent to 6/12 acuity.
  - Move patient back and forth slightly in the chair, helping them get into focus or place combinations of lenses adding up to plano in a trial frame to help magnify their image.

iv **Field defects**
  - *Constricted field (On kinetic perimetry)*
    - These field defects show steep margins
    - Remains same regardless of size of object and test distance from screen (tunnel vision).
    - The degree of functional constriction may vary in the same patient from one examination to the next. This may be demonstrated in malingering using tangent screen.
    - Marks used to outline the patient's visual field are moved to new positions closer to fixation when the patient is absent.
    - When the test is repeated, the new field will confirm to new pin arrangement.
  - *Monocular hemianopias*
    Field testing monocularly and binocularly—fields overlap.
  - *Paracentral field defect*
    In this malingering can be detected with the help of red Amsler grid test.

CHAPTER
8

Orbit

8.1. ECTROPION

1. **What is ectropion?**

   Ectropion is an eyelid malposition characterized by an outward turning of the eyelid margin away from the globe accompanied by separation between the eyelid and the globe.

2. **What is the surgical anatomy of the eyelid?**

   Eyelid is a bilamellar structure.

   Anterior lamella consists of:

   i. Skin
   ii. Thin areolar subcutaneous connective tissue
   iii. Orbicularis oculi: It is a striated muscle, which is anatomically divided into 3 parts, viz. orbital, preseptal and the pretarsal.

   Posterior lamella consists of:

   i. Tarsal plate
      - Dense fibrous tissue
      - 25–29 mm long
      - 1–1.5 mm thick
      - Upper tarsus: 8–12 mm in height
      - Lower tarsus: 4–5 mm in height
   ii. Conjunctiva.

3. **What are the upper lid and lower lid retractors?**

   i. These lie between the anterior and the posterior lamella.
   ii. *Upper lid retractors:*
      - Levator palpebrae superioris
      - Muller's muscle
   iii. *Lower lid retractors:*
      Capsulopalpebral fascia
      Sympathetically innervated inferior tarsal muscle.

4. **What is capsulopalpebral fascia?**
    i. **Origin:** as capsulopalpebral head from delicate attachments to inferior rectus muscle.
   ii. Extends anteriorly and splits into two and surrounds the inferior oblique muscle.
  iii. Again rejoins to form the Lockwood's ligament and fascial tissue anterior to this forms the capsule palpebral fascia.
   iv. **Insertion:** on the inferior fornix along with inferior tarsal muscle and on inferior border of tarsus.

5. **How are the eyelids attached to the bony orbit?**
   Eyelids are attached to bony orbit via the medial and lateral tendons.
   Medial canthal tendon: 2 limbs
    i. Anterior (superficial)—attached to the anterior lacrimal crest
   ii. Posterior (deep)—attached to the posterior lacrimal crest
  iii. Lacrimal sac is enclosed between the two.
   iv. Common canaliculus lies immediately posterior to the anterior limb.
   Lateral canthal tendon:
    i. Laterally the tarsal plate becomes fibrous strands that form the crura of lateral canthal tendon.
   ii. The crura of upper and lower lid fuse to form common lateral canthal tendon.
  iii. It is about 1–3 mm thick and 5–7 mm long.
   iv. Insertion is 1.5 mm inside the lateral orbital rim on the Whitnall's tubercle as a part of the lateral retinaculum.
      Laxity of lateral canthal tendon is due to stretching and redundancy of the free portion of tendon between the tarsal plate and the tubercle.

6. **How is ectropion classified?**
   Classification:
   Upper lid ectropion
   Lower lid ectropion—more common
    i. Medial
   ii. Lateral
  iii. Total
   Etiologically
    i. Involutional
   ii. Cicatricial
  iii. Paralytic
   iv. Mechanical
    v. Congenital.

7. **How do we stage the severity of ectropion?**

    Staging

    i. *Mild:* Posterior lid margin just falls away from contact with globe
    ii. *Moderate:* Complete eversion of lid margin exposing the conjunctiva
    iii. *Severe:* Complete eversion of lid (tarsal ectropion).

8. **What are the clinical features of ectropion?**

    Clinical features:

    Can be asymptomatic

    i. **Punctal eversion:** This leads to decrease tear drainage and disuse punctal atrophy → epiphora → constant wiping → eczematous changes in the skin → further aggravation of the ectropion.
    ii. **Conjuctival exposure:** This leads to keratinization, hyperemia, xerosis → punctal stenosis and chronic conjunctivitis → chronic irritation and foreign body sensation.
    iii. **Corneal exposure:** It is due to improper closure of the lids → keratitis → pain, photophobia and decreased vision.

9. **How to clinically evaluate ectropion?**

    Clinical evaluation: Aim is → find type,

    i. Underlying mechanism and
    ii. Decide the appropriate treatment.

    It is done in 3 parts:

    i. *Ocular:*
    ii. *Local:* look for:
        – Herpes zoster dermatitis
        – Surgical scars
        – Traumatic scars
        – Facial anatomy and symmetry
        – Facial function
    iii. *Systemic:* look for:
        – Skin disorders, e.g. lamellar ichthyosis
        – Actinic dermatitis
        – Parkinsonism.

10. **How do you test for the following?**

    i. *Lid laxity:* 2 tests:
        – *Pinch/retraction/distraction test:* If central portion of lower lid can be pinched (between index finger and the thumb) and is able to be pulled >6 mm from the globe, significant lid laxity is present.
        – *Snap back test:* Central portion of lid is pulled and released; failure to snap back in its original position indicates lid laxity.

ii. ***Canthal tendon integrity:***
  – ***Lateral tendon:***
    • Rounding of the lateral canthal angle
    • Horizontal shortening of the palpebral fissure
    • Decrease in distance between temporal limbus and lateral canthal angle
    • Direct palpation of inferior crus of the lateral canthal tendon with simultaneous medial traction.
  – ***Medial tendon:***
    • Look for position of the punctum during lateral traction of the lid. Movement of punctum lateral to nasal limbus or displacement >3 mm indicates partial dehiscence
    • Rounding of the medial canthal angle
    • Direct palpation of the medial canthal tendon with simultaneous lateral traction.
iii. ***Orbicularis muscle tone:*** Ask the patient to squeeze the eyes tightly and try and open the eyes against resistance.
iv. ***Lower lid retractor disinsertion:***
  – Inferior fornix deeper than the normal
  – Higher resting position of the lower lid
  – Diminished excursion of lower lid in the downgaze.
  – Disinserted edge of the retractors may be seen as a whitish band in the inferior fornix below the inferior edge of the tarsus.
v. ***Lacrimal apparatus:*** Look for:
  – Direction of the punctum
  – Stenosis of the punctum
  – Patency of lacrimal drainage system
vi. ***Cicatricial component:*** Grasp the lower lid margin and pull superiorly; if it does not reach 2 mm above the inferior limbus → vertical deficiency present.
vii. ***Inferior scleral show:*** This is seen if associated with lid retraction. In such cases mere lid shortening procedures will aggravate the retraction and have to be combined with free full thickness skin graft.
viii. ***Orbitotarsal disparity:*** When contact and thereby pressure is inadequate between orbital contents and eyelid, there is lid instability.
ix. ***Corneal sensations:*** decreased sensations esp. in case of paralytic ectropion indicates early surgical intervention.
x. ***Lagophthalmos.***

11. What is involutional ectropion and the mechanisms of it?
  i. Involutional ectropion:
    – Most common
    – Gradual onset

- Most common in lower lid
- Earliest symptom: tearing
- Earliest sign: inferior punctal eversion

ii. Mechanisms:
- Laxity of both medial and lateral canthal tendon
- Partial dehiscence of the canthal tendon
- Orbicularis muscle undergoes ischemic changes due to microinfarcts → laxity
- Fragmentation of elastic and collagenous tissue within the tarsus leads to thinning and instability.
- Dehiscence of lower lid retractors.

12. **What is the management of involutional ectropion?**

Medical management:

i. To relieve tearing and inflammation, lubricating antibiotic ointment can be used.
ii. Antibiotic—steroid combination can be used preoperatively for 2–3 weeks to decrease eyelid edema and hyperemia.

Punctal ectropion: Following procedures can be done:

i. **Suture technique:**
- 2 double armed 5-0 chromic sutures are taken
- The first suture is taken at the inferior border of tarsus at junction of nasal and medial 1/3rd of lid
- The second is taken at similar position at junction of medial and lateral 1/3rd of lid
- Both emerge through skin at level of infraorbital rim

Advantage:

Useful in debilitated patients

Disadvantage:
- Temporary method
- Recurrence
- Foreshortening of the inferior fornix

ii. **Medial spindle procedure:** Also called as the tarsoconjunctival excision
- The lower punctum is inverted by vertically shortening the posterior lamella and tightening the lower lid retractors.
- Diamond shaped area (6 mm × 3 mm) of tarsoconjunctiva is excised below the punctum. Closed with absorbable sutures from upper apex to lower apex including the lower lid retractors.

iii. **Electrocautery:**
- Several deep burns placed 2 mm apart along the entire lower lid at the junction of conjunctiva and the lower margin of the tarsus

- Effect can be titrated by depth and duration of cauterization
- Recurrence is common

iv. **Punctoplasty:**
- Done in combination with ectropion, if associated with punctal stenosis
- One snip, two snip procedures can be employed

v. **Otis Lee procedure:**
- Done in case of severe punctal ectropion or in atonic medial ectropion involving both upper and lower puncta
- Horizontal incision at the junction of skin and conjunctiva medial to the puncta
- Lids joined with nonabsorbable suture
- Excess of skin is removed.

vi. **Smith's lazy-T procedure:**
- Done when medial ectropion is associated with horizontal lid laxity.
- Done when medial canthal tendon is firm
- Pentagonal wedge of excess horizontal eyelid tissue is resected 4 mm lateral to the punctum.
- This is coupled with excision of diamond of tarsoconjuctiva below the punctum to invert it.
- Conjunctiva is closed horizontally with interrupted catgut sutures
- Eyelid is closed.

vii. **Medial canthal tendon plication:**
- Indicated in excess medial tendon laxity
- Canalicular part of medial canthal tendon is shortened by suturing the medial end of lower tarsal plate to the main part of medial canthal tendon with nonabsorbable suture.

viii. **Pentagonal wedge resection:**
- Generalized ectropion with horizontal lid laxity
- No excess of skin is seen
- A full thickness pentagon is resected to correct the excess of horizontal lid laxity
- Done usually 5 mm from the lateral canthus or at the maximum lid laxity
- Lid defect is repaired

ix. **Smith's modification of Kuhnt–Szymanowski procedure:**
- Done when medial canthal tendon is firm
- Associated with horizontal lid laxity and excess of skin
- Subciliary blepharoplasty incision is made
- Pentagonal wedge resection is done to correct horizontal lid laxity

- Excess of skin is removed as a triangular flap
- Both skin and lid are closed.

x. **Lateral tarsal strip procedure:**
  - Done when ectropion is associated with horizontal lid laxity and lateral tendon laxity.
  - A subciliary incision is made from the lateral 2/5th of eyelid up to the lateral canthus and extending posteriorly.
  - Lateral canthotomy is done.
  - Inferior crux of lateral tendon is incised.
  - Tarsal strip is made by excising the mucosa cilia orbicularis and skin at the lateral end.
  - Lid is shortened by removing the excess tarsus.
  - Tarsal strip is sutured to lateral orbital tubercle.
  - Excess of skin is removed.

xi. **Edelstein–Dryden procedure:**
  - Done when ectropion is associated with mid facial trauma involving the lacrimal system.
  - Associated with detached posterior horn of medial tendon
  - Periosteal flap is made from nasal bone and everted and hinged medially to lacrimal sac fossa and sutured to nasal margin of the tendon.
  - Thus, a new posterior horn is created.

13. **What is cicatricial ectropion?**
  i. Seen in both upper and lower lid.
  ii. Associated with vertical shortening within the anterior lamella of lid.

Etiology:
  i. Trauma—mechanical, thermal, chemical, radiation
  ii. Actinic dermatitis
  iii. Herpes zoster dermatitis
  iv. Basal cell carcinoma
  v. Lamellar ichthyosis
  vi. Iatrogenic, e.g. post-blepharoplasty.

Management:
Medical: Ocular lubricants, soft contact lens, air humidification,
Digital massage of the scar
Steroids injection in the scar
Wait for 6 months post-trauma for scar to soften before surgery.
Surgical:
  i. **Z-plasty:**
    - Done for localized vertical scar crossing the skin tension lines.
    - Initial incision made along the scar and another incision at each end of the central line at an angle of 60°.

- Scar tissue is excised.
- Two flaps of skin are transposed which increase the length of the skin in the line of scar contraction at the expense of shortening the skin at right angles to it.
- It also alters the line of the scar.

   ii. **V-Y plasty:**
- Done for localized vertical scar but with minimal skin shortening.
- V shaped incision with apex of V at the base of scar
- Scar tissue is excised and V is closed as Y thereby lengthening the lid vertically.

   iii. **Skin replacement:**
- Indicated in generalized shortage of the skin
- Can be a transposition flap from the upper lid (if excess skin is present) or a thin full thickness skin graft (in case of extensive scarring).
- Skin graft can be taken from upper eyelid, retroauricular skin, supraclavicular area.

14. **What is paralytic ectropion?**
    i. Due to facial nerve palsy, a loss of orbicularis tone → tarsal instability and an ectropion
   ii. Preexisting involutional changes make the condition more pronounced
  iii. Associated with failure of lacrimal pump function
   iv. Other features of facial nerve palsy are seen.

15. **What is the management of paralytic ectropion?**
    Management: Primary goal is to protect cornea.
    i. *Medical:* apart from lubricants, moisture chambers, Donaldson's patch can be used.
   ii. *Surgical:* indications are
- Progressive corneal deterioration
- Permanent facial paralysis
- Corneal anesthesia
- Dry eye
- Lack of good Bell's phenomenon
- Monocular vision on the paralytic side

    Medial canthoplasty:
    i. Indicated in paralytic medial ectropion
   ii. Eyelids are sutured together medial to lacrimal puncta to reduce the increased vertical interpalpebral distance at the medial canthus

caused by the unopposed action of the lid retractors and to bring the lacrimal puncta into the tear film.

iii Excess of skin is cut.

Lateral canthal sling:

i. Usually combined with medial canthoplasty

ii. Indicated in generalized lid laxity.

Temporary suture tarsorrhaphy:

Facial sling:

Used to support the lid when large bulk of atonic midfacial tissue continues to drag down the lower lid. Commonly fascia lata is used.

Temporalis transfer:

Reserved for most severe cases that have recurred after previous surgery and in permanent facial nerve damage.

16. **What is mechanical ectropion?**

   i. Secondary to mechanical factor which either displaces the lid or pulls the lid out of its normal position against the globe.

   ii. For example, large lid tumors, conjunctival chemosis from orbital inflammatory conditions, severe lid edema.

   iii. *Management:* Treat the cause.

17. **What is congenital ectropion?**

   i. Rare, familial, but no Mendelian inheritance

   ii. Due to deficiency of eyelid skin → vertical shortening → ectropion

   iii. Associated with blepharophimosis syndrome

   iv. At rest the lids are apposed, but on attempt to look up or close the lids → eversion

   v. Treatment is horizontal lid tightening with free full thickness skin grafting.

18. **What are the features of upper lid ectropion?**

   i. Rare, congenital, common in black male infants, associated with trisomy-21

   ii. Usually bilateral

   iii. Can also be seen in cicatricial conditions, e.g. lamellar ichthyosis

   iv. Mechanisms: vertical shortening of anterior lamella, vertical lengthening of posterior lamella, failure of fusion between septum and levator aponeurosis and spasm of orbicularis.

   v. *Treatment:* Pressure patch over re-inverted lids
   Lid reconstruction procedures.

8.2. ENTROPION

1. **Define entropion.**

    Inward rotation of the eyelid margin such that the cilia brush against the globe.

2. **How do you classify entropion?**
    i.   Involutional entropion (senile entropion)
    ii. Cicatricial entropion
    iii. Congenital entropion
    iv. Spastic

3. **What is the pathophysiology of involutional entropion?**

    It affects mainly lower lid because upper lid has a wider tarsus and is more stable.

    Pathogenesis:
    i.   Horizontal lid laxity/medial and lateral tendon laxity.
    ii. Over riding of preseptal over pretarsal orbicularis during lid closure.
    iii. Lower lid retractor weakness (excursion decreased of lower lid in downgaze).

4. **What are the causes of cicatricial entropion?**

    Caused by severe scarring of the palpebral conjunctiva which pulls the lid margin toward the globe.

    Causes:
    i. **Infection**
        – Trachoma
        – Chronic blepharoconjunctivitis
        – Herpes zoster ophthalmicus
    ii. **Trauma**
        – Chemical
        – Mechanical
        – Radiation
    iii. **Immunological**
        – Erythema multiforme
        – Ocular cicatricial pemphigoid
        – Cicatricial vernal conjunctivtis
        – Dysthyroid.

5. **What is congenital entropion?**
    i. It is caused by the improper development of retractor aponeurosis insertion into inferior border of the tarsal plate.
    ii. It is extremely rare.

iii. Inversion of entire tarsus and lid margin

iv. Epiblepharon and horizontal tarsal kink are to be differentiated.

6. **How is congenital entropion classified?**

Classification is based on severity.

Kemp and Collin classification

i. **Minimal**
   - Apparent migration of meibomian glands
   - Conjunctivilization of lid margin
   - Lash globe contact on upgaze.

ii. **Moderate**

   Same features plus

   - Lid retraction
   - Thickening of tarsal plate.

iii. **Severe**

   Lid retraction (incomplete closure)

   - Gross lid retraction
   - Metaplastic lashes
   - Presence of keratin plaques.

7. **What are the examinations to be done in a case of entropion?**

i. *Lid margin and ocular surface*—look for signs of punctate kerato-pathy due to blepharitis, meibomianitis, trichiasis, foreign bodies, dry eyes, corneal disease

ii. *Lid instability*—forceful lid closure

   Excursion of the lower lid in downgaze usually 3–4 mm—loss of movement indicates retractor weakness/disinsertion

iii. *Lid laxity*—pinch test

iv. *Lid elasticity*—snap test

v. *Medial canthal tendon (MCT) laxity*

vi. *Cicatricial component*—see directly by everting the lids. It can also be ascertained by pulling the lid superiorly. If it does not reach 2 mm above the lower limbus, lid is vertically deficient.

vii. Syringing

viii. Jones dye test

ix. Schirmer's test.

8. **What are the preoperative evaluation tests to be done in a case of entropion?**

Preoperative evaluation/testing

i. **Assessment of capsulopalpebral fascia**
   - Higher eyelid resting position in primary gaze
   - Presence of white infratarsal band

- Increased depth of inferior conjunctival fornix
- Reduction in vertical eyelid excursion from upgaze to down gaze.

ii. **Assessment of horizontal eyelid laxity**
- Passive horizontal eyelid distraction.
- Hills test—central eyelid pulled >6 mm between eyelid and cornea—abnormal.

iii. **Enophthalmos**
- Assessment of relative enophthalmos—exophthalmometry.

iv. **Assessment of preseptal orbicularis muscle override**
- Subjective assessment—done in primary gaze/forceful eyelid closure/spontaneous blink.
- Thick appearance of eyelid.

v. **Assessment of posterior lamellar support**
- Height of tarsal plate

vi. **Presence of cicatrizing conjunctival disease**
- Trachoma
- Stevens–Johnson syndrome
- Ocular cicatricial pemphigoid
- Chronic meibomian gland dysfunction
- Chemical injury/topical medication

vii. **Corneal/conjunctival status**

viii. **Lash position/lacrimal and meibomian gland function.**

9. **What are the nonsurgical management of entropion?**
   i. Taping
   ii. Treatment of associated blepharitis, meibomianitis, corneal disease
   iii. Lubricants
   iv. Botulinum toxin injection
   v. Bandage contact lenses.

10. **What are the temporary surgical measures in involutional entropion?**
   i. *Transverse sutures* are placed through the lid to prevent the upward movement of the preseptal orbicularis muscle.
   ii. *Everting sutures* are placed obliquely to shorten the lower lid retractors and transfer their pull to the upper border of the tarsus.
   iii. *Transverse sutures*—3 doubled armed 4-0 catgut sutures are taken through the lid from the conjunctiva to the skin in the lateral two thirds of the lid. Start below tarsus and make each needle emerge through the skin about 2 mm apart, just below the level at which they entered the conjunctiva.
   iv. *Everting sutures*—they are similar but start lower in the fornix and emerge nearer to the lashes.
   v. Sutures are removed after 10–14 days

11. What are the principles of permanent treatment in involutional entropion?

Strengthening the lid retractors as in Jones, Reeh, Wobigs and modified Jones procedure where the inferior lid retractors are plicated or attached to the tarsus.

Shortening the anterior lamina by suturing the preseptal orbicularis to pretarsal orbicularis so as to prevent migration of orbicularis, forming a cicatrix between the two parts of orbicularis.

Removal of horizontal lid laxity if present by tarsal strip procedure, where small strip of lid margin, conjunctiva and skin are removed to create a free end of the tarsal plate that functions as the canthal ligament.

12. What is Weiss procedure?

 i. Transverse lid split + everting sutures.

 ii. This is indicated in cases with minimum horizontal lid laxity when long term results are required.

13. What is Quickert procedure?

 i. Transverse lid split + everting sutures + horizontal lid shortening.

 ii. This is a long term procedure for cases where horizontal lid laxity also presents.

14. What is Jones procedure?

Plication of lower lid retractors.

Indication: Recurrence after Quickert's procedure

15. What are the steps of modified Jones procedure?

 i. Mark a subciliary incision along the length of the lid. If there is lengthening the amount of shortening required should be marked.

 ii. Incision is made into the skin—muscle upto the tarsal plate. The tarsal plate is exposed.

 iii. Blunt dissection is continued at inferior margin of tarsus. The stretched is dehisced. Retractors will be visible.

 iv. Three double armed 6-0 vicryl sutures are passed; the retractors may be plicated or simply reattached. The 3 sutures are tightened and correction observed. The straightening of margin is immediately seen. The end point is when the posterior margin is just apposed to the globe.

 v. The skin and muscle lamina usually needs to be shortened and is excised in a spindle manner.

 vi. Associated lengthening—by excising the lid in full thickness pentagonal shape (Bick's procedure)

 vii. Sutures are removed in 6–7 days

16. **What is the surgical procedure for congenital entropion?**

    Hotz procedure

    Minimal ellipse of skin and orbicularis is excised from medial two thirds of the lower lid.

    Skin is fixed to lower edge of the tarsus.

17. **What is the management of cicatricial entropion?**

    Marginal incision and grafting

    Tarsal fracture and margin rotation—Tenzel procedure—indicated when lid retraction is <1.5 mm from the limbus.

    Posterior lamellar grafting in cases of posterior lamellar shortening—indicated when lid retraction is >1.5 mm from the limbus.

    Tarsal wedge resection—common procedure used in cases with trachomatous scarring (especially if tylosis is present).

18. **What are the various materials used as posterior lamellar grafts?**
    i. Conchal cartilage
    ii. Nasal chondromucosa
    iii. Palatal mucoperichondrium
    iv. Buccal mucosa
    v. Tarsoconjunctival composite graft
    vi. Mucous membrane graft
    vii. Amniotic membrane transplant—now becoming more popular

19. **What are the complications after surgery for entropion?**
    i. *Recurrence*—it is the most common complication of surgical correction of entropion.
    ii. *Ectropion*—possible mechanisms include excessive skin removal, over advancement of the retractors onto the anterior face of the tarsal plate. Shortening of the septum, hematoma and excessive scar formation.
    iii. *Lagophthalmos*—shortened septum—warm compresses and massage with corticosteroid ointment may correct mild cases.
    iv. *Lid necrosis*—margin rotation techniques commoner.
    v. *Lid infection, wound dehiscence*
    vi. *Graft complications*—symblepharon, corneal injury induced by rough posterior eyelid surface.

8.3. PTOSIS

1. **What is the definition of blepharoptosis?**

   Drooping or inferior displacement of upper eyelid.

2. **How will you classify blephroptosis?**

   Two classification systems.

   According to onset:
   i. Congenital
   ii. Acquired

   According to cause:
   i. Neurogenic
      - Third nerve palsy
      - Third nerve misdirection
      - Horner's syndrome
      - Marcus Gunn jaw-winking syndrome
   ii. Myogenic
      - Myasthenia gravis
      - Myotonic dystrophy
      - Ocular myopathies
      - Simple congenital
      - Blepharophimosis syndrome
   iii. Aponeurotic
      - Involutional attenuation
      - Repetitive traction like rigid contact lenses
   iv. Mechanical
      - Plexiform neuroma
      - Hemangioma
      - Acquired neoplasm

3. **What are the components of ptosis workup?**

   i. Palpebral fissure height
   ii. Margin reflex distance
   iii. Margin crease distance
   iv. LPS action
   v. Lagophthalmos
   vi. Bell's phenomenon
   vii. Marcus Gunn phenomenon
   viii. Tarsal height
   ix. Pupillary reaction
   x. Corneal sensation
   xi. Ocular movements

xii. Fatigability test
xiii. Cogan's lid twitch sign
xiv. Ice pack test

4. **How can we classify the amount of ptosis based on relationship between upper lid level and pupil?**
    i.   Mild—upper eyelid margin just above the upper border of pupil
    ii. Moderate—upper eyelid margin at the upper border of pupil or covering half of the pupil
    iii. Severe—upper eyelid margin at or below the lower border of pupil

5. **How to classify amount of blephroptosis?**
    The difference in marginal reflex distance (MRD) 1 of the two sides in unilateral cases
    Or
    The difference from normal in bilateral cases gives the amount of ptosis.

    Amount of ptosis may be classified as:
    i.   Mild ptosis   — 2 mm or less
    ii. Moderate ptosis   — 3 mm
    iii. Severe ptosis   — 4 mm or more

6. **What is the normal position of the upper lid?**
    The upper lid margin covers 1–2 mm of the superior cornea

7. **What is the Whitnall's ligament?**
    Whitnall's (superior transverse) ligament is a sleeve of elastic fibers around the levator muscle located in the area of transition from levator muscle to levator aponeurosis. It functions to convert the anterior-posterior vector force of the levator to a superior-inferior direction during eyelid movement

8. **What is MRD1 and its significance?**
    Margin reflex distance (MRD)
    The distance between the center of the lid margin of the upper lid and the light reflex on the cornea in primary position would give the MRD1.
    i.   If the margin is above the light reflex, the MRD1 has a **positive value**.
    ii. If the lid margin is below the corneal reflex in cases of very severe ptosis the MRD1 would have a **negative value**. The latter would be calculated by keeping the scale at the middle of upper lid margin and elevating the lid till the corneal light reflex is visible. The distance between the reflex and the marked original upper lid margin would be the MRD1.
    iii. MRD1 is the single most effective measurement in describing the amount of ptosis.

Margin reflex distance 1 (MRD1): Normal 4–5 mm

The mean measurement in Indian eyes is 4.1 ± 0.5

It must be remembered that ptotic lid in unilateral congenital ptosis is usually higher in down gaze due to the failure of levator to relax.
The ptotic lid in acquired ptosis is invariably lower than the normal lid in down gaze.

9. **What is margin reflex distance 2 (MRD2)?**

   MRD2 is the distance from corneal light reflex to lower eyelid margin.

10. **What are various methods to evaluate levator function?**

    i. **Berke's method (lid excursion)**

    Measures the excursion of the upper lid from extreme down gaze to extreme upgaze with action of frontalis muscle blocked.
    The patient is positioned against a wall while the surgeon's hands press the forehead above the eyebrows ensuring that there is no downward or upward push. The patient is then asked to look at extreme downgaze and then in extreme upgaze and the readings are recorded in millimeters. Crowell Beard reported normal eyelid excursion to be between 12–17 mm.

    ii. **The levator function is classified as:**

    | 8 mm or more | — Good |
    | 5–7 mm | — Fair |
    | 4 mm | — Poor |

    iii. **Putterman's method**

    This is carried out by the measurement of distance between the middle of upper lid margin to the 6'o clock limbus in extreme upgaze. This is also known as the margin limbal distance (MLD).
    Normal is about 9.0 mm.
    The difference in MLD of two sides in unilateral cases
    (Or)
    The difference with normal in bilateral cases multiplied by three would give the amount of levator resection required.

    iv. **Assessment in children**

    Measurement of levator function in small children is a difficult task. The presence of lid fold and increase or decrease on its size on movement of the eyelid gives us a clue to the levator action. Presence of anomalous head posture like the child throwing his head back suggests a poor levator action.

    v. **Iliff test**

    This is another indicator of levator action. It is applicable in first year of life. The upper eyelid of the child is everted as the child looks down. If the levator action is good, the eyelid reverts back on its own.

11. **What is palpebral fissure height?**

    i. It is the distance between the upper and lower lid margins, measured in pupillary plane.

    ii. The upper lid margin normally rests about 2 mm below the upper limbus and the lower lid margin rests 1 mm above or at the level of lower limbus.

        Normal value

        Males   : 7–10 mm

        Females   : 8–12 mm

    iii. It is measured after negating the frontalis action.

12. **What is the margin crease distance (MCD)? What is its significance?**

The MCD is the distance from the central eyelid margin to the central upper lid skin crease with the upper lid in the down gaze and skin fold slightly elevated to expose the crease

Normal values: Varies with race and gender

In Indians,

Male—5–7 mm

Female—7–9 mm

The insertion of the fibers from the levator muscle into the skin contributes to the formation of the upper eyelid crease. The significance is twofold:

    i. The crease is usually elevated in patients with involutional ptosis and is often shallow or absent in patients with congenital ptosis.

    ii. MCD helps in marking the incision site on the eyelid.

13. **What is Bell's phenomenon?**

It is the involuntary protective reflex producing upward rotation of eyeball on closure of the eye. This is referred to as Bell's phenomenon.

Confirmation of presence of Bell's phenomenon is important before undertaking any surgical procedure to avoid risk of postoperative exposure keratopathy.

14. **How do we grade Bell's phenomenon?**

Good—less than one third of the inferior part of the cornea visible

Fair—one third to one half of the inferior part of the cornea visible

Poor—more than one half of the inferior part of the cornea visible

15. **What are the different types of Bell's phenomenon?**

    i. Normal: Upward and outward movement of eyeball.

    ii. Inverse: Upward and inward movement of eyeball.

    iii. Reverse: Downward movement of eyeball.

    iv. Perverse: Lateral movement of eyeball.

16. How is tarsal height measured and what is its significance?

The upper lid is everted and the vertical height of the tarsus is measured over the central portion of the lid with a calliper. This measurement is usually between 10 and 12 mm in Caucasians and between 6.5 mm and 7.5 mm in Asians. This is the range between low, medium and high crease height.

The height of the tarsus determines the overall central position of the crease during blepharoplasty. The shaved–off tip of wooden cotton tip applicator dipped with methylene blue is ideal for drawing a thin crease line. The crease height is carefully transcribed onto the external skin surface over the central part of the eyelid skin.

This point directly overlies the superior tarsal border and will serve as a reference point for the overall crease height along the central one third of the eyelid, whether the crease shape is to be nasally tapered, parallel or laterally flared.

For those patients who already have a crease the tarsal height still has to be measured to confirm the apparent crease seen is indeed the correct crease line to use.

17. What is pseudoptosis?

Pseudoptosis is false impression of eyelid drooping. It may be caused by:

   i. *Lack of support* of lids by the globe as in artificial eye, microphthalmos, phthisis bulbi or enophthalmos.
   ii. Contralateral lid retraction
   iii. *Ipsilateral hypotropia.* The pseudoptosis will disappear when hypotropic eye assumes fixation on covering the normal eye.
   iv. *Brow ptosis* due to excessive skin on brow or seventh nerve palsy.
   v. *Dermatochalasis* in which excessive upper lid skin overhangs the eyelid margin.

18. What is Marcus Gunn jaw winking syndrome?

It is the most common type of congenital synkinetic neurogenic ptosis. About 5% of congenital ptosis manifests this phenomenon.

This synkinesis is thought to be caused by aberrant connection between motor division of cranial nerve 5 and levator muscle.

Signs:

Retraction of ptotic lid in conjunction with stimulation of the ipsilateral pterygoid muscles by chewing, sucking, opening the mouth or contralateral jaw movement.

Jaw winking does not improve with age, although patient may learn to mask it.

Treatment:

No surgical treatment is entirely satisfactory.

Management depends on the cosmetic significance of the jaw winking, where jaw winking is not significant the choice of procedure depends on the amount of ptosis and the levator action is carried out as in any case of congenital simple ptosis. A larger levator resection is necessary and under correction is common. In case with significant jaw winking bilateral levator excision with a fascia lata, sling surgery is the procedure of choice.

19. How is Marcus Gunn phenomenon graded?

Elevation of upper lid on jaw movement	Degree of Marcus Gunn phenomenon
Symmetrization with opposite eye	Mild
To upper lid	Moderate
Beyond upper limbus	Severe

Retraction of lid	Degree of Marcus Gunn phenomenon
2 mm	Mild
2–5 mm	Moderate
More than 5 mm	Severe

20. How do you differentiate congenital ptosis from acquired ptosis?

Characteristics	Congenital ptosis	Acquired ptosis
Cause	Myogenic (poorly developed levator muscle)	Aponeurotic (stretching or even disinsertion of levator aponeurosis)
Palpebral fissure height	Mild-to-severe ptosis	Mild-to-severe ptosis
Upper lid crease	Weak or absent crease in normal position	Higher than normal crease
Levator function	Reduced	Near normal
Downgaze	Eyelid lag	Eyelid drop
Amblyopia	Commonly seen in 20%	uncommon
Marcus Gunn jaw winking phenomenon	May or may not be present.	Absent

21. What is BPES?

The blepharophimosis–ptosis–epicanthus inversus syndrome is an auto-somal-dominant condition with marked hypoplasia of the tarsal plate. Blepharophimosis is a reduction in the maximum vertical distance between the upper and lower eyelids combined with short palpebral fissure.

Two clinical types:

BPES 1: Transmission through males only. Associated menstrual irregularity and infertility due to ovarian failure

BPES 2 : No associated infertility and transmitted through both sexes.

22. **What are the precautions to be undertaken before administering local anesthesia for ptosis surgery?**

After appropriate marking, the upper eyelid is typically infiltrated with a small volume of local anesthetic, typically 1–1.5 mL of 1–2% lidocaine mixed with epinephrine, in a subcutaneous plane. The anesthetic paralyses the orbicularis oculi muscle and the epinephrine can stimulate the Muller's muscle, rendering the intraoperative eyelid position higher than what is expected post-operatively. To avoid this, some surgeons will set the eyelid height 1 to 1.5 mm higher than the desired postoperative position. Care should be taken not to pierce the orbital septum while injecting local anesthesia as excess anesthesia can weaken the levator making intraoperative assessment difficult. Allowing the epinephrine 7–10 minutes to work, increases its hemostatic effect allowing better visualization of tissue planes

23. **What are various options for ptosis repair?**

Ptosis repair is a challenging oculoplastic surgical procedure.

Nonsurgical treatment—are unusual but may include devices called eyelid crutches that are attached to eyeglass frames. They are occasionally useful in patients with neurogenic or myogenic ptosis in whom surgical correction can lead to severe, exposure related corneal problems.

It is advisable to wait till 3–4 years of age for surgical correction when the tissues are mature enough to withstand the surgical trauma and a better assessment and postoperative care is possible due to improved patient cooperation. There should be no delay in surgical management in cases of severe ptosis where pupil is obstructed and the possibility of the development of amblyopia is high.

Surgical approach depends on whether
  i. Ptosis is unilateral or bilateral
 ii. Severity of ptosis
iii. Levator action
 iv. Presence of abnormal ocular movements, jaw winking phenomena or blepharophimosis syndrome.

The choice of surgical procedure is as follows:

Fasanella–Servat operation
  i. Mild ptosis (<2 mm or less)
 ii. Levator action >10 mm
iii. Well defined lid fold—no excess skin

Levator resection

  i. Mild/moderate/severe ptosis

 ii. Levator action ≥4 mm

Brow suspension ptosis repair

  i. Severe ptosis

 ii. Levator action <4 mm

iii. Jaw-winking ptosis or blepharophimos is syndrome

Bilateral ptosis

In cases of bilateral ptosis, simultaneous bilateral surgery is preferred to ensure a similar surgical intervention in the two eyes. However in cases where gross asymmetry exists between the two eyes, the eye with a greater ptosis is operated first and the other eye is operated after 6–8 weeks when the final correction of the operated.

24. **What are the indications and contraindications of various ptosis repair procedures?**

Fasanella–Servat operation

Indications:

   i. Ptosis <2 mm

  ii. Levator function >10 mm

 iii. Mild congenital ptosis

  iv. Horner's syndrome

   v. Senile (involutional) ptosis

  vi. Minor contour adjustment, after previous ptosis or other upper lid surgery

 vii. Well defined lid fold—no excess skin

Contraindications:

  i. Dry eye syndromes

 ii. Corneal diseases

iii. Bleb

Levator resection

Indications:

  i. Mild/moderate/severe ptosis

 ii. Levator function ≥4 mm

Contraindications:

   i. Levator function <4 mm

  ii. Poor Bell's phenomenon

 iii. Decreased corneal sensation

  iv. Decreased tear production

Brow suspension

Indications:

i. Severe ptosis
ii. Levator function <4 mm
iii. After levator excision surgery (done previously)
iv. Blepharophimosis
v. Jaw winking
vi. Infants where levator function is not assessable (to prevent amblyopia)

Contraindications:

i. Mild to moderate ptosis with good levator function
ii. Absent Bell's phenomenon
iii. Restricted elevation (do under correction)

(e.g. CPEO, ocular myopathies, long-standing III nerve palsy)

25. **What are the various surgical steps in the different techniques for ptosis correction?**

Modified Fasanella–Servat Surgery:

It is done for:

i. Mild ptosis (<2 mm or less)
ii. Levator action >10 mm

It is the excision of tarsoconjunctiva, Muller's muscle and levator.

Xylocaine with adrenaline is used for local anesthesia in adults but general anesthesia is necessary for children.

Surgical steps

i. Three sutures are passed close to the folded superior margin of the tarsal plate at the junction of middle, lateral and medial one-third of the lid.
ii. Three corresponding sutures are placed close to the everted lid margin starting from conjunctival aspect near the superior fornix in positions corresponding to the first 3 sutures.
iii. Proposed incision is marked on the tarsal plate such that a uniform piece of tarsus, decreasing gradually towards the periphery is excised.
iv. A groove is made on the marked line of incision and the incision is completed with a scissor. The first set of sutures help in lifting the tarsal plate for excision.
v. The tarsal plate not more than 3 mm in width is excised.

Levator Resection

This is the most commonly practised surgery for ptosis correction. It may be performed through skin or conjunctival route.

Surgical steps

i. The proposed lid crease is marked to match the normal eye considering the margin crease.
ii. Incision through the skin and orbicularis is made along the crease marking.
iii. The inferior skin and orbicularis are dissected away from the tarsal plate.
iv. The upper edge is separated from the orbital septum.
v. The fibers of the aponeurosis are cut from their insertion in the inferior half of the anterior surface of the tarsus.
vi. The levator is freed from the adjoining structures.
vii. The lateral and the medial horn are cut whenever a large resection is planned.
viii. Care should be taken that Whitnall's ligament is not damaged.
ix. A double armed 5-0 vicryl is passed through the center of the tarsal plate by a partial thickness bite.
x. It is then passed through the levator aponeurosis at height judged by the preoperative evaluation. Intraoperative assessment is made.
xi. Two more double armed vicryl 5-0 sutures are passed through the tarsus about 2 mm from the upper border in the center and at the junction of central third with the medial and lateral thirds.
xii. These sutures are then placed in the levator and intraoperative assessment made.
xiii. Excess levator is excised.
xiv. Four to five lid fold forming sutures are placed.

Brow suspension repair

This surgery is the procedure of choice in simple congenital ptosis with a poor levator action. A number of materials like nonabsorbable sutures, extended polytetrafluoroethylene (ePTFE), muscle strips, banked or fresh fascia lata strips have been used for suspension.

Temporary sling

Thread sling is carried out in very young children with severe ptosis where prevention of amblyopia and uncovering the pupil is the main aim.

The suture sling procedures have a relatively higher recurrence rate of or may show formation of suture granuloma. Definitive surgery may be performed at a later date when a fascia lata sling is carried out.

Fascia lata sling

It is considered in children above four years of age having severe congenital simple ptosis with poor levator action. Even in cases of unilateral severe ptosis a bilateral procedure is preferred because a unilateral surgery causes marked asymmetry in downgaze. Results of bilateral surgery are more acceptable.

26. **How will you estimate the amount of levator resection?**

Degree of ptosis	LPS function	Amount of levator resection needed	Ideal postoperative correction
Mild (<2 mm)	Good (>8 mm)	Small (10–13 mm) Moderate (14–17 mm)	Undercorrect by 1–3 mm
Moderate (3 mm)	Moderate (5–7 mm) Poor (<5 mm)	Large (18–22 mm) Maximum 23 mm or more)	Match the normal lid; Fully correct the ptosis
Severe (>4 mm)	Poor (<5 mm)	Supra-maximal (>27 mm)	Overcorrect by 1–2 mm

27. **How do we manage a patient with ptosis and strabismus?**

Vertical strabismus—strabismus surgery first followed by ptosis correction after 3 months. For example, hypotropia can cause pseudoptosis. In such condition, correction of the squint corrects the ptosis also.

Horizontal Strabismus—can be done at the same sitting

28. **Timing of surgery for congenital ptosis:**

Correct ptosis by 5 years of age. If possible it is advisable to wait till 3–4 years of age in cases of congenital ptosis. The following advantages are obtained:

  i. Better assessment is possible
 ii. Tissues are better developed to withstand surgical trauma
iii. Better postoperative care is possible due to better cooperation

However, exception to this timing are bilateral or unilateral ptosis where there is complete obscuration of the visual axis.

29. **Two techniques of brow suspension surgery?**

  i. Crawford's technique
 ii. Fox's technique

30. **Points to present in a case of ptosis.**

		Normal
1	Vertical palpebral fissure height	9–10 mm
2	Marginal reflex distance 1	4–5 mm
3	Marginal reflex distance 2	4–5 mm
4	Levator function	12–17 mm
5	Margin crease distance	Males—5–7 mm Females—7–9 mm
6	Bell's phenomenon	
7	Lagophthalmos	
8	Marcus–Gunn phenomenon	

8.4. EYELID RECONSTRUCTION

1. **What are the common causes of eyelid defects?**

   Eyelid tissue loss is usually the result of trauma or resection of a patho-logic process such as tumor or segmental trichiasis.

   i. **Defects due to trauma**

   Eyelid wounds, especially those resulting from trauma, tend to gape widely giving the unnerving appearance of a large amount of tissue loss. Fortunately, the eyelid is quite elastic and a large majority of these defects can be repaired with direct closure.

   ii. **Defects due to surgical resection of tumor**

   Reconstruction of the eyelid is simplified by the technique of resec-tion. Resection of a lesion of the eyelid should be made with full thickness incisions.

2. **What are the principles of eyelid reconstruction?**

   i. The repair depends on its size and position and the state of surround-ing tissues.

   ii. Components which require consideration include the posterior lamella, the anterior lamella, both lamella or a full-thickness defect, the medial and lateral canthi and the lacrimal drainage system.

   iii. The approach should proceed by considering direct repair first, fol-lowed by lateral cantholysis and then a tissue transfer procedure using either a flap and/or a graft.

3. **What is the anesthesia required?**

   i. Local anesthesia for repair of eyelid lacerations is best obtained by performing a regional block. Anesthesia of most of the lower eyelid can be obtained by injecting 1cc of anesthetic into the infraorbital foramen.

   ii. Anesthesia of the upper lid is obtained by blocking the supraor-bital nerve. Again, additional anesthesia may be necessary laterally because of the lacrimal nerve. Anesthesia to the medial canthal area and lacrimal sac is obtained by blocking the infratrochlear nerve.

4. **What are the preoperative preparations?**

   i. The eye should be anesthetized with xylocaine eye drops. A corneal shield lubricated with antibiotic ointment is useful. The surrounding skin should be prepped with betadine but the solution should not be used to cleanse the wound. The wound should be irrigated profusely with warmed saline. All dirt and foreign particles should be cleansed, especially embedded dirt which can cause permanent discoloration and tattooing.

ii. Wound edges should be minimally debrided of all necrotic tissue. Irregular edges should be freshened to allow for straight surgical margins to suture together. Identifiable landmarks such as eyebrows or eyelid margins should be sutured first.

5. **Classify common reconstruction options of periocular defects.**

Region and defect	Closure option	Indication
Eyelids		
Partial thickness (anterior lamellar)	Primary closure Local skin and myocutaneous flap Full-thickness skin graft	
Full-thickness	Primary closure	Defects <15 mm or <25% of lid margin
	Primary closure + lateral canthotomy + cantholysis	Defects 25–50% of lid margin
	Tenzel semicircular flap	Defects of 50–75% of lid margin
	Hughes tarsoconjunctival flap + full-thickness skin graft or local flap	Lower eyelid defects >75% of lid margin
	Cutler–Beard technique	Upper eyelid defects >75% of lid margin
	Free graft for posterior lamella + local flap for anterior lamella	Defects >75% of lid margin
	Mustarde rotating cheek and opposing lid flaps	Large lid defects >75%
	Composite lid grafts	Defects <8 mm of lid margin
Medial canthus		
	Local flaps (e.g. nasoglabellar transposition flap	
	Paramedian forehead flap	
	Full-thickness skin grafts	
	Combination of above	
Lateral canthus		
	Local flaps	
	Full-thickness skin grafts	

6. **What are the procedures for repairing anterior lamellar defects?**
   i. Direct skin closure
   ii. Skin flaps
   iii. Skin graft: (a) full thickness; (b) partial thickness.

7. How is direct skin repair done?

Wounds involving a small loss of partial thickness eyelid skin with an intact eyelid margin can usually be closed primarily. Skin can be closed with 6-0 or 7-0 silk in adults and 7-0 chromic gut in children. If tissue closure results in some tension, the wound should be closed with horizontal tension rather than vertical tension to try avoiding ectropion. Sutures can be removed at 5–7 days and scar massage beginning in one week after suture removal.

8. What are the various types of skin flaps used?

   i. *V-Y plasty*—to lengthen structures, e.g. telecanthus repair and close defects. Glabellar flap is its variant.

   ii. *Rhomboid flap*—used in closure of medial and lateral periorbital defects. The rhombic flap is useful for non-marginal lesions where vertical tension on the eyelids can be avoided.

   iii. *Z-plasty*—to increase the length of skin and to change the direction of scar.

9. What are the various type of skin grafts used for anterior lamellar repair?

   i. **Full-thickness skin grafts**

A full-thickness skin graft contains both epidermal and dermal components. For eyelid reconstruction, the contralateral eyelid is the best donor site. If not enough tissue can be obtained from there, the postauricular region and supraclavicular region are also good choices. All donor sites should be hairless to avoid trichiasis.

After harvesting the full-thickness graft in the standard way, the graft is sewn into place. A standard bolster is then placed. The dressing may be removed in five days.

   ii. **Split-thickness skin grafts**

A split-thickness skin graft (STSG) is composed of epidermal components only. STSGs have a poor texture and color match with eyelid skin and tend to contract more than full-thickness grafts. They, therefore, are not used very much in eyelid reconstruction unless there is no other alternative (e.g. a badly burned patient without full-thickness skin to harvest). Usually taken from inner arm or thigh.

10. What are the various procedures for posterior lamellar reconstruction?

Posterior lamellar graft:

   i. Tarsal rotation

   ii. Hughes procedure

   iii. Ear cartilage graft

   iv. Mucous membrane graft

   v. Tarsoconjunctival graft.

11. What is the principle of posterior lamellar graft?

The posterior lamella consists of tarsus and conjunctiva. In cases of posterior lamellar shortening grafts like sclera, cartilage, mucosa graft can be used to lengthen posterior lamella. In upper lid, grafts are placed between tarsus and LPs. In lower lid grafts are placed between tarsus and lower lid retractors.

12. What is free tarsoconjunctival graft?

For full-thickness defects that are too large to close primarily, a graft taken from the posterior surface of the ipsilateral or contralateral upper eyelid will provide both conjunctiva and tarsus to reconstruct the posterior lamella. The donor site is left to granulate. The graft is sutured to the residual tarsus or canthal tendons in the recipient site and then covered by a sliding myocutaneous flap to reconstruct the anterior lamella. This technique works equally well for the lower or upper eyelid.

13. What is Hughes tarsoconjunctival flap and skin graft procedure?

The Hughes procedure is a two-staged operation for reconstruction of total or near total lower eyelid defects. As with the free tarsoconjunctival graft, a block of tarsus and conjunctiva is marked out on the ipsilateral upper lid. However, the upper border is left attached superiorly and a conjunctival flap is dissected off of the underlying Müller's muscle to the superior fornix. The tarsal flap is advanced down into the lower lid defect and sutured to residual tarsus or canthal tendons and the lower lid retractors. The anterior lamella is reconstructed with a skin graft or myocutaneous flap. After three weeks the conjunctival flap is cut off along the new lower lid margin.

14. How to repair eyelid defects with eyelid margin involvement?

i. The wound edges should be sharply trimmed (minimally). A 6-0 or 7-0 silk is first placed through a meibomian gland 3 mm from eyelid margin to depth of 3 mm. The suture is brought out of the laceration and into the other side 3 mm deep to the lid margin emerging 3 mm from the laceration. The second suture is placed in a similar fashion through the posterior lash line. The third is placed between these in the gray line. They are tied anteriorly and left long.

ii. The tarsus is then closed by placing absorbable suture through 3/4th to 7/8th of the tarsal thickness. Full thickness bites of the tarsus in the upper lid would expose to the conjunctival surface and most likely cause a corneal abrasion. Heavier suture should be used for the lower lid tarsus (5-0 chromic) than the upper lid tarsus (6-0 chromic) because there is greater tension on the lower lid.

iii. The skin can then be closed with 6-0 or 7-0 interrupted silks with the eyelid margin sutures tucked under the eyelash margin sutures to keep from touching the cornea. Skin sutures can be removed in 5–7 days, while the eyelid margin sutures should remain for 10–14 days.

15. What is lateral cantholysis?

For full-thickness defects with moderate loss of tissue, closure may be obtained by performing a lateral canthotomy with cantholysis. The lateral canthotomy is performed by making a horizontal cut from the lateral canthus to the orbital margin using a straight Stevens scissors. This maneuver splits the tendon into an upper and lower limb. An additional 3–5 mm of length can be obtained by cutting either limb (depending on which eyelid is involved). The eyelid margin can then be closed. The skin of the lateral canthotomy can be closed with 6-0 silk.

16. How will you classify full thickness lid defect repair?

1. *Horizontal extent of defect*
   Can be classified as
   i. <30%
   ii. 30–50% defect
   iii. >50% defect

2. *Assess the vertical extent of the defect*
   i. Vertically shallow (5–10 mm)
      • Skin mobilization and posterior lamellar reconstruction
   ii. Intermediate (10–15 mm)
      • Skin flap and posterior lamellar reconstruction
   iii. Large vertical (>15 mm)
      • Rotation flap + posterior lamellar reconstruction.

17. How is the procedure of semicircular flap of Tenzel done?

i. This flap is a variation of the lateral cantholysis. It adds rotation to the lateral advancement. A full thickness semicircular flap of skin and orbicularis muscle which is high arched, [i.e. vertical diameter (22 mm) is more than horizontal diameter (19 mm)] is fashioned superior to the lateral canthal angle for lower eyelid defects and inferior to the lateral canthal angle for upper eyelid defects.

ii. After cantholysis and wide undermining is performed, the flap is rotated to close the defect with minimal tension. Again, it is important to secure the deep orbicularis musculature to the periosteum to prevent drooping of the lateral canthal angle.

18. **What are the various skin muscle flaps used for full thickness eyelid reconstruction?**
     i. Temporal advancement flap
     ii. Semicircular flap of Tenzel
     iii. Mustarde cheek rotation flap
     iv. Median forehead flap
     v. Temporal forehead or frickle flap
     vi. Cutler–Beard flap
     vii. Glabellar flap.

19. **What is Cutler–Beard or bridge procedure?**
     i. The Cutler–Beard procedure is used for repair of large full-thickness defects of the upper lid.
     ii. The true width of the defect should be determined by grasping the cut tarsal edges with a forceps.
     iii. The horizontal width of the defect is then marked on the lower lid 1–2 mm below the inferior tarsal border. This avoids compromising the marginal artery of the lower eyelid.
     iv. The horizontal incision is placed through skin and conjunctiva. Vertical incisions (usually 1–2 cm) are made full-thickness into the lower fornix until enough laxity exists to allow the flap to advance.
     v. The flap is then brought beneath the bridge of the lower eyelid margin and tarsus to cover the globe. It is then sutured into the upper lid defect.
     vi. The dressing is important for the success of this flap. It is important to avoid any pressure on the inferior margin bridge of tissue. A protective shield should be worn until the flap is taken down 6–8 weeks later. This is accomplished by severing the flap about 2 mm from the desired lid margin. Again, the conjunctival side should be longer than the skin side so that it can wrap around and create a new lid margin.

20. **What is the Mustarde cheek rotation flap?**
     i. It is useful for reconstruction of very large lower eyelid defects, especially if the defect extends into the cheek tissue.
     ii. The flap is created by making an incision at the lateral canthus which extends superolaterally then curving inferiorly to just in front of the ear. Wide undermining is then done (beware of facial nerve branches) to allow the flap to rotate.
     iii. This flap is not used as much anymore because the thick cheek skin does not make a good match with the eyelid skin. Additionally, it

has the potential for numerous complications including facial nerve paralysis, sagging of the lateral canthal angle, ectropion, pseudotrichiasis from facial skin hairs and cheek flap necrosis.

21. **What is glabellar flap?**
    i. It is used for repair of defects involving medial canthus and medial part of upper lid. In it, a V-Y flap is advanced and rotated from glabellar region.
    ii. An inverted V incision is made in midline of the brow. The flap is undermined and is sutured into the defect.

22. **What are the precautions to be employed before closure of wounds?**
    i. Ensure complete hemostasis and remove all blood clots
    ii. Eliminate tension in wound edges by adequate undermining
    iii. There should be no dead space
    iv. Meticulous wound closure in layers. Adequate closure of deeper tissues using inverted mattress suture.
    v. Ensure eversion of wound edges and no overlapping.

23. **What are the important points to be kept in mind while suturing non marginal lid defects?**
    i. Smaller defects can be sutured without undermining.
    ii. Round defect should be converted into elliptical shape.
    iii. All vertical tension on lid margins should be eliminated by adequate undermining.
    iv. Incisions should be parallel to lines of tension/lid margin.
    v. Defect should be sutured in three layers.
    vi. For larger defects local skin flaps/grafts indicated.

24. **What are the basic differences between upper and lower lid reconstruction?**

S.no.	Upper eyelid reconstruction	Lower eyelid reconstruction
1.	More important than lower lid due to cornea closure	Less important for corneal protection
2.	Should be done on priority if both lids are missing	Can wait
3.	Incision should be parallel to lines of tension and lid margin, preferably at lid crease	Wound parallel to lines of tension and lid margin would result in scleral show/ectropion. Hence wound should be converted perpendicular to lid margin
4.	Gravitational effect and lid laxity does not cause adverse effects	Can cause ectropion, retraction, scleral show
5.	Thinner skin	Thicker
6.	Height of tarsus: 8–9 mm	Height : 5 mm
7.	Less important for tear drainage	More important for tear drainage

25. How is the full thickness lid margin defects managed?

   i. **Less than 30% defect**
- Direct closure
- Direct closure with canthotomy and cantholysis

  ii. **30–50% defect**
- Direct Closure with canthotomy and cantholysis
- Rotational flaps like Tenzy semicircular flap

 iii. **Greater than 50% defect**
- Cutler–Beard technique—for upper lid
- Reverse Cutler–Beard technique for lower lid
- Hughes tarsoconjunctival flap
- Mustarde's cheek rotational flap

 iv. **Total loss of upper lid**
- Mustarde's switch flap
- Transposition cheek flap
- Fricke temporal forehead transposition flap
- Posterior lamellar graft is necessary for lining all these flaps.

  v. **Total loss of upper lid and partial loss of lower lid**
- *If total loss of lower lid is associated with presence of lateral part of lower lid:* This part of lower lid is used as a switch flap for upper lid (Mustarde operation). Remaining part of lower lid is reconstructed with temporal frontal pedicle flap lined by mucous membrane.
- *If total loss of UL is associated with presence of medial part of LL:* This need not be transferred to UL. UL is formed by supraorbital/forehead flap and LL formed by cheek rotation flap is lined by mucus membrane.

 vi. **Absence of both lids with intact eyeball:**
Protection of cornea: By suturing the remnants of conjunctiva over it.
                               By free mucosal grafts

26. What are the techniques for upper eyelid reconstruction?

    i. Direct closure
   ii. Tenzel's lateral semicircular rotation flap
  iii. Cutler–Beard bridge flap
  iv. Tarsoconjunctival flap
   v. Free tarsoconjuctival graft
  vi. Mustarde's marginal pedicle rotation flap
 vii. Composite eyelid graft
viii. Local myocutaneous flap with posterior lamellar graft
  ix. Periorbital flaps with posterior lamellar grafts.
     Inclusion of few fibers of LPS while forming lid crease is essential.

27. What are the techniques for lower eyelid reconstruction?

    i. Direct closure
   ii. Lateral semicircular rotation flap
  iii. Reverse Cutler–Beard operation
  iv. Free tarsoconjunctival graft with myocutaneous advancement flap
   v. Hughes tarsoconjunctival advancement flap
  vi. Mustarde's cheek rotation flap
 vii. Temporal forehead flap with posterior lamellar grafts
viii. Composite eyelid graft

8.5. BLEPHAROPHIMOSIS SYNDROME

1. **What is blepharophimosis syndrome?**

   Approximately 6% of children with congenital ptosis demonstrate the typical findings of blepharophimosis syndrome.

   Clinical features commonly seen are:

   i. There is severe bilateral ptosis with poor levator function.
   ii. The palpebral fissures are horizontally shortened (blepharophimosis)
   iii. Epicanthus inversus
   iv. Telecanthus—the intercanthal distance is more than half the inter-pupillary distance. It occurs due to increase length of medial canthal tendons.
   v. True hypertelorism is occasionally present.
   vi. Lateral ectropion of lower lids.
   vii. High arching of eyebrows.

   Associated features may include tarsal plate hypoplasia and poorly developed nasal bridge. Some patients demonstrate low-set, "lop" ears.

   Blepharophimosis is a dominantly inherited condition, although the severity of findings varies among affected family members. Sporadic cases also occur.

   Blepharophimosis is associated with primary amenorrhea in some family lines.

   Treatment of blepharophimosis usually requires a staged approach.

   Mustarde's double "Z" plasty or Y-V plasty with transnasal wiring is done as a primary procedure. This gives a good surgical result both in terms of correction of telecanthus as well as deep placement of the medial canthus. The results are long lasting.

   Brow suspension is carried out 6 months after the first procedure for correction of ptosis.

8.6. THYROID-RELATED ORBITOPATHY (TRO) AND PROPTOSIS

1. **What is the volume of the orbit?**

   30 mL.

2. **Why is the new terminology of thyroid orbitopathy preferred over the older thyroid-related ophthalmopathy?**

   It is a disease in which orbit is the primary site of involvement in which the following changes take place:
   i. Increase in the volume of extraocular muscles.
   ii. Increased fat synthesis.
   iii. Associated primary lacrimal gland dysfunction.
   iv. Compression of the orbital part of the optic nerve.

3. **What is the difference in the terminology of exophthalmos and proptosis?**

   i. **Exophthalmos** is an active or a dynamic disease characterized by the forward protrusion of the eyeball, classically seen in thyroid-related orbitopathy and hence usually bilateral.
   ii. **Proptosis** is a passive protrusion of the eyeball classically seen in retro-orbital space occupying lesions and hence usually unilateral.

4. **What is physiological proptosis?**

   It is seen in infants, owing to the fact that orbital cavities do not attain their full volume as rapidly as the eyeball. It is also seen in conditions such as bending forwards or during straining/strangulation.

5. **What are the accepted exophthalmometry values to determine proptosis or enophthalmos?**

   Proptosis >21 mm
   Enophthalmos <10–12 mm

6. **Mention few causes of acute proptosis.**
   i. Orbital emphysema
   ii. Orbital hemorrhage
   iii. Orbital cellulitis.

7. **Mention a few causes of intermittent proptosis.**
   i. Orbital varices (90%)
   ii. Highly vascular neoplasms like hemangioma or lymphangioma
   iii. Recurrent orbital hemorrhages
   iv. Due to vascular congestions such as:
   - strangulation, suffocation
   - intense muscular efforts

– constriction of jugular veins in cases of cavernous sinus thrombosis.
v. Periodic orbital edema (particularly angioneurotic edema)
vi. Intermittent ethmoiditis
vii. Recurrent emphysema.

8. Mention causes of pulsating proptosis.

It may be vascular or cerebral in origin.

Vascular pulsations
i. Aneurysm of carotid or ophthalmic artery
– A-V aneurysms (most common—carotid-cavernous communications 90%)
– Saccular aneurysms
– Circoid aneurysm of orbit
ii. Venous dilatations
Orbital varix—rarely pulsates
iii. Thrombosis of cavernous sinus
iv. Vascular tumors in orbit—hemangioma, lymphangioma (rarely).

Cerebral pulsations
Transmission pulsation present when there is orbital wall defect.
i. Orbital root defect associated with meningocele or encephalocele
ii. Neurofibromatosis associated with large dehiscence in orbital wall
iii. Traumatic hiatus.

9. What is the anatomical basis for increase in proptosis with straining or internal jugular venous or carotid artery compression?

i. Acutely raised pulmonary artery pressure may be transmitted to the veins of the head and neck including facial vein.
ii. The facial vein lacks valves, so that raised facial venous pressure may in turn be transmitted to orbit through its anastomosis with superior ophthalmic vein (principal venous drainage of orbit). This is the probable anatomical basis for congestive expansion of the orbit.

10. What are the causes of unilateral proptosis?

The causes can be divided into following causes:
i. Thyroid related orbitopathy
ii. Deformities of the cranium and asymmetric orbital size
iii. Inflammatory lesions
– Acute inflammations
• Inflammation of orbital tissue
• Lacrimal gland
• Whole globe (panophthalmitis)

- Para nasal sinuses
- Eyelids
- Cavernous sinus
    - Chronic inflammations
      - Granulomas
      - Tuberculoma
      - Gummas
      - Sarcoidosis
      - Chronic dacryoadenitis.
iv. Circulatory disturbances
    - Varicoceles
    - Retrobulbar hemorrhage
      - Trauma
      - Hemophilia
    - Aneurysms
v. Cysts
    - Dermoid cyst
    - Parasitic cyst
    - Implantation cyst
    - Cyst of optic nerve
    - Cyst of lacrimal gland
    - Congenital cystic eyeball
vi. Tumors
    - Primary orbital tumors
    - Lacrimal gland tumors
    - Optic nerve tumors
    - Secondaries
vii. Traumatic
    - Retrobulbar hemorrhage
    - Retained intraocular foreign body
    - Emphysema
viii. Associated with general disorders
    - Lymphatic deposits in leukemia
    - Lipogranulomatous deposits as in histiocytosis
    - Localized amyloidosis.

11. What do you mean by orbitotonometry or piezometry?

Assessment of compressibility of orbital contents or the "tension of orbit" is called piezometry.

i. It is of diagnostic value
ii. It gives idea of effectivity of treatment. For example, orbitonometer of Cooper.

12. What are the different types of exophthalmometry?

They are:

i. Clinical exophthalmometry

ii. Stereophotographic method of exophthalmometry

iii. Radiographic exophthalmometry.

Clinical methods are:

i. Zehender's exophthalmometer

ii. Gormaz exophthalmomter

iii. Luedde exophthalmometer (used in children)

iv. Hertel exopthtalmometer (used for axial proptosis)

v. Davenger's exophthalmometer

vi. Watson's ocular topometer (in eccentric proptosis)

vii. Measurement of displacement of globe with persplex ruler.

13. What are the causes of bilateral proptosis?

i. Thyroid orbitopathy

ii. Developmental anomalies of the skull

- Craniofacial dysostosis
- Generalized osteodysplasia

iii. Osteopathies

- Infantile cortical hyperostosis
- Fibrous dysplasia
- Osteoporosis
- Rickets
- Acromegaly

iv. Enchephalocele in the ethmoidal region

v. Edema

- Angioneurotic edema
- Cavernous sinus thrombosis

vi. Neoplasms

- Symmetric lymphoma
- Chloromas
- Malignancy of nasopharynx
- Metastatic neuroblastoma

14. What is the most common cause unilateral proptosis in adults?

Thyroid orbitopathy.

15. What is the most common cause of bilateral proptosis in adults?

Thyroid orbitopathy.

16. What is the most common cause of unilateral proptosis in children?

Orbital cellulitis.

17. What do you mean by pseudoproptosis?

It is the clinical appearance of proptosis where in no real forward displacement of the globe takes place.

18. What are the causes of pseudoproptosis?

It can be classified as:
  i. *When globe is enlarged*
     – Congenital buphthalmos/congenital cystic eyeball
     – High axial myopia
     – Staphyloma
     – Unilateral secondary glaucoma in childhood
 ii. *Retracting lids*
     – Microblepharon
     – Dermatosis or ichthyosis or from scarring
     – Sympathetic overaction such as Graves' disease or Parkinson's disease
iii. *Lower lid sagging*
     – Facial palsy
     – Retraction of inferior rectus
     – Following recession of inferior oblique
 iv. *Deformation of orbit or facial asymmetry*
     – Asymmetry of bony orbit
     – Progressive facial hemiatrophy (Parry–Rombergs' syndrome)
     – Harlequin orbit
     – Hypoplastic supraorbital ridges as in trisomy 18
     – Shallow orbit as in Crouzon's disease (craniofacial dysostosis)
  v. *Opposite eye enophthalmos.*

19. What are the causes of enophthalmos?

Causes of enophthalmos are:
  i. Microphthalmos
 ii. Phthisis bulbi
iii. Blowout fracture
 iv. Subluxation of the globe
  v. Age-related absorption of the fat.

20. Classify proptosis.

Proptosis can be classified based on different criteria:
  i. Unilateral or bilateral
 ii. Axial or eccentric
iii. Acute, chronic, recurrent, intermittent
 iv. Pulsatile or nonpulsatile.

21. What do you mean by axial proptosis?

Axial proptosis is caused by any space occupying lesion in the muscle cone or any diffuse orbital inflammatory or neoplastic lesions. For example, optic nerve glioma, cavernous hemangioma, meningioma, schwanomma, metastatic tumors from CA—breast, lung or prostate.

22. What do you mean by eccentric proptosis?

Proptosis caused by any extraconal lesion or fracture displacement of orbital bones protruding inwardly.

23. Give a few causes of non-axial proptosis.

i. *Lateral displacement of globe/down and out:*
  - Ethmoidal mucocele
  - Frontal mucocele
  - Lacrimal sac tumors
  - Nasopharyngeal tumors
  - Rhabdomyosarcoma

ii. *Down and in:*
  - Lacrimal gland tumors
  - Sphenoid wing meningoma

iii. *Upward:*
  - Tumors of floor of orbit
  - Maxillary tumors
  - Lymphoma
  - Lacrimal sac tumors

iv. *Downward:*
  - Fibrous dysplasia
  - Fibrous mucocele
  - Lymphoma
  - Neuroblastoma
  - Neurofibroma
  - Schwannoma
  - Subperiosteal hematoma

24. What is the DD for a palpable mass in the superonasal quadrant?

i. Mucocele
ii. Mucopyocele
iii. Encephalocele
iv. Neurofibroma
v. Dermoid cyst
vi. Lymphoma.

25. What is the DD for a palpable mass in the superotemporal quadrant?

   i. Prolapsed lacrimal gland

   ii. Dermoid cyst

  iii. Lacrimal gland tumor

  iv. Lymphoma

   v. Nonspecific orbital inflammation

26. What are the important causes of proptosis in the following age group?

It can be divided into following categories:

Newborn

  i. Orbital sepsis

 ii. Orbital neoplasm

Neonates

Osteomyelitis of maxilla

Infants

   i. Dermoid cyst

  ii. Dermolipoma

 iii. Hemangioma

 iv. Histocytosis X

   v. Orbital extension of retinoblastoma

Children

    i. Dermoid cyst

   ii. Teratoma

  iii. Capillary hemangioma

  iv. Lymphangioma

   v. Orbital nerve glioma

  vi. Plexiform neurofibroma

 vii. Rhabdomyosarcoma

viii. Acute myeloid leukemia

  ix. Histocytosis

   x. Neuroblastoma

 xi. Wilms' tumor

 xii. Ewing's tumor

Adults

    i. Thyroid orbitopathy

   ii. Cavernous hemangioma

  iii. Orbital varices

  iv. Optic nerve meningoma

   v. Schwannoma

  vi. Fibrous histocytoma

 vii. Lymphoma

viii. Secondaries from breast, lung, prostate carcinoma.

27. What is proptometry?

It is the measurement of the distance between apex of the cornea and the bony point usually taken as deepest portion of the lateral orbital rim with the eye looking in primary gaze.

28. Which instruments are used for measuring eccentric proptosis?

    i. Topometer of Watson
   ii. Persplex ruler
  iii. Luedde exophthalmometer

29. How to palpate in case of proptosis?

Insinuation of the orbital margins are done using the little finger and patient is asked to look down to palate the orbital rim since the down position would relax the orbital septum

30. What are the types of exophthalmometry?

Types of exophthalmometry are:

    i. Absolute exophthalmometry: The amount of proptosis is compared with a known normal value.
   ii. Comparative exophthalmometry: The reading is compared from time to time in the same eye.
  iii. Relative exophthalmometry: The reading is compared between two eyes.

31. Which age group is commonly affected and what is the sex preponderance in TRO?

    i. Average age of onset is in 40s
   ii. Females are 3–6 times more affected than males

32. What refractive errors are associated with TRO?

    i. Astigmatism due to lid retraction
   ii. Induced hyperopia as a result of flattening of posterior pole due to retrobulbar mass.

33. What is the reason of dilated vessels over muscles?

With increasing inflammation of muscles, the anterior radials of the muscular vessels become engorged, producing characteristic dilated and visible vessels subconjunctivally over the insertions.

34. What is the sequence of muscle involvement in TRO?

    i. Inferior rectus
   ii. Medial rectus
  iii. Superior rectus
  iv. Lateral rectus

35. Why inferior rectus is most commonly involved in TRO?

   i. Inferior rectus involvement occurs due to well-developed connective tissue system around inferior oblique and inferior rectus muscles, which also have good septal connections with adjacent periorbita.

   ii. Also inferior rectus contains high concentration of macrophages (CD4+ memory T cells, CD8 T cells) which may account for disease activity in muscles.

36. What are the reasons for restricted ocular movements in TRO?

It can be divided into causes due to:

   i. Edematous muscle—this occurs in active stage caused by imbibitions of fluid into the muscle belly, which causes increase in size of the muscle. This causes restriction of contraction of the muscle.

   ii. Fibrosed muscle—this occurs following chronic disease.

   iii. Fibrosis causes contracture and restriction of the muscle movements.

37. What are the causes of muscle enlargement in TRO?

   i. Increased glycosaminoglycans with secondary water retention

   ii. Immunologic response meditated through antigen, target cells and cytokines

   iii. Destruction of muscle fibers and infiltration by mature fat cells.

   iv. Fibrosis of muscle

38. What are systemic associations of TRO?

Autoimmune or immunoregulatory diseases:

   i. Myasthenia gravis

   ii. Pernicious anemia

   iii. Vitiligo.

39. What is Braley's test?

   i. Also known as differential tonometry or positional tonomerty

   ii. It refers to an increase in IOP measured during upgaze

   iii. An increase in IOP of more than 6 mm Hg is significant

   iv. Normal—2 mm Hg

   v. Increase in IOP more than 9–10 mm Hg suggests optic neuropathy.

40. What are the clinical signs in thyroid eye disease?

   i. **Facial signs:**
     – Joffroy's sign: Absent crease on upper forehead on upgaze.

   ii. **Eyelid signs:**
     – Kocher's sign: Staring appearance
     – Vigoroux sign: Eyelid fullness or puffiness
     – Rosenbach sign: Tremors of eyelid (when closed)
     – Riesman sign: Bruit over the eyelids.

- **Upper eyelid signs:**
  - von Graefes sign: Upper lid lag on downgaze
  - Dalrymple sign: Upper eyelid retraction
  - Stellwag's sign: Incomplete and infrequent blinking
  - Grove sign: Resistance to pulling the retracted upper lid
  - Boston sign: Uneven jerky movements of upper lid on inferior gaze
  - Gellinek's sign: Abnormal pigmentation on upperlid
  - Gifford's sign: Difficulty in everting the upper lid
  - Means sign: Increased superior scleral show on upgaze
- **Lower eyelid signs:**
  - Enroths sign: Edema of the lower lid
  - Griffith's sign: Lower lid lag on upgaze
iii. **Extraocular movements sign:**
  - Moebius sign: Inability to converge eyes
  - Ballet's sign: Restriction of one or more extraocular muscles
  - Suker's sign: Poor fixation on abduction
  - Jendrassik's sign: Paralysis of all extra ocular muscles
iv. **Conjunctival signs:**
  - Goldzieher sign: Conjunctival injection
v. **Pupillary involvement sign:**
  - Knies sign: Uneven pupillary dilatation
  - Cowen's sign: Jerky contraction of pupil to light.

41. What is the reason of increase in IOP in TRO?

i. Enlargement of recti interferes with uveoscleral drainage in various positions of gaze.

ii. Increased tension due to resistance of inferior rectus opposing supra-duction, provoking compression of eye and elevation in IOP in upgaze.

42. What are the causes of increase in IOP in upgaze?

i. TRO

ii. Fractures

iii. Myositis

iv. Irradiation

v. Orbital metastasis.

43. Are all patients with TRO hyperthyroid?

Approximately 80% of the patients with TRO are hyperthyroid at the time of diagnosis or develop hyperthyroid status within 6 months of the disease.

10% are hypothyroid and the rest 10% are euthyroid.

44. What is the most significant environmental factor causing TRO?

Smoking: Smokers with TRO have more severe disease than nonsmokers.

45. What are the causes of upper lid retraction in TRO?

The causes of upper lid retraction in TRO are:

  i. Fibrotic contracture of the levator associated with adhesion with overlying orbital tissue.
 ii. Sympathetic overstimulation of Muller's muscle.
iii. Secondary overaction of levator superior rectus complex in response to hypophoria produced by fibrosis of inferior rectus muscle.

46. What are the causes of lower lid retraction?

Fibrosis of the inferior lid retractors (capsulopalpebral head).

47. How do you grade lid retraction?

  i. Mild—intersection of lid at superior limbus, 1–2 mm of superior sclera show, MRD 1: 6 mm
 ii. Moderate—2–4 mm of superior sclera show, MRD 1: 6–10 mm
iii. Severe—> 4 mm of superior sclera show, MRD 1: >10 mm

48. What is the importance of measuring lid retraction?

If surgical correction is mandatory for lid retraction, size of spacer graft depends on amount of lid retraction.
1 mm of lid retraction = 3 mm of spacer graft.

49. When does one get ptosis instead of lid retraction in TRO?

  i. When there is apical compression and congestion of orbit as in tight orbit syndrome
 ii. Severe proptosis may cause disinsertion of aponeurosis of elevators of lids leading to ptosis
iii. Ptosis may be associated with myasthenia gravis.

50. What are the causes of vision loss in TRO?

   i. Exposure keratopathy
  ii. Diplopia due to involvement of extraocular muscles
 iii. Optic nerve traction
  iv. Optic nerve compression (by enlarged EOM)
   v. Macular edema
  vi. Macular scar
 vii. Glaucomatous optic neuropathy (systemic steroid induced).
viii. Posterior subcapsular cataract secondary to steroids used in the treatment of TRO.

51. Where is the site of compression of optic nerve by enlarged extraocular muscles?

Orbital apex caused by the crowding of the enlarged muscles.

52. What is the earliest and most sensitive indicator of optic nerve damage and why?

   i. Color vision: pseudoisochromatic plates and Fansworth Munsell Hue test.
   ii. Color vision is affected earlier because axons that precede macula are most sensitive to damage.
   iii. Pattern reversal visual evoked potential: also sensitive for detecting early damage.

53. What are the visual field defects seen in optic neuropathy due to TRO?

   i. Central scotoma
   ii. Inferior altitudinal defect.

Less commonly

   i. Enlarged blind spot
   ii. Paracentral scotoma
   iii. Nerve fiber bundle defect
   iv. Generalized constriction.

54. What are the causes of exposure keratopathy in TRO?

   i. Severe proptosis preventing mechanical closure of eyelids.
   ii. Retraction of the upper and lower eyelids.
   iii. Decreased secretion of tears due to primary lacrimal gland dysfunction.

55. What are Sallmann's folds?

These are choroidal folds seen in macula in case of retrobulbar mass. Seen in TRO.

Other conditions where choroidal folds may be seen are:

   i. Idiopathic
   ii. Retrobulbar tumors
   iii. Choroidal melanomas
   iv. Ocular hypotony
   v. Posterior scleritis
   vi. Post scleral buckling.

56. What are racoon eyes? Where it is seen in context of orbit?

Dark purple discoloration/periorbital ecchymoses giving an appearance similar to that of a racoon/panda.

Otherwise seen in following conditions:

    i. Bilateral proptosis due to metastatic neuroblastoma.

    ii. Fracture of base of skull.

    iii. Amylodosis.

    iv. Kaposi's sarcoma.

    v. Multiple myeloma.

57. What do you mean by temporal flare in a patient with TRO?

The upper eyelid retraction in Graves' disease has a characteristic temporal flare, with a greater amount of sclera visible laterally as compared with medially.

58. What is the cause of temporal flare in TRO?

The results of inflammation, resultant adhesions and fibrosis clearly affect the lateral horn of the levator aponeurosis.

    i. The lateral horn of the levator aponeurosis is much stronger than the medial horn, and its insertion through the lateral orbital retinaculum at the lateral orbital tubercle is much more defined than its medial insertion. The lateral fibers of the muscular portion of the levator muscle, proximal to Whitnall's ligament, blend with the superior transverse ligament as it courses to the lateral orbital attachment, exerting a strong pull on the lateral aspect of the eyelid through the aponeurosis, the suspensory ligament of the fornix and the conjunctiva.

    ii. Müller's muscle, an involuntary muscle, may develop over reaction or be enlarged secondary to a direct inflammatory infiltrate in thyroid-related orbitopathy. An involved Müller's muscle, with its substantial lateral extensions, contributes to and may cause more temporal flare than in those patients with thyroid-related orbitopathy but without this muscle involvement.

59. Which is the most common extraocular muscle involved in TRO and why?

Inferior rectus (second most common muscle involved is medial rectus).

Inferior rectus involvement occurs due to well-developed connective tissue system around it and also because it has the greatest number of septal connections with adjacent periorbita.

60. Mention a few conditions which are associated with extraocular muscle enlargement.

It can be classified as:

Inflammatory:

    i. Graves' orbitopathy

ii. Myositis
iii. Orbital cellulitis
iv. Sarcoidosis
v. Vasculitides

Neoplastic:
  i. Rhabdomyosarcoma
  ii. Metastasis
  iii. Lymphoid tumors

Vascular:
  i. Carotid-cavernous fistula
  ii. A-V malformation
  iii. Lymphoid tumors

Miscellaneous:
  i. Acromegaly
  ii. Amyloidosis
  iii. POEMS syndrome
  iv. Trichinosis
  v. Lithium therapy.

61. What is differential tonometry?

It refers to an increase in the intraocular pressure measured during upgaze. This is caused by the compression of the globe by fibrosed inferior rectus. An increase in IOP of >6 mm of Hg is significant.

62. What is the significance of retinoscopy in a case of proptosis?

  i. To identify any high axial myopia which manifests as pseudoproptosis.
  ii. Axial length may be decreased in a case of retrobulbar mass causing hyperopic shift due to compression of the posterior pole.

63. What is the difference between von Graefe's sign and pseudo-von Graefe's sign?

von Graefe's sign: It is seen in thyroid orbitopathy due to retarded descent of the globe on downgaze.

Pseudo-von Graefe's sign: It is seen in III cranial nerve palsy with aberrant regeneration of the nerve where there is lid retraction on attempted downgaze.

64. What is the cause of increase in the volume of extraocular muscles?

In a patient with TRO, there is a 100-fold increase in the synthesis of GAGs (glycosaminoglycans) by the preadipocyte fibroblasts, which causes imbibition of water into the muscles causing the thickness to increase.

65. What is the type of hypersensitivity reaction in thyroid orbitopathy?

Type V hypersensitivity reaction.

66. **What is the significance of ultrasonography in a patient with suspected TRO?**

It can detect early thyroid disease in a case with unequivocal laboratory tests.

i. It helps differentiate TRO from pseudotumor.
ii. It can predict whether the disease in active or inactive. The amount of internal reflectivity is less in a patient with active disease.

67. **What is the frequency of orbital ultrasound?**

8–15 MHz.

68. **How do you differentiate between enlarged muscles in myositis from that of TRO on USG?**

In myositis there is a typical enlargement of the tendinous insertion of the muscles whereas in TRO there is a fusiform enlargement of the muscle belly.

69. **How do you clinically differentiate active and an inactive disease?**

Features	Active disease	Inactive disease
Accompanying signs of inflammation like chemosis and congestion	More	Less (usually eye will be quiet)
Amount of proptosis	Severe	Less
Restriction of extraocular movements	1 or 2 gazes	May be in all gazes

Inflammatory score (Activity of the disease)		
1.	ORBITAL PAIN	
	No pain	0
	At gaze	1
	At rest	2
2.	CHEMOSIS	
	Not beyond gray line	1
	Beyond gray line	2
3.	EYELID EDEMA	
	Present but no overhanging of tissues	1
	Roll in eyelid skin like festoons	2
4.	CONJUNCTIVAL INJECTION	
	Absent	1
	Present	2
5.	EYELID INJECTION	
	Absent	1
	Present	2
	Total	0–8

If the score is <3/8 and there is no deterioration then management is conservative with cool compresses, head elevation and NSAIDs.

If the score is >4/8 or if there is evidence of progression then the management is oral or IV steroids, radiotherapy or immunosuppressive agents.

70. What do you mean by VISA?

It is a new classification of TRO which helps in grading and planning management at all the levels of TRO, where VISA stands for:

V: Vision

I: Inflammation

S: Strabismus

A: Appearance.

71. What is the best investigation for early diagnosis of compressive optic neuropathy in Graves' disease?

MRI.

72. What are the indications of orbital imaging in a patient with TRO?

i. Suspicion of optic nerve compression

ii. Evaluation before orbital decompression surgery

iii. Orbital irradiation

iv. To rule out pseudotumor.

73. What is the significance of CT scanning in a patient of TRO?

i. CT scan allows reliable identification of even minimally enlarged recti muscles.

ii. In patients with unilateral proptosis, it can detect subclinical enlargement of extraocular muscles EOM in contralateral eye.

iii. Can detect patients with risk of developing optic neuropathy as depicted by

– Severe apical crowding

– Dilated superior ophthalmic vein.

74. What are the characteristic findings of CT scan in TRO?

Fusiform enlargement of extraocular muscles which is usually bilateral and symmetric with sharply defined borders and sparing the tendinous insertions.

75. What is the best cross-sectional view in CT scan to visualize enlarged muscle?

Coronal section.

76. What are the laboratory tests done in TRO?

i. Thyroid timulating hormone (TSH)

ii. Thyroxine (total and free T4)

iii. Triiodothyronine (T3)

iv. Thyroid stimulating immunoglobulin.

77. How will you treat TRO?

The treatment has to be done in conjunction with management of the underlying thyroid disease by an Endocrinologist

    i. Topical lubrication with artificial tears
   ii. Lid taping at bedtime
  iii. Cold compresses in the morning and head elevation in the night
  iv. Punctual occlusion for more severe dry eye symptoms
   v. Lateral tarsorrhaphy useful in cases of lateral chemosis or widened lateral palpebral fissure or to prevent exposure together
  vi. Surgical eyelid recession (lengthening) for eyelid retraction after 6 months
 vii. If diplopia is present then oral steroids, Fresnel prism or strabismus surgery as indicated
viii. For threatened optic nerve involvement, oral steroids and orbital decompression

78. Which wall should not be decompressed?

Removal of the inferior wall is avoided if possible due to higher incidence of induced diplopia

79. What are the indications of orbital decompression surgery?

    i. Compressive optic neuropathy
   ii. Exposure keratopathy
  iii. Cosmetically unacceptable proptosis.

80. What is the most common site of orbital wall decompression?

Deep lateral wall.

81. What are principles/goal of orbital decompression?

    i. Expanding orbital volume (bony expansion)
   ii. Reducing orbital soft tissue (fat decompression).

82. What is approach for orbital decompression?

    i. For exophthalmometry <22 mm
       Lateral wall + fat decompression
   ii. For exophthalmometry—22–25 mm
       Lateral wall + fat + medial wall decompression
  iii. For exophthalmometry >25 mm
       Lateral wall + fat + medial wall decompression + posterior orbital floor decompression + lateral rim advancement.

83. What are the complications of orbital decompression?

    i. Most common is worsening of diplopia or new double vision.
   ii. Infraorbital hyperesthesia.
  iii. Risk of visual loss.
  iv. Bleeding and infection.

84. What are the indications of extraocular muscle surgery and which surgery is preferred for the same?

  i. Diplopia in primary gaze
  ii. Quiescent disease and stable angle of deviation for a minimum of 6 months.
     The preferred surgery to correct diplopia is recession of inferior oblique muscle with adjustable sutures.

85. How long will you wait for strabismus surgery in TRO and why?

We wait for 6 months as diplopia tends to get resolved with prisms and/or systemic corticosteroids in the acute phase. Also TRO tend to be progressive, and hence we wait for 6 months so that strabismus measurement stabilizes.

86. How does strabismus surgery affect eyelid retraction?

Recession of tight inferior rectus often improves upper eyelid retraction. Superior rectus had to work against tight inferior rectus, thus associated levator muscles was overactive, causing eyelid retraction.
When inferior rectus is recessed, overactivity ends.

87. What should be the sequence of surgery in patients with thyroid orbitopathy?

The evaluation and treatment of thyroid-related orbitopathy may require one or multiple stages of surgery, depending on the severity and manifestation of the disease process. Each stage will affect the decision making for subsequent stages, and therefore the surgery should be staged in a specific sequence, with orbital decompression, then strabismus surgery if indicated and finally eyelid repositioning and removal of excess fat and skin.

Any of the stages may be skipped when deemed unnecessary or not indicated, but maintaining the correct order reduces the number of procedures to a minimum.

Orbital decompression can result in a change in the extraocular muscle position and function relative to the globe, displacement of the muscle cone, and alteration of the muscle pulley system, which may result in postoperative phorias or diplopia.

Recession or resection of the vertical extraocular muscles for the correction of hypertrophies, especially large deviations, may increase the retraction of the eyelids secondary to alterations of the anatomical connectivity between the retractor complex and the vertical extraocular muscles. This is avoidable by careful and meticulous dissection of the extraocular muscles. Orbital decompression can also change the position of the eyelids.

88. Differentiate between orbital pseudotumor and graves orbitopathy.

Features	Idiopathic pseudotumor	Graves orbitopathy
Sex—F:M ratio	Equal	3:1
Mode of onset	Acute, subacute or chronic	Chronic
Pain	Often present. May be severe	Painless (unless keratitis or orbital congestion present)
Laterality	Usually unilateral	Usually bilateral
Lid signs	Lid edema, lid erythema, ptosis	Lid and periorbital edema, lid retraction, lid lag and lagophthalmos
Systemic symptoms	Malaise	Generally well. Associated symptoms of thyroid disease
Laboratory findings	Elevated ESR	Abnormal thyroid functions
Radiography	▪ Infiltrate or a mass ▪ Uveoscleral enhancement ▪ Extraocular muscle enlargement including tendon	▪ Spindle shaped extraocular muscle enlargement ▪ Sparing tendon ▪ Inferior and medial recti most commonly involved
Ultrasonography	▪ Uveoscleral thickening ▪ Sub-Tenon's effusion	▪ Extraocular muscle enlargement detected before CT scan

89. Which neuroimaging test is best to evaluate the etiology of proptosis?

CT scan is superior in most cases.

MRI may be desirable in certain cases when optic nerve dysfunction is present.

90. What are the indications for CT scan in proptosis?

 i. Acute proptosis
 ii. Progressive proptosis
 iii. When there is RAPD
 iv. Orbital fracture
 v. Orbital foreign body.

91. What is Coca-cola sign?

It is CT scan finding seen in coronal section where there is bilateral bowing of lamina papyracea/medial wall of the orbit due to bilateral medial rectus enlargement in TRO.

92. **What are the indications of biopsy in proptosis?**
    i. Pseudotumor refractory to medical treatment.
    ii. Suspected lymphoma or other malignancies.

93. **How is orbital bruit best examined?**
    Place the stethoscope bell over the closed eyelids and ask the patient to gently open the eyelids.

94. **What are the bones comprising the walls of the orbit?**
    i. **Medial wall (weakest wall)**
       (from front to back)
       – Frontal process of maxilla
       – Lacrimal bone
       – Orbital plate of ethmoid
       – Body of sphenoid
    ii. **Inferior wall**
       – Orbital surface of maxilla (medially)
       – Orbital surface of zygomatic (laterally)
       – Palatine bone (posteriorly)
    iii. **Lateral wall (strongest wall)**
       – Zygomatic bone (anteriorly)
       – Greater wing if sphenoid (posteriorly)
    iv. **Roof**
       – Orbital plate of frontal bone (anteriorly)
       – Lesser wing of sphenoid (posteriorly).

95. **What are the approaches to the orbital surgery?**
    Surgical approaches can be:
    i. Superior orbitotomy
    ii. Medial orbitotomy
    iii. Lateral orbitotomy
    iv. Inferior orbitotomy
    v. Transcranial approach
    vi. Transnasal endoscopic approach
    vii. Transantral approach

    Anterior can also be divided as:

    Inferior orbitotomy
    i. Extraperiosteal approach—subciliary incision
    ii. Conjunctival incision in inferior fornix for orbital floor fracture repair
    Superior orbitotomy
    i. Coronal approach
    ii. Conjunctival incision

iii. Subbrow incision

iv. Eyelid crease incision

Anterior orbitotomy—superomedial lesion–lid split incision

Medial orbitotomy

  i. Inferomedial lesion—DCR like incision

 ii. Medial orbitotomy—conjunctival approach for central and peripheral space

iii. Endoscopic approach

iv. Lateral orbitotomy

 v. Transfrontal orbitotomy.

96. What is lateral orbitotomy?

Lateral approach is used for deeper orbital lesions that cannot be reached through an anterior incision. The type of skin incisions include:

  i. S-shaped (Stallard–Wright)

 ii. Horizontal canthal crease

iii. Eyelid crease incision.

The skin is cut with a scalpel blade, and dissection is extended through orbicularis muscle

↓

Periosteum is cut elevated from the lateral orbital wall till zygomatic bone and greater wing of sphenoid is exposed

↓

The bone is cut with oscillating saw or small holes can be drilled, and the bone is fractured out.

↓

Thin bone of greater wing of sphenoid is removed to provide adequate retrobulbar exposure

↓

Periorbita is opened with scissors by making a cut just inferior to lateral rectus muscle.

↓

The orbital fat dissected, the lesion identified and dissected out, hemostasis achieved

↓

Periorbita closed with interrupted 6-0 vicryl, lateral orbital rim replaced, sutured with 4-0 prolene

↓

Periostium closed with 4-0 vicryl, orbicularis with 6-0 chromic catgut and the skin with 6-0 nylon or silk vertical mattress sutures.

97. What are the surgical spaces of the orbit?

These spaces include:

  i. Central surgical space (intraconal space)

 ii. Peripheral surgical space (extraconal space)

iii. Subperiosteal space
iv. Preaponeurotic space
v. Tenon's space
vi. Periorbital tissues.

98. What are the TRO signs?

The signs of TRO were given by Werner's classification and grading of thyroid orbitopathy.

Class	Grade	Mnemonic	Suggestions for grading
0		N	No physical signs or symptoms
1		O	Signs only
2		S	Soft-tissue involvement
	0		Absent
	A		Minimal
	B		Moderate
	C		Marked
3		P	Proptosis of 3 mm or more
	0		Absent
	A		3–4 mm
	B		5–7 mm
	C		8 mm or more
4		E	Extraocular muscle involvement
	0		Absent
	A		Limitation of motion at extremes of gaze
	B		Evident restriction of motion
	C		Fixation of globe
5		C	Corneal involvement
	0		Absent
	A		Punctate lesions
	B		Ulceration
	C		Necrosis or perforation
6		S	Sight loss (due to optic nerve)
	0		Absent
	A		20/20–20/60
	B		20/70–20/200
	C		Worse than 20/200

99. What are the differences between optic nerve glioma and optic nerve sheath meningioma?

Optic nerve glioma	Optic nerve sheath meningioma
1. Age: Children and young girls	1. Middle aged adults, mostly women
2. Arise from astrocytes of the optic nerve	2. Arise from meningoendothelial cells of arachnoid villi
3. Visual loss followed by proptosis	3. Proptosis presents first followed by visual loss
4. CT: Fusiform enlargement of optic nerve	4. Tubular thickening of optic nerve ("Tram-tracking")
5. X-ray shows regular enlargement of optic foramen	5. Irregular enlargement

8.7. BLOWOUT FRACTURES OF THE ORBIT

1. **Who were the first to describe orbital blowout fractures?**

   Smith and Regan in 1957.

2. **What is the mechanism of a blowout fracture?**

   A blowout fracture of the orbital floor is typically caused by a sudden increase in the orbital pressure by an impacting object which is greater in diameter than the orbital aperture (about 5 cm), such as a fist or tennis ball so that the eyeball itself is displaced and transmits rather than absorbs the impact. Since the bones of the lateral wall and the roof are usually able to withstand such trauma, the fracture most frequently involves the floor of the orbit along the thin bone covering the infraorbital canal.

3. **What are the theories explaining the mechanism of the blowout fracture?**

   Two theories have been proposed to explain the mechanism of the blowout fracture:

   i. Hydraulic theory
   ii. Buckling theory.

4. **What is the hydraulic theory?**

   In hydraulic theory the external injury is supposed to cause an increase in the intraorbital pressure which causes the thin orbital floor medial to the infraorbital groove and the medial wall to give way and help in absorbing the impact of the injury and thereby protect the globe from injury.

5. **What is the buckling theory?**

   In the buckling theory the stress of the initial injury is transmitted directly from the orbital rim to the orbital floor and results in the fracture.

6. **How are blowout fractures classified?**

   The blowout fractures is classified into two types:

   i. Pure blowout fracture
   ii. Impure or complex blowout fracture
      - A **pure blowout** fracture is fracture of the orbital wall without involvement of the orbital rim.
      - **Impure blowout** fracture is a variety in which the orbital rim and the adjacent facial bones are involved.

7. **How are pure blowout fractures classified?**

   i. Trapdoor refers to cases in which either edge of the inferior orbital wall is attached to its original position (teardrop sign).
   ii. Non-trapdoor refers to cases in which the inferior orbital wall is completely separated from its original position and the periorbital tissue has escaped into the maxillary sinus.

8. **What are the symptoms in blow out fracture?**
   i. Pain with vertical eye movement
   ii. Binocular diplopia
   iii. Eyelid edema
   iv. Crepitus, particularly after nose bleeding

9. **What are the clinical signs seen in a patient with blowout fracture?**

   Eyelid signs: Ecchymosis and edema of eyelids, occasionally subcutaneous emphysema.

   Infraorbital nerve anesthesia involving the lower lid, cheek, side of nose, upper lip, upper teeth and gums is very common because the fracture frequently involves the infraorbital canal.

   Diplopia with limitation of upgaze, downgaze or both:

   Diplopia may be caused by one of the following mechanisms:
   i. Hemorrhage and edema in the orbit may cause the septa connecting the inferior rectus and inferior oblique muscles to the periorbita to become taut and thus restrict movement of the globe. Ocular motility usually improves as the hemorrhage and edema resolve.
   ii. Mechanical entrapment within the fracture of the inferior rectus or inferior oblique muscle, or adjacent connective tissue and fat. Diplopia typically occurs in both upgaze and downgaze (double diplopia).
   iii. In these cases forced duction and the differential intraocular pressure tests are positive. Diplopia may subsequently improve if it is mainly due to entrapment of connective tissue and fat, but usually persists if there is significant involvement of the muscles themselves.
   iv. Direct injury to an extraocular muscle is associated with a negative forced duction test. The muscle fibers usually regenerate and normal function returns within about 2 months.

   Enophthalmos may be present if the fracture is severe, although it tends to manifest only after a few days as the initial edema resolves. In the absence of surgical intervention, enophthalmos may continue to increase for about 6 months as post-traumatic orbital degeneration and fibrosis develop.

10. **What are the differential diagnosis of muscle entrapment in orbital fracture?**
    i. Orbital edema and hemorrhage
    ii. Cranial nerve palsy.

11. **Why are pediatric patients particularly vulnerable to trapdoor fracture?**

    Since their bones tend to be cartilaginous and bendable

12. What is "white eyed blowout fracture"?

It is a well described entity especially in the pediatric group which presents with signs of entrapment of the extraocular muscles with a relatively white eye which reveals minimal signs of inflammation. These patients can also have symptoms suggestive of oculocardiac reflex with resultant bradycardia and nausea.

13. What are the causes of vision loss following a blowout fracture?

In patients with orbital floor fractures, vision loss can result from injury to the optic nerve or increased orbital pressure causing a compartment syndrome.

14. What is the initial management of blowout fractures?

The majority of blowout fractures do not require surgical intervention. Initial treatment is conservative with antibiotics; ice packs and nasal decongestants may be helpful. The patient should be instructed not to blow the nose, because of the possibility of forcing infected sinus contents into the orbit. Systemic steroids are occasionally required for severe orbital edema, particularly if this is compromising the optic nerve.

15. What are the indications of surgery in cases of blowout fracture?

i. Diplopia with limitation of upgaze and/or downgaze within 30 degrees of the primary position with a positive traction test result 7–10 days after injury and with radiologic confirmation of a fracture of the orbital floor.

ii. Enophthalmos that exceeds 2 mm and that is cosmetically unacceptable to the patient.

iii. Large fractures involving at least half of the orbital floor, particularly when associated with large medial wall fractures.

16. When is surgery indicated as an emergency in blow out fracture?

Urgent surgery (<24 hours) is indicated in pediatric cases with entrapment

17. How do we manage white eyed blowout fracture?

The "white-eyed" fracture requires urgent repair to avoid permanent neuromuscular damage. Release of the entrapped muscle should be done to avoid restriction and fibrosis.

18. What are the preoperative investigations done?

i. Visual acuity testing, papillary reflex
ii. Ocular motility evaluation using Hess chart/Lees screen
iii. Hertel exophthalmometry
iv. Slit-lamp biomicroscopy
v. Applanation tonometry

vi. Fundus ophthalmoscopy

vii. Evaluation of sensitivity in the distribution of infraorbital nerve

viii. Forced duction test (FDT)—to confirm mechanical restriction

ix. Imaging—CT scan of the orbit (2 mm slice) in axial, coronal and sagittal planes to identify the extent of fracture.

x. Determining the nature of maxillary antral soft tissue densities which may represent prolapsed orbital fat, extraocular muscles, hematoma or unrelated antral polyps.

CT scan is the imaging of choice in orbital fractures.

19. What are the various approaches to orbital floor during surgical management?

For orbital floor fractures, surgical procedures are routinely performed via:

i. Transorbital approach

ii. Transantral approach

iii. Endoscopic endonasal approach.

20. Explain about the transorbital approach.

Most anterior fractures are managed by the transorbital route which can be via:

i. Transcutaneous incision

ii. Transconjunctival incision

   – Inferior forniceal (to approach floor)

   – Transcaruncular (to approach medial wall).

21. What are the approaches to posterior and medial fractures?

The transantral approach is used to approach posteriorly placed fractures which might be difficult to approach through anterior approach.

The endoscopic approach is in managing medial wall fractures.

22. What are the steps done in surgical management of blowout fractures?

i. Open reduction of the fracture

ii. Release of entrapped tissues

iii. Repositioning of the herniated orbital soft tissue within the orbit

iv. Repair of the post traumatic defect with an orbital implant as needed.

23. Describe about the transcutaneous approach.

i. In transcutaneous approach the skin incision is made in the lower eyelid at 3–4 mm below the subciliary fold following the natural curve of the lid.

ii. A dissection is then carried down until the periosteum is reached at the level of the orbital rim.

iii. The incision is then carried through the periosteum just below the orbital rim.

iv. The reflection of the periosteum is made over the rim using a periosteal elevator until the fracture is visualized.

v. To relieve any orbital structure entrapment and to restore the orbital contents to their original place, a forced traction of the globe is made.

vi. The implant is then cut to the appropriate size and then placed to bridge the fracture site and is anchored anteriorly with screws in case there is no posterior support.

vii. The periosteum is closed with 5-0 chromic catgut and the subcutaneous tissue approximated.

viii. The 6-0 silk is used to close the skin.

24. What is the transconjunctival approach?

In transconjunctival approach the orbital rim periosteum is reached via the inferior fornix incision in case of floor fractures and transcaruncular incision for medial wall fractures.

25. What are orbital implants?

The orbital implant restores the structural integrity of the orbital wall by bridging the defect and preventing orbital contents from herniating into the adjacent periorbital sinuses. The implant also prevents extraocular motility limitations by minimizing scar tissue adhesions with orbital contents. These implants can also serve to augment the orbital volume by compressing the intraorbital contents to correct enophthalmos.

26. What are the current orbital implants?

They include:

i. Autogenous bone grafts

ii. Human donor grafts

iii. Xenografts

iv. Alloplastic implants.

27. What are the properties of an ideal alloplastic implant?

The ideal alloplastic implant should be readily sizable, sterilizable, strong, inert, nonallergenic, durable, noncarcinogenic, easily manipulated, shaped and suitable for single stage reconstruction.

Also the implant should be accepted and well integrated into the surrounding tissues with minimal inflammatory response, foreign body reaction, or risk of infection.

The implant should provide mechanical support strong enough to hold up the orbital contents, and have the stability to be easily anchored to the surrounding bone to prevent migration and extrusion.

Finally, it should be readily available in larger quantities if necessary at reasonable cost.

28. What are the various materials used as orbital implants?

    i. Autogenous bone grafts (iliac crest/rib)

   ii. Silastic sheets

 iii. Porous polyethylene (MEDPOR)—the porous polyethylene implants are available as sheets which can be cut, channel implants which have provisions for inserting a plate which can be fixed to the orbital rim with screws and with titanium sheets (TITAN).

 iv. Titanium implant—these are available as titanium sheets which can be cut or preshaped models.

29. What are the complications of blowout fracture surgery?

    i. Decreased visual acuity

   ii. Diplopia

 iii. Undercorrection/overcorrection of enophthalmos

 iv. Lower eyelid retraction

   v. Infraorbital nerve hypoesthesia

 vi. Infection

 vii. Extrusion of implant

viii. Chronic sinusitis

 ix. Dacryocystitis

  x. Chronic skin orbital floor fistulas/maxillary sinus orbital fistulas

 xi. Loss of lacrimal pump mechanism

 xii. Intraorbital hemorrhage

8.8. ORBITOTOMIES

1. **What are the walls of the orbit?**
   i. Medial wall
   ii. Inferior wall (floor)
   iii. Lateral wall
   iv. Roof.

2. **What are the contents of medial wall?**
   It is quadrilateral in shape, and the thinnest wall of the orbit and consists of:
   i. The frontal process of maxilla
   ii. Lacrimal bone
   iii. Orbital plate of ethmoid bone
   iv. Body of sphenoid.

3. **What is the most common complication in these surgeries?**
   Hemorrhage is the most common due to injury of ethmoid vessels, medial-palpebral, frontal and dorsal-nasal arteries.

4. **What are the contents of floor of the orbit?**
   It is triangular in shape; consists of
   i. Orbital surface of the maxillary bone medially
   ii. Orbital surface of the zygomatic bone laterally
   iii. Palatine bone posteriorly.

5. **What are the contents passing through the infraorbital foramen?**
   Infraorbital nerve, artery and the vein.

6. **What are the contents of the lateral wall of the orbit?**
   It is triangular in shape and consists of
   i. Zygomatic bone anteriorly
   ii. Greater wing of sphenoid posteriorly.
      Posterior part of the wall there is a small projection called spina recti lateralis, which gives origin to a part of lateral rectus muscle.

7. **What is the importance of the lateral wall?**
   i. It protects the posterior part of the eyeball.
   ii. Palpation of retro-orbital tumors is easier.
   iii. Lateral orbital surgeries are more popular.
   iv. It is devoid of foramina, so hemorrhage is less.
   v. It is the strongest portion of orbit.
   vi. Once sawed open has direct access to superolateral, inferolateral and retrobulbar contents.

8. **What are the contents of the roof?**

It is triangular and consists of:
   i. Orbital plate of frontal bone,
   ii. Behind this is lesser wing of sphenoid.
   iii. The anterolateral part has a depression called fossa for lacrimal gland.

9. **What are the surgical approaches?**
   i. Superior approach
   ii. Inferior approach
   iii. Medial approach
   iv. Lateral approach.

10. **What are the incisions for the superior approach?**
   i. Transcutaneous
   ii. Transconjunctival
   iii. Vertical eyelid splitting.

11. **How is transcutaneous incision made?**
   i. Upper eyelid crease incision is made.
   ii. Access to superior orbital rim by dissecting superiorly in the postorbicularis fascial plane anterior to the orbital septum.
   iii. Incision is made in the arcus marginalis of the rim, and a periosteal elevator is then used to separate the periosteum from the frontal bone of the orbital roof.
   iv. The periorbita is kept intact to prevent orbital fat from obscuring the vision.

12. **How is transconjunctival incision made?**

Incision in the superior conjunctiva can be used to reach the superonasal, episcleral, intra- or extra-conal spaces; but dissection must be performed medial to the levator muscle to prevent postoperative ptosis.

13. **How is vertical eyelid splitting made?**

Incise the eyelid and levator aponeurosis vertically to expose the superomedial intraconal spaces.

It allows extended transconjunctival exposure for the removal of superomedial intraconal tumors.

14. **What are the types of inferior approach and how are they made?**

It is suitable for masses that are visible or palpable in the inferior conjunctival fornix of the lower eyelid, as well for deeper inferior extraconal masses.

Transcutaneous incisions
   i. Infraciliary blepharoplasty incision is made in the lower eyelid and dissection beneath the orbicularis muscle to expose the inferior orbital septum and inferior orbital rim.

ii. For access to the inferior subperiosteal space, an extended subciliary incision or an incision in the lower eyelid crease with downward reflection of the skin and orbicularis muscle allows exposure of the rim.

Transconjunctival incision

i. To reach the extraconal surgical space and the orbital floor, incision is made through the inferior conjunctiva and the lower eyelid retractors.
ii. Exposure to the globe is optimized when this incision is combined with a lateral canthotomy and cantholysis.
iii. The intra conal-space may be reached by opening the reflected periosteum and the retracting the muscle and intraconal fat.

15. What are the types of medial approach and how are they made?

While dissecting the medial orbit care should be taken to avoid damaging,

i. Medial canthal tendon
ii. Lacrimal canaliculi and sac
iii. Trochlea
iv. Superior oblique tendon
v. Inferior oblique muscle
vi. Sensory nerves and vessels.

Types of incision

Transcutaneous incisions (Lynch or frontoethmoidal incision)

i. Tumors within or near the lacrimal sac, the frontal or ethmoidal sinus, and the medial rectus muscle can be approached.
ii. Skin incision is placed vertically just medial to the incision of the medial canthal tendon.
iii. Mainly used to enter the subperiosteal space.

Transconjunctival incision

i. An incision in the bulbar conjunctiva allows entry into the extraconal or episcleral surgical space.
ii. If the medial rectus is detached, one can enter the intraconal surgical space to expose the region of the anterior optic nerve for examination biopsy or sheath fenestration.
iii. If the posterior optic nerve or muscle cone needs to be seen, combined lateral/medial orbitotomies can be performed.
iv. Lateral orbitotomy with removal of lateral orbital wall displaces the globe temporally, maximizing medial access to deeper orbit.

Transcaruncular incision

i. An incision through the posterior third of the caruncle or the conjunctiva immediately lateral to it allows excellent exposure of the medial periosteum.
ii. Medial dissection just posterior to the lacrimal sac allows access to the subperiosteal space along the medial orbital wall.

   iii. Incision and elevation of the medial periorbita has advantage of providing better cosmetic results than the traditional Lynch incision.

   iv. The combination of transcaruncular route with an inferior transconjunctival incision allows extensive exposure of the inferior and medial orbit.

   v. This approach provides access for repair of medial wall fractures, for medial orbital bone decompression, for drainage of medial subperiosteal abscess.

16. How is the lateral approach done?

   i. It is used when a lesion is located within the lateral intraconal space, behind the equator of the globe or in the lacrimal gland fossa.

   ii. The traditional "S" shaped Stallard–Wright skin incision extending from beneath the eyebrow laterally and curving down along the zygomatic arch allows good exposure of the lateral rim.

   iii. It has been replaced by upper eyelid crease incision or lateral canthotomy incision.

   iv. Dissecting through the periorbita and then the intermuscular septum, either above or below the lateral rectus and posterior to equator provides access to retrobulbar space.

   v. If the lesion is too big, the bone of the lateral rim is removed.

   vi. Tumors can be prolapsed by application of gentle pressure of the eyelid.

17. What are the complications?

   i. Hemorrhage

   ii. Optic nerve injury

   iii. Damage to vessels and nerves

   iv. Damage to muscles and tendons

   v. Injury to lacrimal gland

8.9. BOTULINUM TOXIN

1. **What is botulinum toxin (Botox) ?**

   Botulinum toxin is a protein produced by the bacterium *Clostridium botulinum*, and is considered the most powerful neurotoxin.

2. **When was it discovered and by whom?**

   The German physician and poet **Justinus Kerner (1786–1862)** first developed the idea of a possible therapeutic use of botulinum toxin, which he called "**sausage poison**."

3. **What is the mechanism of action of botox?**

   Botulinum toxin acts by binding presynaptically to high-affinity recognition sites on the cholinergic nerve terminals and decreasing the release of acetylcholine, causing a neuromuscular blocking effect.

4. **What is the structure of Botox?**
   i. They are proteins that are produced by several different clostridial bacterial species and are related to tetanus toxin.
   ii. The neurotoxin proteins are synthesized along with hemagglutinin and nontoxin hemagglutinin proteins that together form a protein complex progenitor toxin.

5. **What is the concern with the use of Botox?**

   The formation of blocking antibodies leading to non-response of subsequent botox injections, called as "**secondary nonresponders**."

6. **What are the preparations used?**
   i. Botox (Allergan Irvine, USA)
   ii. Dysport (Ipsen, France)
   iii. Myobloc (Elan Pharma, USA).

7. **Contents of 1 vial.**

   Each vial contains 100 Units (U) of *C. botulinum* neurotoxin complex,
   i. 0.5 mg human albumin
   ii. 0.9 mg sodium chloride.
   All these in sterile vacuum dried solid without preservatives.

8. **Botulinum toxin concentration with various amount of diluents used.**

Diluent added (0.9% NaCl) (mL)	Botox used (U/0.1 mL) (U)	Dysport dose (U/0.1) (U)
1	10	50
2	5	25
4	2.5	12.5
8	1.25	6.25

9. **Dose recommendations for common therapeutic indications of botulinum toxin in ophthalmic plastic surgery?**

Clinical condition	Approx dose of botox required (U)
Benign essential blepharospasm	30–40
Hemifacial spasm	15–20
Chemotarsorrhaphy	5–10
Upper eyelid retraction	5–25
Lower eyelid senile entropion	10–20
Injection to the lacrimal gland	2.5–5

10. **What are the common complications?**
    i. Upper eyelid ptosis
    ii. Lagophthalmos
    iii. Entropion
    iv. Ectropion
    v. Functional epiphora due to lacrimal pump failure
    vi. Diplopia
    vii. Eyelid hematoma.

8.10. LACRIMAL SECRETORY AND DRAINAGE SYSTEMS

1. **How is tear produced from lacrimal gland?**

   Afferent pathway: Ophthlamic branch of the trigeminal nerve
   Efferent pathway: Lacrimal fibers via the superior branch of the zygomatic nerve (VII nerve).

2. **What is the cause of the upper and lower canaliculi?**

   They run 2 mm vertically and then turn 90° and run 8–10 mm medially to connect with the lacrimal sac.

3. **Which structure prevents tear reflux from the sac back into the canaliculi?**

   Valve of Rosenmuller.

4. **In any lacrimal sac distension, why does it distend more inferiorly than superiorly?**

   Because superiorly, the sac is lined with fibrous tissue.

5. **Where does the angular artery and vein lie?**

   7–8 mm, medial to the medial canthal angle.

6. **What are the key points with regard to the nasolacrimal duct?**

   i. It is 12 mm in length.
   ii. It travels through bone within the nasolacrimal canal in an inferior, lateral and posterior direction.
   iii. It open into the nose through an ostium under the inferior meatus
   iv. This ostium is 2.5 cm posterior to the naris.

7. **What are the factors involved in the normal tear drainage?**

   i. Action of the orbicularis muscle
   ii. Negative pressure produced in the lacrimal sac during eyelid opening
   iii. When the eyelids are fully open, the puncta open and the negative pressure draws tear into the canaliculi.

8. **What are the common symptoms in congenital lacrimal drainage obstruction?**

   i. Constant tearing with minimal micropurulence: Block is at the upper level caused by punctal or canalicular dysgenesis.
   ii. Constant tearing with frequent micropurulence and matting of lashes: Complete obstruction of the nasolacrimal duct (NLD).
   iii. Intermittent tearing with micropurulence: Intermittent obstruction of the NLD as a result of a swollen inferior nasal turbinate.

9. **What are "soft stops" and "hard stops" during probing performed for congenital lacrimal duct obstruction?**

   a. Soft stops: This implies a resistance to passage of the probe along with medial movement of the eyelid soft tissue and signifies canalicular obstruction.

   b. Hard stops: If the probe advances successfully through the common canalicular system and across the lacrimal sac, the medial wall of the lacrimal sac and adjacent lacrimal bone will be encountered as a hard stop.

10. **What is the distance from the punctum to the level of inferior meatus in an infant?**

    20 mm.

11. **How is the syringing test interpreted?**

    i. Difficulty in advancing the irrigating cannula and an inability to irrigate fluid: Total canalicular obstruction.

    ii. If saline can be irrigated successfully but it reflexes through the upper canalicular system with no distension of lacrimal sac: Complete blockage of the common canaliculus.

    iii. If mucoid material reflexes through the opposite punctum with palpable lacrimal sac distension: Complete nasolacrimal duct obstruction

    iv. A combination of saline reflux through the opposite canaliculus: Partial NLD stenosis.

12. **What are the different types of punctual plugs used for conserving tears?**

    i. Temporary plugs: Collagen (dissoluble)

    ii. Permanent plugs: Silicon.

13. **What is dacryocystorhinostomy (DCR)?**

    Dacryocystorhinostomy surgery consists of making a permanent opening from the lacrimal sac into the nasal space through which tears will drain freely, resulting in the relief of epiphora and discharge.

14. **What are the indications and contraindications of external DCR?**

    Indications:

    Obstruction of the lacrimal sac or the nasolacrimal duct distal to the internal opening of the common canaliculus.

    i. Primary congenital nasolacrimal duct obstruction.

    ii. Secondary nasolacrimal duct obstruction, e.g. dacryolithiasis, endonaal surgery, inflammatory sinonasal disease or prior midfacial injury.

   iii. Persistent congenital NLDO (after unsuccessful probing or intubation)

   iv. Recurrent dacryocystitis

   v. Chronic dacryocystitis

Contraindications:

   i. Tuberculosis of the sac

   ii. Malignancies of the sac

   iii. Unstable systemic condition

   iv. Atrophic rhinitis (relative contraindication)

   v. Presence of a canalicular block (Conjunctival DCR indicated).

15. What are the types of DCR?

   i. Conventional

   ii. Endonasal.

16. What are the surgical steps of external DCR?

   i. Done under local anesthesia or general anesthesia.

   ii. In both cases nose is premedicated with a decongestant—naphazoline

   iii. Patient is placed in reverse Trendelenburg position to reduce venous congestion.

   iv. Lacrimal duct syringing and probing is repeated on table to confirm NLDO.

   v. Skin incision—a medial incision 8 mm medial to the medial canthus, 2 mm above the medial palpebral ligament tendon or a tear trough incision along the lacrimal crest can be made.

   vi. Exposure of the Medial canthal tendon and anterior lacrimal crest: Skin separated from underlying orbicularis muscle and blunt dissection is done until the medial canthal tendon and periosteum are identified and divided as far as the spine on the anterior lacrimal crest.

   vii. Dissection of the lacrimal sac: The periosteum along with the sac is reflected with a periosteal elevator laterally as far as the posterior lacrimal crest exposing the floor of lacrimal fossa.

   viii. Exposure of the nasal mucosa: Traquair's periosteal elevator is used to separate the suture between the lacrimal bone and frontal process of maxilla or between the lacrimal bone and ethmoid thus exposing the nasal mucosa. A bone trephine, drill, hammer and chisel can also be used. The nasal mucosa is detached with the periosteal elevator.

   ix. Kerrison's bone punches used to enlarge the opening of the rhinostomy.

   x. The anterior lacrimal crest along with the frontal process of maxilla are removed.

   xi. Sac lumen identified by passing a probe via the canaliculus and medial wall incised vertically extended upwards upto the fundus, downwards into the NLD. Flaps are made by converting the vertical incision to H shaped.

xii. Nasal flaps are created by a similar vertical incision converted to H shaped.

xiii. The anterior nasal mucosal flap is sutured to that of the sac with the 6-0 vicryl followed by suturing of posterior flaps.

xiv. The skin is then closed with 6-0 silk/nylon.

17. What are the advantages of external DCR?

i. Direct visualization of the lacrimal sac abnormalities like stones, foreign bodies, tumors.

ii. Sutured apposition and primary intention healing of mucosal flaps.

iii. Large osteotomy facilitates future closed placement of glass canalicular bypass tubes if required.

iv. Ready access for management for canalicular disease—like canaliculo-DCR, intubation, canalicular bypass tube.

18. What are the techniques helping vasoconstriction and hemostasis?

Local anesthesia:

i. Nasal packing with paraffin oaked gauzes or nasal decongestants like naphazoline.

ii. Supplementary intramucosal injection of local anesthetic with 1:200,000 epinephrine.

General anesthesia:

i. 3 intranasal cotton tip buds moistened with 1:1,000 epinephrine placed at and above the anterior end of middle turbinate.

ii. Infiltration with LA at the site of incision.

iii. Controlled systemic hypotension—BP maintained at 90/60 mm Hg.

General measures:

i. Reverse Trendelenburg position to reduce venous congestion

ii. Continuous suction device to help maintain a bloodless field

iii. Gentle diathermy of cut edges and respect for surgical planes.

19. What are the indications for intubation in DCR?

Conditions predisposing to fibrosis or closure of the rhinostomy:

i. Repeat DCR

ii. Failed DCR

iii. Traumatic NLDO

iv. Chronic inflammatory mucosal conditions—sinonasal disease, Wegener's disease

v. Absent mucosa/sac

vi. Poor flap construction

20. What are the indications and contraindications of endonasal DCR?

Indications:

   i. When obstruction is in the lower drainage system and the canaliculi are anatomically normal
  ii. Chronic epiphora due to acquired dacryostenosis
 iii. Chronic dacryocystitis
  iv. Recurrent dacryostenosis in children despite probing and lacrimal intubation
   v. Functional NLDO.

Contraindications:

   i. History of midfacial trauma
  ii. Lacrimal sac neoplasms
 iii. Septal anomalies; large middle turbinate; nasal polyps; tight nostrils
  iv. Granular inflamed nasal mucosa.

21. What are the surgical steps of endonasal DCR?

   i. Preparation and anesthesia
  ii. Identification of sac area
 iii. The fibreoptic probe is passed through the canaliculus into the sac and visualized in the nasal cavity
  iv. A mucosal incision made in the lateral wall of nasal cavity, just anterior to the ridge formed by frontal process of the maxilla called the "axilla". It is extended 10 mm vertically and inferiorly.
   v. Posterior incisions made at the superior and inferior margins of the flap using Yasargil scissors and free periosteal elevator is used to reflect the nasal flaps medially exposing the lacrimal bone
  vi. Osteotomy is done with the help of Kerrison's rongeur removing the frontal process of maxilla and lacrimal bone exposing the lacrimal sac.
 vii. The sac is filled with methylcellulose and medial wall is incised vertically. The sac is massaged at the inner cathus to view the fundus and aid in removal of any dacryolith.
viii. The nasal mucosal flaps are mobilized laterally so that the flaps stay in close apposition and form a mucosal lined fistula from the sac to the nose.
  ix. Bicanalicular intubation is done with silicone tubes.

22. What is the postoperative care after endonasal DCR?

   i. Saline spraying of the nostrils—3 or 4 times a day for 1 week.
  ii. Antibiotic steroid combination eye drops—TDS or QID—1 week.
 iii. Lacrimal system is irrigated at 1 week and 1 month postoperatively.
  iv. Tube removal done at the end of 1 month

v. Endoscopy at 1 month to confirm adequate healing at the surgical site

vi. Final follow up—at 3 months to confirm the patency of lacrimal passage.

23. **What are the advantages and disadvantages of endoscopic surgery?**

Advantages

i. No scar
ii. Less bleed
iii. Less chances of injury
iv. Less time consuming
v. Less postoperative morbidity

Disadvantages

i. Less success rate
ii. Experience required is more
iii. Expensive equipment.

24. **What are the complications of dacryocystorhinostomy surgery?**

Early complications

i. Wound infection
ii. Bleeding
iii. Tube lateral displacement
iv. Infranasal synechiae
v. Delayed healing

Intermediate complications

i. Rhinostomy fibrosis
ii. Granulomas
iii. Corneal erosions from tube

Late complications

i. Webbed facial scar
ii. Chronic fistula
iii. Persistent intranasal synechiae

25. **What is functional failure?**

Instead of anatomical patency of lacrimal drainage system, there occurs persistent epiphora after DCR surgery with the absence of any attributable problems in the eyelids and ocular surface. This is known as functional failure.

26. **What are the causes for functional failure?**

i. Canalicular obstruction
ii. Small lacrimal sac (mostly in primary nasolacrimal duct obstruction)
iii. Narrow nasal cavity

iv. Thick maxilla

v. Severe anteriorization of ethmoid sinus

vi. Absence of mucous dacryocystitis.

27. How does distal canalicular or canalicular block affect functional success?

Distal canaliculi or common canaliculi is the narrowest portion of lacrimal drainage system after DCR. So it may act as bottleneck in the tear drainage pathway.

28. How does lacrimal sac size cause functional failure?

Cicatrized and contracted sac impinges upon the transmission of hydrostatic pressure resulting in a decrease in lacrimal pump activity.

29. What is sump syndrome?

The surgical opening in the lacrimal bone is too small and too high. Thus there is a dilated lacrimal sac lateral to and below the level of inferior margin of the ostium in which the secretions collect and are unable to gain access to the ostium and thence the nasal cavity.

30. What are the bones that are broken during DCR?

i. Lacrimal fossa

ii. Lacrimal bone

iii. Frontal process of maxillary bone

iv. Part of ethmoid bone

v. Part of the nasal bone.

8.11. CONTRACTED SOCKET

1. **Define contracted socket.**

   Contracted socket is defined as decrease in depth of fornices and orbital volume which results in an inability to retain a prosthesis.

2. **What important past history you will ask a patient with contracted socket?**

   i. Nature of assault that lead to loss of sight (e.g. trauma, tumor, congenital, etc.)

   ii. Any history of pain, redness watering in other eye (to R/O sympathetic ophthalmia)

   iii. Any family history positive (to R/O cancers like RB)

3. **What are the morphological types of contracted socket?**

   Four types:

i. Anophthalmic:	Seen after evisceration and enucleation and is most common type.
ii. Microphthalmic:	Seen in presence of a phthisical eye .
iii. Ophthalmic:	seen following chemical, thermal and radiation injuries, leading to symblepharon and ankyloblepharon
iv. Hypoplastic:	Seen when there is congenital under development of bony socket .

4. **What are features of contracted socket?**

   i. Volume reduction and redistribution leading to post enucleation syndrome comprising

   – Contraction of Tenon's capsule and retraction of extra ocular muscles leading to back shift of muscle cone and retrusion of posterior wall.

   – Shifting and retraction of levator muscle leading to superior sulcus depression.

   – Change in the axis of action of the levator muscle from vertically upward to horizontally backward.

   ii. Conjunctival shortening with shallowing of fornices.

5. **What are the underlying precipitating causes that lead to socket disorders?**

   i. Congenital and developmental

   – Congenital anophthalmos

   – Microphthalmos with cyst

   – Facial and orbital hypoplasia

ii. Aging

Deficiency of orbital volume

iii. Iatrogenic
  - Poor enucleation
  - Multiple operations on socket
  - Alloplastic material in socket

iv. Traumatic
  - Mechanical
  - Chemical
  - Thermal
  - Radiation induced.

6. **Classify contracted socket and brief the management of each class.**

Grade	Character of socket	Management
0	Normal socket with adequate roomy fornices lined by healthy conjunctiva and no lid abnormality.	Prosthetic eye (custom fit prosthesis)
1	Posterior lamina shortening leading to entropion. Shallowing or shelving of the lower fornix.	Correction of entropion. Inferior fornix forming mattress sutures over a silastic stent (closed method) or undermining of conjunctiva with excision of prolapsed fat and inferior fornix forming sutures (open method)
2	Absence of the lower fornix and pulling down of the fundus of the socket. Superior fornix may show contracture.	Mucous membrane grafting with fornix forming sutures.
3	Grade 2 plus absence of medial and lateral fornices.	Mucous membrane/amniotic membrane grafting.
4	Grade 3 plus severe shrinkage due to scarring leading to reduction of palpebral aperture in all directions. Absence of conjunctival lining of the socket	Split thickness skin grafting
5	Inoperable socket	Spectacle prosthesis

7. **What is the use of dermis fat graft in anophthalmic socket?**

Dermis fat graft is used to replace volume.

Indications are:

i. As a primary implant after primary enucleation
ii. As a secondary implant after orbital implant migration or extrusion.
iii. After evisceration it may be placed within the scleral shell
iv. For superior sulcus deformity.

The preferred site is the upper and outer quadrant of the gluteal region because it is not a weight bearing area and less chance of injuring sciatic nerve.

8. **What are the problems associated with dermis fat graft?**
   i. Atrophy of the graft
   ii. Necrosis of the graft
   iii. Central ulceration of the graft
   iv. Growth of the fatty tissue leading to proptosis of the artificial eye.
   v. Pyogenic granuloma.

9. **What is the important problem in outcome of anophthalmic socket of a child?**
   There is an increased chance of facial dysmorphism in case of a child.

10. **What is the age when facial bone growth completes?**
    14 years

8.12. ORBITAL IMPLANTS AND PROSTHESIS

1. **What are the requirements of a functionally and cosmetically acceptable anophthalmic socket?**
    i.   An orbital implant of adequate volume centered within the orbit
    ii. Eyelids with adequate tone and normal appearance to support a prosthesis.
    iii. A socket lined with conjunctiva or mucous membrane with fornices deep enough to hold a prosthesis
    iv. Good transmission of motility from the implant to the overlying prosthesis
    v.   Comfortable prosthesis similar to the normal eye

2. **What are orbital implants?**
    Orbital implants are:
    i.   They replace the volume lost by the enucleated eye,
    ii. Impart motility to the prosthesis,
    iii. Maintain cosmetic symmetry with the fellow eye.

3. **Classify orbital implants**

Type	Definition	Example
Nonintegrated	No direct or indirect integration of the synthetic implant with the orbital structures or with the prosthesis.	PMMA or Silicon implants
Semi-integrated	Indirect (mechanical) integration of the synthetic implant with the orbital structures but not with the prosthesis	Allens, Iowa, Universal, Castroveijo
Integrated	Indirect (mechanical) integration Of the synthetic implant with orbital structures and with prosthesis	Cutler's implant
Biointegrated	Direct (biological) integration of a natural or a synthetic implant with the orbital structures with or without integration with the prosthesis.	Hydroxyapatite (Bio eye) Porus polyethylene (Medpore) Aluminum oxide (Bioceramic)
Biogenic	An autograft or allograft of a natural tissue with direct (biological) integration with orbital structures but not with the prosthesis.	Dermis fat graft Cancellous bone

4. **What are the commonly used orbital implants in clinical practice?**
    Nonintegrated implants like PMMA and silicon implants.

5. **How will the implant motility can be improved in case of nonintegrated implants?**
    By wrapping it with a donor sclera and attaching the extra ocular muscles of the host to the sclera.

6. **What are advantages and disadvantages of non-integrated implants?**

Advantages:
   i. Cheaper, affordable especially in developing countries
   ii. Easier to perform surgery

Disadvantages:
   i. Implant motility not good
   ii. Increased chance of extrusion

7. **What are advantages and disadvantages of Biointegrated implants?**

Advantages:
   i. Better implant motility
   ii. Better stability

Disadvantages:
   i. High cost factor
   ii. Implant exposure

8. **What is motility peg insertion?**

It is an indirect attachment of the implant to the prosthesis, enhancing prosthesis motility. Pegging of hydroxyl apatite implant can sometimes be performed as early as 6 months after surgery, pending confirmation of vascularization. Pegging may however increase risk of implant exposure and infection.

9. **How is the implant size calculated?**
   i. Implants provide about 65–70% of volume replacement of anophthalmic socket and the rest 35–30% by the prosthesis.
   ii. A smaller implant has a higher tendency to displace or migrate and develop superior sulcus deformity. A larger implant is known to improve both cosmesis and motility. However an inappropriately large implant may result in wound gap and implant exposure.
   iii. Implant sizing has mostly been empirical and is often decided in the operating room.
   iv. Generally a 16–18 mm implant is used for infants, 18–20 mm in older children, 20–22 mm in adults.
   v. There are implant sizers that help gauge the appropriate size.
   vi. Axial length of the other eye can also be taken as a guide (axial length in mm−2 = implant diameter in mm). An additional 2 mm is deducted from the axial length if the implant is traditionally wrapped.

10. **What are the advantages of implant wrapping?**

Advantages:
   i. An additional barrier, so decreased chance of implant exposure.
   ii. Enables easy attachment of extra ocular muscles, thus providing better prosthesis motility.

iii. Entails a smooth external surface. Thus making the process of implant insertion easier.

iv. Helps in volume augmentation by adding around 1.5 mm to the implant diameter.

11. What are the materials used for implant wrapping?

   i. Donor sclera (most popular)

  ii. Donor processed pericardium and fascia lata (commercially available)

iii. Autologous sclera (if the cause of enucleation is other than suspected tumor)

iv. Synthetic materials (polyglactin-910 mesh, polytetrafluoroethylene sheet)

12. What are the special steps to take when enucleation is done for children?

   i. A large adult size implant should be used to replace orbital volume

  ii. Autogenous dermis fat grafts are preferred as anophthalmic implants

8.13. MISCELLANEOUS OCULAR SURGERIES

Enucleation

1. **Define enucleation**

   Enucleation is the removal of the eyeball with the covering sclera and cornea along with a stump of optic nerve.

2. **What are the indications of enucleation?**

   i. Absolute indication:
      - Intra ocular malignancy (nontreatable)
      - Possibility of sympathetic ophthalmia

   ii. Relative indication:
      - Extensively traumatized globes with uveal tissue loss, retinal damage, disorganization of globe
      - Irritable painful, deformed, or disfigured globes with or without atrophy, secondary to RD, absolute glaucoma etc.
      - Phthisis bulbi, especially painful
      - Blind globes with staphyloma
      - Severe buphthalmos with painful blind eye
      - Blind eyes with inextractable foreign bodies.

3. **Name the various enucleation techniques:**

   i. Enucleation without insertion of an implant
   ii. Enucleation with exposed integrated implant
   iii. Enucleation with implant inserted within Tenon's capsule
   iv. Enucleation with wrapped implant (with sclera, fascia lata graft or synthetic material)
   v. Enucleation with incorporation of dermis fat graft.

4. **What is the important step doing before enucleation surgery?**

   Identify the patient and confirm the eye to be enucleated. Also check the signature of two senior doctors advising enucleation.

5. **What are the special steps to undertake when enucleation is performed for an intraocular tumor?**

   i. In case of retinoblastoma, a long segment of optic nerve should be cut to increase the chance for the tumor to be completely removed
   ii. Avoid penetrating the globe and to manipulate the globe gently to minimize the risk of tumor dissemination

Evisceration

1. **Define evisceration.**

   Evisceration is defined as the complete removal of the ocular contents through an opening in the cornea or sclera, leaving the optic nerving and sclera intact along with the attached extraocular muscles.

   The procedure may be performed with or without removal of cornea.

2. **What are indications of evisceration?**
     i. Endophthalmitis, virulent enough and resistant to antibiotic therapy
    ii. Panophthalmitis
   iii. Expulsive choroidal hemorrhage
    iv. Bleeding anterior staphyloma
     v. Globe injury with intact sclera shell
    vi. Blind eye due to absolute glaucoma, uveitis, corneal scarring with or without pain
   vii. Chemical burn with severe disfigurement.

3. **What are the contraindications of evisceration?**
     i. Intra ocular tumor
    ii. Phthisis bulbi
   iii. Advanced degeneration of globe
    iv. Pathological examination of ocular contents desired
     v. Chronically inflamed eye
    vi. Nystagmus in the eye planned for destructive surgery.

4. **What are the advantages of evisceration over enucleation?**
     i. Less disruption of orbital anatomy: Thus, the chance of injury to extra ocular muscles and nerves and atrophy of fat is reduced with less dissection within the orbit. Good motility of the prosthesis is obtained.
    ii. Prevention of orbital spread: Evisceration is preferred in cases of endophthalmitis because extirpation and drainage of the ocular contents can occur without invasion of the orbit. The chance of contamination of the orbit with possible subsequent orbital cellulitis or intracranial extension is therefore theoretically reduced.
   iii. A technically simpler procedure: Performing this less invasive procedure may be important when general anesthesia is contraindicated or when bleeding disorders increase the risk of orbital dissection.
    iv. *Lower rate of migration, extrusion and reoperation.*
     v. *Good motility of the prosthesis*

5. What are the disadvantages of evisceration?

  i. Cannot be performed for intraocular tumors
  ii. Theoretical increased risk of sympathetic ophthalmia
  iii. Inadequate specimen for pathologic examinations

Exenteration

1. Define exenteration.

Exentration is defined as the removal of all the soft tissues of orbit i. e. the globe, extraocular muscles, fat and other orbital contents along with the periobita lining the orbital cavity.

2. What are indications of exenteration?

  i. Destructive tumors extending into the orbit from the sinuses, face, eyelids, conjunctiva, or intracranial space.
  ii. Intraocular melanomas or retinoblastomas that have extended outside the globe (if evidence of distant metastases is excluded). When local control of the tumor would benefit the nursing care of the patient exenteration is indicated.
  iii. Malignant epithelial tumors of the lacrimal gland. Although the procedure is some~what controversial, these tumors may require extended exenteration with radical bone removal of the roof, lateral wall and floor.
  iv. Sarcomas and other primary orbital malignancies that do not respond to nonsurgical therapy. Some tumors such as rhabdomyosarcomas that were previously treated by exenteration are now initially treated by radiation and chemotherapy.
  v. Fungal infection. Subtotal or total exenteration may be necessary for the management of orbital zygomycosis which occurs most commonly in patients who are diabetic or immunosuppressed. However, attention is now being focalized on achieving control through more limited debridement of involved orbital tissues.

3. What are the types of exenteration surgeries?

Subtotal: The eye and adjacent intraorbital tissues are removed such that the lesion is locally excised (leaving the periorbita and part or all of the eyelids). This technique is used for some locally invasive tumors, for debulking of disseminated tumors, or for partial treatment in selected patients.

Total: All intraorbital soft tissues, including periorbita, are removed, with or without the skin of the eyelids.

Extended: All intraorbital soft tissues are removed, together with adjacent structures (usually bony walls and sinuses).

CHAPTER
9

Pediatric Ophthalmology and Strabismus

9.1. PEDIATRIC–OPHTHALMIC MANAGEMENT

1. **What is the visual acuity during infancy?**

1 month of age	: 6/120
6 months	: 6/30
12–18 months	: 6/48–6/12
36 months	: 6/12–6/6

2. **How can we estimate visual acuity by examining the fixation of a child?**
   i. Central steady fixation: 6/6–6/9
   ii. Central steady fixation with strong dominance to other eye: 6/12–6/24
   iii. Central fixation but unsteady: 6/36–6/60
   iv. Unsteady fixation: Less than 6/60
   v. Gross eccentric fixation to no fixation: Vision less than 6\60.

3. **What are the drugs used in refraction for children?**
   i. Cyclopentolate (0.5–2%) combined with tropicamide
   ii. Combination of Phenyl ephrine 2.5% with 0.5% cyclopentolate in premature babies upto 6 months
   iii. Homide 2% (preferred in children with history of seizures)
   iv. Atropine 1% in ointment form (used 1-2 times daily for three days prior to retinoscopy to produce complete cycloplegia).

4. **What is the amount to be subtracted from retinoscopy findings to take into account the working distance?**

Working distance (in m)	Diopters to be subtracted
1.0	1.00
0.75	1.33
0.66	1.50

   0.5 M as it is what used in young children substitute 2 D

5. **What are the general principles with regard to prescription of spectacles in various refractive errors?**

    In general, correction of refractive errors depends upon its association with strabismus

    Hypermetropia:
    i. With strabismus—full correction if esotropia, under correct if exotropia
    ii. Without strabismus—subjective acceptance/optimum correction.

    Myopia:
    i. With strabismus—full correction if exotropia, under correct if esotropia
    ii. Without strabismus: The weakest concave spherical lens giving good distance vision should be prescribed.

    Astigmatism: Under correction below 3 years of age, full correction in older children.

6. **What is amblyopia?**

    It is a reduction of best corrected visual acuity that cannot be attributed directly to the structural abnormality of the eye. It is often unilateral but can also occur bilaterally.

7. **What are the types and causes of amblyopia?**
    i. Strabismic amblyopia—develops in a deviated eye
    ii. Refractive amblyopia
        Anisometropic—develops when there is a difference in refractive error between the two eyes of 1.5 D hyperopia, 3 D myopia or 2 D astigmatism
        Ametropic amblyopia is bilateral seen in hyperopia more than 4–5 D and myopia more than 5–6 D
    iii. Visual deprivation amblyopia—occurs due to lesions that obscure the visual axis, such as ptosis, corneal opacities, cataract and vitreous hemorrhage.

8. **How do you manage a case of amblyopia?**
    i.   Exclude other causes of poor vision by performing a comprehensive eye examination.
    ii. Clear the media
    iii. Correct refractive errors fully
    iv. Occlusion of the better eye
    v.   Penalization of the better eye (pharmacological penalization with atropine/optical penalization with high plus lens)
    vi. Visual stimulation of the amblyopic eye
    vii. Dichoptic stimulation (computer-based binocular stimulation).

9. **What is a horopter?**

   It is an imaginary plane in space in which all corresponding retinal points are seen singly.

10. **What are the factors which are required for the presence of binocular single vision (BSV)?**

    i. Clear visual axis in both eyes
    ii. Eyes in Orthophoria
    iii. Ability of the cerebral cortex to fuse the images.

11. **What are the three grades of BSV?**

    i. Simultaneous macular perception
    ii. Fusion
    iii. Stereopsis

12. **What are the compensatory mechanisms which happen when BSV is interrupted?**

    i. Abnormal head posture
    ii. Suppression
    iii. Anomalous retinal correspondence
    iv. Blind spot syndrome.

13. **What are synergists?**

    Muscles that are paired to achieve movement in the same direction are called as yoke muscles or synergists.
    Ipsilateral synergists: Synergist muscles in the same eye (e.g. right SR and right IO in dextroelevation)
    Contralateral synergists: Synergist muscles in opposite eyes (e.g. right LR and left MR in dextroversion).

14. **What are yoke muscles?**

    These are otherwise called as contralateral synergists. They are pairs of muscles, one in each eye that produces conjugate ocular movements. For example, left lateral rectus is the yoke muscle for right medial rectus in levoversion.

15. **What is Sherrington's law?**

    This law (also called as the law of reciprocal innervation) states that the increased innervation and contraction of an extraocular muscle (e.g. right lateral rectus) is accompanied by a reciprocal decrease in innervation and contraction of its antagonist (right medial rectus).

16. **What is Hering's law?**

    This law (also called as the law of motor correspondence) states that equal and simultaneous innervations flows to the yoke muscles concerned with the direction of gaze.

17. What are the various supranuclear control systems for eye movement?

    i. Saccadic system

    ii. Smooth pursuit system

    iii. Vergence system

    iv. Optokinetic nystagmus

    v. Vestibular ocular reflex.

18. What are the steps in evaluation of strabismus?

    i. History

    ii. Inspection
  - Head posture
  - Asymmetry of Face\ skull
  - Palpebral fissure and lids
  - Anterior segment

    iii. Vision assessment

    iv. Corneal reflex (Hirschberg test)

    v. Sensory tests
  - Binocular vision—worth 4-dot test, Bagolini
  - Stereopsis—TNO, Langs, Titmus fly test

    vi. Cover test
  - Cover–uncover test
  - Alternate cover test
  - Prism cover test
  - Simultaneous prism cover test

    vii. Modified Krimsky (when vision is low in one eye)

    viii. Ocular movements

    ix. Special tests
  - Four prism test (to assess microtropia)
  - Patch test (for IXT)
  - Parks three step test (in vertical deviations)
  - AC/A ratio (in convergence excess esotropia)
  - Forced duction test (to differentiate muscle palsy and restriction)
  - Synoptophore (especially to measure the deviation in all cardinal gaze positions)

    x. Tests for diplopia
  - Diplopia charting
  - Hess charting/Lees test
  - Goldmann perimetry—to assess field of binocular vision

    xi. Tests for torsion
  - Double Maddox rod
  - Lancaster red green

    xii. Cycloplegic refraction

    xiii. Fundus evaluation (to assess retina and torsion).

19. **What are the causes of pseudosquint?**

    i. Flat, broad nasal bridge

    ii. Prominent epicanthal folds

    iii. Narrow or very wide interpupillary distance

    iv. Positive/negative angle kappa

    v. Asymmetry of face

    vi. Deep set eyes.

20. **What are phorias and tropias?**

    i. *Phoria:* A latent deviation in which fusional control is always present

    ii. *Tropia:* A manifest deviation in which fusional control is not present.

21. **What are the causes for abnormal head postures?**

    Nonocular causes:

    i. Torticollis

    ii. Deafness

    iii. Disorders of the cervical spine

    iv. Habitual

    Ocular causes:

    i. Diplopia

    ii. Limitation of ocular movements

    iii. Nystagmus

    iv. One eyed (to expand field of vision).

22. **What are the components of a head posture?**

    i. Head tilt/turn to the right or left shoulder

    ii. Face turn to right or left side.

    iii. Chin elevation or depression.

23. **What are the reasons for a head tilt in a case of strabismus?**

    The head is tilted for two reasons:

    i. *Vertical deviation:* The head is tilted to the side of the lower eye to elevate the diplopic images and make fusion possible.

    ii. *Torsional deviation:* Normally, if the head is tilted to the right shoulder, the right eye will intort and the left eye will extort. However, in case like a left IV nerve palsy, where the left eye is already extorted, the head is tilted to the right to compensate the extorsion.

24. **What is the reason for a face turn in a case of squint?**

    The face turned either to left or right to place the eyes away from the field of main action of the paralyzed muscle and into the position of least deviation. For example, in a case of right sixth nerve palsy, the face is turned to the right to place the eyes in left gaze.

25. **What are the reasons for change in chin position?**

The chin is elevated or depressed in cases of vertical strabismus for the following reasons:
  i. To place the eyes away from the field of action of the paretic muscle.
  ii. To place the eyes in a position in which the deviation can be controlled.
  iii. To avoid discomfort.

26. **What is angle kappa?**

It is the angle formed between the optical axis and the visual axis.

27. **What are the tests based on light reflex to test for ocular alignment?**
  i. **Hirschberg test:** This test is based on the principle of the corneal light reflex (Purkinje image 1). Normally light reflex will fall just nasal to the center of the pupil. 1 mm of decentration of the corneal light reflex corresponds to about 7° or 15 prism of ocular deviation. If the light reflex is seen at the border of the pupil, it is a 15° or a 30 prism D deviation. If the light reflex is seen in the mid-iris region which is about 4 mm from the center of the pupil, corresponds to 30° or 60 prisms of ocular deviation.
  ii. **Krimsky test:** It involves placing prisms before the deviated eye. The prisms are adjusted to center the corneal reflection in the deviated eye and the amount of prism required is taken as a quantitative measure. Modified Krimsky test is commonly employed, wherein the prisms are placed in front of the normal eye, to make the observation easier in the deviating eye.
  iii. **Bruckner test:** The direct ophthalmoscope is used from an arm's distance to obtain a red reflex simultaneously in both the eyes. The deviated eye will have a brighter reflex.

28. **What are the various cover tests?**
  i. *Cover–uncover test:* The cover test is to detect tropia while the uncover test is to detect phorias. The patient is asked to fix a distant target. The fixing eye is closed and the eye suspected of deviation is observed. No movement indicates that the eye is orthotropic. Now, the cover is removed and the movement of the eye behind the cover is looked for movement. No movement indicates that the eyes are orthophoric.
  ii. *Alternate cover test:* It is a test to assess the deviation suspending the fusion mechanisms by placing the cover alternately in front of both eyes and observe the movement in both eyes.
  iii. *Prism cover test:* It is a test to quantitatively measure the angle of deviation. After performing the alternate cover test, prisms of increasing strength are placed in front of an eye with the base opposite the direction of the deviation. The alternate cover test is performed with

increase in prism strength until the deviation is neutralized and no movement is seen.

29. How many types of cover tests are there?

There are 3 types of cover tests. They are:

i. Cover uncover test
ii. Alternate cover test
iii. Simultaneous prism and cover test

All can be performed fixating at near and distance.

30. What are the pre-requisites for cover test?

i. Good visual acuity
ii. Should have central fixation which is maintained
iii. Should have reasonably good ocular movements.

31. How do you perform the monocular cover uncover test?

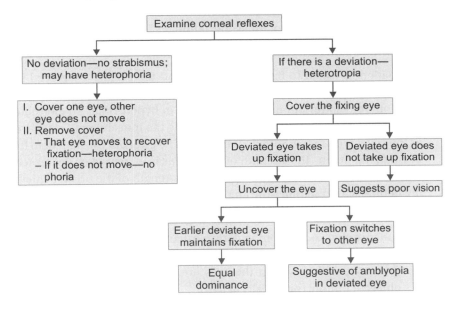

In this test, one eye is covered and then uncovered. During the process, the movement of the eye under cover is noted as the cover is taken away. In heterophoria, the eye behind the cover deviates, then straightens as the cover is removed. The phoria is graded as good, fair or poor control depending upon the force at which the deviated eye takes up fixation.

32. What is alternate cover test?

In this test, the cover is changed from one eye to the other and back several times. In cases of phoria it gives information on the type of phoria.

In case of tropia, it gives information on the type of deviation, whether it is constant/intermittent, unilateral/alternating.

33. What do you mean by alternation of squint and what does it imply?

The deviation is seen in both eyes with equal dominance.

On cover test both eyes take up fixation equally well in presence of other eye deviation.

Implies equal vision in both eyes (no amblyopia).

34. How do you place prisms in front of the eye to measure deviation?

Plastic prisms: Placed in the frontal position, i.e. parallel to the infraorbital margin

Glass prisms: Prentice position—posterior face of the prism is perpendicular to the line of sight.

Plastic prisms are commonly used.

Apex of the prism is placed in direction of the deviation in front of the squinting eye, e.g. base out for esodeviation.

35. How will you quantify the amount of deviation?

The patient is asked to fixate on a target and the prisms are placed in front of the squinting eye. The prism is placed base-in for exodeviations, base-out for esodeviations and base-down in hypertropia. An alternate cover test is then performed while observing the movement of each eye as the cover is changed. Sufficient time must be given for the patient to fix through the prism. The strength of the prisms is increased or decreased until there is no refixation movement. The strength of the prism achieving neutralisation signifies the amount of deviation.

36. How do you assess ocular motility?

Versions are checked first binocularly particularly paying attention to the nine cardinal positions of gaze. The nine positions of gaze are follows:
   i. Primary position—when the eyes are fixing straight ahead on an object at infinity (practically at 6 m).
   ii. Cardinal positions are the 6 positions of gaze, the movement of which is made by yoke muscles.
   iii. Midline positions—straight up and straight down from the primary position (they do not isolate any one muscle as 2 elevators and 2 depressors are involved in the midline positions).

If versions are limited in any direction duction (uniocular) movement should be assessed for each eye separately.

37. How do you test for convergence?

The near point of convergence is tested by keeping the fixation object at 40 cm in the midsagittal plane of the patient's head. As the patient fixates, the target is moved closer and the point at which one eye loses fixation and turns outwardly is tested. RAF ruler is used for the same purpose. Normal value is 8–10 cm or less.

38. What is Parks–Bielchowsky three-step test used for?

It is an objective test used to know whether a cyclovertical muscle is involved in a patient with vertical deviation.

39. What are the principles on which the Parks three-step test is based on?

i. Torsional imbalance when a single cyclovertical muscle is paretic.

ii. Vertical recti have the maximum vertical action in abduction and obliques in adduction.

iii. Head tilt is based on vestibular stimulation which produces a compensatory cyclorotation of the eyes. This is disrupted when a cyclovertical muscle is paralyzed and causes an increase in the vertical deviation.

40. How do you use Maddox rod?

Maddox rod is a device which consists of a series of parellelly arranged cylinders which convert a point source of light (spot light) into a linear image at 90° to the axis of the cylinders. It is usually colored red and used at 6 meters distance. The rod is placed in a trial frame with the ridges horizontal, giving a vertical line. The patient fixes at a spot light at eye level and is asked where he sees the line. Fusion is impossible since the images are dissimilar, the eyes are therefore dissociated making any latent squint to become manifest. In esophoria, the light will be on the same side as the line, in exophoria it will be on the opposite side.

To detect the vertical phoria the rod is placed with the ridges vertically so as to give a horizontal line. The other steps are the same as above.

41. What does the Maddox rod test do?

It dissociates both the eyes, by employing two dissimilar images in front of both the eyes.

42. What is double Maddox rod test?

It is a subjective test to detect and measure the amount of torsion associated with vertical deviation.

43. How do you perform a double Maddox rod test?

Herein two Maddox rods preferably a white and red are placed one in front of each eye to produce two horizontal lines. (ridges placed vertically). The patient is asked if both are straight and parallel or one is tilted. A tilt toward the nose denotes extorsion and a tilt toward the ear denotes intorsion. The side of the tilted line is identified and it is position is adjusted by rotating the concerned Maddox rod in the trial frame until two parallel lines are seen abolishing the tilt. The direction and degrees are read from the readings on the trial frame.

44. What is the use of Maddox wing?

It dissociates both the eyes for near fixation and is used to measure phorias.

45. What is Worth four-dot test?

    i. It is a test used for estimating binocular single vision.

    ii. It dissociates both eyes by red and green goggles.

    iii. It can be used both at near and distance.

    iv. The test consists of four round lights (in a box for distance, in a torch light for near), one red, two green and one white. Patient is asked to view these round lights through a red and green glasses. The colors being complimentary, the red and white lights are seen through the red glass, green and white through the green glass (1 red, 1 white and 2 green).

    v. The following is the interpretation:
- **Normal fusion:** All 4 lights are seen.
- **Anomalous retinal correspondence:** All 4 lights are seen in the presence of a manifest squint.
- **Left suppression:** 2 red lights are seen.
- **Right suppression:** 3 green lights are seen.
- **Diplopia:** 5 lights are seen; 2 red and 3 green indicating a manifest squint with normal correspondence.

46. What are the uses of synoptophore?

Diagnostic:

    i. To determine the grades of BSV estimate the type of suppression, retinal correspondence, fusion range measurement, measurement of angle kappa

    ii. To measure the objective and subjective angle of deviation

    iii. To measure the deviation in all nine positions

    iv. To measure primary and secondary deviation

Therapeutic: Used to treat suppression and intermittent tropias and phorias.

47. What are the types of exotropia?

    i. Concomitant exotropia
- Infantile exotropia
- Intermittent exotropia
- Consecutive exotropia
- Sensory exotropia

   ii. Incomitant exotropia
- Paralytic—oculomotor nerve palsy
- Myasthenia gravis
- Duane's,
- Thyroid eye disease.

48. What are the different types of esodeviation?

   i. Concomitant esotropia
- Infantile esotropia
- Accommodative esotropia:
  - Refractive accommodative esotropia
  - Nonrefractive accommodative esotropia
  - Partially accommodative esotropia
- Late onset or acquired esotropia
  - Basic esotropia
  - Convergence excess esotropia
  - Divergence insufficiency esotropia
- Cyclic esotropia
- Sensory esotropia
- Nystagmus blockade syndrome
- Consecutive esotropia

   ii. Inconcomitant esotropia
  - Paralytic 6th nerve palsy
  - Restrictive Duane's, thyroid, trauma, etc.

49. What are the characteristic features of essential infantile esotropia?

   i. Presents by 4 months of age and persists
   ii. Large angle of deviation
   iii. Free alternation
   iv. Cross fixation
   v. No significant refractive error on cycloplegic refraction
   vi. No neurological defect
   vii. May be associated with IOOA, nystagmus or DVD.

50. What are the variants of essential infantile esotropia?

Ciancia syndrome and Lang's syndrome.

51. What is the timing of surgery in cases of essential infantile esotropia?

Surgical correction is preferred by 6–18 months of age. Most surgeons operate at 12 months of age.
The requirement is:

   i. The deviation is constant with repeated measurements
   ii. Proper assessment of the associated oblique overactions

52. What are the surgical options for this condition?

  i. Monocular recess resect procedure

  ii. Bimedial recession with appropriate management of oblique overaction if present with strabismus.

53. What are the special factors that have to be taken into account while operating in very small children?

  i. Exact measurement of squint is difficult as very young children may not be cooperative.

    In small children, the results obtained per mm of surgery on a muscle is much more than in adults. Results may be less predictable due to this, and the large angle in small eyeballs.

  ii. In children less than 6 months of age posterior segment is still developing so the results might be unpredictable due to growth of the eye ball.

  iii. Distance from the limbus to the rectus may be variable hence measurements may be taken from the limbus.

54. What can be the postoperative outcomes when operating on a child with infantile esotropia?

  i. Optimal outcome—subnormal binocular vision

  ii. Desirable outcome—microtropia

  iii. Acceptable—small residual angle

  iv. Unacceptable—large angle strabismus with suppression.

55. What are the characteristics of refractive accommodative esotropia?

  i. Manifests at 2–3 years of age,

  ii. Hypermetropia 2–6 dioptres

  iii. Ocular deviation at near fixation more than distance fixation

  iv. Normal AC/A ratio.

The deviation gets corrected fully with refractive correction

If not treated promptly, will result in amblyopia in one eye.

56. What is accommodative convergence/accommodation ratio (AC/A) ratio?

It is the amount of convergence in prism dioptre per unit change in accommodation in diopter. It can be measured by two methods:

  i. Gradient method:

    1st step: Patient wears the corrective spectacles and is made to fix at 6 M Snellen letter. Ocular deviation is measured by prism cover test.

    2nd step:—3D lenses are added on both sides and the deviation is again measured.

    3rd step: The first measurement is subtracted from the second measurement and divided by (3D).

The measurement can also be done by making the patient fix for near and adding + 3D lenses in the trial frame.

ii. Heterophoria method: IPD + (deviation for near—deviation for distance) / Fixation distance in diopter.

57. When is AC/A ratio tested?

When there is a disparity in the near and distance deviation, especially if a patient is more exotropic or less esotropic for near then a low AC/A ratio is suspected.

If esotropia is more for near and less for distance, then a high ratio should be suspected.

An abnormally high AC/A ratio can less for distance be managed optically, medically or surgically.

58. What is Duane's syndrome?

i. It is a disorder of ocular motility, in which there is limitation of horizontal ocular movements and changes in height of palpebral fissure due to retraction of globe. Up/down shoots of the globe may be present during attempted adduction.

ii. Huber's classification
   - Type I: Limitation in abduction
   - Type II: Limitation in adduction
   - Type III: Limitation in abduction and adduction

59. What are the disorders associated with Duane's syndrome?

i. Systemic association:
   - Epilepsy
   - Deafness
   - Maldevelopment of the genitourinary system
   - Goldenhar's syndrome
   - Klippel–Feil syndrome

ii. Ocular association:
   - Ptosis
   - Dermoids
   - Nystagmus
   - Myelinated nerve fibers
   - Crocodile tears.

60. What is Brown syndrome?

It is also called as superior oblique tendon sheath syndrome. The characteristic features are:

i. Limitation of the active and passive elevation in adduction.

ii. Downdrift of the affected eye on contralateral version.

   iii. Predominance of a V pattern

   iv. Positive forced-duction test

   v. Hess chart shows a limitation of movement but with a normal lower field.

61. What are the types of Brown syndrome?

   i. Congenital:

   ii. Acquired:
- Trauma to the trochlea or superior oblique tendon
- Inflammation of the tendon due to inflammatory conditions such as rheumatoid arthritis, scleritis, etc.

62. What is Mobius syndrome?

It is a congenital disorder characterized by bilateral facial weakness, bilateral VI nerve palsies and horizontal gaze palsies (bilateral 7th and 6th nerve paralysis).

63. What are the indications for squint surgeries?

   i. To restore BSV

   ii. To correct abnormal head posture

   iii. To treat diplopia and confusion.

   iv. For cosmetic purposes

64. What are the surgical procedures which cause weakening of the recti muscles?

   i. Recession

   ii. Retroequatorial myopexy (Faden's procedure)

   iii. Marginal myotomy

   iv. Myectomy

   v. Free tenotomy.

65. What is the principle of recession?

In this procedure, the muscle is disinserted and reinserted to a point closer to its origin, inducing a laxity in the muscle action.

66. What are the maximal limits of recession?

   i. Adults: 6 mm for medial rectus and 9 mm for lateral rectus

   ii. Children: 5.5 mm for medial rectus and 8 mm for lateral rectus.

67. What is the principle of resection?

A resection strengthens the muscle function. Herein a segment of the muscle near the insertion is removed and the posterior end of the cut muscle is reattached to the insertion. The muscle is strengthened by making it shorter and taut.

68. Why does surgery (recession or resection) performed on the inferior rectus muscle result in alteration of the palpebral fissure width?

Recession of the inferior rectus causes widening of the palpebral fissure while resection causes narrowing. This is because the inferior rectus is bound to the lower eyelid by inferior palpebral ligament.

69. What is Faden's procedure?

It is a retroequatorial myopexy without disinsertion of the muscle. In this surgery, the muscle is sutured to the sclera well posterior to its insertion, thus considerably weakening the muscle in its field of action. The indications are:

  i. Non-refractive accommodative esotropia

 ii. Nystagmus blockade syndrome

iii. Dissociated vertical deviations.

9.2. DIPLOPIA CHARTING

1. **What is diplopia charting?**

   It gives a pictorial record of diplopia in cases where there is separation of two images, changing with the position of gaze.

2. **What is the principle of diplopia charting?**

   Each retinal point has its own value of direction in gazes.

3. **What are the indications for diplopia charting?**

   In patients with incomitant deviation, it can be an aid for diagnosis and for follow-up.

4. **What are the data derived from diplopia charting?**
   i. The areas of single vision and diplopia
   ii. The distance between the two images in the areas of diplopia
   iii. Whether the images are on the same level or not
   iv. Whether one image is tilted or both are erect
   v. Whether the diplopia is crossed or uncrossed

5. **What are the prerequisites for doing diplopia charting?**
   i. Patient should have binocular vision.
   ii. Good visual acuity.
   iii. Patient should be cooperative.

6. **What are the materials required for diplopia charting?**
   i. A pair of red and green glasses.
   ii. Linear light source.

7. **Why linear light?**

   Linear light is preferable since it allows the patient to see a tilted image in the presence of cyclotropia.

8. **Explain the procedure.**
   i. The patient is seated comfortably.
   ii. The procedure is explained to the patient in detail.
   iii. It is made sure that the head is held straight for the whole procedure.
   iv. Goggles are fitted such that the red glass is in front of the right eye.
   v. The linear light is held vertically in the primary position at a distance of about 50 cm and the patient is asked about the diplopia.
   vi. Patient is asked which colored image appears straight in front of him and on which side does he see the second image.
   vii. Ask if the image is higher/lower and if it is straight/tilted.
   viii. If the patient is cooperative, he can be given two pencils and asked to hold them apart exactly as he sees the two lights in different gazes.

9. **What are the precautions to be followed during the procedure?**
   i. Patient must not be allowed to turn his head to look in any position of gaze
   ii. The light source must be moved as far as possible in each direction of gaze checking that it is visible to both the eyes.
   iii. If the patient says that he sees only one light indicating possible binocular single vision the examiner must make sure that the line image has not moved out of the visual field.

10. **How do we record the results?**
    i. Patient's right and left side to be clearly labeled
    ii. Which eye projects the red image and green image to be noted
    iii. Record the separation of images and tilted images as described by the patient using red and green colors.

11. **How do we interpret the charting?**
    i. If two images are joined together—no diplopia.
    ii. If images are separated—confirms diplopia.
    iii. Maximum separation is in the quadrant in which the muscle is restricted/paralyzed.
    iv. If horizontal separation with uncrossed images—esodeviation.
    v. If horizontal separation with crossed images—exodeviation.
    vi. If vertical separation with uncrossed images—oblique muscles involved.
    vii. If vertical separation with crossed image—vertical recti muscle involved.

12. **What are the disadvantages of diplopia charting?**
    i. It is mainly a subjective test.
    ii. Needs a cooperative patient.
    iii. Test is not reproducible.
    iv. In many cases the patients are uncooperative or their intelligence is obscured by intracranial disease or contracture of the antagonistic muscles may have set in.
    v. The test may give false interpretations if the paresis unmasks a latent squint or the patient starts fixing with the paralyzed eye, especially if this eye has the greater visual acuity.

13. **What are the causes of uniocular dioplopia?**
    i. Light defraction—decentred IOL, Ectopia Lentis, Polycoria
    ii. Metamorphopsia—due to macular lesion
    iii. Cerebral polyopic—due to occipital lobe lesions.

9.3. HESS CHARTING

1. **What is the clinical significance of Hess charting?**
    i. The Hess screen test is an important diagnostic modality that helps in the diagnosis and prognostication of incomitant strabismus.
    ii. It provides an accurate clinical method of determining the position of each visual axis in different directions of gaze.
    iii. It provides a permanent and accurate record which may be compared with the results of subsequent examinations.
    iv. May help to differentiate recent onset paralysis from long standing one.
    v. May enable to differentiate paretic squint caused by neurological pathology from restrictive myopathy like thyroid eye disease or blowout fracture of the orbit.

2. **Describe in detail about Hess chart.**

    The electrically operated Hess screen has largely replaced the original Hess screen.

    The hess screen consists of a grey scale with grid of intersecting lines at 15 and 30 degree with a controlled switch panel for illumination of red dots. The red dots form fixation points and plotting is aided by a movable illuminated green indicator.
    i. A light source is present behind each red light aperture, the illumination of which is controlled from a control unit.
    ii. Each of the red fixation spot lights can be switched on in turn by the insertion of a plug into the switch board, the apertures of which correspond to the circular apertures of the Hess screen.
    iii. The patient holds a green spotlight, the color of which is identical with that of the green eyepiece of red green glasses.
    iv. Each eye has to be tested separately. This can be done by changing the side of red and green glasses.
    v. The eye behind the green glass is the testing eye. The patient tries to place a green light tip pointer on each of the red points in turns. The place indicated by the patient is recorded on a chart printed with similar marking. The recorded points are joined to form an inner and outer square.
    vi. For interpreting the results of the Hess test, it is important to be aware of the muscle sequelae that follow paralytic strabismus and the laws that govern them.

3. **What are the principles of Hess chart?**
    i. Foveal projection
    ii. Hering's law

iii. Dissociation of eyes

iv. Haplascopic principle.

4. **What are the indications of Hess chart?**

    i. Patient with incomitant squint.

    ii. Patients with divergence weakness type of esotropia to exclude mild sixth nerve palsy.

    iii. To differentiate divergence palsy from sixth nerve palsy.

5. **What are the stages in the development of muscle sequelae?**

    i. Overaction of contralateral synergist according to Hering's law.

    ii. Overaction of ipsilateral antagonist as its action is unopposed by the parallel muscle.

    iii. Secondary underaction of the contralateral antagonist. However, in long standing palsies, there is the spread of comitance and these stages cannot be easily discerned.

6. **What are the prerequisites for Hess charting?**

There are certain prerequisites required before conducting a Hess charting:

    i. Full understanding of the procedure.

    ii. Good vision in both eyes.

    iii. Central fixation.

7. **Describe the procedure.**

    i. The patient is seated at 50 cm facing the screen being plotted.

    ii. Head erect and eyes in primary position with the head centered on the fixation spot.

    iii. The patient wears red and green glasses.

    iv. Patient instructed to shine the green spotlight upon each red fixation light as it is illuminated.

    v. With green glasses in front of left eye he fixes red dots with his right eye, indicator shows deviation of left eye and then glasses are reversed.

8. **What are the features of the Hess chart used for interpretation?**

General guidelines

    i. The central dot in each field indicates the deviation in the primary position.

    ii. Smaller field belongs to the paretic eye.

    iii. Inward displacement of the dots indicates underaction. The eye cannot move far enough to plot in normal position.

  iv. Outward displacement of dot indicates overaction (or contracture). Excessive movement of eye causes dots to be plotted beyond the normal position.

  v. Equal sized fields indicate that muscle sequelae have developed. Underaction of the affected muscle, overaction of the contralateral synergist, contracture of ipsilateral antagonist of paretic muscle, secondary underaction of the contralateral synergist of contracted muscle. The paresis is therefore long standing or congenital.

  vi. The outer fields should be examined for small under and overactions which may not be apparent on inner fields.

  vii. If the outer field is very close to the inner field, a mechanical cause for the limited movement is likely.

  viii. Each small square subtends 5°. The inner square therefore measures 15° movement from the primary position to each position of gaze. The outer square measures 30° of movement.

  ix. When the right eye fixes the red dots, the field of movement of the left eye is plotted and vice versa. The fixing eye determines the amount of innervation sent to non-fixing eye.

  x. Number of lights in the Hess chart is 24.

Interpretation of Hess chart

  i. Compare the size of the two fields.

  ii. Examine the smaller field (paretic eye) and note position of maximum inward displacement which will be in the direction of main action of paretic muscle.

  iii. In the side with smaller field, note if there is outward displacement in the direction of action of the ipsilateral antagonist of the affected muscle. Outward displacement indicates contracture shown as overaction.

  iv. Examine the larger field and note position of maximum outward displacement, indicating overaction of contralateral synergist of paretic muscle.

  v. In the side with larger field, note if there is inward displacement of the antagonist of the overacting muscle, indicating secondary underaction (this muscle is contralateral synergist of the contracted muscle).

  vi. Look at the relationship between the inner and outer field.

  vii. Look at the position of center dots (inward displacement indicate esotropia).

  viii. Equal sized fields indicate either symmetrical limitation of movement in both eyes or a concomitant strabismus.

  ix. Sloping fields denote A or V pattern.

9. **What are the features of neurogenic defects?**
   i. The smaller field has a proportional spacing between the outer and inner fields.
   ii. Muscle sequelae is common.
   iii. The Hess chart between the two eyes tend to become more similar in size with time.

10. **What are the features of mechanical defects?**
    i. Compressed field either vertically or horizontally
    ii. The most obvious feature of a mechanical defect is normally the marked overaction of the contralateral synergist.
    iii. There is not normally an obvious overaction of the direct antagonist, nor underaction of the contralateral antagonist.

11. **What are the uses of the Hess chart?**
    i. Diagnosis of a muscle palsy.
    ii. Assessing progress.
    iii. Planning muscle surgery.
    iv. Evaluating results of incomitant strabismus.
    v. Provides a permanent and accurate record which may be compared with the results of subsequent examinations.

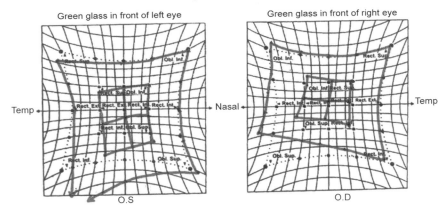

Right eye has a smaller field—affected eye
Right hypertropia of less than 5°
Proportional spacing between inner and outer squares
Limitation of right depression in adduction (right superior oblique underaction)
Extorsion of field of the right eye
Above point to right superior oblique palsy

Overaction of right inferior oblique and left inferior rectus (muscle sequel).

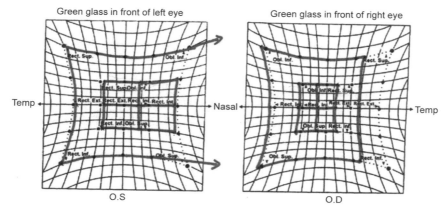

Diagnosis–right lateral rectus palsy

Right eye has a smaller field—affected eye

Right esotropia of 5° in primary position (one small square)

Right abduction restriction

Proportional spacing between inner and outer squares

Left medial rectus overaction (muscle sequalae)

Optics and Refraction

1. **Classify the types of optical defects of the eye.**

   It can be classified as **physiological and pathological.**

   i. Physiological can be of the following types:
      - Diffraction of light
      - Chromatic aberration
      - Spherical aberration
      - Decentering
      - Peripheral aberrations

   ii. Pathological optical defects are of three main types. Subclassifications have been described later.
      - Myopia
      - Hypermetropia
      - Astigmatism
        - **Diffraction of light:** Property of light waves is to deviate after passing through an aperture. Smaller the aperture (pupil) more is the diffraction.
        - **Chromatic aberration:** Light of different wavelength i.e. different color gets refracted differently. Shorter wavelengths (blue) are refracted more than longer wavelengths (red) light. More chromatic aberration takes place with larger pupil size.
          Normally, the eye focuses light of the greatest intensity, yellow, which is in middle of spectrum. So, images formed by light of longer and shorter wavelength are less intense and are neglected.
          The eye is hypermetropic for red and myopic for blue light.
        - **Spherical aberration:** Periphery of an optical lens has more refracting power than the center. So, the peripheral rays are brought to focus at a point earlier than the central rays. This is seen only when the pupil is widely dilated. Small pupil cuts off the peripheral rays.

- **Decentering:** The centering of the eye as an optical system is never exact. The various optical axes and center of lenses do not coincide with each other. But these variations are so small that they are functionally negligible.
- **Peripheral aberrations:** There are several optical phenomena which combine to make the image formed at the peripheral retina less clear than the central image. The most important of these are—oblique astigmatism and distortion of image. Most of these are neutralized by the peculiar shape of the eye.

2. **What are the causes of pathological optical defects?**
   i. Positions of the elements of the system
      - Shorter anteroposterior (AP) diameter—axial hypermetropia
      - Longer AP diameter—axial myopia
      - Lenticular displacement—forward—myopia; backward—hypermetropia
   ii. Anomalies of the refractive surfaces
      - Decreased curvature of cornea—curvature hypermetropia
      - Increased curvature of cornea—curvature myopia
      - Irregular curvature—astigmatism
   iii. Obliquity of the elements of the system
      - Lenticular obliquity/subluxation—astigmatism
      - Retinal obliquity—irregular image formation (e.g. staphyloma)
   iv. Abnormalities of the refractive index (RI)
      - If RI of aqueous is too low or that of vitreous too high—index hypermetropia
      - If RI of aqueous is too high or that of vitreous too low—index myopia
      - RI of lens too low as a whole—index hypermetropia
      - RI of lens too high as a whole—index myopia
      - RI of cortex increases and equals the nucleus—index hypermetropia
      - RI of nucleus increases—index myopia
   v. Absence of lens—aphakia—extreme form of hypermetropia.

3. **What are the important axes related to refraction?**
   i. Optical axis: The line passing through the center of curvature of the cornea and lens
   ii. Visual axis: The line joining the object or fixation point with the fovea and passing through the nodal point is called the visual axis
   iii. Fixation axis: Line joining the object and center of rotation (which lies on the optical axis)
   iv. Pupillary Line: Used as a substitute for the optical axis because clinically it is easier to determine the center of pupil than the center of cornea. Pupillary center is determined by a light reflex and the line drawn perpendicular to it is the pupillary line.

4. **What are the important angles in relation to refraction?**

    i. Angle alpha: This is the angle formed between the visual axis and the optical axis at the nodal point.

    Normally the visual axis cuts the cornea nasally this is denoted as positive angle alpha. If it cuts temporally it is negative alpha and if optical and visual axes coincide, the angle alpha is nil.

    ii. Angle gamma: Angle formed between optical axis and fixation axis at the center of rotation

    iii. Angle kappa: Angle formed between the pupillary line and visual axis. Substituted for angle alpha as it can be measured clinically.

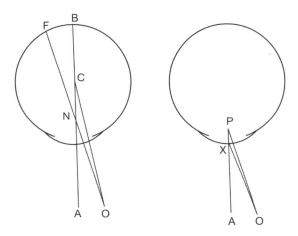

Definition of angles:

C-center of rotation; F-fovea; N-nodal point;

O-point of fixation; P-center of pupil;

X-point of cornea that lies in the central pupillary line;

AB-optical axis; AP-central pupillary line;

OC-fixation axis; OF-visual axis;

angle ONA-angle alpha;

angle OCA-angle gamma;

angle OPA-angle kappa;

angle OPA-angle kappa, as measured clinically.

5. **Define hypermetropia.**

    Definition: A form of refractive error in which parallel rays of light coming from infinity are brought to focus some distance behind the sentient layer of the retina when the accommodation is at rest.

    The image formed is made up of circles of diffusion of considerable size and is blurred.

6. **What are the causes of hypermetropia?**
    i. Axial hypermetropia—1 mm shortening of AP diameter = 3 D of hypermetrpia
        - As a part of growth and development of the eye, hypermetropia is the most common of all refractive anomalies.
        - Pathologically due to orbital tumour or inflammatory mass indenting the posterior pole.
        - Intraocular neoplasm or edema may displace the retina forward.
    ii. Curvature hypermetropia—1 mm increase in radius of curvature = 6 D of hypermetropia
        Cornea plana, flattening due to trauma or disease
    iii. Index hypermetropia—due to decrease in the effective refractivity of the lens. Seen in old age and pathologically in diabetics under treatment
    iv. Backward displacement of lens, congenital or traumatic, leads to positional hypermetropia
    v. Aphakia—extreme form of hypermetropia in the absence of crystalline lens

7. **What are the optical changes of hypermetropia?**
    i. Image formed behind the retina
    ii. Image size smaller than in emmetropia
    iii. Rays emerging from the eye is divergent and tend to meet at a virtual point behind the eye.

8. **What are the clinical features of hypermetropia?**
    i. Eyes are typically small—AP diameter, small cornea, shallow AC.
    ii. At risk for angle closure glaucoma.
    iii. Fundus shows a peculiar sheen or reflex effect called silk-shot retina.
    iv. Pseudopapillitis of the optic disk—resembles optic neuritis. Hyperemic with irregular borders.
    v. This leads to large positive angle kappa—apparent divergent squint.
    vi. Accommodative convergent squint.
    vii. Accommodative asthenopia and ciliary muscle spasm

9. **What are the components of hypermetropia?**
    i. Latent hypermetropia—is overcome physiologically by the tone of the ciliary muscles.
    ii. Manifest hypermetropia—uncorrected at resting state of the eye
        - Facultative hypermetropia—can be overcome by increasing accommodation
        - Absolute hypermetropia—cannot be overcome by accommodation
    Thus, total hypermetropia = Latent + Manifest = Latent + Facultative + Absolute.

10. **Define myopia**

Myopia is that form of refractive error where parallel rays of light come to a focus in front of the sentient layer of the retina when accommodation at rest.

11. **What are the types and causes of myopia?**

    i. Axial Myopia occurs when the AP diameter is long. 1mm lengthening corresponds to 3 D of myopia.
    ii. Curvature myopia—associated with increased curvature of the cornea or both the surfaces of the lens. 1 mm increased curvature induces 6 D of myopia. This is accompanied by astigmatism. For example, keratoconus, keratoglobus, lenticonus, spasm of accommodation.
    iii. Index myopia—seen in incipient cataract where the RI of the lens nucleus increases. Decreased RI of lens cortex may play a role in diabetic myopia.

    Axial myopia may be divided as simple and pathological. Simple is further classified as physiological and intermediate.

12. **Describe the optical changes of myopia.**

    i. Parallel rays come to focus at a point in front of the retina.
    ii. The furthest at which objects can be seen distinctly is called the far point or punctum remotum. More the myopia, closer is the far point.
    iii. As the nodal point is further away from the retina, the image formed is larger than that of an emmetropic eye.
    iv. The negative angle Kappa leads to an apparent convergent squint.

13. **What are the clinical features of myopia?**

    i. Anteroposterior elongation of the eye, limited to the posterior pole. Anterior part is relatively normal.
    ii. Deep AC, sluggish pupil, atrophy of the circular ciliary muscles due to absence of any stimulus for accommodation.
    iii. Fundus—generalized atrophy of the retina and choroid. Tessellated or tigroid retina with visible choroidal vessels.
    iv. Temporal crescent and supertraction crescent nasally.
    v. Posterior staphyloma
    vi. Cystoid degeneration at the ora serrata
    vii. Weiss reflex streak
    viii. Foster Fuchs fleck—caused by proliferation of the pigmentary epithelium associated with an intrachoroidal hemorrhage or thrombosis. It is thought to be a precursor of CNVM.
    ix. PVD and liquefaction of vitreous leading to muscae volitantes

14. **What is astigmatism?**

It is the refractive error in which the refraction varies in different meridia of the eye.

15. **Classify astigmatism.**

Astigmatism can be classified based on:
   i. Position and steepness of the principle meridians
   ii. Position of the image formed on the retina/position of the principle foci.
   - Based on the principle meridians it is of the following types.
     - Regular astigmatism: Where the principle meridians (steepest and flattest axes) are perpendicular to each other.
       o With-the-rule astigmatism: The vertical meridian is steepest (a rugby ball or American football lying on its side).
       o Against-the-rule astigmatism: The horizontal meridian is steepest (a rugby ball or American football standing on its end).
       o Oblique astigmatism: The steepest curve lies in between 120 and 150° and 30 and 60°.
     - Bioblique astigmatism: Principle meridians are not at 90° to each other.
     - Irregular astigmatism No principle meridians can be determined.
   - Based on principle focus it is of the following types:
     - Simple myopic: One focus is in front and the other is on the retina.
     - Simple hypermetropic: One focus is behind and the other is on the retina.
     - Compound myopic: Both the foci are in front of the retina.
     - Compound hypermetropic: Both the foci are behind the retina.
     - Mixed: The foci are on either sides of the retina.

16. **Define Sturm's conoid.**

The configuration of the rays refracted through the toric surface is called Sturms conoid. In this one principle meridian is more curved than the other.

Unlike a point focus of spherical lens, it consists of two line foci which are at right angles to each other. The distance between them is known as the interval of Sturm.

17. **What is circle of least diffusion?**

The circle of least diffusion or the circle of least confusion is where the section between the two principal media are circular. In this the divergence of vertical rays is exactly equal to the convergence of horizontalrays. It lies dioptrically midway foci. For example, if the foci are D1 and D2, the circle of least confusion will be at (D1 + D2)/2 diopters or 2/(D1 + D2) meter away from the lens. The diameter of the circle of least confusion decreases as the two line foci come closer. The spherical equivalent represents the dioptrical midpoint and corresponds to the circle of least diffusion.

18. What are the effect of lenses on the conoid of Sturm?

A plus or convex lens brings the line foci closer to the lens, decreasing the interval of Sturm. A minus or concave lens pushes the line foci away from the lens, increasing the interval of Sturm. In both cases, the distal focus moves more than the proximal focus. The cylindrical power, however, remains unchanged.

A cross cylinder has the effect of contracting or expanding the interval of Sturm about the fixed circle of diffusion depending on the axis.

19. What is presbyopia?

The amplitude of accommodation declines steadily with age. This is due mainly to sclerosis of the fibers of the crystalline lens and changes in its capsule. This inadequacy of accommodation is called presbyopia.

20. How do you calculate for presbyopic correction?

The amount of presbyopic correction necessary for a given patient can be calculated if the remaining amplitude of accommodation is determined (from his near point) and the desired working distance is specified.

In order to achieve comfortable near vision he must keep one third to half of this in reserve. (Elkington says 1/3rd in reserve, AAO BCSC advises half in reserve).

For example:

  i. Assume an emmetrope with near point = 50 cm. Therefore amplitude of accommodation = 2 D.
 ii. Target near distance = 33 cm. This needs 3 D of accommodation.
iii. If we give him +1 D of near correction, he will be able to read at 33 cm, but he will be using full accommodation to do so and this will lead to symptoms of eye strain.
 iv. For comfortable near vision he should have one-third (Elkington) or half (AAO BCSC) of accommodation in reserve.
  v. So we should keep 0.67 D (1/3 of 2 D) or 1.0 D (1/2 of 2 D) in reserve and give correction accordingly.
 vi. So an ideal correction would be +1 D + 0.67 D or +1 D + 1 D i.e. +1.75 D (rounded to nearest practical value) or +2 D

21. What are the prerequisites for prescribing presbyopic glasses?

  i. Existing amplitude of accommodation
 ii. Reading distance or near work distance. Might be less than 33 cm for example with goldsmiths or watchmakers.
iii. Purpose of near glasses. An executive bifocal or near vision alone is better suited for occupational work. People with desk-jobs do better with PALs.
 iv. Age of patient.
  v. Preexisting refractive error.
 vi. Lens status—pseudophakic or phakic.

22. What are the various treatment options for myopia, hypermetropia and presbyopia?

Method	Myopia	Hyperopia	Presbyopia	Astigmatism
A: Noninvasive				
Spectacles	+	+	+	+
Contact Lens	+	+	+	+
B: Invasive				
IA: Corneal—Incisional				
a. Radial keratotomy	+	–	–	–
b. Astigmatic keratotomy	–	–	–	+
c. Hexagonal keratotomy	–	+	–	–
IB: Excimer laser				
a. PRK	+	+	+	+
b. LASEK	+	+	+	+
c. LASIK (includes femto)	+	+	+	+
d. Epi-LASIK	+	+	+	+
IC: Intrastromal corneal ring segments	+	–	–	–
ID: Conductive keratoplasty	–	+	–	+
IIA: Intraocular—phakic				
a. Phakic ACIOL	+	–	–	–
b. Phakic Iris fixated IOL	+	–	–	–
c. Phakic PCIOL	+	–	–	–
IIB: Intraocular—pseudophakic				
Refractive lens exchange—multifocal/accommodating	+	+	+	–
Refractive lens exchange—toric	+	+	–	+

23. Define accommodation.

The ability of the eye to focus the diverging rays from the near object on the retina is called accommodation.

24. What is far point?

The *far point* of distinct vision is the position of an object such that its image falls on the retina in the relaxed eye, i.e. in the absence of accommodation. The far point of the emmetropic eye is at infinity.

25. What is near point?

The *near point* of distinct vision is the nearest point at which an object can be clearly seen when maximum accommodation is used.

26. What is range of accommodation?

The *range of accommodation* is the distance between the far point and the near point.

27. What is amplitude of accommodation?

The *amplitude of accommodation* is the difference in dioptric power between the eye at rest and the fully accommodated eye.

28. What is schematic eye and its dimensions?

Schematic eye is a way to represent the complex refracting system of the human eye. It was given by Gullstrand. In the schematic eye the refracting system is expressed in terms of its cardinal points in mm from the anterior corneal surface.

First principal point	P1	1.35
Second principal point	P2	1.60
First nodal point	N1	7.08
Second nodal point	N2	7.33
First focal point		−15.7
Second focal point		24.4
Refractive power		+58.64 D

29. What is the reduced eye and its dimensions?

It is a simplified version of the schematic eye and was given by Listing. It assumes a single principle point and a single nodal point. The values are measured from the anterior corneal surface.

Principal point	P	1.35
Nodal point	N	7.08
First focal point		−15.7
Second focal point		24.13
Refractive power		+58.6 D

30. What is anisometropia?

Inequality of refractive status of both eyes.

31. What are the types of anisometropia?

  i. Simple
    – Myopic
    – Hypermetropic
 ii. Compound
    – Myopic
    – Hypermetropic
iii. Mixed—antimetropia
iv. Simple astigmatic
 v. Compound astigmatic.

32. What is aniseikonia?

Inequality in the image sizes perceived in two eyes in presence of binocularity.

33. What is the etiology of aniseikonia?

   i. Optical aniseikonia

  ii. Retinal aniseikonia

 iii. Cortical aniseikonia.

34. What are the clinical types?

  i. Symmetrical
- Overall
- Meridional

 ii. Asymmetrical
- Regular
- Irregular
- Pin cushion.

35. What are the symptoms of aniseikonia?

   i. Asthenopia

  ii. Depth perception difficulty

 iii. Obliquity

 iv. Watering

  v. Pain

 vi. Focusing difficulty.

36. What is an eikonometer?

Instrument for measuring aniseikonia.

37. What are the types of eikonometer?

  i. Standard eikonometer

 ii. Space eikonometer.

38. What are the treatment options for aniseikonia?

  i. Optical type:
- Aniseikonic glasses
- Contact lens
- Lenticular surgeries
- Corneal procedures

 ii. Retinal & Cortical types
- Treat cause.

39. What are Purkinje–Sanson images?

Purkinje–Sanson images or catoptric images are formed by the partial reflection of light from the refracting interfaces of the eye.

The interfaces forming these images are—anterior and posterior corneal surface and anterior and posterior lens surfaces.

40. **What is the nature of these images?**

Images 1, 2 and 3 are formed by convex surface and are erect and virtual.

Image 4 is formed by a concave surface and is inverted and real.

41. **What is a prism?**

A prism is a transparent triangular piece of glass or plastic. It has two plane (flat) refracting sides, one apex (top) and a base (bottom). A ray of light incident to a prism always bend towards the base of the prism. The image formed appears displaced toward its apex.

42. **What is the image formed in a prism?**

The image formed by a prism is erect, virtual and *displaced towards the apex of the prism.* In contrast, the rays are always displaced towards the base of the prism.

43. **What are the positions for keeping a prism?**

   i. **Position of minimum deviation**—deviation is reduced to a minimum when light passes through the prism symmetrically.
   ii. **Prentice position**—in the Prentice position one surface of the prism is normal to the ray of light so that all the deviation takes place at the other surface of the prism. The deviation of light in the Prentice position is greater than that in the position of minimum deviation, because in the Prentice position the angle of incidence does not equal the angle of emergence.

44. **Classify prisms based on the deviation they produce**

   i. Right-angled prism—deviates by 90°
   ii. Porro prism—deviates by 180°, image gets inverted but there is no right-left transposition.
   iii. Dove prism—no deviation, image is inverted but not transposed left to right.

45. **What are the ways of prism notation?**

   i. **The prism diopter:** A prism of one prism diopter power produces a linear apparent displacement of 1 cm, of an object situated at 1 m.
   ii. **Angle of apparent deviation:** The apparent displacement of the object O can also be measured in terms of the angle q, the angle of apparent deviation. Under conditions of ophthalmic usage a prism of 1 prism diopter power produces an angle of apparent deviation of $1/2°$. Thus 1 prism diopter = $1/2°$.

iii. **The centrad:** This unit differs from the prism diopter only in that the image displacement is measured along an arc 1m from the prism.

iv. **Refracting angle:** A prism may also be described by its refracting angle. However, unless the refractive index of the prism material is also known, the prism power cannot be deduced.

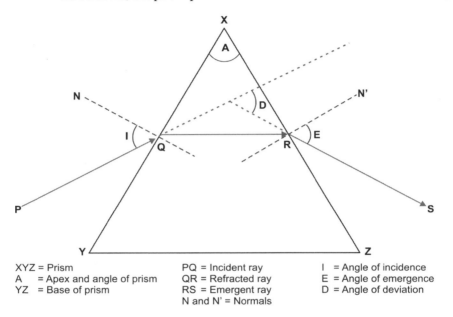

XYZ = Prism	PQ = Incident ray	I = Angle of incidence
A = Apex and angle of prism	QR = Refracted ray	E = Angle of emergence
YZ = Base of prism	RS = Emergent ray	D = Angle of deviation
	N and N' = Normals	

46. What are the uses of prism?

There are three main uses of prism in ophthalmology:

i. **Diagnostic prisms**
  – Assessment of squint and heterophoria.
    • Measurement of angle objectively by prism cover test.
    • Measurement of angle subjectively by Maddox rod and Risley prism
    • To assess likelihood of diplopia after proposed squint surgery in adults.
    • Measurement of fusional reserve.
    • The four-diopter prism test. This is a delicate test for small degrees of esotropia (microtropia)
  – Assessment of simulated blindness.

  Forms of prism used in assessment include single prisms, the prisms from the trial lens set and prism bars.

ii. **Therapeutic prisms**
- Convergence insufficiency. The most common therapeutic use of prisms in the orthoptic department is in building up the fusional reserve of patients with convergence insufficiency. The prisms are used base-out
- To relieve diplopia in certain cases of squint. These include decompensated heterophorias, small vertical squints and some paralytic squints with diplopia in the primary position.
- To reduce nystagmus & to improve near vision in a case of nystagmus with dampening on convergence.
- Can also be used in small paretic deviations to improve the binocularity thereby improving the headposture eg SO palsy, Brown's

Forms of therapeutic prism
- Temporary wear—used as clip-on spectacle prisms for trial wear. An improvement on these are Fresnel prisms which consists of a plastic sheet of parallel tiny prisms of identical refracting angle.
- Permanent wear—permanent incorporation of a prism into a patient's spectacles.

iii. **Prisms in optical instruments**
Instruments in which prisms are used include the slit lamp microscope, operating microscope, the applanation tonometer keratometer, ophthalmoscope, Gonio, synoptophore, etc.

47. **What are the uses of curved mirror?**
The theory of curved mirrors has a major clinical application. The anterior surface of the cornea acts as a convex mirror and is used as such by the standard instruments employed to measure corneal curvature e.g. keratometer.

48. **What is Prentice rule?**
Prentice rule or formula is used to calculate the prismatic power induced by decentering a spherical lens.
It is given as $P = F \times D$
where P = prismatic power in prism diopters, F = lens power in diopters and D = Decentration in centimeters.

49. **How do you do simple transposition of cylindrical lenses?**
This is a change in the description of a toric astigmatic lens so that the cylinder is expressed in the opposite power.
Steps are:
i. Sum: Algebraic addition of sphere and cylinder gives new power of sphere.
ii. Sign: Change sign of cylinder, retaining numerical power.
iii. Axis: Rotate axis of cylinder through 90°. (Add 90° if the original axis is at or less than 90°. Subtract 90° from any axis value greater than 90°.)

Examples of transposition:

i. +1.0 DS/+2.0 Dcyl × 75°
New sphere = Sum = +1.0 + (+2.0) = +3.0 DS
New cylinder = Reverse sign = −2.0 Dcyl
Axis = Rotate by 90° = 75 + 90 = 165°
Answer = +3.0 DS/−2.0 Dcyl × 165°

ii. −2.5 DS/−1.5 Dcyl × 90°
New sphere = Sum = −2.5 + (−1.5) = −4.0 DS
New cylinder = Reverse sign = +1.5 Dcyl
Axis = Rotate by 90° = 90 + 90 = 180°
Answer = −4.0 DS/ +1.5 Dcyl × 180°

iii. +1.0 DS/−2.0 Dcyl × 150°
New sphere = Sum = +1.0 + (−2.0) = −1.0 DS
New cylinder = Reverse sign = +2.0 Dcyl
Axis = Rotate by 90° = 150 − 90 = 60°
Answer = −1.0 DS/ +2.0 Dcyl × 60°

iv. +3.0 DS/−0.5 Dcyl × 60°
New sphere = Sum = +3.0 + (−0.5) = +2.5 DS
New cylinder = Reverse sign = +0.5 Dcyl
Axis = Rotate by 90° = 60 + 90 = 150°
Answer = +2.5 DS/ +0.5 Dcyl × 150°

v. −2.5 DS/+1.0 Dcyl × 180°
New sphere = Sum = −2.5 + (+1.0) = −1.5 DS
New cylinder = Reverse sign = −1.0 Dcyl
Axis = Rotate by 90° = 180−90 = 90°
Answer = −1.5 DS/−1.0 Dcyl × 90°

vi. −1.0 DS/ +3.0 Dcyl × 135°
New sphere = Sum = −1.0 + (+3.0) = +2.0 DS
New cylinder = Reverse sign = −3.0 Dcyl
Axis = Rotate by 90° = 135−90 = 45°
Answer = +2.0 DS/−3.0 Dcyl × 45°

vii. +2.5 Dcyl × 50°
New sphere = Sum = 0 + 2.5 = 2.5 DS
New cylinder = Reverse sign = −2.5 Dcyl
Axis = Rotate by 90° = 50 + 90 = 140°
Answer = +2.5 DS/−2.5 Dcyl × 140°

viii. −3.75 Dcyl × 160°
New sphere = Sum = 0 + (−3.75) = −3.75 DS
New cylinder = Reverse sign = +3.75 Dcyl
Axis = Rotate by 90° = 160 − 90 = 70°
Answer = −3.75 DS/ + 3.75 Dcyl × 70°

50. Why is cylinder power transposed?

    i. A minus cylinder (concave) makes the lens thinner thereby making it lighter and more cosmetic.

    ii. Also, it reduces some amount of aberrations.

    iii. It is difficult to manufacture a plus cylinder than a minus cylinder. Though now with the advent of machines, it is a lesser concern.

    iv. A plus cylinder is often difficult to adjust to for the wearer.

51. How do you calculate the spherical equivalent of a toric lens?

Spherical equivalent gives the closest spherical power of a sphero-cylindrical lens. The *spherical equivalent* power is calculated from the toric lens prescription by algebraic addition of the spherical power and half the cylindrical power. The signs are left unchanged

Spherical Equivalent (SE) = DS + (Dcyl/2)

Eg. = SE of + 2.0 DS/−1.50 Dcyl × 90° = 2 + (−1.5/2) = 1.25 DS

52. What is an achromatic lens?

Lenses made with glasses of different refractive indices and different dispersions to form a compound lens to cancel out the effects. Flint (u = 1.7) has double the dispersion of crown glass (u = 1.5). Thus an achromatic lens can be made by combining a convex crown lens with a concave flint lens of half power.

53. What is an aplanatic or aspheric lens?

If the lens is grinded in such a way that the curvature gradually decreases from the center to the periphery, the spherical aberration can be eliminated. These are aplanatic lenses. Other way of diminishing spherical aberration is by using meniscus or periscopic lenses where the anterior curvature is more than the posterior.

54. What are the steps in refraction? (*marked ones are essential)

    i. External examination in diffuse light*

    ii. Examination of motility of light

    iii. Cover test to detect squint and heterophoria

    iv. Uncorrected visual acuity—uniocularly and binocularly for near and distance*

    v. Vision with pinhole*

    vi. Visual acuity for near and distance with existing glasses*

    vii. Objective refraction: Autorefraction and retinoscopy*

    viii. Subjective refraction: Trial frame and lenses*

    ix. Refining of spheres with duochrome test and fogging*

    x. Refining of cylinder with JCC, astigmatic fan or dial*

    xi. Testing of muscle balance for distance with full correction

    xii. Determination of near point of accommodation and convergence with full correction

xiii. Addition for near work based on age and reading distance*

xiv. Testing of muscle balance for near with full correction

xv. Final glasses prescription*

xvi. Cycloplegic refraction when indicated

55. Define retinoscopy.

Retinoscopy or skiascopy is an objective method of determining the refractive state of an eye based on the movement of shadow in the pupillary area.

56. What are the types of retinoscopes?

  i. Based on light source:
  - Reflecting retinoscope
  - Self-illuminating type
  ii. Based on type of beam
  - Spot retinoscope
  - Streak retinoscope.

57. What are the types of mirrors in a retinoscope?

A retinoscope uses a plane mirror and concave mirror.

In newer retinoscopes, there is a plane mirror and a movable convex lens. The distance between them can be adjusted by pushing the handle up or down to convert it between a concave and a plane mirror.

  i. When the sleeve is moved to the lowest position, it acts as a plane mirror.
  ii. At the highest position it acts as a concave mirror.

58. What are the stages of retinoscopy?

There are three stages of retinoscopy:

  i. Illumination stage: Patch of subject's retina is illuminated
  ii. Reflex stage: The image of the retina is formed at the subject's far point
  iii. Projection stage: The observer locates this image by moving the illumination across the fundus and noting the behavior of the luminous reflex.

59. What is the principle of retinoscopy?

The principle of retinoscopy is to convert the far point of the subject's eye to the nodal point of the observer's eye. At this point, the reflex is uniform and there is no change with movement of illumination. This is known as the point of neutrality or point of reversal. Correcting lenses are placed in front of the subject till this point is reached.

60. What is working distance?

Working distance is the distance between the eyes of the subject and the observer. Theoretically, the further the distance, the more accurate the results are. But practically, it is difficult to see the reflex clearly on stretching one's arms. Usually 2/3 m or 67 cm is taken as a comfortable working distance.

This corresponds to the far point of the subject's eye at neutrality. This induces a myopia of 3/2 = 1.5 D and that must be corrected from all the retinoscopic values obtained.

(All discussions here assume working distance of 2/3 m.)

61. What does direction of movement of reflex imply? (Working distance = 2/3 m)

   i. With movement implies myopia of <1.5 D or emmetropia or hypermetropia
   ii. No movement of reflex means myopia of 1.5 D
   iii. Against movement of reflex means myopia of >1.5 D.

62. What are the characteristics of the retinoscopic reflex?

   i. Speed: Large refractive errors have slow reflex whereas small refractive errors have faster reflex.
   ii. Brilliance: Reflex is dull when far point is away from the observer and becomes clearer as it comes closer to neutrality. Against reflexes are usually dimmer than with reflexes.
   iii. Width: Streak is narrow when the far point is away, becomes wider and at neutrality it fills the entire pupil. This holds true only for with movement reflexes.

63. What are the characteristics of a cylindrical streak reflex?

   i. Break—is seen when the streak is not oriented to the principle axes and disappears when it is rotated correctly.
   ii. Width—varies with the angle of the streak. It is narrowest when the streak aligns with the axis.
   iii. Intensity—brighter when oriented with the correct axis
   iv. Skew—is the oblique motion of the reflex. The intercept or streak moves slightly differently than the reflex when the axes are not aligned. It can be used to refine axis in small cylinders.

64. What is the difference between static and dynamic refraction?

The dioptric power of the resting eye is called its *static* refraction. The dioptric power of the accommodated eye is called its *dynamic* refraction.

65. What are the difficulties faced while performing retinoscopy?

   i. Maintaining a steady working distance for all examinations

  ii. Subject accommodating during examination. This can be addressed with fogging or by using cycloplegics.

 iii. Bizarre reflex in dilated retinoscopy. Only the central reflex should be considered.

 iv. Faint reflex due to hazy media or very high refractive errors

  v. Scissor reflex caused by aberrations or keratoconus.

66. What are the methods of refining the cylindrical refraction?

   i. Astigmatic fan or dial

  ii. Jackson cross cylinder

 iii. Stenopeic slit.

67. What is astigmatic dial?

It is a test chart with radially arranged lines which is used to determine the axis of astigmatism. The spokes that are parallel to the principle meridian of the eye appears sharpest.

68. What are the steps used in astigmatic dial refraction for refining cylinder?

   i. Best visual acuity with spheres

  ii. Fog with plus sphere

 iii. Ask the patient to locate the sharpest line in the astigmatic dial

 iv. Add minus cylinder with axis parallel to this line until all lines appear equal

  v. Reduce the plus sphere till best visual acuity is obtained with Snellen chart.

69. What is Jackson's cross cylinder?

JCC is a type of toric lens used during refraction. It is a spherocylindrical lens in which the power of the cylinder is twice the power of the sphere and of the opposite sign. Eg. +1 Dcyl combined with −0.50 Dsph

The net result is thus the same as superimposing two cylindrical lenses of equal power but opposite sign with their axes at right angles. The lens is mounted on a handle which is placed at 45° to the axes of the cylinders.

Cross-cylinders are named by the power of the cylinder, and this is marked on the handle.

70. How is it used to check correct axis?

To check the axis, the cross-cylinder is held before the eye with its handle in line with the axis of the trial cylinder. The cross-cylinder is turned over and the patient asked which position gives a better visual result. The cross-cylinder is held in the preferred position and the axis of the trial cylinder rotated slightly towards the axis of the same sign on the cross-cylinder. This is repeated till there is no difference on flipping the JCC.

71. How is used to check correct power?

To check the power of the trial cylinder the cross-cylinder is held with first one axis and then the other overlying the trial cylinder. If the patient sees better at a certain orientation, cylinder power corresponding to the JCC axis is increased.

72. What are the methods of refining spherical refraction?

   i. Duochrome test

  ii. Fogging.

73. What is the duochrome test?

Duochrome or bichrome or red-green test is a subjective method of refining spherical power. A split red-green filter is used which makes the background appear as vertical red half and green half. Because of chromatic aberration, the shorter green wavelength is focused in front than the longer red wavelength. The eye normally focuses on yellow which is between red and green. Each eye is tested separately. As it is based on chromatic aberration, it can be used in color blind individuals.

   i. If the power is accurate, the red and green halves should appear equally sharp.

  ii. If the red side appears sharper, it implies the eye is over-plused and minus power is added.

 iii. If the green half appear sharper, the eye is over-minused and plus power is added.

(A useful mnemonic is RAM-GAP—red add minus, green add plus.)

74. What are the uses for the different cells in a trial frame?

From behind to front the four cells are used for

   i. High power lenses

  ii. Spheres

 iii. Cylinders

 iv. Specials like Maddox Rod, stenopic slit, prisms and presbyopic adds

75. What are the lenses in a trial set?

   i. Spheres (both positive and negative)

     At 0.25 D interval till 4 D

     At 0.50 D interval till 6 D

     At 1.0 D interval till 14 D

     At 2.0 D interval till 20 D

ii. Cylinders (both positive and negative)

At 0.25 interval till 2 D

At 0.50 interval till 6 D

iii. Prisms ½, 1, 2, 3, 4, 5, 6, 8, 10, 12

iv. Specials

  – Occluder

  – Pinhole

  – Stenopic slit

  – Maddox rod

  – Red-green lenses.

76. What is the principle of pinhole?

Theoretically, the pinhole allows only a single ray from each point of the object to pass through and a clear image is formed irrespective of the position of the screen. Similarly, when placed in front of an ametropic eye, a clear image is formed on the retina regardless of the refractive state.

77. What is the size of ideal pinhole?

Clinically, the ideal pinhole is 1.2 mm diameter (and is able to correct errors between +5.0 D and −5.0 D). If it is made any smaller, the blurring due to diffraction is more than the pinhole effect.

78. When do you use a multiple-pinhole?

i. There are five pinhole sizes in the multi-pinhole from 0.8 mm to 1.5 mm.

ii. The smaller pinholes provide routine acuity testing while the larger pinholes provide for testing for suspected reduced vision due to decreases in retinal illumination.

iii. The multi-pinhole can also be used in visual acuity testing in mydriatic patients where the multi-pinhole compensates for the inability to contract the iris, thus assisting the eye in obtaining a retinal projection similar to that of a noncycloplegic eye.

iv. Also, it can be used to see vision improvement in patients with central lens opacities or central retinal pathology.

79. How do you measure interpupillary distance (IPD)?

IPD can be measured in two ways:

i. A millimetre rule is rested across the bridge of the patient's nose and the patient asked to look at the examiner's left eye. The zero of the rule is aligned with the nasal limbus of the patient's right eye. The patient is then instructed to look at the examiner's right eye and the position of the temporal limbus of the patient's left eye is noted, giving the anatomical interpupillary distance.

(The limbus to limbus measurement excludes inaccuracy due to differences or changes in pupil size.)

ii. Alternatively, a fixation light may be held in front of each of the examiner's eyes in turn and a similar procedure followed, the distance between the corneal light reflexes on the patient's eyes being measured.

80. Cycloplegics used in refraction along with some common properties

Drug	Concentration	Onset of maximum cycloplegia	Duration of cycloplegia
Atropine Sulphate	1.0	1–2 hr	7–14 days
Scopolamine HBr	0.25	30–60 min	3–4 days
Homatropine HBr	2.0; 5.0	30–60 min	1–2 days
Cyclopentolate HCl	0.5; 1.0; 2.0	20–60 min	1–2 days
Tropicamide	0.5; 1.0; 2.0	20–40 min	4–6 hr

81. How much correction will you make for each?

1 D is deducted for atropine, 0.5 D for other cycloplegics.

For phenylephrine and Tropicamide no correction is necessary.

82. What are the indications for a cycloplegics refraction? (Duane's)

The indications for a cycloplegics refraction are:

    i. Accurate refraction in young children

    ii. Distinguish true myopia from pseudomyopia

   iii. Diagnose accommodative spasm

   iv. All forms of strabismus, particularly esotropia

    v. Pharmacologic occlusion therapy in amblyopia

   vi. Latent hyperopia

  vii. Mentally disabled or uncooperative patient

 viii. Visual acuity not consistent with manifest refraction

   ix. Suspected malingering or hysteria

    x. Opacities in the ocular media

   xi. Preoperative refractive laser patients.

83. What is postmydriatic test? When is it done?

Postmydriatic test refers to repeating the refraction after the effect of cycloplegia has worn off.

Ideally, it should be done in all cases where a cycloplegics refraction was done.

Practically it is done when there is a difference in the correction in dry and cycloplegics refraction

The next visit depends on the cycloplegics agent used. Eg. for atropine it is done after 2 weeks, for homatropine and cyclopentolate it is done after 2–3 days.

84. How will you reverse mydriasis?

Ideally, it should be allowed to reverse spontaneously depending on action of the drug.

Pharmacologically, it can be reversed by using

  i. Pilocarpine—parasympathomimetic
 ii. Dapiprazole hydrochloride—alpha-adrenergic antagonist

It is used to reverse mydriasis caused by alpha agonist like phenylephrine or by sympatholytic like tropicamide.

85. What are some of the factors taken into account while prescribing glasses for children?

Prescribing spectacles for children has the following goals:

  i. Providing a focused retinal image
 ii. Achieving an optimal balance between accommodation and convergence
iii. Allowing for normal growth and emmetropization of the eye.

For myopia:

  i. Cycloplegic refraction mandatory
 ii. Full refractive correction including cylinder should be given
iii. Intentional overcorrection may help with controlling intermittent exodeviations but it leads to accommodative stress and asthenopic symptoms.
 iv. Contact lens may be tried in older children to avoid the problem of minification of images.

For hypermetropia:

  i. Minimal hyperopia may be left uncorrected if there is no esodeviation or complaints of reduced vision. This is physiological and usually corrects with growth of eyeball.
 ii. In hyperopia with esotropia, give full cycloplegics correction.

For anisometropia, give full cycloplegics correction for both eyes irrespective of age, presence of squint and degree of anisometropia. This is to prevent development of amblyopia.

86. What are the properties commonly considered when choosing the lens material for spectacles?

  i. Refractive index—higher RI means thinner lenses
 ii. Specific gravity or density—lower specific gravity means lighter lenses
iii. Abbe number—this value indicates the degree of chromatic aberration or distortion that occurs due to dispersion of light at the periphery. Higher Abbe number implies better quality lenses.
 iv. Impact Resistance—indicates the durability/fragility of lenses.

87. What are the materials used commonly?

i. Standard glass—usually made of crown glass.
  - Advantage—superior optics, scratch resistant
  - Disadvantage—low impact resistance, heavy, increased thickness

ii. Standard Plastic—made of hard resin or CR-39. Most common material.
  - Advantage—light weight, UV absorption
  - Disadvantage—scratches easily, average thickness, average shatter resistance

iii. Polycarbonate
  - Advantage—thinner, lighter lenses due to higher refractive index and lesser specific gravity, very high impact resistance.
  - Disadvantage—high chromatic aberrations, scratches easily

iv. Trivex
  - Advantage—high impact resistance, light weight, good optics, blocks UV
  - Disadvantage—not very thin lenses, scratches easily

v. High-Index material—a lens with refractive index more than 1.60 is referred to as a high-index lens. Can be either glass or plastic. Plastics are made of thiourethanes.
  - Advantage—thinner, more cosmetic lenses, good shatter resistance
  - Disadvantage—chromatic aberrations are more in high-index plastic.

88. What is antireflection coating?

It is a thin layer added on the lenses to reduce glare and reflection of light from the surface. It uses the principle of destructive interference.

89. What are the materials used?

Commonly used materials are magnesium fluoride, silicon monoxide and yttrium fluoride. Other metal oxides can also be used.

90. What are the materials used to make photochromatic lenses?

- Glass lenses—silver halides usually Silver chloride (a photochemical reaction changes silver halide salts to elemental silver)
- Plastic lenses—organic photochromatic molecules like oxazines and naphthopyrans (photochemical reaction alters between cis- and trans chemical structures).

91. What are the types of bifocal glasses?

i. Split lens or Benjamin Franklin type
ii. Cemented bifocal
iii. Fused bifocals
  - Round top or kryptok
  - Flat top
  - Curved top
  - Ribbon segment

iv. Executive type

v. One piece type, e.g. Ultex-type.

92. In a bifocal spectacles, where is the center of near segment located?

The center of near segment is located 8–10 mm inferior and 1.5–3 mm nasal to the optical center of the distance lens. Commonly 8 mm below and 2 mm nasal is used.

93. How do you apply Prentice rule in bifocal glasses?

The image displacement due to Prentice Rule can be compensated by using certain type of bifocal designs.

i. With a plus lens, round top bifocal segment is used

ii. With a minus lens, a flat top bifocal segment is used.

94. What is PAL? What are its advantages and disadvantages?

PAL stands for progressive addition lenses. It is a type of multifocal lens where there is a gradual change of power from distance to near as one looks from top to bottom.

Advantages

i. Gradual change of power

ii. No abrupt image shifts

iii. Clear vision at all focal distances

iv. Cosmetically better—no visible demarcation line.

Disadvantages

i. Peripheral distortion. This aberration is caused by combined astigmatism resulting from the changing aspheric curves.

ii. Distortion is maximum in lower inner and outer quadrants.

iii. PAL spectacles take some time to get used to.

95. What are the different parts of a PAL?

There are four parts of a PAL

i. Spherical distance zone

ii. Reading zone

iii. Transition zone or corridor

iv. Zones of peripheral distortion

96. What are the types of PAL spectacles?

i. Soft design—long progression and soft periphery

ii. Hard design—short progression and hard periphery.

97. What are the parts of a spectacles frame?

Rims, bridge, side-pieces, joints, nose-pads.

98. What are the types of spectacle frames?

    i. Full-rim

    ii. Half-rim

    iii. Rimless

    iv. Nylon supra—half rim with a thin nylon thread supporting the lenses at the bottom.

99. What materials are used?

    i. Metal—titanium, aluminum, nickel, stainless steel, gold.

    ii. Plastic—perspex, cellulose nitrate, cellulose acetate, newer polymers

    iii. Tortoise shell—made of hawk-bill turtle shell.

CASE SHEET WRITING

Optics and Refraction

Simple Myopia

    i. Patient details—Mr ABC, 25 years, male

    ii. Patient complaints—both eyes defective distance vision × 6 months

    iii. UCVA—RE –6/60; LE –6/36

    iv. Vision with own spectacles—if present. Also neutralize and determine spectacle power.

    v. Vision with pinhole RE –6/12; LE –6/9

    vi. Check for Phorias; mention if present

    vii. Objective refraction with retinoscopy. Working distance = 2/3 m (66 cm) hence correction = –1.5 D

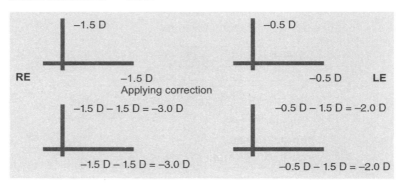

    viii. Subjective refraction
- Confirming with trial frame and loose lens
  Start with exact power obtained from retinoscopy.
  - For myopes decrease power till patient can read clearly with minimum minus power, e.g. Start with –3.0 D in RE and try with –2.75, –2.50 and so on
  - For hypermetropia increase power till patient reads clearly with maximum plus power.
    RE 6/60 with –3.0 DS = 6/6
    LE 6/36 with –2.0 DS = 6/6
- Refining of power (optional)
  - Duochrome test—to avoid over or undercorrection
  - Fogging with plus lenses

ix. Check for near vision (at 33 cm)
- RE N6 Nil glass
- LE N6 Nil glass

x. Optional, but mention these when asked in viva:
- Binocular balancing with four prism diopter kept base up and base down
- Back vertex distance for power more than +/−5 D
- Cycloplegic correction factor based on the drug used for dilatation. In this case 0.5 D is deducted from each value.
- Muscle balance with full correction
- Decide to call for PMT if pre- and post-cycloplegic refraction is different

xi. Interpupillary distance or mean pupillary distance for each eye.
RE 34 mm, LE 34 mm

xii. Will full correction, ask patient to walk around and check comfort level

xiii. Final Prescription including lens type and design, frame type.
Comment: No drug correction for minus spheres

RE	Sph	Cyl	Axis	VA	LE	Sph	Cyl	Axis	VA
DV	−3.0 D	–	–	6/6	DV	−2.0 D	–	–	6/6
NV	–	–	–	N6	NV	–	–	–	N6

Distance vision only
Plastic lens, photochromatic
MPD: RE 34 mm   LE 34 mm

Hypermetropia with Presbyopia

i. Patient details—Mr TGFBR, 45 years, male

ii. Patient complaints—both eyes defective vision for near and distance × 6 months

iii. UCVA – RE – 6/36; LE – 6/24 || RE – N18; LE – N12

iv. Vision with own spectacles—partly improving.
- Vision with own PG: RE = 6/9 p; LE = 6/9 || BE N9
- Existing PG power: RE = +1.0 DS; LE = +0.5 DS || BE Add +1.0

v. Vision with pinhole—RE −6/9; LE −6/6p

vi. Check for phorias; mention if present

  vii. Objective refraction with retinoscopy.

      Working distance = 2/3 m (66 cm) hence correction = −1.5 D

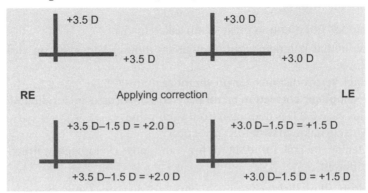

  viii. Subjective refraction
- Confirming with trial frame and loose lens
  Start with exact power obtained from retinoscopy.
  - For myopia decrease power till patient can read clearly with minimum minus power
  - For hypermetropia increase power till patient reads clearly with maximum plus power.
    e.g. Start with +2.0 D in RE and try with +2.25, +2.50 and so on
    RE 6/36 with +2.0 DS = 6/6
    LE 6/24 with +1.75 DS = 6/6
- Refining of power (optional)
  - Duochrome test—to avoid over or under-correction
  - Fogging with plus lenses (in this case, put a plus lens greater than the correction, e.g. +4.0 D)

  ix. With distance correction in place, check for near vision at patient's reading/working distance.
- RE Add +1.5 D N6 at 33 cm
- LE Add +1.5 D N6 at 33 cm

  x. Optional, but mention these when asked in viva:
- Binocular balancing with four prism diopter kept Base up and base down
- Back vertex distance for power more than +/−5 D
- Presbyopic correction is checked in undilated pupil. Hence, cycloplegics correction is not required.
- Muscle balance with full correction
- Decide to call for PMT if pre- and post-cycloplegic refraction is different

- Interpupillary distance or mean pupillary distance for each eye.
  - RE 32 mm; LE 32 mm
- Will full correction, ask patient to walk around and check comfort level.

  Final prescription including lens type and design, frame type.

RE	Sph	Cyl	Axis	VA	LE	Sph	Cyl	Axis	VA
DV	+2.0 DS	–	–	6/6	DV	+1.5 DS	–	–	6/6
NV (Add)	+1.5 DS	–	–	N6	NV (Add)	+1.5 DS	–	–	N6

RE	Sph	Cyl	Axis	VA	LE	Sph	Cyl	Axis	VA
DV	+2.0 DS	–	–	6/6	DV	+1.5 DS	–	–	6/6
NV	+3.5 DS	–	–	N6	NV	+3.0 DS	–	–	N6

Bifocal design—Kryptok or PAL
Plastic lens
MPD: RE 32 mm   LE 32 mm

Some examiners do not prefer the "Add" in prescription. In that case write the sum of spheres in the NV section.

Compound Myopic Astigmatism

i. Patient details—Ms APMPPE, 30 years, female

ii. Patient complaints—both eyes defective vision for near and distance × 6 months

iii. UCVA – RE – 6/60; LE – 6/24

iv. Vision with own spectacles—partly improving.
   - Vision with own PG: RE = 6/12; LE = 6/9
   - Existing PG Power:
   RE = −1.0 DS/−0.5 Dcyl × 90°;
   LE = −0.5 DS/−0.5 Dcyl × 90°

v. Vision with pinhole – RE – 6/9; LE – 6/9

vi. Check for phorias; mention if present

vii. Objective refraction with retinoscopy.
   Working distance = 2/3 m (66 cm) hence correction = −1.5 D

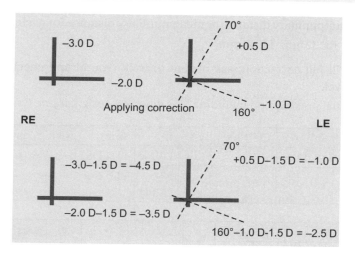

Power = –4.5 Dsp/+1.0 Dcyl × 90°   **Power = –2.5 Dsp/+1.5 Dcyl ×**
160°

Transposing = –3.5 Dsp/–1.0 Dcyl × 180°   **Transposing = –1.0 Dsp/**
–1.5 Dcyl × 70°

viii. Subjective refraction
- Confirming with trial frame and loose lens:
  Start with exact power obtained from retinoscopy.
  - For myopia decrease power till patient can read clearly with minimum minus power
  - For hypermetropia increase power till patient reads clearly with maximum plus power.
  - For astigmatism, correct sphere first to give best vision and then correct cylinder.

  In this case, after putting a –3.0 D Sph in RE for BCVA of 6/9p, then start correcting the cylindrical power.
- Refining:
  In case of astigmatism, refining is done in following order:
  - Cylinder axis with JCC (align the cross-cylinder axes 45° from the principal meridians)
  - Cylinder power with JCC (align the cross-cylinder axes with the principal meridians of the correcting cylinder)
  - Sphere power by fogging or duochrome
- contd. For example, after subjective refraction and refining, the final power is as follows
  RE = –3.5 Dsp/–1.0 Dcyl × 180°
  LE = –1.0 Dsp/–1.5 Dcyl × 70°

ix. With distance correction in place, check for near vision at patient's reading/working distance.

RE N6 Nil glass

LE N6 Nil glass

x. Optional, but mention these when asked in viva
   - Binocular balancing with four prism diopter kept base up and base down
   - Back vertex distance for power more than +/−5 D
   - Cycloplegic correction factor based on the drug used for dilatation. In this case 0.5 D is deducted from each value.
   - Muscle balance with full correction
   - Decide to call for PMT if pre- and postcycloplegic refraction is different

xi. Inter pupillary distance or mean pupillary distance for each eye.

RE 32 mm; LE 32 mm

xii. Will full correction, ask patient to walk around and check comfort level. It is vitally important for spheres to confirm acceptance.

xiii. Final prescription including lens type and design, frame type.

Comment: No drug correction for minus spheres

RE	Sph	Cyl	Axis	VA	LE	Sph	Cyl	Axis	VA
DV	−3.50	−1.0	180°	6/6	DV	−1.0	−1.5	70°	6/6
NV	–	–	–	N6	NV	–	–	–	N6

Distance vision only

Plastic lens, with ARC

MPD: RE 30 mm   LE 30 mm

Examples of Retinoscopy Problems

Example 1: 40 yrs/Phenylephrine

$$\frac{\qquad}{\Big|} \begin{array}{l} +3.5 \\ +2.5 \end{array}$$

<u>**8 steps for prescription**</u>

1. Power cross

$$\frac{\qquad}{\Big|} \begin{array}{l} +3.5 \\ +2.5 \end{array}$$

2. Distance correction

$$\frac{\quad}{\quad} \Big|\begin{array}{l} +2.5 \\ +1.5 \end{array}$$

3. Subjective

$$\frac{+1.5 \text{ D sph}}{+1\text{D cyl} \times 180}$$

4. Transposition

$$\frac{+2.5 \text{ D sph}}{-1 \text{ D cyl} \times 90}$$

5. Drug correction—nil

6. Near vision add +1

7. Glass prescription

Sph	Cyl	Axis	Vn
+2.5	−1	90	6/6
+3.5	−1	90	N6

8. Diagnosis: Compound hypermetropic astigmatism against rule with presbyopia

Example 2: 25 yrs/homatropine

$$\frac{\quad}{\quad} \Big|\begin{array}{l} -1.5 \\ +/- \end{array}$$

8 steps for prescription

1. Power cross

$$\frac{\quad}{\quad} \Big|\begin{array}{l} -1.5 \\ +/- \end{array}$$

2. Distance correction

$$\frac{\quad}{\quad} \Big|\begin{array}{l} -2.5 \\ -1 \end{array}$$

3. Subjective

$$\frac{-1\text{D sph}}{-1.5\text{D cyl} \times 180}$$

4. **Transposition**

$$\frac{-2.5D \text{ sph}}{+1.5D \text{ cyl} \times 90}$$

5. **Drug correction—nil**

6. **Near vision—nil**

7. **Glass prescription**

Sph	Cyl	Axis	Vn
−1	−1.5	180	6/6
			N6

8. **Diagnosis: Compound Myopia Astigmatism with Rule**

Donder's rule for near vision

Reads @ 67 cm
Needs @ 25 cm

1.	Available power NV @ 67 cm	–	1.5 D
2.	Power needed at 25 cm	–	4 D
3.	1/3 reserve and remaining 1.5–1	–	1 D
4.	Give required power 4–1	–	3 D

When signs are opposite in sphere and cylinders, how to make a diagnosis?

Diagnosis

1. +2.75 DS/−2.5 DC 180
2. +2.75 DS/−3.0 DC 180
3. +2.75 DS/−2.75 DC 180

Transpose

1. +0.25 DS/+2.5 DC 90	i. CHA
2. −0.25 DS/+ 3.0 DC 90	ii. MA
3. +0 DS/+2.75 DC 90	iii. SA

When spherical power is more than cylinder—compound astigmatism
When cylinder is more than sphered—mixed astigmatism
When sphere and cylinder are same—simple astigmatism

Astigmatism

1. **How can astigmatism be corrected?**

   i. Eye glasses
   ii. Contact lenses, preferably RGP
   iii. Toric contact lenses
   iv. Refractive surgery
   v. Toric intraocular lenses.

2. **What are the factors affecting the refractive outcomes following cataract surgery?**

   The factors affecting are:

   i. The accuracy of biometry measurements
   ii. Surgical techniques with respect to wound construction and placement,
   iii. Consistency of capsulotomy size
   iv. Circularity and centration
   v. IOL type (especially with regard to a constant) and rotational stability (especially with toric IOL)
   vi. Correlation between predicted and actual effective IOL position.

3. **What are the surgical techniques of correcting astigmatism alongside cataract surgery?**

   i. Site of the incision (Incision on the steeper meridian is preferable.)
   ii. Size of the incision (A larger incision induces more astigmatism.)
   iii. Astigmatic keratotomy
   iv. Limbal Relaxing incisions (LRIs)
   v. Toric IOLs.

4. **What are the advantages of toric IOLs?**

   i. The lenses are introduced through a small incision and hence recovery is quick.
   ii. The incision is unlikely to induce irregular astigmatism.
   iii. There is potential for correcting high amounts of astigmatism even up to 5 D.

5. **What are the disadvantages of toric IOLs?**

   i. They do not correct astigmatism at the source (cornea), so distortion may be induced, even if astigmatism is fully nullified
   ii. Residual astigmatism with toric lenses is usually oblique
   iii. They are not useful for correcting asymmetric bowtie astigmatism
   iv. The results also are dependent on the rotational stability of the lens.

6. **What are the advantages of limbal relaxing incisions (LRIs)?**

   i. The technique is easy to learn and perform.
   ii. LRIS can be quickly performed adding minimal time to cataract surgery.

   iii. LRIs correct problem at the source (cornea).
   iv. There is no issue of rotation unlike toric IOLs.
    v. LRIs can work well for asymmetric corneal astigmatism

7. What are the disadvantages of limbal relaxing incisions (LRIs)?

   i. The incisions are longer and possibly more irritating than a phako incision would be.
   ii. Large incisions are less predictable, occasionally gape, can be difficult to hydrate and sometimes require sutures.
   iii. LRIs cannot be used in patients with keratoconus.

8. What is astigmatic keratotomy?

This refers to making transverse or arcuate cuts in the mid periphery perpendicular to the steepest meridian.

9. What is the mechanism of astigmatic keratotomy?

The incised meridian flattens while the meridian 90° away steepens to nearly same amount.

10. How much astigmatism can be corrected by astigmatic keratotomy?

It can correct astigmatism up to 4–6 D.

11. What are the risks involved in doing astigmatic keratotomy?

Irregular astigmatism, microperforations and overcorrection.

12. How much astigmatism can be corrected by Limbal Relaxing incisions (LRIs)?

It can correct up to −1.00 to −2.00 astigmatism.

13. Describe the technique of astigmatic keratotomy?

   i. Transverse incisions—done in pairs along the steepest meridian, and may extend for about 3 mm.
   ii. Arcuate incisions—clear corneal incisions are made which remains at a constant distance from the center of the pupil.

14. How to place the toric IOL?

The toric IOL must be aligned with the appropriate steep meridian of the astigmatism.

15. How much astigmatism can clear corneal incisions correct?

   i. A 3 mm temporal CCI induces between 0.28 and 0.53 D of temporal flattening.
   ii. A 3 mm superior or superotemporal CCI induces a flattening of up to 1.2 D.
   iii. For correcting astigmatism greater than 1.20 D, a wide incision or an additional opposite clear corneal incision are needed.

iv. Opposite clear corneal incisions are self-sealing, require no extra surgical equipment and are reported to correct 0.50–2.0 D

16. **How much rotation of toric IOL is tolerated?**
    i. Rotation of 15° decreases the astigmatic correction to ≈50%.
    ii. Rotation of 30° decreases astigmatic correction to close to zero with a large shift in the astigmatic axis.
    iii. Rotation greater than 30° can increase astigmatism and change its axis.

Miscellaneous

11.1. VITAMIN A DEFICIENCY

1. **What is vitamin A?**

    It is a fat soluble vitamin stored in the liver. Vitamin A, in strictest sense refers to retinol. However the oxidized metabolites, retinaldehyde, and retinoic acid are also biologically active compounds.

2. **What are available forms of vitamin A?**

    There are four forms:
    - i.   Acid—retinoic acid
    - ii. Aldehyde—retinaldehyde
    - iii. Alcohol—retinal
    - iv. Ester—retinyl ester.

3. **What is role of retinaldehyde and retinoic acid in normal body?**

    Retinaldehyde—is required for normal vision.

    Retinoic acid—is necessary for normal morphogenesis, growth, and cell differentiation.

4. **What are sources of vitamin A?**

    Vitamin A is available from both plant and animal sources as retinyl palmitate and carotene respectively.

    Animal sources—meat, milk, liver, fish, cod liver oil.

    Plant sources—green leafy vegetable, carrots, fruits especially yellow fruits (mango and papaya).

5. **What are requirement of vitamin A?**

Adults	300–750 µg/day
Lactating female	1150–4600 µg/day.

6. What is the role of vitamin A in the body?

Role in general

   i. Maintenance of mucus secreting cells of epithelia of body.

  ii. Normal morphogenesis, growth, and cell differentiation.

 iii. Role in iron utilization.

 iv. Role in humoral immunity, T-cell-mediated immunity, natural cell killer activity, and phagocytosis.

Role in eye

   i. Precursor of photosensitive visual pigment (rhodopsin)

  ii. Maintain conjunctival mucosa and corneal stroma.

 iii. Outer segment turnover epithelium.

7. What is the blood level of vitamin A?

It is made by measurement of serum retinol.

Normal range—   30–65 µg/dL or
                        150–300 IU/dL.

8. What is etiology of vitamin A deficiency?

   i. Primary vitamin A deficiency: This is due to deficient dietary intake of vitamin A and other micronutrients.

  ii. Secondary vitamin A deficiency: It is due to defect in absorptions and utilization. It occurs in the following conditions.

For example:

   i. Malabsorption syndrome

  ii. Chronic liver disease

 iii. Severe infection

 iv. Chronic pancreatitis.

9. What are the risk factors of vitamin A deficiency?

    i. Age: preschool children (2–3 years of age)

   ii. Sex: males>females

  iii. Social economic status: low social class

  iv. Physiological status: pregnant and lactating women are vulnerable to low vitamin A content in breast milk

   v. Diet: rice dependent communities in most tropics

  vi. Seasons: dry summer

 vii. Breast feeding: highly protective, weaning diet highly crucial

viii. Cultural: dietary habits in some communities

  ix. Infectious diseases: some diseases predispose to vitamin A deficiencies.

For example, diarrhea, intestinal parasites, AIDS, measles.

10. **What is WHO classification of xerophthalmia?**
    i. XN Night blindness
    ii. X1A Conjunctival xerosis
    iii. X1B Conjunctival xerosis ± Bitot's spot
    iv. X2 Corneal xerosis
    v. X3A Corneal ulceration/keratomalacia/involving <1/3rd of corneal surface
    vi. X3B Corneal ulceration/keratomalacia/involving >1/3rd of corneal surface
    vii. XS Corneal scars
    viii. XF Xerophthalmia fundus.

11. **What is xerophthalmia?**

    The term used to describe irregular, lusterless, and poorly wettable surface of the conjunctiva and cornea associated with vitamin A deficiency.

12. **Describe night blindness.**

    One of the most common and earliest manifestation.
    i. It is reversible.
    ii. It is due to inadequate or slow recovery of rhodopsin in retina after exposure to bright light.
    iii. Occurs because retinol is essential for production of rhodopsin by rod photoreceptor.
    iv. With oral replacement night blindness may disappear in 48 hours.

13. **Describe conjunctival xerosis.**

    Characteristic changes are usually confined to bulbar conjunctiva.
    i. Changes are dryness, lack of wettability, loss of transparency, thickening, wrinkling and pigmentation.
    ii. Histopathology
       – Metaplasia of normal columnar cells to stratified squamous.
       – Prominent granular layer.
       – Formation of metaplastic, keratinized surface.

14. **What is Bitot's spot?**

    It is a classic sign of xerophthalmia.
    i. It is described as a paralimbal grayish plaques of keratinized conjunctival debris, frothy foamy cheese in appearance and not wetted by tear.
    ii. Pathologically, it is a tangle of keratinizing epithelial cells mixed with saprophytic bacteria and sometimes fungi, fatty debris over edema of mucosa and submucosa.

15. **What is site of occurrence of Bitot's spot?**

Site in decreasing order of frequency,

Temporal → nasal → inferior → superior

More significant diagnostically if nasal in position.

16. **Describe corneal xerosis.**

Usually associated with conjunctival xerosis.

Torch light examination shows

 i. Roughened and lusterless surface.
 ii. Peau "d" orange appearance.

Slit lamp examination

 i. Stromal edema.
 ii. Superficial punctate keratitis.
 iii. Keratinization.
 iv. Fluorescein shows pooling between plaques and keratinized epithelia—tree bark appearance.

17. **What are the subclinical signs of vitamin A deficiency?**

 i. Dark adaptometry—abnormal rod threshold
 ii. Vision restoration test—delayed response after blanching
 iii. Pupil constriction—failure to constrict in low illumination
 iv. Conjunctival impression cytology—abnormal epithelial and goblet cell pattern.

18. **Describe corneal ulceration in vitamin A deficiency.**

They occur mostly in inferior or nasal part.

 i. Ulcer has very sharp margin as if cut with a trephine.
 ii. More severe lesions results in frank necrosis or sloughing of stroma known as keratomalacia.
 iii. It is generally not reversed with treatment.

19. **Describe xerophthalmic fundus.**

Whitish yellow changes in pigment epithelium.

 i. Both eyes are affected.
 ii. Corresponds to areas of temporary visual field loss.
 iii. Appear to be window defect in fundus fluorescein angiogram (FFA).
 iv. Known as Uyemura's syndrome.

20. **How do you diagnose vitamin A deficiency?**

Diagnosis depends on:

 i. Clinical signs, symptoms
 ii. Serum vitamin A level
 iii. Conjunctival impression cytology for mucin secreting cells, goblet cells, and epithelial cells.

21. How do you treat a patient with vitamin A deficiency?

| Children— | <1 year of age or <8 kg in wt | 100,000 IU—immediately
100,000 IU—next day
100,000 IU—after 4 months. |
| Children— | 1–6 yr of age | 200,000 IU—immediately
—next day
—after 4 months. |

   i. It will take care of acute manifestation of vitamin A deficiency.
  ii. They should also be treated with both vitamin and protein calorie supplement.
 iii. Maintenance of adequate corneal lubrication and prevention of infection and corneal melting is essential.

22. What is prophylactic treatment for prevention of vitamin A deficiency?

Nutritional fortification.

   i. Children—   <1 year of age   100,000 IU every 6 months.
                    <8 kg of wt
  ii. Children—   1–6 years 200,000 IU every 6 months.

23. What are the measures for eye care?

Immediate parenteral/oral supplementation of vitamin A is the first step. The ocular conditions can then be cotreated as follows:

   i. For conjunctival xerosis—artificial tears every 3–4 hours
  ii. For keratomalacia—broad spectrum antibiotics
      Atropine eye ointment two times a day
      Subconjunctival injection of gentamicin with atropine can be given.

11.2. LOCALIZATION OF INTRAOCULAR FOREIGN BODIES

1. **Intraocular foreign body (IOFB) occurs more commonly in:**
   i. Males
   ii. Age 20–40 years
   iii. In the work setting
   iv. Mostly are the results of hammering metal on metal.

2. **What history should be elicited from the patient having IOFB?**
   i. Circumstance and mechanism of injury
   ii. Nature of material
   iii. Any likelihood of contamination
   iv. Force with which it hit the eye.

3. **Classify the different types of foreign bodies.**

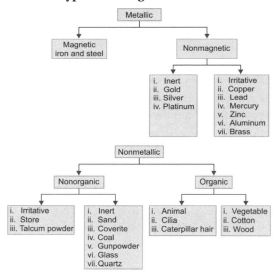

4. **How does the entrance of the foreign body into the eye cause damage?**
   i. By mechanical effects
   ii. By introduction of infection
   iii. By specific action (chemical and otherwise) on the tissue.

5. **Where can the foreign body be embedded in the anterior chamber?**
   i. It can either fall to the bottom and if very small embedded in the angle.
   ii. It can get embedded in the iris.

6. **How can the foreign body pass into the vitreous?**
   i. Through the cornea, iris, and lens when there will be a hole in the iris and traumatic cataract.
   ii. Through the cornea, pupil, and lens
   iii. Through the cornea, iris, and zonule
   iv. Through the sclera directly.

7. **What changes does the foreign body cause in the vitreous?**

   The foreign body may be suspended for some time and ultimately sinks to the bottom of the vitreous cavity due to degenerative changes in the gel, which lead to liquefaction partial or complete. The track of the foreign body through the vitreous is seen as a gray line.

8. **How can the foreign body penetrate the retina?**

   Mostly the particle has enough energy to carry it directly into the retina where it may ricochet once or even twice before it comes to rest. Occasionally, it pierces the coats of the eye to rest in the orbital tissues (double perforation).

9. **How does the foreign body look if lodged in the sclera?**

   The foreign body often appears black with a metallic lusture. It is surrounded by white exudates and red blood clot. Eventually fibrous issue usually encapsulates it and retina in the neighborhood becomes heavily pigmented.

10. **What degenerative changes does the foreign body cause in the posterior segment?**
    i. There may be widespread degeneration but most frequently fine pigmentary disturbances at the macula → often the result of concussion.
    ii. Vitreous turns fluid usually
    iii. Bands of fibrous tissue may traverse along the path of the foreign body
    iv. Hemorrhage may be extensive
    v. Retinal detachment may follow.

11. **What is the reaction of the ocular tissue to the nonorganic materials?**
    i. They are inert.
    ii. Excite a local irritative response, which leads to formation of fibrous tissue and results in encapsulation.
    iii. Produce a suppurative reaction.
    iv. Cause specific degenerative changes.

12. **What do organic materials produce?**

    They cause a proliferation reaction characterized by formation of granulation tissue.

13. What is siderosis?

Iron contamination of intraocular tissues causes a characteristic picture called siderosis (so does steel in proportion to its ferrous content). The condition is due to electrolytic dissociation of the metal, especially trivalent ion by the current of rest in the eye, which disseminates the material throughout the tissues and enables it to combine with the cellular proteins, thus killing cell causing atrophy.

14. What are the features of siderosis?

i. A rusty staining of cornea—Coats' white ring when deposits are at the level of Bowman's membrane.
ii. Brown colored iris, mid-dilated pupil, nonreactive due to damage to dilator muscle.
iii. Deposition of iron in the anterior capsules of the lens as a rusty deposit, arranged radially corresponding with the dilated pupil.
iv. The ring becomes stained first greenish and then reddish brown.
v. Eventually this leads to development of cataract.
vi. Retinal degeneration with attenuation of vessels.
vii. Secondary glaucoma of chronic type is a complication due to iron deposition in trabecular meshwork.
viii. Powerful oxidants like superoxide, hydrogen peroxide, which causes lipid peroxidation, leading to enzyme inactivation and cell membrane damage.

15. How are the deposits of iron revealed pathologically?

They are revealed by the Prussian blue reaction with Perl's microchemical stain. The characteristic blue pigmentation is found particularly in the corneal corpuscles, in the trabecular meshwork, on the inner surface of the ciliary body, and in the retina where the whole retinal vasculature system is clearly marked out.

16. What is the reaction of copper?

If the metal is pure, a profuse formation of fibrous tissue occurs which is followed by a suppurative reaction and eventually shrinkage of globe. If the metal is alloyed (bronze/brass), a milder reaction occurs called chalcosis. It gets deposited where resistance to its migration is offered by a continuous membrane. So it has a tendency to get deposited on basement membranes like Descemet's membrane, anterior lens capsule, and internal limiting membrane. The typical sites are:

i. Deep parts of cornea more in the periphery causing the appearance of golden brown Kayser–Fleischer ring.
ii. Under the lens capsule where it is deposited to form a brilliant golden green sheen aggregated in radiating formations like petals of a flower → sunflower cataract.

iii. On the retina at the posterior pole where lustrous golden plaques reflect the light with a metallic sheen.

iv. Greenish discoloration of iris.

v. Impregnation on zonular fibers.

vi. Brownish red vitreous opacities.

17. What is the reaction of lead?

One of the commonest form of foreign body.

It is rapidly covered by layer of insoluble carbonate, which prevents its diffusion. It produces few changes in the anterior chamber, and liquefaction and opacification of vitreous gel can occur. If the metal lies on retina or choroid, it causes an exudative reaction, partly purulent and partly fibrinous.

18. What is ophthalmia nodosa?

Caterpillar hair may penetrate the eye inciting a severe iridocyclitis characterized by the formation of granulomatous nodules.

19. What are the methods for localization of foreign body?

i. Clinical methods for direct visualization.

ii. Special methods for indirect visualization.

20. What will you look for in direct visualization?

i. Wound of entry

ii. Associated corneal, scleral, iris tear

iii. Penetrating tract in iris, vitreous

iv. Gonioscopy for angle recession

v. Any signs of siderosis or chalcosis.

21. What are the clinical signs of importance?

i. Localized tenderness

ii. Mydriasis 3–6 weeks after an accident

iii. Undue persistence of irritation

iv. Delayed occurrence of unexplained uveitis.

22. What are the special methods for investigation?

i. Those depending on magnetic property of the foreign body

ii. Those depending on electrical conductivity and induction

iii. Those depending on chemical analysis

iv. Radiology including X-ray, CT, MRI

v. USG

vi. ERG.

23. What are the instruments used for detection of foreign body based on electrical conduction?

i. Bermann's locator: The detecting range for magnetic foreign body is ten times the diameter of the foreign body. For nonmetallic foreign body it ranges between 1–2 times. Nonmagnetic foreign body can be detected only if they are more than 3 mm in diameter.

ii. Roper Hall's locator: Also called electroacoustic foreign body detector, metallic foreign body is continuous while nonmetallic foreign body is intermittent.

iii. Carnay's locator.

iv. Ophthalmometalloscope of Hale.

24. What is the sensitivity for foreign body in radiographic methods?

i. 0.5 mm diameter will be evident in X-rays. (All metals except aluminum, which has an equal bone density. So bone-free method is used.)

ii. Only 40% are located with plain films and they can be difficult to locate accurately.

25. What are the views most suitable for demonstration of foreign body?

i. **True lateral**—affected side toward the film.

ii. **Posteroanterior**—face against the film.
   – Nose and chin in contact with film.
   – Tube is centered to middle of orbit.

26. What are the different radiological methods used?

i. Direct methods

ii. Methods depending on relational movements of eye

iii. Methods on geometric projection

iv. Bone-free methods

v. Stereoscopic methods

vi. Methods based on delineation of globe using contrast media.

27. What is the direct radiographic method?

i. Two exposures—posteroanterior and lateral are taken

ii. The foreign body is located in relation to a marker bearing a known relation to the globe.

28. What are the limitations of direct radiographic method?

i. Errors may arise from movement of marker

ii. Markers cannot be kept in a badly damaged eye.

iii. Eyeball is thought to be 24 mm which is not always true.

29. What are the principle of methods depending on rotation of globe?

i. Head and X-ray tube remain fixed.

ii. Several exposures with eye moving in different directions.

iii. Three exposures in lateral view with eye looking straight upward and downward.

iv. Position of foreign body calculated with amount and direction of displacement with reference to center of rotation of globe.

30. **What are its limitations?**
    i. There is no true center of rotation of the globe.
    ii. The calculations are made in reference to a schematic eye 24 mm.

31. **What is the principle of methods depending on geometric construction?**

    Sweet's Method
    i. Eye and head remain fixed.
    ii. Two X-rays are taken with X-ray tube in known position.
    iii. Two metal indicators are used.
    iv. Foreign body position localized with reference to fixed indicators.

32. **Different methods based on geometric construction are:**
    i. Mackinzie Davidson
    ii. Sweet's method (ingenious and very accurate)
       Indicators: – Center of cornea
                    – Temporal side
    iii. Dixon's method

       Modified by Bromley
       ↓
       Modified by McGregor.

33. **What are its limitations?**
    i. Measurements are incorrect if the patient does not fix properly.
    ii. Measurements on schematic eye of 24 mm axial length.

34. **What is the principle in stereoscope methods?**
    i. Two X-ray are positioned at two fixed angles with markers attached to globe eye in different position.
    ii. Foreign body is calculated with reference to displacement of its shadow from the radiopaque marker.

35. **How do you delineate the globe by using contrast media?**

    Injecting air or dye (thorotrast, lipiodol, diodrast) in the Tenon's space.

36. **What are the disadvantages?**
    i. Air embolism if air is used.
    ii. Tissue reaction to eye.

37. **What is the principle in bone free or Vogt's method?**

    Dental film is held over and perpendicular to inner canthus of eye and the ray are directed from the side so that a shadow of the profile of the anterior segment of the eye (8–12 mm) is recorded on the film.

38. What are the indicators for Vogt's method?

    i. Useful when a small foreign body is in anterior segment of eye.

    ii. Foreign body density equals to that of bone.

39. How is the limbal ring used to detect foreign body?

    i. This was introduced by Stallard and Somerset.

    ii. In this method, a metallic ring 11–14 mm in diameter half the diameter of the schematic eye, is sutured to limbus and X-ray. PA view and lateral view are taken.

    iii. Precaution:

        Image of the ring on PA view should be circular.

        Image of ring on lateral view should be vertical.

    iv. On PA view:

        The center of the ring formed by the limbal ring is marked.

        A schematic eye of 24 mm is drawn from center.

        If the foreign body falls within the schematic eye it is intraocular, otherwise it is extraocular.

        A vertical corneal axis is drawn passing through the center of the ring and the distance of the foreign body nasal or temporal to this axis is noted and measured.

    v. On lateral view:

        A horizontal corneal axis is drawn.

        Distance of the foreign body above or below this axis is also noted and the distance of foreign body from behind limbal ring is also noted. To measure the AP measurement from the front of cornea, 3 mm should be added to the measurement from the limbal ring.

        Finally the position of the foreign body is charted on a Bromley's chart or Cridland graticule.

40. What are the limitations of the limbal ring test?

    i. Errors may arise from movement of ring and its inaccuracy of its fit.

    ii. Inaccurate orientation of globe can occur.

    iii. The ring cannot be sutured to a badly damaged eye.

    iv. Standard eyeball size is taken as 24 mm which is not always true.

41. What is the contact lens method?

Comberg's method

It utilizes a contact lens with radiopaque markers (lead) in all four quadrants.

A PA exposure is taken with the central ray focused on the anterior pole of the eye and lateral exposure where central ray passes through the limbus.

From the frontal X-ray the anterior pole of the eye is indicated by intersection of the diagonals joining the markers and the distance of the foreign body from this point is determined. Its position in the sagittal plane is obtained from lateral view by measurement of the distance of the foreign body behind the markers.

Worst Lovac contact lens: This contact lens is held in constant position during filming by a partial vacuum produced between the contact lens and cornea. It has a central opening which is connected to a metal tube which is attached to a rubber suction bulb. PA and lateral view are taken.

42. What are the disadvantages of contact lens method?
    i. It is assumed that the eyeball size is 24 mm.
    ii. The marker may superimpose on the foreign body.
    iii. It is an additional trauma to the eye.
    iv. Improper positioning of lens can occur due to chemosis and AC deformation.
    v. Sometimes, a poor contact lens fit will allow movement of lens and so false limbal reference points may be identified.

43. What is the frequency of ultrasonogram used to detect foreign bodies?
8–10 MHz. In the presence of severe inflammation, then 5 MHz is used.

44. What are the two modes used?
    i. **A-scan**
       – One-dimensional method
       – It may reveal orbital foreign body posterior to sclera
       – Foreign body appears as steeply rising echospike.
    ii. **B-scan two-dimensional, more valuable than A-scan**
       – Foreign body appears as acoustically white (opaque).

45. What is quantitative echography used in the detection of a foreign body?
    i. The reflectivity of a foreign body echospike is extremely high reaching 100% with lowest gain.
    ii. This allows a comparison with scleral signal.

46. What are the advantages of USG?
    i. Can detect foreign body even in opaque medium
    ii. Can detect the presence of retinal detachment or vitreous hemorrhage
    iii. Gives axial length of eyeball
    iv. Can localize nonmetallic foreign body
    v. Can precisely localize intraocular or extraocular foreign body.

47. What are the disadvantages of USG?
    i. Hazardous in open globe
    ii. Information only in two dimensions
    iii. More anterior part of globe may not be directed in USG.

48. What is the relevance of ERG in the detection of foreign bodies?

  i. In siderosis bulbi—early ERG changes include an increased amplitude of the "a" wave and a normal "b" wave. Late changes include a diminished b wave and ultimately an extinguished ERG.

  ii. In chalcosis, ERG shows initial a wave amplitude and later a decreased "a" wave and a "b" wave amplitude.

49. What are the advantages of CT scan?

  i. It is extremely sensitive

  ii. No globe manipulation is required

  iii. Multiple foreign bodies can be localized

  iv. Little patient cooperation is required

  v. Allows detection of smaller foreign body 0.5 mm or more

  vi. Distinguish metallic from nonmetallic and identifies composition of nonmetallic.

50. What are the suggested cuts for CT scan?

Thin axial cuts (≥1.5 mm) and direct coronal cuts are used.

51. What are the limitations of MRI?

  i. If there is a magnetic foreign body, they have been shown to move on exposure to the magnetic field.

  ii. Visual loss and vitreous hemorrhage have been attributed to movement of occult foreign body after MRI and hence they are contraindicated for magnetic foreign bodies.

52. Management of intraocular foreign bodies.

Intravitreal	Well-visualized	Poorly visualized
a. Magnetic	External magnet	Vitrectomy, forceps/REM
b. Nonmagnetic	Vitrectomy/forceps	Vitrectomy/forceps
Intraretinal		
a. Magnetic	Transcleral "trapdoor" or vitrectomy forceps/REM	Vitrectomy forceps/REM
b. Nonmagnetic	Transcleral "trapdoor" or vitrectomy forceps/REM	Vitrectomy forceps/REM

53. What are the types of magnets?

  i. Hand-held magnet

  – It is small and low powered. Applicable only when the foreign body is within 1 mm of its tip.

  ii. Giant magnet or Bronson's electromagnet

  – This magnet has a strong magnetic field.

  – It is of two types

  • The Haab's type of electromagnet.

  • The ring method.

  iii. Intraocular magnet.

54. What is the "Lancaster's working criteria for a magnet?"

The rule states that to be effective, a giant magnet should pull steel bale of 1 mm diameter with a force of over 50 times its weight at a distance of 20 mm.

55. What can be the associated complication with foreign bodies?

i. Vitreous hemorrhage
ii. Retinal tears
iii. Retinal detachment
iv. Endophthalmitis
v. Traumatic cataract
vi. Iridocyclitis
vii. Subluxated lens with zonular dialysis, etc.

56. What is the treatment of siderosis?

i. First remove the foreign body
ii. Galvanic deactivation
iii. Administration of IV EDTA
iv. Subconjunctival injection of adenosine triphosphate
v. Administration of desferrioxamine, which traps the free ions and converts it nontoxic chelate.

57. What is the treatment of chalcosis?

i. Sodium thiosulfate
ii. Sodium hyposulfate
iii. BAL (British anti-Lewisite).

11.3. GENETICS

1. **What are genes?**

   Genes are the basic units of inheritance, and they include the sequence of nucleotides that codes for a single trait or a single polypeptide chain and its associated regulatory regions. Approximately 20,000–25,000 genes are found among the 23 pairs of known chromosomes.

2. **What are chromosomes?**

   Genes are located primarily in the cell nucleus, where they are assembled into chromosomes of varying sizes. Each normal human somatic cell has 46 chromosomes composed of 23 homologous pairs. Of the 46 chromosomes, 44 are called autosomes because they provide information on somatic characteristics; the remaining 2 chromosomes are X and Y.

   Females have 2x chromosomes. Males have both an X and a Y chromosome. The male parent contributes his only X chromosome to all his daughters and his only Y chromosome to all his sons. Among these Y chromosomal genes is the testis-determining factor (TDF also called sex-determining region Y, SRY).

3. **What do you mean by the following terminologies: Hereditary, genetic, familial, congenital?**

   Hereditary indicates that a disease or trait under consideration results directly from an individual's particular genetic composition (or genome) and it can be passed from one generation to another.

   Genetic denotes that the disorder is caused by a defect of genes, whether acquired or inherited.

   Familial: A condition is familial if it occurs in more than one member of a family. It can be caused by common exposure to infectious agents, excess food intake, or environmental agents.

   Congenital refers to characteristics present at birth. These characteristics may be hereditary or familial, or they may occur as an isolated event, often as the result of infection or a toxic agent.

4. **What are the characteristic features of autosomal dominant disease?**

   i. Affected individuals usually have an affected parent.
   ii. Disease does not usually skip a generation, unless there is nonpenetrances.
   iii. Affected individuals have a 50% risk of having affected offspring.
   iv. Males and females are equally affected.
   v. Males and females have an equal likelihood of transmitting the disorder to offspring.

5. **Name some autosomal dominant disorders of eye.**
    i. Retinitis pigmentosa
    ii. All corneal dystrophies except three AR types
    iii. Retinoblastoma
    iv. von-Hippel Lindau disease
    v. CFEOM type 1 and 3 [congenital fibrosis of extraocular muscles]
    vi. Best disease
    vii. Neurofibromatosis 1 and 2
    viii. Familial exudative vitreoretinopathy (FEVR)
    ix. Cavernous hemangioma
    x. Wagner disease
    xi. Osteogenesis imperfecta
    xii. Tuberous sclerosis
    xiii. Aniridia
    xiv. Myotonic dystrophy
    xv. Familial radial drusen
    xvi. Marfan's syndrome
    xvii. Blepharophimosis syndrome
    xviii. CHARGE syndrome
    xix. Axenfeld Rieger syndrome
    xx. Blepharophimosis syndrome
    xxi. Stickler syndrome
    xxii. Treacher–Collins syndrome
    xxiii. Waardenburg syndrome
    xxiv. Gorlin syndrome (nevoid basal cell carcinoma syndrome).

6. **What are the characteristic features of autosomal recessive disease?**
    i. Affected individuals are born to unaffected parents.
    ii. Offsprings are rarely affected, unless there is consanguinity.
    iii. Males and females are equally affected.
    iv. There is a 25% risk to each subsequent child of parents with one affected child.

7. **Name some autosomal recessive disorders.**
    i. Retinitis pigmentosa
    ii. Macular dystrophy, lattice dystrophy type 3, CHED type 2
    iii. All sphingolipidoses except Fabry disease
    iv. All mucopolysaccharidosis except Hunter's syndrome
    v. CFEOM type 2 and unclassified type
    vi. Stargardt disease
    vii. Fundus albipunctatus
    viii. Leber congenital amourosis
    ix. Gyrate atrophy of choroid and retina

    x. Oguchi disease

    xi. Refsum disease

    xii. Wilson disease

    xiii. Congenital achromatopsia

    xiv. Usher syndrome

    xv. Bardet–Biedl syndrome

    xvi. Weill–Marchesani syndrome

    xvii. Wolfram syndrome (DIDMOAD)

    xviii. Goldmann–Favre syndrome

    xix. Homocystinuria

    xx. Ectopia lentis et papillae.

8. What are the characteristic features of a X-linked recessive disease?

    i. Affects males or males are generally more severely affected than females

    ii. Affected males have unaffected sons, but all daughters are carriers

    iii. A female carrier has a 50% risk of her son being affected or her daughter being a carrier.

9. What is the distinctive feature of X- linked inheritance?

The distinctive feature of X-linked inheritance, both dominant and recessive, is the absence of father to son transmission. Because the male X chromosome passes only to daughters, all daughters of an affected male will inherit the mutant gene.

10. Name some X-linked recessive disorders.

    i. Retinitis pigmentosa

    ii. Megalocornea

    iii. Fabry disease

    iv. Hunter's syndrome

    v. Lowe syndrome

    vi. Alport syndrome

    vii. Incontinenta pigmenti

    viii. Norrie disease (X-linked FEVR)

    ix. Choroideremia

    x. Congenital stationary night blindness

    xi. X-linked juvenile retinoschisis.

11. What are the characteristic features of mitochondrial inheritance?

    i. Mitochondrial DNA is derived exclusively from the ovum and hence the inheritance is maternal.

    ii. Children of affected females all have the mutation, but may not be affected due to nonpenetrance and variable expressivity.

12. Name some mitochondrial inheritance disorders of eye.

    i. Neuropathy, ataxia, retinitis pigmentosa (NARP) syndrome

    ii. Chronic progressive external ophthalmoplegia (CPEO)

   iii. Kearns–Sayre syndrome

   iv. Leber hereditary optic neuropathy (LHON).

13. What are chromosomal disorders?

Chromosomal disorders result from an abnormal chromosome number or structure rearrangement. They can result from nondisjunction, deletions, or translocations. Aneuploidy denotes an abnormal number of chromosomes in cells. Trisomy 21 syndrome or Down syndrome is the most common chromosomal syndrome in humans with an overall incidence of 1:1800 live births.

14. What are the ocular findings in Down syndrome?

     i. Almond-shaped palpebral fissures

    ii. Upslanting (mongoloid) palpebral fissures

   iii. Prominent epicanthal folds

   iv. Blepharitis, usually chronic, with cicatricial ectropion

    v. Nasolacrimal duct obstruction

   vi. Strabismus, usually esotropic

  vii. Nystagmus, typically horizontal

 viii. Keratoconus

   ix. Iris stromal hypoplasia

    x. Brushfield spots

   xi. Cataract

  xii. Aberrant retinal vessels (at disk)

 xiii. Optic atrophy

 xiv. Myopia.

15. What are the ophthalmically important chromosomal aberrations?

Long arm 13 deletion (13q14) syndrome: Retinoblastoma

Short arm 11 deletion (11p13) syndrome: Aniridia.

16. What is Knudson's two-hit hypothesis?

Rb1 (Retinoblastoma gene), a tumor suppressor gene is located on long arm of chromosome 13. Both copies of the gene present on homologous loci on the two chromosomes must be abnormal to initiate oncogenesis. In the heritable forms, one copy is defective by birth. If the other copy is damaged by environmental factors, the tumor is formed. In the sporadic form, the hypothesis is that both copies of the gene are damaged due to environmental influences.

17. **What are the characteristic features of aniridia?**

Aniridia is a panophthalmic disorder characterized by the following features:

     i. Subnormal visual acuity
    ii. Congenital nystagmus
   iii. Strabismus
   iv. Keratitis due to limbal stem cell failure
    v. Iris absence or severe hypoplasia
   vi. Cataracts (usually anterior polar)
  vii. Ectopia lentis
 viii. Glaucoma
   ix. Optic nerve hypoplasia
    x. Foveal or macular hypoplasia.

18. **What is the significance of PAX6 gene?**

     i. PAX6 gene product is a transcription factor required for normal development of the eye. Mutations of PAX6 have been reported in aniridia, Peter's anomaly, autosomal dominant keratitis, and dominant foveal hypoplasia.
    ii. The genes responsible for these disorders participate in the development of periocular mesenchyme. These developmental disorders are inherited as autosomal dominant traits.
   iii. Axenfield–Reiger syndrome: Mutations in PITX2 gene and FOXC1 gene.
   iv. Aniridia: mutation in PAX6 gene.
    v. Nail–patella syndrome: mutation in LMX1B gene.

19. **What are the genes associated with glaucoma?**

Disease	Gene
Juvenile open-angle glaucoma Adult open-angle glaucoma	Myocilin (TIGR) (1q25)
Congenital glaucoma	CYP1B1 (2p16)
Normal-tension glaucoma	Optineurin (10p15)

20. **Name the genes associated with corneal disease.**

Disease	Gene
Dominant corneal dystrophies (lattice, macular, Avellino, Reis–Bucklers')	Keratoepithilin (5q31)
Meesmann's corneal dystrophy	Keratin K3 (12q12-q13)
Fuch's endothelial dystrophy	Collagen type VIII (1q25)
Cornea plana (type 2 AR)	KERA (12q)

21. Name the genes affected in congenital ocular genetic disorders.

Disorder	Gene affected
Blepharophimosis syndrome	FOXL2X
Crouzon/Apert	FGFR2
Treacher–Collins	TCOF1
Marfan syndrome	FBN1
Ataxia telangiectasia	ATM
Oculocutaneous albinism type1	TYR
Oculocutaneous albinism type 2	OCA2
Stickler syndrome	COL9A1,COL11A1,COL11A2
Aniridia	PAX6, WT
Peter's anomaly	PAX6,PITX3,CYP1B1
Microphthalmos	PAX6
Cataract	PAX6, BMP 4,7
Chediak–Higashi syndrome	LYST
Retinitis pigmentosa	CRB1
X-linked retinoschisis	XLRS1
X-linked congenital idiopathic nystagmus	FRMD7

22. What is pharmacogenetics?

The study of heritable factors that determine how drugs are chemically metabolized in the body is called pharmacogenetics. This field addresses genetic differences among population segments that are responsible for variations in both the therapeutic and adverse effects of drugs.

23. What are the commonly used techniques for genetic testing?

  i. Karyotyping analysis
 ii. Restriction fragment length polymorphism (RFLP)
iii. Single strand conformation polymorphism (SSCP)
 iv. Linkage analysis.

24. What is genetic counseling?

Genetic counseling is a communication process which deals with human problems associated with the occurrence or risk of occurrence of a genetic disorder in a family. This process involves:

  i. Interpretation of family and medical histories to assess the chance of disease occurrence or recurrence
 ii. Education about inheritance, testing, management, prevention, resources and research
iii. Counseling to promote informed choices and adaptation to the risk or condition.

11.4. COMMUNITY OPHTHALMOLOGY

1. **What is the WHO definition of blindness?**
   i. **Based on visual acuity**
      WHO defined blindness as visual acuity less than 3/60 or its equivalent in the better eye with best possible refractive correction (best corrected visual acuity <3/60).
   ii. **Based on visual field**
      Visual field less than 10° in the better eye, irrespective of the level of visual acuity.

2. **How will you categorize visual impairment and blindness?**

   WHO classification (1992)

CATEGORY	BCVA
0 —normal	6/6–6/18
1 —visual impairment	6/24–6/60
2 —severe visual impairment	< 6/60–3/60 (economic blindness)
3 —blind	< 3/60–1/60 (social blindness)
4 —blind	< 1/60–PL+ (legal blindness)
5 —blind	NO PL (complete/total blindness)

3. **What is the population of India?**
   As per the 2011 census, it is 1.21 billion and is estimated to grow at 1.6% annually.

4. **What is the percentage of pediatric patients?**
   <16 years: 29%

5. **What is the percentage of population above the age of 40?**
   30%

6. **What is the Indian definition of blindness?**
   Best Corrected Visual Acuity (BCVA) less than 6/60 or its equivalent in the better eye or diminution of the field of vision to 20° or less in the better eye.

7. **What is avoidable blindness?**
   i. **Preventable** blindness which can be easily prevented by attacking the causative factor at an appropriate time, e.g. corneal blindness due to vitamin A deficiency and trachoma.
   ii. **Curable** blindness which vision can be restored by timely intervention, e.g. cataract blindness.

8. **What is the magnitude of blindness?**
   Global—45 million blind and 180 million visually disabled.
   India—9 million blind (1/5th of the world)
         Prevalence of blindness in India is 1.1% (NPCB 2001–2002)

9. **What are the causes of blindness in Indian scenario?**

The causes of blindness in Indian scenario:

NPCB survey (2001–2001), presenting vision < 6/60

Cataract	—	62.6%
Refractive error	—	19.7%
Glaucoma	—	5.8%
Posterior segment pathology	—	4.7%
Corneal opacity	—	0.9%
Surgical complications	—	1.2%
Others	—	4.1%

10. **What is cataract surgery rate (CSR)?**

It is the number of cataract surgeries performed per million population.

According to 2005 statistics, CSR for India was 5200 per million populations.

Highest is in Gujarat (13,108) and lowest in Sikkim (339).

11. **What is the management of ophthalmia neonatorum?**

   i. **Prophylaxis**

   Antenatal—treat genital infection

   Intranatal—hygienic delivery

   Postnatal—1% tetracycline eye ointment (or) 1% silver nitrate (Crede's method) (or) 2.5% povidone-iodine immediately into the eyes of the babies after birth.

   ii. **Curative**

   Conjunctival swab for culture sensitivity and cytology taken. Patient is started on broad spectrum antibiotic like topical fluoro-quinolone till the reports arrive, following which specific treatment is started.

Neonatal conjunctivitis (Ophthalmia neonatorum)

Infection	Treatment
Chlamydia trachomatis	Oral erythromycin 50 mg/kg in four divided dose for 14 days
Gram-positive bacteria	Erythromycin 0.5% e/o QID
Gram-negative bacteria (gonococcal)	Systemic: Inj. ceftriaxone 25–50 mg/kg IV or IM single dose × 7 days or Inj. cefotaxime 100 mg/kg IV or IM single dose × 7 days Topical: saline lavage hourly, bacitracin eye ointment qid, or penicillin drops 5,000–10,000 U/mL
Others	Topical gentamicin or tobramycin
HSV	Topical and systemic antivirals

12. **What are the prophylaxis and treatment options in vitamin A deficiency?**

Prophylaxis

i. Immunization (e.g. measles)
ii. Vitamin A supplements
iii. Nutritional education to mothers
iv. Fortified foods.

These prophylactic measures can be observed under following strategies.

Short-term strategies

i. WHO recommendation: 6 monthly supplementation of high dose of vitamin A
   Children (age—1-6 years)—2 lakh IU orally every 6 months.
   Infants 6–12 months old—1 lakh IU orally every 6 months.
   Infants < 6 months—50,000 IU orally.
ii. Indian recommendation: CSSM (Child survival and safe motherhood)
   First dose (1 lakh IU)—at 9 months along with measles vaccine
   Second dose (2 lakh IU)—at 18 months along with booster dose of DPT/OPV
   Third dose (2 lakh IU)—at 2 years of age.

Medium-term strategies

i. Food fortification (salt, dalda)
ii. Food supplementation

Long-term strategies

i. Improve intake of vitamin A in daily diet
ii. Nutritional health education to school children.

Treatment

keratomalacia reflects very severe vitamin A deficiency and should be treated as medical emergency to reduce child mortality

i. **Systemic**
   - Systemic treatment of xerophthalmia involve oral or intramuscular vitamin A
   - Multivitamin supplements and dietary sources of vitamin A are also administered.
   - Vitamin A doses:
     Age >1 year   —2 lakh IU on days 0,1,14.
     Age 6 months to 1 year   —1 lakh IU on days 0,1,14.
     Age <6 months   —50,000 IU on days 0,1,14.

ii. **Local**
  - Intense lubrication
  - Topical retinoic acid may promote healing but is not sufficient without systemic supplements
  - Emergency surgery for corneal perforation may be necessary.

13. **What are the objectives of vision 2020? What are eye diseases covered under the same?**

Vision 2020: The right to sight

It is a global initiative launched by WHO in Geneva on February 18, 1999 in a broad coalition with the international NGOs to combat the problem of blindness.

Objectives

To intensify and accelerate present prevention of blindness activities so as to achieve the goal of eliminating avoidable blindness by the year 2020.

Implementation:

Through four phases of five-year plans, the first one started in 2000.

Strategic approaches:

The five basic strategies of this initiative are:
  i. Effective disease prevention and control
  ii. Training of eye health personnel
  iii. Strengthening of existing eye care infrastructure
  iv. Use of appropriate and affordable technology
  v. Mobilization of resources

Priority diseases

Globally five conditions have been identified for immediate attention for achieving goals of vision 2020. They are:
  i. Cataract
  ii. Trachoma
  iii. Onchocerciasis
  iv. Childhood blindness
  v. Refractive error and low vision
     In Indian scenario in addition to aforementioned conditions, emphasis to be laid on
     - glaucoma
     - diabetic retinopathy
     - corneal blindness.

14. **Comment briefly upon National Programme for Control of Blindness (NPCB).**

National Programme for Control of Blindness (NPCB) was launched in the year 1976. It is a 100% centrally sponsored scheme with the goal of reducing the prevalence of blindness to 0.3% by 2020. Rapid Survey on Avoidable Blindness conducted under NPCB during 2006–7 showed reduction in the prevalence rate of blindness from 1.1% (2001–2) to 1% (2006–7).

The main objectives of the program are:
  i. To reduce the backlog of blindness through identification and treatment of blind;
 ii. To develop comprehensive eye care facilities in every district;
iii. To develop human resources for providing eye care services;
 iv. To improve quality of service delivery;
  v. To secure participation of voluntary organizations/private practitioners in eye care;
 vi. To enhance community awareness on eye care.

The program objectives are to be achieved by adopting the following strategy:
   i. Decentralized implementation of the scheme through District Health Societies (NPCB);
  ii. Reduction in the backlog of blind persons by active screening of population above 50 years, organizing screening eye camps and transporting operable cases to eye care facilities;
 iii. Involvement of voluntary organization in various eye care activities;
  iv. Participation of community and Panchayat Raj institutions in organizing services in rural areas;
   v. Development of eye care services and improvement in quality of eye care by training of personnel, supply of high-tech ophthalmic equipments, strengthening follow-up services, and regular monitoring of services;
  vi. Screening of school-age group children for identification and treatment of refractive errors with special attention in under-served areas;
 vii. Public awareness about prevention and timely treatment of eye ailments;
viii. Special focus on illiterate women in rural areas. For this purpose, there should be convergence with various ongoing schemes for development of women and children;
  ix. To make eye care comprehensive, besides cataract surgery, provision of assistance for other eye diseases like diabetic retinopathy, glaucoma management, laser techniques, corneal transplantation, vitreoretinal surgery, treatment of childhood blindness, etc.;
   x. Construction of dedicated eye wards and eye OTs in District Hospitals in NE states and few other states as per need;
  xi. Development of mobile ophthalmic units in NE states and other hilly states linked with tele-ophthalmic network and few fixed models;
 xii. Involvement of private practitioners in sub-district, blocks and village levels.

15. **What is the prevalence of corneal blindness? How much is the requirement of cornea?**

In India, there are around 120,000 corneally blind. This number is increasing by 25,000–30,000 each year.

Total number of corneal tissues procured in India per year: 50,000

Total number of corneal tissues utilized in India per year: 22,000 (roughly 45% utilization rate)

Best performing states in India in corneal donation: Tamil Nadu and Gujarat

Causes of corneal blindness

   i. *Infective*
      - Trachoma
      - Infective keratitis
      - Onchocerciasis
      - Ophthalmia neonatorum
      - Leprosy
   ii. *Nutritional*
      - Vitamin A deficiency
   iii. *Trauma*
      - Penetrating trauma
      - Chemical injury
   iv. *Inflammatory*
      - Mooren's ulcer
      - Sjogren's syndrome
   v. *Inherited*
      - Stromal dystrophies
      - Fuch's endothelial dystrophy
      - CHED
   vi. *Degenerative*
      - Keratoconus
   vii. *Traditional eye medicines*
      - Milk, blood, saliva, dried plant powder.

16. **How many eye banks are there in India?**

Approximately 800.

17. **Prevalence and causes of childhood blindness?**

It is estimated that 1.5 million children suffer from severe visual impairment and blindness and of these 1 million live in Asia.

Causes of childhood blindness

Hereditary : Chromosomal disorders, single-gene defects

Intrauterine : Congenital rubella, fetal alcohol syndrome

Perinatal   : Ophthalmia neonatorum, retinopathy of prematurity, birth trauma

Childhood   : Vitamin A deficiency, measles, trauma

Unclassified: Impossible to determine the underlying cause.

18. **Recommendations for screening of children for eye diseases.**

    i. *At birth*
       - Buphthalmos
       - Cataract
       - Ophthalmia neonatorum
       - Microphthalmia or anophthalmos
       - Nystagmus
       - Squint
       - Retinopathy of prematurity

    ii. *Preschool*
       - Squint and amblyopia
       - Retinoblastoma
       - Vitamin A deficiency

    iii. *School*
       - Refractive error.

19. **What is trachoma? How does it cause blindness?**

    Trachoma is a leading cause for blindness in developing countries in Africa. Six million people are blind.

    Trachoma is caused by *Chlamydia trachomatis*. Spread by fomites, house, and flies.

    It results in conjunctival scarring leading to entropion, trichiasis, secondary corneal infections, and scarring.

    Treatment:
    i. Tetracycline eye ointment BD for 6 weeks
    ii. Oral erythromycin, azithromycin

    Prevention:
    SAFE strategy:
    i. **S**urgery to correct lid deformity and prevent blindness
    ii. **A**ntibiotics to acute infections and community control
    iii. **F**acial hygiene
    iv. **E**nvironmental change.

20. **How does onchocerciasis spread? Its treatment?**

    Onchocerciasis is a parasitic infestation by *Onchocerca volvulus*, a filarial worm. Endemic in Africa, Central America, Yemen.

    Definitive host—man

    Intermediate host—blackfly *Simulium*.

Blindness results from corneal scar, glaucoma, retinopathy, and optic atrophy.

Treatment: Oral ivermectin 150 mg/kg body weight

Available as Mectizan 6 mg per tablet in market.

21. **Functions of an eye bank?**
    i. Promotion of eye donation
    ii. Registration of the pledger for eye donation
    iii. Collection of the donated eyes from the deceased
    iv. Receiving and processing the donor eyes
    v. Preservation of the tissue for short-, intermediate-, long-, or very long- term
    vi. Distribution of the donor tissue to the corneal surgeons
    vii. Research activities.

22. **Contraindications to the use of donor cornea?**
    i. *Systemic* conditions potentially hazardous to eye bank personnel and fatal, if transmitted:
       – AIDS or HIV seropositivity
       – Rabies
       – Active viral hepatitis
       – Creutzfeldt–Jacob disease

    Other contraindications
    – Subacute sclerosing panencephalitis
    – Progressive multifocal leukoencephalopathy
    – Reye's syndrome
    – Death from unknown cause including unknown encephalitis
    – Congenital rubella
    – Active septicemia including endocarditis
    – Intravenous drug abusers
    – Leukemia
    – Lymphoma and lymphosarcoma
    ii. *Ocular*
       – Intrinsic eye disease
         • Retinoblastoma
         • Active inflammatory diseases
         • Congenital abnormalities
         • Central opacities
         • Pterygium
       – Prior refractive procedures
         • Radial keratotomy scars
         • Lamellar inserts
         • Laser photoablation
       – Anterior segment surgical procedures.

23. What is the Utilization percentage of donor corneas for optical keratoplasty?

50%

24. How many corneas are retrieved per year in India?

50,000 corneas.

Number of corneas required per year to meet the demand—2 lakh corneas per year (as per vision 2020).

25. How many eye banks are there in India?

252

26. How many keratoplasties are performed in India?

In the year 2013–2014 (compiled data of top 10 eye banks)

Optical penetrating keratoplasty—4737

Therapeutic keratoplasty—3209

DSEK—1245

DALK—436

11.5. TRAUMATIC HYPHEMA AND GLAUCOMA

1. How does hyphema cause raised intraocular pressure?

Hyphema cause a secondary glaucoma which can be either open angle or closed angle glaucoma

i. Open angle glaucoma causes—
   - Obstruction of trabecular meshwork by red blood cells, fibrin, debris, or inflammatory cells
   - Obstruction of trabecular meshwork by melanin which is released into the anterior chamber during trauma
   - Associated injury to the trabecular meshwork
   - Recurrent hemorrhage
   - Angle recession
   - Ghost cell glaucoma

ii. Angle closure glaucoma causes—
   - Pupillary block—due to clot formation of 8-ball hyphema
   - Peripheral anterior synechiae
   - Posterior synechiae with iris bombe

2. What is an 8-ball hyphema?

Formation of a big blood clot in AC along with degenerated red blood cells from an associated vitreous hemorrhage which impedes aqueous outflow.

3. What is the frequency of rebleed after a traumatic hyphema?

4%–35%

4. When is rebleed common?

It is common during first week after initial injury usually the fourth day because normal lysis and retraction of clot occurs during that time. Hence it is essential to follow up with these patients till that time post injury.

5. How do you evaluate a patient with hyphema due to trauma?

   i. Vision
   ii. Examine for other associated ocular injuries
   iii. Size of hyphema
       - Height in mm
       - Percentage of AC filled with blood
       - Number of clock hours of involvement
       - Presence of clot
       (Any increase in the size of hyphema which is suggestive of a rebleed)
   iv. Intraocular pressure

   v. Corneal blood staining
  vi. Gonioscopy (if possible in a case of trauma)
     – To look for an anterior synechiae
     – Angle recession (in follow-up cases of traumatic glaucoma)
 vii. Fundus evaluation—for signs of preexisting optic nerve head damage
viii. Examination of other eye—specifically for fundus evaluation. If media is not clear for fundus examination in traumatized eye.

6. What are the laboratory investigations performed in traumatic hyphema cases?
   i. Hb electrophoresis
  ii. LFT
 iii. PT, CT, BT
 iv. Platelet count
  v. RFT.

7. What are the complications of traumatic hyphema?
   i. Rebleeding
  ii. Glaucoma
 iii. Corneal blood staining.

8. What are the risk factors for rebleeding?
   i. Initial size of hyphema—if total hyphema occurs
  ii. Degree of reduced visual acuity
 iii. Delayed medical attention
 iv. Use of drugs like aspirin which inhibit platelet clotting action
  v. Increased IOP
 vi. Hypotony
 vii. Sickle cell trait/anemia.

9. How do you manage a case of traumatic hyphema?
   i. Investigations—mentioned above
  ii. Aim of management
     – To resorb existing hyphema
     – To prevent rebleeding
Resorption of hyphema:
   i. Conservative management
     – Bed rest
     – Patch
     – Avoid use of aspiring/NSAIDS
  ii. Medical treatment if IOP is elevated—to prevent optic nerve damage
     – Aqueous suppressant—topical beta blockers
     – Topical steroids—1% prednisolone acetate QID
     – Atropine 1% e/o BD
     – To avoid: aspirin (which has propensity to cause rebleed)

Miotics

Adrenergics

(Miotics and adrenergics are associated with increased intraocular inflammation)

Antifibrinolytic agents

– Tranexamic acid
– Aminocaproic acid
  • Used when clot is present
  • Systemic or topical
  • Help in preventing rebleeding

iii. Surgical:
   – AC washout
     Evaluation of suspended AC cells and debris through corneal paracentesis
   – Clot removal by
     • Cryoextraction
     • Ultrasonic emulsification and extraction
     • Removal with vitrectomy cutting—aspiration instrument
       Clot removal is usually done between 4 and 7 days post-trauma because clot reaches maximum consolidation and retraction at this time so can be expressed out easily
   – Trabeculectomy and iridectomy with irrigation of AC in recalcitrant cause of increased IOP.

10. Mention the surgical indications in a case of traumatic hyphema.

   i. Corneal blood stain
   ii. Raised intraocular pressure:
      – >50 mm Hg for 5 days
      – >35 mm Hg for 7 days
      – Total or near total hyphema with IOP >25 mm HD for 5 days
   iii. Total hyphema not resolving by day 5
   iv. Clots persisting for >10 days.

11. Comparison between aminocaproic acid and tranexamic acid for better one to prevent rebleeding.

   i. According to studies there is no difference between the two antifibrinolytic agents for preventing chances of a rebleed
   ii. However side effects of systemic aminocaproic acid limits its use
      – Light headedness
      – Nausea, vomiting
      – Systemic hypotension
      – Increased IOP with accelerated clot dissolution.

12. What is the mechanism of action of antifibrinolytic agents?

They competitively inhibit conversion of plasminogen to plasmin which degrades the fibrin in the clot.

There is a reduction in the rate of clot lysis. Thereby giving the injured vessel more time to heal.

13. What are the side effects and contraindications of aminocaproic acid?

   i. Side effects are:
- Nausea, vomiting
- Postural hypotension
- Light headedness

  ii. Contraindicated in:
- Active intravascular clotting disorders
- Pregnancy
- Hepatitis patients
- Renal disease

[Hence the need to check for LFT, RFT in a case of traumatic hyphema if antifibrinolytic drugs have to be administered.].

14. Why is it important to treat a patient of sickle cell trait/anemia having traumatic hyphema/glaucoma aggressively?

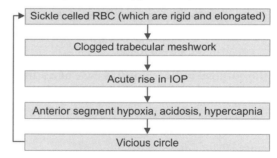

In these patients the vascular system is already sludged with elongated, rigid sickled RBCs leading to ischemia and vaso occlusion.

Further if IOP rises (even if to a minimal extent of 25 mm Hg) it would lead to development of CRAO and rapid optic nerve damage.

Hence the need to monitor closely and treat aggressively.

15. What special care is given to sickle cell anemic patients with a traumatic hyphema?

Aggressive treatment is provided with close monitoring to prevent rise in IOP

   i. Hospitalize the patient

  ii. Manage with medical treatment first

 iii. If IOP is >25 mm Hg for >24 hours—surgery is done

iv. Other modalities for sickle cell anemia patient—use of hyperbaric

v. Oxygen—intracameral or transcorneal (humidified O_2—1–3 L/min)

16. Which anti-glaucoma agent is contraindicated in sickle cell anemia and why?

Carbonic anhydrase inhibitor

Because these agents increase the concentration of ascorbic acid in the aqueous humor leading to more sickling of RBCs in the AC.

17. What are the various mechanism by which traumatic glaucoma occurs?

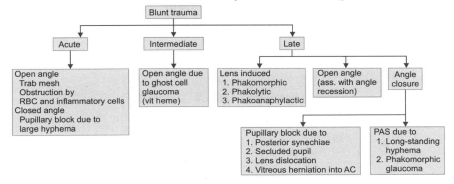

18. What is ghost cell glaucoma?

A form of glaucoma in which degenerated RBCs (ghost cells) develop in the vitreous cavity and then subsequently enter the AC through a disrupted anterior hyaloid and obstructs aqueous outflow.

19. What are ghost cells?

In the vitreous cavity, fresh RBCs get degenerated and are transformed from typical biconcave, pliable nature to tan or khaki colored, spherical less pliable structures called ghost cells.

20. How do ghost cells in AC cause glaucoma?

Ghost cells are nonpliable, spherical RBCs having thin wall and contain only denatured hemoglobin called Heinz bodies within it. These nonpliable cells are unable to pass through the trabecular meshwork readily, thereby causing an obstruction in the outflow.

21. What is "candy-stripe sign"?

Large quantities of ghost cells in AC layer out inferiorly creating pseudohypopyon which is occasionally associated with a layer of fresh RBC—called as candy stripe sign when seen in slit lamp biomicroscope.

22. What are the differential diagnosis for ghost cell glaucoma?

i. Hemolytic glaucoma

ii. Hemosideric glaucoma

iii. Neovascular glaucoma.

23. How do you confirm presence of ghost cells in AC?

It is confirmed by examination of aqueous aspirate under either phase contrast microscopy or routine light microscopy of a paraffin embedded specimen stained with hemotoxylin and eosin which will reveal presence of cells.

24. Mechanism of glaucoma post-penetrating injury?

   i. Inflammation
   ii. Hemorrhage
   iii. Intumescent/swollen lens—angle closure
   iv. Cyclitic membrane
   v. Lens subluxation
   vi. Forward displacement of lens iris diaphragm with pupillary block and iris bombe.

25. How can a penetrating trauma cause hypotony?

A decrease in IOP post-penetrating injury could be due to—

   i. An open wound
   ii. Associated iridocyclitis.

26. How do you manage glaucoma post-penetrating trauma?

   i. Treatment of penetrating wound is important—mostly surgical
   ii. Removal of incarcerated portion of uveal tissue
   iii. Aspiration of lens matter
   iv. Anterior vitrectomy
   v. Removal of foreign body
   vi. Meticulous closure of any corneal—scleral wound
   vii. Anterior chamber formation.

Post-initial wound management, glaucoma can be controlled by steroids (for reducing inflammation) and anti-glaucoma medications.

27. What is angle recession?

Angle recession is an irregular widening of ciliary body band seen on gonioscopy. Histologically, it is a tear present between longitudinal and circular muscles of ciliary body.

11.6. STERILIZATION

1. **Define sterilization and disinfection?**

    Sterilization is defined as the complete absence of any viable microorganisms including spores

    Disinfection is reducing the number of viable microorganisms, but not inactivating all viruses and bacterial spores

2. **What are the steps in sterilization?**
    i. Cleaning
    ii. Packaging
    iii. Sterilization
    iv. Storage
    v. Indicators of sterilization.

3. **What are the types of cleaning?**
    i. Manual cleaning with running water followed by drying
    ii. Mechanical cleaning using ultrasonicator.

4. **What are the different methods of sterilization?**
    i. Autoclaving (steam under pressure)
    ii. Hot air oven (dry heat)
    iii. Chemical sterilization such as ethylene oxide gas or glutaraldehyde 2% solution.

5. **What are the usual components of handwash disinfectants?**
    i. Iodophor
    ii. Chlorhexidine fluconate.

6. **What is the preferred autoclaving parameter?**
    i. Pressure 15 pounds
    ii. Temperature: 121° C
    iii. Time: 30 minutes.

7. **Use of various sterilization techniques.**
    i. Dry heat (Hot air oven): For bulk power, petroleum products, reusable glass, metal instruments oil, and ointments
    ii. Autoclaving:
        – Do not load liquids with instruments because sterilization time is different
        – Instruments are placed in a perforated tray to allow stream penetration
        – Sharp and delicate instrument are kept at the top of the tray
        – Loose packing and space between items are very important for easy circulation and penetration of stream
        – All detachable items in the instruments are disassembled. Oil and lubricants are to be wiped well

iii. Ethylene oxide sterilization (ETO): Used for vitrophage, cryoprobe, fiber-optic light, IOL's sutures, plastics
Timing: At 5 psi—12 hours
At 10 psi—6 hours.

8. **What is the mechanism of action of each method?**

i. Steam: It kills organism by coagulation of the cell protein

ii. ETO: It is a very effective alkylating agent which reacts with DNA and destroys the ability of microorganisms to metabolize or reproduce it.

9. **What are the different agents used as chemical disinfectant?**

i. ETO

ii. Glutaraldehyde

iii. Formaline for OT sterilization

iv. 70% isopropyl alcohol

v. 10% povidone iodine.

10. **How will you monitor the effectiveness of sterilization?**

i. Mechanical indicators: the time, temperature, and pressure recording devices

ii. Chemical indicators: For testing ETO, dry heat, and steam processes

iii. Biological indicators: Use heat resistant bacterial endospores to demonstrate whether or not sterilization has been achieved.

11.7. LANDMARK STUDIES IN OPHTHALMOLOGY

Cornea

1. **Herpetic Eye Disease Study (HEDS) 1.**

    Questions asked

    i.   What is the role of topical steroids in treating herpes simplex stromal keratitis in conjunction with topical antivirals?

    ii. What is the role of oral acyclovir in treating herpes simplex stromal keratitis in patients receiving concomitant topical corticosteroids and antivirals?

    iii. What is the efficacy of oral acyclovir in treating herpes simplex iridocyclitis in combination with topical steroids and antivirals?

    Results

    The study conducted three randomized controlled trials where in patients were examined for a 16-week period. A treatment failure was defined as worsening of stromal keratitis or uveitis at any scheduled visit, no change in stromal inflammation in the first 2 weeks or 3 later consecutive weeks, or occurrence of an adverse event

    i.   The patients who received Prednisolone phosphate 1% drops had faster resolution of the stromal keratitis and fewer treatment failures. Delaying the initiation of corticosteroid treatment did not affect the eventual outcome of the disease.

    ii. On adding oral acyclovir 400 mg five times a day for 10 weeks to topical corticosteroids and trifluridine, no benefit was noted in stromal keratitis and a mild benefit was noted in iridocyclitis.

    Conclusions

    Topical steroids are useful in the treatment of HSV viral stromal keratitis. Systemic acyclovir is not useful in stromal keratitis.

    Herpetic Eye Disease Study (HEDS) II.

    Questions asked

    i.   Does early treatment with oral acyclovir for HSV epithelial keratitis prevent progression to the complications of stromal keratitis and iridocyclitis?

    ii. What is the efficacy of oral acyclovir in preventing recurrences in patients with previous episodes of herpetic eye disease?

    iii. Is there any role of external or behavioral factors in the induction of ocular recurrences of HSV infections?

Results

i. There was no benefit from the addition of oral acyclovir to topical trifluridine in preventing the development of stromal keratitis or iritis. Also, the study found that the risk of stromal keratitis or iridocyclitis was quite low in the year following an episode of epithelial keratitis treated with topical trifluridine alone.

ii. There are no statistically significant external or behavioral factors leading to recurrence.

Conclusion

Oral acyclovir is not recommended during an active episode of epithelial keratitis.

2. **Mycotic Ulcer Treatment Trial.**

MUTT 1

Questions asked

i. To compare the safety and efficacy of topical 5% natamycin and topical 1% voriconazole in filamentous fungal keratitis?

ii. What role do the above-mentioned drugs play in *Fusarium* and *Aspergillus* keratitis?

Results

MUTT was a randomized controlled trial for smear positive filamentary fungal keratitis comparing natamycin 5% and voriconazole 1% with the primary outcome being best spectacle-corrected visual acuity at 3 months; secondary outcomes included corneal perforation and/or therapeutic penetrating keratoplasty.

i. Natamycin treatment was associated with significantly better clinical and microbiological outcomes than voriconazole

ii. Voriconazole-treated cases were more likely to have a perforation

iii. Fusarium cases fared much better with natamycin than with voriconazole

Conclusions

Natamycin is superior to voriconazole in the treatment of filamentary fungal keratitis. This difference is even more pronounced in keratitis caused by *Fusarium*. Voriconazole is not recommended as a monotherapy in filamentous keratitis.

MUTT II

Questions asked

What is the role of oral voriconazole in fungal keratitis?

Results

There was no difference in the rate of corneal perforation or the need for TPK between oral voriconazole vs placebo and patients who received oral voriconazole experienced a lot of adverse events

Conclusion

Oral voriconazole is not found to be useful in the treatment of severe filamentous fungal keratitis.

3. **Steroids in corneal ulcer trial (SCUT).**

Questions asked

Does the addition of topical corticosteroids to antibacterials as adjunctive therapy for bacterial keratitis improve clinical outcomes?

Results

It was a randomized controlled trial comparing 1.0% Prednisolone sodium phosphate to placebo in the treatment of bacterial keratitis with culture-positive ulcers receiving 48 hours of moxifloxacin eye drops before randomization

Although the steroid-treated group had a significant delay in re-epithelialization, steroids were not associated with a statistically significant difference in BSCVA or infiltrate/scar size

Conclusions

It is left to the discretion of the treating ophthalmologist to add steroids as per the case. Central large ulcers caused by *Pseudomonas* may benefit from adjunctive topical steroid therapy along with moxifloxacin. Ulcers caused by *Nocardia* should not be treated with steroids.

4. **Collaborative Corneal Transplantation Studies (CCTS).**

Questions asked

Is there a role of histocompatibility matching (HLA matching) of corneal transplant donors and recipients in reducing the incidence of graft rejection in high-risk patients?

Results

It conducted two studies—the Crossmatch Study and the Antigen Matching Study to assess the effectiveness of cross matching and HLA-A, -B, and -DR donor-recipient matching in preventing graft rejection among high-risk patients with and without lymphocytotoxic antibodies respectively.

HLA matching or cross matching doesn't reduce or increase the likelihood of corneal graft failure. Instead ABO blood group matching, may be effective in reducing the risk of graft failure.

Conclusion

HLA matching does not change the prognosis.

5. **Corneal Transplant Epidemiological Study (CORTES).**

   Questions asked

   Mention the changing trends for indications, patient demographics and surgical techniques from the CORTES study.

   Results

   This study aimed to examine evolving indications and changing trends for corneal transplantation in Italy. Keratoconus, regraft, and pseudophakic bullous keratopathy were the leading indications for PK, with keratoconus and regraft showing higher indications for ALK, whereas pseudophakic bullous keratopathy and regraft were the major indications for EK.

   Conclusion

   There is an important shift in managing corneal diseases toward more conservative surgeries and changes in indications in corneal transplantation.

6. **Dry Eye Workshop Study (DEWS).**

   DEWS (2007)

   Questions asked

   What is DEWS and what changes did it bring about in ocular surface disease?

   Results

   A new definition of dry eye was developed by the DEWS committee to reflect current understanding of the disease, and recommended a three-part classification system. The first part is etiopathogenic and illustrates the multiple causes of dry eye. The second is mechanistic and shows how each cause of dry eye may act through a common pathway. Finally, a scheme is presented, based on the severity of the dry eye disease (DED), which is expected to provide a rational basis for therapy. Risk factors for dry eye and morbidity of the disease are identified, and the impact on quality of life and visual function are outlined.

   Conclusion

   It recognizes the multifactorial nature of the dry eye.

   DEWS II (2017)

   Questions asked

   Brief note on tear-film ocular surface (TFOS) DEWS II.

Results

There is a revised definition of the dry eye with addition of the phrase "loss of homeostasis and neurosensory abnormalities." Tear film instability, hyperosmolarity, and ocular surface inflammation and damage were determined to be important etiologies. It also takes neurotrophic conditions and neuropathic pain into consideration.

Conclusion

Loss of homeostasis of the tear film is the central pathophysiological concept and differentiating between aqueous-deficient and evaporative dry eye disease was critical in selecting the most appropriate management strategy.

7. **Corneal Donor Study (CDS)**

   Questions asked

   What role does the age of donor cornea play in the success of penetrating keratoplasty done for corneal endothelial disorders?

   Results

   This study was undertaken over a period of 10 years to assess the success rate of penetrating keratoplasty for endothelial disorders like Fuchs and pseudophakic corneal edema. There was no significant difference in success rates comparing donors aged 12–65 years with those aged 66–75 years.

   Conclusion

   Age of donor cornea is not related to the long-term success rate of penetrating keratoplasty for endothelial disorders.

Retina

Retinal Detachment Studies

1. **Silicone Oil Study (1985–91).**

   Purpose

   Evaluate and compare silicone oil vs long acting gas in RD with PVR.

   Inclusion Criteria

   PVR of Grade C-3 or greater according to the Retina Society Classification and visual acuity of light perception or better.

   Outcome Measure

   Visual acuity of 5/200 or greater and macular reattachment for 6 months.

   Result/Conclusion

   No significant differences in the rates of complete retinal attachment, VA, corneal abnormalities or glaucoma were found between treatment groups. Gas-treated eyes had more hypotony. Anterior PVR was more prevalent than was posterior PVR and had a worse prognosis.

2. **SPR (Scleral buckling vs Primary Vitrectomy in RRD)—Phakic Subtrial (1998–2003).**

Purpose

Scleral buckling vs primary vitrectomy in RRD.

Inclusion Criteria

Phakic patient with clear break situation.

Outcome Measure

Change in VA, postoperative development of PVR and cataract and retinal reattachment rate at 1 year.

Result/Conclusion

SB achieved greater improvement in final VA than those who underwent primary PPV.

Cataract progression was more with PPV. There is a benefit of SB in phakic eyes with respect to BCVA improvement.

3. **SPR (Scleral buckling vs Primary vitrectomy in RRD)—Pseudophakic Subtrial: (1998–2003)**

Purpose

Scleral buckling vs primary vitrectomy in RRD.

Inclusion Criteria

Medium-severe RRD not treatable with a single 7.5 × 2.75 mm silastic sponge, aphakic/pseudophakic patients with an unclear whole situation.

Outcome Measure

Change in VA, postoperative development of PVR and cataract and retinal reattachment rate at 1 year.

Result/Conclusion

No significant difference between the groups in terms of functional outcome. Primary anatomical success rate was significantly higher in the primary PPV group compared to the SB group. Primary vitrectomy is recommended in these patients.

DIABETIC RETINOPATHY

Epidemiological Studies

1. **WESDR (Wisconsin Epidemiological Study of Diabetic Retinopathy) (1979).**

   Purpose

   Prevalence, incidence, and progression of diabetic retinopathy and its component lesions along with visual loss.

   Inclusion Criteria

   Patients with diabetes diagnosed before 30 years of age and diabetics diagnosed at 30 years of age or older.

   Results and Conclusions

   71% of younger-onset persons had retinopathy. In the older-onset group, 50% had retinopathy 6% of the younger and 5% of the older-onset subjects had CSME Both the frequency and severity of retinopathy and CSME increased with increasing duration of diabetes.

2. **DCCT (Diabetes Control and Complications Trial) (1983).**

   Purpose

   Effect of tight glycemic control on complications of diabetes for persons with type 1 diabetes.

   Inclusion Criteria

   ID DM, age 13–39 years, absence of hypertension, hypercholesterolemia, and severe diabetic complications.

   Outcome Measures

   Appearance and progression of retinopathy and other complications over 6.5 years.

   Results and Conclusions

   Intensive therapy delays the onset and slows the progression of microvascular complications of diabetes (diabetic retinopathy, nephropathy, and neuropathy) in IDDM.

3. **EDIC (Epidemiology of Diabetes Interventions and Complications).**

   Purpose

   To examine the persistence of the original treatment effects 10 years after the DCCT.

   Inclusion Criteria

   Patients aged 19–45 years, who were participants of the DCCT.

Outcome Measures

Appearance of micro- and macrovascular complications (presently in 13th year follow-up).

Results and Conclusions

The persistent difference in diabetic retinopathy between former intensive and conventional therapy continues for at least 10 years but may be waning.

4. **UKPDS (United Kingdom Prospective Diabetes Study) (1977).**

   Purpose

   Improved blood glucose and blood pressure control in type 2 diabetes for preventing the complications of diabetes.

   Inclusion Criteria

   Newly diagnosed type 2 diabetes patients.

   Outcome Measures

   Follow up of patients to major fatal and nonfatal clinical endpoints.

   Results and Conclusions

   Intensive blood-glucose control and tight blood pressure control reduces the risk of diabetic complications, the greatest effect being on microvascular complications.

5. **ABCD (Appropriate Blood Pressure Control in NIDDM) (1993).**

   Purpose

   Intensive BP control vs moderate control in the prevention and progression of nephropathy, retinopathy, cardiovascular disease, and neuropathy in NIDDM.

   Inclusion Criteria

   Hypertensive subjects with NIDDM were included.

   Outcome Measures

   Glomerular filtration rate as assessed by 24 hours creatinine clearance

   Result/Conclusion

   The more intensive blood pressure control decreased all-cause mortality.

Landmark Studies

1. **DRS (Diabetic Retinopathy Study) (1971).**

   Purpose

   Photocoagulation in preventing severe visual loss from PDR efficacy and safety of argon vs xenon.

Inclusion Criteria

BCVA of 20/100 or better in each eye and the presence of PDR in at least one eye or severe NPDR in both eyes.

Results and Conclusions

i. Photocoagulation reduced the risk of severe visual loss by 50% compared with no treatment.
ii. Xenon laser resulted in more harmful effects than Argon laser.
iii. Defined high risk PDR. Eyes with high-risk PDR should receive prompt PRP.

2. **ETDRS (Early Treatment Diabetic Retinopathy Study)(1979).**

Purpose

Determine best time to initiate PRP in DR efficacy of photocoagulation in DME effectiveness of aspirin in altering course of DR.

Inclusion Criteria

Patients with moderate or severe NPDR or mild PDR in both eyes and with visual acuity of 20/40 or better (20/200 or better if macular edema was present)

Results and Conclusions

i. Focal laser is useful for clinically significant macular edema.
ii. Scatter treatment is not indicated for eyes with mild to moderate NPDR and should be considered in severe NPDR or early PDR.
iii. Aspirin had no effect on DR.

3. **DRVS (Diabetic Retinopathy Vitrectomy Study) (1976).**

Purpose

Early vitrectomy vs conventional management for recent severe vitreous hemorrhage.

Inclusion Criteria

At least one eye with recent severe vitreous hemorrhage and visual acuity of 5/200 or less Extensive active neovascular or fibrovascular proliferations and visual acuity of 10/200 or better.

Outcome Measures

Visual acuity was main outcome measure. Visual acuity of 10/20 or better was considered "good vision" while less than 5/200 was "poor vision."

Results and Conclusions

Early vitrectomy provided a greater chance of prompt recovery of visual acuity, especially in type 1 diabetics and if vision is poor in the fellow eye. Early vitrectomy is of benefit especially in those with both fibrous proliferations and at least moderately severe new vessels, in which extensive scatter photocoagulation has been carried out or is precluded by vitreous hemorrhage.

Anti-VEGFs for DME

1. **READ-2 (Ranibizumab for Edema of the Macula in Diabetes: a phase 2 study) (2006).**

   Purpose

   Compare RBZ with focal/grid laser or combination of both in DME.

   Inclusion Criteria

   DME with CFT ≥250 μ, VA ≤20/40 but ≥20/320

   Outcome Measures

   Change from baseline in BCVA.

   Results and Conclusions

   At 6 months, RBZ injections had a better visual outcome than focal/grid laser RBZ provided benefit in DME for at least 2 years. A combination of this treatment with focal/grid laser was even more beneficial in clearing the amount of residual edema and reducing the frequency of injections needed.

2. **RIDE and RISE (A Study of Ranibizumab Injection in Subjects with Clinically Significant Macular Edema with Center Involvement Secondary to Diabetes Mellitus) (2007).**

   Purpose

   Efficacy and safety of intravitreal RBZ in DME patients.

   Inclusion Criteria

   Adults with DME with CFT ≥275 microns, BCVA of 20/40 to 20/320 and HbA1C ≤12%.

   Results and Conclusions

   BZ rapidly and sustainably improved vision, reduced the risk of further vision loss, and improved macular edema in patients with DME, with low rates of ocular and nonocular harm.

3. **RESOLVE (Safety and Efficacy of Ranibizumab in Diabetic Macular Edema with Center Involvement) (2005).**

   Purpose

   Safety and efficacy of RBZ in DME involving the foveal center.

   Inclusion Criteria

   Adults, type 1 or 2 diabetes, CFT ≥300 μm, and BCVA of 73–39 ETDRS letters.

Outcome Measures

Efficacy in terms of BCVA and CFT and safety at 12 months.

Results and Conclusions

RBZ is effective in improving BCVA and is well tolerated in DME.

4. **RESTORE (Ranibizumab monotherapy or combined with laser vs laser monotherapy for diabetic macular edema) (2008).**

   Purpose

   Superiority of RBZ 0.5 mg monotherapy or combined with laser over laser alone in DME.

   Inclusion Criteria

   Adults, type 1 or 2 DM and visual impairment due to DME.

   Outcome Measures

   Mean average change in BCVA from baseline to month 1 through 12 safety.

   Results and Conclusions

   RBZ monotherapy and combined with laser provided superior visual acuity over laser in patients with DME.

5. **BOLT (A prospective randomized trial of intravitreal Bevacizumab or Laser Therapy in the management of diabetic macular edema) (2007).**

   Purpose

   Bevacizumab vs Macular Laser Therapy (MLT) in CSME.

   Inclusion Criteria

   Patients with center-involving CSME, at least 1 prior MLT, BCVA 20/40 to 20/320.

   Outcome Measures

   Difference in BCVA at 12 months between the bevacizumab and laser arms.

   Results and Conclusions

   The study supports the use of bevacizumab in patients with center-involving CSME without advanced macular ischemia.

6. **DA VINCI (DME and VEGF Trap-Eye: Investigation of Clinical Impact) (2008).**

   Purpose

   VEGF Trap-Eye vs laser in DME.

Inclusion Criteria

Adults >18 years, CSME with central involvement, BCVA 20/40 to 20/320.

Outcome Measures

Change in BCVA at 24 weeks and at 52 weeks.

Results and Conclusions

VEGF Trap-Eye produced a statistically significant and clinically relevant improvement in BCVA compared with macular laser in DME at 24 and 52 weeks.

7. **VISTA (VEGF Trap-Eye in Vision Impairment Due to DME) and VIVID DME (2011).**

Purpose

Efficacy of VEGF Trap-Eye on BCVA in DME with central involvement.

Inclusion Criteria

Adults >18 years, DME and BCVA 20/40 to 20/320.

Outcome Measures

Mean change in visual acuity from baseline (ETDRS).

Results and Conclusions

In Both VISTA and VIVID, VEGF Trap-Eye was superior to Macular laser photocoagulation for BCVA and anatomical outcomes.

8. **FAME (Fluocinolone Acetonide in Diabetic Macular Edema) (2011).**

Purpose

To assess the efficacy of low dose and high dose fluocinolone acetonide implant (FA) in DME.

Inclusion Criteria

Persistent DME despite at least 1 macular laser treatment.

Outcome Measures

Percentage of patients with improvement from baseline BCVA in ETDRS letter score of ≥15 at 36 months.

Results and Conclusions

FA inserts improved BCVA over 2 years, and the risk-to-benefit ratio was superior for the low-dose insert. Almost all phakic patients in the FA groups developed cataract. The incidence of incisional glaucoma surgery at month 36 was 4.8% in the low-dose group and 8.1% in the high-dose insert group.

9. **RETAIN (Ranibizumab 0.5 mg treat-and-extend regimen for diabetic macular edema) (2013).**

Purpose

To demonstrate the noninferiority of ranibizumab treat and extent with/without Laser to ranibizumab (PRN) for BCVA in patients with DME.

Inclusion Criteria

DME with VA between 20/32–20/160.

Outcome Measures

Mean average change in BCVA from baseline to months 1–12 (primary), Mean BCVA change from base line to months 12 and 24, treatment exposure and safety profile.

Results and Conclusion

Both treat and extent regimens (with/without laser) were non-inferior to PRN based on BCVA.

Steroids for DME

1. **MEAD (Dexamethasone intravitreal implant in patients with diabetic macular edema) (2012).**

Purpose

To evaluate the safety and efficacy of Dexamethasone implant 0.7 and 0.35 mg for DME.

Inclusion Criteria

Patients with DME, BCVA 20/50-20/200 CRT >= 300 microns.

Outcome Measures

Improvement of more than 15 letters in BCVA from base line, study of adverse events.

Results and Conclusion

Dexamethasone implant 0.7 and 0.35 mg resulted in >= 15-letter gain in BCVA and side effects were acceptable.

2. **OZLASE Study (Comparison of a combination of repeated intravitreal Ozurdex and macular laser therapy vs macular laser only in center-involving diabetic macular edema) (2015).**

Purpose

To evaluate the efficacy and safety of combined repeated Ozurdex and macular laser therapy (MLT) compared with MLT monotherapy in center involving DME.

Inclusion Criteria

Patients with center involving DME.

Outcome Measures

Mean change in BCVA at week 56.

Results and Conclusions

Visual outcome following combination therapy did not differ from MLT alone in the center involving DME despite a significant decrease in CST likely due to an entry level ceiling effect and cataract development.

3. **OZDRY Study (Comparison of fixed vs pro-re-nata dosing of Ozurdex in refractory diabetic macular edema) (2015).**

    Purpose

    To compare the clinical effectiveness and safety of 5 monthly fixed dosing vs PRN ozurdex treatment in patients with refractory DME.

    Inclusion Criteria

    Refractory DME, BCVA 20/40–20/200, CRT >=300 microns.

    Outcome Measures

    Primary outcome measures—change in BCVA (Non-inferiority margin of 5 letters). Secondary outcome measures—change in Patient-Reported Outcome Scores (PROMS), macular thickness, morphology, retinopathy and safety profile.

    Results and Conclusions

    The mean Change in BCVA in 5-monthly fixed dosing of Ozurdex was non-inferior to OCT-guided PRN dosing.

4. **PLACID STUDY (Dexamethasone intravitreal implant in combination with laser photocoagulation for the treatment of diffuse diabetic macular edema) (2013).**

    Purpose

    To evaluate Ozurdex (dexamethasone intravitreal implant [DEX implant]; Allergan, Inc, Irvine, CA) 0.7 mg combined with laser photocoagulation compared with laser alone for treatment of diffuse diabetic macular edema (DME).

    Inclusion Criteria

    Patients with DME.

    Outcome Measures

    Change in BCVA of more than 10 letters.

Results and Conclusion

Equal percentage of patients gained more than 10 letters between the two groups; however, greater improvement in BCVA occurred in DEX with laser group than laser alone.

Anti-VEGF and Steroids for DME

1. **BEVORDEX: Efficacy of dexamethasone vs bevacizumab on regression of hard exudates in diabetic maculopathy: data from the BEVORDEX randomized clinical trial.**

   Purpose

   To report the effect of bevacizumab vs dexamethasone on hard exudates (HEX) in diabetic macular edema (DME).

   Inclusion Criteria

   Eyes with center-involving DME resistant to or unlikely to benefit from macular laser therapy were included.

   Outcome Measures

   Change in area of HEX and distance of closest HEX to center of fovea.

   Results and Conclusions

   Bevacizumab and DEX were effective in reducing area of HEX in eyes with DME. DEX provided more rapid regression of HEX from the foveal center although bevacizumab-treated eyes started to catch up by 24 months.

Anti VEGF for PDR

1. **CLARITY Study (Clinical efficacy of intravitreal aflibercept vs panretinal photocoagulation for best corrected visual acuity in patients with proliferative diabetic retinopathy at 52 weeks): 2017.**

   Purpose

   To report the safety and efficacy of intravitreal Aflibercept for PDR.

   Inclusion Criteria

   Type 1 or type 2 DM patients with PDR (untreated or previously laser treated active).

   Outcome Measures

   Change in BNCVA at week 52.

   Results and Conclusion

   Aflibercept was superior to PRP.

DRCR.net

1. **Protocol-I: Laser-Ranibizumab-Triamcinolone Study for DME.**

   Purpose

   To evaluate intravitreal 0.5 mg ranibizumab or 4 mg triamcinolone combined with focal/grid laser compared with focal/grid laser alone for treatment of DME.

   Inclusion Criteria

   VA of 20/32 to 20/320 and DME involving the fovea.

   Outcome Measures

   BCVA and safety at 2-year.

   Results and Conclusion

   Intravitreal ranibizumab with prompt or deferred laser is more effective at 2 years compared with prompt laser alone for the treatment of DME involving the central macula. In pseudophakic eyes, intravitreal triamcinolone + prompt laser seem more effective than laser alone but frequently increase the risk of IOP elevation.

2. **Protocol-S: Panretinal Photocoagulation vs Intravitreous Ranibizumab for Proliferative Diabetic Retinopathy: A Randomized Clinical Trial.**

   Purpose

   Compare ranibizumab vs PRP for PDR.

   Inclusion Criteria

   Patients with PDR.

   Outcome Measures

   Primary: mean visual acuity change at 2 years (5-letter noninferiority margin; intention-to-treat analysis).

   Secondary: visual acuity area under the curve, peripheral visual field loss, DME development, neovascularization, vitrectomy, and safety.

   Results and Conclusion

   Among eyes with PDR, treatment with ranibizumab resulted in visual acuity that was non-inferior to (not worse than) PRP treatment at 2 years.

3. **Protocol-T Aflibercept, Bevacizumab, or Ranibizumab for Diabetic Macular Edema; 2-Year Results from a Comparative Effectiveness Randomized Clinical Trial.**

Purpose

To provide 2-year results comparing anti vascular endothelial growth factor (VEGF) agents for center-involved diabetic macular edema (DME) using a standardized follow-up and retreatment regimen.

Inclusion Criteria

Patients with DME.

Methods

Randomization to 2.0-mg aflibercept, 1.25-mg repackaged (compounded) bevacizumab, or 0.3-mg ranibizumab intravitreous injections performed up to monthly using a protocol-specific follow-up and retreatment regimen. Focal/grid laser photocoagulation was added after 6 months if DME persisted. Visits occurred every 4 weeks during year 1 and were extended up to every 4 months thereafter when VA and macular thickness were stable.

Main Outcome Measures

Change in VA, adverse events, and retreatment frequency.

Conclusions

All three anti-VEGF groups showed VA improvement from baseline to 2 years with a decreased number of injections in year 2. Visual acuity outcomes were similar for eyes with better baseline VA. Among eyes with worse baseline VA, aflibercept had superior 2-year VA outcomes compared with bevacizumab, but superiority of aflibercept over ranibizumab, noted at 1 year, was no longer identified. Higher Anti-Platelet Trialists' Collaboration (APTC) event rates with ranibizumab over 2 years warrants continued evaluation in future trials.

RVO studies

1. **BVOS (Branch Vein Occlusion Study) (1984).**

Purpose

To assess the efficacy of scatter argon photocoagulation for prevention of NV and vitreous hemorrhage and improving visual acuity in eyes with macular edema reducing vision to 20/40 or worse.

Inclusion Criteria

Major BRVO without NV Major BRVO with NV BRVO with macular edema and reduced vision.

Outcome Measures

Visual acuity and development of NV or vitreous hemorrhage.

Result and Conclusion

Scatter argon photocoagulation prevents the development of NV and vitreous hemorrhage but should be applied after the development of NV. Argon laser improved visual outcome in eyes with BRVO and visual acuity reduced from macular edema to 6/12 or worse.

2. **CVOS (Central Vein Occlusion Study) (1988).**

   Purpose

   i. To study the effects of Early PRP for prevention of INV in ischemic CRVO.
   ii. To compare Early PRP vs PRP at first identification of INV Grid-pattern photocoagulation for loss of central visual acuity due to macular edema.

   Inclusion Criteria

   Patients of CRVO, age 21 or older, visual acuity of light perception or better, IOP <30 mm Hg and sufficient clarity of the ocular media.

   Outcome Measures

   Visual acuity, fundus evaluation, fluorescein angiography, and INV.

   Result and Conclusion

   i. Prophylactic PRP did not prevent the development of INV. It is safe to wait for the development of early INV and then apply PRP.
   ii. Macular grid photocoagulation was effective in reducing angiographic evidence of macular edema but did not improve visual acuity.
   iii. Patients with CRVO are recommended to have frequent follow up examination every 1 month for first 6 months to look for NVI.

3. **SCORE (Standard care vs COrticosteroid for REtinalvein occlusion Study) (2004).**

   Purpose

   Standard care vs intravitreal injection(s) of Triamcinolone Acetonide for macular edema of CRVO and BRVO.

Inclusion Criteria

Center-involving macular edema secondary to either CRVO or BRVO, <24 month old, VA ≥19 letters and ≤73 letters, retinal thickness >250 microns in the central subfield.

Outcome Measures

Improvement by 15 or more letters from baseline in best-corrected ETDRS visual acuity score at the 12-month visit

Result and Conclusion

Intravitreal triamcinolone is superior to observation for treating vision loss associated with macular edema secondary to CRVO but not in BRVO. 1mg dose has a safety profile superior to that of the 4mg dose.

4. **BRAVO (Ranibizumab for the Treatment of Macular Edema Following Branch Retinal Vein Occlusion: Evaluation of Efficacy and Safety) (2007).**

Purpose

Intravitreal Ranibizumab vs sham injections in patients with macular edema due to BRVO

Inclusion Criteria

Macular edema involving foveal center due to BRVO, CFT ≥250 μm on OCT and BCVA of 20/40 to 20/400.

Outcome Measures

Mean change in BCVA letter score at month 6 from baseline.

Result and Conclusion

Ranibizumab provided rapid and effective treatment for macular edema following BRVO with low rates of ocular and nonocular safety events.

5. **CRUISE (Central Retinal Vein Occlusion Study: Evaluation of Efficacy and Safety) (2007).**

Purpose

Intravitreal Ranibizumab vs sham injections in patients with macular edema due to CRVO.

Inclusion Criteria

Macular edema involving foveal center due to CRVO, CFT ≥250 μm on OCT, and BCVA of 20/40 to 20/320.

Outcome Measures

Mean change in BCVA letter score at month 6 from baseline.

Result and Conclusion

Ranibizumab provided rapid improvement in 6-month visual acuity and macular edema following CRVO, with low rates of ocular and nonocular safety events.

6. **GENEVA (Global Evaluation of Implantable dExamethasone in Retinal Vein Occlusion with Macular Edema) (2004).**

   Purpose

   Dexamethasone intravitreal implant vs sham in vision loss due to macular edema due to BRVO or CRVO.

   Inclusion Criteria

   Decreased VA due to ME associated with either CRVO or BRVO, BCVA of between 34 and 68 letters, central subfield $\geq$300 µm on OCT.

   Outcome Measures

   Time to achieve a $\geq$15-letter improvement in BCVA

   Result and Conclusion

   Dexamethasone intravitreal implant can both reduce the risk of vision loss and improve the speed and incidence of visual improvement in eyes with macular edema secondary to BRVO or CRVO.

7. **COPERNICUS (Controlled Phase 3 Evaluation of Repeated Intravitreal Administration of VEGF Trap-Eye In Central Retinal Vein Occlusion: Utility and Safety).**

   Purpose

   Intravitreal VEGF Trap-Eye in eyes with macular edema secondary to CRVO.

   Inclusion Criteria

   Center-involved macular edema secondary to CRVO for no longer than 9 months, central subfield thickness $\geq$250 µm, BCVA of 20/40 to 20/320.

   Outcome Measures

   Proportion of eyes with a $\geq$15-letter gain BCVA at week 24.

   Result and Conclusion

   Intravitreal VEGF Trap-Eye for macular edema secondary to CRVO resulted in a significant improvement in visual acuity.

8. **GALILEO (General Assessment Limiting Infiltration of Exudates in Central Retinal Vein Occlusion with VEGF Trap-Eye).**

   Purpose

   Intravitreal VEGF Trap-Eye in patients with macular edema secondary to CRVO.

   Inclusion Criteria

   Center-involved macular edema secondary to CRVO for no longer than 9 months, central subfield thickness $\geq$250 µm, BCVA of 20/40 to 20/320.

   Outcome Measures

   Percentage of eyes which gained $\geq$15 letters at week 24.

   Result and Conclusion

   Intravitreal VEGF Trap-Eye was efficacious in CRVO with an acceptable safety profile.

9. **VIBRANT (Intravitreal Aflibercept for Macular Edema Following Branch Retinal Vein Occlusion) (2016).**

   Purpose

   To determine efficacy and safety outcomes in eyes with macular edema after BRVO treated with 2 mg intravitreal aflibercept injection (IAI) compared with grid laser.

   Inclusion Criteria

   Treatment-naïve eyes with macular edema after BRVO if the occlusion occurred within 12 months and BCVA was between 20/40 and 20/320.

   Outcome Measures

   Percentage of eyes with improvement from BCVA letter score >= 15 at week 24 and 52.

   Results and Conclusions

   After 6 monthly IAI, injections every 8 weeks maintained control of macular edema and visual benefits through week 52. In the laser group, rescue IAI given from week 24 onward resulted in substantial visual improvements at week 52.

10. **MARVEL (Study of the Efficacy and Safety of Intravitreal Bevacizumab vs Ranibizumab in the Treatment of Macular Edema due to Branch Retinal Vein Occlusion) – Report 1: 2015.**

    Purpose

    To assess the efficacy and safety of intravitreal bevacizumab (IVB) compared with ranibizumab (IVR) in the treatment of macular edema due to branch retinal vein occlusion (BRVO).

Inclusion Criteria

BRVO with macular edema.

Outcome Measures

The primary outcome measure was the difference in mean changes in best-corrected visual acuity (BCVA) at 6 months. Secondary outcome measures included mean change in central retinal thickness (CRT), the proportion of patients improving by >15 letters and the proportion of patients developing neovascularisation

Results and Conclusion

This study demonstrated significant gain in visual acuity in eyes with BRVO treated with either bevacizumab or ranibizumab.

11. **SCORE-2 (Study of Comparative Treatments for Retinal Vein Occlusion 2) Effect of Bevacizumab vs Aflibercept on Visual Acuity Among Patients With Macular Edema due to Central Retinal Vein Occlusion (2017).**

Purpose

To study whether bevacizumab is non-inferior to aflibercept for visual acuity in eyes with macular edema due to central retinal or hemiretinal vein occlusion.

Inclusion Criteria

Patients with macular edema due to central retinal or hemiretinal vein occlusion.

Main Outcomes and Measures

The primary outcome was mean change in visual acuity (VA) letter score (VALS) from the randomization visit to the 6-month follow-up visit, based on the best-corrected electronic ETDRS VALS (scores range from 0–100; higher scores indicate better VA).

Conclusions and Relevance

Among patients with macular edema due to central retinal or hemiretinal vein occlusion, intravitreal bevacizumab was noninferior to aflibercept with respect to visual acuity after 6 months of treatment.

ROP Studies

1. **CRYO-ROP (Cryotherapy for Retinopathy of Prematurity Cryotherapy for Retinopathy of Prematurity) (1986).**

Purpose

To assess the safety and efficacy of trans-scleral cryotherapy in infants with ROP.

Inclusion Criteria

Premature infants weighing <1,251 grams at birth and had survived the first 28 days of life with threshold ROP.

Outcome Measures

Fundus photo and VA at 1 year of age.

Result/Conclusion

Cryotherapy reduces the risk of unfavorable retinal and functional outcome (by half) from threshold ROP. The benefit of was maintained across 15 years of follow-up.

2. **ET-ROP (Early Treatment for Retinopathy of Prematurity Study) (2000).**

    Purpose

    To compare the Early vs conventional timing of treatment in ROP.

    Inclusion Criteria

    Infants <1,251 grams birth weight, examined by 42 days of life and with prethreshold ROP.

    Outcome Measures

    Functional (primary) and structural (secondary) outcome at 9 months.

    Result/Conclusion

    Early treatment significantly reduced unfavorable outcomes in both primary and secondary measures. Retinal ablative therapy is recommended for type I ROP; observation is recommended for type II ROP.

3. **BEAT-ROP (Bevacizumab Eliminates the Angiogenic Threat of Retinopathy of Prematurity) (2008).**

    Purpose

    Efficacy of intravitreal bevacizumab in ROP and compare it with conventional laser in ROP.

    Inclusion Criteria

    Infants ≤1500 grams at birth and ≤30 weeks gestation who develop stage 3 + ROP in zone I or posterior zone II.

    Result/Conclusion

    Intravitreal bevacizumab monotherapy, compared with conventional laser therapy showed a benefit for zone I but not zone II disease. Trial was too small to assess safety.

4. **STOP-ROP (Supplemental Therapeutic Oxygen for Prethreshold Retinopathy of Prematurity) (1994).**

   Purpose

   To assess the supplemental oxygen in moderately severe ROP (prethreshold ROP).

   Inclusion Criteria

   Newborns with prethreshold ROP in one or both eyes.

   Outcome Measures

   Adverse endpoint was progression to threshold ROP. Favorable endpoint was regression of the ROP into zone 3 or complete retinal vascularization.

   Result/Conclusion

   Supplemental oxygen did not cause additional progression of prethreshold ROP but also did not significantly reduce the need of peripheral retinal ablative surgery. Supplemental oxygen increased the risk of adverse pulmonary events.

5. **HOPE-ROP (High Oxygen Percentage in Retinopathy of Prematurity Study) (1996).**

   Purpose

   Rate of progression from prethreshold to threshold ROP in infants excluded from STOP-ROP.

   Inclusion Criteria

   Newborns with prethreshold ROP in one or both eyes.

   Outcome Measures

   Adverse endpoint was progression to threshold ROP. Favorable endpoint was regression of the ROP into zone 3 or complete retinal vascularization.

   Result/Conclusion

   HOPE-ROP infants progressed from prethreshold to threshold ROP less often than STOP-ROP infants.

6. **LIGHT-ROP (Effects of Light Reduction on Retinopathy of Prematurity (LIGHT-ROP) (1995).**

   Purpose

   To study the effect of ambient light reduction on the incidence of ROP.

   Inclusion Criteria

   Premature infants weighing <1,251 grams at birth and having a gestational age of <31 weeks.

Outcome Measures

Development of ROP or full vascularization.

Result/Conclusion

Reduction in the ambient-light exposure does not alter the incidence of ROP.

7. **PHOTO-ROP (Photographic Screening for Retinopathy of Prematurity Study) (2000).**

Purpose

Digital fundus imaging compared to indirect ophthalmoscopy to screen for ROP.

Inclusion Criteria

Premature infants <31 weeks postmenstrual age at birth and <1,000 g birth weight.

Outcome Measures

Sensitivity, specificity, positive, and negative predictive values of reading center image interpretations compared to clinical impressions based on bedside indirect ophthalmoscopy.

Result/Conclusion

Remote digital fundus imaging is unlikely to supplant bedside ophthalmoscopy due to limitations in diagnostic sensitivity, specificity, and accuracy when image quality is poor. However, fundus imaging is useful adjunct to indirect ophthalmoscopy especially when image quality is good.

8. **RAINBOW Study (RAnibizumab Compared With Laser Therapy for the Treatment of INfants BOrn Prematurely With Retinopathy of Prematurity).**

Purpose

To determine if intravitreal ranibizumab is superior to laser ablation therapy in the treatment of retinopathy of prematurity (ROP).

Inclusion Criteria

BW less than 1,500 g
Bilateral ROP with 1 of the following retinal findings in each eye:
  i. Zone I, stage 1+, 2+, 3 or 3+ disease or
  ii. Zone II, stage 3+ disease or
  iii. Aggressive posterior ROP.

Primary Outcome Measures

Absence of active ROP and unfavorable structural outcome (Time frame: 24 weeks after starting investigational treatment).

To achieve this outcome, patients must fulfill all the following criteria, i. survival, ii. no intervention with a second modality for ROP, iii. absence of active ROP, and iv. absence of unfavorable structural outcome.

Secondary Outcome Measures

i. Requirement for intervention with a second modality for ROP (Time frame: 24 weeks after starting investigational treatment).

ii. Time to intervention with a second modality for ROP or development of unfavorable structural outcome or death (Time frame: 24 weeks after starting investigational treatment).

iii. Recurrence of ROP (Time frame: 24 weeks after starting investigational treatment).

iv. Number of patients having any ocular adverse event (Time frame: 24 weeks after starting investigational treatment).

v. Systemic ranibizumab levels (Time frame: Within 24 hours, 14 days, and 28 days after ranibizumab treatment).

vi. Systemic Vascular Endothelial Growth Factor (VEGF) levels (Time frame: Before investigational treatment, 14 days, and 28 days after investigational treatment).

vii. Number of ranibizumab administrations (Time frame: 24 weeks after starting investigational treatment).

viii. Number of patients having any systemic adverse event (Time frame: 24 weeks after starting investigational treatment).

Laser Photocoagulation in Choroidal Neovascularization (CNV)

1. **MPS (Macular Photocoagulation Study)—Argon study (1979).**

   Purpose

   To evaluate laser treatment of CNV (well-demarcated classic).

   Inclusion Criteria

   Extrafoveal CNV in AMD, POH (presumed ocular histoplasmosis), INVM (idiopathic neovascular membranes) with VA ≥20/100.

   Outcome Measures

   Change in BCVA from baseline.

   Conclusion

   Laser is beneficial in extrafoveal and juxtafoveal well-demarcated classic CNV.

2. **MPS (Macular Photocoagulation Study)—Krypton study (1979).**

   Purpose

   To evaluate laser treatment of CNV (well-demarcated classic).

Inclusion Criteria

Juxtafoveal CNV in AMD, POH (presumed ocular histoplasmosis), INVM (idiopathic neovascular membranes) with VA ≥20/400.

Outcome Measures

Change in BCVA from baseline.

Conclusion

Laser is beneficial in extrafoveal and juxtafoveal well-demarcated classic CNV.

3. **MPS (Macular Photocoagulation Study)—Foveal study (1979).**
   Purpose

   To evaluate laser treatment of CNV (well-demarcated classic).

   Inclusion Criteria

   Subfoveal new (<4 disk areas) or recurrent (<6 disk areas) CNV in AMD with VA 20/320 to 20/40.

   Outcome Measures

   Change in BCVA from baseline.

   Conclusion

   Laser is beneficial in subfoveal classic CNV (especially if small) and in conditions with worse initial VA.

Photodynamic Therapy (PDT) in CNV

1. **TAP (Treatment of ARMD with Photodynamic Therapy) (1998).**
   Purpose

   To evaluate PDT in subfoveal CNV in AMD.

   Inclusion Criteria

   Subfoveal classic CNV, size ≤ 5,400 µ, VA ≥20/100.

   Outcome Measures

   Eyes with <15 letters VA loss at 2 years.

   Conclusion

   PDT is beneficial in predominantly classic subfoveal CNV.

2. **VIP (Verteporfin in Photodynamic Therapy)—Myopic CNV (1998).**
   Purpose

   To evaluate PDT in subfoveal CNV in myopia.

   Inclusion Criteria

   Subfoveal CNV, size ≤ 5,400 µ, VA ≥20/100

Outcome Measures

Eyes with <8 letters VA loss.

Conclusion

PDT is beneficial in subfoveal CNV in myopia.

3. **VIP (Verteporfin in Photodynamic Therapy)—CNV in AMD (1998).**

Purpose

To evaluate PDT in subfoveal CNV in AMD, occult or classic with good VA.

Inclusion Criteria

Subfoveal CNV, size ≤5,400 μ, occult—VA ≥20/100 with recent progression; classic—VA >20/40.

Outcome Measures

Loss of 15 letters, that is, moderate vision loss.

Conclusion

Occult CNV should be treated with PDT if <4 disk areas, VA <20/50 or if classic features develop.

4. **VIM (Visudyne in minimally classic choroidal neovascularisation) (2001).**

Purpose

To evaluate SF (standard fluence)/RF (reduced fluence) PDT in subfoveal minimally classic CNV in AMD.

Inclusion Criteria

Subfoveal, minimally classic, VA ≥20/250, lesion size <6 MPS disk areas

Outcome Measures

Loss of 15 letters.

Conclusion

PDT is beneficial in small subfoveal minimally classic CNV in AMD.

Submacular Surgery Trials (SST)

1. **SST (Submacular Surgery Trial)—H (1997).**

Purpose

To compare surgical removal of subfoveal CNV in OHS (ocular histoplasmosis syndrome) or INVM (idiopathic Neovascular membrane) vs observation.

Inclusion Criteria

Subfoveal CNV (new or recurrent after laser), <9 MPS disk areas, VA 20/50 to 20/800.

Outcome Measures

Improvement in VA or retention of VA.

Conclusion

There is no benefit of performing surgery.

2. **SST (Submacular Surgery Trial)—B (1997).**

    Purpose

    To compare surgical removal of subfoveal CNV in AMD vs observation.

    Inclusion Criteria

    Large hemorrhages from subfoveal CNV (area of hemorrhage >CNV on FA), VA of 20/100 to light perception.

    Outcome Measures

    Improvement in VA or retention of VA.

    Conclusion

    Submacular surgery did not improve VA, but reduced the risk of severe VA loss compared to observation.

3. **SST (Submacular Surgery Trial)—N (1997).**

    Purpose

    To compare surgical removal of subfoveal CNV in AMD vs observation.

    Inclusion Criteria

    New subfoveal CNV due to AMD, <9 MPS disk areas, with poorly demarcated boundaries, VA of 20/100 to 20/800.

    Outcome Measures

    Improvement in VA or retention of VA.

    Conclusion

    Submacular surgery did not improve or preserve VA is not recommended.

4. **VISION (VEGF Inhibition Study in Ocular Neovascularisation).**

    Purpose

    To assess the efficacy of pegaptanib sodium in early subfoveal CNV secondary to AMD.

    Inclusion Criteria

    All angiographic CNV lesion compositions of AMD

    Outcome Measures

    Proportion of patients avoiding three lines of vision loss at 1 year.

    Result/Conclusion

    There is a benefit in receiving therapy with pegaptanib in year 2. The safety profile of was favorable.

5. **ANCHOR (Anti-VEGF Antibody for the Treatment of Predominantly Classic Choroidal Neovascularization in AMD).**

Purpose

To compare Ranibuzimab (RBZ) vs PDT in predominantly classic neovascular AMD.

Inclusion Criteria

Predominantly classic, subfoveal CNV not previously treated with PDT or antiangiogenic drugs, total size <5,400 µm, BCVA of 20/40 to 20/320

Outcome Measures

Percentage losing <15 letters and percentage gaining >or = 15 letters from baseline.

Result/Conclusion

RBZ over a 24-month period was effective, and superior to PDT treatment, in maintaining or improving VA and lesion characteristics.

6. **MARINA (Minimally Classic/Occult Trial of the Anti-VEGF Antibody Ranibizumab in the Treatment of Neovascular ARMD)**

Purpose

To assess the efficacy of RBZ in minimally classic/occult neovascular ARMD.

Inclusion Criteria

BCVA 20/40 to 20/320; primary or recurrent subfoveal CNV due to AMD, minimally classic or occult with no classic CNV; maximum lesion size of 12 DA, and presumed recent progression.

Result/Conclusion

RBZ for nonclassic neovascular AMD had substantially better VA outcomes compared to sham injections. RBZ treatment showed stabilization of lesion size.

7. **PIER (Phase IIIb, Multicenter, Randomized, Double-Masked, Sham Injection-Controlled Study of Efficacy and Safety of Ranibizumab (RBZ) in Subjects with Subfoveal CNV with or without Classic CNV secondary to AMD).**

Purpose

To assess the efficacy of RBZ given monthly for 3 months and then quarterly in patients with subfoveal CNV due to AMD.

Inclusion Criteria

All lesion types due to ARMD if the active CNV accounted for at least 50% of the total lesion.

Outcome Measure

Mean change from baseline visual acuity at month 12th and 24th.

Result/Conclusion

RBZ provided significant VA benefit. With quarterly dosing, there was a steady decline in VA during months 4 through 24 in PIER compared to the VA stabilization achieved in ANCHOR and MARINA with monthly injections.

8. **EXCITE (Efficacy and Safety of Ranibizumab Inpatients with Subfoveal CNV Secondary to AMD).**

Purpose

To assess the Quarterly vs monthly regimen of RBZ in subfoveal CNV secondary to AMD (PIER vs MARINA/ANCHOR) regimen.

Inclusion Criteria

Classic and nonclassic subfoveal neovascular AMD.

Outcome Measures

Mean change in BCVA central retinal thickness (CRT) from baseline to month 12.

Result/Conclusion

At month 12, BCVA gain in the monthly regimen was higher than that of the quarterly regimens.

9. **PrONTO (Prospective Optical Coherence Tomography Imaging of Patients with Neovascular AMD Treated with intra-Ocular Ranibizumab).**

Purpose

OCT-guided, variable dosing regimen RBZ for patients with neovascular AMD.

Inclusion Criteria

AMD patients with subfoveal CNV and a CRT of at least 300 microns.

Outcome Measures

Change in VA scores and OCT measurements from baseline at 24 months.

Result/Conclusion

OCT-guided variable-dosing regimen with RBZ resulted in VA outcomes similar to results from the Phase III MARINA and ANCHOR studies.

10. **SUSTAIN (Study of Ranibizumab in Patients with Subfoveal CNV Secondary to AMD).**

Purpose

To assess the Individualized RBZ (PRN regime) in patients with neovascular AMD.

Inclusion Criteria

AMD patients with subfoveal CNV naïve to RBZ treatment.

Outcome Measure

Frequency of adverse events, monthly change of BCVA and CRT from baseline.

Result/Conclusion

Like PrONTO, results from the SUSTAIN trial showed a rapid increase in VA in the first 3 months, which deteriorates slightly, but not nearly as much as in PIER, over the 9 months of PRN dosing.

11. **HARBOR (Phase III, double-masked, multicenter, randomized, Active treatment-controlled study of the efficacy and safety of 0.5 mg and 2.0 mg Ranibizumab administered monthly or on an as-needed Basis (PRN) in patients with subfoveal neOvasculaR age-related macular degeneration).**

Purpose

RBZ 0.5 mg and 2.0 mg monthly vs on PRN basis in treatment-naïve subfoveal neovascular AMD.

Inclusion Criteria

Subfoveal CNV due to ARMD, lesions <12 disk areas and BCVA 20/40–20/320.

Outcome Measures

Mean change from baseline in BCVA at month 12th.

Result/Conclusion

RBZ 0.5 mg dosed monthly provides optimum results in patients with wet AMD. There is no additional benefit from the high dose in treatment-naïve wet AMD.

12. **SAILOR (Safety Assessment of Intravitreal Lucentis for AMD).**

Purpose

RBZ in a large population of subjects with neovascular AMD.

Inclusion Criteria

Angiographically determined subfoveal CNV secondary to AMD.

Outcome Measures

Safety outcomes included the incidence of ocular and nonocular adverse events efficacy outcomes included changes in BCVA.

Result/Conclusion

Intravitreal RBZ was safe and well tolerated in a large population with neovascular AMD. Although the risks of arterial thrombotic events related to RBZ are low, they were similar to that observed in previous RBZ studies and ophthalmologists should be aware of these risks.

13. **HORIZON (Extension Trial of Ranibizumab for Neovascular Age-Related Macular Degeneration).**

Purpose

Long-term safety and efficacy of RBZ injections in patients with CNV secondary to AMD.

Inclusion Criteria

Patients who completed the controlled treatment phase of 1 of 3, 2-year clinical trials (ANCHOR, MARINA, or FOCUS).

Outcome Measures

Incidence and severity of ocular and nonocular adverse events.

Result/Conclusion

The incidence of serious ocular and nonocular adverse effects during the 2-year study period of HORIZON trial were low and consistent with those observed during the 24 months of treatment in the prior phase III trials.

14. **SANA (Systemic bevacizumab (Avastin) Therapy for Neovascular Age-related macular degeneration).**

Purpose

Systemic bevacizumab (BVZ) for the treatment of subfoveal CNV in neovascular AMD.

Inclusion Criteria

AMD with subfoveal CNV, BCVA letter scores of 70–20 and a central retinal thickness of 300 microns.

Outcome Measures

Safety assessments, changes from baseline in VA scores, OCT measurements, and angiographic lesion characteristics.

Result/Conclusion

Systemic BVZ for neovascular AMD was well tolerated and effective for all 18 patients through 24 weeks, with an improvement in VA, OCT, and angiographic outcomes.

15. **ABC (Avastin (R) (Bevacizumab) for Choroidal neovascularisation trial).**

Purpose

To compare Intravitreal BVZ vs PDT (for classic) or pegaptanib (for occult/minimally classic) for the treatment of neovascular AMD.

Inclusion Criteria

Predominantly classic or occult or minimally classic type neovascular AMD.

Outcome Measures

Proportion of patients gaining $>/= 15$ letters of visual acuity at 1 year.

Result/Conclusion

BVZ retreatment regimen is superior to standard care (pegaptanib sodium, verteporfin, sham), with low rates of serious ocular adverse events. Treatment improved visual acuity on average at 54 weeks.

16. **CATT (Comparison of Age-related Macular Degeneration Treatments Trials).**

Purpose

To compare RBZ vs BVZ administered monthly or as needed for 2 years in neovascular ARMD.

Inclusion Criteria

Active, subfoveal CNV, fibrosis <50% of total lesion area, VA 20/25- 20/320 and at least 1 drusen in either eye or late AMD in fellow eye.

Outcome Measures

Mean change in visual acuity at 1 year.

Result/Conclusion

RBZ and BVZ had similar effects on visual acuity over a 2-year period. Treatment as needed resulted in less gain in visual acuity. No differences between drugs in rates of death or arteriothrombotic events.

17. **IVAN (Inhibit VEGF in Age-related Choroidal Neovascularisation).**

Purpose

To compare RBZ vs BVZ intravitreal injections to treat neovascular AMD.

Inclusion Criteria

Untreated subfoveal neovascular AMD in the study eye with VA ≥ 25 letters.

Outcome Measures

Distance visual acuity (efficacy) and arteriothrombotic events or heart failure (safety).

Result/Conclusion

The comparison of visual acuity at 1 year between BVZ and RBZ was inconclusive. Visual acuities with continuous and discontinuous treatment were equivalent.

18. **CLEAR—IT 2 (Phase 2, Randomized, Controlled Dose-and-Interval-Ranging Study of Intravitreal VEGF Trap Eye in Patients with Neovascular Age-Related Macular Degeneration).**

Purpose

VEGF Trap-Eye for neovascular AMD.

Inclusion Criteria

Subfoveal CNV secondary to wet AMD.

Outcome Measure

Change in central retinal/lesion thickness (CR/LT), change in total lesion and CNV size, mean change in BCVA, proportion of patients with 15-letter loss or gain, time to first PRN injection, reinjection frequency, and safety at week 52nd.

Result/Conclusion

PRN dosing with VEGF Trap-Eye at weeks 16–52 maintained the significant anatomic and vision improvements established during the 12-week fixed-dosing phase with a low frequency of reinjections.

19. **VIEW 1 and 2 (VEGF Trap-Eye: Investigation of Efficacy and Safety in Wet AMD).**

Purpose

Monthly and every-2-month dosing of intravitreal VEGF Trap-Eye vs monthly RBZ in subfoveal CNV secondary to ARMD.

Inclusion Criteria

Subfoveal CNV secondary to ARMD.

Outcome Measures

Non-inferiority (margin of 10%) of the VEGF Trap-Eye regimens to RBZ in the proportion of patients maintaining vision at week 52nd.

Result/Conclusion

VEGF Trap-Eye dosed monthly or every 2 months after 3 initial monthly doses produced similar efficacy and safety outcomes as monthly RBZ.

20. **FOCUS (RhuFab V2 Ocular Treatment Combining the Use of Visudyne to Evaluate Safety).**

Purpose

RBZ combined with verteporfin PDT in predominantly classic CNV in AMD.

Inclusion Criteria

Predominantly classic CNV in AMD (PDT was performed 7 days before initial RBZ or sham treatment).

Outcome Measures

Proportion of patients losing fewer than 15 letters from baseline visual acuity at 12 months.

Result/Conclusion

A combination of RBZ and PDT were more efficacious than PDT alone for treating neovascular AMD, though RBZ treatment increased the risk of serious intraocular inflammation.

21. **PROTECT**

Purpose

To assess the safety of same-day administration of verteporfin PDT (standard fluence) and RBZ.

Inclusion Criteria

Predominantly classic or occult CNV secondary to AMD.

Outcome Measures

Incidence of severe vision loss (BCVA loss > or = 30 letters).

Result/Conclusion

Same-day verteporfin and RBZ was safe and not associated with severe vision loss or severe ocular inflammation.

22. **TORPEDO**

Purpose

To assess the efficacy of one-time reduced fluence-PDT followed by RBZ on a variable dosing regimen in neovascular AMD.

Inclusion Criteria

Previously untreated, active neovascular AMD.

Outcome Measures

Improvement in BCVA over 2 years.

Result/Conclusion

Combined PDT and RBZ injection the same day was well tolerated in all patients. 84% of patients had stable or improved vision at month 24th.

23. **DENALI (Verteporfin plus ranibizumab for choroidal neovascularization in age-related macular degeneration).**

Purpose

To compare RBZ in combination with verteporfin PDT vs RBZ monotherapy in subfoveal CNV in AMD.

Inclusion Criteria

Subfoveal CNV in AMD, lesion size <9 DA, naïve to AMD treatment, and a BCVA letter score of 73–24.

Outcome Measures

Mean change in BCVA from baseline at month 12th.

Result/Conclusions

RBZ monotherapy or combined with verteporfin PDT improved BCVA at month 12. Verteporfin reduced fluence did not confer clinical benefits over verteporfin standard fluence.

24. **MONT BLANC (Verteporfin plus ranibizumab for choroidal neovascularization in Age-related macular degeneration).**

    Purpose

    To compare same-day verteporfin PDT and intravitreal RBZ vs RBZ monotherapy in neovascular AMD.

    Inclusion Criteria

    Subfoveal CNV secondary to AMD, lesion size <9 DA, naïve to AMD treatment, and a BCVA letter score of 73–24.

    Outcome Measures

    Mean change in BCVA from baseline to month 12th.

    Result/Conclusion

    The combination was effective in achieving BCVA gain comparable with RBZ monotherapy. Study did not show benefits with respect to reducing the number of RBZ retreatment over 12 months.

25. **EVEREST (Efficacy and safety of verteporfin photodynamic therapy in combination with ranibizumab or alone vs ranibizumab monotherapy in patients with symptomatic macular polypoidal choroidal vasculopathy).**

    Purpose

    To compare verteporfin PDT combined with RBZ or alone vs RBZ monotherapy in symptomatic macular PCV.

    Inclusion Criteria

    PCV with BCVA letter score between 73 and 24, greatest linear dimension of the total lesion area <5,400 μm.

    Outcome Measures

    Proportion of patients with ICGA assessed complete regression of polyps at month 6th.

    Result/Conclusion

    At month 6th, verteporfin combined with RBZ or alone was superior to RBZ monotherapy in achieving complete polyp regression.

26. **RADICAL (Reduced Fluence Visudyne-Anti-VEGF-Dexamethasone in Combination for AMD Lesions).**

Purpose

To compare RF PDT + RBZ vs either of two regimens of RF PDT + RBZ + Dexamethasone vs RBZ monotherapy.

Inclusion Criteria

Treatment-naïve subfoveal CNV due to AMD, GLD <9 DA, BC VA score of 25–73 letters.

Outcome Measures

Mean number of retreatments and the mean change in BCVA from baseline at 24 months.

Result/Conclusion

Significantly fewer retreatment visits were required with combination therapies than with RBZ monotherapy. Mean VA change from baseline was not statistically different among the treatment groups.

27. **CABERNET (The Choroidal Neovascularisation Secondary to AMD Treated with Beta Radiation Epiretinal Therapy).**

Purpose

To estimate the safety and efficacy of epimacular brachytherapy (EMBT) for the treatment of CNV in neovascular AMD.

Inclusion Criteria

Predominantly classic, minimally classic, or occult with no classic lesions, secondary to AMD, with a total lesion size of <12 DA, and a GLD ≤5.4 mm.

Outcome Measure

Proportion of patients losing fewer than 15 letters from baseline and the proportion gaining more than 15 letters.

Result/Conclusion

The 2-year efficacy data do not support the routine use of EMBT for treatment-naïve wet AMD, despite an acceptable safety profile.

28. **AREDS (Age-related Eye Disease Study) (1992).**

Purpose

Determine clinical course, prognosis, and risk factors of AMD and cataract. Evaluate effects of high doses of antioxidants and zinc on the progression of AMD, cataract, and vision loss.

Inclusion Criteria

Extensive small drusen, intermediate drusen, large drusen, noncentral GA, or pigment abnormalities in one or both eyes, or advanced AMD or vision loss due to AMD in one eye. At least one eye had best-corrected visual acuity of 20/32 or better.

Outcome Measure

Increase from baseline in nuclear, cortical, or posterior subcapsular opacity grades or cataract surgery moderate visual acuity loss from baseline.

Result/Conclusion

Patients with extensive intermediate-sized drusen, at least one large drusen, noncentral GA in one or both eyes, or advanced AMD or vision loss due to AMD in one eye should consider taking a supplement of antioxidants plus zinc. Use of a high-dose formulations of vitamin C, E, and beta carotene in well-nourished older adult cohort had no apparent effect on the 7-year risk of development or progression of age-related lens opacities.

29. **AREDS (Age-related Eye Disease Study)-2 (2006).**

Purpose

Evaluate effect of the two dietary xanthophylls and two omega-3 fatty acids (LCPUFAs), on progression to AMD and/or moderate vision loss in people at moderate to high risk for progression.

Inclusion Criteria

Persons aged 50–85 with bilateral intermediate AMD or advanced AMD in one eye.

Outcome Measure

Progression to advanced AMD.

Result/Conclusion

Awaited.

30. **CAPT (Complications of Age-related Macular Degeneration Prevention Trial) (1999).**

Purpose

Low-intensity laser of eyes with drusen in the macula for preventing later complications of AMD.

Inclusion Criteria

Male or female, aged at least 50, vision in each eye 20/40 or better with at least 10 large (>125 μm) drusen in each eye.

Result/Conclusion

Low-intensity laser treatment did not demonstrate a clinically significant benefit for vision. Risk factors for CNV and GA stated.

Endophthalmitis Vitrectomy Study (EVS).

EVS (1990–1995)

Purpose

To assess the role of early PPV vs intravitreal antibiotics and intravenous antibiotics in postoperative endophthalmitis.

Inclusion Criteria

Patients with endophthalmitis following cataract surgery or IOL implantation with VA<20/50 and > light perception (LP).

Outcome Measures

Visual acuity (VA) by ETDRS chart and media clarity.

Follow-up

3 and 9 months.

Results Follow-up

VA was better with PPV in patients with LP vision results were comparable when initial vision was HM or better. Intravenous antibiotics did not affect outcome.

Conclusion

Immediate vitrectomy is not necessary in patients with better than light perception vision at presentation while results are better with PPV in patients in whom VA is light perception only.

CLINICAL TRIALS IN GLAUCOMA

1. **Ocular Hypertension Treatment Study (OHTS).**

   Questions asked

   i. Does medical reduction of IOP prevent or delay the onset of optic nerve damage and visual field loss in patients with ocular hypertension?

   ii. Who are the people more likely to develop glaucoma, and therefore perhaps benefit from treatment; and which people with increased IOP are unlikely to develop glaucoma and therefore could probably be followed without treatment?

   Results

   i. The results of OHTS proved that topical anti-glaucoma medication reduces the incidence of glaucoma.

   ii. The cumulative probability of developing POAG was 4.4% in the medication group and 9.5% in the observation group.

   iii. Medical treatment reduced the development of glaucoma by more than 50% at the end of 5 years.

   iv. The predictive factors found included increasing age, increasing IOP, decreased thickness of the cornea, and increased cup/disk ratio.

   v. The risk of developing glaucoma is variable. It may be as low as 1–2% in some ocular hypertensive patients and as high as 25–35% in some patients over 5 years.

   Conclusion

   Patients receiving topical anti-glaucoma medications had a lower risk of developing POAG than patients receiving no medication. The risk can be determined by analyzing the following parameters like increasing patient's age, IOP, corneal thickness, cup/disk ratio, and higher pattern standard deviation.

2. **Early manifest glaucoma trial (EMGT).**

   Questions asked

   i. What is the effect of immediate therapy to lower the IOP vs late or no treatment on the progression of early, newly detected open angle glaucoma?

   ii. What is the extent of IOP reduction attained by treatment and what are the factors that influence glaucoma progression?

   Results

   i. Multicenter randomized controlled clinical trial comparing observation with betaxolol and laser trabeculoplasty for open angle glaucoma.

   ii. Early signs of advancing disease were detected earlier in the untreated group when compared to the treated group.

   iii. No factors, aside from exfoliation glaucoma, were related to longitudinal changes in IOP.

   iv. A 25% decrease of IOP from baseline reduced the risk of progression by 50%.

   v. Risk of progression decreased 10% with each 1 mm Hg IOP reduction from baseline to the first follow up visit.

Conclusion

Untreated patients had twice the glaucoma progression risk of patients who received treatment, and those with the greatest IOP lowering enjoyed the most benefit.

3. **Collaborative Normal Tension Glaucoma Study (CNTGS).**

Question asked

What is the role of IOP control in preventing the progression in normal-tension glaucoma (NTG).

Results

   i. One eye of each eligible subject was randomized either not to be treated (control group) or to have intraocular pressure lowered by 30% from baseline by surgical and/or medical means.

   ii. Mean IOP in the treatment group was 10.6 mm Hg and untreated group was 16.0 mm Hg.

   iii. Survival analysis showed statistically significant difference in disease progression in the two groups when examining for specifically defined endpoint criteria of optic disk appearances and field loss.

   iv. The incidence of cataract was higher in the treated arm, with the highest incidence in those whose treatment included filtration surgery.

Conclusion

Slower rate of incidence of visual field loss was seen in cases with 30% or more lowering of intraocular pressure in normal tension glaucoma. Progression of visual field loss was faster in women, in patients with migraine headaches, and in the presence of disk hemorrhages.

4. **European Glaucoma Preventing Study (EGPS).**

Question asked

How effective is the reduction of IOP by dorzolamide in preventing or delaying POAG in patients affected by ocular hypertension (OHT).

Results

   i. Patients were randomized to treatment with dorzolamide or placebo (excipients of dorzolamide).

   ii. Dorzolamide reduced IOP by 15–22% throughout the 5 years of the trial.

iii. Same predictors for the development of POAG in OHTS and EGPS: baseline older age, higher IOP, thinner central corneal thickness, larger vertical cup-to-disk ratio, and higher Humphrey visual field pattern standard deviation

Conclusion

EGPS failed to detect statistical difference between the chosen medical therapy and placebo, either in IOP lowering effect, or in the rate of progression to POAG.

5. **Collaborative Initial Glaucoma Treatment Study (CIGTS).**

Question asked

Are patients with open angle glaucoma best managed with initial topical medication or by initial filtration surgery?

Results
   i. Newly diagnosed open angle glaucoma were randomized to either medication or trabeculectomy (with or without 5-fluorouracil).
   ii. There was no significant difference in visual field loss between the two groups.
   iii. Patients randomized to surgery had initially poorer quality of life and underwent cataract surgery more than twice as often as patients in the medically treated group.
   iv. The average visual acuity in the two groups after 4 years was about equal.
   v. IOP reduction was greater with surgery than with medical therapy (48% vs 35%).

Conclusion

Initial medical treatment and initial filtering surgery were both effective at preserving vision; there was a slight advantage for the medication arm, in terms of comfort.

6. **Advanced Glaucoma Intervention Study (AGIS).**

Question asked

How are outcomes in open angle glaucoma affected by the sequence of treatment with ALT and trabeculectomy?

Results
   i. Eyes were randomized to receive either ALT followed by trabeculectomy 1 and trabeculectomy 2 (ATT sequence) or trabeculectomy 1 followed by ALT and then trabeculectomy 2 (TAT sequence).
   ii. Younger age and higher preoperative IOP were associated with increased failure rates for both groups.

iii. In black patients, the average percent of eyes with visual field loss was less in ATT sequence than in TAT sequence.

iv. In white patients, the average percent of eyes with visual field loss was less in TAT sequence.

Conclusion

Long-term visual function outcomes were better for the ATT sequence in black patients and better for the TAT sequence in white patients.

7. **Tube vs Trabeculectomy Study (TVT).**

Question asked

Trabeculectomy or Tube shunt surgery: which is safer and effective in lowering the IOP in eyes with previous intraocular surgery?

Results

i. Patients with previous cataract and/or failed glaucoma surgery and uncontrolled glaucoma on maximum tolerated medical therapy were randomized to receive either nonvalved tube shunt surgery (Baerveldt implant) and/or trabeculectomy with application of mitomycin C for 4 minutes.

ii. After 3 months, both procedures produced sustained pressure reduction to the low teens throughout the 5-year duration of the study.

iii. Trabeculectomy had a higher long-term failure rate (47% vs 30% after 5 years)

iv. The tube shunt surgery group had a lower rate of early postoperative complications.

v. The rates of visual loss and of late or serious complications were similar between the two groups.

Conclusion

Tube shunt had higher success rate compared to trabeculectomy with MMC during 5 years of follow-up. Both procedures were associated with similar IOP reduction and use of supplemental medical therapy at 5 years. Additional glaucoma surgery was needed more frequently after trabeculectomy with MMC than tube shunt placement.

8. **The Glaucoma Laser Trial (GLT).**

Question asked

How safe and effective is argon laser trabeculoplasty (ALT) as an alternative to treatment with topical anti-glaucoma medication for controlling intraocular pressure in patients with newly diagnosed, previously untreated primary open angle glaucoma?

Results

i. Each patient had one eye randomly assigned to ALT (laser first [LF] eye) and the other eye assigned to timolol maleate 0.5% (medication first [MF] eye).

ii. LF eyes had lower mean IOPs than MF eyes.

iii. Fewer LF eyes than MF eyes required simultaneous prescription of two or more medications to control IOP.

Conclusion

There were no major differences between the two treatment approaches with respect to changes in visual acuity or visual field over the 2 years of follow-up.

9. **Glaucoma Laser Trial Follow-up Study (GLTFS).**

Question asked

What are the differences between the two treatment groups of the Glaucoma Laser Trial with respect to intraocular pressure, visual fields, optic disk cupping, and therapy for primary open-angle glaucoma?

Results

i. This was a follow-up study of patients who enrolled in the Glaucoma Laser Trial and the median duration of follow-up was 7 years (maximum 9 years).

ii. Eyes initially treated with laser trabeculoplasty had 1.2 mm Hg greater reduction in intraocular pressure and 0.6 dB greater improvements in the visual field when compared to eyes initially treated with anti-glaucoma medications.

iii. The overall difference between eyes with regard to change in ratio of optic cup area to optic disk area indicated slightly more deterioration for eyes initially treated with medication.

Conclusion

Initial treatment efficacy with argon laser trabeculoplasty was comparable to initial treatment with topical anti-glaucoma medication.

10. **Fluorouracil Filtering Surgery Study (FFSS).**

Question asked

i. Does postoperative subconjunctival injections of 5-fluorouracil (5-FU) increase the success of trabeculectomy in patients at risk for trabeculectomy failure?

ii. What are the risk factors for failure of surgery?

Results

i. Patients with medically uncontrolled glaucoma after previous cataract extraction or unsuccessful filtering surgery, or both, were randomized to a trabeculectomy alone (standard treatment), or to trabeculectomy with adjunctive 5-FU injections.

ii. The study demonstrated improved surgical control of glaucoma using 5-FU in patients at high risk for trabeculectomy failure.

iii. After 5 years, 51% of eyes that received 5 FU and 74% of the eyes that did not receive 5 FU had failed trabeculectomies.

iv. Risk factors other than treatment that clearly affect success are preoperative IOP, number of previous ocular procedures with conjunctival incision, the number of procedures with conjunctival incisions and Hispanic ethnicity.

v. The development of late onset bleb leak was more likely to occur in the 5-FU group than in standard therapy group.

Conclusion

Adjuvant 5 FU improved the success rates of trabeculectomy when followed up for 5 years, especially in eyes with poor prognosis.

11. **The Ahmed vs Baerveldt Study (AVB).**

Question asked

To compare two frequently used aqueous shunts for the treatment of glaucoma.

Results

i. Both implants were effective in lowering IOP. Ahmed group had a lower mean IOP in the early postoperative period. Baerveldt group had a greater IOP reduction than the Ahmed group at all follow-up visits beginning at 1 year and continuing to 5 years.

ii. After 5 years of follow-up, the Ahmed group had a higher failure rate of 53% compared with 40% in the Baerveldt group.

iii. The two groups had similar complication rates (Ahmed 63%, Baerveldt 69%) and intervention rates.

iv. Hypotony resulted in failure in five patients in the Baerveldt group compared with none in the Ahmed group.

Conclusion

Both implants were effective in reducing IOP and the need for glaucoma medications. The Baerveldt group had a lower failure rate and a lower IOP on fewer medications than the Ahmed group, but had a small risk of hypotony that was not seen in the Ahmed group.

12. **Ahmed Baerveldt Comparison Study (ABC).**

Question asked

What is the relative efficacy and complications of the Ahmed glaucoma valve (AGV) and the Baerveldt glaucoma implant (BGI) in refractory glaucoma.

Results

i. The BGI group had a statistically significant lower mean IOP than the AGV group at most of the annual study visits, including at 5 years.

ii. Mean number of medications in the AGV and BGI groups did not vary significantly at any of the annual follow up visits.

iii. Similar rates of surgical success were observed with both implants during 5 years of follow up, but the reasons for treatment failure were different.

iv. Failure after AGV was usually due to high IOP endpoints, while failure with the BGI was most commonly related to safety endpoints (hypotony, implant explantation, and loss of light perception).

Conclusion

Similar rates of surgical success were observed with both implants at 5 years. BGI implantation produced greater IOP reduction and a lower rate of glaucoma reoperation than AGV implantation but BGI implantation was associated with twice as many failures.

13. **United Kingdom Glaucoma Treatment Study (UKGTS).**

Question asked

Does treatment with a topical prostaglandin analog, compared with placebo, reduce the frequency of visual field (VF) deterioration events in patients with open-angle glaucoma (OAG)?

Results

i. Patients were randomly assigned to treatment with latanoprost 0.005% or placebo.

ii. Visual field preservation was significantly longer in the latanoprost group than in the placebo group.

iii. The intraocular-pressure reduction compared with baseline was 3.8 mm Hg in the latanoprost group and 0.9 mm Hg in the placebo group.

iv. A visual field endpoint was reached by 24 months in 34% of participants in the untreated group vs in 20% of participants in the treated group.

Conclusion

The study provides evidence of the vision-preserving benefits of topical prostaglandin analogs.

UVEITIS STUDIES

1. **SITE Study (Systemic Immunosuppressive Therapy for Eye diseases)**

   Question: To compare the occurrence of malignancy in patients with severe ocular inflammatory disease treated with systemic corticosteroids alone or with systemic immunosuppressive drugs with or without systemic corticosteroids.

   Result: It was a retrospective cohort study comparing ocular inflammatory disease treated with systemic steroids or immunosuppressive chemotherapy. The rate of malignancy in the immunosuppressant group was not significantly different from the rate in the corticosteroids alone group (p >0.90).

   Conclusion: These findings do not support the hypothesis of an increased risk of malignancy in patients with severe ocular inflammatory disease who are treated with systemic immunosuppressive agents compared with patients treated with systemic corticosteroids.

2. **MUST Study (The Multicenter Uveitis Steroid Treatment Trial).**

   Question: Whether systemic corticosteroids plus immunosuppression when indicated (systemic therapy) is relatively more effective than fluocinolone acetonide implant (implant therapy) for noninfectious intermediate, posterior, or pan uveitis.

   Result: This was a randomized controlled parallel superiority trial for 24 months.

   In each treatment group, mean visual acuity improved over 24 months, with neither approach superior to a degree detectable with the study's power.

   Implant-assigned eyes had a higher risk of cataract surgery, treatment for elevated intraocular pressure, and glaucoma.

   Systemic-assigned patients had more prescription-requiring infections without notable long-term consequences.

   Conclusion: The specific advantages and disadvantages identified should dictate selection between the alternative treatments in consideration of individual patients' particular circumstances. Systemic therapy with aggressive use of corticosteroid-sparing immunosuppression was well-tolerated, suggesting that this approach is reasonably safe for local and systemic inflammatory disorders.

3. **SAVE Study (Sirolimus as a Therapeutic Approach Uveitis Study).**

   Question

   To determine the efficacy and safety of repeated intravitreal and subconjunctival administrations of sirolimus in patients with noninfectious uveitis—1 year.

Result

Open-label, prospective, and randomized interventional clinical trial in which patients with noninfectious intermediate, posterior, or panuveitis were randomized 1:1 to receive sirolimus intravitreal or subconjunctival injection. Sirolimus was administered at days 0, 60, and 120. At month 6, all subjects were allowed to receive sirolimus at intervals greater than or equal to 2 months and until month 12. Changes in vitreous haze (VH), visual acuity (VA), and retinal thickness at month 12 were compared with baseline.

At the end of 1 year, no statistical differences in efficacy were found between intravitreal and subconjunctival groups. No serious adverse events were determined to be secondary to sirolimus.

Conclusion

Repeated subconjunctival/intravitreal injections of sirolimus appear to be tolerated by patients with noninfectious uveitis over 12 months. The intravitreal route, however, was better tolerated.

4. **Shield, Insure, Endure Study.**

   Question

   To determine the efficacy and safety of different doses of secukinumab, a fully human monoclonal antibody for targeted interleukin-17A blockade, in patients with noninfectious uveitis.

   Result

   Three multicenter, randomized, double-masked, placebo-controlled, dose-ranging phase III studies: SHIELD, INSURE, and ENDURE.

   A total of 118 patients with Behçet's uveitis (SHIELD study); 31 patients with active, noninfectious, non-Behçet's uveitis (INSURE study); and 125 patients with quiescent, noninfectious, non-Behçet's uveitis (ENDURE study) were enrolled.

   Main endpoint is reduction of uveitis recurrence or vitreous haze score during withdrawal of concomitant immunosuppressive medication (ISM). Other endpoints included best-corrected visual acuity, ISM use, and safety outcomes.

   Conclusion

   The primary efficacy end-points of the three studies were not met. The secondary efficacy data from these studies suggest a beneficial effect of secukinumab in reducing the use of concomitant ISM.

5. **HURON Study**

   Question

   To evaluate the safety and effectiveness of an intravitreal implant of dexamethasone for the treatment of noninfectious intermediate or posterior uveitis.

Result

In this 26-week trial, eyes with noninfectious intermediate or posterior uveitis were randomized to a single treatment with a 0.7-mg/0.35-mg DEX implant, or sham procedure.

The main outcome measure was the proportion of eyes with a vitreous haze score of 0 at week 8.

i. The proportion of eyes with a vitreous haze score of 0 at week 8 was better with the 0.7-mg DEX implant, followed by 0.35-mg DEX implant, and less with the sham; this benefit persisted through week 26.

ii. A gain of 15 or more letters from baseline best-corrected visual acuity was seen in significantly more eyes in the DEX implant groups than the sham group at all study visits.

Conclusion

In patients with noninfectious intermediate or posterior uveitis, a single dexamethasone implant significantly improved intraocular inflammation and visual acuity persisting for 6 months. Dexamethasone intravitreal implant may be used safely and effectively for treatment of intermediate and posterior uveitis.

6. **MACRT Study (Monoclonal Antibody CMV Retinitis Trial).**

Question

Whether intravenous human monoclonal antibody to cytomegalovirus (CMV), MSL-109, is effective and safe as an adjuvant treatment for CMV retinitis.

Result

Two hundred nine patients with acquired immunodeficiency syndrome and active CMV retinitis were enrolled in a multicenter, randomized, placebo-controlled clinical trial. Patients received adjuvant treatment with MSL-109, 60 mg intravenously every 2 weeks, or placebo.

Conclusion

Intravenous MSL-109, every 2 weeks, appeared to be ineffective adjuvant therapy for CMV retinitis and the mortality rate was higher in the MSL-109-treated group.

7. **HPCRT Study (HPMPC Peripheral CMV Retinitis Trial).**

Question

Whether two doses of intravenous cidofovir (HPMPC) is effective and safe in short- and long-term treatment of small peripheral cytomegalovirus (CMV) retinitis lesions.

Result

It was a multicenter, randomized, controlled clinical trial.

Patients were randomly assigned to one of three groups: the deferral group, in which treatment was deferred until retinitis progressed; the low-dose cidofovir group (5 mg/kg once weekly for 2 weeks), then maintenance therapy once every 2 weeks; or the high-dose cidofovir group, which received cidofovir (5 mg/kg once weekly for 2 weeks), then maintenance therapy once every 2 weeks.

Progression of retinitis, the amount of retinal area involved by CMV; the loss of visual acuity were evaluated.

Conclusion

Intravenous cidofovir, high- or low-dose, effectively slowed the progression of CMV retinitis.

8. **CRRT Study (CMV Retinitis Retreatment Trial).**

Question

To assess the safety and efficacy of three therapeutic regimens (foscarnet, ganciclovir, or the combination) for recurrent or persistent AIDS-related cytomegalovirus (CMV) retinitis.

Result

Patients were randomized to receive foscarnet, ganciclovir, or a combination of the two drugs.

Initially, patients undergo single or multiple cycles of induction therapy for 14 days followed by maintenance therapy. Patients in whom the retinitis continues to progress or who are intolerant of the initial treatment switch to the alternative drug for further cycles of induction and maintenance.

Patients on the combination arm in whom retinitis continues to progress were given further cycles of the combination at an increased dose, or, if one drug is causing toxicity, are given further cycles with the alternative drug. Patients were followed monthly for 6 months and then every 3 months thereafter.

Although no difference could be detected in visual acuity outcomes, visual field loss and retinal area involvement on fundus photographs both paralleled the progression results, with the most favorable results in the combination therapy group.

Conclusion

For patients with AIDS and CMV retinitis whose retinitis has relapsed and who can tolerate both drugs, combination therapy appears to be the most effective therapy for controlling CMV retinitis.

9. **FGCRT Study (Foscarnet-Ganciclovir CMV Retinitis Trial).**

    Question

    To evaluate the relative safety and efficacy of ganciclovir and foscarnet as initial treatment of patients with cytomegalovirus (CMV) retinitis.

    Result

    The FGCRT was a multicenter, randomized, controlled clinical trial comparing foscarnet and ganciclovir as initial therapy for CMV retinitis.

    Patients with previously untreated CMV retinitis were randomized to therapy with either intravenous ganciclovir or intravenous foscarnet. The outcome measures of this trial were survival, retinitis progression.

    i. Excess mortality in the ganciclovir group (as compared with the foscarnet group) led the Policy and Data Monitoring Board to recommend suspension of the treatment protocol 19 months after the trial started.
    ii. There was no difference between the two treatment groups in the rate of progression of retinitis.

    Conclusion

    These results suggest that for patients with AIDS, and cytomegalovirus retinitis, treatment with foscarnet offers a survival advantage over treatment with ganciclovir.

10. **COMA Study (The Collaborative Ocular Melanoma Study).**

    Question

    To compare the effectiveness of brachytherapy to enucleation for treatment of medium-size choroidal melanomas.

    Result

    The Collaborative Ocular Melanoma Study (COMS) is a three-arm study that includes two multicenter randomized clinical trials designed to compare the effectiveness of brachytherapy to enucleation for treatment of medium-size choroidal melanomas, and the effectiveness of enucleation with and without preoperative external-beam radiotherapy for large choroidal melanomas. The third arm is an observational study of small choroidal melanomas.

    Conclusion

    Similar rates of mortality after treatment with enucleation and brachytherapy shift the emphasis of selection of therapy to secondary outcomes such as preservation of vision.

11. FAUS Study (Fluocinocone Acetonide Uveitis Study).

Question

The purpose of this study was to evaluate the safety and efficacy of a 0.59- and 2.1-mg FA intravitreal implant in patients with noninfectious posterior uveitis.

Result

A prospective, multicenter, randomized, double-masked, dose-controlled study was performed. Patients were randomized to the 0.59- or 2.1-mg FA intravitreal implant and were evaluated at visits through 3 years. Outcomes included uveitis recurrence rate, best-corrected visual acuity (BCVA), use of adjunctive therapy, and safety.

Conclusion

The FA intravitreal implant significantly reduced uveitis recurrence rates and led to improvements in visual acuity and reductions in adjunctive therapy. Lens clarity and intraocular pressure require monitoring.

PEDIATRIC OPHTHALMOLOGY

1. **Amblyopia Treatment Study (ATS)**

   Questions asked

   i. What is more effective patching or atropine as treatment for moderate amblyopia in children less than 7 years of age?

   ii. How many hours of patching should be given for severe amblyopia (vision—6/60 to 6/120)?

   iii. How many hours of patching should be given for moderate amblyopia(vision—6/24 or better)?

   iv. Should amblyopia be treated after 7 years of age?

   v. Can amblyopia recur once the treatment has been stopped?

   vi. Do near activities enhance the effect of patching on visual acuity improvement in amblyopia?

   vii. Is levodopa/carbidopa therapy effective in amblyopia treatment?

   Results

   The Pediatric Eye Disease Investigator Group (PEDIG) is a collaborative network dedicated to facilitating multicenter clinical research in strabismus, amblyopia, and other eye disorders that affect children. It has conducted 20 amblyopia treatment studies since 1997.

   In ATS 01 419 children <7 years with amblyopia and VA in the range of 6/12 to 6/60 were assigned to receive either patching or atropine. VA improved in both groups by 3.16 lines in patching and 2.84 lines in atropine group, which was statistically not significant

   In ATS 2A 175 children <7 years with amblyopia in the range of 6/60 to 6/120 (severe amblyopia) were recruited and were assigned to full-time patching (all hours) or 6 hours of patching per day and VA in the amblyopic eye after 4 months was noted. There was an improvement in the amblyopic eye VA from baseline to 4 months averaged 4.8 lines in the 6-hour group and 4.7 lines in the full-time group.

   In ATS 2B 189 children <7 years with amblyopia in the range of 6/12 to 6/24 (moderate amblyopia) were assigned to 2 hours or 6 hours of daily patching and VA in the amblyopic eye after 4 months was noted. The improvement in the visual acuity of the amblyopic eye from baseline to 4 months averaged 2.40 lines in each group.

   ATS 06 recruited 425 children 3–<7 years with amblyopia (6/12 to 6/120) and found that performing common near activities does not improve visual acuity outcome when treating anisometropic, strabismic, or combined amblyopia with 2 hours of daily patching

   ATS 14 enrolled amblyopic patients and added levodopa in one of two doses randomly assigned with equal probability (0.51 or 0.76 mg/kg/tid, referred to as lower dose and higher dose, respectively) and it showed promising results with improvement in visual acuity with both doses.

Conclusions

i. Atropine treatment is as effective as patching in the initial active treatment of amblyopia.

ii. There was no demonstrable advantage to a greater number of hours of prescribed patching (more than 2 hours in moderate and 6 hours in severe amblyopia) either in the magnitude of improvement or the rate of improvement.

iii. For patients aged 7–12 years, prescribing 2–6 hours per day of patching with near visual activities and atropine can improve visual acuity even if the amblyopia has been previously treated.

iv. For patients 13–17 years, prescribing patching 2–6 hours per day with near visual activities may improve visual acuity when amblyopia has not been previously treated.

v. Performing common near activities does not improve VA when treating anisometropic, strabismic, or combined amblyopia with 2 hours of daily patching.

vi. Approximately one fourth of successfully treated amblyopic children experience a recurrence within the first year off treatment. For patients treated with 6 or more hours of daily patching, risk of recurrence is greater when patching is stopped abruptly rather than when it is reduced to 2 hours per day prior to cessation.

vii. Levodopa/carbidopa therapy for residual amblyopia in older children and teenagers is well tolerated and may improve visual acuity.

2. **Infant Aphakia Treatment Study (IATS)**

Questions asked

i. To compare the visual outcomes of patients optically corrected with contact lenses vs IOLs following unilateral cataract surgery during early infancy.

ii. After what age IOL placement in pediatric patients is recommended?

Results

A multicenter randomized clinical trial of 114 infants with unilateral congenital cataract in referral centers who were between ages 1 and 6 months at surgery. Cataract surgery with or without primary IOL implantation was performed. Contact lenses were used to correct aphakia in patients who did not receive IOLs.

At 4.5 years of age, the median logMAR visual acuity was not significantly different between the treated eyes in the two treatment groups. However, since the initial cataract surgery, significantly more patients in the IOL group have had at least one additional intraocular surgery (contact lens, 21%; IOL, 72%; P < .001).

Conclusions

i. There was no significant difference between the median visual acuity of operated eyes in children who underwent primary IOL implantation and those left aphakic. However, there were significantly more adverse events and additional intraoperative procedures in the IOL group.

ii. When operating on an infant younger than 7 months of age with a unilateral cataract, leaving the eye aphakic and focusing the eye with a contact lens was recommended.

3. **Atropine for the Treatment of Myopia Study (ATOM)**

Questions asked

i. Is atropine 1% eye drops effective in controlling myopic progression? (ATOM 1)

ii. What concentrations of atropine can be used to treat myopia and which one is most efficacious with least side-effects? (ATOM 2)

Results

In ATOM 1, 400 children 6–12 years old with myopia of at least −2 diopter and astigmatism of −1.5 D or less were recruited. One eye was administered 1% atropine once at night and the other eye was untreated.

In ATOM 2, 400 children aged 6–12 years with myopia of at least −2 diopter and astigmatism of −1.5 D or less were recruited and randomly assigned in a 2:2:1 ratio to 0.5%, 0.1%, and 0.01% atropine to be administered once nightly for 2 years.

ATOM 1 showed a 77% reduction in mean progression of myopia in 2 years with atropine 1% eye drops. However, side-effects like pupil dilation, glare, loss of accommodation were noted. Also, there was a significant rebound of myopia progression upon cessation of atropine 1% eye drops.

ATOM 2 compared efficacy and visual side-effects of three lower doses of atropine: 0.5%, 0.1%, and 0.01% and found that 0.01% atropine is clinically similar to 0.1%, 0.5%, and 1.0% in efficacy, as compared to placebo and had a negligible effect on accommodation and pupil size, and no effect on near visual acuity.

Conclusions

i. Atropine eye drops reduces myopia progression and axial elongation in children in a dose-related manner, but a rebound phenomenon occurs with the higher doses of atropine

ii. Atropine eye drops are safe, with no serious adverse events, but in the higher doses, the side-effects of pupil dilatation, loss of accommodation, and near vision limits practical use

iii. Atropine 0.01% has the best therapeutic index, with clinically insignificant amounts of pupil dilatation, near vision and accommodation loss, and yet is as effective as the higher doses

iv. Atropine 0.01% appears to retard myopia progression by 50%, and retreatment after a period of treatment cessation still appears to be equally effective.

4. **The Correction of Myopia Evaluation Trial (COMET)**

Questions asked

Do progressive addition lenses (PALs) reduce the rate of myopia progression by reducing retinal blur in myopic children?

Results

After 5 years of follow–up the adjusted progression of myopia (mean ± se) was −1.97 ± 0.09 D in children wearing PALs and −2.10 ± 0.09 D in children wearing SVLs, resulting in a difference of 0.13 ± 0.10 D, which was not statistically significant.

Conclusion

The progression of myopia is similar between children wearing progressive addition lenses and single vision lenses.

STUDIES IN NEURO-OPHTHALMOLOGY

1. **Optic Neuritis Treatment Trial (ONTT)**

   Questions asked

   i. To assess the beneficial and adverse effects of corticosteroid treatment for optic neuritis.
   ii. To determine the natural history of vision in patients who suffer optic neuritis.
   iii. To investigate the relationship between optic neuritis and multiple sclerosis (MS).

   Methodology

   Patients were randomized to one of the three following treatment groups at 15 clinical centers:

   i. Oral prednisone (1mg/kg/day) for 14 days.
   ii. Intravenous methylprednisolone (250 mg every 6 hours) for 3 days followed by oral prednisone (1mg/kg/day) for 11 days.
   iii. Oral placebo for 14 days.

   Results

   i. Intravenous methylprednisolone followed by oral prednisone accelerated the recovery of vision. However, at 6 months, there was no significant difference in visual acuity, visual fields, color vision, or contrast sensitivity when compared with placebo.
   ii. Oral prednisone alone was found to increase the risk of recurrent optic neuritis.
   iii. Treatment with IV steroids followed by oral steroids reduced the rate of development of MS during the first 2 years.
   iv. By 3 years, the treatment effects subsided.

   Inference

   i. There is no role for oral prednisolone alone as a treatment modality for optic neuritis.
   ii. IV methylprednisolone followed by oral prednisone accelerates the visual recovery but the long-term visual outcome is the same as placebo.
   iii. IV steroid regimen reduced the risk of MS in the first 2 years but the efficacy is lost by the third year.
   iv. MRI should be obtained in all cases on optic neuritis to assess the risk of MS.
   v. Chest X-ray, blood tests, and lumbar puncture are not necessary to evaluate patients with typical clinical features of acute optic neuritis.

2. **Longitudinal Optic Neuritis Study (LONS)**

Questions asked

i. What is the risk of developing MS after optic neuritis?
ii. What are the factors predictive of high and low risk of developing MS?

Results

i. The probability of developing MS by 15 years was 50%.
ii. Development of MS has a strong relation to the presence of lesions on a non-contrast enhanced baseline brain MRI. Higher number of lesions do not appreciably increase the risk.
iii. After 10 years, the risk of developing MS was very low for patients without baseline lesions but remained substantial for those with lesions.
iv. The factors with lower risk for developing MS were male gender, optic disk swelling and certain atypical features of optic neuritis like
    – No light perception
    – Absence of pain
    – Opthalmoscopic findings of severe optic disk edema, peripapillary hemorrhages or retinal exudates.

Inference

i. The presence of brain MRI abnormalities at the time of an optic neuritis attack is a strong predictor of the 15-year risk of MS.
ii. In the absence of MRI lesions, male gender, optic disk swelling, and atypical clinical features of optic neuritis are associated with a low likelihood of developing MS.

3. **Idiopathic Intracranial Hypertension (IIH) Treatment Trial.**

(Multicenter, randomized, double-masked, placebo-controlled study)

Questions asked

i. To determine whether acetazolamide is beneficial in improving vision when added to a low-sodium weight reduction diet in patients with IIH and mild visual loss.
ii. Does vitamin A play a role in the development of IIH?
iii. Do optic disk hemorrhages have any correlation to visual outcome in idiopathic intracranial hypertension (IIH).

Results

i. There was significant improvement in Frisén papilledema grade associated with acetazolamide treatment in the study eye and in the fellow eye.
ii. Acetazolamide-treated participants also experienced significant improvement in quality-of-life measures, including the VFQ-25 total score.

iii. No significant treatment effects were noted with respect to headache disability or visual acuity.
iv. At study entry, of the vitamin A metabolites, only serum ATRA was significantly different in IIHTT subjects and controls. Except for alpha-carotene and CSF all-trans retinoic acid (ATRA), no other vitamin A measures were significantly altered over 6 months in either the acetazolamide or placebo group.
v. 71% of subjects that met criteria for treatment failure had nerve fiber layer hemorrhages in at least one eye. Subjects with nerve fiber layer hemorrhages had a higher cerebrospinal fluid pressure.

Inference
i. In patients with IIH and mild visual loss, the use of acetazolamide with a low-sodium weight-reduction diet resulted in modest improvement in visual field function.
ii. Acetazolamide appears to have an acceptable safety profile at dosages up to 4 g/d in the treatment of idiopathic intracranial hypertension.
iii. Vitamin A toxicity is unlikely a contributory factor in the causation of IIH.
iv. Nerve fiber layer hemorrhages are common in patients with IIH with mild visual loss and correlate with the severity of the papilledema. They occur more frequently in treatment failure subjects and therefore may be associated with poor visual outcomes.

4. **The Longitudinal Idiopathic Hypertension Trial.**
To determine whether the beneficial effects of acetazolamide (ACZ) in improving vision at 6 months continues to month 12 in participants of the Idiopathic Intracranial Hypertension Treatment Trial (IIHTT).

Results
i. In the IIHTT, subjects were randomly assigned to placebo-plus-diet or maximally tolerated dosage of acetazolamide-plus-diet. At 6 months, some subjects from the placebo group were transitioned from placebo to acetazolamide.
ii. At 12 months, papilledema grade, quality of life (QoL), and headache disability scores showed significant improvements in the group transitioned from placebo to acetazolamide.

Conclusion and Inference
Improvements in papilledema grade, headache, and QoL measures continued from month 6 to month 12 of the IIHTT in all treatment groups, most marked in the placebo group transitioned to ACZ.

5. **The International Optic Nerve Trauma Study.**

   Questions asked

   i. To compare the visual outcome of patients of traumatic optic neuropathy treated with
      – corticosteroids
      – optic canal decompression surgery
      – observed without treatment.

   Results

   Visual acuity by > or = 3 lines in 32% of the surgery group, 57% of the untreated group and 52% of the steroid group.

   Inference

   There is no clear benefit for either corticosteroid therapy or optic canal decompression surgery in traumatic optic neuropathy.

6. **Champs Study (The Controlled High Risk Avonex Multiple Sclerosis Trial).**

   Questions asked

   To determine whether interferon beta (Avonex) treatment would benefit patients who had experienced a first acute demyelinating event involving the optic nerve, brain stem/cerebellum, or spinal cord, and who displayed MRI brain signal abnormalities that have previously predicted a high likelihood of future MS-like events.

   Results

   i. The Avonex-treated group demonstrated a 44% reduction in the 3-year cumulative probability of developing clinically definite multiple sclerosis.

   ii. Among placebo-treated patients, 82% had developed a new subclinical MRI signal abnormality by the eighteenth month after study entry.

   Inference

   This study supports the efficacy of Avonex therapy in significantly reducing the 3-year likelihood of future neurologic events and worsening of the brain MRI in patients with a first acute CNS demyelinating event.

7. **A Randomized Placebo-Controlled Trial of Idebenone in Leber's Hereditary Optic Neuropathy (LHON).**

   (Multicenter double-blind, randomized, placebo-controlled trial)

Questions asked

To determine the efficacy and safety of idebenone in LHON (idebenone is a potent antioxidant and inhibitor of lipid peroxidation, interacting with the mitochondrial electron transport chain and facilitating mito-chondrial electron flux in bypassing complex I).

Results

i. The primary endpoint was the best recovery in visual acuity. The main secondary endpoint was the change in best visual acuity. Other secondary endpoints were changes in visual acuity of the best eye at baseline and changes in visual acuity for both eyes in each patient.

ii. The primary endpoint did not reach statistical significance in the intention to treat population. However, post hoc interaction analysis showed a different response to idebenone in patients with discordant visual acuities at baseline; in these patients, all secondary endpoints were significantly different between the idebenone and placebo groups.

Inference: This trial provides evidence that patients with discordant visual acuities are the most likely to benefit from idebenone treatment, which is safe and well tolerated.

CATARACT SURGERY

1. **Intracameral antibiotics and barriers during cataract surgery—evidence and barriers.**

    Questions asked
    i.   Is intracameral (IC) moxifloxacin prophylaxis effective in decreasing the rate of endophthalmitis in cataract surgery?
    ii. Does PCR increases rate of endophthalmitis in patients?
    iii. Is intracameral (IC) moxifloxacin prophylaxis effective in decreasing the rate of endophthalmitis in cataract surgery complicated by PCR?
    iv. What are the barriers and concerns in the prophylactic intracameral use of antibiotics during cataract surgery?

    Results
    Approximately half of the eyes did not receive IC moxifloxacin and half of the eyes did and approximately half of the eyes that had PCR receive IC moxifloxacin and half did not
    i.   There was a significant decline in the endophthalmitis rate with IC moxifloxacin as compared to without IC moxifloxacin prophylaxis.
    ii. PCR increased the endophthalmitis rate nearly seven fold.
    iii. IC moxifloxacin reduced the endophthalmitis rate with PCR.
    iv. Barriers and concerns are:
         - Lack of a commercially approved preparation in most countries.
         - Using pharmacies to compound antibiotics raises the theoretical risk of introducing intraocular contaminants or adjuvants that can cause toxic anterior segment syndrome (TASS).
         - Concerns that routine intraocular antibiotic prophylaxis can lead to increasing bacterial drug resistance

    Conclusions
    Routine IC moxifloxacin prophylaxis reduced the overall endophthalmitis rate. There was also a statistical benefit for eyes complicated by PCR, and IC antibiotic prophylaxis should be strongly considered for this high-risk population. Considering the association of hemorrhagic occlusive retinal vasculitis with vancomycin and the commercial unavailability of IC cefuroxime in many countries, moxifloxacin appears to be an effective option for surgeons electing IC antibiotic prophylaxis.

2. **Long-Term Posterior Capsule Opacification Reduction with Square-Edge Polymethylmethacrylate Intraocular Lens**

    Questions asked
    i.   Is there any difference in long-term PCO formation and Nd:YAG capsulotomy rate of a square-edge (SE) PMMA IOL modification in comparison with a round-edge (RE) PMMA IOL?

ii. Is there any difference in long-term PCO formation and Nd:YAG capsulotomy rate of a square-edge (SE) PMMA IOL in comparison with SE hydrophobic acrylic IOL (SE-Acrylic)?

Results

The patients were randomized into two groups—one with SE single-piece PMMA IOL in one eye and an RE single-piece PMMA IOL in the fellow eye and other group received an SE single-piece PMMA in one eye and an SE single-piece hydrophobic acrylic IOL in the fellow eye. Nine-year follow-up was achieved

i. The mean PCO score was significantly lower in the SE-PMMA IOL eyes compared with the contralateral RE-PMMA eyes at all follow-up visits.

ii. The mean PCO score was statistically lower in the SE-PMMA IOL eyes compared with the contralateral SE-Acrylic IOL eyes.

iii. Nine-year Nd:YAG capsulotomy rates were less for SE-PMMA IOLs as compared to RE-PMMA IOLs and they were also less for SE-PMMA IOL as compared to SE-Acrylic IOLs.

iv. The RE-PMMA PCO rate did not plateau and continued to increase throughout the 9-year study period.

Conclusions

This prospective, 9-year fellow eye comparison study suggests that an inexpensive PMMA IOL design modification—a squared optic edged-could significantly reduce the burden of vision-impairing secondary membrane in developing countries.

3. **Accuracy of Intraocular Lens Power Calculation Formulas for Highly Myopic Eyes.**

Questions asked

Which is the most accurate intraocular lens (IOL) power calculation formulas for eyes with an axial length (AL) greater than 26.00 mm?

Results

i. The Barrett Universal II formula had the lowest mean absolute error (MAE) and SRK/T and Haigis had similar MAE, and the statistical highest MAE were seen with the Holladay and Hoffer Q formulas.

ii. The Barrett Universal II formulas yielded the highest percentage of eyes within ±1.0 D and ±0.5 D of the target refraction in this study.

Conclusions

Barrett Universal II formula produced the lowest predictive error and the least variable predictive error compared with the SRK/T, Haigis,

Holladay, and Hoffer Q formulas. For high myopic eyes, the Barrett Universal II formula may be a more suitable choice.

4. **Combination of toric and multifocal intraocular lens implantation in bilateral cataract patients with unilateral astigmatism.**

Questions asked

What is the quality of binocular visual function in bilateral cataract patients with unilateral astigmatism after combined implantations of toric with multifocal intraocular lens (IOL) as compared to toric and monofocal IOL implantation?

Results

i. Mean near vision for patient satisfaction was statistically significantly higher in toric/multifocal IOL group patients vs than that in toric/monofocal group.
ii. The stereopsis of toric/multifocal IOL eyes decreased slightly monofocal IOL group. Visual disturbance was not noticed in either group.

Conclusion

Although the combination of toric and multifocal IOL implantation results in compromising stereoacuity, it can still provide patients with high levels of spectacle freedom and good overall binocular visual acuity.

5. **Phakoemulsification vs manual small-incision cataract surgery for white cataract.**

Questions asked

What is the safety and efficacy of phakoemulsification as compared to manual small-incision cataract surgery (SICS) to treat white cataracts?

Results

Approximately half of the patients were randomized to the phakoemulsification group and half to the manual SICS group.

i. On the first postoperative day, the manual SICS group had less corneal edema than the phakoemulsification group.
ii. The mean time was statistically significantly shorter in the manual SICS group than in the phakoemulsification group.

Conclusions

Both techniques achieved excellent visual outcomes with low complication rates. Because manual SICS is significantly faster, less expensive, and less technology dependent than phakoemulsification, it may be a more appropriate technique in eyes with mature cataract in the developing world.

6. **Double-flanged-haptic and capsular tension ring or segment for sutureless fixation in zonular instability.**

Questions asked

Is sutureless management of zonular dialysis greater than 120° using a capsular tension segment (CTS) or a modified capsular tension ring (m-CTR) possible?

Result

A successful sutureless IOL implantation with a double flanged m-CTR/CTS technique.

Conclusion

This double-flanged m-CTR/CTS technique allows suture-free option for managing zonular weakness or dialysis while performing cataract surgery.

7. **Safety, efficacy, and intraoperative characteristics of *DisCoVisc* and *Healon* ophthalmic viscosurgical devices for cataract surgery.**

Question asked

What is the safety and efficacy of *DisCoVisc* ophthalmic viscosurgical device as compared to *Healon* OVD?

Results

i. DisCoVisc OVD group and the Healon OVD group had statistically similar outcomes for IOP and for endothelial cell loss.

ii. Viscosity of Healon OVD was most often rated "cohesive" and DisCoVisc OVD most often rated "both dispersive and cohesive."

iii. Workspace most frequently rated "full chamber maintained" when using DisCoVisc OVD and most frequently rated "workspace maintained" when using Healon OVD. "Flat" or "shallow" workspace ratings occurred only in the Healon OVD group.

Conclusion

DisCoVisc OVD had both cohesive and dispersive properties, and was safe and effective for every stage of cataract surgery.

8. **Advanced Phako Systems: Developments such as high-tech fluidics improve outcomes and safety for microincision cataract surgery.**

Questions asked

What are the advances made in phako machines to facilitate smaller incisions and raise the bar for safety and efficiency?

Results

Centurion Vision System

i. The Centurion's Intrepid Balanced Tip provides a uniquely efficient tip motion. Because of that, movement at the shaft is relatively reduced so the chance for thermal effect at the incision is reduced.

ii. The fluidics capabilities of the Centurion give less concern about complications, such as intraoperative floppy iris syndrome (IFIS) and also easy to operate on small pupils. Turbulence is reduced and pupils don't come down.

iii. Two computer-controlled plates squeeze the BSS bag gently to provide a constant IOP rather than relying on gravity and a hanging bottle.

WHITESTAR Signature System

i. The system has the ability to sequentially use true peristaltic and true venturi pumps for different steps. The design allows us to utilize the holding power of the peristaltic pump during lens disassembly then switch over to venturi fluidics to draw the pieces safely to the phako tip.

ii. Uses elliptical phacoemulsification technology. The longitudinal and lateral energies blend into a smooth elliptical movement. There is less repulsion at the tip, so we can use lower fluidic parameters.

Vision Stellaris Enhancement System

i. Has high-performance vacuum-based pump technology.

ii. It has forced infusion pressure, rather than a gravity-based hanging bag, which gives very precise pressure control.

Conclusions

phako tip design is enabling surgeons to give patients all the benefits of microincision surgery. Elliptical phacoemulsification permits them to use lower pressure, which is in turn supported by advances in fluidics. Fluidics based on pumps, rather than gravity, give physicians greater control for easier removal of both soft and hard cataracts. They experience complications, such as IFIS or rupture of the posterior capsule, less often.

Management Summary of Commonly Kept Examination Cases

NONPROLIFERATIVE DIABETIC RETINOPATHY (NPDR) WITH CLINICALLY SIGNIFICANT MACULAR EDEMA (CSME)

The aim of my treatment is to improve vision by reducing macular edema and prevent further progression of retinopathy.

Management

This treatment has to be in conjunction with the physician to have good glycemic control and control of associated systemic factors such as hypertension and dyslipidemia.

Apart from above mentioned measures, I would like to do **fluorescein angiography:**

1. For identifying areas of focal and diffuse leakage
2. For identifying pathologic enlargement of foveal avascular zone (FAZ) since the management differs based on the above factors.

I would like to do optical coherence tomography (OCT)

1. To detect subtle edema
2. To look for serous macular detachment
3. For the purpose of follow up after treatment.

There are various options to treat CSME:

1. Laser photocoagulation
2. Intravitreal/sub-Tenon's steroids
   Triamcinolone acetonide: 2 mg in 0.05 mL/4 mg in 0.1 mL
3. Intravitreal anti-VEGF:

   – Bevacizumab (Avastin): 1.25 mg in 0.05 mL
   – Ranibizumab (Lucentis): 0.3 mg in 0.05 mL
   – Pegaptanib sodium: 0.3 mg in 90 µL
4. Pars plana vitrectomy (PPV)

What to look for in FFA

1. Look for type of leakage: discrete or diffuse
2. Look for macular ischemia since laser photocoagulation is harmful in ischemic maculopathy.

What to look for in OCT

1. Vitreomacular interface abnormality
2. Thickness of macula
3. Subclinical serous macular detachment
4. Foveal contour.

First-line therapy includes either laser photocoagulation (focalmodified ETDRS grid).

Or

Intravitreal pharmacotherapy +/–laser photocoagulation.

The decision is made based on FFA and OCT findings.

1. **I would like to do laser photocoagulation in cases of:**
   - Parafoveal edema
   - Discrete areas of leakage in FFA
   - Mild to moderate retinal thickening on OCT
   - No vitreomacular interface abnormalities.

2. **I would prefer intravitreal injections in cases of:**
   - Foveal edema (where foveal contour is altered)
   - Diffuse leakage on FFA
   - Moderate-to-severe retinal thickening in OCT
   - Serous macular detachment on OCT.

   Anti-VEGF agents are preferred over steroids. Patient might require three to four anti-VEGF injections, one every month, to dry out the macula.

3. **I would like to do PPV in cases of:**
   - Taut posterior hyaloid face
   - Vitreomacular traction.

Combination therapy

It is an alternative therapy where first an intravitreal injection is given to bring down the edema and then it is followed by grid laser.

Follow-up

Patients are re-evaluated three months after laser treatment. If the patient is given intravitreal anti-VEGF therapy then the patient is reviewed after 1 month.

During follow up,

If CSME is persistent or in cases of recurrent CSME

I would like to do:

1. Repeat photocoagulation
2. Give intravitreal triamcinolone acetonide or intravitreal anti-VEGF agent.

If CSME is refractory to photocoagulation and pharmacotherapies, then I would like to do pars plana vitrectomy (PPV).

1. **No vitreomacular traction**: PPV with ILM peeling is done
2. **Taut posterior hyaloid face or vitreomacular traction syndrome (VMT)**: PPV.

PROLIFERATIVE DIABETIC RETINOPATHY (PDR) MANAGEMENT

The aim of my management is essentially three fold:

1. To retard and stop the proliferation of new vessels (*Neovascularization*), so that complications such as vitreous hemorrhage and retinal detachment could be prevented.
2. I would like to use adjuvant pharmacological agents, if indicated to treat associated macular edema.
3. I would also like to work closely with the general physician to achieve good metabolic control and also to sensitize him about the necessity for regular screening for diabetic nephropathy, since both these conditions have a high frequency of occurrence in the same individuals.

After confirmation of my diagnosis, I would aim and advise for systemic control of diabetes mellitus followed by ocular management of PDR which involves:

1. Medical management: Intravitreal anti-VEGF agents, Triamcinolone acetonide, dexamethasone implants (Ozurdex).
2. Laser treatment: Scatter PRP Focal grid LASER
3. Surgical management: PPV with Endolaser PRP.

My mainstay of treatment for PDR involves the use of thermal laser photocoagulation in a panretinal pattern to induce regression of new vessel formation i.e., neovascularization of disk (NVD) or elsewhere (NVE) and to avoid its complications.

Also, I would perform PRP in (PDR) in any of the following associated findings:

1. NVD or NVE of any degree if associated with preretinal or vitreous hemorrhage.
2. Rubeosis with or without neovascular glaucoma.
3. Moderate-to-severe NVE alone, particularly in juvenile diabetic patients.
4. Widespread retinal ischemia and capillary drop-out on fluorescein angiography.
5. PDR developing in pregnancy, particularly with the institution of tight metabolic control.
6. Preproliferative retinopathy in the second eye of a juvenile diabetic patient with severe PDR in the other eye.

And I would do Focal Grid laser in case of associated diabetic macular edema/ clinically significant macular edema (CSME) in presence of the following criteria:

1. Retinal edema located at or within 500 microns of the center of the macula.
2. Hard exudates at or within 500 microns of the center of the macula, if associated with thickening of adjacent retina.

3. A zone of thickening larger than 1 disk area if located within 1 disk diameter of the center of the macula.

I would do an urgent panretinal photocoagulation (PRP) along with intravitreal anti-VEGF therapy, if the PDR is at the high-risk stage (i.e., if NVD is extensive or vitreous/ preretinal hemorrhage has occurred recently).

I would start intravitreal Anti-VEGF therapy like *ranibizumab* (**Lucentis**) **0.3-0.5 mg/0.05 mL** or *bevacizumab* (**Avastin**) **1.25 mg/0.05 mL**, or *pegaptanib* (**Macugen**) 0.3 mg/0.09 mL, or *aflibercept* (**Eylea**) **2 mg /0.05 mL** to temporarily decrease leakage and cause regression of diabetic neovascularization and also as an adjunct to vitrectomy for diabetic traction retinal detachment by reducing intraoperative bleeding and allowing for easier dissection when administered preoperatively.

Also, in the presence of associated macular edema, I would administer triamcinolone acetate **1 mg or 4 mg** intravitreal injection (IVTA) or dexamethasone intravitreal implant (Ozurdex) which contains Dexamethasone **350 µL or 700 µL** available as a biodegradable slow release implant.

I would advise surgical management with PPV in case of:

1. Development of sequelae of advanced PDR like dense, non-clearing persistent vitreous hemorrhage despite maximal PRP
2. Tractional retinal detachment (macula-threatening)
3. Combined traction-rhegmatogenous retinal detachment
4. Vitreous hemorrhage with coexisting rubeosis iridis
5. Presence of diffuse DME associated with posterior hyaloidal traction
6. Severe progressive fibrovascular proliferation
7. Anterior segment neovascularization with media opacities preventing photocoagulation
8. Dense premacular (subhyaloid) hemorrhage.

I would follow up the patients according to the type of PDR as follows:

Severity of PDR	Follow-up (months)	Panretinal photocoagulation scatter laser	Focal/ grid laser	Intravitreal anti-VEGF therapy/IVTA	Surgery (pars plana vitrectomy)
Non-high-risk PDR	4	If needed	No	No	Not always
High risk PDR	4	Highly recommended	No	Beneficial	Recommended
Diabetic macular edema	4	Recommended	If needed, Yes	If needed, Yes	If needed in chronic DME
Clinically significant macular edema	1	Recommended	If needed, Yes	If needed, Yes	If needed, in vitreomacular traction

RHEGMATOGENOUS RETINAL DETACHMENT

The main aim of my management is to achieve the anatomical restoration of the detached retina with the choroid with the ultimate aim being to restore the maximum possible visual acuity. In addition, I would also like to treat the other eye prophylactically for any predisposing lesions.

Steps

1. The definitive treatment is surgery, but before intervening we should determine visual potential and explain the prognosis very clearly to the patient. (The patient should understand that in some cases, there may not be any improvement in vision postoperatively. And in even rarer cases there is a drop in existing vision.)
2. The most important step is to do a thorough indirect ophthalmoscopic examination of the affected eye to find the extent of the RD, locate the breaks and predisposing lesions. The fellow eye should also be examined to search for such predisposing lesions.
3. The choice of procedure is based on certain factors:
    i. Location and extent of the RD and breaks
    ii. Presence or absence of PVR changes
    iii. Age of the patient
    iv. Lens status
4. The principles of surgery are:
    i. Find all breaks (see the lesion)
    ii. Create chorioretinal adhesion around each break (seal the lesion)
    iii. Bring the retina and choroid close together for a sufficient duration so that a chorioretinal adhesion is formed which will close the subretinal space permanently. This is done from outside by scleral buckling and inside by intraocular gases or silicon oil.

The procedures done are:

1. **Laser demarcation:** Indicated in small peripheral RDs with no risk of progression. Usually in young myopes with clear media.

    The aim is to create a band of effective chorioretinal adhesion which surrounds the detached area completely.
2. **Pneumatic retinopexy:** Done in RRDs in phakic eyes with superior breaks, not extending beyond 2 clock hours, and without any PVR changes.

    An expanding gas (C_3F_8 or SF_6) is injected in the retina. Cryo or laser is done to induce chorioretinal adhesion once the retina is reattached. Patient should be compliant and willing to maintain specific head position postoperatively.
3. **Scleral buckling:** Indicated in RRDs with breaks which are close together without any PVR changes.

The aim of buckling is to create an indentation of the sclera beneath the retinal break.

4. **Vitrectomy:** Indicated in eyes with extensive detachment, multiple breaks, or breaks inaccessible to buckling (like posterior breaks), media opacities, PVR changes, and vitreous traction.

   Usually combined with a cataract surgery in phakic eyes because chance of postoperative cataract development is very high.

   The aim of primary vitrectomy is to remove vitreous attachments to the retinal breaks, drain the subretinal fluid, tamponade the breaks with air, gas or silicon oil, and create chorioretinal adhesion using endolaser photocoagulation or cryopexy.

   A supplemental scleral buckle can be combined along with primary vitrectomy in very extensive RDs, where complete clearance of vitreous is not possible, or in cases with risk of PVR changes in the future.

RETINITIS PIGMENTOSA (RP)

Aim

The main aim of my management is to provide visual rehabilitation by appropriate management of comorbid ocular conditions and providing low vision devices with the ultimate aim of achieving maximum possible visual acuity.

In addition, I would like to exclude/manage systemic associations by multidisciplinary approach and also provide genetic counseling, updated information of treatment options, psychological support and counseling.

Treatment Modalities

Although RP is currently incurable, the morbidity associated can be reduced by a multidisciplinary approach. These patients require annual ophthalmic evaluation which includes visual acuity assessment, ocular examination, color vision. Periodic ERG may be considered for prognostic value.

Systemic examination is important to rule out syndromes associated with RP like Usher's syndrome, Waardenburg syndrome, Refsum's disease, Abetalipoproteinemia, Mucopolysaccharidosis, Bardet–Biedl syndrome, Alport syndrome, Alstrom syndrome, Kearn–Sayre syndrome, essential gyrate atrophy.

Counseling the patient regarding prognosis and progressive nature of the disease is important.

Medical Treatment

Considering the neurodegenerative etiopathogenesis, various antioxidant formulations may be prescribed on empirical basis like

Vitamin A – 15,000 IU/day
Beta-carotene – 25,000 IU/day
Docosahexanoic acid – 400 mg/day
Lutein/zeaxanthin – 6–20 mg/day (increases macular pigment).

These nutritional supplements may help in preventing further retinal damage and in slowing down the progression of disease.

Cataract in RP

Many RP patients develop visually significant cataract at younger age. If the patients have a recent onset gross defective vision in daylight as well and if there is a significant central cataract, I would like to perform the cataract extraction after explaining the guarded visual prognosis. The patient needs continuous monitoring for development of CME and PCO. These patients are at more risk of developing anterior capsular phimosis.

CME in RP

In cases of RP with macular edema, I would like to start topical carbonic anhydrase inhibitor such as dorzolamide (2%) e/d TDS. If the patient does not respond, I would like to proceed to oral Acetazolamide, an induction dose of 500 mg/day, followed by maintenance dose of 250 mg/day.

If the patient is not responsive to carbonic anhydrase inhibitors, I would like to give intravitreal injection of triamcinolone acetonide 2 mg in 0.05 mL/ 4 mg in 0.1 mL. Ozurdex (dexamethasone intravitreal implant) 0.7 mg can also be tried.

Low Vision Aids

I would like to provide low vision devices by:
1. Best refraction and simple magnification – magnifiers and closed circuit television for near work
2. Control of glare by using dark glasses during outdoor activities – CPF (corning photochromatic filters)
3. Use of night vision scopes and high intensity lantern for night vision
4. Use of field enhancement procedures such as
    i. Mirrors and prisms mounted on spectacles
    ii. Reverse Gallilean telescopes
    iii. Image intensifiers.

Counseling

The aim of **genetic counseling** is to educate patients about the hereditary nature of the disease. I would like to examine other family members to know the extent of manifestation, expected rate of progression, and to establish the mode of inheritance.

I would like to provide **psychological and vocational counseling** to the patient for functional and emotional wellbeing.

Recent advances in the treatment of RP includes:

Retinal transplantation: Involves transplanting fetal retinal cells along with attached RPE which provides nourishment to photoreceptor cells of the patient.

Photoreceptor transplantation: Involves using adult human cadaver allogenic photoreceptor sheets harvested with the excimer laser within 24 hours of death.

Neuroprosthetic devices: Controlled electrical stimulation of retina releases growth factors which may delay degeneration of retina from RP.

Pharmacologic agents: Neurotrophic factors like basic fibroblast growth factor, ciliary neurotrophic factor and anti-Parkinson drugs have been tried based on their antiapoptotic properties.

Retinal Prosthesis

- **ARGUS II**: Artificial silicone retina of 2 mm diameter silicone chip implanted in subretinal space which stimulates the contacting retinal cells upon exposure to light.
- **EPI–RET 3 implants:** An extraocular camera fitted to spectacle lenses transmits images wirelessly to a receiver placed in anterior vitreous. This receiver in turn stimulates an epiretinal implant via a connecting microcable.

Intravitreal or subretinal gene therapy: Adenoviral or lentiviral vector is used to replace the defect in identified forms of RP.

CENTRAL RETINAL VEIN OCCLUSION

The aim of my treatment would be:

1. To identify and treat the underlying systemic disorders to prevent recurrence.
2. To identify and differentiate ischemic and nonischemic type of central retinal vein occlusion (CRVO) to predict the progression and treatment.
3. To identify and treat the vision threatening conditions like macular edema and neovascular glaucoma promptly.

Treatment Schedule

1. First step is to do a complete ophthalmic examination including slit lamp examination for neovascularization of iris, fundus examination for the severity of hemorrhage, and to look for macular edema, gonioscopy for neovascularization of the angles and intraocular pressure for NVG. Poor presenting visual acuity and RAPD are simple tools in predicting ischemic type.
2. To diagnose and treat underlying systemic disorders like diabetes, hypertension, cardiovascular disorders, dyslipidemia. In younger age group, hypercoagulable diseases like sickle cell anemia, leukemia, polycythemia by doing a complete blood count, prothrombin time, partial thromboplastin time, ESR, antinuclear antibodies have to be ruled out. To instruct the patient to avoid smoking and use of drugs like oral contraceptive agents.
3. OCT is done to quantify and monitor macular edema.
4. FFA is not done routinely but it can be done to confirm the ischemic type with capillary non-perfusion areas. If it has to be done, it has to be performed after 6 weeks after the resolution of the blood. ERG also can help in diagnosing ischemic type in doubtful cases (b-wave amplitude reduction).
5. Macular edema if present can be treated with intravitreal anti VEGF agents like bevazizumab (Avastin) – 1.25 mg in 0.05 mL, ranibizumab (Lucentis) – 0.5 mg in 0.05 mL, aflibercept (Eyelea) – 2 mg in 0.05 mL or intravitreal steroids like triamcinolone acetonide 4 mg in 0.1 mL, or steroid implants like Ozurdex (dexamethasone 0.7 mg).
6. Neovascularization if present should be treated with prompt PRP. Intravitreal anti VEGF agents can also be tried for neovascular glaucoma along with topical and systemic antiglaucoma therapy. Medically unmanageable NVG cases are candidates for glaucoma drainage devices, trab with MMC or in poor visual prognosis eyes with cyclodestructive procedures like DLCP, cyclo-cryo.
7. Radial optic neurotomy is a surgical mode of treatment with varying results, not commonly done.

Follow-up: The patient should be reviewed every month for the first 6 months, every two months up to 1 year after diagnosis and every 4 months for 2 years.

OPTIC ATROPHY

Aim

My aim is to treat the underlying cause, preserve the existing vision, and rehabilitate the patient for daily activities.

Treatment

Optic atrophy is irreversible. Early diagnosis and appropriate treatment of the underlying cause can prevent further damage and the development of optic atrophy and vision loss.

1. **Primary Optic Atrophy**

    i. **Retrobulbar optic neuritis**

       – Injection methyl prednisolone 1 g IV × 3 days followed by tapering doses of oral prednisolone

    ii. **Compressive lesions of the optic nerve**

       Pituitary tumors
       Meningiomas } Surgical removal of the tumors
       Gliomas

    iii. **Traumatic optic atrophy**

       – Optic atrophy occurs 3–6 weeks after injury
       – Intravenous methyl prednisolone given within 8 days of injury causes improvement in vision
       – optic nerve decompression

    iv. **Toxic optic neuropathy**

       Alcohols: Methanol, ethylene glycol.

       The essential therapy of methanol poisoning is adequate alkalinization and methanol administration. Ethanol competes with methanol for the enzyme alcohol dehydrogenase in the liver, thereby preventing the accumulation of toxic metabolites in the body. Ethanol is given as 10% solution in 5% dextrose solution intravenously. A loading dose of 0.6 g/kg followed by an IV infusion of 0.007–0.16 g/kg/hr. Dialysis is recommended in those patients who have visual disturbances, blood methanol of 50 mg% or more, ingestion of more than 60 mL of methanol and severe acidosis not corrected by sodium bicarbonate administration.

       The following drugs can cause optic neuropathy. Patients need to stop the drugs and use multivitamin supplementation.

       Antibiotics: Chloramphenicol, sulfonamides, linezolid

       Antimalarials: Chloroquine, quinine

Antitubercular drugs: Isoniazid, ethambutol, streptomycin

Antiarrhythmic agents: Digitalis, amiodarone

Heavy metals: Lead, mercury

Others: Carbon monoxide, tobacco.

2. **Secondary Optic Atrophy**

   i. **Papillitis:** IV methyl prednisolone 1g od × 3 days followed by tapering doses of oral prednisolone.

   ii. **Papilledema:** Findout the cause for raised intracranial pressure by doing neuroimaging and treatment of the cause.

   In case of idiopathic intracranial hypertension-weight reduction, T. Acetozolamide 500 mg bd oral glycerol, corticosteroids

   Optic nerve decompression, repeated lumbar puncture, lumbo-peritoneal shunt.

3. **Consecutive Optic Atrophy**

   i. **Central retinal artery occlusion:** If the patient presents early as soon as loss of vision occurs and immediate treatment done to re-perfuse the retina, can prevent optic atrophy. The treatment options include:
      – Ocular massage: Digital Gonio massage
      – Anterior chamber paracentesis
      – IOP lowering drugs: Acetazolamide 500 mg, 20% IV mannitol, 50% oral glycerol
      – Carbogen inhalation
      – Retrobulbar or systemic vasodilators like papavarine or tolazoline
      – Sublingual nitroglycerine
      – Fibrinolytic agents
      – Injection urokinase into internal carotid artery by femoral artery catheterization
      – Systemic thrombolysis using plasminogen
      – Systemic pentoxifylline.

   ii. **Retinitis pigmentosa**
      – Treatment of allied conditions
      – Low vision aids
      – Genetic counseling
      – Psychological and vocational counseling.

4. **Cavernous Optic Atrophy**

   Glaucoma

   i. IOP lowering drugs
   ii. Filtering surgeries

iii. Treating the cause of secondary glaucoma

iv. Regular follow-up

v. Screening of patients with family history of glaucoma.

5. **Segmental Optic Atrophy**

   i. **Temporal pallor**

      – **Toxic amblyopia** (tobacco, ethyl alcohol)

      Stop smoking, abstinence from alcohol

      Injections of hydroxycobalamine 1000 µg intramuscularly. The dose should be repeated 5 times at interval of 4 days.

      – **Nutritional amblyopia**

      It is due to atrophy of papillomacular nerve fibres caused by deficiency of vitamin B12, B6, B1, B2, and Niacin

      Treatment-balanced diet, multivitamin supplements.

   ii. **Altitudinal pallor**

      – Acute ischemic optic neuropathy-IV methyl prednisolone 1 g × 3 days followed by tapering doses of oral prednisolone.

   iii. **Wedge-shaped pallor**

      Branch retinal artery occlusion—same as CRAO.

6. **Hereditary Optic Atrophy**

   i. Congenital optic atrophy

   ii. Lebers' optic atrophy   } Genetic counseling

   iii. Behrs' optic atrophy

Rehabilitation

Generally magnification and illumination control are used to enhance visual function.

1. **Reading**

   i. Strong reading glasses

   ii. Optical and electronic magnifiers

   iii. Software to enlarge text on computer screens.

2. **Illumination control**

   Tinted wraparound sun glasses—reduce brightness but increase contrast.

3. **Distance vision**

   Handheld or spectacle mounted telescopic devices.

Prognosis

Prognosis depends on many features. They are:

1. **Pallor and optic atrophy**

   Pallor does not signify optic atrophy unless there is demonstrable defect in visual acuity, color vision and field.

2. **Attenuation of arteries**

   It is always a sign of poor prognosis.

3. **Papilledema combined with pallor**

   Poor visual prognosis.

Recent Trial

Intravitreal stem cell transplantation

Neural progenitor cells delivered to the vitreous can integrate into the ganglion cell layer of the retina, turn on neurofilament genes and migrate into the host optic nerve.

Stem beads

Activation of endogenous stem cells that remains dormant within the optic nerve by implantation of biodegradable beads that release cell activating growth factor.

MANAGEMENT OF PAPILLEDEMA

1. **Aim of Management**

   My primary aim would be to look for treat the cause for increased intracranial pressure by either medical management or surgical management.

   Since papilledema is the result of raised intracranial pressure, which in turn could be caused by various aetiology like:

   i. Idiopathic intracranial hypertension (most common)
   ii. Mass Lesion or tumors
   iii. Drugs
   iv. Cavernous sinus thrombosis and arteriovenous malformations.

   I would do an urgent neurologic evaluation and neuroimaging (MRI or CT with contrast) to rule out:

   i. Intracranial mass lesion, hemorrhage, hydrocephalus or venous thrombosis
   ii. MR venography – if venous clot is suspected
   iii. MR angiography – if dural arteriovenous malformation is considered

   If the neuroimaging turns out to be normal I would do a lumbar puncture:
   - To rule out infections
   - Document for CSF opening pressure
   - Look for normal CSF composition.

2. **Treatment**

   I would treat the patient depending on the etiology causing the raised intracranial pressure.

3. **Mass Lesions**

   If the raised intracranial pressure is due to a mass lesion blocking either the ventricular system or venous outflow, I would refer the patient to neurosurgeon manage the condition by removal of the lesion or if the mass lesion cannot be removed a ventriculoperitoneal shunt or a lumboperitoneal shunt can be done.

4. **Idiopathic Intracranial Hypertension (IIH)**

   If the neuroimaging is normal then a diagnosis of IIH has to be made and the following treatment given.

   i. **General measures**
      - If there is presence of inciting factors like drugs, I would advise the patient to discontinue those medications.
      - If the patient is obese, reduction in weight of the patient, as well control of cholesterol as a general measure yields a good progress in the treatment of IIH.

ii. **Medical treatment for IIH**

I would start the patient on Carbonic anhydrase inhibitors like aceta-zolamide 250 mg bd and slowly increase it to 1 g so as to bring down the raised intracranial pressure.

iii. **Surgical treatment**

– **Indications**
  - Progressive loss of vision despite maximal medical therapy.
  - Severe or rapid vision loss at onset including the development of an afferent pupillary defect or signs of advanced optic nerve dysfunction.
  - Severe papilledema causing macular edema or exudates.

– **Surgical options**
  - Optic nerve sheath decompression
  - Shunt procedures

iv. **Other causes**

If any thrombus, hematoma (which could be secondary to trauma), arteriovenous malformations are found out as a causative factor, I would promptly refer the patient to a neurosurgeon as it is a medical emergency.

Conditions like Sarcoid (which can give rise to a granuloma which can in turn obstruct the CSF outflow), tuberculosis and syphilis needs to be addressed with a combined approach of the ophthalmolgist rheumatologist (for sarcoid), and neurologist.

THIRD NERVE PALSY

Aims of Treatment

1. Identifying the cause and treating them:
   i. **Pupil involving 3rd nerve palsy is** a surgical emergency.

      Most common cause of pupil involving 3rd nerve palsy is intracranial aneurysm and it requires immediate referral to neurosurgery for the relevant surgical rehabilitation such as clipping, gluing, coiling or wrapping of the aneurysm.
   ii. In case of **Pupil sparing 3rd nerve palsy** ischemia is the most common cause. The cause for the ischemia is usually a vascular disorder such as diabetes and hence it should be looked for and controlled. With good metabolic control, the palsy will resolve spontaneously in 6 to 8 weeks.
2. To relieve patient's discomfort and treat symptomatically conservative treatment:

Treatment during symptomatic interval is directed at alleviating symptoms, mainly pain and diplopia.

Nonsteroidal anti-inflammatory drugs are the first line of treatment of choice for the pain. Diplopia is not a problem when ptosis occludes the involved eye.

When diplopia is from large angle divergence of the visual axes, patching one eye is the only practical short-term solution.

When the angle of deviation is smaller, fusion in primary position often can be achieved by using horizontal or vertical prism or both.

Since the condition is expected to resolve spontaneously within a few weeks, most physicians would prescribe the Fresnel prism.

Surgical Treatment

It is ideal to wait for at least 6–8 months before contemplating any surgery.

Patients who do not recover from 3rd cranial nerve palsy after 6–8 months may become candidates for surgical treatment.

Goals of Surgery

1. To improve alignment in primary gaze
2. To produce or enlarge some degree of binocular single vision.

Surgical Procedures

1. Eye muscle (MEDIAL RECTUS) resection or (LATERAL RECTUS) recession to treat persistent and stable angle diplopia.

2. Some of these patients also may require some form of lid lift surgery like frontalis sling for persistent ptosis that restricts vision or is cosmetically unacceptable to the patient.
3. Botulinum toxin injection to lateral rectus muscle can relieve the eye for better fusion in some patients with mild involvement.

TREATMENT OF SIXTH NERVE PALSY

The aim of my treatment is to identify and treat the primary cause for this problem. Till that time, to provide symptomatic relief for the patient and to avoid accidental injuries, I would give monocular occlusion of the affected eye or use prisms.

Treatment Options

1. **Isolated 6th nerve palsy >50 years of age:** In such instances the most common cause is vascular ischemia. I would like to work closely with the patient's physician to control their systemic condition like diabetes and hypertension. I will explain to the patient that there is a high chance for spontaneous recovery within 3–4 months and also explain to them in advance, that in case that the recovery does not happen, then we would have to proceed with further investigations like neuroimaging.

2. **Isolated 6th nerve palsy <50 years of age (young patients):** Since the patient is young, I would like to look for varied causes. I would like to do neuroimaging apart from the blood investigations such as TC, DC, ESR, FBS, PPBS. I will also rule out systemic hypertension. If all these parameters are normal, then I will reassure the patient, that this condition will be self-limiting in around 3 months and would review the patient periodically.

3. If the 6th nerve palsy is associated with other neurologic involvement or other cranial nerve involvement, then a routine neuroimaging of the brain (MRI) is performed.

4. Surgical: In case, the strabismus does not improve, then surgery can be considered, after waiting for at least 8 to 10 months. The surgeries performed will be ipsilateral weakening of medial rectus and strengthening of the ipsilateral lateral rectus.

5. Botulinum toxin injection can be considered as a chemodenervation of the antagonist medial rectus to provide transient symptomatic relief. However, it may mask the progression of the lesion and the involvement of the other extraocular muscles.

MYASTHENIA GRAVIS

Aim of My Treatment

The aim of my treatment is to provide symptomatic relief to the patient from ptosis and diplopia and achieve remission of the disease by treating the underlying aetiology, which is autoimmunity.

Treatment Protocol

Management can be divided into:

1. Symptomatic therapy
2. Disease modifying agents.

First, for symptomatic therapy I will start the patient on acetylcholinesterase inhibitors, pyridostigmine bromide or neostigmine bromide, thereby increasing the availability of acetylcholine at the neuromuscular junction. Pyridostigmine being the preferred agent due to its longer duration of action is started at a low dose: **30 mg TDS** (onset of action occurs within 30 minutes and peaks at 1–2 hours).

He is then observed for the improvement of ptosis and relief from diplopia.

If improvement is seen he can be maintained in with the same dose. If there is no symptomatic relief, the dose can be increased until desired result is achieved.

If the patient is not showing any improvement even with increased dose of pyridostigmine, the next line of management ie, corticosteroids are added at the lowest possible dose (T prednisolone 10 mg/day).

This is slowly increased by 10 mg every 4 days to a dose of 1 mg/kg/day (60 mg/day) as a morning dose.

Once remission is achieved the dose can be tapered slowly. If during tapering, exacerbation is seen, the patient is started with the previous high dose.

In situations where steroids are avoided / side effects not tolerated by the patient, Immunosuppressive can be given. Most common, T. Azathioprine, is initiated as a dose of 50 mg/day and increased by 50 mg every week to 150–200 mg/day.

THYROID-RELATED ORBITOPATHY

The aim of my treatment is to halt disease progression and to reduce disease activity:

The decision on whether thyroid-related ophthalmopathy must be treated and requires what type of treatment relies on activity and severity of the disease. Active disease is defined as progression of any of the VISA parameters or CAS of 4 or more (max score = 8). The level of activity can be further divided into mild (CAS 4 or less without deterioration), moderate to severe (CAS 5 or more, or progressive disease), or vision threatening. From the endocrine perspective, the goal of treatment for patients with Graves' disease is the achievement of a euthyroid state. Patients should be counseled regarding the risks of smoking and the benefits of smoking cessation.

The order of treatment follows the sequence in the **V-I-S-A** grading system.

1. **V**ision threatening TRO – Due to dysthyroid optic neuropathy or corneal ulceration is treated first.
2. **I**nflammation is the next priority treated with conservative measures, corticosteroids, steroid-sparing immunosuppressives and/or radiotherapy.
3. **S**trabismus is managed medically (e.g., Fresnel prisms) until the inflammation subsides. Later strabismus surgery can be planned if required.
4. **A**ppearance-proptosis, eyelid retraction, dermatochalasis, and fat prolapse can be managed surgically.

Mild TRO (CAS<3)

The main of my treatment would be to alleviate the patient of his dry eye symptoms and to closely observe him for worsening of the disease. I would prescribe ocular lubricants and advise him to wear glasses for wind avoidance and to elevate the head end of the bed to reduce the periorbital swelling.

Moderate/Severe (CAS>4)

The aim of my treatment is to halt disease progression and to reduce disease activity.
My first choice would be:
IV dosage: 500 mg of IV methylprednisolone given weekly for 6 weeks followed by 250 mg of IV methylprednisolone weekly for 6 more weeks

Caution: Hepatic Dysfunction

Alternatively oral corticosteroids T. Predisolone at a dose of 1–1.5 mg/kg and tapered slowly depending on the response. Usually, the dose is tapered at 10 mg/week until 20 mg/day is reached, then reduced by 5 mg/week.

Caution: Blood Sugar Levels, Osteoporosis

Pulse-Steroid Therapy In Dysthyroid Optic Neuropathy

Adults: IV Methylpredisolone

1 g od 3 days (or)

500 mg bd 3 days.

Followed by rapid tapering of oral steroids.

Rituximab is a new promising drug with comparable results in active thyroid ophthalmopathy.

Cyclosporine is rarely useful individually but can be used along with steroids.

Radiotheraphy

Beneficial only for moderate or worse active disease or with confirmed disease progression. The standard dosing regimen is 20 Gy/orbit in 10 fractions administered over 2 weeks. A temporary worsening of inflammation often occurs after Orbital Radiation (OR) and can be prevented with concurrent glucocorticoid use. OR is relatively contraindicated in diabetic patients and those with concurrent vascular disease due to the risk of worsening retinal microvascular function, and should be used with caution in patients under 35 years of age due to the theoretic risk of secondary malignancy.

Surgery for Throid Related Orbitopathy

In active disease

Urgent indication: Prompt orbital decompression in dysthyroid optic neuropathy is usually done if response to intravenous steroids is poor. Post decompression patient may require steroid therapy. Medial wall decompression is more preferred but balanced medial plus lateral wall decompression can be done.

In inactive disease

1. Inactive disease: Defined as no activity or progression over 6–12 months.
2. The sequence of surgery for inactive TRO, if necessary, is typically decompression, followed by strabismus surgery, and finally eyelid repair.
3. Medial wall removal (especially posteriorly) is most effective in relieving orbital apex crowding.
4. Strabismus surgery is aimed at correcting diplopia in the primary position and downgaze by recessing the restricted muscles, frequently with adjustable sutures to improve postoperative alignment.
5. Eyelid surgery may involve recession of the upper eyelid retractors, recession of the lower eyelid retractors with or without a spacer graft, and conservative blepharoplasty.

ENTROPION

The **aim** of the treatment is to relieve the symptoms, preserve the cornea, and maintain lid integrity.

The patients are started on medical management first with lubricants, ideally without preservatives. Bandage contact lenses may be used as a temporary measure especially to protect the cornea. Botulinum toxin may be used in spastic entropion.

Surgical Treatment

Congenital Entropion (Epiblepharon, Tarsal Kink Syndrome)

The principle is to hold the two lamella together by full thickness eyelid eversion sutures

Upper Eyelid Entropion (Kemp And Collin Classification)

Degree of entropion	Procedure
Minimal	anterior lamellar +/–lid split at grey line
Moderate	anterior lamellar reposition + lid split + tarsal wedge resection or lamellar division
Severe	lamellar advance or rotation of terminal tarsoconjunctiva and posterior lamellar graft

Aquired Entropion

The principles are to:
1. Create a scar tissue between preseptal and pretarsal muscles
2. Tightening or shortening the lower lid retractors
3. Shortening lid tendons. All the described surgeries use either one or more principles.

    i. Involutional entropion

       No horizontal laxity: Wies type procedure (transverse lid split and everting suture)

       With horizontal laxity: Quickert procedure (Wies procedure + horizontal lid shortening)

       Jones procedures: Lower lid retractor reinsertion

    ii. Cicatricial entropion

       Needs to be treated without delay to prevent corneal complications

       Mild to moderate-tarsal wedge resection / tarsal fracture procedures

       Severe-scar tissue excision + posterior lamellar graft

    iii. Spastic entropion

       Immediate treatment: Quickert–Rathbun sutures

       Botulinum toxin injection relieves the spasm of orbicularis oculi but action is delayed.

ECTROPION

The aim of the treatment is to relieve the symptoms, preserve the cornea, and maintain lid integrity.

Congenital Ectropion

Mild cases—topical lubricants

Severe cases—skin grafting to avoid permanent corneal scarring

Aquired Ectropion

Medical Treatment

Lubricant drops and ointment.

Taping, goggles, bandage contact lens to protect ocular surface.

Surgical Treatment

1. Involutional ectropion
     i. Treatment depends on
    ii. degree and location
   iii. degree of horizontal laxity
    iv. laxity of medial and lateral tendon
     v. tone of orbicularis oculi

   – Generalized lid laxity with normal skin-full thickness resection
     With excess skin: Kuhnt symanowksi procedure (horizontal shortening and blepharoplasty)
   – Lateral laxity: Lateral canthal suture lateral tarsal strip
   – Medial laxity: Medial canthal suture medial canthal resection.

2. Paralytic ectropion

   Depends on location

   Generalized–full thickness resection or lateral canthoplasty

   Lateral – lateral canthal elevation for mild and lateral tarsorrhaphy for severe types

   Medial – Lee medial canthoplasty for mild and medial tarsorrhaphy for severe types

3. Cicatricial ectropion

   Mild cases – simple lid tightening procedure like Z-plasty

   Severe cases – scar excision and lengthening of anterior lamella by skin grafting / flaps

4. Mechanical ectropion

   Elimination of specific cause like excision of lid mass/ treating lid edema.

LAGOPHTHALMOS

The aims of the treatment are:

1. To prevent exposure keratopathy
2. To protect the ocular surface
3. To re-establish eyelid function
4. To ensure cosmetically acceptable appearance.

Treatment

If the lagophthalmos is mild with good Bells phenomena and if the patient is asymptomatic, then I would like to offer reassurance and monitor the patient with frequent observational schedules.

The treatment of the symptomatic patient can be medical or surgical, depending on the severity and the longevity of the lesion.

I would like to start the patient on preservative free artificial tear supplements, 4 times a day. Ointments can be applied to the cornea at bed time. Protective goggles have to be worn throughout the day. At night time, it is better to tape the lids or patch the eye closed, to prevent accidental rubbing the cornea during sleep.

If the patient does not improve with time, then the following surgeries can be considered. A temporary lateral tarsorrhaphy can be done to narrow the interpalpebral fissure and to protect the cornea. Gold weights have been suggested to be implanted in the upper lid for paralytic lagophthalmos. Recession of the upper eyelid retractors (levator and Mullers' muscle) can be done in lagophthamos caused by TRO due to upper lid retraction.

If there is a *cicatricial/post surgical lid shortening*, then a combination of full-thickness skin grafts, advancement flaps, tarsal-sharing procedures, and release of scar bands can be performed.

In cases of facial nerve palsy and floppy eyelid syndrome, presence of lagophthalmos due to laxity can be corrected by lateral tarsal strip which will improve apposition of the lower lid to the globe and decrease tearing.

If the patients continue to have exposure of the cornea then the lower eyelid retractor muscles recession and an additional spacing graft may be sutured in the lid to achieve further elevation. Autologous ear cartilage, nasal cartilage, or hard palate grafts are often used.

In cases of severe lagophthalmos, facial reanimation procedures include temporalis muscle transposition/transfer, nerve grafts and anastomoses, palpebral springs, soft tissue repositioning, and suborbicularis oculi fat lifts can be done.

PTOSIS

Aim

The primary aim of treatment is to improve superior visual field and prevent amblyopia while obtaining a cosmetically appealing and symmetrical eyelid height and contour.

Functional Point of View

The goals of surgery are to elevate the eyelid margin above the pupillary axis for improvement in superior visual field and prevent amblyopia. There should also be adequate mobility of the lid when blinking, a normal lid fold and no diplopia.

Cosmetic Point of View

The goals of surgery are to achieve a smooth curvature of the eyelid margin (normal contour), symmetry in eyelid margin height, and symmetry in the soft tissues of the eyelid and eyebrow, particularly the amount of tarsal platform show (TPS).

Management of Ptosis

Non-Surgical Treatment

1. Lid crutches may be used to support a drooping lid mechanically. The type used is a wire support in the form of a semi lunar soldered to the upper part of the rims of a pair of spectacles.
2. Haptic contact lens with a shelf on which the margin of upper lid rests may be used.
3. Elevation of the lid by a mechanical force: a strip of highly magnetic metal is implanted in the upper lid and a magnet is placed behind the upper rim of the frame.

When to Correct Ptosis Surgically

1. Correction of mild to moderate ptosis in a child can often be delayed until the patient is several years old, although consistent chin up positioning / complete ptosis may justify early surgery.
2. In general, congenital ptosis should be repaired when accurate measurements are obtainable and before the child begins school. Most children can undergo repair around 4–5 years of age.
3. Severe ptosis, which may cause amblyopia, must be surgically repaired as soon as possible to preserve normal vision.

4. An acquired ptosis from a traumatic injury or a third nerve palsy should not be operated on before 6 months of age, because often some levator function will return.

5. Any other acquired ptosis may be repaired when the cause has been determined. Specially myasthenia gravis must be ruled out.

Indications for Surgery in Congenital Ptosis

In most instances the primary reason for correcting congenital ptosis is cosmetic. In case of unilateral congenital ptosis of such severity that normal visual development is compromised by total occlusion of visual axis, surgical intervention may be indicated shortly after birth.

In cases of severe bilateral ptosis that interferes with the child's learning walk, surgery may be indicated early. The levator action in these children is always so poor that a frontalis sling procedure is necessary. In general, ptosis causing significant stimulus deprivation or head posturing must be surgically treated without fail. Milder degrees of ptosis need to be corrected only if the patient desires good cosmesis.

Contraindications for Surgery

1. Poor orbicularis muscle function may produce lagophthalmos and corneal exposure.

2. Loss of blink reflex or corneal sensitivity, paralysis of orbicularis or significant keratitis sicca are definite contraindications for ptosis surgery.

3. Total ophthalmoplegia may also result in postoperative corneal exposure as the cornea is exposed during sleep.

Choice of Surgery for Ptosis

In general there are three major groups of ptosis surgery:

1. External levator resection (including aponeurotic repair) for >4 mm for levator function.

2. Posterior tarso muller muscle resection (not generally used in congenital ptosis unless due to congenital horners).

3. Frontalis suspension: For unilateral ptosis with poor levator function, unilateral frontalis sling is a good option.

4. Beard's technique (Chicken Beard technique): In this procedure, a bilateral frontalis sling procedure is performed but the unaffected levator is not disinserted. This technique has the advantage of maintaining better symmetry in downgaze than a unilateral sling.

Principles of Surgical Correction

1. One inherent drawback to all ptosis procedures is that perfect cosmetic and functional results cannot be expected in every case.

2. In general, final result depends on the nature of ptosis, the type of operation selected and the skill with which operation is performed.
3. Levator resection is performed on all levator maldevelopment (congenital dysmyogenic) ptosis cases with levator action of 4 or more whereas frontalis sling is performed when the levator action is 3 mm or less.

Surgical Approach Depends on

1. Ptosis is unilateral or bilateral
2. Severity of ptosis
3. Levator action
4. Presence of abnormal ocular movements, jaw-winking phenomena or blepharophimosis syndrome.

Fasanella Servat Operation

1. Mild ptosis (<2 mm or less)
2. Levator action >10 mm
3. Well defined lid fold – no excess skin.

Levator Resection

1. Mild/moderate/severe ptosis
2. Levator action ≥4 mm.

Brow Suspension Ptosis Repair

1. Severe ptosis
2. Levator action <4 mm
3. Jaw-winking ptosis or blepharophimosis syndrome.

Bilateral Ptosis

In cases of bilateral ptosis, simultaneous bilateral surgery is preferred to ensure a similar surgical intervention in the two eyes. However in cases where gross asymmetry exists between the two eyes, the eye with a greater ptosis is operated first and the other eye is operated after 6–8 weeks when the final correction of the operated.

Modified Fasanella Servat Surgery

It is done for:
1. Mild ptosis (<2 mm or less)
2. Levator action >10 mm.

It is the excision of tarsoconjunctiva, Muller's muscle and levator. Xylocaine with adrenaline is used for local anaesthesia in adults but general anaesthesia is necessary for children.

Surgical Steps

1. Three sutures are passed close to the folded superior margin of the tarsal plate at the junction of middle, lateral and medial one-third of the lid.
2. Three corresponding sutures are placed close to the everted lid margin starting from conjunctival aspect near the superior fornix in positions corresponding to the first three sutures.
3. Proposed incision is marked on the tarsal plate such that a uniform piece of tarsus, decreasing gradually towards the periphery is excised.
4. A groove is made on the marked line of incision and the incision is completed with a scissor. The first set of sutures help in lifting the tarsal plate for excision.
5. The tarsal plate not more than 3 mm in width is excised.

Levator Resection

This is the most commonly practiced surgery for ptosis correction. This technique involves shortening of the levator-aponeurosis complex through a lid crease incision. It may be performed through skin or conjunctival route.

Surgical Steps

1. The proposed lid crease is marked to match the normal eye considering the margin crease.
2. Incision through the skin and orbicularis is made along the crease marking.
3. The inferior skin and orbicularis are dissected away from the tarsal plate.
4. The upper edge is separated from the orbital septum.
5. The fibres of the aponeurosis are cut from their insertion in the inferior half of the anterior surface of the tarsus.
6. The levator is freed from the adjoining structures.
7. The lateral and the medial horn are cut whenever a large resection is planned.
8. Care should be taken that Whitnall's ligament is not damaged.
9. A double armed 5-0 vicryl is passed through the center of the tarsal plate by a partial thickness bite.
10. It is then passed through the levator aponeurosis at height judged by the preoperative evaluation. Intraoperative assessment is made.
11. Two more double armed vicryl 5-0 sutures are passed through the tarsus about 2 mm from the upper border in the center and at the junction of central third with the medial and lateral thirds.
12. These sutures are then placed in the levator and intraoperative assessment made.
13. Excess levator is excised.
14. Four to five lid fold forming sutures are placed.

Brow Suspension Repair

This surgery is the procedure of choice in simple congenital ptosis with a poor levator action. A number of materials like non-absorbable sutures, extended polytetrafluoroethylene (ePTFE), muscle strips, banked, or fresh fascia lata strips have been used for suspension.

Temporalis Sling Repair

1. Thread sling is carried out in very young children with severe ptosis where prevention of amblyopia and uncovering the pupil is the main aim.
2. The suture sling procedures have a relatively higher recurrence rate of or may show formation of suture granuloma.
3. Definitive surgery may be performed at a later date when a fascia lata sling is carried out.

Fascia Lata Sling

1. This procedure is designed to augment the patient's lid elevation through brow elevation.
2. It is considered in children above four years of age having severe congenital simple ptosis with poor levator action.
3. Even in cases of unilateral severe ptosis a bilateral procedure is preferred because a unilateral surgery causes marked asymmetry in downgaze.
4. Results of bilateral surgery are more acceptable.
5. This procedure produces lagophthalmos in most cases.

BLEPHAROPHIMOSIS PTOSIS EPICANTHUS SYNDROME (BPES)

Aims

The aim of treatment is to:

1. Correction of ptosis to improve superior visual field and prevent amblyopia while obtaining a cosmetically appealing and symmetrical eyelid height and contour.
2. Correct telecanthus to reduce the intercanthal distance thus reducing the pseudo squinting.
3. Correct epicanthus to achieve good cosmesis and reduce pseudo-esotropia.

Indications for Surgery in BPES

1. Cosmetic
2. Ptosis causing significant stimulus deprivation or head posturing
3. Severe ptosis, which may cause deprivational amblyopia.

Management

1. Management of BPES is primarily surgical if indicated.
2. Care should be given to treat associated amblyopia.
3. The usual sequence of surgical treatment is correction of the epicanthic folds at about the age of 3 to 4 years and correction of the ptosis about 9–12 months later.
4. However, when ptosis is severe, surgical repair is recommended before the age of 3 years.
5. Frontalis sling is the procedure of choice for ptosis correction as BPES is usually associated with poor levator function.
6. Correction of lateral ectropion of the lower lids, if necessary, with a full thickness skin graft in the teenage years.
7. Early surgery may be necessary for amblyopia.
8. The treatment of blepharophimosis syndrome requires coordination among oculoplastic surgeons, paediatric ophthalmologists, paediatric endocrinologists, gynaecologists and genetic counselors.
9. Systemic treatment of associated primary ovarian failure and hormone replacement therapy.
10. Optometric management:
    Detailed evaluation of ptosis, amblyopia and correction of associated refractive errors are essential.
11. Genetic counseling is an essential component in the management of BPES.

Surgical Management

Epicanthus Fold and Telecanthus

Medial canthoplasty by double Z or Y-Z plasties, transnasal wiring of the medial canthal tendons.

Ptosis

Generally, it is corrected with brow suspension procedure—frontalis sling.

MEDIAL CANTHOPLASTY

Double Z-Plasty (Mustarde)

Principle

A double Z and a Y-V plasty are combined. The double Z lengthens and changes the position of the epicanthic fold and the Y-V plasty, by shortening of the medial canthal tendon, corrects the telecanthus.

Indication

A marked epicanthic fold associated with telecanthus, especially if there is entropion caused by traction from the fold.

Method

1. Make a mark on the skin at the site of the present medial canthus and at the site of the proposed medial canthus.
2. Join these lines and from center draw two lines extending laterally at an angle of approximately 60 degrees. These form the main limbs of Z-plasty.
3. From the end of each limb draw a nearly horizontal line which angles slightly towards the proposed new medial canthus at approximately 45 degrees to the main limb of the Z.
4. Draw a line laterally from the present medial canthus close to the upper and lower lid margin. This completes the skin marks in the figure of a "flying man."
5. Cut through the skin along these marks.
6. Excise the underlying subcutaneous tissue until the medial canthal tendon is exposed. In the blepharophimosis syndrome the tendon is usually elongated, thin and buried under abnormal tissue.
7. Shorten the medial canthal tendon if required.
8. Suture the subcutaneous tissues in the region of old medial canthus to the subcutaneous and deep tissues in the region of the new medial canthus.
9. Transpose the skin flaps.
10. Suture the skin flaps with 6 '0' nylon.

MEDIAL CANTHAL TENDON SHORTENING WITH TRANSNASAL WIRE

Principle

The intercanthal distance is reduced by removing bone and wiring the two medial canthal tendons together across the nose.

Indications

Severe telecanthus and hypertelorism associated with BPES when bone must be removed bilaterally to reduce the intercanthal distance.

Methods

1. Expose and resect the medial canthal tendons.
2. Reduce the bone of the anterior lamellar crest and reflect the lacrimal sac laterally.
3. Pass a Mustarde awl (name of the instrument used in transnasal wiring) across the nose with a wire and a 4 '0' nylon suture.
4. Leave a loop of wire across the nose and one 4 '0' nylon suture.
5. Withdraw the awl with another 4 '0' nylon suture and the end of the wire leaving a loop behind.
6. Suture the resected medial canthal tendons to the transnasal wire loop.
7. Twist the wire to tighten it and correct the telecanthus.
8. Pass the 4 '0' nylon sutures through the medial canthoplasty flaps. Tie them together over bolsters to keep pressure on the wound.
9. Remove the sutures after 5 days.

BROW SUSPENSION/FRONTALIS SLING

Principle

1. The frontalis normally lifts the eyebrow and contributes to eyelid elevation.
2. This action of lifting the lid is enhanced by connecting the frontalis muscle and eyebrow to the lid with a subcutaneous "sling."
3. For definitive cosmetic procedure it is preferable to do a bilateral suspension.

Indications

1. Ptosis with less than 4 mm of levator function.
2. Prevention of amblyopia in an infant with severe ptosis in whom an assessment of levator function is not possible.
3. Following a levator excision.

Methods

1. Make a medial, central and lateral horizontal skin mark on the eyelid about 2–3 mm from the lash line. The skin crease will form here. Make two marks just above the eyebrow, one vertically above and a little lateral to the lateral eyelid mark, and the other vertically above and a little medial to the medial eye mark. Make a forehead mark above and between these two brow marks to complete an isosceles triangle. Preferably mark and operate on both the lids at the same time to ensure symmetry.
2. Make stab incisions through all the marks, widening the three forehead incisions a little.
3. Use a Wright's fascial needle to pass each strip of fascia.
4. Pull up the two triangles of fascia to give a symmetrical lid curve. If there is a normal Bell's phenomenon, raise the lid level as high as possible but stop if it reaches the limbus or if the lid starts to leave the globe. Tie the fascia and reinforce the knot with a 6 '0' absorbable suture.
5. Pull one fascial strip each eyebrow incision through the forehead incision. Tie the strips together and reinforce the knot with a 6 '0' absorbable suture.
6. Close the forehead and eyebrow incisions with 6 '0' nylon sutures. Leave the eyelid incisions open.
7. If required tape a lower lid traction suture top the brow. Remove it at the first dressing 12–48 hours postoperatively. Remove the skin sutures at 5 days.
8. Use lubricant and antibiotic drops and ointment.

TRAUMATIC CATARACT

Aim of Management

The management of traumatic cataract is essentially surgical, however I would like to first control intraocular inflammation, maintain integrity of eyeball and then try to restore maximum useful vision and to prevent infection.

I would like to classify into preoperative, intraoperative and postoperative management.

I would like to first evaluate the patient for the type of ocular injury, look carefully for zonular dehiscence in a dilated pupil, subluxation of lens in supine position, associated complications of trauma, intraocular inflammation, and intraocular pressure and also evaluate the other eye for sympathetic ophthalmia in penetrating trauma. Also I would like to explain the guarded visual prognosis associated with traumatic cataract.

Intraoperative Management

Blunt Injury with Traumatic Cataract

1. **Traumatic cataract without associated complications**

   Choice of surgery: Phacoemulsification or manual SICS

   IOL: three piece acrylic, **in the bag** implantation.

2. **Traumatic cataract with zonular dehiscence**
   i. **Choice of surgery**: Phako or manual SICS
   ii. **Grading of zonular dialysis**
      – **<3 clock hours of ZD:** In the bag implantation of IOL, with haptics stabilizing the weak zones.
      – **3-5 clock hours:** Cataract extraction with CTR, IOL implantation in the bag
      – **5-7 clock hours:** Cataract extraction with CTR/ Cionni ring, IOL implantation in the bag
      – **>7 clock hours:** Cataract extraction with CTR/ Cionni ring / CTS/ iris or scleral fixated IOL.

   iii. **Subluxation of lens**

      Anterior subluxation: Limbal approach, cataract extraction with sulcus implantation/scleral fixated three piece acrylic IOL.
      Posterior subluxation: Pars plana approach with vitrectomy, lensectomy, scleral fixated IOL.

3. **Traumatic cataract with vitreous disturbance**
   i. Minimal: Manual/automated anterior vitrectomy, sulcus implantation of three piece IOL.
   ii. Gross: Pars plana approach with vitrectomy, lensectomy, scleral fixated IOL.

PENETRATING INJURY WITH TRAUMATIC CATARACT

Indications for Primary Cataract Extraction

Corneal tear repair with cataract extraction with or without IOL implantation.

Hyphema (<50%): anterior chamber wash with cataract extraction with IOL implantation.

IOFB induced cataract, especially iron requires an early intervention due to risk of ocular siderosis.

ADVANTAGES: Early visual rehabilitation, better visual outcome, single procedure

Indications for Secondary Cataract Extraction

Severe corneal edema with tear

High IOP with hyphema (>50%)

Disadvantages: Poorer visual outcome, repeated manipulation-increased risk of infection.

MARFAN SYNDROME WITH SUBLUXATION OF LENS

The aim of my management is to give the best possible visual acuity by surgical and nonsurgical means and to prevent amblyopia in young patients.

Steps of Management

The choice of treatment depends on the following factors:

1. Severity or extent of subluxation with respect to visual axis and undilated pupil
2. Age of the patient

Preoperative Evaluation

1. Undilated examination to see if the lens margin is crossing the pupillary region.
2. Prone position or head tilt to rule out posterior subluxation.
3. Examination of retina and cornea as Marfan syndrome is associated with higher incidence of retinal detachment and keratoconus.

Spectacle correction is given in two situations

1. Minimal subluxation with pupillary area being phakic.
2. Severe subluxation when the pupillary area being aphakic.

Indications for Surgery

1. Lens margin in the pupillary region
2. Risk of amblyopia
3. Anterior or posterior displacement of subluxated lens.

Surgical Options

1. **Intracapsular lens extraction with anterior vitrectomy followed by spectacles or contact lens correction:** This is preferred in younger children. IOL power prediction is difficult because of varying refraction. And since Marfan patients are usually myopic, aphakic correction is not very high and well tolerated.
2. **Intracapsular lens extraction with anterior vitrectomy and IOL implantation:** Scleral fixation with glue or haptic tucked in pockets is preferred over sutured SFIOL or sutured IFIOL. Surgeries are done in younger people and the lifespan results of sutures are not known. (If sutured 9-0 prolene or 8-0 goretex is preferred.)
3. **Lens aspiration with bag preservation using CTR/CTS/Cionni's Ring with PCIOL implantation:** This can be done in adult or older children with moderate subluxation. Since the subluxation may progress, CTS or Cionni's ring is preferred over CTR to stabilize the bag. A 3-piece PCIOL is kept in the bag. The 3-piece gives the option of future scleral fixation or iris-fixation should the need arise.

4. **If the lens is displaced posteriorly, pars plana lensectomy with vitrectomy is done.** Followed by silicone fixation IOL with glue or with haptics tucked in pockets.

5. **Other eye surgery:** Most patients will require the second eye surgery. The timing is based on the severity of subluxation and risk of amblyopia development. In children we should wait till GA fitness is allowed for the second time.

Systemic Consideration

We should also ask for a cardiologist opinion because Marfan's syndrome is associated with mitral valve prolapse, aortic dissection and aortic aneurysms.

ACTIVE UVEITIS IN RIGHT EYE AND UVEITIS WITH COMPLICATED CATARACT IN LEFT EYE

The aim of my treatment would be to:

1. Effectively control inflammation,
2. Relieve pain
3. Prevent complications
4. To treat the causative aetiology, if possible.

Right Eye (Active Uveitis)

Treatment of Uveitis

I would like to start the patient on topical 1% prednisolone acetate 6–8 times a day at regular intervals along with a short acting cycloplegic drug like 1% homatropine twice a day. I would review the patient periodically and titrate the dose of the topical steroids depending on the response. If there is a documented reduction of inflammation I would taper the dosage to 4 times, 3 times, 2 times, and 1 time at weekly intervals.

If there is no adequate improvement, I would like to add oral prednisolone acetate 1mg/kg body weight, after ascertaining that the patient does not have systemic contraindications such as diabetes mellitus or gastritis. The patient is examined periodically and if good improvement is seen, the systemic steroids are tapered and the patient is continued only on topical steroids.

Posterior sub-Tenon triamcinolone acetonide (40 mg) can be considered in cases of chronic uveitis with posterior segment involvement.

If the patients is not responding to oral and topical steroids or develops steroid induced ocular or systemic complications, I would like to switch over to immunosuppressive therapy. Considering the cost of the treatment and also the better compliance to the drug due to once-a-week regimen my first choice would be Tablet methotrexate. Dose: 7.5–25 mg/week in a single dose (15 mg/week), folate (1 mg/day) is administered concurrently to minimize nausea. Considering the bone marrow and hepatic toxicity of the drug I would like to monitor the patients' blood counts and liver function tests every 1–2 months.

Indications for Immunosuppressive Use

1. Severe, sight – threatening steroid resistant uveitis
2. Patients with steroid induced complications
3. As a first line drug in patients where long term remission or cure has been shown to be achieved with immunosuppressants, e.g.; Behcets diseses, Wegener's

Left Eye (Uveitis with Complicated Cataract)

If the eye has been quiet for at least 3 months, I would like to go ahead with performing a cataract extraction with IOL implantation after taking proper preoperative and intraoperative precautions. I would also explain the guarded visual prognosis and consequences to the patient. Preoperatively depending on the chronicity and severity of the inflammation, I would like to start the patient on topical 1% prednisolone acetate 6 times a day at least 1 week before the surgery and if needed I would add oral prednisolone 20 mg/day which can be tapered according to the severity of the postoperative inflammation. Intraoperatively, I would be prepared to handle poor view due to band-shaped keratopathy, small pupil, and posterior synechiae and would also expect zonular weakness. I would use intracameral adrenaline (1.5%) to facilitate pupillary dilatation. Alternatively, I will perform multiple small sphincterotomies or use an iris hook to get adequate pupillary dilatation. I would prefer "in the bag" implantation of a three-piece monofocal acrylic intraocular lens, or if available a heparin coated intraocular lens. Care would be taken to take out the cortex and the residual viscoelastics completely. At the end of the surgery, I would give a subconjunctival injection of dexamethasone (0.4 mL of 4 mg/mL) or preservative free intracameral dexamethasone (0.1 mL of 4 mg/mL) Postoperatively I would continue the topical prednisolone and taper it depending on the response. I would also like to add a short acting cycloplegic like 1% homatropine twice a day for at least 15 days and NSAIDs like 0.5% ketorolac 3 times a day for at least 6 weeks to prevent cystoid macular edema. I would also review the patient more often than normal to look for reactivation of the uveitis and also look for early occurrence of posterior capsular opacification.

MANAGEMENT OF PTERYGIUM

Aim of the Treatment

The aim of the treatment is to relieve the patient of the symptoms caused by pterygium either by medical therapy or surgical excision with tissue supplementation with an intention to prevent further recurrence.

Management of Pterygium

1. Medical therapy

- To manage mild irritation, topical lubricants or a mild topical antihistamine vasoconstrictor like 0.1% naphazoline QID are used.
- In case of inflammation of pterygium, mild topical corticosteroid like 0.1% fluoromethalone or loteprednol QID is used for a short period of time.
- Secondary dellen is treated using preservative free lubricating ointments and temporary patching for 24 hours.

2. Surgical management

i. Surgical intervention is indicated in the following cases:
  - Reduced visual acuity due to induced astigmatism or encroachment onto the visual axis
  - Marked discomfort and irritation not relieved by medical management
  - Limitation of ocular motility secondary to restriction
  - Cosmetic reasons

ii. The various surgical approaches are:
  - Pterygium excision
  - Conjunctival flaps and conjunctival autografts
  - Lamellar keratoplasty and penetrating keratoplasty-in case of significant corneal thinning
  - Mucous membrane grafts and amniotic membrane grafts.

My ideal treatment of choice would be the surgical excision of pterygium and supplementing the raw area with autologous conjunctival transplantation. This can be performed with local infiltration anesthesia. I would like to specifically remove as much as subconjunctival tissue as possible, beneath the head of the pterygium, with minimal removal of the conjunctival tissue. The surface of the cornea can be smoothed by a mechanical burr or by using a 15 blade with short superficial shaving movements. I will prepare the conjunctival graft, as thin as possible, by clearing off the underlying Tenon's capsule. The conjunctival graft is secured with proper orientation, either by sutures or fibrin glue. If the sutures are used, then the limbal side of the conjunctival graft is anchored with the peripheral cornea using a 10-0 nylon interrupted suture and the conjunctival side is attached with 8-0 vicryl sutures. If the glue is used, care is taken to dry the bed before the application of the glue. If enough conjunctiva is not available, then amniotic membrane supplementation can be considered, but the recurrence rate with amniotic membrane is higher.

TREATMENT OF KERATOCONUS

The aim of the treatment is to try and arrest the progression of keratoconus and try to achieve the best possible visual acuity for the patient.

Towards this, I will prescribe spectacles or soft toric contact lenses for the patient. If this visual rehabilitation is inadequate, then I will prescribe rigid gas permeable contact lenses (RGP) contact lenses to correct the irregular astigmatism.

If there is a documented progression of keratoconus, as seen by serial topography, then corneal collagen cross linking (C3R) can be done with the aim to prevent or slow down further progression, the residual refractive error may be corrected with RGP contact lenses, 3 months after the C3R procedure.

Intracorneal rings segments (INTACS) are sometimes used in mild or moderate cases to improve tolerance to contact lens wear.

In patients in whom there is corneal scarring or complete contact lens intolerance or not being able to be fit with contact lenses, then corneal transplantation should be considered. DALK is the preferred surgical option. However, in cases of severe deep stromal scarring, PKP is performed.

TREATMENT OF MACULAR CORNEAL DYSTROPHY

(Also Known As Groenouw Type II Dystrophy)

The definitive treatment is corneal transplantation in both eyes. However, in milder cases initial symptomatic treatment is given to provide relief of symptoms.

The management includes:

1. I will recommend the use of tinted glasses to minimize the photophobia.
2. If there are recurrent erosions, I will treat it in the following manner.
   i. Acute episode
      - Use of antibiotic drops to reduce the risk of infection.
      - Control of pain with use of cycloplegic agents, topical non-steroidal anti-inflammatory drugs and oral analgesics.
      - Promote epithelial healing by patching of eye and using therapeutic soft contact lenses.
      Usually heals in 2–3 days, but I would like to follow up the patient closely to ensure erosions are healing.
   ii. Prevention of subsequent erosions
      - Use of Hypertonic solutions such as 5% sodium chloride; especially in the form of eye ointment at bed time. Patient is asked to continue them for several months.
      - Instillation of Lubricating eye drops.
      - Bandage soft contact lenses protect epithelial surface from further damage.
      - Control of concomitant ocular surface conditions if present e.g.: dry eye syndrome.
3. Surgical therapy: The choice of procedure depends on the extent of corneal involvement.
   i. For dystrophies involving the anterior 3rd of stroma, phototherapeutic keratoplasty can be done.

      Phototherapeutic Keratoplasty (PTK) uses excimer laser. The goal is to aim for a central clearing of the opacities and thereby postpone or avoid lamellar/penetrating keratoplasty rather than achieve a totally clear cornea. It removes superficial corneal opacities, smoothens corneal surface and allows epithelium to adhere more tightly. The procedure produces significant visual improvement in these patients. The dystrophy may recur after PTK, in case of which a repeat PTK or a PKP may be necessary.
   ii. For dystrophies involving anterior half of stroma, deep anterior lamellar keratoplasty (DALK) is preferred.

iii. If visual acuity worsens and opacities are deep, a full thickness corneal transplant (PKP) has to be performed. Most patients require a penetrating keratoplasty by 4th decade of their life. The eye which is more affected is operated first followed by the second eye after a time gap of 6 months.

Although the success rate is high, macular dystrophy recurs in the graft over years and re-graft is necessary in such cases.

Genetic counseling: I would also like to educate the patients about the hereditary nature of the disease. Patients are less likely to have an affected child due to its autosomal recessive inheritance.

MANAGEMENT OF BACTERIAL CORNEAL ULCER

Aim of Treatment

Rapid cessation of replication and elimination of infecting organism and thereby preventing the structural damage to cornea with selection of appropriate therapy with minimal toxicity.

Initially, I would like to start with broad spectrum antibiotics monotherapy [gatifloxacin 0.3% or moxifloxacin] on an hourly basis during waking hours for 3 days which later can be modified according to culture results, antibiotics susceptibility, and clinical response.

I also would like to add mydriatics like homatropine 2% in [cyclopentolate 1% or atropine 1%] in the affected eye twice daily to prevent ciliary spasm and dangerous results of iritis e.g., posterior synechiae. I would like to give oral pain relievers like paracetomol to relieve the pain and make the patient comfortable.

There is no need to change the initial therapy if this has induced a favourable clinical response, even if cultures show a resistant organism.

If there is an evidence of grams positive organism, I would like to start with topical chloramphenicol 5 mg/mL or Cefazolin 5% initially hourly for 2 days as a loading dose and then I will modify the regimen depending on the therapeutic responses.

In case of grams negative organisms, I would like to start with topical gentamicin 1.5% hourly or fluroquinolones like 0.3% ciprofloxacin or ofloxacin for 2 days and then modify the regimen depending on therapeutic response.

In severe cases, I would like to start with combination therapy with fortified preparations as duotherapy.

Most common combination used is cephalosporin and aminoglycoside to cover both gram positive and gram negative bacteria.

Positive Signs of Clinical Improvement

1. Decreased pain
2. Decreased discharge
3. Decreased consolidation of corneal infiltrate
4. Decreased anterior chamber reaction
5. Decreased in hypopyon size
6. Corneal re-epithelization
7. Blunting of edges of perimeter of stromal infiltrate
8. Cessation in corneal thinning.

Subconjunctival antibiotics are only indicated if there is poor compliance with topical treatment.

General Principles

1. If inflammation is severe and persist after the infection is controlled, then topical steroids prednisolone 0.5 to 1% – 4 times a day will help to promote healing and prevent vascularization
2. If still no improvement after a further 48 hours then suspension of treatment for 24 hours then re-scraping performed with inoculation on a broader range of media and additional staining techniques requested.
3. If culture remains negative, it may necessary to perform corneal biopsy for histology and culture.
4. If still no improvement seen and ulcer progress I would like to do therapeutic keratoplasty with a plan to perform a later optical keratoplasty if possible.
5. If the ulcer heals with residual scar it may cause surface irregularity and irregular astigmatism I will proceed depending on the situation:
   i. In case of nebular opacity, vision can be improved with rigid gas permeable contact lens.
   ii. If scar is dense n visual potential is present corneal graft [optical keratoplasty] can be done.
   iii. If scar is present and no visual potential then I will advise for cosmetic contact lens or tattooing.
6. If perforation occurs and if it is small over iris, adhesions to cornea will occur by formation of pseudocornea by laying down of fibrin and collagenase and the defect will heal as adherent leukoma.
7. If perforation fails to heal I would like to proceed according to size of ulcer.
8. If the size is less than 2 mm tissue adhesive n-butyl 2-ethyl cyanoacyrlate to seal the gap can be used
9. If the size is 2 to 4 mm then either corneal patch graft or tenoplasty can be done.
10. If size is more than 4 mm, then we have to do tectonic
11. If severe ulcer with opaque media I would like to do ultrasonography to look for exudates in vitreous which suggest of endophthalmitis.

Management of fungal corneal ulcer

In case of filamentous fungi, I would like to start patient with 5% topical natamycin hourly initially, during the waking hours for at least 48 hours.

If no improvement seen topical azole [fluconazole 2% or miconazole 1%] can be added.

Or

Topical itraconzole 1% can be added as it is effective against broad range of filamentous fungi.

Or

Topical voriconazole can be added.

In case of deep invasion of cornea or anterior chamber involvement, I would like to start oral voriconazole 200 mg bd [after performing baseline liver function test]. I also would like to add oral doxycycline 100 mg bd if significant thinning seen.

I also would like to check intraocular pressure digitally.

If ulcer progress despite pharmacological treatment therapeutic keratoplasty is considered as alternative.

Injections voriconazole 50 µg/0.1 mL intrastromal can also be tried.

Indications for therapeutic keratoplasty in acute phase of infection in case of fungal ulcer
1. Progression of infection despite appropriate and adequate pharmacological treatment
2. Impending OR actual perforation
3. Progression of infection to involve limbus and adjacent sclera.

Technique of keratoplasty
1. Size of trephination should include all the infected area and at least 1–1.5 mm of the surrounding clear zone as well
2. Interrupted sutures with slightly longer bites to avoid cheese wiring of suture
3. Anterior chamber irrigation to flush out all the septic material
4. Excise affected intraocular structure and try to preserve lens if possible.

If intraocular structure involvement/endophthalmitis suspected

Intracameral Antifungals should be injected at the time of keratoplasty

Amphotericin 5 µg/0.1 mL

Miconazole 25 µg/0.1 mL

After penetrating keratoplasty continue topical antifungals to prevent recurrence. Do not use topical steroids in the postoperative period

If ulcer progress towards limbus involves sclera [fungal keratoscleritis]

Then I would then like to do start oral antifungals and oral analgesic [to relieve pain n inflammation] and cryotherapy [retinal cryoprobe] to ulcer edges with excision of the sclera.

Or

Corneoscleral graft.

Systemic antifungals indications
1. Severe deep keratitis
2. When lesion is near limbus
3. Scleritis
4. Endopthalmitis

Various systemic antifungals

T. voriconazole 400 mg bd for 1 day

Then 200 mg bd

Or

T. itraconazole 200 mg daily then reduce to 100 mg daily

Or

T. fluconazole 200 mg bd

Or

Tetracycline [doxycycline] for its collagenase activity.

MANAGEMENT OF HERPES SIMPLEX VIRUS KERATITIS

Aim of the Treatment

1. To control and eliminate the infection
2. To relieve the pain and
3. To promote re-epithelization and
4. Prevent recurrence of infection with minimal drugs with minimal toxicity.

Epithelial Keratitis

Initially, I would like to debride the epithelial lesion under topical anesthesia. I would like to start patient with topical antivirals 3% aciclovir ointment 5 times a day for 2 weeks with:

1. Topical lubricants to relieve discomfort
2. Topical cycloplegic if required
3. Topical antivirals should not be continued after two weeks.
4. Debridement can be used for dendrite ulcer to reduce the viral load but not in geographic ulcer.
5. In case with slow healing or frequent recurrence or resistant case, I would like to add oral acyclovir 400 mg 5 times a day for 10 days
6. If frequent recurrence seen, I would like to prescribe oral acyclovir 400 mg 12 hourly for 6 months to year or longer.

Stromal keratitis [including diskiform keratitis, endothelitis, and iridocyclitis]

Initially, I would like to start with topical steroids with antiviral cover 4 times a day [HEDS STUDY].

As improvement occurs I would like to taper and subsequently prednisolone 0.5 to 1% may be used once daily safe dose at which antiviral cover can be stopped.

Topical cyclosporine 0.05% can be used in case to facilitate tapering of steroid such as in steroid related raised intraocular pressure.

Nectrotizing stromal keratitis

I would like to add oral acyclovir 400 mg bd for 10 days.

Herpes-zoster ophthalmicus

I would like to start with oral acyclovir 800 mg 5 times a day for 10 days as soon as possible preferably no longer than 4 days after onset of rash.

I will advise cold compress and strong analgesics.

Patient with shingles can transmit the disease to immunodeficient individual and patient not immune [pregnancy] should be asked to avoid contact.

Other oral antivirals:

1. Valaciclovir 1 g tid
2. Famciclovir 500 mg tid
3. Brivudine 125 mg bd.

Postherpetic neuralgia:

I will advise cold compress and topical capsaicin 0.025% or 0.075% cream for 3 weeks.

Or

Local anesthesia

If not relieved, I will add oral drugs:

1. Simple analgesics paracetamol up to 4 g daily
2. Stronger analgesics codeine 250 mg daily
3. Amitriptyline 10–25 mg at night can be increase up to 75 mg
4. Carbamazepine 400 mg daily for lancinating pain.

Acute eye disease

1. Skin and eyelid involvement: 3% acyclovir + 5% acyclovir ointment for the skin lesions
2. Acute epithelial keratitis: Topical antivirals
3. Episcleritis: mild non-steroidal anti-inflammatory drugs
4. Scleritis: oral flurbiprofen 100 mg 3 times a day

Or

5. Topical dexamethasone 0.1% hourly and antiviral ointment 3% aciclovir 5 times a day and steroid ointment at night.

MANAGEMENT OF ACANTHAMOEBA KERATITIS

Aim of Treatment

1. Not to misdiagnose the ulcer
2. Eradicate the cyst as well as tropozoites
3. Prevent the recurrence
4. With minimal drugs with minimal toxicity.

The treatment is a prolonged one and it would take months for the ulcer to heal. I would like to start patient on topical polyhexamethyl biguanide 0.02% as first line therapy 6–24 times a day (no corneal toxicity) (it is available as 20% parent solution, which is diluted 1000 times with saline/sterile water.

If needed, I would like to do debridement of ulcer so better penetration of drugs can be facilitated.

I also would like to add analgesic flurbiprofen 100 mg 3 times a day.

Despite if ulcer fails to heal I would like to do keratoplasty

If limbitis or scleritis develop I will start prednisolone 1 mg/kg/day or cyclosporine 3.5.to 7.5 mg/kg/day which can be tapered.

Indications of Keratoplasty

1. Non healing ulcer in spite of appropriate antiamebicidal therapy
2. Fulminant corneal abscess
3. Intumescent cataract.

Rationale to eliminate recurrence of acanthamoeba in recipient corneal graft:

Cryotherapy/rapidly freeze cornea used either with or without penetrating keratoplasty.

The sterile pentamidine isethionate powder can be mixed with artificial tears and applied topically as recommended for brolene solution.

0.15% dibrompropamidine [brolene ointment]

0.1% propamidine isethionate [brolene solution]

Miconazole [10 mg/mL]

Clotrimazole [1.0%]

Oral administration of ketoconazole 200–600 mg/day.

PRIMARY OPEN-ANGLE GLAUCOMA

Treatment Protocol

My goal would be to set a target IOP to achieve it with the least possible medication, so that any further progression of the glaucoma is arrested. My first drug of choice would be latanoprost 0.005% eye drops, once a day, preferable at night time to blunt the early morning spike of the intraocular pressure. In case, this drug is contraindicated, then my second choice would be to use 0.5% timolol maleate, twice a day, as a monotherapy.

If the target IOP is not achieved at a month by either of these medications on their individual capacity, then I will use both these drugs as a combination therapy. If the target IOP is still not achieved with these two drugs, then I will add the third drug. The choice of the third drug can be either brimonidine tartrate 0.2%, 3 times a day or dorzolamide 2%, 3 times a day.

Since some studies have shown that adding a second medication decreased adherence to glaucoma treatment, I will advise a fixed combination therapy (combining two or more antiglaucoma drugs into a single preparation) in order to improve compliance. The commonly available fixed combination drugs are:

1. Timolol + Brimonidine
2. Timolol + PG analog
3. Brimonidine + PG analog
4. Topical Carbonic Anhydrase Inhibitors + PG analog
5. Topical Carbonic Anhydrase Inhibitors + Timolol

I will avoid using PG analog with pilocarpine because while prostaglandins relax ciliary muscle and increase uveoscleral outflow, pilocarpine contracts and decreases trabecular outflow.

If the target IOP is still not achieved, after the usage of all three medications, then I will advise the patient to undergo trabeculectomy with or without mitomycin. If there is a high chance for the trabeculectomy to fail, then I would consider performing shunt surgeries using aqueous drainage devices.

The most important thing is to make the patient comply with the treatment protocol. I will counsel the patient about the nature of the disease, the importance of routine follow up, the necessity to adhere to medication in order to stop the disease progression and also the need to screen family members.

POST-FILTER CASE: BE, RE (FUNCTIONING FILTER), AND LE (NONFUNCTIONING FILTER)

Aim

The aim of my management will be to achieve and maintain the TARGET IOP in both the eyes, so as to preserve vision and thereby the quality of life of my patient.

Management

Right eye (Functioning filter)

1. I will check whether target IOP is reached with the functioning filter (extent of optic nerve damage, progression of field defects, along with the age of the patient and central corneal thickness will decide the target IOP)
2. If the target IOP is achieved, then I will ask the patient to follow up every 3–6 months (depending on the stage)
3. If the target IOP is not achieved with the functioning filter, I will add a topical antiglaucoma medication like Timolol maleate 0.5% bd dosage to aid in achieving the TARGET IOP and I will review the patient after a month and decide about the need for HFA-GPA as per the stage of his disease.

Left eye (non-functioning filter)

1. The type of glaucoma and the conjunctival status are the two most important factors in determining the success of filtering surgery
2. IOP and bleb morphology are the important things to be looked at after trabeculectomy surgery
3. Blebs can be graded based on their size, elevation, vascularity, and structure.

Size : (in mm)
> Grade I: 1–3 mm
> Grade II: 3–4 mm
> Grade III: > 4 mm

Elevation from scleral surface:
> Nil, mild moderate and large.

Vascularity: l Grade 0 Nil
> Grade I: Few small vessels
> Grade II: Normal conjunctival vascularity
> Grade III: Locally congested
> Grade IV: Large vessels on bleb site

Structure: Type I: Localized encysted
> Type II: Diffuse microcysts or
> Type III: Loculated thin bleb

1. ***Early failure*** (Immediate post-trab)
   i. I will check the IOP (management is different for too high or too low)
   ii. If it is too high, I will start topical antiglaucoma medications and if needed, oral antiglaucoma medications (carbonic anhydrase inhibitors)
   iii. I will do a GONIOSCOPY to look whether

   - the ostium is patent

   - the peripheral iridectomy is larger than the ostium

   If there is a clot at the ostium, I would observe if the clot is small for it will resolve in a few days or if the clot is large and threatening the optic nerve I would do an anterior chamber wash.

   If the iris is occluding the ostium, a low energy argon laser or Nd YAG laser can be used to disrupt the iris tissue at the ostium.

   - Other important steps include:
     - Hourly steroids topically
     - Digital pressure/massage: Constant and firm digital compression is applied over inferior aspect of globe through the patient's lower lid while the eye is upturned. Duration of each compression shouldn't last for more than 10 seconds
     - Laser suturolysis/releasing sutures
     - Bleb needling (with lignocaine, 5-FU, viscoelastics) in cases of subconjunctival adhesions and fibrosis
     - Regular IOP check along with fields (HFA GPA) are mandatory during this period
     - Repeat filtering procedure with antimetabolites (success rates 50% if done in Primary glaucomas)-higher dose (mitomycin C 0.4%) for a longer duration (up to 3 min)
   - Glaucoma drainage devices to be considered for patients with secondary glaucoma where the chances of failure of repeat trabeculectomy are very high (e.g. NVG, uveitic glaucoma, Sturge–Weber syndrome)

2. ***Late failure:***
   i. Repeat filtering procedure with antimetabolites (success rates 50% if done in primary glaucomas)
      - higher dose (mitomycin C 0.4%) for a longer duration (up to 3 min)
   ii. Glaucoma drainage devices to be considered

If the secondary trabeculectomy also fails or the patients is a poor candidate

   i. young <40 years of age

  ii. previous scleral buckle

 iii. chronic conjunctival inflammation

 iv. previous penetrating keratoplasty

  v. aphakia

 vi. pseudophakia

 vii. post sclera buckle for retinal detachment

viii. previous conjunctival surgery.

Postoperatively, **atropine 1% and scopolamine 0.25%** to be given to relax the ciliary muscle and tighten the zonular-lens-iris diaphragm and in turn to deepen the anterior chamber.

Postoperative evaluation of the eye for the following should be done after repeat trabeculectomy:

   i. Extent and height of the bleb

  ii. Presence or absence of microcysts

 iii. presence or absence of bleb leak

 iv. visibility of scleral flap sutures

  v. IOP

 vi. clarity of cornea

 vii. AC depth

viii. AC inflammation

 ix. Hyphema

  x. Optic disk and macular appearance.

Conclusion

1. IOP and bleb morphology gives valuable information about the functionality of the filter, if needed topical antiglaucoma medications to be started to achieve target IOP and regular follow up with HFA GPA is essential.

2. So, achieving target IOP is the primary goal to improve the quality of life and to preserve vision.

PSEUDOEXFOLIATION GLAUCOMA RE WITH IMC

In a patient with pseudoexfoliation (PXF) and IMC, I would like to manage the glaucoma very carefully, because the glaucoma in PXFG tends to be more aggressive in terms of optic nerve head damage and they also have a poor response to antiglaucoma medications. I would also like to measure the IOP at various time points, since the diurnal variations in PXF tends to be significantly more.

Before planning the treatment I would first like to evaluate whether it is a case of
1. PXFG with open angles.
2. PXFG with narrow/occludable angles.(by doing a gonioscopy)

PXFG with closed/narrow angles: I would like to first do a YAG peripheral iridotomy, control the pressures medically and then treat it like a case of PXFG with open angles.

In PXFG (open angles) with IMC one can do either of the three procedures depending on the clinical condition
1. Cataract extraction with IOL implantation
2. Trabeculectomy
3. Combined cataract extraction with IOL implantation and trabeculectomy (glaucoma triple procedure).

The choice of procedure depends on:
1. Severity of glaucoma in terms of optic neuropathy and visual field defect;
2. Intraocular pressure (IOP) control;
3. Number of glaucoma medications needed for IOP control;

Before surgery, I would like to get an automated visual field analysis done to explain the visual prognosis following the surgery.

Cataract Surgery Alone

This can be performed, if the IOP is well under control with medications and there is no progressive optic neuropathy. Temporal section is preferred and the superior conjunctiva is preserved for future filtering surgery, if necessary. Since the pupillary dialation may be sluggish, intracameral adrenaline or sphincterotomies or iris hooks are used to dilate the pupil. Also, an anterior capsular staining with trypan blue may be useful to delineate the difference between the anterior capsule and the PXF deposition. Zonular dialysis is very common in this group and hence we need to be ready to handle this with a capsular tension ring if necessary.

Trabeculectomy Alone

In conditions of early cataract and when the glaucoma is uncontrolled despite maximum tolerable medical therapy and advanced glaucomatous optic disk changes the surgical procedure of choice is trabeculectomy (which has the greatest chance of providing immediate and long-term IOP control).

Temporal clear corneal phakoemulsification can be done after 3-6 months after the control of IOP.

Combined Procedure

1. Done in cases with moderate glaucoma and visually significant cataract
2. Long-term IOP control is greater with combined procedures than with cataract extraction alone
3. Phakotrabeculectomy single site or twin site (superior trabeculectomy with temporal Phakoemulsification) can be performed.

MANAGEMENT OF NVG

My aim of management is:

1. To treat the underlying disease that initiated the anterior segment neovascularization
2. To reduce the intraocular pressure
3. To reduce the inflammation
4. To give rest to the ciliary body and relieve pain

First of all, I would like to obtain a detailed systemic history from the patient.

In comprehensive ocular examination, I would like to carefully examine pupillary reaction, pupillary margin under high magnification to rule out NVI and undilated gonioscopy to look for presence or absence of NVA.

Management of NVG

In all cases of NVG, systemic disease (e.g. hypertension, diabetes mellitus) have to be controlled and I will work in conjunction with the physician to ensure the same.

Before planning the treatment I would first like to evaluate whether it is a case of:

1. **NVG with *NORMAL* IOP and ocular media clear/hazy**: In case where NVI/NVA has already developed but the IOP is still normal, the primary goal of treatment is to reduce the retinal/ocular ischemia causing regression and involution of anterior segment neovascularization.

   i. **If media clear:** PRP (number of burns, 1200–1500 burns, spot size 200–500 microns, one burn width apart applied to the retina) with or without anti-VEGF (bevacizumab, intavitreally 1.25 mg/mL or intracamerally 0.25 mg/0.02 mL, after ruling out systemic contraindications) is the procedure of choice.

   ii. **In patients with hazy media**-anti-VEGF (bevacizumab) intravitreal 1.25 mg/0.05 mL or intracameral 0.25 mg/0.02 mL alone is given.

2. **NVG with *RAISED* IOP and ocular media clear/hazy**

   i. Osmotic agents (i.v.mannitol 1–2 mg/kg or isosorbide orally 1.5 g/kg) may provide acute but transient lowering of IOP by reducing vitreous volume.

   ii. Further control of elevated IOP is usually accomplished with aqueous suppressants like beta blockers (timolol 0.5%), carbonic anhydrase inhibitors (dorzolamide2%), and alpha 2 agonist (brimonidine 0.1%)

   iii. Inflammation is controlled by topical prednisolone acetate 1% suspension and is titrated accordingly based on the therapeutic response.

iv. Atropine 1% to decrease the ocular pain and Topical corticosteroids (prednisolone suspension 1%) can be used for inflammation.

After the corneal edema resolves and inflammation subsides adjunct combination of intravitreal bevacizumab and PRP should be done in case of clear media.

When media is hazy intravitreal 1.25 mg/0.05 mL or intracameral 0.25 mg/0.02 mL alone is given.

Surgical management: In cases of late stages of NVG where medical management often fails to control IOP and with extensive synechial angle closure surgical intervention is usually required.

1. **Trabeculectomy:** This procedure is reserved in eyes that have potential for useful vision and when extent of PAS >180 degree and performed when the inflammation has been adequately controlled.

   Use of antimetabolites (MMC 0.2 mg/mL applied under the sclera flap for 3 min or 5-FU 50 mg/mL for 5 min or subconjunctivally 5 mg, 180 degrees away from the trabeculectomy site, twice daily, injected in first postoperative week and once daily in second postoperative week) may improve the outcome.

   Preoperative PRP treatment, with anti-VEGF, should be done wherever possible to cause regression of NVI.

2. **Aqueous drainage implants:** Indicated when conventional trabeculectomy fails or is not possible because of excessive conjunctival scarring.

   Molteno, Baerveldts, Ahmed, AADI implants can be used.

   Use of anti-VEGF intravitreally or intracamerally is recommended at least 24 hours prior to surgery.

3. **Cyclodestruction:** Reserved for the end stage NVG with poor visual prognosis, or when all methods have failed to control IOP and when control of pain becomes the primary therapeutic aim.

   These procedures can be done by cyclocryotherapy or Direct laser cyclophotocoagulation or trans-scleral photocoagulation to destroy the ciliary body to reduce aqueous humor production.

4. **Retrobulbar alcohol injection 3 mL:** Painful blind eyes who do not respond to medical/surgical treatment, can be considered for this option.

5. **Enucleation:** if all the above surgical modalities fail to control pain enucleation may be consider, as a last resort.

MANAGEMENT OF AN ACUTE ATTACK OF ANGLE CLOSURE GLAUCOMA

(This narrative is given intentionally in active tense to familiarize the resident in the art of presentation in a viva)

Management of angle closure glaucoma is essentially surgical. However, I would like to control the intraocular pressure as much as possible, by medical means before planning surgery.

If the intraocular pressure is very high (above 50 mm Hg), pressure induced ischemia of the iris leads to paralysis of sphincter muscle and hence miotic therapy does not help. For this reason, the first line of defense is to administer drugs which will promptly reduce the intraocular pressure.

I will start him on 20% intravenous mannitol in a dose of 1–2 g/kg/body wt. over a period of 20–30 minutes.

In the absence of nausea or vomiting, I would like to use oral acetazolamide tablets, 250 mg, 4 times a day or oral hyperosmotic agents like 50% oral glycerol in a dose of 1–1.5 g/kg body weight, after ruling out diabetes mellitus. Apraclonidine 0.5% can be used to reduce the IOP quickly.

After bringing the intraocular pressure below 40 mm Hg, I will start my patient on 2% topical pilocarpine hydrochloride 4 times over 30 minutes and then once every 6 hours (which by causing pupillary miosis, tightens the peripheral iris pulls it away from the trabecular meshwork and relieves the pupillary block). Additionally, I will also use a combination therapy of topical beta blockers like 0.5% timolol maleate, twice a day with alpha 2 adrenergic agonist like 0.2% brimonidine tartrate, thrice a day with a time interval of 10 minutes.

I would like to use topical steroids like 1% prednisolone acetate, 4 times a day, to control the associated intraocular inflammation. Additionally, I would like to give analgesics like oral Ibuprofen 500 mg twice a day to control the pain.

I shall review the patient on an hourly basis. I will record the intraocular pressure and if the cornea is clear I will do gonioscopy of both the affected eye and fellow eye.

Besides the medications, I will perform some maneuvers like axially depressing the central cornea with a goniolens, which may force open the angle temporarily breaking the acute attack.

If the eye is uninflamed and cornea clear with reduced intraocular pressure, I will do primary peripheral iridotomies using Nd:YAG in both the affected and the fellow eye prophylactically.

If the cornea is not clear and if the gonioscopy reveals angle closure of less than 2/3rd. I will perform a surgical iridectomy for the affected eye and do a YAG iridotomy for the fellow eye.

If the angle closure is more than 2/3rd or if there is persistent inflammation with edematous cornea and high intraocular pressure, then I will contemplate primary trabeculectomy.

Repeat or serial gonioscopy is essential for follow-up of the patient to be certain that the angle has adequately opened.

Case Sheet Writing

The following description attempts to train a resident in describing various abnormalities of the fundus in a case of diabetic retinopathy.

Fundus of Mr C aged 70 years.

HIGH–RISK PROLIFERATIVE DIABETIC RETINOPATHY (PDR) WITH CLINICALLY SIGNIFICANT MACULAR EDEMA (CSME) (RIGHT EYE)

Fundus examination of the right eye:

Distant direct ophthalmoscopy at one arms distance showed a good red glow.

Direct ophthalmoscopy close to face revealed a clear media.

Disk was vertically oval, normal in size, pink in color, with well-defined margins, and having a cup–disk ratio of 0.3 with a healthy neuroretinal rim.

Vessels arise from the center of the disk, branching dichotomously maintaining an arteriovenous ratio of 2:3.

Fine, lacy frond of vessels occupying 1 o'clock hour area of the disk superiorly and 3 o'clock hours inferonasally suggestive of neovascularization of the disk are noted.

A whitish, elevated semilunar-shaped fibrous band about 1 disk diameter inferonasal to the disk containing fine tufts of vessels suggestive of neovascularization elsewhere is seen.

Background retina shows numerous red pinhead-shaped lesions not continuous with the blood vessels suggestive of dot hemorrhages in all four quadrants.

A single streak-shaped red lesion at the inferotemporal margin of the disk suggestive of a flame-shaped hemorrhage is seen.

A tortuosity of the vein in the superotemporal arcade suggestive of venous looping is seen.

Localized caliber changes of the veins in the superonasal and superotemporal arcades suggestive of venous beading is seen.

Yellowish, waxy lesions with distinct margins suggestive of hard exudates arranged in clumps at the posterior pole, inferior, nasal, and temporal to the fovea with adjacent retinal thickening are seen.

A dark red, well-defined accumulation of blood in the inferior retina obscuring the view of the underlying retinal vasculature suggestive of a vitreous hemorrhage is seen.

On slit-lamp biomicroscopy with a +90 D lens retinal thickening is seen at the macular area and the above findings are confirmed. Indirect ophthalmoscopy showed the peripheries to be normal.

FUNDUS EXAMINATION OF THE LEFT EYE

Diagnosis: Severe NPDR with CSME

Distant direct ophthalmoscopy at one arms distance showed a good red glow.

Direct ophthalmoscopy close to face revealed a clear media.

Disk was normal in size, vertically oval, pink in color, with well-defined margins and having a cup disk ratio of 0.3 with a healthy neuroretinal rim.

Vessels arise from the center of the disk, branching dichotomously maintaining an arteriovenous ratio of 2:3.

Background retina shows numerous pinhead-shaped red lesions suggestive of dot and blot hemorrhages in all four quadrants.

A streak-shaped red lesion inferior to the fovea suggestive of a flame-shaped hemorrhage is seen.

Yellowish, waxy lesions with distinct margins arranged in clumps along the superior and inferior temporal arcades suggestive of hard exudates are seen.

A yellowish lesion with distinct margins, 2 disk diameter (DD) from the temporal disk margin, surrounded by an area of retinal thickening suggestive of a hard exudates plaque is seen.

A yellowish fluffy lesion with indistinct margins inferior to the disk suggestive of a cotton wool spot is seen.

A few atrophic hypopigmented chorioretinal scars along the inferotemporal arcade suggestive of old laser marks are seen.

On slit-lamp biomicroscopy with a +90 D lens, the above findings are confirmed. Indirect ophthalmoscopy showed the peripheries to be normal.

EXAMINATION OF A LONG CASE: PROPTOSIS

Guidelines

1. Duration of the complaints should be in chronological order.
2. Elaboration of the complaint should have an onset (insidious, sudden, etc.) and a progress mode (rapid, slow, etc.) and any relieving nature (e.g. pain relieved with closing the eyes).

Mr M, a 57-year-old male, farmer by occupation, hailing from Madurai presented to us with complaints of:

1. Prominence of right eye of 4 months duration.
2. Swelling and pain of right eye of 1 month duration.

History of Present Illness

The patient was asymptomatic till 4 months back when he noticed prominence of right eye which was insidious in onset, progressive in nature and more worse in the morning. The prominence was associated with mild discomfort and dryness of the right eye. He consulted a local ophthalmologist and was prescribed some eye drops which provided some symptomatic relief.

The patient then developed swelling of right eye of both upper and lower lid associated with pain and redness of the right eye which was progressive in nature and worse in the morning. The pain was dull aching in nature more of retrobulbar discomfort, typically described by the patient as something pushing behind the eye. The pain was nonradiating, present both at rest and with movements of the eye.

The above symptoms were associated with gritty foreign body sensation of both eyes.

H/o loss of weight with good appetite associated with increased sweating, tremors, and palpitations since past 2 years.

He gives h/o swelling in the neck for past 2 years.

No h/o diplopia.

No h/o defective vision or blackouts or transient loss of vision or defective color perception.

No h/o hyperpigmentation of lids/eyes.

No h/o postural variation (bending forwards).

No h/o variation with sneezing or coughing or straining.

No h/o photophobia, discharge, or colored halos.

No h/o any other swelling in the body.

No h/o dysphagia, dysphonia, easy fatigability, drooping of eyelids.

No h/o radiation therapy or chemotherapy in the past.

No h/o skin discoloration in the past.

No h/o fever, headache, nausea, vomiting.

No h/o nasal block, frequent respiratory tract infection, epistaxis.

No h/o trauma.

Past History

H/o taking tablet Carbimazole 5 mg BD for past 2 years.

No h/o diabetes mellitus, hypertension, cardiac disease.

Personal History

Patient consumes mixed diet.

He is a chronic smoker, consumes average of 6–7 cigarettes per day.

He occasionally consumes alcohol.

Family History

No h/o similar complaints in the family.

General Examination

Patient is averagely built and nourished.

Pulse—90/min, regular in rhythm and volume.

Respiratory rate was 18/min.

Blood pressure was 130/80 mm Hg taken in left upper arm in the supine position.

Higher functions are normal.

No pallor, cyanosis, icterus, and clubbing.

No evidence of any regional or generalized lymphadenopathy.

No evidence of any skin changes or dryness.

Examination of the neck revealed small midline swelling 3 × 5 cm which moved with deglutition and did not move with protrusion of the tongue suggestive of a thyroid swelling.

Fine tremors were noted when the patient was asked to stretch his arms and spread out his fingers.

Tremors were not present at rest.

There was no evidence of dysdiadochokinesia and finger.

Nose past pointing test was negative.

Central nervous system was within normal limits. There was no signs of confusion or dementia, lethargy.

Cardiovascular system was normal without any murmurs.

Respiratory system examination revealed normal vesicular breath sounds in both lungs on auscultation.

Per abdominal examination was normal with no evidence of any palpable intra-abdominal mass.

ENT examination—anterior rhinoscopy was normal with no evidence of sinus tenderness.

Ocular Examination

Visual acuity in both eyes is 6/12p improving to 6/6 with +1.50 D sphere with 2.50 D sphere for near vision.

Parameter	Right eye	Left eye
	Axial proptosis	Normal
Lids	Periorbital edema	Normal
Conjunctiva	Congestion nasally and temporally, mild chemosis, decreased tear film height, decreased tear film breakup height (<10 seconds)	Normal
Cornea	Few punctate epithelial erosions	Clear
Anterior chamber	Normal depth	Normal depth
Iris	Normal color and pattern	Normal color and pattern
Pupil	4 mm, briskly reacting to both direct and consensual light reflex	4 mm, briskly reacting to both direct and consensual light reflex
Lens	Clear	Clear
EOM	Full	Full
Fundus	Normal	Normal

The above findings were confirmed with slit-lamp biomicroscopy and fundus examination with 90 D examination revealed normal findings with no evidence of Sallmann macular folds.

Evaluation of Proptosis

1. Head posture is normal.
2. Facial asymmetry is present.
3. Corneal reflex: Eyes are orthophoric.

Inspection

1. Axial proptosis of the right eye is noted.
2. Nafziger's sign (protrusion of the eye beyond the orbital rim when examined from above and behind the patient) was positive on the right side.
3. On inspection, eyebrows were normal with no evidence of madarosis.
4. Lids revealed periorbital edema of both upper and lower lids.

Right Eye

Inspection

1. In the right eye, lid margins were 3 mm from the superior and inferior limbus suggestive of moderate lid retraction.

2. Temporal flare was present.
3. Lid lag was present on downgaze.
4. There was minimal lagophthalmos with good Bell's phenomenon in the right eye.
5. No variation of proptosis was observed in the right eye with posture especially on bending forwards and with Valsalva's maneuver.
6. The proptosis was nonpulsatile.
7. There was no evidence of engorged veins/corkscrew vessels in the right eye.

Palpation

1. Orbital margins were intact.
2. Insinuation with fingers was possible in all four margins.
3. Resistance to retropulsion was present.
4. Proptosis was noncompressible and nonreducible.
5. No thrills or pulsations felt.
6. There was no evidence of warmth or tenderness over the right eye.
7. No change in the size of the proptosis with jugular vein compression or carotid artery compression.

Left Eye

Inspection

1. Temporal flare was present
2. Lid margins were 1 mm from superior limbus and 2 mm from inferior limbus respectively suggestive of mild lid retraction.
3. Lid lag was present on downgaze.
4. There was minimal lagophthalmos with good Bell's phenomenon.

Palpation

1. Orbital margins were intact.
2. Resistance to retropulsion was present.

Auscultation

No bruits were heard in both eyes.

Measurements

Hertel's Exophthalmometry (Base at 105)

1. Right eye — 22 mm
2. Left eye — 18 mm

Applanation Tonometry

1. Tension by applanation tonometry was 16 mm Hg in the right eye and 18 mm Hg in the left eye in primary gaze.
2. Tension by applanation tonometry was 26 mm Hg in the right eye and 24 mm Hg in the left eye in upgaze.

3. *Schirmer's test:* At the end of 5 minutes revealed 12 mm of Whatmann's strip wetting in the right eye and 15 mm in the left eye suggestive of mild dry eye.
4. Color vision testing with Ishihara's pseudoisochromatic plate was normal in both eyes.
5. Central fields testing with Bjerrum's screen was normal in both eyes.
6. Anterior rhinoscopy was within normal limits. Sinus examination was normal.

Provisional Diagnosis

Right eye unilateral axial proptosis due to acute inflammatory stage of thyroid-related orbitopathy.

Differential Diagnosis

1. Thyroid-related orbitopathy
2. Cavernous hemangioma
3. Idiopathic inflammatory pseudotumor
4. Orbital cellulitis.

Frequently Asked Questions during Presentation

1. **What is the rationale for asking history of radiation therapy or chemo-therapy in the past?**

   To rule out any neoplasm elsewhere in the body which might have metastasized to the orbit.

2. **What is the rationale for asking history of skin discoloration in the past?**

   To rule out thyroid-related skin changes (thyroid myxedema) and also eurofibromatosis (pigmented birthmarks).

3. **What is the rationale for asking history of hyperpigmentation of lids/ eyes?**

   To rule out metastatic neuroblastoma (raccoon eyes).

4. **What is the rationale for asking history of fever, headache, nausea, vomiting?**

   To rule out orbital cellulitis, cavernous sinus thrombosis.

5. **What is the rationale for asking history of nasal block, frequent res-piratory tract infection, epistaxis?**

   To rule out sinusitis and nasopharyngeal carcinoma.

6. **What is the rationale for asking history of trauma?**

   To rule out orbital hematoma and retrobulbar hemorrhage in cases of acute proptosis.

7. **What is the rationale for asking history of dysphonia, dysphasia, easy fatigability in a patient with proptosis?**

   To rule out associated myasthenia gravis.

THIRD NERVE PALSY—MODEL CASE SHEET

Mr G, a 52-year-old male came with the chief complaints of double vision for the past 5 days.

History of Present Illness

1. He was asymptomatic till 5 days ago, when he experienced sudden double vision when he was leaving for work. It was acute in onset, present binocularly, with progressive and horizontal separation of images.
2. There was no diurnal variation and not increasing in any particular gaze.
3. He noticed some restricted movement of the right eye, but was not associated with pain.
4. He was also able to appreciate that while occluding either eye the diplopia subsided.

No drooping of eyelids/defective vision or any history suggestive of defective field of vision.

1. No h/o headache/vomiting
2. No h/o fever/trauma/surgery
3. No h/o diurnal variation
4. No h/o weakness of one side of face/limb weakness/tremors
5. No h/o mental/sleep disturbances
6. No h/o anosmia/hard of hearing/nasal regurgitation/nasal twang
7. No h/o altered bowel/bladder habit
8. No h/o scalp tenderness/jaw claudication
9. In children—rule out postvaccination.

Past History

No similar episodes in the past.

Medical Treatment History

1. He gives history of diabetes mellitus for the past 8 years, and is on irregular medications.
2. He also gives history of systemic hypertension for the past 5 years and on irregular medications.
3. No h/o surgeries in the past.

Personal History

1. Non smoker/non alcoholic
2. Normal bowel and bladder habits
3. Consuming a balanced diet.

General Examination

1. Conscious, oriented to place and time
2. Moderately built and nourished
3. No pallor

4. Icterus
5. Cyanosis
6. Clubbing
7. Lymphadenopathy
8. Pedal edema.

Vitals

1. Afebrile
2. Pulse—80 beats/min—regular rhythm, with normal volume and character.
3. Blood pressure—140/90 mm Hg recorded in supine position over the left arm.
4. Respiratory rate—18 mm times/min.

Systemic Examination

1. CVS—S1 S2 + heard. No murmurs
2. RS—normal vesicular breath sounds heard. No added sounds.
3. Abdomen—soft. No organomegaly.

Ocular Examination

1. Best corrected visual acuity 6/9 in both eyes
   (Distance)
   (Near) N6 at 33 cm with +2.0 DS.
2. No characteristic head posture noted
3. Hirschberg's test revealed 30' exotropia in the (RE)
4. On torch light examination:

Parameter	Right eye	Left eye
Lids/adnexa	Normal	Normal
Conjunctiva	Normal	Normal
Cornea	Clear	Clear
Anterior chamber	Normal depth	Normal depth
Iris	Normal color pattern	Normal color pattern
Pupil	3 mm round-D+-C+	3 mm round-D+-C+
Accommodation reflex present		
Lens	Early lens changes	Early lens changes

5. Extraocular movements: RE
   Restricted adduction, elevation and depression.
   Abduction is present
   Intorsion is present
   The movements of the left eye are normal.
6. The above findings were confirmed using a slit-lamp biomicroscopy with additional inference of
   (BE) - lens—grade I nuclear sclerosis

7. Fundus examination: Using a direct ophthalmoscope:
   i. Revealed a clear media, with normal disk and vessels, with a healthy macula FR –/+
   ii. The above findings were confirmed using a slit-lamp biomicroscopy and 90 D lens.
   iii. The peripheries were examined using an indirect ophthalmoscope and 20 D lens were found to be normal.
8. Corneal sensations (BE)—normal
9. Color vision (BE)—normal (using Ishihara's chart)
10. Tension (BE) by noncontact tonometer—16 mm of Hg
11. No signs of aberrant regeneration
12. Examination of other cranial nerves:
    i. Olfactory nerve
    ii. Optic nerve
    iii. Trigeminal nerve
    iv. Facial nerve
    v. Vestibule cochlear nerve
    vi. Glossopharyngeal nerve
    vii. Vagus nerve
    viii. Accessory nerve
    ix. Hypoglossal nerve
13. Motor system examination—normal
14. Sensory system examination—normal
15. Reflexes
    i. Superficial
    ii. Deep normal
16. Gait—normal
17. Cerebellar function tests—normal

Diagnosis

Right eye, pupil sparing, infranuclear incomplete third nerve palsy, due to an ischemic microangiopathy with probable etiology being DM/HM.

Explanation to the history taking and examination of the model case sheet

1. **Diplopia**
   i. Onset—acute, subacute, insidious in onset
   ii. Progression—progressive or regressive
      Progressive—all neoplasms, myasthenia, TRO
      Regressive—inflammatory, infection causes.
   iii. Horizontal/Vertical –
      Horizontal diplopia—lateral rectus/medial rectus involved
      Vertical diplopia—elevators/depressors involved.

    iv. Diplopia for near or far –

       Near: Trochlear nerve is involved.

       Far: Abducent nerve is involved.

    v. Increases in which gaze—diplopia increases on looking toward the side of paralyzed muscle

    vi. Diurnal variation—to rule out myasthenia gravis

    vii. Diplopia worsens in the evening: Myasthenia gravis

    viii. Diplopia worsens in the morning: Thyroid orbitopathy due to venous stasis and accumulation of glycosaminoglycans.

2. **Conditions causing ophthalmoplegia + pain**

    i. Tolosa–Hunt syndrome

    ii. Giant cell arteritis

    iii. Retrobulbar neuritis

    iv. Migraine

    v. Caroticocavernous fistula

    vi Intrinsic lesions of 3rd nerve—schwannomas/cavernous hemangiomas.

3. **History of drooping of lids**

To know the involvement of LPS—to differentiate a nuclear from an infranuclear palsy.

4. **History of defective vision**

Orbital apex syndrome—optic nerve is affected.

5. **History of defective field of vision**

To know the status of cortical function.

6. **Negative history**

    i. H/o headache/vomiting signs of raised intracranial tension.

    ii. H/o fever/fits to rule out typhoid/tick fever/glandular fever.

    iii. H/o trauma/surgery lumbar puncture can predispose to uncal herniation syndrome/other FESS and neurosurgeries too.

    iv. H/o diurnal variation myasthenia/TRO.

    v. H/o weakness at one side of face/limb weakness/tremors (to rule out involvement of other cranial nerves and the syndromes associated with third nerve palsy)

    vi. H/o epistaxis (raised blood pressure)

    vii H/o vesicular eruption on one side of face—herpetic ophthalmoplegia can predispose to third nerve palsy.

    viii H/o anosmia/nasal regurgitation/nasal twang—to rule out involvement of other cranial nerves.

    ix. H/o altered bowel/bladder habits—(involvement of autonomic nervous system).

    x. H/o scalp tenderness/jaw claudication—giant cell arteritis xi For children—can cause postvaccination neuritis

xii R/o past vaccination.

7. **Significance of medical treatment history?**

Diabetes mellitus and systemic hypertension are the most common causes of pupil sparing third nerve palsy.

8. **History of smoking and alcoholism?**

Smoker—predisposed to thromboembolism

Alcoholic—Wernicke's encephalopathy/trauma.

9. **Importance of contact to tuberculosis?**

Tuberculous meningitis can predispose to third nerve palsy.

10. **Relevance of fundus examination?**

Look for papilledema

11. **Causes of decreased corneal sensations?**

    i. Herpes simplex keratitis
    ii. Neuroparalytic keratitis
    iii. Leprosy
    iv. Herpes zoster ophthalmicus
    v. Absolute glaucoma
    vi. Acoustic neuroma
    vii Neurofibroma.

12. **Examination of other cranial nerves**

    i. *Olfactory*—using asafetida, coffee, beans, check each nostril separately.
       Optic nerve—visual acuity
       Pupil examination
       Visual fields
       Color vision
    ii. *Trigeminal nerve*—motor muscles of mastication/jaw deviates toward paralyzed side
       Sensory—corneal sensations
       Sensations over face.
    iii. *Facial nerve*—motor-orbicularis oculi
       Wrinkling of forehead orbicularis oris (whistling) smile and dense (mouth deviated to healthy side) inflate mouth with air.
       Sensory—test in anterior 2/3rd of tongue.
    iv. *Vestibule cochlear:*
       For cochlear function use 512 Hz because higher frequency—less accurate in finding difference between air and bone conduction.
       - Lower frequency—vibrations produced may be misinterpreted as sound.

    – Rinne's test: Normal sensory neural hearing loss—lateralized to normal ear conductive loss—lateralized to deaf ear.
    – For vestibular functions we check:
- Nystagmus
- Positional vertigo
- Romberg's test.

v. *Glossopharyngeal nerve*—taste in post 1/3rd of tongue palatal reflex.

vi. *Vagus*—gag reflex

vii. **Spinal accessory nerve**—sternomastoid/trapezius muscle

viii. *Hypoglossal nerve*—tongue deviates to paralyzed side.

GLAUCOMA—MODEL CASE SHEET

A 56-year-old gentleman came to us for complaints of:

Defective vision of the right eye (RE)—1 year duration and left eye (LE) of 6 months duration.

History of Present Illness

On elaboration, he revealed he had been suffering from defective vision for the past 1 year. He had consulted an ophthalmologist at his place who said he had raised pressures in both his eyes, and put him on topical medications, twice a day regime for both his eyes. He was not compliant to his medicines, and on his follow-up visit, his doctor had advised surgery for his right eye. He underwent the surgery to reduce his eye pressures. He feels that vision is unsatisfactory in both his eyes and has come for a second opinion.

No history of night blindness

No h/o frequent change of glasses

No h/o headache

No h/o colored haloes

No h/o redness/watering/pain

No h/o injury/trauma.

Past History

Known diabetic for the past 15 years on oral hypoglycemic agents and an asthmatic on inhalational therapy whenever symptomatic.

Apart from the medications which he has been using for both his eyes, twice daily for the past 1 year and surgery to lower pressure in his right eye 6 months back, there is no other medical or surgical history.

Personal History

Smoker, smokes 2–3 beedis per day for the past 30 years.

Not an alcoholic.

Family History

No history of diabetes or ocular diseases amongst/among the family members.

General Examination

Well-built and nourished.

Pulse rate—76/min, regular in rhythm and volume.

Blood pressure—130/70 mm of Hg

Cardiovascular, respiratory, and central nervous system examination within normal limits.

Ocular Examination

Parameter	Right eye	Left eye
Distance		
Unaided vision	6/60	6/24
With pin hole	6/12	6/9
Near vision	N8 at 33 cm with +2D	N6 at 33 cm with +2D

No Facial Asymmetry

Parameter	Right eye	Left eye
Lids and adnexa	Normal	Normal
Conjunctiva	A flat, diffuse translucent bleb, extending from 11 o'clock to 2 o'clock position superiorly above the limbus, with dilated tortuous vessels over its surface and subconjunctival fibrosis obscuring the underlying details was seen	Normal
Cornea	Clear	Clear
Anterior chamber	Normal in depth centrally and in the periphery	Normal in depth centrally and in the periphery
Iris	A single, peripheral triangular defect measuring 2 mm in size seen superiorly at the 12 o'clock position close to the limbus, suggestive of a surgical iridectomy is seen. Retroillumination was positive	Normal in color and pattern
Pupil	4 mm, round and reacting sluggishly to light, with grade 3 RAPD	Normal in size and shape, reacting well to direct, indirect being slightly sluggish
Lens	Nuclear sclerosis, grade 2	Nuclear sclerosis, grade 2
EOM	Full	Full

Fundus Examination

Parameter	Right eye	Left eye
Media	Clear	Clear
Disk	Vertically oval disk with well-defined margins. Cup disk ratio was 0.9 with a diffuse, circumferential loss of neuroretinal rim. Bayonetting of vessels and laminar dot sign was present. Surrounding nerve fiber layer seen with the help of a red-free filter showed a diffuse loss of RNFL	Vertically oval disk with well-defined margins. Cup disk ratio being 0.75 with a focal notching superior and corresponding thinning of neuroretinal rim was seen. An arcuate defect was seen superiorly in the nerve fiber layer with the help of a red-free filter corresponding to the superior notch
Posterior pole	Foveal reflex present and background retina was normal	Foveal reflex was present and background retina was normal

Gonioscopy

Right eye	Left eye
Trabecular meshwork seen in all four quadrants with a patent ostium and peripheral iridectomy seen superiorly	Trabecular meshwork seen in all four quadrants

Intraocular Pressures

Recorded with Goldmann's applanation tonometer showed

Right eye	Left eye
26 mm of Hg	24 mm of Hg

Diagnosis

Right eye: Primary open-angle glaucoma status post-trabeculectomy with failed bleb and grade 2 nuclear sclerosis.

Left eye: Primary open-angle glaucoma and grade 2 nuclear sclerosis.

1. **Why do we ask for history of night blindness?**
   i. Defective dark adaptation is a feature of open-angle glaucoma
   ii. Use of miotics will accentuate night blindness.

2. **What is the cause for frequent change of glasses?**
   i. Patients experience more difficulty for near vision since constant high pressure over zonules and ciliary body impairs accommodation
   ii. Patients tend to confuse defective field of vision with defective vision and hence repeatedly change glasses.

3. **What can cause sudden loss of vision in a glaucoma patient?**
   i. Acute IOP rise resulting in corneal edema
   ii. Central retinal vein occlusion
   iii. Post-trabeculectomy in advanced glaucoma—snuff out phenomena.

4. **What are the structural abnormalities you will look for in a case of glaucoma?**
   i. **Lids and adnexa**
      - Hemangioma (Sturge–Weber)
      - Hypertrichosis (use of latanoprost)
      - Periocular pigmentation (use of epinephrine).
   ii. **Conjunctiva**
      - Dilated tortuous episcleral vessels (Sturge–Weber)
      - Bleb (location, extent, presence of microcysts, vascularity, visibility of scleral flaps, infection, presence of aqueous leak, sub-conjunctival fibrosis)
      - Circumcorneal congestion (In acute congestive glaucoma).

iii. **Cornea**
   - Edema
   - Descemet's folds
   - Keratic precipitates
   - Pigments on the endothelium (Krukenberg's spindle in pigmentary glaucoma)
   - Pseudoexfoliation on the endothelium
   - Prominent Schwalbe's line—congenital glaucoma
   - Peripheral anterior synechiae
   - Megalocornea
   - Cornea plana
   - Sclerocornea
   - Congenital corneal opacity (Peter's anomaly)
   - Prominent corneal nerves (neurofibromatosis).

iv. **Anterior chamber**
   - Depth—peripheral and central
   - Reactions—flare and cells
   - Hyphema
   - Hypopyon.

v. **Iris**
   - Aniridia
   - Atrophic patches (following acute attack)
   - Nodules
   - Holes
   - Pseudoexfoliation material
   - Transillumination defects
   - Peripheral iridectomy (number, position, patency, surgical/laser)
   - Iris cysts
   - Nevus
   - Ectropion uvea.

vi. **Pupil**
   - Size
   - Shape
   - Number
   - Reaction to light—direct and indirect
   - Resistant to dilatation
   - Seclusion or occlusion papillae.

vii. **Lens**
   - Pseudoexfoliation on anterior lens capsule
   - Glaucomflecken
   - Cataract—intumescent/dislocated/subluxated

- Zonular dialysis
- Spherophakia.

5. **What are the management strategies for the following scenarios?**

   i. **Primary open-angle suspect**

   Baseline investigations

   - Tension applanation
   - Central corneal thickness
   - Baseline fundus photo
   - Nerve fiber analysis—GDx
   - HFA-SITA SWAP—glaucoma progression analysis
   - OCT—macular thickness analysis, i.e. ganglion cell complex.

   Treatment

   - Observe the patient if no risk factors.
   - Follow-up after 2 months. If progression is documented, start antiglaucoma therapy.

   ii. **Established primary open-angle glaucoma**

   Baseline investigations

   - Tension applanation
   - Central corneal thickness
   - Baseline fundus photo
   - Nerve fiber analysis—GDx (role controversial in established glaucoma)
   - HFA-24-2
   - OCT—macular thickness analysis, i.e. ganglion cell complex.

   Treatment

   - Calculate the target pressure: This is done using the following formula

     $$TP = IP\,(1-IP/100)-Z+/-2$$

     where: TP = *target pressure*
              IP = *initial pressure*
              Z = *functional status*
              (disk damage/field changes)

     Z-0 *Glaucoma suspect (Low risk)*
     Z-0 *Glaucoma suspect (High risk)*
        Z-1 *Early glaucoma*
        Z-3 *Moderate glaucoma*
        Z-5 *Severe glaucoma*
        Z-7 *End-stage glaucoma*
   - Start on single drug therapy (Prostaglandin analogs are the first choice or else beta-blockers, alpha adrenergic agonists can be started).

– Review after 2 months and see if target pressure is maintained. If not consider substituting or adding another drug.
– Follow-up, and in spite of maximal tolerated medical therapy if the pressures are still not under control, then consider trabeculectomy.

iii. **POAG with significant cataract**

The following considerations should be taken into account while performing surgery in a glaucoma patient:

– Miotic pupils
– Posterior synechiae
– Exfoliation—zonular weakness
– Congested eyes—bleeding
– Prior surgery—scarring/filtering bleb
– Systemic diseases—diabetes, hypertension
– Ocular conditions—myopia, shallow chamber
– Increased incidence of postoperative IOP rise
– Suprachoroidal hemorrhage.

- **Cataract alone can be performed in the following scenario:**
  - Acceptable IOP control with one or two medications
  - No significant visual field loss or disk damage
  - Older age
  - Conditions where compliance and drug intolerance are not an issue
  - Higher target IOP.

  Advantages of doing cataract alone:
  - Single procedure
  - Technically easier
- Short surgical time
- Reduced operative and postoperative complications
- Temporal clear corneal approach enables preserving viable conjunctiva.

Disadvantages of doing cataract alone:
- Early postoperative spike of intraocular pressure
- Long-term IOP control questionable
- Subsequent filtering surgery prone for failure.

- **Combined surgery (Cataract and filtering surgery) can be performed in the following scenario:**
  - Multiple medications required to control IOP
  - Use of glaucoma medications restricted by cost, intolerance, compliance issues
  - Significant glaucomatous visual loss
  - Presence of ocular risk factors—exfoliation, pigment dispersion, angle recession

○ Monocular status—earlier visual recovery
○ Two separate procedures not feasible.

Advantages of combined surgery:

○ Restore vision promptly
○ Single procedure
○ Reduced glaucoma medications
○ Early postoperative IOP control
○ Long-term IOP control
○ Antimetabolite use possible to enhance success
○ Facilitate assessment of disk and visual fields.

Disadvantages of combined surgery:

○ More complications—shallow chamber, bleb leak, choroidal effusion/hemorrhage, hypotony, infection, astigmatism
○ Visual recovery longer than in cataract alone
○ Intensive postoperative care requirements than cataract alone
○ Less IOP control than filtering surgery alone—success of filtering compromised by filtering surgery
○ Glaucoma medications postoperative.

A CASE OF UNILATERAL OLD RHEGMATOGENOUS RETINAL DETACHMENT (RRD)

RE—Subtotal RRD
LE—lattice with hole S/P barrage laser

Right Eye

Distant direct ophthalmoscopy: shows a gray reflex.

Direct ophthalmoscopy close to face

1. Media is clear.
2. Disk appears normal in size, vertically oval, pink in color having a cup–disk ratio of 0.3 with a healthy neuroretinal rim. The margins are well defined.
3. The vessels are seen arising from the center of the disk, branching dichotomously, and tortuous in nature.
4. A convex shallow smooth membrane is seen superonasal, inferonasal, and inferotemporal to the optic disk involving the macula, suggestive of retinal detachment with macula off (focused using high plus power).

On slit-lamp examination

1. PCIOL with PCR present
2. AVF examination shows pigments or tobacco dust.

On Indirect ophthalmoscopy

1. Media is clear
2. Disk appears normal in size, vertically oval, pink in color having a cup–disk ratio of 0.3 with a healthy neuroretinal rim.

3. The vessels are seen arising from the center of the disk, branching dichotomously, and tortuous in nature.

4. A convex shallow smooth elevation of the retina with loss of underlying choroidal pattern is seen. This undulating membrane in the vitreous cavity extends from 2 o'clock to 9 o'clock involving the macula, suggestive of subtotal RRD with macula off. Minimal shifting fluid is present.

5. A wedge-shaped area of retina superotemporal to the optic disk appears to be attached.

6. A retinal tear with the ends pointing toward ora suggestive of horse shoe tear is seen at 2 o'clock position in the equatorial zone. Rolled edges and wrinkling of surface is noted.

7. Full thickness fixed puckering of the detached retina with overlying preretinal membrane spanning 2 o'clock hours at the end of inferotemporal arcade is suggestive of star folds.

8. Intraretinal cyst is seen 1 disk diameter away from the disk at 3 o'clock.

9. Linear yellow areas beneath the surface of retinal detachment suggestive of subretinal bands with demarcation line are present in the inferotemporal area.

Left Eye

Distant direct ophthalmoscopy: shows red glow.

Direct ophthalmoscopy close to face

1. Media is clear

2. Disk appears normal in size, vertically oval, pink in color having a cup–disk ratio of 0.3 with healthy neuroretinal rim.

3. The vessels is seen arising from the center of the disk, branching dichotomously maintaining an arteriovenous ratio of 2:3.

4. Macula appears normal and the foveal reflex is seen.

5. The background retina appears normal.

On slit-lamp examination: the above findings are confirmed.

On indirect ophthalmoscopy: on sclera indentation

1. The peripheral retina shows a sharply demarcated spindle-shaped area of retinal thinning spanning 3 o'clock hours, parallel to the ora, in the periphery of inferotemporal quadrant with vitreous condensation at the margin, suggestive of lattice degeneration.

2. A full thickness defect in the retina surrounded by two rows of regular, equally spaced pigmented lesions indicative of lasered retinal hole is seen adjacent to the lattice.

Rhegmatogenous Retinal Detachment (Fresh)

Fundus examination of right eye

1. Distant direct ophthalmoscopy at one arm distance showed a dull glow/gray reflex.

2. Direct ophthalmoscopy close to face revealed a clear media.
3. Retina could be seen with high "plus" power of the direct ophthalmoscope.
4. Upon further examination with slit-lamp biomicroscopy with 90D and indirect ophthalmoscopy with scleral indentation, the following findings were seen.
5. Brown pigmented tobacco dust like pigments were seen dispersed in the anterior vitreous suggestive of Shafer sign.
6. A bullous, convex elevation of the retina with corrugated appearance and convexity facing toward the disk with loss of underlying choroidal pattern was seen from 1 o'clock hour to 10 o'clock hours position suggestive of subtotal retinal detachment which was extending from ora serrata toward disk area.
7. The disk could be visualized amidst the detached retinal folds and it was vertically oval, larger in size, pink in color with a tilted conformation and well-defined margins having a cup–disk ratio of 0.4 with healthy neuroretinal rim.
8. Peripapillary chorioretinal atrophy was seen.
9. The vessels over the detached retina appeared darker than in the flat retina and hence the venules and arterioles could not be differentiated.
10. The detached retina was seen undulating with eye movements.
11. The highest point of the detached retina was noted supero nasally near 1 o'clock position.
12. Macula was off.
13. A superior wedge of attached retina was seen from 10 o'clock to 1 o'clock hour.
14. A red color horse shoe-shaped tear with the ends pointing toward the ora was seen in the equatorial zone of the retinal surface superiorly between 1 and 2 o'clock position.

Fundus examination of the other eye (left eye)

1. Indirect ophthalmoscopy with scleral indentation of left eye showed the following findings.
2. The disk was vertically oval, larger in size, pink in color with a tilted conformation and well-defined margins having a cup–disk ratio of 0.4 with healthy neuroretinal rim.
3. Peri papillary chorioretinal atrophy was seen.
4. Vessels arise from the center of the disk branching dichotomously maintaining an arteriovenous ratio of 2:3.
5. Background retina showed a pale tessellated tigroid appearance with visibility of large choroidal vessels.
6. Foveal reflex was dull due to retinal pigment degeneration at macular region.
7. An island of sharply demarcated, circumferentially oriented, spindle-shaped area of retinal thinning suggestive of lattice degeneration was

seen from 12 o'clock to 2 o'clock hours zone between the equator and ora serrata with some condensed vitreous at the margin.

8. No holes were found within the lattice.

Diagnosis

1. Right eye Fresh Subtotal Rhegmatogenous Retinal Detachment-Macula off in Myopic Phakic eye

2. Left eye Myopic fundus with lattice degeneration in Phakic eye.

Bilateral Retinitis Pigmentosa with Consecutive Optic Atrophy

Fundus examination of both eyes

1. Distant direct ophthalmoscopy at one arm distance showed a faint red glow

2. Direct ophthalmoscopy close to face revealed a clear media

3. On direct ophthalmoscopy close to the face, the following findings were seen

4. Fine dust like pigmented cells, cotton ball, and spindle-shaped opacities suggestive of vitreous condensations (not in all cases)

5. Disk was normal in size, vertically oval shaped, CDR was 0.3 with well-defined golden ring or yellowish halo with waxy pallor suggestive of consecutive optic atrophy

6. Vessel arising from the center of the disk and branching dichotomously. There is marked arteriolar attenuation and the ratio is altered to 1:3

7. Background retina showed multiple scattered star-shaped pigment deposits in all the four quadrants more in the superotemporal quadrant. In addition, there were multiple hypopigmented patches along the major vascular arcades, more in the midperiphery. The vessels could be traced over the lesion characteristic of intraretinal bony spicules suggesting retinal pigment epithelial atrophy and intraretinal migration of RPE.

8. Upon indentation using the indirect ophthalmoscope, similar bony spicules could also be seen close to ora serrata.

9. There was diffuse mottling and granularity of retinal pigment epithelium

10. Overall gray fundus appearance (advanced stage) with greater visibility of underlying choroidal vessels.

Macular findings (any of the signs could be seen)

1. Healthy macula with a good foveal reflex (early disease)

2. Increased luster with whitish wavy lines suggestive of preretinal fibrosis

3. Tapetal like reflex (bright sheen) seen in the foveal or parafoveal region (classical of X linked RP)

4. Loss of foveal reflex with diffuse thickening of surrounding retina with cyst like spaces (seen with red-free filter) suggestive of cystoid macular edema.

A CASE OF RE–MACULAR DYSTROPHY AND LE–ACUTE CORNEAL GRAFT REJECTION

A 35-year-old female patient presented to us with complaints of

1. **Redness, pain in LE X 10 days**
2. **Defective vision in LE X 1 week.**

History of Presenting Illness

The redness and pain started in her left eye around 10 days back. Initially, the redness was limited only to the lower part of the right eye, but it slowly involved the entire eye. The pain was pricking in nature, constant throughout the waking hours and relieved while keeping the eye closed. After 3 days of pain and redness, she noticed gradual defective vision in her left eye. The defective vision is more in the early morning hours, especially after getting up from sleep and gets slightly better as the day progresses. The defective vision is the same for both the distance and near.

1. No h/o trauma
2. H/o photophobia present
3. No h/o discharge from the eyes
4. H/o of an eye surgery performed in her left eye, around 2 years back for defective vision and had reasonably good vision until the present episode.

Past History

The patient gives a history of mild defective vision of both her eyes from the adolescent age from around 17 years of age in both her eyes. She used to get constant irritation and watering, which used to subside on its own. After around 2 years, these episodes become more and more regular and the visual acuity deteriorated significantly. She consulted her local ophthalmologist, who advised her to use lubricant eye drops and protective eye wear and advised her to consider surgery, whenever she could not do her normal day-to-day activities.

The patient persisted with this regimen until around 2 years back when she underwent surgery for her left eye, because of profound defective vision. She mentions this surgery as an "eye transplantation" and was hospitalized for a period of 10 days.

Subsequently she was regular with her follow-up treatment. She felt that her visual acuity in her operated eye significantly improved over a period of 12 months. She used to get irritation on and off in her left eye and visited the hospital regularly. In some of these follow up, some sutures were removed in her left eye. Since her visual acuity in her left eye had improved and since she did not develop any irritation or pain, she has discontinued all medications for the past 3 months.

1. N/K/C/O DM, hypertension, IHD, BA.
2. No other systemic illness.

Personal History: Veg, non smoker, and non alcoholic.

Family History

Mother and elder sister had similar complaints. The mother had undergone two eye surgeries, one in each eye, while the sister had undergone surgery for her left eye.

General Examination

Well-built and nourished.

PR: 78 BPM, regular in rhythm and volume.

BP: 120/ 80 mmHg.

CVS : S1 and s2 heard. No murmurs.

RS: NVBS

P/A: Soft. No organomegaly.

CNS: NAD.

Ocular Examination

Features	RE	LE
BCVA	6/24	1/60
With PH	6/18p	Nip

No facial asymmetry noted.

Features	RE	LE
Lids and adnexa	Normal	Normal No dystichiasis-predisposes to graft rejection due to constant irritation
Conjunctiva	Normal	Circumciliary congestion present, more in the inferior half
Cornea		A centrally placed **Edematous corneal graft** of about **8 mm** present secured to the recipient cornea which has numerous deposits with interrupted sutures. 8 10-0 nylon **sutures present. Of these,** 3 are loose and are seen in the 3, 5, and 7 o'clock positions.

(Continued)

(Continued)

Features	RE	LE
		Three other sutures (at 8, 10, and 11 o'clock positions) have **sutural infiltrates** seen predominantly in the donor part. Around 10 suture marks are seen in other areas, from where sutures would have been removed earlier. **Graft Host Junction Edematous** between 9 and 12 o'clock position and 5 to 7 o'clock position. **Superficial blood vessels** seen extending from 2 to 8 o'clock position. They are loosely branched **Two areas of deep vascularization** seen, one at 10 o'clock position extending about 4 mm toward the center of the donor graft and the second at 4 o'clock position extending upto 6 mm toward the center of the graft.
Epithelium	Few tiny **epithelial erosions—** 2 centrally, 3 along the periphery at around 7 o'clock position, 3 mm away from the temporal limbus seen.	**Epithelial edema** present. No epithelial rejection line and epithelial defect seen.
Stroma	Diffusely hazy from the center to the periphery. In this generalized haziness, there are some areas of irregular, raised grayish white deposits, seen more in the central part of the cornea. **There are no intervening clear spaces and there is a diffuse stromal haze.**	**Diffuse stromal edema** extending throughout the graft, more prominently seen at the central 360 degree extending upto 5 mm toward the graft host junction and peripherally between 9 and 12 o'clock position and 5-7 o'clock position. **Full thickness stromal haze** seen peripherally in and around 10 o'clock position, adjacent to the **deep corneal vascularization.**

(Continued)

(*Continued*)

Features	RE	LE
Descemet's membrane		Multiple **DM Folds** seen on the donor graft.
Endothelium	Multiple **guttaes** are seen temporally, 4 mm away from the limbus, extending between 7 and 9 o'clock	Multiple **Keratic precipitates** arranged linearly, starting peripherally at around 4 o'clock position and extending upto the center, accompanied by corneal vascularization. (Suggestive of the pathognomic **"ENDOTHELIAL REJECTION LINE OF KHODADOUST".**) Few scattered Keratic precipitates are seen on the endothelium. The peripheral cornea of the recipient reveals a similar picture of hazy cornea like that of the fellow eye.
Anterior chamber	Normal depth, quiet	2 Plus **flare** 2 Plus **cells** Seen
Iris	NCP	Hazy view
Pupil	3 mm, round, reacting to light	Hazy view
Lens	Clear	Hazy view
EOM	Full	Full
Fundus Distant direct Ophthalomoscopy	Revealed red glow	Revealed a dull glow

Diagnosis

Right eye: Macular dystrophy
Left eye: Post-pkp acute endothelia
               Graft rejection

CORNEA PROFORMA FOR A CASE OF KERATOCONUS IN ONE EYE AND A CLEAR CORNEAL GRAFT IN THE OTHER EYE

A 25-year-old male patient came to us with complaints of defective vision in the right eye for the past 7 years.

History of Presenting Illness

He was apparently normal, 7 years back, when he started noticing defective vision in both his eyes. This was insidious in onset and gradual in progression. It was painless and more for distant vision than for near.

He was prescribed spectacles for the same. While he was satisfied for the first 6 months, his distant vision once again deteriorated and he was once again prescribed a change of prescription. This did not improve his vision and thereafter he was advised to wear contact lenses. He wore the same for 2 years, and after some time became intolerant to contact lenses in his left eye. He was then advised surgery for the left eye and following surgery, his vision improved in the left eye.

1. H/o frequent change of glasses for his right eye.
2. H/o irritation and pain on and off in the right eye after even 4 hours of contact lens use.
3. No h/o itching and frequent rubbing of the eyes (rules out ocular allergy and VKC).
4. No h/o episodes of ocular pain associated with redness and sudden decrease in vision (rules out acute hydrops).
5. No h/o double vision (rules out monocular diplopia).

Past History

1. H/o/o ocular surgery in the left eye 4 years back following which he was on regular medication for 2 years.
2. He gives history of repeated suture removals in the left eye on and off for the past 4 years. The last episode was around 3 months back.

Systemic History

No h/o systemic disorders like atrophy or asthma or joint deformities (rules out syndromic associations).

Family History

No h/o similar complaints among parents or siblings (keratoconus has autosomal dominant mode of inheritance).

Personal History

Takes mixed diet. Nonsmoker and nonalcoholic.

General Examination

Height and weight (r/o malformations associated with syndromes).

Vitals

Pulse rate, blood pressure.

Systemic Examination

CVS; S1S2, presence of cardiac murmurs (r/o cardiac abnormalities associated with syndromes)

Ocular Examination

1. Vision with pinhole in RE—6/60 and 6/9 in the left eye
2. Scissoring reflex on retinoscopic examination.

Torch light examination

Features	Right eye	Left eye
Facial symmetry	Normal	Normal
Lids	"V"-shaped configuration of the lower lid on downgaze suggestive of Munson sign. Look for ptosis (to rule out LPS disinsertion due to RGP wear). edema, excoriations, congestion (rules out of allergy)	Normal. e/o trichiasis, entropion, lagophthalmos (predispose to graft rejection) e/o lid edema, congestion
Sclera	Normal (rules out blue sclera)	Normal
Conjunctiva	e/o bulbar and palpebral congestion (rules out allergy and hydrops)	e/o congestion or chemosis (rules out signs of rejection, graft infection)
Cornea	Conical reflection on the nasal cornea on shining the torch from temporal aspect suggestive of Rizzuti sign	A central clear corneal graft present secured to the recipient peripheral cornea by interrupted sutures
Ant. chamber	Normal depth	Normal depth
Iris	Normal in color and pattern. (no e/o aniridia)	Iris normal in color and pattern
Pupil	3 mm size, circular in shape, brisk, regular, sustained reaction to direct and consensual light reflex	3 mm size, circular in shape, brisk, regular, sustained reaction to direct and consensual light reflex
Lens	Clear	Clear
EOM	Full and free	Full and free

SLIT-LAMP examination: the above findings on torch light examination were confirmed on slit-lamp evaluation.

Ocular findings	Right eye	Left eye
Lids	Normal	Normal
Sclera	Normal	Normal
Conjunctiva	Normal. e/o papillae	Normal. Tear film height appears normal
Cornea	Epithelium: —deposition of iron pigments in a semi-circular pattern in the mid peripheral area. —on examining with a cobalt blue filter it was better delineated, well-defined inferiorly, nasally and temporally deficient superiorly s/o of Fleischers ring.	—a full thickness central clear disk of donor corneal tissue of around 8 mm in diameter, round in shape is seen anchored to the peripheral recipient host cornea. 10-0 nylon interrupted sutures with

(Continued)

(*Continued*)

Ocular findings	Right eye	Left eye
	—e/o subepithelial scarring (r/o previous hydrops). Bowmans membrane: e/o prominent corneal nerves. Stroma: Conical protrusion of the cornea is noted along the central and inferior midperipheral aspect, of around 7 mm diameter suggestive of corneal steepening. —stromal thickness reduced by around 1/3rd in the central area of the corneal steepening as compared to the adjacent areas suggestive of corneal thinning. The area of thinning is similar to the area of steepening-fine, vertical lines present at the level of deep stroma in the central aspect of the corneal steepening and disappear on gentle pressure over the lids suggestive of Vogt's striae. Endothelium: appears normal	their knots buried in the donor side is seen. None of it is loose. There are no areas of infiltration or vascularization. Additionally, 10 other areas of old suture marks are also seen. —the graft host junction appears well secure with good wound apposition. The stroma, Descemet's membrane, and endothelium are normal. There is no evidence of any keratic precipitates
Anterior chamber	Normal depth. No e/o cells or flare	Normal depth. No e/o cells or flare
Iris	Normal color and pattern	Normal
Pupil	Normal	Normal
Lens	Clear	Clear
Fundus	Distant direct ophthalmoscopy revealed an oil droplet sign	Distant direct ophthalmoscopy revealed a red glow
	Close to face examination showed an —optic disk size, shape, margins, cup–disk ratio, neuroretinal rim, and vessels. —foveal reflex and background retina (r/o lebers and retinitis pigmentosa)	Close to face examination showed an —optic disk size, shape, margins, cup–disk ratio, neuroretinal rim, and vessels. —foveal reflex and background retina

Diagnosis

RE—keratoconus

LE—a full thickness clear corneal graft s/p optical keratoplasty.

Papilledema—case presentation proforma

Fundus right eye	Fundus left eye
Distant direct ophthalmoscopy at one arm distance showed a good red glow	Distant direct ophthalmoscopy at one arm distance showed a good red glow
Direct ophthalmoscopy close to face revealed a clear media	Direct ophthalmoscopy close to face revealed a clear media
Size and shape of the disk could not be assessed due to blurring of disk margins and elevation of disk	Size and shape of the disk could not be assessed due to blurring of disk margins and elevation of disk
Disk was markedly hyperemic	Disk was markedly hyperemic
Margins were ill-defined throughout, blurred, and obscured	Margins were ill defined throughout, blurred and obscured
Gross elevation of the optic nerve head measuring +6 D equivalent in the direct ophthalmoscopic evaluation corresponding to about 2 mm elevation from the retinal surface	Gross elevation of the optic nerve head measuring +6 D equivalent in the direct ophthalmoscopic evaluation corresponding to about 2 mm elevation from the retinal surface
Physiological cup was obliterated	Physiological cup was obliterated
Vessels were arising from the center of the disk with an arteriovenous ratio of 2:4. The normal dichotomous branching was not appreciated	Vessels were arising from the center of the disk with an arteriovenous ratio of 2:4. The normal dichotomous branching was not appreciated
Retinal veins were congested, dilated, tortuous, and engorged. The engorgement was more marked adjacent to the disk. The arteries appeared normal	Retinal veins were congested, dilated, tortuous, and engorged. The engorgement was more marked adjacent to the disk. The arteries appeared normal
Areas of apparent venous discontinuity was noted, more in the temporal aspect of the disk	Areas of apparent venous discontinuity was noted
Spontaneous venous pulsation over the optic nerve head was absent	Spontaneous venous pulsation over the optic nerve head was absent
Segments of the major blood vessels seemed obscured as they cross the disk margin	Segments of the major blood vessels seemed obscured as they cross the disk margin
A peripapillary halo was seen	A peripapillary halo was seen
Blurring, edema, and opacification of the peripapillary retinal nerve fiber layer was seen	Blurring, edema, and opacification of the peripapillary retinal nerve fiber layer was seen
Reflexes from the peripapillary retinal nerve fiber layer were distorted	Reflexes from the peripapillary retinal nerve fiber layer were distorted
Numerous flame-shaped hemorrhages were seen adjacent to the disk margins more marked superiorly from 10 o'clock to 12 o'clock position and at 6 o'clock position	Numerous flame-shaped hemorrhages were seen adjacent to the disk margins more marked superiorly from 10 o'clock to 12 o'clock position and at 6 o'clock position

(Continued)

(*Continued*)

Fundus right eye	Fundus left eye
Numerous grayish white fluffy lesions with indistinct margins were seen adjacent to the disk margins suggestive of cotton wool spots	Numerous grayish white fluffy lesions with indistinct margins were seen adjacent to the disk margins suggestive of cotton wool spots
Circumferential retino-choroidal folds were seen for 360° around the disk more marked nasally suggestive of Paton's lines	Circumferential retinochoroidal folds were seen for 360° around the disk more marked nasally suggestive of Paton's lines
Foveal reflex was dull	Foveal reflex was dull
No hemorrhages/hard exudates/macular fan/macular star seen at the macula	No hemorrhages/hard exudates/macular fan/macular star seen at the macula

On slit-lamp biomicroscopy with 90 D lens, the above findings were confirmed. The elevation of the optic nerve head was clearly demonstrated using this method.

On indirect ophthalmoscopy, the retinal peripheries were normal.

Diagnosis

In both eyes: Established papilledema.

UVEA: MODEL CASE SHEET

Mr X, 40-year-old male, tailor by occupation, presented to us with chief complaints of pain, redness, watering in right eye for 1 week.

History of Presenting Illness

He complaints of pain, redness, watering in right eye for 1 week which was sudden in onset and progressive in nature. The pain was dull aching, non-radiating, continuous in nature. There were no aggravating or relieving factors. Associated with blurring of vision.

1. H/o difficulty in seeing bright light for 5 days
2. H/o defective vision in right eye for 1 year
3. Which was insidious in onset
4. Progressive in nature
5. No h/o discharge
6. No h/o headache
7. No h/o floaters
8. No h/o trauma
9. No h/o fever/chronic cough/loss of weight
10. H/o low backache on and off for 1 year
11. No h/o joint pain
12. No h/o skin problems/hair problems
13. No h/o mouth ulcers
14. No h/o genital ulcers
15. No h/o ringing in ears/hearing loss.

Past History

He gives history of similar pain and redness in right eye—three episodes in the past 1 year. Last episode was around 4 months back. All episodes resolved with some topical medications. Details were not available.

1. No h/o eye surgeries
2. No h/o diabetes/hypertension
3. No h/o any other systemic disorders.

Personal History

1. Takes mixed diet
2. Non smoker/nonalcoholic
3. No h/o bladder/bowel disturbances
4. No h/o bath in river/pond/pool
5. No h/o contact with pet animals/livestock.

Family History

1. No h/o similar complaints among family members
2. No h/o tuberculosis/diabetes/other autoimmune disorders among family members.

General Examination

1. Patient well-built and nourished
2. Conscious and oriented
3. No pallor/icterus/cyanosis/clubbing
4. No lymphadenopathy/pedal edema.

Vital Signs

1. Afebrile
2. Pulse rate–80/min; respiratory rate–18/min
3. Blood pressure–110/80 mm Hg
4. Cardiovascular, respiratory, and central nervous system examination were within normal limits.

Ocular Examination

1. Best corrected visual acuity
2. RE 6/24 with PH 6/12
3. LE 6/6
4. No abnormal head posture
5. No facial asymmetry
6. Corneal reflex: Appears orthophoric by Hirschberg's test
7. Extraocular movements: Full range.

On torch light examination:

Parameter	Right eye	Left eye
Lids and adnexa	Normal	Normal
Conjunctiva	Circumciliary congestion	Normal
Cornea	Clear	Clear
Anterior chamber	Normal depth	Normal depth
Iris	Normal in color and pattern	Normal in color and pattern
Pupil	4 mm, irregular, sluggishly reacting to light	4 mm, round, reacting to light
Lens	Cataractous lens	Clear

On torch light examination:

Parameter	Right eye	Left eye
Lids and adnexa	Normal No poliosis No madarosis	Normal
Conjunctiva	Dilated, congested vessels arranged radially around limbus suggestive of circumcorneal congestion	Normal
Cornea	Around 20–25 fresh, small sized, non-confluent, non-pigmented, keratic precipitates were seen on the inferior aspect of corneal endothelium in base down triangular pattern	Clear
Anterior chamber	Normal depth Around 10–20 cells were seen corresponding to grade 2+ Associated flare noted and iris and lens details were hazy corresponding to grade 3+	Normal depth
Iris	Normal color. But the pattern was lost. No iris atrophic patches. No iris nodules seen	Normal color and pattern
Pupil	4 mm, irregular, sluggishly reacting to light. Posterior synechiae seen from 3 o'clock to 5 o'clock	4 mm, round, reacting to light
Lens	Posterior subcapsular cataract suggestive of complicated cataract	Clear
Anterior vitreous face	Quiet	Quiet

Fundus examination

Direct ophthalmoscopy	Right eye	Left eye
At arm's distance	Central dark shadow with peripheral red glow due to central PSCC	Good red glow
Close to face	Media hazy due to anterior chamber reaction and posterior subcapsular cataract. Vertically oval disk Normal in size and shape. Cup–disk ratio 0.3.vessels arising from the center of disk branching dichotomously maintaining A:V ratio of 2:3 Foveal reflex (+) Background retina appears normal	Media clear. Vertically oval disk Normal in size and shape. Margins well defined. Cup–disk ratio 0.3. Vessels arising from the center of disk branching dichotomously maintaining A:V ratio of 2:3 Foveal reflex (+) Background retina normal

The above findings were confirmed using slit-lamp biomicroscopy and 90 D lens

The peripheries examined using an indirect ophthalmoscope and 20 D lens were found to be normal.

Intraocular Pressure

Recorded with Goldmann's applanation tonometer (at 9:00 am) showed.

Right eye	Left eye
19 mm Hg	18 mm Hg

Clinical Summary

Mr X, 40-year-old male came with complaints of pain, redness, watering, photophobia in the right eye for 1 week. He had h/o defective vision in the same eye for 1 year.

On examination, right eye showed circumciliary congestion with non-granulomatous keratic precipitates on endothelium. Anterior chamber showed 2+ cells with 3+ flare along with posterior synechiae and posterior subcapsular cataract. Left eye was within normal limits.

Fundus examination of both eyes were within normal limits.

Anatomical Diagnosis

1. Right eye—acute on chronic nongranulomatous anterior uveitis with complicated cataract
2. Left eye—normal.

Differential Diagnosis

1. HLA B27 associated uveitis
2. Tuberculosis
3. Syphilis
4. Viral

Index

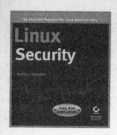

LINUX SECURITY (CRAIG HUNT LINU...

RAMÓN J. HONTAÑÓN

ISBN: 0-7821-2741-X   512 p...

This is the most complete, most advanced guide to Linux security you'll find anywhere. Written by a Linux security expert with over a decade of experience, *Linux Security* teaches you, step-by-step, all the standard and advanced techniques you need to know to keep your Linux environment safe from threats of all kinds. Hundreds of clear, consistent examples illustrate these techniques in detail.

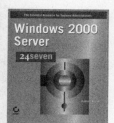

WINDOWS® 2000 SERVER 24SEVEN™

MATTHEW STREBE

ISBN: 0-7821-2669-3   672 pages   US $34.99

For experienced network administrators. At last, here's the book that you and other Windows 2000 administrators have been waiting for. Starting where other books and training courses end and the real world begins, *Windows 2000 Server 24seven* provides the detailed information that will make you a true expert. Inside, Windows 2000 expert Matthew Strebe delivers the advanced coverage and targeted information you need to get the most out of your Windows 2000 network.

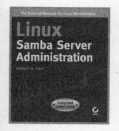

LINUX SAMBA SERVER ADMINISTRATION (CRAIG HUNT LINUX LIBRARY)

RODERICK W. SMITH

ISBN: 0-7821-2740-1   656 pages   US $39.99

Linux Samba Server Administration is the most complete, most advanced guide to Samba you'll find anywhere. Written by a leading Linux expert, this book teaches you, step-by-step, all the standard and advanced Samba techniques you'll need to make Linux and Unix machines operate seamlessly as part of your Windows network. Throughout, scores of clear, consistent examples illustrate these techniques in detail.

SECURITY COMPLETE

SECOND EDITION

SAN FRANCISCO ▸ LONDON

Associate Publisher: Neil Edde

Acquisitions and Developmental Editor: Maureen Adams

Compilation Editor: Mark Lierley

Editor: Tiffany Taylor

Production Editor: Lori Newman

Book Designer: Maureen Forys, Happenstance Type-o-Rama

Electronic Publishing Specialist: Interactive Composition Corporation

Proofreaders: Amey Garber, Emily Hsuan, Nelson Kim, Dave Nash, Laurie O'Connell, Yariv Rabinovitch, Nancy Riddiough, Monique van den Berg

Indexer: Nancy Guenther

Cover Designer: Design Site

Cover Photographer: Neil Leslie

Library of Congress Card Number: 2002108072

ISBN: 0-7821-4144-7

Internet screen shot(s) using Microsoft Internet Explorer 6.0 reprinted by permission from Microsoft Corporation.

Microsoft, the Microsoft Internet Explorer logo, Windows, Windows NT, and the Windows logo are either registered trademarks or trademarks of Microsoft Corporation in the United States and/or other countries.

SYBEX is an independent entity from Microsoft Corporation, and not affiliated with Microsoft Corporation in any manner. This publication may be used in assisting students to prepare for a Microsoft Certified Professional Exam. Neither Microsoft Corporation, its designated review company, nor SYBEX warrants that use of this publication will ensure passing the relevant exam. Microsoft is either a registered trademark or trademark of Microsoft Corporation in the United States and/or other countries.

This study guide and/or material is not sponsored by, endorsed by or affiliated with Cisco Systems, Inc. Cisco®, Cisco Systems®, CCDA™, CCNA™, CCDP™, CCNP™, CCIE™, CCIP™, CCSI™, CSS1™, the Cisco Systems logo and the CCIE logo are trademarks or registered trademarks of Cisco Systems, Inc. in the United States and certain other countries. All other trademarks are trademarks of their respective owners.

TRADEMARKS:

SYBEX has attempted throughout this book to distinguish proprietary trademarks from descriptive terms by following the style used by the trademark holder wherever possible.

The author and publisher have made their best efforts to prepare this book, and the content is based upon final release software whenever possible. Portions of the manuscript may be based upon pre-release versions supplied by software manufacturer(s). The author and the publisher make no representation or warranties of any kind with regard to the completeness or accuracy of the contents herein and accept no liability of any kind including but not limited to performance, merchantability, fitness for any particular purpose, or any losses or damages of any kind caused or alleged to be caused directly or indirectly from this book.

Manufactured in the United States of America

10 9 8 7 6 5 4 3 2 1

CONTENTS AT A GLANCE

CONTENTS

Part III ▶ Firewalls   371

Chapter 11 ▫ Understanding Firewalls   373

Chapter 12 ▫ Packet Filtering   405

Part IV ▶ Cisco Security Specialist (CSS1) Highlights   531

INTRODUCTION

*S*ecurity Complete, Second Edition, is a one-of-a-kind computer book—valuable both for the breadth of its content and for its low price. This compilation of information from some of the very best Sybex books provides comprehensive coverage of the hottest topics in information security today. This book, unique in the computer book world, was created with these goals in mind:

▶ To offer a thorough guide covering all the aspects of computer and network security at an affordable price

▶ To acquaint you with some of our best authors—their writing styles and teaching skills, and the level of expertise they bring to their books—so you can easily find a match for your interests as you delve deeper into computer security

Security Complete, Second Edition, will take you from security basics, to encryption, to protecting yourself against computer crime, to securing specific network platforms, to choosing a firewall, to configuring a Virtual Private Network. This book provides the essential information you'll need to further your information security knowledge while also inviting you to explore greater depths and wider coverage in the original books.

If you've read other computer "how-to" books, you've seen that there are many possible approaches to the task of showing how to use software effectively. The books from which *Security Complete* was compiled represent a range of the approaches to teaching that Sybex and its authors have developed—from the concise and specific *Craig Hunt Linux Library* style to the wide-ranging, thoroughly detailed *Mastering* style. These books also address readers at different levels of computer experience. As you read through various chapters of this book, you'll see which approach works best for you. You'll also see what these books have in common: a commitment to clarity, accuracy, and practicality.

You'll find in these pages ample evidence of the expertise of Sybex's authors. Unlike publishers who produce "books by committee," Sybex authors are encouraged to write in individual voices that reflect their own experience with the software at hand and with the evolution of today's personal computers. Nearly every book represented here is the work of a single writer or a pair of close collaborators, and you are getting the benefit of each author's direct experience.

In adapting the various source materials for inclusion in *Security Complete*, Second Edition, the compiler preserved these individual voices and perspectives. Chapters were edited only to minimize duplication and update or add cross-references so that you can easily follow a topic across chapters. A few sections were also edited for length so that other important security information could be included.

Who Can Benefit from This Book?

Security Complete, Second Edition, is designed to meet the needs of any administrator or enthusiast charged with securing their network environment. The Contents and Index will guide you to the subjects you're looking for.

How This Book Is Organized

Security Complete, Second Edition, has five parts, consisting of 25 chapters and a glossary.

Part I: Network Security Fundamentals: These first four chapters introduce readers to the essential information they need to lay the groundwork for building a secure environment. Coverage includes understanding how your network system communicates, as well as authentication and encryption.

Part II: Operating Systems and Servers: These six chapters explore the special issues involved with securing specific network platforms. We'll discuss Windows 2000, Windows XP, NetWare 6, and Linux.

Part III: Firewalls: The six firewall chapters will help readers identify which firewall is best for their needs and how to configure and launch it into an existing network. Coverage includes packet filtering, network address translation, and platform-specific firewall solutions.

Part IV: Cisco Security Specialist (CSS1) Highlights: These next six chapters discuss the challenges of setting up secure access using popular Cisco products. Coverage includes setting up PIX firewalls, Virtual Private Networks, and Cisco IDS intrusion sensors.

Part V: Security-Related MCSE Highlights: Our final three chapters give readers a taste of how Microsoft tests security professionals through its highly respected MCSE (Microsoft

Certified System Engineer) program. Exam highlights include Windows 2000 security basics, design, and implementation.

A Few Typographical Conventions

When a Windows operation requires a series of choices from menus or dialog boxes, the ➢ symbol is used to guide you through the instructions, like this: "Select Programs ➢ Accessories ➢ System Tools ➢ System Information." The items the ➢ symbol separates may be menu names, toolbar icons, check boxes, or other elements of the Windows interface—any place you can make a selection.

This typeface is used to identify Internet URLs and code, and **boldface type** is used whenever you need to type something into a text box.

You'll find these types of special notes throughout the book:

TIP

You'll see a lot of these—quicker and smarter ways to accomplish a task, which the authors have based on many, many months spent securing networks and individual desktop computers.

NOTE

You'll see these Notes, too. They usually represent alternate ways to accomplish a task or some additional information that needs to be highlighted.

WARNING

In a few places you'll see a Warning like this one. When you see a warning, do pay attention to it.

YOU'LL ALSO SEE "SIDEBAR" BOXES LIKE THIS

These boxed sections provide added explanation of special topics that are noted briefly in the surrounding discussion but that you may want to explore separately. Each sidebar has a heading that announces the topic, so you can quickly decide whether it's something you need to know about.

For More Information...

See the Sybex Web site, www.sybex.com, to learn more about all of the books that went into *Security Complete*, Second Edition. On the site's Catalog page, you'll find links to any book you're interested in. Also be sure to check the Sybex site for late-breaking developments about the applications themselves.

We hope you enjoy this book and find it useful. Good luck in your security endeavors!

Part I
NETWORK SECURITY FUNDAMENTALS

Chapter 1

A SYSTEMS APPROACH TO INFORMATION NETWORKS

We all probably have an idea about what the word *system* means. For those of us who work in information technology, the term has become a catch-all that covers everything from an operating system on a single computer to the Internet itself. Now, we know you're probably thinking that we're going to spend a whole chapter convincing you that because your network is complex, securing it will also be complex. You would be right!

But we're going to do more than that. We're going to give you a small tour through the idea of complexity and how it relates to anything that gets labeled a "system." The goal is to give you several principles that you can apply to any complex system— whether that system is a network, a data recovery procedure, or a security decision tree—in order to build one or more models. These models not only provide a common reference for author

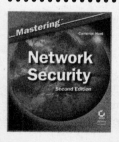

Adapted from *Mastering™ Network Security*,
Second Edition by Chris Brenton and Cameron Hunt
ISBN 0-7821-4142-0 $49.99

and reader, but are valuable tools in their own right in understanding, planning, implementing, and managing any complex group of interrelating, dynamically operating parts. And if anything fits that description, it's a computer network (the thing we're trying to secure, remember?).

An Introduction to Systems Analysis

Systems analysis is the formal term for the *process* (which we cover in Chapter 2) that uses systems principles to identify, reconstruct, optimize, and control a system. The trick is, you have to be able to walk through that process while taking into account multiple objectives, constraints, and resources. Simple, but what's the point? Well, ultimately you want to create possible courses of action, together with their risks, costs, and benefits. And that, in a nutshell, is what network security is all about—choosing among multiple security alternatives to find the best one for your system, given your constraints (technical or financial, typically).

The principles that make up systems analysis come from several theories of information and systems. Let's look at Information Theory first. In its broadest sense, the term *information* is interpreted to include any and all messages occurring in any medium, such as telegraphy, radio, or television, and the signals involved in electronic computers and other data-processing devices. Information Theory (as initially devised in 1948 by Claude E. Shannon, an American mathematician and computer scientist) regards information as *only* those symbols that are unknown (or uncertain) to the receiver.

What's the difference between symbols that are known and symbols that are unknown? First, think of long distance communication a little more than a century ago, in the days of Morse Code and the telegraph. Messages were sent leaving out nonessential (predictable or known) words such as *a* and *the*, while retaining words such as *baby* and *boy* (defined as unknown information in Information Theory). We see the same kind of behavior in today's text messaging—minimal words and abbreviations come to stand for entire phrases.

Shannon argued that unknown information was the only true information and that everything else was redundant and could be removed. As a result, the number of bits necessary to encode information was called the *entropy* of a system. This discovery was incredibly important because it gave scientists a framework they could use to add more and more bandwidth (using compression, or the removal of redundant information) to the same medium. For example, modems increased their speed to the point they were transmitting 56,000 bits of information per second, even though the physical medium of the phone line could represent only 2400 changes (known as *bauds*) per second.

We point out Information Theory and Shannon's definition of information is to illustrate a central concept of understanding systems: You don't have to know *everything* about a system to model it; you only need to know the unknown or nonredundant parts of a system (the information) that can affect the operation of a system as a whole. You can ignore everything else; for all practical purposes, it doesn't exist.

System analysis also draws heavily from another discipline, Systems Theory. Traditional Systems Theory tends to focus on complex (from the Latin *complexus*, which means "entwined" or "twisted together") items such as biological organisms, ecologies, cultures, and machines. The more items that exist and are intertwined in a system, the more complex the system is. Newer studies of systems tend to look not only at items that are complex, but also at items that are also *adaptive*. The assumption is that underlying principles and laws are general to any type of complex adaptive system, principles that then can be used to create models of these systems. The following are some of these principles:

Complexity   Systems are complex structures, with many different types of elements that influence one another. For example, a computer network encompasses software, different layers of protocols, multiple hardware types, and, of course, human users—all interacting with and influencing one another.

Mutuality   The elements of a system operate at the same time (in real time) and cooperate (or not). This principle creates many simultaneous exchanges among the components. A negative example of this is a positive feedback loop! Imagine a computer that creates a log entry every time the CPU utilization is greater than 50 percent. Now, imagine the consequences that will occur if every time the system writes an error log, it forces the CPU to be used greater than—you guessed it—50 percent.

Complementarity   Simultaneous exchanges among the elements create subsystems that interact within multiple processes and structures. The result is that multiple (hierarchical) models are needed to describe a single system.

Evolvability   Complex adaptive systems tend to evolve and grow as the opportunity arises, as opposed to being designed and implemented in an ideal manner. Now, this definitely sounds like most computer networks we've been privy too— patchworks of various brands, capabilities, and complexities, implemented in pieces as time and resources allow.

Constructivity   Systems tend to grow (to scale), and as they do so, they become bound (in the sense of heritage) to their previous configurations (or models) while gaining new features. Anyone who has worked at an organization over an extended period of time has seen this happen. No matter how large the network grows (unless there was a major overhaul somewhere), it still seems to fundamentally reflect the small, original network it originated from, even with additional capabilities and features added over the life of the system.

Reflexivity   Both positive and negative feedback are at work. Because this feedback affects both static entities and dynamic processes, the system as a whole begins to reflect internal patterns. You'll notice that the physical network begins to reflect the way you use that network.

The original Systems Theory was developed in the 1940s by Ludwig von Bertalanffy (1901–72), a biologist, who realized that there were no effective models to describe how biological organisms worked in their environment. Physicists at the time could make a small model of the solar system (through a process of both analysis and reductionism, breaking the components and functions down to their smallest, simplest parts) that would accurately predict planetary orbits while ignoring the universe at large. Biologists, however, could not completely separate an organism from its environment and still study it; it would die of starvation, cold, or boredom. As a result, the systems approach tries to combine the analytic and the synthetic methods, using both a holistic and reductionist view.

Again, think of how this concept applies to a computer network. Systems inside and outside the network make up the environment of the network itself. Although we can break down the parts and functions of a network, we can truly understand it only by looking at the dynamic interaction of the network with other components, whether those components are other networks or human beings.

To identify a system means to identify a boundary. The reality, especially in our connected world, is that boundaries are often arbitrarily dictated and defined, not necessarily created through physical reality. Placing a firewall between your business LAN and the Internet may or may not establish a boundary between two systems. It all depends on the model—the way in which you view your network.

Assuming that we *have* defined a boundary between the system and its environment, we can add some concepts that define how a system interacts with that environment. In the following illustration, *input* is defined as any information added into the system from the environment. *Throughput* is defined as those changes made to the input by the system. *Output,* of course, is what leaves the system and crosses the boundary back into the environment.

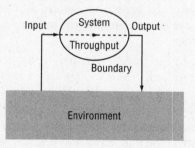

Of course, the environment itself is made up of one or more systems, and we rapidly reach the conclusion that defining a system (which really means defining a boundary between one system and its environment) is really a matter of scale and perspective—a concept that lets us begin to see systems in a hierarchical order (more on this later). Whereas you might view the Internet and your internal LAN as two separate systems, that model no longer functions as effectively when you consider remote workers accessing your network through a VPN (virtual private network) or even a web mail session secured through SSL (Secure Sockets Layer).

If you look at a system as a whole, you don't necessarily need to be aware of all its parts. This perspective is called the *black box view*—seeing a system as something that takes in input and produces output, with us being ignorant of the throughput. (Seeing the innards would then be called a *white box view.*) Although the black box view doesn't necessarily satisfy your inner control freak, it's not always necessary to see the innards of a process in order to implement and maintain it. (Remember the definition of *information* according to Information Theory?) This approach is common in the complex world of information technology, where we often work with black box abstractions of data operations.

In the realm of object-oriented programming languages such as C# and Java, reducing a code object to a black box is considered a primary strength. You are able to use the functionality of a code object (written by another programmer) in programs of your own without knowing *how* the object does the work. As long as the methods used to access the capabilities of the object or its accessible properties don't change, the authors can change, update, or rework their object in any way they desire. Your code can stay the same!

The challenge in dealing with information technology, as well as in dealing with *any* complex adaptive system, is to identify when you should use black or white approaches. And the capability of using both black and white approaches illustrates another principle that we mentioned earlier: Systems are hierarchical. At the higher (or unified) level, you get an abstraction of the system as a whole. At the lower (reduced) level, you see many interrelating components, but you don't necessarily know how they fit together.

According to the traditional analytic approach (the one that existed before von Bertalanffy came along), that low-level view is all that is necessary to understand a system. In other words, if you know the precise state of every component in the system, you should be able to understand how the system functions. Anyone who has ever tried to optimize an operating system for a given task (such as a web server or a database server) knows how limiting this model can be, simply because performance rarely scales in a linear fashion. In other words, increasing the number of users by a specific amount doesn't always guarantee the same rate (proportional or not) of resource utilization.

In the same fashion, doubling the amount of RAM doesn't automatically increase RAM-based performance by the same percentage. Computer components don't (often) exist in simple, linear, cause-and-effect relationships; rather they exist in complex networks of interdependencies that can only be understood by their common purpose: creating the functionality of the system as a whole. Looking at RAM or disk I/O or a CPU as individual elements isn't sufficient to understand resource utilization until you understand the relationship each of these elements has to the others—something not readily apparent by simply dissecting their design.

All this might seem like common sense, and if you've spent any time dealing with computer networks, you've probably come to the belief that these ideas are true, even if you haven't known *why* they are true. Most IT workers have an emotional reaction (and not necessarily a positive one) to the overwhelming complexity and unpredictability normally experienced by trying to understand, let alone manage, a complex system. Add in the feedback (in the *systems* sense of the word) of human users (each with their own method of interacting and altering that system), and we now have to struggle with a complex *adaptive* system.

But we're not done yet. Remember that we said systems have hierarchies? Understanding that systems can affect the structure and functionality of subsystems and, likewise, that subsystems can influence the behavior of a parent system or systems (both directions of influence occurring simultaneously and repeatedly over a period of time) is crucial in Systems Theory. This theory also states that systems tend to mimic (in a general sense) the structures and the functions of their parent systems.

Let's look at a biological example. The cells in your body have boundaries (the cell wall), inputs (the structures on the cell wall that bind to proteins and usher them into the body of the cell), and outputs (internal cell structures that eject waste through the cell wall to the outside). Your body as a whole has inputs (your mouth and nose), outputs, and a boundary (the skin). Both your body, as a parent system, and your cells, as subsystems, have to take in nourishment. Both transform that input into an output. Although the specifics are different, the functions are the same: to allow sustenance, growth, and repair.

Similar structures also exist in the hierarchy of systems. The inputs on your body serve not only to transport nourishment, but also to analyze and prepare it for the body. Likewise, the inputs on the cell (located on the cellular wall itself) identify and "format" the proteins for the use of the cell. Systems Theory, ultimately, asserts that there are universal principles of organization that hold for all systems (biological, social, or informational) and that we can use these principles to understand, build, and manipulate those systems.

Now that you have a better understanding of the theory of information and systems, you need a practical way not just to understand a complex system, but to predict how the system will respond to changes. Such a method allows you not only to understand the security risks a computer network might face, but the consequences (especially the unforeseen ones) of trying to mitigate that risk. The name given to this practical method of managing systems is *systems analysis, decision analysis,* or even *policy analysis.* We'll use the traditional term *systems analysis.*

The systems analysis model is a multidisciplinary field that includes programming, probability and statistics, mathematics, software engineering, and operations research. Although you don't need a background in any of these areas to use the model, understanding the background will help you use the tools. The typical systems analysis process goes something like this:

1. Define the scope of a problem.

2. Determine the objectives, constraints, risks, and costs.

3. Identify alternative courses of action.

4. Evaluate the alternatives according to the constraints (feasibility), the fixed costs (cost-effectiveness), the ratio of benefits to cost (cost-benefit), or the ratio of benefits to risk (risk-benefit).

5. Recommend an alternative that will meet the needs of a decision maker (without violating the constraints of the system).

Sounds easy enough, right? You're creating a model of the system. This model allows you to apply metrics (measurable behaviors of the components, their behaviors, and relationships) in order to make decisions about what courses of actions will allow you to meet your objectives.

Two major challenges are associated with systems analysis of network security. The first is to assign realistic values to the frequency of threats. As we'll illustrate later, the frequency of a threat is one of the primary ways you determine the actual risk to a system. The second challenge is to decide which evaluation criteria to use (the items from step 4). Traditional computer network security has attempted to use all the criteria in the decision-making process, while giving the greatest weight to cost-benefit.

Now that we have a list of the steps in the systems analysis process, let's walk through each of them in more detail.

Define the Scope of the Problem

In systems analysis, a *problem* is something in the system or its environment that requires the system to change. The *scope* of network security includes protecting the system from data corruption and ensuring the availability of data, no matter where the threat originates. The result of this definition of scope is that even if you have no external environmental threat from hackers, you still need to determine if the design of a network itself could put your data at risk—for example, by not providing sufficient levels of data redundancy.

In a practical sense for any individual involved in network security, defining the scope of the problem comes down to two questions: what and why? The first question is essentially about responsibility: What assets (or systems) are you in charge of protecting? This quickly moves beyond a technical arena into the specifics of your business, job, or role within a security effort. Once you clarify the *what* of your work, you can start to define the *why*. In other words, you can evaluate the current state of the system (*state* being formally defined as the current value of any variable element in a system) and decide what needs to be changed.

We'll introduce the formal security process in Chapter 2, but you can probably guess that in an ideal, formal setting, you receive a document that clarifies the areas (or systems) of your responsibility. You then attempt to determine the current state of the system, followed by an analysis of the problem. In network security specifically, this process means identifying and quantifying the risks to your data, including the systems that process, store, and retrieve that data.

Determine Objectives, Constraints, Risks, and Cost

In systems analysis, an *objective* is simply the outcome desired after a course of action is followed. Because objectives (like systems) usually exist in a hierarchy (descending from general to specific, nonquantified to highly quantified), we usually refer to higher-level, abstract objectives as *goals*. Specific quantifiable objectives are referred to as *targets*.

An example of a goal/target combination is a corporate website. The *goal* is to maintain the functionality and integrity of the website as a whole. A *subgoal* is to protect against web page defacement. Two specific *targets* that support that subgoal (which, in turn, supports the overall goal) are to apply vendor security patches to the web server within five hours of release and to create a secure, mirrored content server that over-writes the master website with correct content every five minutes.

Nice and easy, right? The problem comes when you have multiple objectives that are contradictory or competitive (also known as conflict-ing objectives). You usually see conflicting objectives when more than one party is responsible for the state (remember the definition of state?) of a system. You probably already know how rampant conflicting objectives are in the security world, because implementing security almost always comes down to restricting behavior or capability (or increasing cost).

Unfortunately, restricting system capability tends to conflict with the central purpose of information systems, which is to enable and ease behavior or capability. For example, think of how quickly you find notes hidden under keyboards when password complexity and length requirements are enforced in an organization!

Fortunately, systems analysis gives you a method for resolving conflicts by providing hierarchical decision makers. Because the means of achieving your goal of system security might conflict with the accountant's goal of maintaining a low cost of the system, a decision maker at a higher level is usually required to determine either which goal takes precedence or (more commonly in the real world) how to change the constraints of each goal so that they are no longer in opposition. In other words, executive-level decisions are often required to reach a compromise between two competing goals.

A byproduct of conflict resolution is the creation of *proxy* objectives—replacing generalized objectives with those that can be measured in some quantifiable way. An example of proxy objectives is illustrated by multiple security plans, each with a quantified cost/benefit ratio, that are presented to senior management who make the final decision based on how much risk they are willing to accept (the greater the risk, the lower the *initial* cost).

So what are constraints? According to systems analysis, a *constraint* is a limit in the environment or the system that prevents certain actions, alternatives, consequences, and objectives from being applied to a system. A simple, but limited way to understand this idea is to think of the difference between what is *possible* to do in a system and what is *practical*. Thinking of a constraint this way makes it easier to identify the consequences of any given course of action on a system.

A good example is a requirement mandating that biometric security devices (such as a fingerprint scanner) be used on every desktop computer in an organization. Although using a fingerprint scanner would achieve a major goal of network security (and is technically possible in most cases), you could easily run into constraints—initial equipment cost, client enrollment (storing authenticated copies of every employee's fingerprints), and non-biometric capable access devices (such as a Palm Pilot or other PDA) that make the solution unworkable according to other goals (such as maintaining your security within a certain budget).

We know this sounds complicated, and it is. Using systems analysis to guide you in your security process has great rewards, but it also requires you to have a thorough knowledge of your network inventory (hardware, software, and configuration), business procedures and policies, and even some accounting. Using formal worksheets and checklists to guide you through the process is highly recommended, as is hiring a consultant who specializes in systems analysis in a security context.

Once you identify your objectives and initial constraints (additional constraints usually show up when you are defining various courses of action), you need to identify risk. *Risk*, in systems analysis, can mean several things. For our purpose, we'll choose *risk assessment*, which is a two-part process. The first part is identifying the impact (measured, from a security perspective, in cost) of a threat (defined as a successful attack, penetration, corruption, or loss of service); the second part is quantifying the probability of a threat.

We can use the web page defacement example to illustrate risk assessment. You begin by identifying the threat (a successful web page defacement) in terms of the cost to the organization. Now things become difficult to quantify. How much money does an organization lose when investor and customer confidence is lowered (or lost) when a page is defaced? What if the particular page was interactive and the defacement breaks or inhibits commercial interactions?

You could even break the threat down to finer details, assigning cost to each individual defaced page, varied by the amount of time the page was defaced; the time of day, month, and year the defacement took place; the amount of publicity received; and the functionality that was broken.

You must also consider another type of impact: Does the system state change after a threat? In other words, the process needed to deface your web page most likely results in the attacker having some level of control over your system. This, according to strictly defined systems analysis, has changed the state of your system, especially if you extend your concept of your system to include those individuals who are authorized to use your system. Once your system state has changed (for better or worse), new threats are possible, requiring a repeat of the entire risk assessment process. This recursive, hierarchical analysis helps you to establish a multilayered defense—something we'll refer to as *defense in depth*.

Once impact is quantified, you have to assess the probability of a threat (remembering our definition of a threat as an *actual occurrence* of a specific negative event, not just a possible one). You can begin to assess the probability of a threat against a system by using simple comparison: Identify all the known characteristics of systems that have succumbed to that threat in the past. In our web page defacement example, you compare your system (including operating system, web server configuration, level of dynamic code, public exposure and opinion of the website, and so on) to those that have been defaced before.

This process sounds relatively straightforward, but you can't stop here. You also need to attempt to weigh those system characteristics in susceptibility to the threat. Using an example from history, which factor contributed more to the Department of Justice website defacement (the one that left then-Attorney General Janet Reno with a Hitler-like mustache!)— the operating system or the type of web server running on the operating system? The answer is a little more difficult to determine and takes experience along with knowing *how* the threat was carried out. We quickly come to the conclusion that we need another hierarchy: a hierarchy of threats. Although the end threat is still web page defacement, an attacker could use multiple methods to deface a page. The threat probability is then a combination of which methods of attack are the most popular, along with which system configurations are most susceptible to those popular attacks.

Remember that we're speaking of system configuration in the systems analysis sense of the term. Part of your website system is the *environment* in which it operates, including the popularity and publicity associated with that site. If you are, say, a U.S. military organization, the state of your system guarantees a higher level of interest. That raised interest can translate into a higher frequency and sophistication of attack. In this example, not only has the *frequency* of the threat possibly changed, but also the nature of the threat *itself*.

Once you identify your objectives, constraints, and risks, you're ready to decide on *courses of action*—nothing more than the ways in which an objective will be met. Multiple courses of action are defined as *alternatives*, and then only if they are mutually exclusive. For example, an objective requires a standard biometric authentication device across an organization. If the decision makers in the organization are trying to decide between fingerprint scanners and iris scanners, they are said to be selecting from two alternatives. If the organization decides that it could use both alternatives together in a standardized fashion—fingerprint scanners for desktops, iris scanners for server rooms (or combine elements from two mutually exclusive alternatives)—a new, distinct alternative has been created (and possibly a new objective, depending on how strictly that objective was originally defined).

Defining an alternative means to establish the feasibility, costs, benefits, and risks associated with a course of action—a process that usually occurs repeatedly, starting with a multitude of alternatives that are gradually integrated and combined until at last you reach a small collection of alternatives. At this point, the process usually stops for a couple of reasons:

- ▸ You don't have sufficient information to continue an evaluation. Perhaps no one has yet conducted a TCO (Total Cost of Ownership) study comparing biometric authentication with centrally stored user profiles against a system using smart dongles that store an encrypted copy of the user's profile in an embedded chip.

- ▸ All the alternatives that could meet the objective are greater than the budget constraint (an objective/constraint conflict), which (as we mentioned earlier) usually requires the intervention of a higher-level decision maker.

And, after all your hard work, all that is left to do is present your proposal to the decision makers. Although it can be bad enough if someone questions your results, it's worse when your decision makers don't understand your methodology.

APPLYING SYSTEMS ANALYSIS TO INFORMATION TECHNOLOGY

Now that we've covered the general theory of systems analysis, let's apply it to IT systems specifically. This approach might seem like unnecessary repetition, but it's actually an attempt to reinforce important concepts while adding details that are specific to issues you'll face in dealing with security.

When you begin to analyze your network (in preparation to secure it), you'll break it down into four general areas:

Data   The nature of the information stored and processed on the system

Technology   The different types of technology used in the system

Organization   How the organization as a whole uses the system

Individuals   Key decision makers and personalities that use the system

The Nature of the Data

Understanding your organization and the type of work it does goes a long way toward understanding the type of data stored and processed on your system. Translating this knowledge into specifics follows a task orientation: What is your system used for? Some smaller organizations primarily process and store groupware—common address books, shared or centrally stored files, and simple databases, along with e-mail and a website or two. Larger organizations tend to break down their network segments, and the network technical divisions begin to mirror the network logical divisions. For example, a company places its Internet-accessible resources (web servers, mail servers, and so on) on a network that is separate from its internal network (for security and performance reasons, among others). In this case, a parent system (the functionality) is driving a change in a subsystem (the technology).

The Types of Technology

Technology itself helps define the structure of the system, but primarily as background. In other words, understanding the technological topology of your system will help you formulate your constraints and identify and quantify your threats, and will ultimately play a big part in formulating your risk assessment.

How the Organization Uses the System

Understanding how your organization uses the system can be easier in larger organizations, in which the network tends to follow organizational lines along centers of power or divisions of labor. However, even in smaller organizations, understanding how the network is used and *perceived* by the organization becomes critical to projecting the consequences of your various courses of action. Those consequences play a primary role in determining which alternatives you choose to solve a problem.

How Individuals Use the System

This task is not just about evaluating the technical ability of individuals in an organization or simply identifying those with the most influence. It also concerns determining the relationship those individuals have with the system and determining their knowledge of how the system as a whole works, even to the point of the organization's relationship with the system.

Models and Terminology

Once you look at your network through these types of filters, you're ready to begin defining the subsystems. Selecting where to draw the border of a subsystem is always difficult, but, again, systems analysis gives you some direction. Object-Oriented Systems Analysis (OSA) takes the concept of the black box discussed earlier and uses it to create object-based models using the components of the network, using three model types:

ORM (Object-Relationship Model)   Defines objects (and classes of objects), how objects relate to classes, and how objects map to real-world components

OBM (Object-Behavior Model)   Defines the actions of objects (used to define how and why an object changes state)

OIM (Object-Interaction Model)   Defines how objects influence one another

Object-Relationship Model

An *object* is a label you apply to a single thing that has a unique identity either physically or conceptually. Here are a few IT objects:

▶ Router #13

▶ www.go-sos.com

▶ An inventory database

▶ The first primary partition of the second hard drive of the web server

In OSA, objects are represented with a lowercase labeled dot:

router #13

Objects can be grouped into one or more *object classes*, such as the following:

▶ Router

▶ URL

▶ Database

▶ Partition

Object classes are represented with a cylinder and a capitalized label:

For an object to be a member of an object class, it has to meet the constraints. That requirement might seem obvious, but think about the Routers class in the previous example. It's easy to think of a dedicated router as belonging to the Router class, but what about a Windows 2000 server that shares files, hosts e-mail, and provides a VPN connection between a small office and corporate headquarters? Although we don't necessarily think of this machine as a router, it acts in that capacity (by routing traffic over the VPN). Including it in the Router class would depend on the constraints of the Router class; in other words, how you define the class determines what objects qualify for membership.

NOTE

Objects can migrate from class to class as class constraints change or as the state of the object changes.

Objects can have a relationship, which is represented by a simple line between them labeled with a sentence that describes the relationship. Usually, however, this relationship reflects a relationship *set* between object classes. Relationships are grouped into sets when they connect to the same object classes and represent the same *logical* connection among objects. To illustrate a relationship set, you draw the two object classes as boxes and connect them:

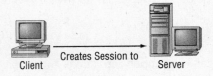

When a relationship set has multiple connections, these connections are referred to as the *arity* of the set. Two connections make a set binary, three connections make a set ternary, and four connections make a set quaternary. Relationships with five or more connections are referred to as *x*-ary, with *x* reflecting the number of connections. When illustrating a relationship set with more than one connection, a diamond is used to interconnect the lines:

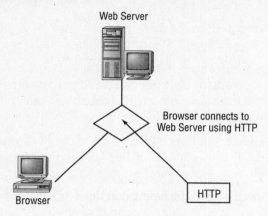

To give an even better level of detail, you can treat the relationship set as an object, which in this case is called Session:

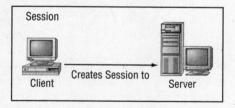

Treating the relationship set as an object allows you to link the Session object to other objects or object classes (in this cases, byproducts or characteristics of the session):

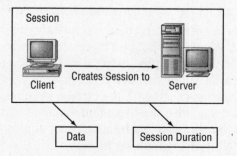

This graphic illustrates that a Session object (really a relationship set) has a relationship between a Data object class and a Session Duration class, much as any network session in the real world has data associated with it, along with an amount of time the session existed.

But something is still missing. When working with relationship sets, you need to clarify the constraints. There are three types:

Participation   Defines (for every connection) how many times an object class or object can participate in the relationship set.

Co-occurrence   Similar to participation, co-occurrence specifies how many times an object can participate in a relationship set with another object. This constraint can also apply to object collections.

General   Defines what is allowed or not allowed in a relationship. This constraint can be expressed as a formal math/logic statement or as a simple statement.

Let's look at an illustrated example of a Participation constraint:

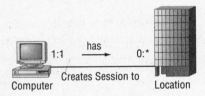

This illustration tells you that a Computer object (belonging to the Computer object class) must have one (but only one) Location object (again, of the Location object class). A Location object, however, doesn't even have to have a single corresponding Computer object, but *can* have an infinite number of Computer objects. For example, if you define a Location object to have a value of Corporate, it is tied to all the Computer objects that are mapped to physical machines at the corporate office (a one-to-many relationship, for all you database programmers).

This makes sense, but you could quickly run into a problem. What happens if you decide to map a laptop (the term *map* in OSA denotes an association between a physical item and a logical object) to the Computer class? Because a Computer object can have only one location (as defined by the Participation constraint), you could have difficulty if you are analyzing objects over time with an expectation that the Location value won't change! You can solve that problem by simply mapping laptops to a Laptop class that doesn't have the same constraint.

The following illustration shows how Co-occurrence constraints can limit the number of objects that can be associated with an object (or a group of objects) in a relationship set:

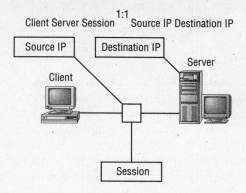

This example is also fairly straightforward. When Client, Server, and Session objects are in a relationship set, there can be only one Source IP and one Destination IP object in that set. This arrangement is similar to real-life network communications, in which the source and destination IP addresses don't change for the duration of a session between a client and a server.

Both of the previous examples illustrate constraints that arise from the workings of the objects themselves (or, in other words, the interaction of the objects *determines* the constraint). However, General constraints often represent constraints imposed on the objects. An example of General constraints is often seen in IT systems in which policies exist about how the system *should* be used, as shown in the following illustration:

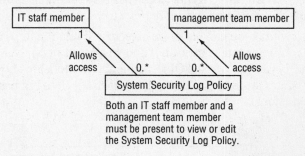

Both an IT staff member and a
management team member
must be present to view or edit
the System Security Log Policy.

This example shows how a simple text sentence is used to create the General constraint. Because IT security policies are all about limiting the use of a system, General constraints are used frequently.

Once you model the objects and their relationships in the system, you're ready to examine their state, defined in OSA through the Object-Behavior

Model as the activity or status of an object. You illustrate state by using an oval and writing the name of the state inside that rectangle:

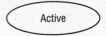

How do you determine all the states an object can have? That's really up to you; you use your experience and understanding of the object you are representing. States are binary—either on or off—and they are activated and deactivated when control (or flow) transitions to another state. Exceptions to this rule are threads (you can turn on multiple threads), prior conjunction (turning off multiple states when one is turned on), and subsequent conjunction (turning multiple states on when one is turned off).

A transition is also formally diagrammed in OSA, sometimes with an identifier, but always with a trigger and an action. The trigger defines the conditions under which a transition fires, along with the resulting action, as shown in the following illustration:

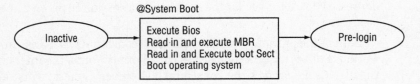

This example uses an event-based trigger (hence the @ sign). Event-triggered transitions execute their action the moment the event becomes true. Conditional triggers (informal statements not preceded with @) cause the transition the *entire time* they are true.

Now that you can illustrate objects and relationships using ORM and use multiple state transitions (known as *state nets*) to show how objects behave, you can use the Object-Interaction Model to show how objects and states are changed through interaction. Here is a basic example of an interaction:

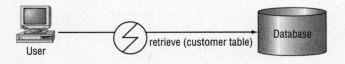

Both User and Database are object classes, with the interaction defined by a circle with a zigzag; *retrieve* is the action, and *customer table* is the object transferred in the transaction. You can use a more complete illustration to show how object class, state changes, and interactions work together:

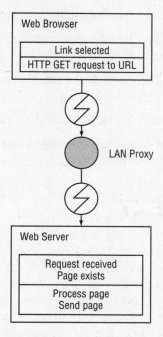

This is a complete (although simplified) example of putting together all the pieces of the OSA to represent your network as a system. Remember also that this is just an introduction to familiarize you with the concepts and symbols. Many specialized security consultants will use these diagrams to document your network, analyze courses of action, and present you with alternatives that meet your criteria and solve your problems. Knowing how to read their documentation will aid you in making better decisions. Although you might not go to the same lengths in analyzing or illustrating your own network, the principles remain the same.

Formal systems analysis makes understanding the environment of a system as important as understanding the system itself. This can be more difficult—especially determining which elements of an environment actually influence the system (particularly those items that remain unknown). Once you begin making a list of items that *might* influence or affect your system, you identify the techniques to determine if they do. Here are some items to look for:

Data   The flow of information streaming into a system

Technology   The limitations and capabilities of other systems that interact with your own

Competition   The capabilities of other organizations

Individuals   People whose activities could influence your system, such as crackers

Capital   The quantity of resources held by systems outside your own

Regulations   The legal limitations faced by all systems

Opportunities   The innovations and capabilities not yet integrated into your own system

WHAT'S NEXT

By formally documenting your system, you can better understand the vulnerabilities and threats it faces. By using the same theory and techniques to document your security alternatives (including their consequences), you can make better choices about *how* to secure your system. In the next chapter, we'll take these techniques and place them in a dynamic context of the security process—an important reminder that security is a constant effort, not just a project to complete!

Chapter 2

SECURITY AS A PROCESS

I n Chapter 1, we talked about understanding information technology as a system that includes the individuals that interact with the technology, as well as the organization that invests in and controls the system. We provided you with some concepts that you can use to define and document your system as a whole. In this chapter, we'll take the static snapshot of a system and move it into a dynamic environment that is constantly changing. Because of constant change, securing your IT resources is no longer a single straightforward action, but a series of continual steps that make up a never-ending process.

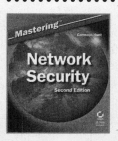

Adapted from *Mastering™ Network Security*,
Second Edition by Chris Brenton and Cameron Hunt
ISBN 0-7821-4142-0 $49.99

SURVIVAL OF THE FITTEST: THE MYTH OF TOTAL SECURITY

Total and complete network security is a myth. Our belief in that statement comes from experience, but *why* total security is a myth really comes from the system model as explained in Chapter 1. If you think of your network as a pseudo-organism that lives in a constantly changing environment, it's not hard to see how your systems are constantly evolving to respond to the demands and threats placed on them and how those threats (again, seen as co-existing organisms in a media and Internet-connected environment) change themselves to be more and more effective.

Let's take a step back for a moment so that we can suggest an idea that might seem like something out of a science fiction movie, but is in reality just another model, another way of looking at your relationship with computer systems: You and your network are one being, one entity, a cyborg. In this model, your network doesn't end at the keyboard, the firewall, or the modem. It ultimately ends in the decision makers who control the funds and direction of your network. In this view, then, your organization's IT budget is as much a part of your computer network as a router or cabling infrastructure, and so are those individuals (or policies) that determine how that budget is employed.

This cyborg entity—your organization (and its information technology)—lives in an environment made up of employees, floods, crackers, and software and hardware vendors, not to mention the business in which you organization is involved. In fact, if we were to borrow a metaphor from a certain visionary of a rather well-known company headquartered in Redmond, Washington, your information technology makes up a digital nervous system for your organization.

Although we like that metaphor (let's say we're embracing it), we see a need to alter it to better fit the topic of this book (let's say we're extending it). You see, the problem with viewing security as just dealing with a *digital* nervous system is that doing so ignores the human beings who also make up that nervous system, whether we're looking at those people as users of the system or as decision makers of the system. In the context of security, both types of individuals can be equally detrimental. For example, suppose an end user unknowingly opens an infected e-mail attachment, and a business executive won't fund an intrusion detection system for a critical web server. Both individuals have quite different levels of interaction with and control over the system, but their (negative) impact is real.

Seeing these two types of users in a biological example can explain how your view of security must be scaled out large enough to see the entire picture. We like to think of the end user as our nose—one that isn't discriminating enough to realize that the milk in the jug is just a little too old to be safely put on our cereal in the morning. The safeguards might be in place, but they are ignored because of some other motivation. For example, an employee ignores virus warnings in order to see the attached dancing reindeer animation, or we occasionally ignore the fact that our expired soy milk can make us just as sick as expired dairy milk.

Sometimes our bodies just don't produce enough white cells. Or, if our white cells don't have experience in fighting a newly introduced disease, we might suffer until they learn how to handle the new invader. The executive who chooses not to fund a key piece of security technology can be seen in this light. And, just like your immune system, all it usually takes is one (nonfatal) failure of security to convince a key decision maker to invest in the appropriate level of protection.

Continuing in this biological model, think of security education as a vaccine—a way of shocking the system into preparing for a potential onslaught. Like a vaccine, the experience can be unpleasant, especially if you are rehearsing (like the body does) for what would happen in a real attack. Although you might suffer an uncomfortable fever while the body adjusts to the dead or deformed bugs used in a vaccine, your company might suffer anything from loss of productive time (for education, meetings, and system reconfiguration) to embarrassment (from the discovery that data recovery procedures don't work) from simulating a cracker attack or computer worm infection.

We can take this model even further. We've all received virus hoaxes in e-mail. The most damaging are those that tell a user to look for a specific virus file (which is actually a critical system component!) in order to delete it. When people take these warnings seriously, they can cause unwarranted damage or reduce their functionality. This is exactly what happens to someone who suffers from diabetes, arthritis, or allergies. Their body is overzealous, sees innocent system components (such as knee joints or a pancreas) or elements of the environment (such as a particular food) as the enemy, and attacks. Likewise, rashly placing extreme security measures (which usually have the dual impact of increasing cost and lowering ease of use and functionality of a system) can limit the system in varying degrees—some of them ultimately crippling, just like diabetes.

Everything seems nice and pat in this biological model. Your system gets an infection; but because you've been inoculated (your antivirus program has a database consisting of virus signatures allowing it to recognize known hostile code in your system), your white blood cells recognize the virus and can kill it. Your users open attachments on a whim, so you start with a company attachment policy and an education program. This could extend to more extreme measures, such as creating a quarantine directory for all e-mail attachments or even prohibiting all files transferred on e-mail! You might be tempted to think that apart from keeping your virus packages updated, you're pretty much done. But again, the biological model works against you. Remember that your network (along with your organization) will experience some level of change, whether through growth, reduction, or just simple age. These changes alter the system state, which means that new threats are possible, and new internal weaknesses could put your information at danger.

At the same time your system is changing, the environment is changing also. Viruses become more sophisticated, and denial of service (DoS) attacks are on the rise. Even new legislation mandating penalties for privacy or data disclosure (not to mention civil lawsuits involving past e-mail) are being enacted with greater frequency. As information technology becomes ubiquitous in the operation of any business—in fact, in any type of social discourse—it becomes more valuable. And things that are valued are stolen, exploited, or fought over in the courts.

Survival of the fittest works right into this model of your network in a big, bad world of hostile threats. If a lawsuit succeeds because incriminating evidence is found in a stored e-mail, future lawsuits will pursue the same avenue of attack. If a highly successful virus is publicized as using an innovative vector (*vector* being the medical term for how a disease is transmitted), other virus writers will embrace and extend that method to make increasingly virulent strains. If there is a trend in the past 10 years of computer security, it is that the number and intensity of attacks have increased even in proportion to the growth of information systems themselves.

Before you start cursing Darwin, realize that many positive benefits are associated with the concept of survival of the fittest, which is known in the IT world as *best of breed*. By allowing products, processes, and concepts to duke it out in an ever-connected world, the overall quality, robustness, capability, and efficiency of our networks are improved. Think of how e-mail and instant messaging have become both a boon and a bane to organizations and have contributed to fundamental changes in how organizations are structured. Even the U.S. military is suffering from an identity crisis brought about by the decentralization offered (or compelled) by quick and inexpensive peer-to-peer communication methods.

How can you, the security expert, keep your network healthy in the face of internal weaknesses and external threats? The same way that biological organisms stay healthy: You evolve in the most efficient manner possible. This evolution touches not just the technology used to process and store information, but also the people, leadership, and procedures themselves. In other words, you have to evolve your entire organization. Don't panic; security professionals face this challenge constantly. The key is to learn how the successful ones do it.

RISK MITIGATION: CASE STUDIES OF SUCCESS AND FAILURE

"Hey, I think we've been hacked!" The phone call, from a network administrator for a local insurance company, came on a Saturday afternoon. We were surprised. We had reviewed this company's production network environment extensively, and the thought that an attack had been successful provided a significant amount of personal discomfort. Like police officers, however, our first thought was to preserve the crime scene.

"Did you unplug the computer from the network?" we asked.

"Yup," he replied.

"Good!" we exclaimed. "Don't turn it off! We'll be there in half an hour."

As we drove, we started reviewing our procedures for isolating a system, identifying its current state, imaging the drive, and conducting a forensic analysis of the contents. We were concerned. This company was a major player in the insurance industry, and Congress was up in arms about financial and medical data and its protection. We knew there could be possible legal ramifications if data had been exposed, not to mention embarrassment.

The company was fortunate: The server was a Windows 2000 server that was deployed on an isolated network with its own Internet access. The server was being used as a test for an upcoming Microsoft Exchange deployment. Its only network service was the web server, which was used to provide Outlook web access functionality. It held no actual sensitive data; even the passwords were specific to that machine.

We took a case history of the machine, which helped explain why it had become victim in a company that was fairly sophisticated in its security—both technically and procedurally. This particular computer had been a backup server, unplugged and stored in a corner for several months, missing the rounds of continual server updates and checks that occurred as a matter of policy in this company. Active (and unpatched) for only three days, it had fallen victim to hostile code known as Solaris/sadmind.worm. Sadmind (also known as sadmin) is a parasitic worm that uses Solaris machines to find unpatched Microsoft web servers and deface them, replacing the default home page with a black background and red words expressing a vulgar and hostile sentiment toward the United States. The company also benefited from timing and obscurity. The web page defacement had been discovered within three hours of the penetration itself, which had occurred on a weekend, and to a system known to and used by only a few select IT staff members.

Even knowing the attack was from a worm, and therefore the result of an automated (and most likely unattended) attack, we still had a concern that the compromised system had been used as a beachhead to explore and attack the network at large. Although the attack signatures of sadmind were in plain view in the log of the web server, no other logging capabilities had been activated on the server. Even the router connecting the network to the Internet lacked intrusion-detection or packet-capturing services.

Fortunately, there were only two other servers on this little test network, and not only were both patched and updated, they also had extensive logging enabled. Through the web logs, we could see the unsuccessful infection attempts by a sadmind worm from an external machine—the same machine that had infected the first test server. We could also see that there had been no communication from the infected server to either of the other test servers. Although we couldn't completely rule out that an attack had been attempted (or was successful) without further time-consuming testing, we were confident that adding a monitoring capability to the test network router (along with setting intrusion-detection alarms) would most likely uncover all but the most sophisticated infection. Along with a complete rebuild (and repatching) of the infected test server, we were almost done. When queried by the network administrator, we told him that the most important correction was not one of a technical nature, but procedural.

"You need to update your checklist and intrusion-detection procedures," we said. "Make sure that before any machine is activated, it has the latest patches and is in line with your company policy about logging, monitoring, and intrusion detection, including setting intrusion alerts and regular review of logs for all machines, not just those in production."

As we said earlier, the company was lucky. The assault was automated, not further exploited, and located on an isolated test system without real data, and the company also had a good foundation to work with. It was only through an oversight, a procedural quirk if you will, that the company fell victim to the worm. This kind of incident—an attack happening despite sound principles and consistent analysis—is a security professional's worst nightmare and unfortunately happens all too often. Understanding why oversights happen can help you catch them, and no example better illustrates this than the tragedy of Apollo 1.

On January 27, 1967, Apollo astronauts Mission Commander Edward White, Command Module Pilot Virgil "Gus" Grissom, and Lunar Module Pilot Roger Chaffee sat in the Apollo Command Module at the Kennedy Space Center, in Cape Canaveral, Florida. While the three space-suited men lay in the conical spacecraft, they participated in a Plugs Out Test, evaluating the capsule as if it were independently operating in the depth of space. As a result, the cabin was filled with pure oxygen at a higher pressure than the air outside the cabin, simulating what it would be like for the astronauts to be traveling in the vacuum of space.

At 6:31 P.M. a cry was heard over the radio: "Fire, I smell fire!" Because the inner door to the capsule only opened inward, the astronauts were trapped, unable to fight against the now-massive internal pressures created by the fire. Within seconds the module ruptured, spitting flame and toxic gases into two levels of the complex. Finally, after five minutes had passed, the workers were able to move through the dense and poisonous smoke to the capsule and begin the process of opening the hatch and removing the dead.

In the investigation that followed, much attention was focused on the pure oxygen environment of the cabin. NASA, however, patiently explained that pure oxygen made the most sense given all the other risk factors (including the decompression sickness that could occur during space walks). Instead, NASA insisted, it had attempted to *mitigate the risk of fire* by reducing the amount of flammable material in the cockpit. But notice in the following quote how NASA went about *determining* that fire risk:

> **"It can be seen in retrospect that attention was principally directed to individual testing of the material. What was not fully understood by ... NASA was the importance of considering the fire potential of combustibles *in a system* of all materials taken together in the position which they would occupy in the spacecraft and in the environment of the spacecraft." (House Committee on Science and Astronautics, Subcommittee on NASA Oversight, Investigation into Apollo 204 Accident Hearings, 3 vols., 90th Cong., 1st session, 10 April to 10 May 1967, pp. 175–76. Italics are mine.)**

In addition, NASA had not adequately planned for how to handle a fire if it did occur, especially on the ground during a testing phase. As one of the NASA astronauts reportedly said, it was "a failure of imagination." This disaster, along with the near-disaster of Apollo 13, began a tradition of multiple layers of redundancy—something that we emulate in network security through the concept of *defense in depth*. It also shows the importance of multilayered contingency plans. What happens when your contingency plan fails or has a problem?

In short, we are arguing that *repetition with recursion* is one of the singular principles of information security. Review a system again and again, looking closer and expanding outward in a never-ending cycle, always seeking more. Of course, the pragmatist will immediately note that this principle runs in direct opposition to that of *resource conservation*. In other words, don't spend money (in the form of time, effort, or capital) unless it would cost more not to—the cost-benefit ratio. Although a balance must be achieved, there is still a lack of awareness of the dynamic nature of systems—a dynamic nature that requires you to continually walk through the security process. Many variations of the security process are possible, but you can get a general model of the process from—where else?—systems analysis!

THE SYSTEMS DEVELOPMENT LIFE CYCLE (SDLC): SECURITY AS A PROCESS FROM BEGINNING TO END

The Systems Development Life Cycle (SDLC) is a method used by system developers and programmers to formalize the implementation of any system-based process—from the initial project definition to the phasing out or replacement of the system. The exact number of steps in the process can vary, but for our purposes we'll use five major phases broken into sublayers:

1. Initiation

   ► Conceptual definition

   ► Functional requirement determination

   ► Protection specifications development

   ► Design review

2. Development and acquisition

   ► Component and code review

   ► System test review

   ► Certification

3. Implementation

   ► Accreditation

4. Operation and maintenance

5. Disposal

Initiation

Initiation is defined as the beginning of the security process. Ideally, of course, security is implemented and integrated along with the full IT system itself. In reality, many times the security process is begun long after a system has been installed and operating. Most security professionals consider this phase the most important and, usually, the most rushed.

Conceptual Definition

Before any work can proceed, you must understand the scope of the security process. You can think of *scope* as defining the boundary of responsibility of the security system or, in other words, the boundary of the system you are charged with protecting. The conceptual definition is also important for another reason: It helps define the responsibility and scope of the individuals involved in the security process. This becomes critical if multiple individuals are involved in the security process, especially if those individuals are from multiple departments (or even from outside companies). You can think of the conceptual definition as the *spirit* of the security system—the guiding ideas and principles that will be made real through the formal and detail-specific implementation plans that will follow in subsequent steps and phases.

Functional Requirement Determination

Although your beginning objectives are initially (and generally) defined in the conceptual definition, in this phase you begins to specify the details of your objectives—from high-level goals to specific targets. In practical terms, this step breaks down into several activities:

Interviews   Interviews serve to clarify and identify what specifically needs to be protected—both data and data processing. Your primary goal is to discover and categorize the data by criticality. As a natural result of this process, you also identify the business processes that are used to store, retrieve, and manipulate that data. The result is that you break your entire network into a series of subsystems whose performance and compliance with your security goals (and targets) can be measured. Measurement is critical, because it provides you with the central indicator of the effectiveness of the security process as a whole—in other words, justifying the expense (in effort and equipment) of performing the security process.

External Reviews   You use a current and historical review of the security environment, along with industry best practices, to establish a benchmark of environmental threats and supports. Visiting sites of organizations that have similar objectives and constraints, along with understanding technology trends and capabilities, are excellent ways to augment this step.

Gap Analysis This step consists of taking the combined information gathered from the internal and external reviews and matching it with the objectives defined originally in the conceptual definition. What remains is the difference between what is and what should be, including identifying which areas of technology, business process, organizational culture, end-user knowledge, and budgeting are necessary to close the gap.

Another term for gap is *risk*, as we defined the term in Chapter 1. The final product created from this phase is a requirements definition: a detailed analysis of what is needed to mitigate those risks identified by comparing your *actual* system state with your *objective* state.

Protection Specifications Development

Once your system is modeled and compared to your objectives, and your risks are defined, you're ready to roll up our sleeves and go to work. At this stage of the process, you create a detailed design of your new system security, starting with a general system model that matches your goals and then burrowing down into matching specific technologies, configurations, procedures, and changes to your various targets.

Because this design is the blueprint for the system, this phase usually produces the most formal documentation, even for the simplest implementations. Oversights or incorrect judgments made at this phase can cripple the success of the project. Some of the typical issues covered in the design (and translated to specific sections of the documentation) are as follows:

Executive Summary This section usually contains a condensed overview of the objectives and constraints used to arrive at the plan. These items are usually referred to as the *selection criteria*, along with the decisions leading to the particular design. Because the repetitive and recursive process of analyzing and combining alternatives might not be apparent to key decisions makers, decision rationale is also included.

Selection Methodology This section spells out your specific criteria, along with how you ranked them based on your initial objectives and constraints. It's also helpful to demonstrate how you evaluated the different combinations of criteria.

Alternatives   Although not every alternative at every level needs to be included, the most contested or competing alternatives should be listed with their respective pros and cons.

Recommendation   The meat of the document, this section contains the specific design details, along with the final rationale criteria.

Design Review

Any good plan needs a final reality check. We find that after being immersed in the discovery, definition, and design steps, we can sometimes miss simple things. Another pair of trusted eyes can help us avoid embarrassment. But more important, the Design Review phase is an opportunity to present your design and its implications to your decision makers. It also serves to clarify job responsibility among all individuals, teams, and organizations involved with the project. The review should reiterate how all the logical pieces are expected to flow together and interoperate.

Development and Acquisition

Get out the credit card. You're going shopping! Once your design is finished and reviewed and the final go-ahead is given, you need to assemble or create your tools, including prototypes and test systems to verify that your configurations function correctly and in the manner that you expect. If your security effort is part of a larger system rollout, you'll have additional tasks, such as reviewing the code or applications that will be installed and testing your security system in the context of the network as a whole.

Component and Code Review

Once you purchase or develop a specific security tool, program, or component, you have to evaluate it in a lab or prototype environment. Although it seems obvious that you want to make sure the components work as advertised, you're also using this time to look for any unknown or unexpected behavior and consequences. Breaking this review into steps helps focus on specific areas of concern:

Component Functionality   This step verifies that a particular security technology works according to your expectations and the requirements of the security system as a whole.

Component Configuration   You also have to test the various configurations of a component to make sure they work as planned. Sometimes you discover additional configurations that might help or harm the system, and naturally you have to determine the implications for the component functionality and the system as a whole if those configurations are activated.

Component Maintenance   This step often provides an opportunity for the groups or individuals responsible for maintaining the component to establish workable procedures and methods for maintaining, updating, and troubleshooting it.

Code Review   A final (and separate) step from the rest, the code review is your last opportunity to explore sensitive or mission-critical areas of program code to look for bugs or fundamental design problems. Because the most common exploits of Internet-exposed network services are due to buffer overflows, finding code that could allow such an attack is the highest priority of this step.

System Test Review

Once you individually prototype and review your tools and technologies, you need to prototype them as a whole system—the lesson that was learned from the Apollo 1 disaster. Although you look at similar issues of functionality, configuration, and maintenance in the component and code review phase, you also use this step as an opportunity to determine the training and implementation efforts necessary to put the system into production. Specifically, prototyping the entire system helps with the following areas:

System Functionality   Assuming that each component functions individually as planned, you must still verify that they will work in concert. This step in the prototype process can reveal negative, unpredicted side-effects of mixing a range of technologies and their various configurations with the established policies, procedures, and business processes of an organization.

System Configuration   Altering the configuration of your components while they are interacting as a system can also highlight hidden problems and weaknesses.

System Maintenance   Understanding the implications of component interactions can also help you develop a detailed plan for maintenance, upgrades, and troubleshooting, including the establishment of a baseline for behavior and performance and an estimated support budget. Again, the emphasis is on issues that present themselves only when the components are interacting.

System Training   What education requirements are necessary for those individuals interacting with the system? Do support staff need to upgrade their technical skills? Do end users need basic training on how to use the system?

System Implementation   One of the most significant benefits of prototyping a security system is learning which obstacles you might encounter in the actual implementation. Being able to document solutions to those implementation problems, along with simple exposure experience to the system itself, is an invaluable investment.

Certification

Similar to having an outside party review your design, certifying your prototype means that you verify a *working* design—a working system that meets your criteria. Once your prototype is verified (your mix of technologies and configurations has been simulated to the most practical degree possible), you can gain the permission to progress to the most dangerous step of all—the implementation.

Implementation

One of the most common IT statistics invoked today (usually used to scare project managers and bean counters everywhere) is that only 70 percent of all IT projects succeed. And when they fail, it's usually in the implementation process. Somehow, somewhere along the path, we inevitably miss things; or, worse, the environment or the system changes enough from the beginning of the security process that our solution no longer meets the objectives, or the objectives themselves change!

Assuming that your design and prototype were sound, there are still great challenges. From our experience, those obstacles usually come in the form of the users of the system. How might you mitigate the risk of acceptance among your users? The usual answer is to provide simple system education. When you teach users how to interact with the new rules and technologies that have been put in place, they will become comfortable with them and accepting of them. Once they understand the system, the users will embrace it and become proactive in carrying the mission of information security into all facets of their work.

Although we believe that education can provide understanding and acceptance, we also believe that there is more to successful internalization and acceptance than simple exposure to the methods and technologies of the new system. Like any of us, users of a system need to understand why the system has changed. In other words, psychologically, they perform their own cost-benefit analysis. Are the changes they have to make in their own established, functional habits worth it?

This is a valid question. Although ideally you could have gained the support of users back in the design stage and augmented it by providing user access and input in the prototype stage, the question inevitability is asked again (even if silently) by every user the moment they have to give up their old way of doing things. You can answer the question in several ways. One way, of course, is to have a high degree of user involvement from the beginning of the security process, as we've mentioned. Additionally, if feasible, you can provide a phased transition from the old system to the new one. And finally, you can resort to tactics used by every successful parent on the planet—bribery and delay!

Start by assuring your users that although their favorite feature might not have made it into this cycle of implementation, you will personally make every effort to include it in the next cycle of system evaluation. By the way, it's helpful to present the users with a schedule of cycles you will be using to reevaluate and reimplement fixes in the security system. By issuing new schedules that list their desired features matched to the expected implementation date, you not only convince users to start the acceptance process, but also provide leverage to management to provide you with the resources necessary to implement that feature. (Bribery works both up and down!)

Although it may seem that we're taking a tongue-in-cheek approach to the problem of user adoption, we're only slightly teasing. Getting end users to accept the system is the only way to reduce your chances that they will misuse it. Consider the Love Bug worm, a viral attachment to an e-mail message that used the address book of the victim to propagate. The worm had a devastating rate of infection, even in organizations that had strict policies about not activating attachments. The reason? Humans' psychological need to be validated (or the curiosity that led them wonder why their boss suddenly expressed an amorous interest in them).

Our final thought is this: The only way to increase the chances that your system will be used as designed is to understand and accept the changes in usability demanded by the most important stakeholders. If you don't do this, you'll spend the rest of the time convincing your users that they don't want the changes they believe they do. Neither approach is easy, and only you can decide which is better for the system as a whole.

Accreditation

There has been a growing trend in the security community to recommend insurance for critical business technology and systems, especially for e-commerce sites. That these sites are often the most visible victims of cracker attacks is certainly a factor, but not the only factor. History has shown that as any specific resource gains value in proportion to the overall value of a product, that resource has been insured, whether it is a building, an actor, or a web server. Although it is easy to put a price on equipment failure, it is an entirely different matter to put a price on an organization's reputation—let alone determine the extent of the damage. In the end, most organizations focus their coverage on immediate and short-term damage to stock prices following such a dramatic incident.

Some feel that insuring a system expresses doubt about the ability of the organization to properly defend it. What they are missing is that this type of insurance isn't usually designed specifically for an external, directed, hostile cracker attack against a computer system; rather, it is an attempt to cover the loss of a critical system against anything that might threaten it, whether that is a web-page defacement, a natural physical disaster, or hardware failure. Seen in this light, insuring a system makes much more sense.

Insurance companies often want to verify that a system meets a reasonable minimum level of security before they will cover it in a policy. As a result, the last step of your implementation should be an accreditation review. Often performed by an outside organization (but not necessarily the insurance company itself), this review verifies that the system meets the design objectives, which means that ideally you have included an insurance company's criteria in your conceptual definition at the beginning of the security process.

Accreditation also helps key stakeholders in the project (think senior management, investors, clients, employees, and so on) have confidence in your efforts. That confidence leads to the most important resource a security professional can maintain—credibility. Having credibility is more important than trust, although credibility encompasses trust. Credibility translates into support. Support translates into providing requested resources, and nothing can hamper a security effort like not dedicating enough to the security budget.

Operation and Maintenance

Like war, this phase can be filled with long stretches of tedium and boredom, followed by brief interludes of sheer terror. Days and days of updates to operating systems, web servers, and virus-scan software can be interrupted by a 2 A.M. page from the firewall that it is about to go under from a massive DDoS (distributed denial of service) attack. Operating a system is more than day-to-day maintenance; you also have to defend and recover the system in the face of threats. Although the sexy battles are with script-kiddy cyberpunks or dissatisfied, disgruntled IT ex-employees, your data is just as endangered by the high temperature levels in the server room, the misconfigured backup tape software, and the executive who insists on deleting key system files to make space for the latest Shakira mp3.

Maintenance is where the security battle is usually lost. Technology and business are both moving fast. Some say that businesses (and even whole economies) are changing in the same duration as dictated by Moore's Law—18 months. While you are scrambling to update your web server with the latest security fixes, you also have to be on the lookout for wireless access points that give someone in the next building local access to your network, and you have to be on call when your CEO loses her PDA (holding the company's not-yet-released earnings report) at the beach.

Ultimately, you will need to take a step back from the day-to-day chaos of your system and evaluate it again from top to bottom. There might even come a time when instead of small fixes, you have to reinvent the security system from the ground up. This is happening more and more frequently as companies grow, merge, acquire, and implement whole new infrastructures. When that day comes, you might have to think not just about what to add, but also what to get rid of.

Disposal

Making the choice about which business procedures and technologies to use is difficult. Sometimes you're presented with a simple choice—the old way or a new way, but not both (at least, not at the same time in the same place). But occasionally you decide that it's just not worth doing what you're doing now. Your old way still functions and still meets the primary objectives, but it begins to conflict with your constraints, especially as they concern cost. This conflict usually occurs when the price of maintaining a system is equal to or greater than the cost to implement and support a new system. You can also be presented with weaknesses that have been discovered in the old way that create or increase a threat against your system. Of course, getting rid of components (or your system as a whole) should never increase the danger level; but, again, that's an ideal.

Steady As It Goes: Putting the "Constant" Back into Vigilance

You have a security system, and you're pretty satisfied. You've had a successful implementation, your maintenance is going well, and you've even scheduled a review of the system process. But you have a little whisper of doubt: What have you missed? Documents, policies, and procedures can only provide some comfort. After all, they are only tools to help the willing.

You know you need to be vigilant; you know you need to be constant. How you accomplish those goals will depend on the uniqueness of you, your system, and its environment. However, may we suggest something we've learned from many long nights of patrol and guard duty observation both in the military and in civilian life? For the watcher, routine is the enemy. Not only does repetition blind you, it also allows a hostile enemy to better plan for your vulnerability. We understand that checklists and standards allow us to work efficiently. And, of course, we've preached against complexity; both of those principles are correct. However, if you are concerned about what you don't know, you need to be prepared to change how and when you look.

This can be a rewarding experience, and on levels beyond the psychological. By evaluating the performance of your system at unusual times, you can learn about issues affecting the system that don't present themselves at other times. Remember that crackers try to disguise their efforts and make inroads in the dead of night or during the busiest times—for example, on a Monday morning when not-yet-caffeinated workers are more likely to fudge a password. But you can also learn that system performance as a whole decreases in unexpected ways during that logon time—something your network administrator might likely be interested in knowing.

One of the ways we like to test our systems is to set up some formal evaluations by external experts, otherwise known as Tiger teams. We provide a strict, agreed-upon set of parameters of what they are allowed or not allowed to do. We establish joint monitoring procedures and set a start and a stop time. Then, as we look over their shoulders, they put our defenses through their paces. Not only do we learn some of the latest cracker techniques, we also get a good idea of what we've done well and what we've been missing. And while we usually finish a little more humble, we also have a lot of fun!

Our final note for this chapter, before we move on to the more technical concepts that make up the meat of this book, is that the sequential process we've outlined is becoming increasingly compressed and less sequential as the rate of system evolution advances. In reality, we either conduct, or prepare to conduct, each phase at the same time, because we rarely implement a network system (let alone a security system) all at once. Although this can be frustrating and potentially dangerous, it also means we can more quickly incorporate the best security tools as they become available and proven. By focusing on providing redundant levels of security for your data and the systems that retrieve, store, and process that data, you increase your tolerance for mistakes—mistakes that are inevitable in your rapidly changing environment, system, and organization.

WHAT'S NEXT

Building on the work of the first chapter, the material we've just covered illustrates how perfect (and effortless) security is a myth. As with any endeavor, you must focus on reducing your risk in the most cost-effective way through a continual cycle of analysis, planning, implementation, and maintenance. Finally, we talked about the need to constantly maintain your alertness. In the next chapter, we'll begin looking at the technical nuts and bolts of how networks function.

Chapter 3

A Bird's-Eye View of Topology *Security*

In this chapter, we will look at the communication properties of network transmissions. You will also see what insecurities exist in everyday network communications and how you can develop a network infrastructure that alleviates some of these problems.

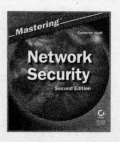

Adapted from *Mastering™ Network Security*,
Second Edition by Chris Brenton and Cameron Hunt
ISBN 0-7821-4142-0 $49.99

UNDERSTANDING NETWORK TRANSMISSIONS

It is no accident that the National Security Agency, which is responsible for setting the encryption standards for the U.S. government, is also responsible for monitoring and cracking encrypted transmissions that are of interest to the government. In order to know how to make something more secure, you must understand what vulnerabilities exist and how they can be exploited.

This same idea applies to network communications. In order to be able to design security into your network infrastructure, you must understand how networked systems communicate with one another. Many exploits leverage basic communication properties. If you are aware of these communication properties, you can take steps to ensure that they are not exploited.

Digital Communication

Digital communication is analogous to Morse code or the early telegraph system: certain patterns of pulses represent different characters during transmission. Figure 3.1 shows an example of a digital transmission. A voltage placed on the transmission medium is considered a binary 1. The absence of a signal is interpreted as a binary 0.

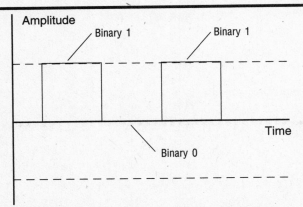

FIGURE 3.1:   A digital transmission plotted over time

Because this waveform is so predictable and the variation between acceptable values is so great, it is easy to determine the state of the transmission. This is important if the signal is electrical, because the introduction of noise to a circuit can skew voltage values slightly. As shown in Figure 3.2, even when there is noise in the circuit, you can still see which part of the signal is a binary 1 and which is a 0.

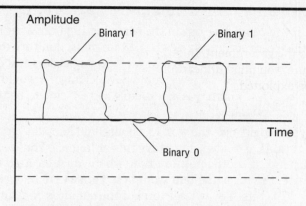

FIGURE 3.2:   A digital transmission on a noisy circuit

This simple format, which allows digital communication to be so noise-resistant, can also be its biggest drawback. The information for the ASCII character *A* can be transmitted with a single analog wave or vibration, but transmitting the binary or digital equivalent requires eight separate waves or vibrations (to transmit 01000001). Despite this inherent drawback, digital communication is usually much more efficient than analog circuits, which require a larger amount of overhead in order to detect and correct noisy transmissions.

NOTE

Overhead is the amount of additional information that must be transmitted on a circuit to ensure that the receiving system gets the correct data and that the data is free of errors. Typically, when a circuit requires more overhead, less bandwidth is available to transmit the actual data. It's like the packaging used for shipping: You didn't want hundreds of little Styrofoam acorns, but they're in the box taking up space to ensure that your item is delivered safely.

When you have an electric circuit (such as an Ethernet network that uses twisted-pair wiring), you need to pulsate your voltage in order to transmit information. This means your voltage state is constantly changing, which introduces your first insecurity: electromagnetic interference.

Electromagnetic Interference (EMI)

Electromagnetic Interference (EMI) is produced by circuits that use an alternating signal, like analog or digital communications (referred to as an *alternating current* or an *AC circuit*). EMI is not produced by circuits that contain a consistent power level (referred to as a *direct current* or a *DC circuit*).

For example, if you could slice one of the wires coming from a car battery and watch the electrons moving down the wire (kids: don't try this at home), you would see a steady stream of power moving evenly and uniformly down the cable. The power level would never change: It would stay at a constant 12 volts. A car battery is an example of a DC circuit, because the power level remains stable.

Now, let's say you could slice the wire to a household lamp and try the same experiment (kids: *definitely* do not try this at home!). You would now see that, depending on the point in time when you measured the voltage on the wire, the measurement would read anywhere between −120 volts and +120 volts. The voltage level of the circuit is constantly changing. Plotted over time, the voltage level resembles an analog signal.

As you watched the flow of electrons in the AC wire, you would notice something interesting. As the voltage changes and the current flows down the wire, the electrons tend to ride predominantly on the surface of the wire. The center point of the wire shows almost no electron movement at all. If you increase the frequency of the power cycle, more and more of the electrons travel on the surface of the wire, instead of at the core. This effect is somewhat similar to what happens to a water skier—the faster the boat travels, the closer to the top of the water the skier rides.

As the frequency of the power cycle increases, energy begins to radiate at a 90° angle to the flow of current. In the same way that water ripples out when a rock breaks its surface, energy moves out from the center core of the wire. This radiation is in a direct relationship with the signal on the wire; if the voltage level or the frequency is increased, the amount of energy radiated also increases (see Figure 3.3).

This energy has magnetic properties and is the basis of how electromagnets and transformers operate. The downside is that the electromagnetic radiation can be measured in order to "sniff" the signal traveling down the wire. Electricians have had tools for this purpose for many years. Most electricians carry a device that they can simply connect around a wire in order to measure the signal traveling through the center conductor.

More sophisticated devices can measure the EMI radiation coming off an electrical network cable and record the digital pulses traveling down the wire. Once a record of these pulses is made, it is a simple matter to convert them from a binary format to a format that humans can read. (Although a serious geek is just as happy reading the information in binary format, we did specifically say "humans.")

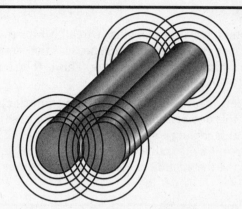

Copper wire conducting AC signal

FIGURE 3.3:   A conductor carrying an AC signal radiating EMI

NOTE

Although twisted-pair cabling has become popular because of its low cost, it is also extremely insecure. Most of today's networks are wired using unshielded twisted pair. Because twisted pair is used for the transmission of electrical signals, EMI is produced. Because the cable does not use any shielding, it is extremely easy to detect the EMI radiating from each of the conductors. Although twisted pair is an excellent choice for general network use, it is not a good selection if the information traveling along the wire needs to remain 100 percent secure.

Your first point of vulnerability, therefore, is your network cables. People typically overlook these when evaluating the security of a network. Although an organization may go to great lengths to secure its computer room, a web of cabling may be running through the ceilings.

This can be even more of a problem if an organization is located in shared office space and cabling runs through common areas. A would-be attacker would never have to go near a computer room or wiring closet to collect sensitive information. A stepladder and a popped ceiling tile are all that's needed to create an access point to your network. A savvy attacker might even use a radio transmitter to relay the captured information to another location. This means that the attacker can safely continue to collect information for an extended period of time.

Fiber-Optic Cable

Fiber-optic cable consists of a cylindrical glass thread center core 62.5 microns in diameter wrapped in cladding that protects the central core and reflects the light back into the glass conductor. This is then encapsulated in a jacket of tough KEVLAR fiber.

The whole thing is then sheathed in PVC (polyvinyl chloride) or Plenum. The diameter of this outer sheath is 125 microns. Because of the diameter measurements, this cabling is sometimes referred to as 62.5/125 cable. Although the glass core is breakable, the KEVLAR fiber jacket helps fiber-optic cable stand up to a fair amount of abuse. Figure 3.4 shows a fiber-optic cable.

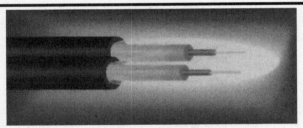

FIGURE 3.4: A stripped-back fiber-optic cable

Unlike twisted-pair cable, fiber-optic cable uses a light source for data transmission. This light source is typically a light-emitting diode (LED) that produces a signal in the visible infrared range. On the other end of the cable is another diode that receives the LED signals. The type of light transmission can take one of two forms: single mode or multimode.

TIP

Never look into the beam of an active fiber-optic cable! The light intensity is strong enough to cause permanent blindness. If you must visually inspect a cable, first make sure that it is completely disconnected from the network. Just because a cable is dark for a moment does not mean it is inactive. The risk of blindness or visual "dead spots" is too high to take risks—unless you know the cable is *completely* disconnected.

LIGHT DISPERSION

You'll see light dispersion if you shine a flashlight against a nearby wall: The light pattern on the wall will have a larger diameter than the flashlight lens. If you hold two flashlights together and shine them both against the wall, you'll get a fuzzy area in the middle where it's difficult to determine which light source is responsible for which portion of the illumination. The farther from the wall you move, the larger this fuzzy area becomes. This is, in effect, what limits the distance on multimode fiber-optic cable (that is, if you can call 1.2 miles a distance limitation for a single cable run). As the length of the cable increases, it becomes more difficult for the diode on the receiving end to distinguish between the different light frequencies.

Single-mode fiber-optic cable consists of an LED that produces a single frequency of light. This single frequency is pulsed in a digital format to transmit data from one end of the cable to another. The benefit of single-mode fiber-optic cable over multimode is that it is faster and will travel longer distances (in the tens-of-miles range). The drawbacks are that the hardware is extremely expensive and installation can be tedious at best. Unless your company name ends with the word *Telephone* or *Utility*, single-mode fiber-optic cable would be overkill.

Multimode transmissions consist of multiple light frequencies. Because the light range does not need to be quite so precise as single-mode, the hardware costs for multimode are dramatically less than for single-mode. The drawback of multimode fiber-optic cable is *light dispersion*—the tendency of light rays to spread out as they travel.

Because multimode transmissions are light-based instead of electrical, fiber-optic cable benefits from being completely immune to all types of EMI monitoring. There is no radiation to monitor as a signal passes down the conductor. Although it might be possible to cut away part of the sheath in order to get at the glass conductor, doing so might cause the system to fail, thus foiling the attacker. However, newer fiber-optic systems are more resilient and, ironically, more susceptible to monitoring from this kind of attack.

Fiber-optic cable has one other major benefit: It can support large bandwidth connections—10MB, 100MB, and even gigabit Ethernet. So, along with security improvements, it offers performance improvements.

This is extremely helpful in justifying the use of fiber-optic cable within your network; you can satisfy both bandwidth and security concerns. If Woolly Attacker is going to attempt to tap into your network in order to monitor transmissions, he will to want to choose a network segment with a lot of traffic so that he can collect the largest amount of data. Coincidentally, these are also the segments where you would want to use fiber-optic cable in order to support the large amount of data flowing though this point in the network. By using fiber-optic cable on these segments, you can help to protect the integrity of your cabling infrastructure.

Bound and Unbound Transmissions

The atmosphere is referred to as an *unbound medium*—a circuit with no formal boundaries. It has no constraints to force a signal to flow within a certain path. Twisted-pair cable and fiber-optic cable are examples of bound media, because they restrain the signal to within the wire. An unbound transmission is free to travel anywhere.

Unbound transmissions bring a host of security problems. Because a signal has no constraints that confine it within a specific area, it becomes that much more susceptible to interception and monitoring. The atmosphere is capable of transmitting a variety of signal types. The most commonly used are light and radio waves.

Light Transmissions

Light transmissions through the atmosphere use lasers to transmit and receive network signals. These devices operate similarly to a fiber-optic cable circuit, but without the glass medium.

Because laser transmissions use a focused beam of light, they require a clear line of sight and precise alignment between the devices. This requirement helps to enhance system security, because it severely limits the physical area from which a signal can be monitored. The atmosphere limits the light transmission's effective distance, however, as well as the number of situations in which it can be used.

Unbound light transmissions are also sensitive to environmental conditions; a heavy mist or snowfall can interfere with their transmission properties. This means it is easy to interrupt a light-based circuit—thus denying users service. Still, light transmissions through the atmosphere make for a relatively secure transmission medium when physical cabling cannot be used.

Radio Waves

Radio waves used for networking purposes are typically transmitted in the 1–20GHz range and are referred to as *microwave* signals. These signals can be fixed frequency or spread spectrum in nature.

Fixed Frequency Signals   A *fixed frequency signal* is a single frequency used as a carrier wave for the information you want to transmit. A radio station is a good example of a single frequency transmission. When you tune in to a station's carrier wave frequency on your FM dial, you can hear the signal that is riding on it.

A *carrier wave* is a signal that is used to carry other information. This information is superimposed onto the signal (in much the same way as noise), and the resultant wave is transmitted into the atmosphere. This signal is then received by a device called a *demodulator* (in effect, your car radio is a demodulator that can be set for different frequencies), which removes the carrier signal and passes along the remaining information. A carrier wave is used to boost a signal's power and to extend the receiving range of the signal.

Fixed frequency signals are easy to monitor. Once an attacker knows the carrier frequency, they have all the information they need to begin receiving your transmitted signals. They also have all the information they need to jam your signal, thus blocking all transmissions.

Spread Spectrum Signals   A *spread spectrum signal* is identical to a fixed frequency signal, except multiple frequencies are transmitted because of the reduction of interference through noise. Spread spectrum technology arose during wartime, when an enemy would jam a fixed frequency signal by transmitting on an identical frequency. Because spread spectrum uses multiple frequencies, it is much more difficult to disrupt.

Notice the operative words "more difficult." It is still possible to jam or monitor spread spectrum signals. Although the signal varies through a range of frequencies, this range is typically a repeated pattern. Once an attacker determines the timing and pattern of the frequency changes, they are in a position to jam or monitor transmissions.

NOTE
Because it is so easy to monitor or jam radio signals, most transmissions rely on encryption to scramble the signal so that it cannot be monitored by outside parties.

Terrestrial vs. Space-Based Transmissions   Two methods can be used to transmit both fixed frequency and spread spectrum signals. These are referred to as *terrestrial* and *space-based* transmissions:

> **Terrestrial Transmissions**   *Terrestrial transmissions* are completely land-based radio signals. The sending stations are typically transmission towers located on top of mountains or tall buildings. The range of these systems is usually line of sight, although an unobstructed view is not required. Depending on the signal strength, 50 miles is about the maximum range achievable with a terrestrial transmission system. Local TV and radio stations are good examples of industries that rely on terrestrial-based broadcasts. Their signals can only be received locally.

> **Space-Based Transmissions**   *Space-based transmissions* are signals that originate from a land-based system but are then bounced off one or more satellites that orbit the earth in the upper atmosphere. The greatest benefit of space-based communications is range. Signals can be received from almost every corner of the world. The space-based satellites can be tuned to increase or decrease the effective broadcast area.

Of course, the larger the broadcast range of a signal, the more susceptible it is to being monitored. As the signal range increases, so does the possibility that someone knowledgeable enough to monitor your signals will be within your broadcast area.

Choosing a Transmission Medium

You should consider a number of security issues when choosing a medium for transferring data across your network. Keep in mind that any security concerns (read: objectives) will have to be balanced by other system objectives such as flexibility and cost. Although it is currently the most maligned network technology, the 802.11b protocol has also enabled rapid and flexible network access for thousands of businesses and individuals. Creative solutions that meet your security requirements while still allowing for the deployment of these popular communications media can be considered a best practice.

How Valuable Is My Data?

As you saw in earlier chapters, typical attackers must feel that they have something to gain by assaulting your network. Do you maintain databases that contain financial information? If so, someone might find the payoff high enough to make it worth the risk of staging a physical attack.

Of course, there is another consideration. Because of the growth in laws (and lawsuits) concerning data privacy and integrity, especially as applied to specific industries (health care) and types of data (financial), you must also consider the compliance levels your network must meet in order to avoid legal liability or retain insurance coverage.

Which Network Segments Carry Sensitive Data?

Your networks carry sensitive information on a daily basis. To protect this information, you need to understand the workflow of how it is used. For example, if you identify your organization's accounting information as sensitive, you should know where the information is stored and who has access to it. A small workgroup with its own local server will be far more secure than an accounting database that is accessed from a remote facility using an unbound transmission medium.

TIP

Be careful when analyzing the types of services that will be passing between your facilities. For example, e-mail is typically given little consideration, yet it usually contains more information about your organization than any other business service. Considering that most e-mail systems pass messages in the clear (if an attacker captures this traffic, it appears as plain text), e-mail should be one of your best-guarded network services.

TIP

Care should also be given to the applications that pass sensitive data. Even the most highly encrypted traffic can be rendered ineffective if the program passing the data is vulnerable to hostile attack—attacks that would lead to the compromise of the system holding the data!

Will an Intruder Be Noticed?

It's easy to spot an intruder when an organization consists of three of four people. Scale this to three or four thousand, and the task becomes proportionately difficult. If you are the network administrator, you may have no say in the physical security practices of your organization. You can, however, strive to make eavesdropping on your network a bit more difficult.

When you select a physical medium, keep in mind that you may need to make your network more resilient to attacks if other security precautions are lacking—especially as our definition of a "local" network logically extends to an Internet-connected laptop half a world away.

Are Backbone Segments Accessible?

If would-be attackers are going to monitor your network, they will look for central nodes where they can collect the most information. Wiring closets and server rooms are prime targets because these areas tend to be junction points for many communication sessions. When laying out your network, pay special attention to these areas and consider using a more secure medium (such as fiber-optic cable) if possible.

Consider these issues carefully when choosing a method of data transmission. Use the risk analysis information you collected in Chapter 2 to cost-justify your choices. Although increasing the level of topology security might appear to be an expensive proposition, the cost may be more than justified when compared with the cost of recovering from an intrusion.

TOPOLOGY SECURITY

Now that you have a good understanding of the transmission media available for carrying your data, let's look at how these media are configured to function as a network. *Topology* is defined as the rules for physically connecting and communicating on given network media. Each topology has its own set of rules for connecting your network systems and even specifies how these systems must "speak" to one another on the wire.

LAN Topologies

The past decade has seen a major change in local area network (LAN) infrastructure, with Ethernet emerging victorious from its battle with Token Ring as the topology of choice. Beginning with the new century, however, wireless technologies are rapidly encroaching and crossing LAN/WAN boundaries, even as speed and security concerns persist.

Ethernet

Let's examine how Ethernet moves information from one system to another across a network. The better you understand network communication properties, the easier it will be to secure your network.

NOTE

Ethernet was developed in the late 1970s by Xerox; it later evolved into the IEEE specification 802.3 (pronounced "eight-oh-two-dot-three"). Its flexibility, high transmission rate (at the time, anyway), and nonproprietary nature quickly made it the networking topology of choice for many network administrators.

Ethernet's ability to support a wide range of cable types, low-cost hardware, and Plug and Play connectivity has caused it to find its way into more corporate (as well as home) networks than any other topology.

Ethernet's communication rules are called *Carrier Sense Multiple Access with Collision Detection* (CSMA/CD). This is a mouthful, but it's simple enough to understand when you break it down:

- *Carrier sense* means that all Ethernet stations are required to listen to the wire at all times (even when transmitting). By "listen," we mean the station should be constantly monitoring the network to see if any other stations are currently sending data. By monitoring the transmissions of other stations, a station can tell if the network is open or in use. This way, the station does not just blindly transfer information and interfere with other stations. Being in a constant listening mode also means that the station is ready when another station wants to send it data.

- *Multiple access* simply means that more than two stations can be connected to the same network, and that all stations are allowed to transmit whenever the network is free. It is far more efficient to allow stations to transmit only when they need to than it is to assign each system a time block in which it is allowed to transmit. Multiple access also scales much more easily as you add more stations to the network.

- *Collision detection* answers this question: "What happens if two systems think the circuit is free and try to transmit data at the same time?" When two stations transmit simultaneously, a *collision* takes place. A collision is similar to interference, and the resulting transmission becomes mangled and useless for carrying data. As a station transmits data, it watches for this condition; if it detects such a condition, the workstation assumes that a collision has taken place. The station will back off, wait for a random period of time, and then retransmit.

Part I

NOTE

Each station is responsible for determining its own random waiting period before retransmission. This helps to ensure that each station is waiting for a different period of time, avoiding another collision. In the unlikely event that a second collision does occur (the station backs off but is again involved in a collision), each station is required to double its waiting period before trying again. Two or more consecutive collisions are referred to as a *multiple collision*.

If you were to chart CSMA/CD, it would look something like Figure 3.5. This process takes place after the ARP (Address Resolution Protocol) decision process.

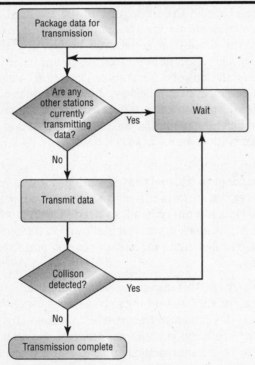

FIGURE 3.5:   A flow chart of Ethernet communication rules

An integral part of Ethernet communications is that each system is constantly monitoring the transmissions of all the other stations on the wire. Unfortunately, this is also Ethernet's biggest security flaw. It is possible to configure a system to read all this information it receives; this is commonly referred to as a *promiscuous mode* system.

A network administrator can leverage promiscuous mode to monitor a network from one central station so that errors and network statistics can be gathered. A network analyzer is effectively a computer operating in promiscuous mode. Because a station is listening to all network traffic anyway, a simple software change allows a system to record all the information it sees.

Unfortunately, the existence of promiscuous mode also means that a not-so-honest person might be able to eavesdrop on network communications or steal sensitive information. This is particularly a problem because most information passed along a computer network is transmitted as clear text. See Figure 3.6 for an example of this output.

```
Packet Number : 13            3:52:02 PM
Length : 66 bytes
ether: ==================== Ethernet Datalink Layer ====================
       Station: Skylar ----> This_Workstation
       Type: 0x0800 (IP)
   ip: ======================= Internet Protocol =======================
       Station:10.1.1.100 ---->10.1.1.25
       Protocol: TCP
       Version: 4
       Header Length (32 bit words): 5
       Precedence: Routine
             Normal Delay, Normal Throughput, Normal Reliability
       Total length: 48
       Identification: 21249
       Fragmentation not allowed, Last fragment
       Fragment Offset: 0
       Time to Live: 128 seconds
       Checksum: 0x9148(Valid)
  tcp: ================= Transmission Control Protocol =================
       Source Port: 258
       Destination Port: 1027
       Sequence Number: 417610
       Acknowledgement Number: 898472
       Data Offset (32-bit words): 5
       Window: 8510
       Control Bits: Acknowledgement Field is Valid (ACK)
             Push Function Requested (PSH)
       Checksum: 0x5DB5(Valid)
       Urgent Pointer: 0
```

FIGURE 3.6:   A packet capture of a network file

To minimize the amount of information that can be collected with a network monitor or analyzer, you can segment network traffic to isolate network communications by using a switch or a router—although many sophisticated techniques exist that can bypass the filtering capability of a switch. These devices (and their limitations) are discussed in the "Basic Networking Hardware" section of this chapter.

Wireless

Both 802.11b and, increasingly, Bluetooth wireless standards can be implemented as LAN technologies, with upcoming upgrades to both promising faster data throughput and increased security. (Bluetooth was originally conceived as more of a "personal" network connecting a PDA to a laptop or a laptop to a printer.) As vendors increasingly integrate wireless capability into network devices ranging from printers to PDAs, the security threats to unsecured wireless access points have reached mythic proportions.

WiFi   Advertised as an 11Mbps half-duplex (meaning that a wireless station can't transmit and receive at the same time) protocol, WiFi (formally known as 802.11b) operates in the 2.4GHz range, which means that some newer cordless phones can interfere with optimal operation. Also, the reality is that most communication occurs between 2.5Mbps and 4.5Mbps, with speeds decreasing as space between the access point and wireless station increases or as barriers (such as walls) are placed between them.

A WiFi topology operates in one of two modes—Ad-Hoc or Infrastructure. In Ad-Hoc mode, all wireless-capable devices talk directly to one another. In Infrastructure mode, all wireless traffic passes through one or more *access points*. Access points are used primarily to provide nonwireless networks (and devices) access to the wireless LAN and vice-versa.

Access points also operate in modes:

NAT   In this mode, the access point acts like a Network Address Translation router, in that traffic can originate from the wireless network and travel to the wired network. Traffic originating from the wired network, however, is not allowed to flow back. This configuration is common when an office or a home network has multiple computers that need to share a single, public IP address on the Internet.

Bridge   Access points acting as bridges transparently connect wireless and wired networks, while still providing the traffic segmentation features found in bridges and switches.

NAT + Bridge   Access points can bridge wired and wireless networks and then use a WAN port to NAT that traffic onto a distinct network. This configuration is common in offices that have a mix of wired and wireless computers that need NAT services.

Security for wireless networks is provided by WEP (Wired Equivalent Privacy). Although WEP includes both low (64-bit) and high (128-bit) encryption modes, several flaws in the WEP infrastructure have rendered it unreliable and vulnerable to attack. Vendors are responding to this problem by providing proven industry-strength encryption on the wireless cards themselves, although not all these devices will interoperate.

802.11a   The 802.11a standard is a sister technology to WiFi (they both use the same Media Access Control [MAC] standard). Although still grouped under the WiFi banner, there are some significant differences—primarily in how the standards use the radio spectrum. The 802.11a standard uses a technology called OFDM (Orthogonal Frequency-Division Multiplexing), a signal modulation technique that uses frequencies in the range of 5GHz. OFDM provides for a greater use of available bandwidth than earlier technologies, which allows the theoretical top speed of 802.11a to approach 54Mbps.

Although the 802.11a components are more expensive and use more power than WLAN devices, the newer technologies (and operating frequencies) mean that they are less susceptible to interference from cordless phones, microwave ovens, Bluetooth networks, and even WiFi networks. Although it is helpful in the United States, 802.11a is not a worldwide standard (WiFi is), 802.11a devices can't communicate with WiFis, and they use the same vulnerable WEP encryption as WiFi. And finally, because higher frequencies are more easily absorbed, the 5GHz signals don't penetrate walls and windows as easily, significantly limiting their range indoors to 50 meters, as opposed to 100 meters for WiFi.

With all these concerns, will 802.11a find a place in today's home and office networks? The most likely scenario is that high-bandwidth multimedia devices will take the most advantage of the higher data rates offered by the protocol. In fact, some vendors see it as the super-fast alternative for Bluetooth; limited range and high resistance against interference are perfect qualities for a transfer mechanism from a digital camera to a laptop.

Bluetooth   Originally designed as a cable replacement technology, Bluetooth technology is being integrated directly into laptops, PDAs, cell phones, and printers, as opposed to 802.11b, which is usually implemented as a distinct network device. With a much more limited range and data throughput (10 meters and 1Mbps as opposed to the 300+ and 11Mbps of 802.11b), Bluetooth is still eight times faster than the average parallel port.

Although the abilities of 802.11b seem dramatic in comparison, Bluetooth embodies fundamental infrastructure improvements, including support for full-duplex communications and a more sophisticated interference immunity provided by a spread spectrum made up of more than 79 (as opposed to the 11 of 802.11b) frequencies.

Bluetooth devices are separated into three classes based on the amount of power they use, as shown in Table 3.1.

TABLE 3.1:   Classes of Bluetooth Devices

CLASS	POWER (IN MILLIWATTS)	RANGE (IN METERS)
1	100	100
2	1–2.5	10
3	1	0.1–10

When two Bluetooth-enabled devices attempt to communicate, they use LMP (Link Manager Protocol) to initiate, authenticate, and manage sessions, along with device power management. When more than two devices communicate in a session, they are said to join a *piconet*. A piconet is a network that operates like 802.11b in Ad-Hoc mode, with the difference that one of the devices will become a master (with the rest remaining slaves) for the purpose of maintaining the frequency hopping in sync. Multiple piconets (as many as 10) can be connected to form *scatternets*, although this arrangement is seen as impractical.

Bluetooth security is broken into three modes for devices:

SM1   This mode is also called promiscuous mode. A device operating in SM1 will allow any other device to initiate a session.

SM2   Security is enforced after a session is initiated. Although it leaves devices vulnerable to an intermediate (man-in-the-middle) attack, SM2 enables flexible security policies to be applied to sessions.

SM3   All sessions, regardless of connection status, are wrapped in an encryption and authentication wrapper.

Additionally, service *levels* are applied to both devices and services. Devices can either be *trusted* or *untrusted*, with trusted devices gaining access to a full range of services. Although untrusted devices can be limited from all services, they can also be granted access to a controlled subset of services.

Services have three security levels:

Authentication/Authorization   To access a service at this level, devices must first authenticate themselves (prove their identity) and then receive authorization (their identity must be on an approved list for access). If a device is trusted, access is granted automatically. Untrusted devices can gain access, but only through user intervention.

Authentication   Services with the authentication service level require only that the identity of the device be assured.

Open   Services at this level are said to be *promiscuous*—open to all devices without restriction.

Most wireless security experts are in agreement that although future weaknesses might be found, Bluetooth is generally secure and provides a level of sophistication lacking in WLAN, as long as vendors continue to implement the security capabilities by default.

Wide Area Network Topologies

Wide area network (WAN) topologies are network configurations that are designed to carry data over a great distance. Unlike LANs, which are designed to deliver data between many systems, WAN topologies are usually point to point. *Point to point* means that the technology was developed to support only two nodes sending and receiving data. If multiple nodes need access to the WAN, a LAN is placed behind it to accommodate this functionality. Here are two of the more common private circuit topologies.

Leased lines are dedicated analog or digital circuits that are paid for on a flat-rate basis. Whether you use the circuit or not, you pay a fixed monthly fee. Leased lines are point-to-point connections that connect one geographical location to another. The maximum throughput on a leased line is 56Kbps. A *T1* is a full-duplex signal (each end of the connection can transmit and receive simultaneously) over two-pair wire cabling.

Part I

This wire pair terminates in a receptacle that resembles the square phone jacks used in older homes. T1s are used for dedicated point-to-point connections in the same way that leased lines are. Bandwidth on a T1 is available in increments from 64Kb up to 1.544Mb. T1s use time division to break the two wire pairs into 24 separate channels. *Time division* is the allotment of available bandwidth based on time increments. This arrangement is extremely useful because a T1 can carry both voice and data at the same time.

Typically, you can deploy leased lines or T1s in two ways:

▶ The circuit constitutes the entire length of the connection between the two organizational facilities (such as a branch office and a main office).

▶ The leased line is used for the connection from each location to its local exchange carrier. Connectivity between the two exchange carriers is then provided by some other technology, such as Frame Relay (discussed in the next section).

The first of these two options creates the more secure connection, but at a much higher cost. Using a private circuit for end-to-end connectivity between two geographically separated sites is the best way to ensure that your data is not monitored. Although it is still possible to sniff one of these circuits, an attacker would need to gain physical access to some point along its path. The attacker would also need to be able to identify the specific circuit to monitor. Telephone carriers are not known for using attacker-friendly labels such as "Bank XYZ's financial data: monitor here."

The second option is simply used to get your signal to the local exchange carrier. From there, data travels over a public network, such as Frame Relay.

Frame Relay

Frame Relay is a *packet-switched* technology. Because data on a packet-switched network can follow any available circuit path, such networks are represented by clouds in graphical presentations such as Figure 3.7.

Frame Relay must be configured as a *permanent virtual circuit* (PVC), meaning that all data entering the cloud at point A is automatically forwarded to point B. These end points are defined at the time the service is leased. For large WAN environments, Frame Relay can be far more cost effective than dedicated circuits because you can run multiple PVCs through a single WAN connection.

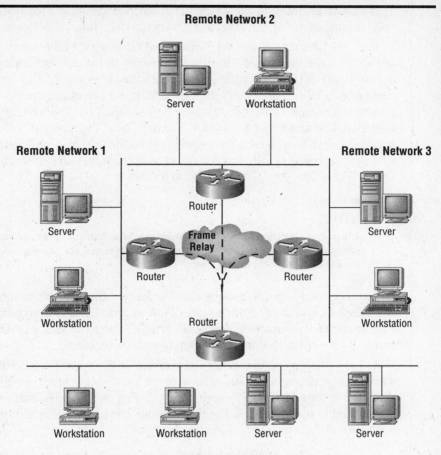

FIGURE 3.7: A WAN Frame Relay cloud connecting three remote networks to a corporate office

For example, let's say you have four remote sites that require a 56Kb connection to the home office. To construct this network out of dedicated circuits, you would need a 56Kb leased line connection at each of the remote sites, as well as four 56Kb leased line connections running into the main office.

With Frame Relay, however, you could replace the four dedicated connections at the main office with one fractional T1 connection and simply activate four channels of the T1 circuit to accept the data. By requiring only a single circuit at the main site, you can reduce your WAN costs.

In fact, nothing says the CIR (Committed Information Rate—the rate per second, under normal conditions, that the frame connection can deliver data) at the main office must equal the CIR value of all your remote sites. For example, let's assume that the connections to your remote site are used strictly for transferring e-mail. If bandwidth requirements are low, you might be able to drop the CIR at the main office from 256Kb to 128Kb. As long as the combined traffic to your four remote sites never exceeds 128Kb, you will not even notice a drop in performance. This would reduce your WAN costs even further.

NOTE

The packet-switched network is a shared medium. Your exchange carrier uses the same network for all PVCs it leases out. In effect, you are sharing available bandwidth with every other client.

Your connection point into the cloud is defined through the use of a *Data Link Connection Identifier* (DLCI). A unique DLCI is assigned to each router that connects to the cloud. The DLCI lets the local exchange carrier know which PVC it should map to your connection.

As long as everyone uses their assigned DLCI, life is good. The problem occurs when someone incorrectly, or with malicious intent, assigns their router the same DLCI as your circuit. Doing so can cause traffic to be diverted to their network. For this to occur, the following conditions must be met:

1. The attacker must be connected to the same local exchange carrier.

2. The attacker must be connected to the same physical switch.

3. The attacker must know your DLCI.

Clearly, this is not the most difficult attack to stage. Although it would be expensive (unless the attacker can gain access to another organization's network and "borrow" that connection), this attack may be well worth the effort if the attacker knows sensitive information will be passing across the link.

Also, a would-be attacker can redirect a PVC to another geographical location. Although doing so would eliminate the need to be connected through the same local carrier and the same switch in order to capture data, the attacker would have to infiltrate the exchange carrier's management system. Although this is not an easy task, it has been done in the past.

Asynchronous Transfer Mode (ATM)

Asynchronous Transfer Mode (ATM) is a point-to-point WAN technology most commonly implemented at speeds ranging from 25 to 622Mbps and beyond. Although ATM was initially very popular as a cost-effective, scalable, and reliable alternative to traditional leased lines, it also has significant vulnerabilities when it comes to user authentication, data integrity, data availability, and data privacy; it has also begun to lose some popularity compared with advancements in other less-expensive technologies. ATM works differently from Frame Relay because it breaks data into fixed-size packets known as *cells*. These cells are quite small (53 bytes), which allows them to transmit video, audio, and computer data over the same network, all the while making sure that no single type of data monopolizes the bandwidth.

The cell-based packets of ATM aren't compatible with packet-filtering firewalls, because these firewalls would have to be considered the endpoint of a point-to-point ATM connection. The overhead of *segmentation and reassembly* (SAR) of ATM packets simply wouldn't be efficient. Also, because ATM services can transfer non-IP traffic, there are vulnerabilities not associated with IP traffic (and therefore not covered by traditional IP-based network security mechanisms).

A cracker could get access to your ATM data two ways. The first method depends on your transport media. Although most ATM is run on fiber-optic cables, this is not necessarily the cracker-showstopper you would think. Crackers have eavesdropped on fiber-optic by pulling away the insulation and then bending the fiber-optic enough to force some of the light out of the transmission path (but not enough to completely terminate the session and thus alert someone to their actions).

The second method takes advantage of the virtual circuit running on a network: switched (SVC) or permanent (PVC). Most SVC management systems have an Add to Call feature that allows any system to join a session currently in progress. If the SVC administrator has not predefined and closed a session, any person can join in and eavesdrop. PVCs are also vulnerable through their management systems, especially if their interfaces are Telnet- or web-based. On these interfaces, a cracker can take advantage of sniffing passwords (in the case of Telnet) or exploiting weaknesses in implementation (web-based utilities).

Once a cracker has access to your network (and can create their own PVC or SVC), they can use the Interim Local Management Interface (ILMI) or Private Network-to-Network Interface (PNNI) to change the routing of your ATM network and send the data directly to a system they control on the Internet.

Wireless

Known as *broadband fixed wireless*, wireless WAN solutions are gaining in popularity as speed increases, hardware prices decrease, and reliability concerns prove to be unfounded. Most commercial providers of wireless WAN services include comprehensive data encryption as part of their service, although the level of encryption can vary among providers.

Although designed to be only a LAN wireless solution, the 802.11b standard has become so popular as an inter- and intraoffice solution that stories abound in the popular media about *whacking*, or wireless hacking. The process involves sensitive but inexpensive directional antennae that are used to locate and exploit wireless hubs physically located inside office buildings, but without encryption or authentication requirements that would keep a cracker from gaining access to the LAN as if they were sitting at a desk inside the building. Adding to the embarrassment is the revelation that the encryption level built into the standard was easily cracked. Vendors are responding to this threat by upgrading their equipment to add strong levels of encryption by default for all wireless communications.

BASIC NETWORKING HARDWARE

These days you must consider a plethora of networking products when planning your network infrastructure. There are devices for everything from connecting computer systems to the network to extending a topology's specifications to controlling network traffic. Sometimes your choices are limited—for example, to connect an office computer to the network, you must have a network card.

Many of these devices, when used correctly, can also help to improve your network security. In this section, we'll take a look at some common networking hardware and discuss which can be used to reinforce your security posture.

Hubs

Hubs are probably the most common piece of network hardware next to network interface cards. Physically, they are boxes of varying sizes that have multiple female RJ45 connectors. Each connector is designed to accept one twisted-pair cable outfitted with a male RJ45 connector. This twisted-pair cable is then used to connect a single server or workstation to the hub.

Hubs are essentially multiport repeaters that support twisted-pair cables in a star typology. Each node communicates with the hub, which in turn amplifies the signal and transmits it out each of the ports (including back out to the transmitting system). Hubs work at the electrical level.

Almost as popular as wire-only hubs and switches, wireless hubs/ switches combine hub and switching functions with a wireless access point. Most current popular models also include a dedicated WAN port (for DSL or cable modem connection) and basic firewall, logging, and NAT functions. Several wireless standards exist, from the highly popular 11MB 802.11b standard to its faster, newer cousin, the 54MB 802.11a.

Bridges

Although bridges as distinct pieces of hardware are relics of the past, their functionality is still retained in today's switches. To better under-stand that functionality, however, it will help to review what bridges *were*. Essentially, a bridge was a small box with two network connectors that attached to two separate portions of the network. A bridge incorporated the functionality of a hub (signal amplification), but it looked at the frames of data, which was a great benefit.

Ethernet data frames describe the information contained within the frame header. Bridges put this header information to use by monitoring the source and destination MAC address in each frame of data. By moni-toring the source address, the bridge learns where all the network systems are located. It constructs a table listing which MAC addresses are di-rectly accessible by each of its ports. It then uses that information to play traffic cop and regulate the flow of data on the network. Let's look at an example.

In the network in Figure 3.8, Betty needs to send data to the server Thoth. Because everyone on the network is required to monitor the network, Betty first listens for the transmissions of other stations. If the wire is free, Betty transmits a frame of data. The bridge is also watching for traffic and will look at the destination address in the header of Betty's frame. Because the bridge is unsure which port the system with MAC address 00C08BBE0052 (Thoth) is connected to, it amplifies the signal and retransmits it out Port B.

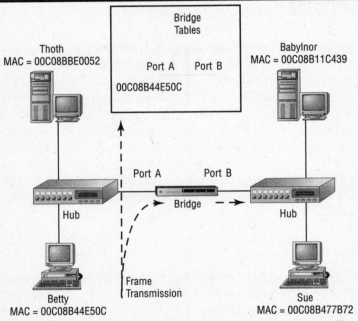

FIGURE 3.8: Betty transmits data to the server Thoth by putting Thoth's MAC address into the destination field of the frame.

When Thoth replies to Betty's request, as shown in Figure 3.9, the bridge looks at the destination address in the frame of data again. This time, however, it finds a match in its table, noting that Betty is also attached to Port A. Because it knows Betty can receive this information directly, it drops the frame and blocks it from being transmitted from Port B. The bridge also makes a new table entry for Thoth, recording the MAC address as being off Port A.

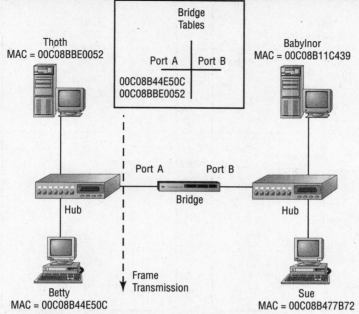

FIGURE 3.9:   Thoth's reply to Betty's message

For as long as the bridge remembers each station's MAC address, all communications between Betty and Thoth are isolated from Sue and Babylnor. *Traffic isolation* is a powerful feature; systems on both sides of the bridge can carry on conversations at the same time, effectively doubling the available bandwidth. The bridge ensures that communications on both sides stay isolated, as if they were not even connected. Because stations cannot see transmissions on the other side of the bridge, they assume the network is free and send their data.

Each system needs to contend for bandwidth only with systems on its own segment. There is no way for a station to have a collision outside its segment. Thus, these segments are referred to as *collision domains*, as shown in Figure 3.10. Notice that one port on each side of the bridge is part of each collision domain. This is because each of its ports will contend for bandwidth with the systems to which it is directly connected. The bridge isolates traffic within each collision domain, so there is no way for separated systems to collide their signals. The effect is a doubling of potential bandwidth.

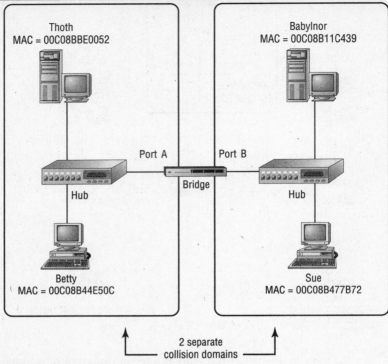

FIGURE 3.10: Two separate collision domains

Also notice that splitting the network into two collision domains has increased the security of the network. For example, let's say that the system named Babylnor becomes compromised. An attacker has gained high-level access to this system and begins capturing network activity in order to look for sensitive information.

Given the network design, Thoth and Betty can carry on a conversation with relative security. The only traffic that will find its way onto Babylnor's collision domain is broadcast traffic. A broadcast frame needs to be delivered to all local systems. For this reason, a bridge will also forward broadcast traffic. By using a bridge in this situation, you get a double bonus light: You have increased not only performance, but security as well.

What happens when traffic needs to traverse the bridge? As mentioned, when a bridge is unsure of the location of a system, it always passes the packet along just in case. Once the bridge learns that the system is located off its other port, it continues to pass the frame along as required.

If Betty begins communicating with Sue, for example, this data crosses the bridge and is transmitted onto the same collision domain as Babylnor. This means that Babylnor can capture this data stream. Although the bridge helped to secure Betty's communications with Thoth, it provides no additional security when Betty begins communicating with Sue.

To secure both of these sessions, you would need a bridge capable of dedicating a single port to each system. This type of functionality is provided in a device referred to as a *switch*.

Switches

Switches embody the marriage of hub and bridge technology. They resemble hubs in appearance, having multiple RJ45 connectors for connecting network systems. Instead of being a dumb amplifier like a hub, however, a switch functions as though it has a miniature bridge built into each port. A switch keeps track of the MAC addresses attached to each of its ports and routes traffic destined for a certain address only to the port to which it is attached.

Figure 3.11 shows a switched environment in which each device is connected to a dedicated port. The switch learns the MAC identification of each station once a single frame transmission occurs (identical to a bridge). Assuming this has already happened, you now find that at exactly the same instant Station 1 needs to send data to Server 1, Station 2 needs to send data to Server 2, and Station 3 needs to send data to Server 3.

There are some interesting things about this situation. First, each wire run involves only the switch and the station attached to it. Each collision domain is limited to these two devices, because each port of the switch is acting like a bridge. The only traffic seen by the workstations and servers is any frame specifically sent to them or to the broadcast address. As a result, all three stations see little network traffic and can transmit immediately. This is a powerful feature that goes a long way toward increasing potential bandwidth. Given our example, if this is a 10Mbps topology, the effective throughput has just increased by a factor of 3. All three sets of systems can carry on their conversations simultaneously, because the switch isolates them from one another. Although the network is still technically 10Mbps Ethernet, potential throughput has increased to 30Mbps.

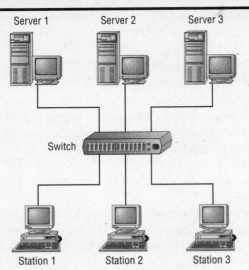

Server 1   Server 2   Server 3

Switch

Station 1   Station 2   Station 3

FIGURE 3.11: A switch installation showing three workstations and three servers that need to communicate

Besides increasing performance dramatically, you have also increased security. If any one of these systems becomes compromised, the only sessions that can be monitored are sessions with the compromised system. For example, if an attacker gains access to Server 2, they will not be able to monitor communication sessions with Servers 1 or 3—only Server 2.

Monitoring devices can only collect traffic that is transmitting within their collision domain. Because Server 2's collision domain consists of itself and the switch port it is connected to, the switch does an effective job of isolating System 2 from the communication sessions being held with the other servers. Although this is a wonderful security feature, it does make legitimate monitoring of your network somewhat cumbersome, which is why many switches include a *monitoring port*.

A monitoring port is simply a port on the switch that can be configured to receive a copy of all data transmitted to one or more ports. For example, you can plug your analyzer into port 10 of the switch and configure the device to listen to all traffic on port 3. If port 3 is one of your servers, you can now analyze all traffic flowing to and from this system.

This situation can also be a potential security hole. If an attacker is able to gain administrative access to the switch (through Telnet, HTTP, SNMP, or the console port), they would have free rein to monitor any system connected to, or communicating through, the switch. To return to our

Part I

example, if the attacker could access Server 2 and the switch itself, they are now in a perfect position to monitor all network communications.

Even without access to the switch's monitoring port, a cracker can still get access to network traffic, if only temporarily. In recent years, a number of sophisticated attacks have been created that force the switch to dump the MAC address table (something that a switch will do on its own if there are a large quantity of network changes in a short amount of time—such as unplugging all the cables and putting them back into different ports). Known as *MAC address poisoning*, the attack involves the cracker sending information to the switch that makes the switch think it has corrupted information in the table associating MAC addresses with network segments.

As a result, the switch *fails open.* It stops filtering network traffic in an attempt to remap which MAC addresses correspond to which network segments, thus allowing the hacker to eavesdrop on all network communication. Of course, once the switch has learned the network, it would normally reenable the switching function, but savvy attackers will continue to confuse the switch by sending it false mapping information, keeping it in a state of perpetual learning. Newer switches include management functions that allow them to report when a MAC address table dump has occurred—an event that can trigger management alarms and alert you to an intruder on your network!

NOTE

Keep in mind that bridges, switches, and similar networking devices are designed primarily to improve network performance, not to improve security. Increased security is just a secondary benefit. These devices have not received the same type of abusive, real-world testing as, say, a firewall or a router product. A switch can augment your security policy, but it should not be the core device to implement it.

Switching introduces a technology referred to as the *virtual local area network* (VLAN). Software running on the switch allows you to set up connectivity parameters for connected systems by workgroup (referred to as *VLAN groups*) instead of by geographical location. The switch's administrator is allowed to organize port transmissions logically so that connectivity is grouped according to each user's requirements. The "virtual" part is that these VLAN groups can span multiple physical network segments, as well as multiple switches. For example, by assigning all switch ports that connect to PCs used by accounting personnel to the same VLAN group, you can create a virtual accounting network.

Think of VLANs as the virtual equivalent of taking an ax to a switch with many ports in order to create multiple switches. If you have a 24-port switch and you divide the ports equally into three separate VLANs, you essentially have three 8-port switches.

Essentially is the key word here, because you still have one physical device. Although this arrangement makes for simpler administration, from a security perspective it is not nearly as good as having three physical switches. If an attacker is able to compromise a switch using VLANs, they might be able to configure their connection to monitor any of the other VLANs on the device.

This situation can be extremely bad if you have one large switch providing connectivity on both sides of a traffic-control device such as a firewall. An attacker may not need to penetrate your firewall; they may find the switch to be a far easier target. At the very least, the attacker now has two potential ways into the network instead of just one.

Routers

A *router* is a multiport device that decides how to handle the contents of a frame, based on protocol and network information. To understand what this means, we must first look at what a protocol is and how it works. Until now, we've been happily communicating using the MAC address assigned to our networking devices. Our systems have used this number to contact other systems and transmit information as required.

The problem with this scheme is that it does not scale well. For example, what if you have 2,000 systems that need to communicate with one another? You now have 2,000 systems fighting one another for bandwidth on a single Ethernet network. Even if you employ switching, the number of broadcast frames will eventually reach a point where network performance will degrade and you cannot add any more systems. This is where protocols such as IP and IPX come in.

Network Protocols

At its lowest level, a *network protocol* is a set of communication rules that provide the means for networking systems to be grouped by geographical area and common wiring. To indicate it is part of a specific group, each of these systems is assigned an identical protocol network address.

Network addresses are kind of like zip codes. Let's assume someone mails a letter, and the front of the envelope simply reads Fritz & Wren,

7 Spring Road. If this happens in a very small town, the letter will probably get through (as if you'd used a MAC address on a LAN).

If the letter were mailed in a city such as Boston or New York, however, the Post Office would have no clue where to send it (although postal workers would probably get a good laugh). Without a zip code, they may not even attempt delivery. The zip code provides a way to specify the general area where this letter needs to be delivered. The postal worker processing the letter is not required to know exactly where Spring Road is located. They simply look at the zip code and forward the letter to the Post Office responsible for this code. It is up to the local Post Office to know the location of Spring Road and to use this knowledge to deliver the letter.

Protocol network addresses operate in a similar fashion. A protocol-aware device adds the network address of the destination device to the data field of a frame. It also records its own network address, in case the remote system needs to send a reply. This is where a router comes in. A router is a protocol-aware device that maintains a table of all known networks. It uses this table to help forward information to its final destination. Let's walk through an example to see how a routed network operates.

A Routed Network Example

Let's assume you have a network similar to that shown in Figure 3.12 and that System B needs to transmit information to System F.

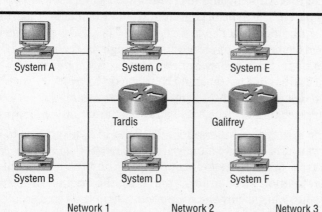

System A   System C   System E

Tardis   Galifrey

System B   System D   System F

Network 1   Network 2   Network 3

FIGURE 3.12:   An example of a routed network

System B begins by comparing its network address to that of System F. If there is a match, System B assumes the system is local and attempts to deliver the information directly. If the network addresses are different (as they are in our example), System B refers to its routing table. If it does not have a specific entry for Network 3, it falls back on its default router, which in this case is Tardis. In order to deliver the information to Tardis, System B ARPs for Tardis's MAC address. System B then adds the network protocol delivery information for System F (the source and destination network numbers) to the data and creates a frame using Tardis's MAC address as the destination. It does this because System B assumes that Tardis will take care of forwarding the information to the destination network.

Once Tardis receives the frame, it performs a cyclical redundancy check (CRC) to ensure the integrity of the data. If the frame checks out, Tardis strips off the header and trailer. Tardis then analyzes the destination network address listed in the frame (in this case, Network 3) to see if it is locally connected to this network. Because Tardis is not directly connected to Network 3, it consults its routing table to find the best route to get there. Tardis then discovers that Galifrey can reach Network 3.

Tardis now ARPs to discover the local MAC address being used by Galifrey. Tardis then creates a new frame around the data packet by creating a header consisting of its MAC address in the source address field and Galifrey's MAC address in the destination field. Finally, Tardis generates a new CRC value for the trailer.

Although all this stripping and re-creating seems like a lot of work, it is a necessary part of this type of communication. Remember that routers are placed at the borders of a network segment. The CRC is performed to ensure that bad frames are not propagated throughout the network. The header information is stripped away because it is only applicable on Network 1. When Tardis tries to transmit the frame on Network 2, the original source and destination MAC addresses have no meaning. This is why Tardis must replace these values with values that are valid for Network 2.

Because the majority of the header (12 of the 14 bytes) needs to be replaced anyway, it is easier to simply strip the header completely away and create it from scratch. As for stripping off the trailer, once the source and destination MAC addresses change, the original CRC value is no longer valid. This is why the router must strip it off and create a new one.

NOTE

A data field that contains protocol information is referred to as a *packet*. Although this term is sometimes used interchangeably with the term *frame*, a packet in fact describes only a portion of a frame.

Tardis has created a new frame around the packet and is ready to transmit it. Tardis transmits the frame out onto Network 2 so that the frame is received by Galifrey. Galifrey receives the frame and processes it in a similar fashion to Tardis. It checks the CRC and strips off the header and trailer.

Galifrey now repeats the earlier ARP process to find the address of System F. Once it has the MAC address, it builds a new frame around the packet and transmits it on the wire.

Protocol Specificity

In order for a router to provide this type of functionality, it needs to understand the rules for the protocol being used. A router is *protocol specific*. Unlike a bridge, which will handle any valid topology traffic you throw at it, a router must be specifically designed to support both the topology and the protocol being used. For example, if your network contains Banyan Vines systems, make sure that your router supports VinesIP.

Routers can be powerful tools for controlling the flow of traffic on your network. If you have a network segment that is using IPX and IP but only IP is approved for use on the company backbone, simply enable IP support only on your router. The router will ignore any IPX traffic it receives.

A wonderful feature of routers is their ability to block broadcasts. Because any point on the other side of the router is a new network, these frames are blocked.

NOTE

A counterpart to this is an *all-networks broadcast* that contains all Fs in both the network and MAC address fields. These frames are used to broadcast to local networks when the network address is not known. Most routers will still block these all-networks broadcasts by default.

Most routers can also filter out certain traffic. For example, let's say your company enters a partnership with another organization. You need to access services on this new network but do not want to allow your partner to access your servers. To accomplish this, simply install a router between the two networks and configure it to filter out any communication sessions originating from the other organization's network.

Most routers use static packet filtering to control traffic flow. For now, just keep in mind that routers cannot provide the same level of traffic control that may be found in the average firewall. Still, if your security requirements are minimal, packet filtering may be a good choice. Chances are you will need a router to connect your networks, anyway.

A Comparison of Bridging/Switching and Routing

Table 3.2 presents a summary of the information discussed in the preceding sections. It provides a quick reference to the differences between controlling traffic at the data link layer (bridges and switches) and controlling traffic at the network layer (routers).

TABLE 3.2: Bridging/Switching vs. Routing

A Bridge (Switch)	A Router
Uses the same network address off all ports	Uses different network addresses off all ports
Builds tables based on the MAC address	Builds tables based on the network layer address
Filters traffic based on MAC information	Filters traffic based on network or host information
Forwards broadcast traffic	Blocks broadcast traffic
Forwards traffic to unknown addresses	Blocks traffic to unknown addresses
Does not modify the frame	Creates a new header and trailer
Can forward traffic based on the frame header	Must always queue traffic before forwarding

Layer-3 Switching

Now that you have a clear understanding of the differences between a switch and a router, let's look at a technology that, on the surface, appears to mesh the two. (In fact, we've talked a lot about this information already, but this is a good review.) The terms *Layer-3 switching*, *switch routing*, and *router switching* are used interchangeably to describe the same devices, and Layer-3 switching has become so popular that even more traditional Layer-2 devices perform the same function.

A switch router is not quite as revolutionary a device as you might think. In fact, these devices are more an evolution of existing router technology. The association with the word *switch* is more for marketing appeal to emphasize the increase in raw throughput these devices can provide.

These devices typically (but not always) perform the same functions as a standard router. When a frame of data is received, it is buffered into memory, and a CRC check is performed. The topology frame is then stripped off the data packet. Just like a regular router, a switch router references its routing table to determine the best route of delivery, repackages the data packet into a frame, and sends it on its merry way.

How does a switch router differ from a standard router? The answer lies under the hood of the device. Processing is provided by application-specific integrated circuit (ASIC) hardware. With a standard router, all processing was typically performed by a single RISC (Reduced Instruction Set Computer) processor. In a switch router, components are dedicated to performing specific tasks within the routing process. The result is a dramatic increase in throughput.

Keep in mind that the real goal of these devices is to pass information along faster than the standard router. To accomplish this, a vendor may choose to do things slightly differently than the average router implementation in order to increase throughput (after all, raw throughput is everything, right?). For example, a specific vendor implementation might not buffer inbound traffic in order to perform a CRC check on the frame. Once enough of the frame has been read in order to make a routing decision, the device might immediately begin transmitting information out the other end.

From a security perspective, this may not always be a good thing. Certainly performance is a concern—but not at the cost of accidentally passing traffic that should have been blocked. Because the real goal of a switch router is performance, it may not be as nitpicky as the typical router about what it passes along.

Layer-3 switching has some growing up to do before it can be considered a viable replacement for the time-tested router. Most of today's routers can process more than one million packets per second. Typically, higher traffic rates are required only on a network backbone. To date, this is why switches have dominated this area of the network.

Switch routing may make good security sense as a replacement for regular switches, however. The ability to segregate traffic into true subnets instead of just collision domains brings a whole new level of control to this area of the network.

Like their router counterparts, some switch routers support access control lists (ACLs), which allow the network administrator to manipulate which systems can communicate between each of the subnets and what services they can access. This is a much higher level of granular control than is provided with a regular switch. Switch routing can help to fortify the security of your internal network without the typical degradation in performance. If your security requirements are light, a switch router might be just the thing to augment your security policy.

WHAT'S NEXT

We've covered a lot of ground in this chapter. We discussed the basics of communication properties and looked at transmission media and hardware from a security perspective. We also discussed what traffic control options are available with typical network hardware.

In the next few chapters, we'll look at authentication and encryption technologies and their importance to network security.

Chapter 4

AUTHENTICATION AND ENCRYPTION

Authentication and encryption are two intertwined technologies that help to ensure that your data remains secure. *Authentication* is the process of ensuring that both ends of the connection are in fact who they say they are. It applies not only to the entity trying to access a service (such as an end user) but also to the entity providing the service (such as a file server or a website). *Encryption* helps to ensure that the information within a session is not compromised. This includes not only reading the information within a data stream, but also altering it.

Although authentication and encryption have their own responsibilities in securing a communication session, maximum protection can only be achieved when the two are combined. For this reason, many security protocols contain both authentication and encryption specifications.

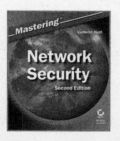

Adapted from *Mastering™ Network Security*,
Second Edition by Chris Brenton and Cameron Hunt
ISBN 0-7821-4142-0 $49.99

THE NEED FOR IMPROVED SECURITY

When IP (Internet Protocol) version 4, the version currently in use on the Internet, was created back in the 1970s, network security was not a major concern. Although system security was important, little attention was paid to the transport used when exchanging information. When IP was first introduced, it contained no inherent security standards. The specifications for IP do not take into account that you might want to protect the data that IP is transporting. This approach will change with IP version 6, but it appears that wide acceptance of this new specification is still many years in the future.

IP currently transmits all data as cleartext, which is commonly referred to as *transmitting in the clear*. Data and authentication information are not scrambled or rearranged; they are simply transmitted in raw form. To see how this appears, let's start by looking at Figure 4.1.

No.	Source	Destination	Layer	Summary	Error	Size	Interpacket Time	Absolute Time
3	0000E82F772A	0020AF247F25	tcp	Port:1067 ---> POP3 SYN		64	323 µs	8:58:38 PM
4	0020AF247F25	0000E82F772A	tcp	Port:POP3 ---> 1067 ACK SYN		64	203 µs	8:58:38 PM
5	0000E82F772A	0020AF247F25	tcp	Port:1067 ---> POP3 ACK		64	372 µs	8:58:38 PM
6	0020AF247F25	0000E82F772A	tcp	Port:POP3 ---> 1067 ACK PUSH		97	49 ms	8:58:38 PM
7	0000E82F772A	0020AF247F25	tcp	Port:1067 ---> POP3 ACK		64	192 ms	8:58:38 PM
8	0000E82F772A	0020AF247F25	tcp	Port:1067 ---> POP3 ACK PUSH		71	326 ms	8:58:38 PM
9	0020AF247F25	0000E82F772A	tcp	Port:POP3 ---> 1067 ACK PUSH		77	7 ms	8:58:38 PM
10	0000E82F772A	0020AF247F25	tcp	Port:1067 ---> POP3 ACK		64	162 ms	8:58:39 PM

```
 0:  00 20 AF 24 7F 25 00 00 E8 2F 77 2A 08 00 45 00    . .$.%.../w*..E.
10:  00 35 87 05 40 00 80 06 EF CC C0 A8 01 3C C0 A8    .5..@........<..
20:  01 64 04 2B 00 6E 00 BF 06 D2 00 0D 0D 56 50 18    .d.+.n.......VP.
30:  22 11 DC 54 00 00 55 53 45 52 20 62 67 61 74 65    "..T..USER bgate
40:  73 0D 0A                                           s..
```

FIGURE 4.1:   A packet decode of an authentication session initializing

Figure 4.1 shows a network analyzer's view of a communication session. A user is in the process of retrieving e-mail with a POP3 (Post Office Protocol, version 3) e-mail client. Packets 3 through 5 are the TCP (Transmission Control Protocol) three-packet handshake used to initialize the connection. Packets 6 and 7 are the POP3 e-mail server informing the client that it is online and ready. In packet 8 we begin finding some interesting information. If you look toward the bottom of Figure 4.1, you will see the decoded contents of the data field within packet 8. A POP3 client uses the USER command to pass the logon name to a POP3 server. Any text following the USER command is the name of the person who is attempting to authenticate with the system.

Figure 4.2 shows the POP3 server's response to this logon name. If you look at the decode for packet 9, you can see that the logon name was accepted. This tells us that the logon name captured in Figure 4.1 is legitimate. If you can discover this user's password, you will have enough information to gain access to the system.

No.	Source	Destination	Layer	Summary	Error	Size	Interpacket Time	Absolute Time
6	0020AF247F25	0000E82F772A	tcp	Port:POP3 ---> 1067 ACK PUSH		97	49 ms	8:58:38 PM
7	0000E82F772A	0020AF247F25	tcp	Port:1067 ---> POP3 ACK		64	192 ms	8:58:38 PM
8	0000E82F772A	0020AF247F25	tcp	Port:1067 ---> POP3 ACK PUSH		71	326 ms	8:58:38 PM
9	0020AF247F25	0000E82F772A	tcp	Port:POP3 ---> 1067 ACK PUSH		77	7 ms	8:58:38 PM
10	0000E82F772A	0020AF247F25	tcp	Port:1067 ---> POP3 ACK		64	162 ms	8:58:39 PM
11	0000E82F772A	0020AF247F25	tcp	Port:1067 ---> POP3 ACK PUSH		74	326 ms	8:58:39 PM
12	0020AF247F25	0000E82F772A	tcp	Port:POP3 ---> 1067 ACK PUSH		91	920 µs	8:58:39 PM
13	0000E82F772A	0020AF247F25	tcp	Port:1067 ---> POP3 ACK		64	172 ms	8:58:39 PM

```
 0: 00 00 E8 2F 77 2A 00 20 AF 24 7F 25 08 00 45 00   .../w*. .$.%..E.
10: 00 3B 1C 00 40 00 20 06 BA CC C0 A8 01 64 C0 A8   .;..@. .......d..
20: 01 3C 00 6E 04 2B 00 0D 0D 56 00 BF 06 DF 50 18   .<.n.+...V....P.
30: 22 2B D3 06 00 00 2B 4F 4B 20 75 73 65 72 20 61   "+....+OK user a
40: 63 63 65 70 74 65 64 0D 0A                        ccepted..
```

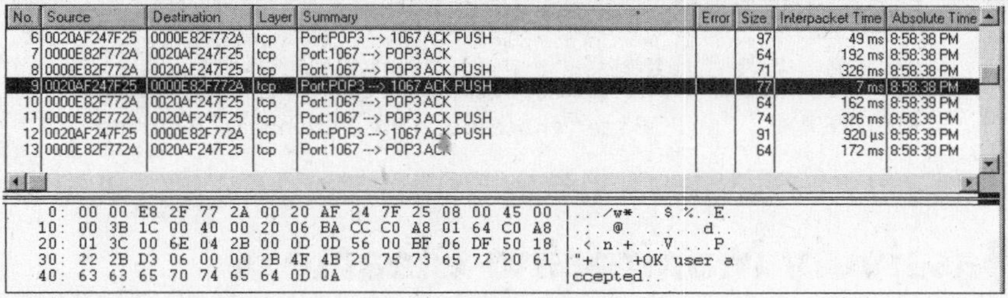

FIGURE 4.2: The POP3 server accepting the logon name

Figure 4.3 shows a decode of packet 11. This is the next set of commands sent by the POP3 e-mail client to the server. The client uses the PASS command to send the password string. Any text that follows this command is the password for the user attempting to authenticate with the system. As you can see, the password is plainly visible.

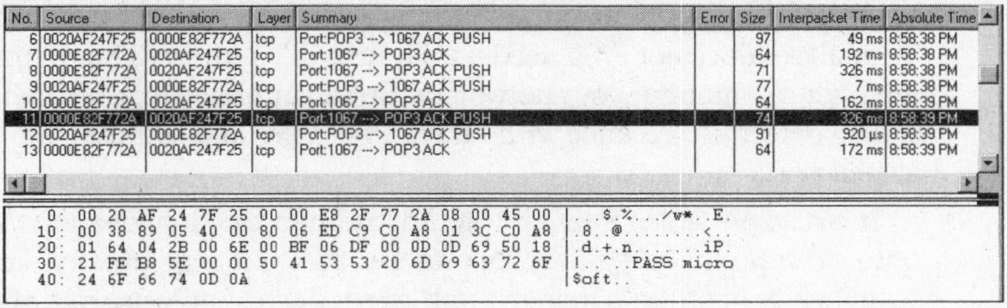

No.	Source	Destination	Layer	Summary	Error	Size	Interpacket Time	Absolute Time
6	0020AF247F25	0000E82F772A	tcp	Port:POP3 ---> 1067 ACK PUSH		97	49 ms	8:58:38 PM
7	0000E82F772A	0020AF247F25	tcp	Port:1067 ---> POP3 ACK		64	192 ms	8:58:38 PM
8	0000E82F772A	0020AF247F25	tcp	Port:1067 ---> POP3 ACK PUSH		71	326 ms	8:58:38 PM
9	0020AF247F25	0000E82F772A	tcp	Port:POP3 ---> 1067 ACK PUSH		77	7 ms	8:58:38 PM
10	0000E82F772A	0020AF247F25	tcp	Port:1067 ---> POP3 ACK		64	162 ms	8:58:38 PM
11	0000E82F772A	0020AF247F25	tcp	Port:1067 ---> POP3 ACK PUSH		74	326 µs	8:58:39 PM
12	0020AF247F25	0000E82F772A	tcp	Port:POP3 ---> 1067 ACK PUSH		91	920 µs	8:58:39 PM
13	0000E82F772A	0020AF247F25	tcp	Port:1067 ---> POP3 ACK		64	172 ms	8:58:39 PM

```
 0: 00 20 AF 24 7F 25 00 00 E8 2F 77 2A 08 00 45 00   . .$.%.../w*..E.
10: 00 38 89 05 40 00 80 06 ED C9 C0 A8 01 3C C0 A8   .8..@........<..
20: 01 64 04 2B 00 6E 00 BF 06 DF 00 0D 0D 69 50 18   .d.+.n.......iP.
30: 21 FE B8 5E 00 00 50 41 53 53 20 6D 69 63 72 6F   !..^..PASS micro
40: 24 6F 66 74 0D 0A                                 $oft..
```

FIGURE 4.3: The POP3 client sending the user's password

Figure 4.4 shows a decode of packet 12. This is the server's response to the authentication attempt. Notice that the server has accepted the logon name and password combination. We now know that this was a valid authentication session and that we have a legitimate logon name and password combination in order to gain access to the system. In fact, if we decoded further packets, we would be able to view every e-mail message downloaded by this user.

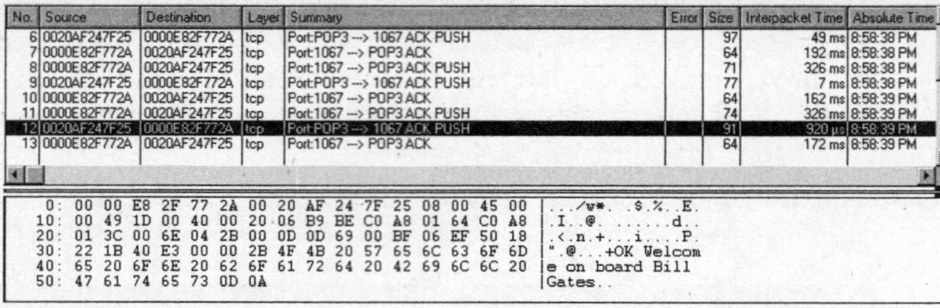

No.	Source	Destination	Layer	Summary	Error	Size	Interpacket Time	Absolute Time
6	0020AF247F25	0000E82F772A	tcp	Port:POP3 --> 1067 ACK PUSH		97	49 ms	8:58:38 PM
7	0000E82F772A	0020AF247F25	tcp	Port:1067 --> POP3 ACK		64	192 ms	8:58:38 PM
8	0000E82F772A	0020AF247F25	tcp	Port:1067 --> POP3 ACK PUSH		71	326 ms	8:58:38 PM
9	0020AF247F25	0000E82F772A	tcp	Port:POP3 --> 1067 ACK PUSH		77	7 ms	8:58:38 PM
10	0000E82F772A	0020AF247F25	tcp	Port:1067 --> POP3 ACK		64	162 ms	8:58:39 PM
11	0000E82F772A	0020AF247F25	tcp	Port:1067 --> POP3 ACK PUSH		74	326 ms	8:58:39 PM
12	0020AF247F25	0000E82F772A	tcp	Port:POP3 --> 1067 ACK PUSH		91	920 µs	8:58:39 PM
13	0000E82F772A	0020AF247F25	tcp	Port:1067 --> POP3 ACK		64	172 ms	8:58:39 PM

```
 0:  00 00 E8 2F 77 2A 00 20 AF 24 7F 25 08 00 45 00    .../w*. .$.%..E.
10:  00 49 1D 00 40 00 20 06 B9 BE C0 A8 01 64 C0 A8    .I..@. ......d..
20:  01 3C 00 6E 04 2B 00 0D 0D 69 00 BF 06 EF 50 18    .<.n.+...i....P.
30:  22 1B 40 E3 00 00 2B 4F 4B 20 57 65 6C 63 6F 6D    ".@...+OK Welcom
40:  65 20 6F 6E 20 62 6F 61 72 64 20 42 69 6C 6C 20    e on board Bill
50:  47 61 74 65 73 0D 0A                               Gates..
```

FIGURE 4.4:   The POP3 server accepting the authentication attempt

Passively Monitoring Cleartext

The POP3 authentication session in Figures 4.1 through 4.4 was captured using a network analyzer. A network analyzer can be either a dedicated hardware tool or a software program that runs on an existing system. You can purchase network analyzer software for less than $1,000 for Windows or Mac platforms, and it is freely available for Windows and Unix.

Network analyzers operate as truly passive devices, meaning that they do not need to transmit any data to the network in order to monitor traffic. Although some analyzers do transmit traffic (usually in an effort to locate a management station), doing so is not a requirement. In fact, an analyzer does not even need a valid network address. Thus, a network analyzer can monitor your network without your knowledge. You have no way to detect its presence without tracing cables and counting hub and switch ports.

It is also possible for an attacker to load network analyzer software onto a compromised system. An attacker does not need physical access to your facility in order to monitor traffic—they can simply use one of your existing systems to capture the traffic. This is why it is so important to perform regular audits on your systems. You clearly do not want a passive monitoring attack to go unnoticed.

In order for a network analyzer to capture a communication session, it must be connected somewhere along the session's path. It could be connected on the network at some point between the system initializing the session and the destination system. It could also connect by compromising one of the systems at either end of the session. This means that an attacker cannot capture your network traffic over the Internet from a remote location. They must place some form of probe or analyzer within your network.

Cleartext Protocols

POP3 is not the only IP service that communicates via cleartext. Nearly every nonproprietary IP service that is not specifically designed to provide authentication and encryption services transmits data as cleartext. Here is a partial list of cleartext services:

FTP (File Transfer Protocol)   Authentication is cleartext.

Telnet   Authentication is cleartext.

SMTP (Simple Mail Transfer Protocol)   Contents of e-mail messages are delivered as cleartext.

HTTP (Hypertext Transfer Protocol)   Page content and the contents of fields within forms are sent as cleartext.

IMAP (Internet Message Access Protocol)   Authentication is cleartext.

SNMPv1 (Simple Network Management Protocol, version 1)   Authentication is cleartext.

WARNING

The fact that SNMPv1 uses cleartext is particularly nasty. SNMP is used to manage and query network devices, including switches, routers, servers, and even firewalls. If the SMTP password is compromised, an attacker can wreak havoc on your network. SNMPv2 and SNMPv3 include a message algorithm similar to the one used with Open Shortest Path First (OSPF). This algorithm provides a much higher level of security and data integrity than the original SNMP specification. Unfortunately, not every networking device supports SNMPv2, let alone SNMPv3. Thus, SNMPv1 is still widely used today.

GOOD AUTHENTICATION REQUIRED

By now, the need for good authentication should be obvious. A service that passes logon information as cleartext is far too easy to monitor. Easily snooped logons can be an even larger problem in environments that do not require frequent password changes, which gives an attacker plenty of time to launch an attack using the compromised account. Also of concern is that most users try to maintain the same logon name and password for all accounts. Thus, if an attacker can capture the authentication credentials from an insecure service (such as POP3), they might now have a valid logon name and passwords to other systems on the network, such as NT and NetWare servers.

Good authentication goes beyond validating the source attempting to access a service during initial logon. You should also validate that the source has not been replaced by an attacking host in the course of the communication session. This type of attack is commonly called *session hijacking*.

Session Hijacking

Consider the simple network drawing in Figure 4.5. A client is communicating with a server over an insecure network connection. The client has already authenticated with the server and has been granted access. Let's make this a fun example and assume that the client has administrator-level privileges. Woolly Attacker is sitting on a network segment between the client and the server and has been quietly monitoring the session, learning which port and sequence numbers are being used to carry on the conversation.

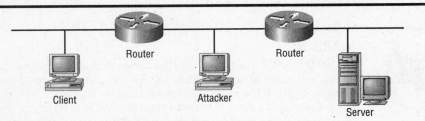

FIGURE 4.5:   An example of a man-in-the-middle attack

Now let's assume that Woolly Attacker wants to hijack the administrator's session in order to create a new account with administrator-level privileges. The first thing he does is force the client into a state where it can no longer communicate with the server. He can crash the client by sending it a Ping of Death or using a utility such as WinNuke. He can also launch an attack such as an ICMP (Internet Control Message Protocol) flood. No matter which type of attack Woolly launches, his goal is to ensure that the client cannot respond to traffic sent by the server.

NOTE

When an ICMP flood is launched against a target, the target spends so much time processing ICMP requests that it does not have enough time to respond to any other communications.

Now that the client is out of the way, Woolly Attacker is free to communicate with the server as if he were the client. He can do this by capturing the server's replies as they head back to the client in order to formulate a proper response. If Woolly has an intimate knowledge of IP, he might even be able to completely ignore the server's replies and transmit port and sequence numbers based on the expected responses from the server. In either case, Woolly Attacker is now communicating with the server—except that the server thinks it is still communicating with the original client.

Therefore, good authentication should also verify that the source remains constant and has not been replaced by another system. This can be done by having the two systems exchange a secret during the course of the communication session. A secret can be exchanged with each packet transmitted or at random intervals during the course of the session. Obviously, verifying the source of every packet is far more secure than verifying the source at random intervals. The communication session would be even more secure if you could vary the secret with each packet exchange. This approach helps to ensure that your session is not vulnerable to session hijacking.

Verifying the Destination

The need to authenticate the source both before and during a communication session is apparent. What may not be apparent is the need to verify the server. Many people take for granted that they will either connect to the intended server or receive some form of host-unreachable message. It may not dawn on them that what they assume is the server may actually be an attacker attempting to compromise the network.

Later versions of Windows (post Windows 95) use stronger types of authentication by default (discussed later in this chapter), culminating in the Kerberos protocol that makes both the client *and* the server authenticate to each other.

DNS Poisoning

Another exploit that displays the need for authentication is *DNS poisoning*. DNS poisoning, also known as *cache poisoning*, is the process of handing out incorrect IP address information for a specific host with the intent to divert traffic from its true destination. Eugene Kashpureff proved this was possible in the summer of 1997 when he diverted requests for

InterNIC hosts to his alternate domain name registry site called AlterNIC.
He diverted these requests by exploiting a known vulnerability in DNS
services.

When a name server receives a reply to a DNS query, it does not validate the source of the reply or ignore information not specifically requested.
Kashpureff capitalized on these vulnerabilities by hiding bogus DNS
information inside valid replies. The name server receiving the reply
cached the valid information, as well as the bogus information. The result
was that if a user tried to resolve a host within the InterNIC's domain
(for example rs.internic.net, which is used for whois queries), they
received an IP address within AlterNIC's domain and were diverted to a
system on the AlterNIC network.

Although Kashpureff's attack can be considered little more than a
prank, it does open the door to some far nastier possibilities. In an age
when online banking is the norm, consider the ramifications if someone
diverts traffic from a bank's website. An attacker, using cache poisoning
to divert bank traffic to an alternate server, could configure the phony
server to appear identical to the bank's legitimate server.

When a bank client attempts to authenticate to the bank's web server
in order to manage their bank account, an attacker captures the authentication information and simply presents the user with a banner screen
stating that the system is currently offline. Unless digital certificates are
being used, the client has no way of knowing they are being diverted to
another site unless they happen to notice the discrepancy in IP addresses.

NOTE
Digital certificates are described in the "Digital Certificate Servers" section
later in this chapter.

It is just as important to verify the server you are attempting to authenticate with as it is to verify the client's credentials or the integrity of the
session. All three points in the communication process are vulnerable to
attack.

ENCRYPTION 101

Cryptography is a set of techniques used to transform information into an
alternate format that can later be reversed. This alternate format is referred

to as the *ciphertext* and is typically created using a crypto algorithm and a crypto key. The *crypto algorithm* is simply a mathematical formula that is applied to the information you want to encrypt. The *crypto key* is an additional variable injected into the algorithm to ensure that the ciphertext is not derived using the same computational operation every time the algorithm processes information.

Let's say the number 42 is extremely important to you, and you want to guard this value from peering eyes. You create the following crypto algorithm to encrypt this data:

```
data / crypto key + (2 x crypto key)
```

This process relies on two important pieces: the crypto algorithm itself and the crypto key. Both are used to create the ciphertext, which is a new numeric value. To reverse the ciphertext and produce an answer of 42, you need to know both the algorithm and the key. There are less secure crypto algorithms known as *Caesar ciphers* that do not use keys, but they typically are not used because they do not have the additional security of a crypto key. You only need to know the algorithm for a Caesar cipher in order to decrypt the ciphertext.

NOTE

Julius Caesar is credited as being one of the first people to use encryption. Using the substitution method, he shifted each letter of his message to the letter three places down in the alphabet. He replaced all his letter As with Ds, Bs with Es, and so on. Because his generals were the only people aware of his algorithm, he considered his messages safe from untrusted messengers. This type of encryption is commonly referred to as the *Caesar cipher*.

Because encryption uses mathematical formulas, a symbiotic relationship exists among the following:

- ▶ The algorithm
- ▶ The key
- ▶ The original data
- ▶ The ciphertext

Knowing any three of these pieces allows you to derive the fourth. The exception is knowing the combination of the original data and the ciphertext. If you have multiple examples of both, you might be able to discover the algorithm and the key.

Methods of Encryption

The two methods of producing ciphertext are:

- ▶ The stream cipher
- ▶ The block cipher

The two methods are similar except for the amount of data each encrypts on each pass. Most of today's encryption schemes use some form of block cipher.

Stream Cipher

Using the *stream cipher* is one of the simplest ways to encrypt data. When a stream cipher is employed, each bit of the data is sequentially encrypted using one bit of the key. A classic example of a stream cipher was the Vernam cipher used to encrypt Teletype traffic. The crypto key for the Vernam cipher was stored on a loop of paper. As the Teletype message was fed through the machine, one bit of the data was combined with one bit of the key in order to produce the ciphertext. The recipient of the ciphertext then reversed the process, using an identical loop of paper to decode the original message.

The Vernam cipher used a fixed-length key, which can be easy to deduce if you compare the ciphertext from multiple messages. To make a stream cipher more difficult to crack, you can use a crypto key that varies in length. A variable-length crypto key helps to mask any discernible patterns in the resulting ciphertext. In fact, by randomly changing the crypto key used on each bit of data, you can produce ciphertext that is mathematically impossible to crack. Using different random keys does not generate any repeating patterns that can give a cracker the clues required to break the crypto key. The process of continually varying the encryption key is known as a *one-time pad*.

Although virtually unbreakable, the one-time pad method is far less common than other methods of encryption because it produces overhead equivalent to the amount of plain text being protected. This, of course, creates additional traffic and decreases the efficiency of your network. However, a cryptographic system doesn't need to be unbreakable to be useful. It needs only to be strong enough to resists attacks by likely enemies for as long your information needs to be protected.

Block Cipher

Unlike stream ciphers, which encrypt every single bit, *block ciphers* encrypt data in chunks of a specific size. A block cipher specification identifies how much data should be encrypted on each pass (called a *block*) as well as what size key should be applied to each block. For example, the Data Encryption Standard (DES) specifies that DES-encrypted data should be processed in 64-bit blocks using a 56-bit key.

You can use a number of different algorithms when processing block cipher encryption. The most basic is to simply take the data and break it into blocks while applying the key to each. Although this method is efficient, it can produce repetitive ciphertext. If two blocks of data contain exactly the same information, the two resulting blocks of ciphertext will be identical, as well. As mentioned earlier, a cracker can use ciphertext that repeats in a nonrandom fashion to break the crypto key.

A better solution is to use earlier results from the algorithm and combine them with later keys. Figure 4.6 shows one possible variation. The data you want to encrypt is broken into blocks labeled DB1 through DB4. An *initialization vector* (IV) is added to the beginning of the data to ensure that all blocks can be properly ciphered. The IV is simply a random character string to ensure that two identical messages will not create the same ciphertext. To create your first block of ciphertext (CT1), you mathematically combine the crypto key, the first block of data (DB1), and the initialization vector (IV).

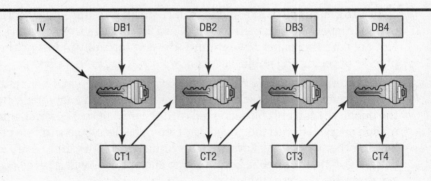

Key + IV + DB1 = CT1
Key + CT1 + DB2 = CT2
Key + CT2 + DB3 = CT3
Key + CT3 + DB4 = CT4

FIGURE 4.6: Block cipher encryption

When you create the second block of ciphertext (CT2), you mathematically combine the crypto key, the first block of ciphertext (CT1), and the second block of data (DB2). Because the variables in your algorithm have changed, DB1 and DB2 could be identical, but the resulting ciphertext (CT1 and CT2) will contain different values. This helps to ensure that the resulting ciphertext is sufficiently scrambled so that it appears completely random. This process of using resulting ciphertext to encrypt additional blocks of data will continue until all the data blocks have been processed.

There are a number of variations on how to mathematically combine the crypto key, the initialization vector, and previously created ciphertext. All these methods share the same goal, which is to create a seemingly random character string of ciphertext.

Public/Private Crypto Keys

So far, all the encryption techniques we have discussed use *secret key algorithms*. A secret key algorithm relies on the same key to encrypt and to decrypt the ciphertext. Thus, the crypto key must remain secret to ensure the confidentiality of the ciphertext. If an attacker learns your secret key, they can unlock all your encrypted messages. This situation creates an interesting Catch-22, because you now need a secure method for exchanging the secret key in order to use the secret key to create a secure method of exchanging information!

In 1976, Whitfield Diffie and Martin Hellman introduced the concept of public cipher keys in their paper "New Directions in Cryptography." Not only did this paper revolutionize the cryptography industry; the process of generating public keys is now known as *Diffie-Hellman*.

In lay terms, a *public key* is a crypto key that has been mathematically derived from a private or secret crypto key. Information encrypted with the public key can only be decrypted with the private key; however, information encrypted with the private key cannot be decrypted with the public key. In other words, the keys are not symmetrical. They are specifically designed so that the public key is used to encrypt data, whereas the private key is used to decrypt ciphertext.

This process eliminates the Catch-22 of the symmetrical secret key, because a secure channel is not required to exchange key information. Public keys can be exchanged over insecure channels while still maintaining the secrecy of the messages they encrypted. If your friend Fred Tuttle wants to send you a private message, all Fred has to do is encrypt it using your public key. The resulting ciphertext can then only be decrypted using your private key.

You can even use Diffie-Hellman to provide authentication. You authenticate by signing a message with your private key before encrypting it with the recipient's public key. *Signing* is simply a mathematical algorithm that processes your private key and the contents of the message. This process creates a unique digital signature that is appended to the end of the message. Because the contents of the message are used to create the signature, your digital signature will be different on every message you send.

For example, let's say you want to send Fred a private message. First you create a digital signature using your private key, and then you encrypt the message using Fred's public key. When Fred receives the message, he first decrypts the ciphertext using his private key and then checks the digital signature using your public key. If the signature matches, Fred knows that the message is authentic and that it has not been altered in transit. If the signature does not match, Fred knows that either the message was not signed by your private key or that the ciphertext was altered in transit. In either event, the recipient knows that he should be suspicious of the contents of the message.

Encryption Weaknesses

Encryption weaknesses fall into three categories:

- ▶ Mishandling or human error
- ▶ Deficiencies in the cipher itself
- ▶ Brute force attacks

When deciding which encryption method best suits your needs, be sure you are aware of the weaknesses of your choice.

Mishandling or Human Error

Although the stupid user syndrome may be an odd topic to bring up when discussing encryption methods, it does play a critical role in ensuring that your data remains secure. Some methods of encryption lend themselves better to poor key management practices than others. When selecting a method of encryption, be sure you have the correct infrastructure required to administer the cipher keys in an appropriate manner.

PROPER KEY MANAGEMENT IS KEY

Back in the 1940s, the Soviet Union was using a one-time pad to encrypt its most sensitive data. As you saw in the section on stream ciphers, it is mathematically impossible to break encryption using a one-time pad. This, of course, assumes that the user understands the definition of "one-time." Apparently, the Soviet Union did not.

Because cipher keys were in short supply, the Soviet Union began reusing some of its existing one-time pad keys by rotating them through different field offices. The assumption was that as long as the same office did not use the same key more than once, the resulting ciphertext would be sufficiently secure. (How many of you can see your pointy-haired boss making a similar management decision?)

Apparently, this assumption was off base: The United States was able to identify the duplicate key patterns and decrypt the actual messages within the ciphertext. For more than five years, the United States was able to track Soviet spying activity within the United States. This tracking continued until information regarding the cracking activity was relayed to a double agent.

Although a one-time pad may be the most secure cipher to use, you must be able to generate enough unique keys to keep up with your data encryption needs. Even if you use a regular secret key cipher, you must make sure that you have a secure method for exchanging key information between hosts. It does little good to encrypt your data if you are simply going to transmit your secret key over the same insecure channel.

Simple key management is one of the reasons that public/private cipher keys have become so popular. The ability to exchange key information over the same insecure channel that you want to use for your data has great appeal. This approach greatly simplifies management: You can keep your private key locked up and secure while transmitting your public key using any method you choose.

WARNING

You must make sure that the public keys you use to encrypt data have been received from the legitimate source and not from an attacker who has swapped in a private key of their own. You can easily authenticate the validity of a public key through a phone call or some other means.

Cipher Deficiencies

Determining whether there are any deficiencies in the cipher algorithm of a specific type of encryption is probably the hardest task a noncryptographer can attempt. You can, however, look for a few things to ensure that the encryption is secure:

▶ The mathematical formula that makes up the encryption algorithm should be public knowledge. Algorithms that rely on secrecy may very well have flaws that can be extorted to expedite cracking.

▶ The encryption algorithm should have undergone open public scrutiny. Anyone should be able to evaluate the algorithm and be free to discuss their findings. Analysis of the algorithm cannot be restricted by confidentiality agreements and cannot be contingent on the cryptographer's signing a nondisclosure agreement.

▶ The encryption algorithm should have been publicly available for a reasonable length of time to ensure that a proper analysis has been performed. An encryption algorithm with no known flaws that has only been publicly available for a few months has not stood the test of time. One of the reasons that many people trust DES encryption is that it has been around since 1976.

▶ Public analysis should have produced no useful weaknesses in the algorithm. This can be a gray area because nearly all encryption algorithms have some form of minor flaw. As a rule of thumb, the flaws within an algorithm should not dramatically reduce the amount of time needed to crack a key beyond what could be achieved by trying all possible key combinations.

By following these simple guidelines, you should be able to make an educated guess about the relative security of an encryption algorithm.

Brute Force Attacks

A brute force attack is simply an attempt to try all possible cipher key combinations in order to find the one that unlocks the ciphertext. This attack is also known as an *exhaustive key search*. The cracker makes no attempt to actually crack the key, but relies on the ability to try all possible key combinations in a reasonable amount of time. All encryption algorithms are vulnerable to brute force attacks.

The preceding paragraph contains a couple of key terms. The first is *reasonable*. An attacker must feel that launching a brute force attack is worth the time. If an exhaustive key search will produce your VISA platinum card number in a few hours, the attack might be worth the effort. If, however, four weeks of work are required to decrypt your father-in-law's chili recipe, a brute force attack might not be worth the attacker's effort.

The other operative word is *vulnerable*. Although all encryption algorithms are susceptible to a brute force attack, some may take so long to try all possible key combinations that the amount of time spent cannot be considered reasonable. For example, encryption using a one-time pad can be broken using a brute force attack, but the attacker had better plan on having many of his descendants carry on the work long after he is gone. To date, the earth has not existed long enough for an attacker to be able to break a proper one-time pad encryption scheme using existing computing power.

Therefore, the amount of time required to perform a brute force attack is contingent on two factors: how long it takes to try a specific key and the number of possible key combinations. The amount of time required to try each key depends on the device providing the processing power. A typical desktop computer can test approximately five keys per second. A device specifically designed to break encryption keys might be able to process 200 keys or more per second. Of course, greater results can be achieved by combining multiple systems.

The number of possible key combinations is directly proportional to the size of the cipher key. Size does matter in cryptography: The larger the cipher key, the more possible key combinations exist. Table 4.1 shows some common encryption methods, along with their associated key size. Notice that as the size of the key increases, the number of possible key combinations increases exponentially.

TABLE 4.1: Methods of Encryption and Their Associated Keys

ENCRYPTION	BITS IN KEY	NUMBER OF POSSIBLE KEYS
Netscape	40	1.1×10^6
DES	56	72.1×10^6
Triple-DES (2 keys)	112	5.2×10^{33}
RC4/128	128	3.4×10^{38}
Triple-DES (3 keys)	168	3.7×10^{50}
Future standard?	256	1.2×10^{77}

Of course, this discussion leads to the question of how long it takes to perform an exhaustive key search on a particular encryption algorithm. The answer should scare you. DES encryption (discussed in the DES section of this chapter) has become somewhat of an industry standard. Over the past few years, RSA Laboratories has staged a DES challenge to see how long it would take for a person or persons to crack a string of ciphertext and discover the message hidden inside.

In 1997, the challenge was completed in approximately five months. In January 1998, the challenge was completed in 39 days. By July 1998, the Electronic Frontier Foundation (EFF) was able to complete the challenge in less than three days.

The EFF accomplished this task through a device designed specifically for brute forcing DES encryption. The cost of the device was approximately $250,000—well within the price range of organized crime and big business. Just after the challenge, the EFF published a book entitled *Cracking DES* (O'Reilly and Associates, 1998), which completely documents the design of the device they used. Obviously, this has put a whole new spin on what key lengths are considered secure.

For more information on the RSA Challenge, which offers prizes ranging from $10,000 to $200,000 for successful decryption of highly secure keys, visit RSA's website at www.rsasecurity.com.

Government Intervention

As you may know, the federal government regulates the export or use of encryption across U.S. borders. These regulations originated during World War II, when the use of encryption was thought to be limited to spies and terrorists. These regulations still exist today, in part because of the efforts of the National Security Agency (NSA). The NSA is responsible for monitoring and decrypting all communication that can be considered of interest to the security of the U.S. government.

Originally, the regulations controlled the cipher key size that could be exported or used across U.S. borders. For many rules, the limitation was a maximum key size of 40 bits, with few exceptions. Organizations that wanted to use a larger key size had to apply to the Department of Commerce and obtain a license to do so under the International Traffic in Arms Regulations (ITAR). Such licenses typically were sought by financial institutions or U.S.-based companies with foreign subsidiaries.

However, on October 19, 2000, the Bureau of Export Administration published a rule that embodied changes made by the Clinton administration earlier that year, which intended to liberalize export policy on not only the length, but also the type of encryption products that could be exported. The major impetus for the change came from the administration's recognition that non-U.S. companies already provided encryption technologies that exceeded the export restrictions. Bowing to pressure not only from U.S. companies, but also from countries in the European Union (EU), the change allows most encryption products to be exported without a governmental review to all 15 EU countries and eight other trading parties.

So, what does this mean for you? Better encryption products domestically, for one thing. Because vendors don't have to produce two versions of their products (with distinct encryption strengths), there is more incentive to include greater encryption as opposed to keeping to the lowest common denominator.

GOOD ENCRYPTION REQUIRED

If you are properly verifying your authentication session, why do you even need encryption? Encryption serves two purposes:

▶ To protect the data from snooping

▶ To protect the data from being altered

In the section on cleartext transmissions earlier in this chapter, you saw how most IP services transmit all information in the clear. This fact should be sufficient justification for using encryption to shield your data from peering eyes.

Encryption can also help to ensure that your data is not altered during transmission. Altering data during transmission is commonly referred to as a *man-in-the-middle attack* (as mentioned earlier), because it relies on the attacker's ability to disrupt the data transfer. Let's assume you have a web server configured to accept online catalog orders. Your customer fills out an online form, which is then saved on the web server in a plain text format. At regular intervals, these files are transferred to another system via FTP or SMTP.

If an attacker can gain access to the web server's file system, they can modify these text files prior to processing. A malicious attacker can then change quantities or product numbers to introduce inaccuracies. The result is a very unhappy client when the wrong order is received. Although this example assumes that the attacker has gained access to a file system, it is also possible to launch a man-in-the-middle attack while information is in transit on the network.

Although such attackers have not stolen anything, they have altered the data—and disrupted your business. Had this information been saved using a good encryption algorithm, this attack would have been far more difficult to stage because the attacker would not know which values within the encrypted file to change. Even if the attacker were a good guesser, the algorithm decrypting the cipher would detect the change in data.

SOLUTIONS

A number of solutions are available for providing authentication and encryption services. Some are products from a specific vendor, and others are open standards. Which option is right for you depends on your specific requirements. The following options are the most popular for providing authentication, encryption, or a combination. Most likely, one of these solutions can fill your needs.

Data Encryption Standard (DES)

DES was, for many years, the encryption standard used by the U.S. government for protecting sensitive, but not classified, data. The American National Standards Institute (ANSI) and the Internet Engineering Task Force (IETF) have also incorporated DES into security standards. DES is by far the most popular secret key algorithm in use today.

The original standard of DES uses a 40-bit (for export) or 56-bit key for encrypting data. The latest standard, referred to as *triple-DES* (3DES), encrypts the plain text three times using two or three different 56-bit keys. This approach produces ciphertext that is scrambled to the equivalent of a 112-bit or 168-bit key, while still maintaining backward compatibility.

DES is designed so that even if someone knows some of the plain-text data and the corresponding ciphertext, they have no way to determine the key without trying all possible keys. The strength of DES encryption–based security rests on the size of the key and on properly protecting the key. Although the original DES standard has been broken in brute force attacks of only 56 hours, the new 3DES standard should remain secure for many years to come.

Part I

Advanced Encryption Standard (AES)

As of May 26, 2002, the new standard used by the U.S government for protecting sensitive, but not classified, data is AES (Advanced Encryption Standard). This new standard was the result of a "best of breed" approach in which multiple encryption algorithms (MARS, RC6, Rijndael, Serpent, and Twofish) were submitted and evaluated on the basis of not only brute protection, but also speed, maintenance, and administration. As a result of this process, the Rijndael algorithm was selected to be the official algorithm of the new standard.

Rijndael (as implemented in AES) is a symmetric block cipher that uses 128-, 192-, and 256-bit keys (in blocks of 128 bits). Although all the algorithms submitted to the government were considered strong enough for AES, Rijndael excelled in areas of performance, efficiency, and flexibility. These areas take on additional importance when you understand that the protocol has to be implemented in hardware/software combinations with less power than traditional desktop computers (such as radios, key/card readers, and other devices).

And what about the IETF's opinion of AES and the AES algorithm? After performing a stuffy review of IETF protocols (including SSL [Secure Sockets Layer], S/MIME [Secure Multipurpose Internet Mail Extension], SSH [Secure Shell], and Kerberos, among others), they reached the conclusion that most protocols that already use encryption can be easily modified to accommodate it. As a result, by the end of 2003, all IETF protocols will be AES-capable, even though DES/3DES will still be supported a little beyond that date.

Digital Certificate Servers

As you saw in the section on public and private cipher keys, you can use a private key to create a unique digital signature. This signature can then be verified later with the public key to ensure that the signature is authentic. This process provides a strong method for authenticating a user's identity. A *digital certificate server* provides a central point of management for multiple public keys. It prevents every user from having to maintain and manage copies of every other user's public cipher key. For example, a Lotus Notes server can act as a digital certificate server, allowing users to sign messages using their private keys. The Notes server can then inform the recipient on delivery whether the Notes server could verify the digital signature.

Digital certificate servers, also known as *certificate authorities* (CAs), provide verification of digital signatures. For example, if Toby receives a digitally signed message from Lynn but does not have a copy of Lynn's public cipher key, Toby can obtain a copy of Lynn's public key from the CA to verify that the message is authentic. Also, let's assume that Toby wants to respond to Lynn's e-mail but wants to encrypt the message to protect it from prying eyes. Toby can again obtain a copy of Lynn's public key from the CA so that the message can be encrypted using Lynn's public key.

You can even use certificate servers to provide single sign-on and access control. You can map certificates to access control lists for files stored on a server in order to restrict access. When a user attempts to access a file, the server verifies that the user's certificate has been granted access. This approach allows a CA to manage nearly all document security for an organization.

NOTE

Netscape Certificate Server is a good example of a CA that supports file-level access control.

The largest benefit comes from using a CA that supports X.509, an industry standard format for digital certificates. This approach allows certificates to be verified and information to be encrypted between organizations. If the predominant method of exchanging information between two domains is e-mail, a CA may be far more cost effective than investing in virtual private networking.

IP Security (IPSec)

IPSec (IP Security) is a set of protocols developed by the IETF to support the encryption and authentication of data at the IP layer of the OSI (Open Standards Interconnect) Reference Model; as a result, it has become a key technology in the deployment of VPNs (virtual private networks). The various protocols include the following:

AH (Authentication Header)   This protocol is used to authenticate and validate packets—in other words, to digitally sign each packet. A receiving station can verify the identity of the sender of the message, and also the integrity of the data (that is, verify that the data hasn't been changed, either through corruption or malicious intent).

ESP (Encapsulating Security Protocol)   This protocol encrypts the data payload of a packet so that only the sender and receiver know the contents.

IPCOMP (IP Compression)   Because encryption can reduce the effectiveness of encryption, IPCOMP works to compress the data and then hands it off to ESP for encryption.

IKE (Internet Key Exchange)   Because AH and ESP use public/private keys to generate and exchange a symmetric session key, IKE is used to negotiate how that process takes place.

IPSec can be used in two modes: transport and tunnel. *Transport mode* simply encrypts communication between two hosts. *Tunnel mode*, however, works to support VPNs by placing the entire encrypted IP packet into an additional IP packet so that the encrypted data is "tunneled" through to the destination. Both AH and ESP can operate in either transport or tunnel mode.

When you implement IPSec, you need to give your system guidelines so that it knows which packets are to be processed by IPSec. You do so by defining an IPSec policy, which really comes down to deciding whether IPSec is applied to a specific type of packet or to a service as a whole.

For example, an IPSec rule applies to all packets being sent to a specific destination network. This approach is most common when an IPSec-aware router is used to establish a secure connection (possibly a VPN, but not necessarily) from one network to another. In this case, all packets, regardless of which service or client they originate from, are encrypted, as long as they are destined for the specific network.

If you want to set up an IPSec-aware service (such as an e-mail server), you can also specify that all packets sent or received on a specific port— regardless of their origin or destination—are processed by IPSec. In this case, IPSec is said to be applied in a *per-server fashion*.

In addition to the flexibility of the functions performed by IPSec, the standard also allows for a choice of encryption algorithms that can be used by AH and ESP, as well as by IKE. This feature is important when you are combining IPSec with other security implementations from various vendors.

Kerberos

Kerberos is another authentication solution that is designed to provide a single sign-on to a heterogeneous environment. Kerberos allows mutual authentication and encrypted communication between users and services. Unlike security tokens, however, Kerberos relies on each user to remember and maintain a unique password.

When a user authenticates to the local operating system, a local agent sends an authentication request to the Kerberos server. The server responds by sending the encrypted credentials for the user attempting to authenticate to the system. The local agent then tries to decrypt the credentials using the user-supplied password. If the correct password has been supplied, the user is validated and given authentication tickets, which allow the user to access other Kerberos-authenticated services. The user is also given a set of cipher keys that can be used to encrypt all data sessions.

Once users are validated, they are not required to authenticate with any Kerberos-aware servers or applications. The tickets issued by the Kerberos server provide the credentials required to access additional network resources. Although the user is still required to remember their password, they only need one password to access all systems on the network to which they have access.

One of the biggest benefits of Kerberos is that it is free. You can download and use the source code without cost. Many commercial applications, such as IBM's Global Sign-On (GSO) product, are also Kerberos-compatible but sport additional features and improved management. A number of security flaws have been discovered in Kerberos over the years, but most, if not all, have been fixed as of Kerberos V.

TIP

Chapter 5 contains more detailed information about Kerberos, in the context of Windows 2000.

PPTP/L2TP

A discussion of encryption techniques would not be complete without at least mentioning PPTP (Point-to-Point Tunneling Protocol) and L2TP (Layer 2 Tunneling Protocol). Developed by Microsoft, PPTP uses authentication based on the Point-to-Point Protocol (PPP) and encryption based on a Microsoft algorithm. Microsoft has integrated support for PPTP into all versions of Windows.

However, although this technology made for rapid and easy deployment of Microsoft VPNs, PPTP has never been considered secure. As a result, Microsoft took the best features of PPTP and merged them with Cisco's L2F (Layer 2 Forwarding) to create L2TP. (This standard was later adopted by the IETF.) L2TP can use IPSec for its authentication and encryption, and because IPSec implementations can choose from among various algorithms, it is more flexible (and secure). There is an additional implementation and maintenance cost, however, because of IPSec's reliance on a public-key infrastructure.

L2TP can operate without IPSec, however, and in this mode it uses the same authentication and access controls of PPP (Point to Point Protocol)—PAP (Password Authentication Protocol) and CHAP (Challenge Handshake Authentication Protocol), along with NCP (Network Control Protocol)—to handle the IP address assignment of the remote VPN client. (The VPN client can appear to the host network to have an IP address on the same, or complementary, subnet.) Microsoft's implementation of L2TP can also use EAP (discussed next) for more flexible and stronger authentication.

EAP (Extensible Authentication Protocol)

EAP is an extension to PPP that allows for multiple authentication methods, including token cards, one-time passwords, public key authentication (using smart cards), and even Kerberos and RADIUS (see the next section). Microsoft provides for both CHAP and TLS (Transport Layer Security) with its implementation of EAP. TLS is a mutual authentication scheme (like Kerberos) that requires both client and server to prove their identity (through certificates) and is simply an extension (and improvement) of SSL.

Remote Access Dial-In User Service (RADIUS)

RADIUS allows multiple remote access devices to share the same authentication database. RADIUS provides a central point of management for all remote network access. When a user attempts to connect to a RADIUS client (such as a terminal access server), they are challenged for a logon name and password. The RADIUS client then forwards these credentials to the RADIUS server. If the credentials are valid, the server returns an affirmative reply, and the user is granted access to the network. If the credentials do not match, the RADIUS server replies with a rejection, causing the RADIUS client to drop the user's connection.

RADIUS has been used predominantly for remote modem access to a network. Over the years, it has enjoyed widespread support from such vendors as 3COM, Cisco, and Ascend. RADIUS is also starting to become accepted as a method for authenticating remote users who are attempting to access the local network through a firewall. Support for RADIUS has been added to Checkpoint's Firewall-1 and Cisco's PIX Firewall.

The biggest drawback to using RADIUS for firewall connectivity is that the specification does not include encryption. Although RADIUS can perform strong authentication, it has no way to ensure the integrity of your data once the session is established. If you do use RADIUS authentication on the firewall, you will need an additional solution in order to provide encryption.

RSA Encryption

The RSA encryption algorithm was created by Ron Rivest, Adi Shamir, and Leonard Adleman in 1977. RSA is considered the de facto standard in public/private key encryption: It has found its way into products from Microsoft, Apple, Novell, Sun, and even Lotus. As a public/private key scheme, it can also perform authentication.

The fact that RSA is widely used is important when considering interoperability. You cannot authenticate or decrypt a message if you are using a different algorithm from the algorithm used to create it. Sticking with a product that supports RSA helps to ensure that you can exchange information with a large base of users. The large installation base also means that RSA has received its share of scrutiny over the years. This consideration is also important when you are selecting an algorithm to protect your data.

RSA Laboratories was the original owner of the algorithm, but in September 2000 it released the algorithm into the public domain. This release further confirms the position of the algorithm and will do nothing but increase its ubiquity in products and services.

Secure Shell (SSH)

SSH is a powerful method of performing client authentication and safeguarding multiple service sessions between two systems. Written by a Finnish student named Tatu Yl nen, SSH has received widespread acceptance within the Unix world. The protocol has even been ported to Windows and OS/2.

Systems running SSH listen on port 22 for incoming connection requests. When two systems running SSH establish a connection, they validate each other's credentials by performing a digital certificate exchange using RSA. Once the credentials for each system have been validated, 3DES is used to encrypt all information that is exchanged between the two systems. The two hosts authenticate each other in the course of the communication session and periodically change encryption keys. This process helps to ensure that brute force or playback attacks are not effective.

SSH is an excellent method of securing protocols that are known to be insecure. For example, Telnet and FTP sessions exchange all authentication information in the clear. SSH can encapsulate these sessions to ensure that no cleartext information is visible.

Secure Sockets Layer (SSL)

Created by Netscape, SSL provides RSA encryption at the session layer of the OSI model. By encrypting at the session layer, SSL can be service independent. Although SSL works equally well with FTP, HTTP, and even Telnet, the main use of SSL is in secure Web commerce. Because the RSA encryption is a public/private key encryption, digital certificates are also supported. Thus, SSL can authenticate the server and optionally authenticate the client.

Netscape includes SSL in its web browser and web server products. Netscape has even provided source code so that SSL can be adapted to other web server platforms. A webmaster developing a web page can flag the page as requiring an SSL connection from all web browsers. This requirement allows online commerce to be conducted in a relatively secure manner.

SSL was the creation of Netscape, which then passed the standard to the IETF. The IETF built TLS from SSL, while still retaining backward compatibility. As a result, HTTPS (Hypertext Transfer Protocol Secure) supports both SSL and TLS.

Security Tokens

Security tokens, also called *token cards*, are password-generating devices that can be used to access local clients or network services. Physically, a token is a small device with an LCD display that shows the current password and the amount of time remaining before the password expires.

Once the current password expires, a new one is generated. This approach provides a high level of authentication security, because a compromised password has a limited lifespan. Figure 4.7 shows a number of security tokens produced by Security Dynamics Technologies. These tokens are referred to as SecurID cards.

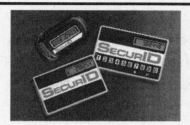

FIGURE 4.7: SecurID cards from Security Dynamics Technologies

Security tokens do not directly authenticate with an existing operating system or application. An agent is required to redirect the logon request to an authentication server. For example, Firewall-1 supports inbound client authentication via SecurID. When a user on the Internet wants to access internal services protected by Firewall-1, they use their SecurID token to authenticate at the firewall. Firewall-1 does not handle this authentication directly; rather, an agent on the firewall forwards the logon request to a SecurID authentication server, known as an *ACE/Server*. If the credentials are legitimate, validation is returned to the agent via an encrypted session, and the user is allowed access to the internal network.

Each security token is identified by a unit ID number. The unit ID number uniquely identifies each security token to the server. The unit ID is also used to modify the algorithm used to generate each password so that multiple tokens will not produce the same sequence of passwords. Because passwords expire at regular intervals (usually 60 seconds), the security token needs to be initially synchronized with the authentication server.

A number of benefits are associated with this type of authentication. First, users are no longer required to remember their passwords. They simply read the current password from the security token and use this value for authentication. This obviously removes the need for users to change their passwords at regular intervals, because it is done automatically by the security token. Also, it is far less likely that a user will give out their password to another individual, because the token is a physical device that needs to be referenced during each authentication attempt. Even if a user does read their password to another user, the consequences are minimized because the password is only valid for a short period of time.

Security tokens are an excellent way to provide authentication. Their only drawback is that they do not provide any type of session encryption. They rely on the underlying operating system or application to provide this functionality. For example, authentication information can still be read as cleartext if an attacker snoops on a Telnet session. Still, the limited lifespan of any password makes it difficult to capitalize on this information.

Simple Key Management for Internet Protocols (SKIP)

SKIP is similar to SSL in that it operates at the session level. Like SSL, SKIP can support IP services regardless of whether the services specifically support encryption. This feature is extremely useful when multiple IP services are running between two hosts.

SKIP is unique because it requires no prior communication in order to establish or exchange keys on a session-by-session basis. The Diffie-Hellman public/private algorithm is used to generate a shared secret. This shared secret is used to provide IP packet–based encryption and authentication.

Although SKIP is extremely efficient at encrypting data, which improves VPN performance, it relies on the long-term protection of this shared secret to maintain the integrity of each session. SKIP does not continually generate new key values, as SSH does. Thus, SKIP encryption is vulnerable if the keys are not protected properly.

WHAT'S NEXT

In this chapter, you saw why good authentication is important and what kinds of attacks can be launched if you do not use it. You also learned about encryption and the differences between secret and public/private algorithms. Finally, you looked at a number of authentication and encryption options that are currently available.

Now that you understand encryption, it is time to evaluate and compare the most popular network operating systems on the market. We will begin with Windows 2000 Server, one of the most popular systems on the market.

Part II
OPERATING SYSTEMS AND SERVERS

Chapter 5

WINDOWS 2000 SECURITY

When Windows NT was first introduced in 1993, security meant keeping authorized users from seeing sensitive information stored on a server, and perhaps using callback security for remote access users so that you could control who was able to dial in to your systems from outside your site. Windows NT was considered secure because it used one-way password hashes for user authentication and inherited security tokens for interprocess security.

The Internet changed all of that. Windows NT 4 was released in 1996 with a new and immature TCP/IP stack, just as the Internet was gaining momentum, and the operating system was unprepared for the Internet-based hacking onslaught that ensued for the four years of its release life. Microsoft created hotfix after hotfix and service pack after service pack, trying to shore up new breaches discovered in Windows NT's services, protocols, and drivers.

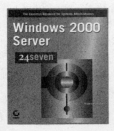

Adapted from *Windows® 2000 Server: 24seven*™ by Matthew Strebe
ISBN 0-7821-2669-3 $34.99

Many of the breaches were caused by new optional components in Windows NT 4, such as Internet Information Server and FrontPage Server Extensions. A big part of the problem was providing Internet service itself: How does a system discriminate between legitimate Web users and a hacker probing the back doors for unauthorized entrance? What is the right balance of useful service and security? How can you be certain of someone's identity when they're connecting from the Internet?

Security in the Internet era means actively blocking sessions from unknown computers, authenticating users based on public key encryption certificates, auditing the use of files and directories, encrypting communications, and preventing legitimate users from unintentionally activating viruses and Trojan horses.

Having learned the lessons of the ill-prepared Windows NT 4, Windows 2000 provides a complex suite of tools to authenticate users, encrypt data, secure connections, block unauthorized access, and manage security holistically. Windows 2000 can be made as secure with its default set of services as any other mass-market operating system—including any version of Unix or Linux—and it's far easier to manage and use in its secure state.

Windows 2000 can't fix everything, however, because Microsoft and third-party software vendors still put ease of use ahead of security in consumer products such as Internet Explorer, Outlook, and Office. All of these programs have serious security flaws because of their built-in scripting engines, so network administrators must remain vigilant. Windows 2000 can help in fixing these problems as well, but until Microsoft places more focus on security in its end-user products, the only way to prevent these programs from causing security problems on your network is to not use them.

In this chapter, I provide you with all the information you need to understand Windows 2000 security mechanisms, along with some management advice and practical walkthroughs. Once you've read this chapter and used the information to design a security architecture for your network, consult the Internet RFCs upon which most of these standards are based for technical details of their operation. You'll find an excellent searchable source for Internet RFCs at www.rfc.net. Microsoft's Resource Kit is the authoritative source for the Microsoft implementation of these mechanisms and should be consulted for configuration-specific information.

SECURITY THEORY

Security is the sum of all measures taken to prevent loss of any kind. A fundamentally secure system is one in which no user has access to anything. Unfortunately, totally secure systems are useless, so it is necessary to accept a certain amount of security risk in order to provide usability. The goal of security management is to minimize the risk involved in providing the necessary level of system usability.

All modern computer security is based upon the fundamental concept of user identity. To gain access to the system, people identify themselves in a manner that the system trusts. This process is called *logging on*. Once the user has logged on to the system, their access to data and programs can be positively controlled based on their identity.

Of course, to keep this system trustworthy, access to the system must never be allowed without logging on. Even in systems that are open to the anonymous public, an account must be used to control what anonymous users have access to. If access cannot be denied to illegitimate users, security cannot be controlled.

In many cases, users must be allowed to operate on sensitive data that they could potentially destroy, either willfully or by accident. Because usability is the opposite of security, access restrictions must be eased for a system to be functional. In these cases, security is replaced by *accountability*. In pure accountability-based systems, users are given free reign with the knowledge that everything they do is being recorded. This arrangement ensures that users will not knowingly cause damage to the system unless they're willing to face the consequences. Because anonymous users cannot be held accountable for their actions, accountability systems cannot function without the ability to correlate a specific person to a user account. In accountability-based systems, every user must have a unique account and no user account can ever be used by more than one person.

Windows 2000 uses a number of mechanisms to secure the local computer against malicious programs, to identify users, and to secure network communications. Here are the major Windows 2000 security mechanisms:

Control Access Absolutely By preventing untrusted computers from connecting to the secure system using packet filtering and Network Address Translation; by ensuring that allowed user sessions cannot be forged, hijacked, or spoofed using Kerberos

Part II

and IPSec; and by preventing programs from violating the address space of another program using memory protection.

Determine the Identity of the User   By using authentication methods such as Kerberos, Message Digest Authentication, smart cards, RADIUS authentication, or third-party authentication protocols such as those that implement biometric methods.

Restrict or Permit Access Based on User Identity   With access control lists for security-managed objects such as printers, services, and NTFS stored files and directories; by encrypting files using the Encrypting File System; by restricting access to operating system features that could be abused using Group Policy; and by authorizing remote users from the Internet or dial-up connections using RRAS policy.

Record User Activity   With audit logs of especially sensitive information and connection logs for public services such as the Web and FTP.

Communicate Privately between Computers   By using IPSec, Point-to-Point Tunneling Protocol (PPTP), or Layer 2 Tunneling Protocol (L2TP) to encrypt the communication stream between computers. PPTP and L2TP are used to enable users to initiate secure communication streams, and IPSec is used to enable two computers to communicate securely over a public medium irrespective of user identity.

Minimize the Risk of Misconfiguration   By grouping similar security mechanisms into policies and then applying those policies to groups of similar users or computers. Windows 2000's Group Policy, RRAS policy, and IPSec policy management tools allow administrators to make sweeping changes to large portions of a secure system without worrying about individual mistakes.

Security must be managed with the entire network system in mind. Enabling individual security features doesn't provide complete security because there are invariably ways to get around individuated security features.

Windows 2000 in its default state is configured to be useful, not secure. Hard disks are created by default to give full control to everyone, no group policies are in place by default, and most intercomputer communications are not secured. No files are encrypted by default, and no packet filters are enabled by default.

To create a secure system, you must enable all important security features (often referred to as *hardening* the OS) and then ease up on security features to provide access to valid users and to improve performance. Coming from an unsecured posture and attempting to enable individual security features will undoubtedly leave numerous security holes.

There is no Enable All Security Features button in Windows 2000. Despite great strides in holistic management, Windows 2000 still has quite a ways to go, in my opinion, to secure the default configuration. But the tools are easy to find and they do work well together to provide a manageable security interface.

A CRYPTOGRAPHIC PRIMER

Cryptography is the study of codes and ciphers. Windows 2000 uses pervasive cryptography to secure everything from stored files to communications streams to user passwords to domain authentication. Because cryptography and encryption are so important to Windows 2000 security, you need to understand the basic mechanisms of cryptography in order to understand Windows 2000 security. This section is an introduction to cryptography and the cryptographic mechanisms discussed later in this chapter.

Part II

NOTE

Bruce Schneier's book *Applied Cryptography* (2nd ed.) is the best mass-market book on cryptography. Consult it for more in-depth information on cryptography.

All of the new security features of Windows 2000 are based on cryptography. In contrast, the first release of Windows NT used cryptography only for password hashing. Over the release life of Windows NT 4, various different cryptographic elements were added to the operating system, but they were not handled in a coherent and secure fashion—they were simply piled on. Windows 2000 changes that situation by using the Active Directory as the container for nearly all security-related configuration and policy applications.

Like any other group of specialists, cryptographers have a language of their own to describe what they do. You don't have to be a theoretical mathematician to evaluate and use cryptography in your network, but it helps to have a general understanding when you are evaluating cryptography options for your network. The "Terminology: Cryptography and Encryption" sidebar defines the terms you should be familiar with.

TERMINOLOGY: CRYPTOGRAPHY AND ENCRYPTION

You should know the precise meanings of these cryptographic terms as they are used in this book:

Algorithm   Detailed steps for performing a function.

Asymmetric Algorithm   An algorithm in which different keys are used for encryption and decryption. Public key algorithms are asymmetric.

Restricted Algorithm   An algorithm that is kept secret to make it more difficult to break.

Symmetric Algorithm   An algorithm in which the same key is used for encryption and decryption. Secret key algorithms are symmetric.

Block Cipher   A cipher designed to operate on fixed-size blocks of data. Block ciphers are used for bulk encryption.

Breakable   A cipher that, given a reasonable amount of time and resources, can be compromised by a competent cryptanalyst.

Computationally Secure   A cipher that, given all the computational power that will be available to the most powerful governments for the foreseeable future, is unlikely to be compromised.

Keyspace   The range of all possible keys for a cipher. A cipher with a large keyspace is harder to crack than one with a smaller keyspace because there are more keys (numbers or combinations of letters) to try.

Secure   A cipher that, even given a reasonable amount of time and resources, most likely cannot be compromised by a competent cryptanalyst.

Stream Cipher   A cipher designed to operate on a continuous stream of data.

Strong   A cipher that, given the computational power that may reasonably be brought to bear on it any time in the near future, is unlikely to be compromised.

Unconditionally Secure   A cipher that, given an unlimited amount of time and an infinitely powerful processor, cannot be compromised.

Windows 2000 uses encryption for three vitally important purposes:

▶ To prove the identity of a security principal

▶ To validate the contents of a message or file

▶ To hide the contents of a data store or stream

A *cipher* is an encryption algorithm; it protects a message by rearranging it or performing modifications to the encoding, rather than the meaning, of the message. A *code* is an agreed-upon way of keeping a secret between two or more individuals. A *key* is a bit of information that is required to decrypt a message, usually in the form of a value that is used with a cipher to encrypt a message. The key must be kept secret in order for the message to remain private.

Encryption Algorithms

One algorithm that was developed in secret but then released for use by the public as well as the government (but only for "Unclassified but Sensitive" information) is the *Data Encryption Standard (DES)*. It is a symmetric algorithm, which means the same key is used for encryption and decryption, and it was designed to use a 56-bit key, although until recently the U.S. government limited export versions of DES to 40 bits. DES is widely used in commercial software and in communication devices that support encryption. There is lingering suspicion, however, that a possible weakness in the DES algorithm could allow the National Security Agency (NSA), which has a vested interest in maintaining its ability to decrypt communications and which cooperated in the development of DES, to more easily break messages encrypted with DES.

RSA (named after its inventors: Rivest, Shamir, and Adleman) is an algorithm that was not developed by a government agency. Its creators exploited the computationally difficult problem of factoring prime numbers to develop an *asymmetric*, or *public key*, algorithm, which can be used for both encryption and digital signatures. RSA has since become a very popular alternative to DES. RSA is used by a number of software companies whose products must negotiate secure connections over the insecure Internet (such as web browsers), including Microsoft, Digital, Sun, Novell, Netscape, and IBM. The patent on RSA recently expired, and its owners have placed it in the public domain.

The ciphers described here are not the only ones available for use in computers and networks today. Other governments (such as the former

Part II

USSR) were just as active as the United States in developing codes and ciphers, and many private individuals (especially in the last decade) have made contributions to the field of cryptography. GOST was developed in the former USSR, FEAL was developed by NTT Japan, LOKI was developed in Australia, and IDEA was developed in Europe. Most of these ciphers use patented algorithms that must be licensed for commercial use, but some (such as Blowfish) do not. Each cipher has strengths and weaknesses.

NOTE
All of the ciphers described in this section have the same weakness: If you know the cipher being used to encode a message but not the key, you can use a number of attacks to attempt to decode the message, including the "brute force" method of trying all the possible keys.

The purpose of ciphers, after all, is to hide information. Hiding information would not be a useful activity (especially for wartime governments that have other pressing areas to spend time and money on) if no one were interested in the information being hidden. The converse of hiding information is attempting to discover what is hidden, and advances in *breaking* codes (or deciphering codes without the key) have progressed hand-in-hand with developments in creating codes. The practice of attempting to break codes is called *cryptanalysis*, and the people who break codes are called *cryptanalysts*. A number of different types of cryptanalytical attacks can be used against secure systems:

Keyspace Attack   This is the hard way to crack an encrypted message. A *keyspace search* involves checking every possible key that might have been used to encrypt the message. Such a search is like trying every possible combination on a bank vault in order to open it. A keyspace search is feasible only when there are not many possible keys. A cryptanalyst might use this technique if the key length is 40 or 56 bits, and perhaps if it were 128 bits and the message were really worth the millions of dollars of hardware that would be required. Keyspace searches of larger keyspaces are impractical at the present level of computing technology.

Known Plain Text   A cryptanalyst can reduce the number of possible keys to be searched for many ciphers if the plain text of the encrypted message is already known. (Why would the cryptanalyst want the key if the message is already out? Perhaps another message is encrypted with the same key.) If even a portion of the message is always the same, especially at the beginning of the message (for example, the headers in an e-mail message are always the same), your cipher text may be vulnerable.

WARNING

In an encrypted file system, if a standard system file is encrypted using the same key as secret documents, it is trivial (for a cryptanalyst) to derive the decryption key using the standard system file. For this reason, you should never encrypt files that were not created by your organization.

Linear and Differential Cryptanalysis A cryptanalyst may also look for mathematical patterns in collections of cipher texts that have all been encrypted with the same key. Some ciphers (not all) are vulnerable to either or both of these kinds of analysis, and a cryptanalyst may then have a much smaller range of keys to search.

The Almost Perfect Cipher

There is one encryption cipher—the *one-time pad*—that cannot be com-promised if you do not have the key, even with all the time left in the universe and all the computational power that is theoretically possible. It is not simply improbable that the key would be discovered or the message retrieved by using brute force; it is impossible. Unfortunately, the require-ments of the cipher make it impractical for use in anything but certain kinds of low-bandwidth communications.

A one-time pad uses a key exactly as long as the message being encoded. The key must be completely random (anything less than random leaves your message open to certain kinds of cryptographic analysis), and no portion of it can be reused without compromising the security of your message. Each letter (or byte) of your message is combined mathematically with an equal-sized portion of the key (often by the XOR mathematical function or the addition with modulus mathematical function) that results in the cipher text and uses up the key.

The one-time pad is so secure because the cipher text being decoded can result in any plain text (of the same length) and associated key. For example, *henryjtillman* encoded with the one-time pad key *lfwpxzgwpoieq* results in the cipher text *tkkhsjafbavfe*. Although the cipher text decoded with the correct key produces the original message, the cipher text can also be decoded using the possible key *swgpnmquypciq*, resulting in the message *andrewjackson*, or using the key *gbywrvwcmlkwz*, resulting in the message *milkandcookie*. The attacker has no way of knowing which key and resulting plain text are correct.

The problem with the one-time pad is that it requires a key as big as the message being sent, and both the sender and the receiver must have the same key. If you must encrypt a 10Mbps Ethernet link, you could use up a CD-ROM's worth of key data in just 10 minutes!

NOTE

Clearly, the one-time pad is best used when communication is infrequent or uses very little bandwidth, such as e-mail messages that must have the most secure encryption possible.

Symmetric Functions

If the same key can be used to encrypt or decrypt the message, then the cipher uses a *symmetric function*. Both the sender and receiver must have that same key. Good symmetric ciphers are fast, secure, and easy to implement using modern microprocessors.

Some ciphers are more secure than others. The XOR cipher, for example, is not very secure. A competent cryptanalyst can decode an XOR-encoded message in short order. Two general features of a symmetric algorithm make it secure:

▶ The algorithm produces cipher text that is difficult to analyze.

▶ The algorithm has a sufficiently large keyspace.

Cryptanalysts test cipher text for correspondences in the text, an uneven distribution of instances of numbers, and essentially anything that differentiates the cipher text from a series of truly random numbers. A good algorithm will produce a cipher text that is as random-seeming as possible. This is where the XOR cipher fails miserably—an XOR-ed message has a lot in common with a regular ASCII text message. Cryptographers will exploit these commonalities to recover the key and decode the whole message.

A cryptanalyst who cannot exploit nonrandomness in the cipher text has little choice but to simply try all the possible key combinations to decode the message. This is a lot like hackers trying to guess the password to your system; if they don't know that the password is a birthday or the name of your dog, then they must try all the possible passwords.

NOTE
Just as a longer password is safer than a shorter one, a longer key is more secure than a shorter key.

A number of symmetric ciphers are used in both software and hardware. You can get a feel for what is available by comparing the following three ciphers:

DES IBM and the U.S. National Security Agency cooperated to develop this cipher. It is resistant to differential cryptanalysis but susceptible to linear cryptanalysis. Its key length is only 56 bits, which makes it increasingly easy to perform a brute-force examination of all the possible keys for an encrypted cipher text. DES is in common use in encryption hardware and software. It is an ANSI standard. Windows 2000 implements both 40-bit DES and 168-bit 3DES (*triple*-DES—DES with three contiguous keys).

IDEA This cipher has a key length of 128 bits—considerably more than DES uses. Although a sufficiently motivated and financed organization or a large cabal of hackers can break a DES-encoded message, the large keyspace makes a brute-force attack on IDEA impractical. IDEA was designed to be immune to linear and differential cryptanalysis, and you can reasonably be assured that not even the NSA can decode an IDEA-encrypted message without the key. IDEA is patented in Europe and the United States.

Blowfish This cipher can use a key from 32 to 448 bits long, allowing you to select how secure you want to make your message. It was designed to be immune to linear and differential cryptanalysis. Its developer, Bruce Schneier, has not sought a patent on the algorithm so that a good, freely implementable algorithm would be available to both private individuals and public sector.

One-Way Functions

When you type your password to log on to Windows 2000, it is encrypted and compared against the stored encrypted value of your password (see "Windows 2000 Local Security" later in this chapter). The password is

Part II

stored using a *one-way function* (also called a *hash*, *trap-door*, *digest*, or *fingerprint*) so that it will be difficult to determine your password even if a hacker has gained access to the operating system's stored settings.

Hash functions can also be used for other purposes. For example, you can use a hash to "fingerprint" files (create a digital fingerprint, or hash, that is unique to that file). A hash function can produce a result that is much smaller than the input text; a hash of a multimegabyte word-processor document, for example, may result in a 128-bit number. A hash is also unique to the file that produced it; it is practically impossible to create another file that will produce the same hash value. You might use this kind of hash to make sure that your Internet-distributed software product is delivered free of viruses and other malicious modifications. You can allow your customers to download the software, and then tell them what the hash value for the software files is. Only your unmodified software files will hash to the same value.

NOTE

One feature of a hash function (especially one that produces short hashes) is that any hash value is equally likely. Therefore, it is practically impossible to create another file that will hash to the same value.

Some hash functions require a key; others do not. Anyone can calculate a hash that does not use a key; this kind of hash is good for distributing software or making sure that files have not been changed without you noticing. A hash function with a key can only be calculated by someone (or something) who has the key.

Public Key Encryption

Whereas symmetric ciphers use the same key to encrypt and decrypt messages (that's why they're called *symmetric*), *public key encryption* (or a *public key cipher*) uses a different key to decrypt than was used to encrypt. This is a relatively new development in cryptography, and it solves many longstanding problems with cryptographic systems, such as how to exchange those secret keys in the first place.

The problem with symmetric ciphers is this: Both the sender and the recipient must have the same key in order to exchange encrypted messages over an insecure medium. If two parties decide to exchange private messages, or if two computers' network devices or programs must establish a secure channel, the two parties must decide on a common key. Either party may simply decide on a key, but that party will have no way to send it to the other without the risk of it being intercepted on its way. It's a chicken-and-egg problem: Without a secure channel, there is no way to establish a secure channel.

In 1976, Witfield Diffie and Martin Hellman discovered a way out of the secure channel dilemma. They found that by using a different key, certain one-way functions could be undone. Their solution (called *public key cryptography*) takes advantage of a characteristic of prime and almost prime numbers—specifically, how hard it is to find the two factors of a large number that has only two factors, both of which are prime. Since Diffie and Hellman developed their system, some other public key ciphers have been introduced. For example, the difficulty of determining quadratic residues (a subtle mathematical construct that few people other than mathematicians and cryptologists really understand) has been exploited to make a public key cipher.

With a public key cipher, one key (the public key) is used to encrypt a message, and the other one (the private key) is the only key that can decrypt the message. This means that you can tell anyone your public key—even complete strangers and NSA agents. Whoever has your key can encrypt a message that only you can decrypt. Even the NSA agent who has your public key cannot decrypt the message.

One problem that plagues secure public key ciphers is that they are slow—much slower than symmetric ciphers. You can expect a good public key cipher to take 1,000 times as long to encrypt the same amount of data as a good symmetric cipher. This can be quite a drag on your computer's performance if you have a lot of data to transmit or receive.

Although it is much slower than symmetric systems, the public key/ private key system neatly solves the problem that bedevils symmetric cryptosystems. When two people (or devices) need to establish a secure channel for communication, one of them can just pick a secret key and then encrypt that secret key using the other's public key. The encrypted key is then sent to the other party, and even if the key is intercepted, only the other party can decrypt the secret key, using the private key. Communication may then continue between the two parties using a symmetric cipher and that secret key. A system that uses both symmetric and public key encryption is called a *hybrid cryptosystem*.

Generating Keys

Most cryptographic systems manage the selection of keys and the negotiation of protocols for you. Systems that do this must be able to select keys that are not easily guessed, because one way to attack a cryptographic system is to predict the keys that might be used in the system. These keys are selected by generating random numbers.

It is difficult for a computer to generate good random numbers. Computers, by their very nature, are extremely predictable, and hundreds of thousands of engineers have labored (collectively) millions of years to make them more so. If you run a computer program twice and give it the same input the second time as you did the first, you will get the same output the second time as you did the first. Because the whole point of a truly random number is not to be able to guess the output based on the input, computers (unassisted) make lousy dice-throwers.

NOTE

An example of the randomness problem existed in early versions of Netscape Navigator. In order to generate a random number for the Secure Socket Layer, Netscape used the system time, which provides a 12-bit number, to generate a 40-bit crypto key. Because there was only 12 bits' worth of unique keys in that 40-bit space, hackers were able to crack and exploit secure sessions in a matter of minutes. A 12-bit key is so short that it's worthless for security. It's about as secure as a two-character password.

The best that computers can do by themselves are *pseudorandom numbers*, which are numbers created by a deterministic means (that is, given identical starting conditions, identical numbers will be produced). Good pseudorandom numbers have a long periodicity (it's unlikely that the same number will be generated repeatedly from different seeds) and satisfy the other conditions of random numbers, such as incompressibility (there is no redundant or repeated information in the number) and having an even distribution (generated numbers are equally likely across the possible range of numbers, rather than being clumped together). *Random numbers*, on the other hand, are unpredictable (an identical series of random numbers cannot be reproduced, even from identical starting conditions). Truly random numbers also satisfy other criteria, such as incompressibility and having an even distribution.

In order to get a good random number (to use as a seed value, for example), the computer must look outside itself, because computers are inherently deterministic. Many sources of randomness exist in the real (noncomputer) world—the weather, ocean waves, lava-lamp wax gyrations, the times between one keystroke and the next—and a computer can measure these events and use them to generate random numbers. Keystroke timing is commonly used to generate secret keys. Another way is to ask the user to type in a paragraph or two of text. There are no published algorithms that will predict arbitrary user input (yet).

If a random number is going to be used as a seed for pseudorandom numbers, it should have enough bits to make it difficult to guess. For example, you don't want to protect a 128-bit cryptosystem that uses IDEA with a password of eight characters or less for a seed—this is effectively only about 48 bits of security if you just use common printable ASCII characters in the password (the characters used in passwords provide about six bits' worth of uniqueness each).

Uses of Encryption

You can use encryption to protect the following types of network data:

- ▶ Private communications
- ▶ Secure file storage
- ▶ User or computer authentication
- ▶ Secure password exchange

You should encrypt any communications containing sensitive or proprietary information that go over an insecure medium such as radio, a telephone network, or the Internet. Use file system encryption to protect sensitive data when operating system features are not effective (when the hard drive has been removed or the operating system has been replaced).

The most common use for encryption with computers is to protect communications between computer users and between communications devices. This use of encryption is an extension of the role codes and ciphers have played throughout history. The only difference is that instead of a human being laboriously converting messages to and from an encoded form, the computer does all the hard work.

Secure File Storage

Encryption can be used to protect data in storage, such as data on a hard drive. All Unix implementations and Windows NT have many sophisticated security features. You may configure your operating system to allow

Part II

only authorized users to access files while the operating system is running, but when you turn your computer off, all those security features go away and your data is left defenseless. An intruder could load another operating system on the computer or even remove the hard drive and place it in another computer that does not respect the security settings of the original computer.

You can use encryption software to encrypt specific files that you want to protect and then decrypt them when you need to access them. The encryption and decryption process can be cumbersome, however, and you may end up having to remember a lot of encryption keys. Using encryption in this manner can also leave behind temporary files or files that are erased but still present on the hard drive containing sensitive information. This is obviously not what you want.

A better approach to security is to have the operating system encrypt and decrypt the files for you. Windows 2000 and Windows XP come with an Encrypting File System (EFS) that will encrypt all the files on your hard drive—even temporary ones created by the applications you use.

To use EFS securely, you must supply the cryptographic key when you start your computer, or use it with a smart card, but otherwise you can treat the files on your hard drive as regular, unencrypted files. EFS doesn't protect your files from being accessed while the operating system is running—that is what the operating system security features are for—but it does keep the data safe, even if someone steals the hard drive.

User or Computer Authentication

In addition to keeping secrets (either stored or transmitted), encryption can be used for almost the opposite purpose—to verify identities. Encryption can authenticate users logging on to computers, ensure that software you download from the Internet comes from a reputable source, and ensure that the person who sends a message is really who they say they are.

When you log on to a Microsoft operating system such as Windows Me, Windows 2000, or Windows XP, the operating system does not compare your password to a stored password. Instead, it encrypts your password using a one-way cryptographic function and then compares the result to a stored result. Other operating systems such as Unix and OS/2 work the same way.

This seems a roundabout way of verifying your identity when you log on, but there is a very good reason for the operating system to do it this way. By only storing the cryptographic hash of your password, the operating system makes it more difficult for a hacker to get all of the passwords in your system when they gain access to the system. One of the first things a hacker goes for in a compromised system (that is, one where the hacker has gotten at least one password) is that computer's password list, so that the hacker can get account names and passwords that may be valid on other computers in your network.

With a one-way cryptographic function, it's easy to generate a hashed value from the password, but it's difficult or impossible to generate the password from the hashed value. Because only the hashed values are stored, even a hacker who has complete access to the computer can't just read out the passwords. The best the hacker can do is to supply passwords one by one and see if they match any of the hashes in the password list. The hacker can run a program to do this instead of typing them all in by hand, but it can take a while if the users of the computer have chosen good passwords.

NOTE

Hackers have combined forces to "precompute" password hashes for all possible LAN Manager passwords. A precomputed hash uses the normal hashing function and records the password and its hash in a database. By dividing the keyspace hashing task among thousands of home computers and running as a background application, hackers have created a complete database of passwords to hashes. Hackers can now simply take the hash value (which Internet Explorer will give to any website that asks) and look it up in this directory to see which password matches that hash. This is why LAN Manager passwords are not secure.

Digital Signatures

Usually, public key encryption is used to transmit secrets encrypted with the public key and decrypted with the private key. You can also do it the other way: encrypt with the private key and decrypt with the public key.

Why would you want to encrypt a message that anyone can decrypt? That seems a bit silly, but there is a good reason to do so: Only the holder of the private key can encrypt a message that can be decrypted with the public key. It is, in effect, a *digital signature*, proving that the holder of the private key produced the message.

Because the purpose of a digital signature is not to conceal information but rather to certify it, the private key is often used to encrypt a hash of the original document, and the encrypted hash is appended to the document or sent along with it. This process takes much less processing time to generate or verify than does encrypting the entire document, and it still guarantees that the holder of the private key signed the document.

Internet e-mail was not designed with security in mind. Messages are not protected from snooping by intermediate Internet hosts, and you have no guarantee that a message actually came from the person identified in the e-mail's From field. Internet newsgroup messages have the same problem: You cannot really tell from whom the message actually came. You can encrypt the body of the message to take care of the first problem, and digital signatures take care of the second.

Digital signatures are useful because although anyone can check the signature, only the individual with the private key can create the signature. The difference between a digital signature and a certificate is that you can check the authenticity of a certificate with a certificate authority.

Secure Password Exchange

When you log on to your network file server, or when you connect to your Internet service provider, you supply a username and password. These two pieces of information control your access to the network and represent your identity on the network. They must be protected from eavesdropping.

Most network operating systems (Windows 2000 and all modern versions of Unix included) protect your username and password when you log on by encrypting the username and password before sending them over the network to be authenticated. The file server (or ISP host) checks the encrypted username and password against the list of legitimate users and passwords. The host can check the password by decrypting it and checking the database of passwords stored in the clear, or it can encrypt the stored password and check the result against what has been sent from the client over the network.

To keep the same encrypted data from being sent every time, the client can also include some additional information, such as the time the logon request was sent. This way your network credentials are never sent unprotected over your local LAN or over the telephone system. Windows 2000 does accept unencrypted passwords from older LAN Manager network clients, however, so you should be careful about allowing older clients on your network.

NOTE

Not every authentication protocol encrypts the username and password. SLIP, for example, does not. Telnet and FTP do not, although the Windows 2000 Telnet service can be configured to work only with Windows NT hashes rather than plain-text passwords. Point-to-Point Protocol (PPP) may, if both the dial-up client and server are configured that way. Windows NT by default requires encrypted authentication. Windows 2000 and Windows XP use secure secret-key-based Kerberos for authentication.

Steganography

Cryptography can be very effective at keeping a secret. With a sufficiently powerful cipher and a sufficiently long key, even major world governments cannot read your diary. What if you don't want people to know that you're keeping secrets, though? After all, an encrypted file or an encrypted hard drive is pretty strong evidence that you're hiding something. *Steganography* is the process of hiding those encrypted files where it is unlikely that anyone will find them.

Encrypted files look like random numbers, so anything that also looks like random numbers can hide an encrypted message. For example, in graphic images that use many colors, the low-order bit for each pixel in the image doesn't make much difference to the quality of the image. You can hide an encrypted message in the graphics file by replacing the low-order bits with the bits from your message. The low-order bits of high-fidelity sound files are another good place for encrypted data. You can even exchange encrypted messages with someone surreptitiously by sending graphics and sound files with those messages hidden in them.

A Word about Passwords

Passwords are secret keys. They can be used to authenticate users, encrypt data, and secure communication streams. Kerberos uses passwords as the secret key to prove client credentials to a Kerberos Key Distribution Center.

Having stressed the necessity for randomness in secret keys, it follows that passwords, being secret keys, must also be secure. Of course, telling people your password compromises it, but you can unintentionally compromise your password in a number of other ways.

The most common way is to choose an easily guessable password, such as an empty password, the word *password* itself, slang words, the

Part II

names of deities, or the names of children or pets. You may think that if a hacker doesn't know you, they won't know the names of your children. Think again. There are only 7,000 baby names at babynames.com. By creating a word list from that site, I was able to crack a web server over the Internet in just 45 minutes—and that's because I'd gotten all the way to *R*. Last names aren't much more secure; lists of registered voters or phone books can provide a complete set. At just one guess per second (the rate at which commonly available NetBIOS-based crack tools operate over the Internet), it would take less than 12 hours to go through the complete list of 40,000 unique last names in the San Diego telephone book—and automated crack tools can run far faster than one attempt per second by opening multiple simultaneous connections. Using words in the English language is even worse. Shakespeare is estimated to have had a vocabulary of 25,000 words. Mine is only about 15,000. Using any word I know as a password yields a crack time of about two hours from over the Internet.

Using truly random passwords yields much better results. Just a 14-character random password using the standard ASCII keyboard set yields 20 million quintillion (1,021) passwords. At one per second, the universe would be cold and dark (or would have collapsed, depending upon which theory is correct) before a hacker got into your network. So the concept of passwords is not fundamentally flawed, but most people choose seriously flawed passwords.

Even if you choose strong passwords, you have probably compromised them many times over. Ever signed up for a service or bought anything off the Web? Sure you have. Ever entered a password to create a new account? Probably. Was it the same password you use everywhere? Probably. How many websites have your password now? Lots.

I use four levels of passwords:

> **Low-Quality Public Password**   Usually an English word, I use this password for public services that I don't care about but which require a password anyway, such as my subscription to news websites. This password is so unimportant to me that I'll print it here: *Action!*, which is the first compiled programming language I learned.

> **Medium-Quality Public Password**   A short but completely random password, I use this on sites where my money could be spent or actual services could be stolen, such as my online credit card billing site, my favorite e-commerce vendors, and so on.

Why just a medium-quality password? Because although it's a hassle, my credit card company is liable for the fraudulent use of my card, not me. I also use this password for nonadministrative access to private networks. This password is seven characters long, yielding about 40 bits of uniqueness.

High-Quality Password   I use this password for private networks where I'm the administrator and where serious harm could be done to a customer if this password leaked out. I never tell this password to anyone, and I never, ever create accounts on public systems with it. I do use this password at multiple customer sites. This password is 12 characters long, yielding about 70 bits of uniqueness.

Extremely High-Quality Password   I use this password to encrypt files and store secrets on my personal computers that would seriously disrupt my life if they leaked out. This password never leaves my own systems and has never been written down or spoken aloud. This password is 14 characters long, yielding about 84 bits of uniqueness.

I don't change my passwords frequently, because frankly, it's really hard to remember good random passwords; and, if you change truly random passwords, you'll never remember old ones if you have to go back to a system you haven't been to in a while. Although changing passwords often is good in theory, forcing users to use heavy password rotation guarantees that you'll have extremely weak passwords on your network. In my opinion, a good, highly random password should only be changed if you've leaked it by accident.

Windows 2000 Local Security

Windows 2000 security is based on user authentication. Before you can use a Windows 2000 computer, you must supply a username and a password. The logon prompt (provided by the WinLogon process) identifies you to the computer, which then provides access to resources you are allowed to use and denies access to things you aren't.

Windows 2000 also provides group accounts. When a user account is a member of a group account, the permissions that apply to the group account also apply to the user account.

NOTE

Even when a group of people does the same job, each user should have an individual account. That way, when one user violates security, you can track the violation back to a specific user rather than to a group of people who use the same account.

User and group accounts are only valid for the Windows 2000 computer on which they are created. These accounts are local to the computer. The only exceptions to this rule are computers that are members of a domain and therefore trust the user accounts created in the Active Directory on a domain controller. Domain security is discussed in the later section "Kerberos Authentication and Domain Security."

Each Windows 2000 computer has its own list of local user and group accounts. When the WinLogon process (which logs you on and sets up your computing environment) needs to refer to the security database, it communicates with the Security Accounts Manager (SAM), which is the Windows 2000 operating system component that controls local account information. If the information is stored locally on the Windows 2000 computer, the SAM will refer to the database (stored in the Registry) and return the information to the WinLogon process. If the information is not stored locally (for example, it pertains to a domain account), the SAM will query the domain controller and return the validated logon information (the *security identifier*) to the WinLogon process.

Irrespective of the source of authentication, access is allowed only to the local computer by the computer's Local Security Authority (LSA). When you access other computers on the network, the local computer's LSA establishes your credentials automatically with the LSA on the foreign computer, effecting a logon for each computer you contact. To gain access to a foreign computer, that computer must trust the credentials provided by your computer.

Security Identifiers

Security principals such as users and computers are represented as *security identifiers* (SIDs). The SID uniquely identifies the security principal to all the computers in the domain. When you create an account using the Local Users and Groups snap-in, a new SID is always created, even if you use the same account name and password as a deleted account. The SID will remain with the account for as long as the account exists. You may change any other aspect of the account, including the username and password, but you cannot change the SID under normal circumstances—if you did, you would create a new account.

Group accounts also have a SID, which is a unique identifier that is created when the group is created. The same rules that apply to account SIDs also apply to group SIDs.

Referring again to user login, if the account name is valid and the password is correct, the WinLogon process will create an Access Token for you. The *Access Token* is composed of the user account SID, the SIDs of the groups the account belongs to, and a Locally Unique Identifier (LUID), which indicates user rights and a specific logon session.

NOTE

An Access Token is created each time you log on to Windows 2000. This is why you must log off and then log back on again after making changes to your user account—you need a new Access Token that will reflect the changes you have made. You can use WhoAmI, a Windows 2000 Resource Kit utility, to view your Access Token.

Special SIDs exist. The *System SID* is reserved for system services; Access Tokens that contain the System SID can bypass all account-based security restrictions. This SID gives system services permission to do things that a regular user account (even the Administrator account) cannot do. The Windows 2000 kernel, not the WinLogon process, starts operating system services, and these services receive the System SID from the kernel when they are started.

Resource Access

Threads (individual chains of execution in a process) must provide an Access Token at each attempt to access a resource. Threads receive their Access Tokens from their parent process when they are created. A user application, for example, usually receives its Access Token from Windows Explorer. Windows Explorer receives its Access Token from the WinLogon process. The WinLogon process is started from a user-generated interrupt (the Ctrl+Alt+Del keyboard interrupt) and is especially able to create new Access Tokens by querying either the local SAM or the Directory Services Agent (DSA) on an Active Directory domain controller.

Through this method, every thread that is started after a user has logged on will have the Access Token that represents the user. Because user mode threads must always provide that token to access resources, there is no way to circumvent Windows 2000 resource security under normal circumstances.

SAGE ADVICE: MANDATORY LOGONS

The foundation of Windows 2000 security is the *mandatory logon*. Unlike in some networking systems, a user cannot do anything in Windows 2000 without providing a user account name and password. Although you can choose to automatically log on with credentials provided from the Registry, a user account logon still occurs.

Although it's not the friendliest of keystrokes, there's a very good reason Windows 2000 requires the Ctrl+Alt+Del keystroke to log on, and it's one of the reasons Windows 2000 is considered secure. Because the computer handles the Ctrl+Alt+Del keystroke as a hardware interrupt, there's literally no way a clever programmer can make the keystroke do something else without rewriting the operating system.

Without this feature, a hacker would be able to write a program that displayed a fake logon screen and collect passwords from unsuspecting users. However, because the fake screen couldn't include the Ctrl+Alt+Del keystroke, users familiar with Windows 2000 would not be fooled.

Because the Access Token is passed to a new thread upon creation, there is no further need to access the SAM database locally or the Active Directory on a domain controller for authentication once a user has logged on.

Inheriting Access Tokens

When you log on to a Windows 2000 server over the network, the Access Token generated by the WinLogon or Kerberos process on the server is not sent back to your client computer. Instead, the Access Token is inherited by a session of the Server service on the Windows 2000 server, which maintains a connection to your client computer and performs the actions on the server (opening files, writing data, printing documents, and so on) for the client computer. Because the Access Token never leaves the

Windows 2000 server, there is no chance it will be intercepted on your LAN, and a malicious program on an insecure operating system such as Windows 95 cannot modify it.

Windows 2000 goes through the following steps when a user logs on locally:

1. The user presses Ctrl+Alt+Del, which causes a hardware interrupt that activates the WinLogon process.

2. The WinLogon process presents the user with the account name and password logon prompt.

3. The WinLogon process sends the account name and encrypted password to the LSA. If the user account is local to that Windows 2000 computer, the LSA queries the SAM of the local Windows 2000 computer; otherwise, the LSA queries a domain controller for the domain in which the computer is a member.

4. If the user has presented a valid username and password, the LSA creates an Access Token containing the user account SID and the group SIDs for the groups of which that user is a member. The Access Token also gets an LUID, which will be described later in this chapter in the "Rights versus Permissions" section. The Access Token is then passed back to the WinLogon process.

5. The WinLogon process passes the Access Token to the Win32 subsystem along with a request to create a logon process for the user.

6. The logon process establishes the user environment, including starting Windows Explorer and displaying the backdrop and Desktop icons.

Objects and Permissions

Windows 2000 maintains security for various types of objects, including (but not limited to) directories, files, printers, processes, and network shares. Each object exposes services that the object allows to be performed upon it: for example, open, close, read, write, delete, start, stop, print, and so on.

The security information for an object is contained in the object's *security descriptor*. The security descriptor has four parts: owner, group,

Discretionary Access Control List (DACL), and System Access Control List (SACL). Windows 2000 uses these parts of the security descriptor for the following purposes:

Owner   This part contains the SID of the user account that has ownership of the object. The object's owner may always change the settings in the DACL (the permissions) of the object.

Group   This part is used by the POSIX subsystem of Windows 2000. Files and directories in Unix operating systems can belong to a group as well as to an individual user account. This part contains the SID of the group of this object for the purposes of POSIX compatibility, as well as to identify the primary group for user accounts.

Discretionary Access Control List   The DACL contains a list of user accounts and group accounts that have permission to access the object's services. The DACL has as many access control entries as there are user or group accounts that have specifically given access to the object.

System Access Control List   The SACL also contains access control entries (ACEs), but these ACEs are used for auditing rather than for permitting or denying access to the object's services. The SACL has as many ACEs as there are user or group accounts that are specifically being audited.

Each access control entry in the DACL and SACL consists of a security identifier followed by an access mask. The *access mask* in the DACL identifies those services of the object that the SID has permission to access. A special type of ACE, called a *deny ACE*, indicates that all access to the object will be denied to the account identified by the SID. A deny ACE overrides all other ACEs. Windows 2000 implements the No Access permission using the deny ACE.

Access is allowed if an Access Token contains any SID that matches a permission in the DACL. For example, if an individual account is allowed read access, and the user account is a member of a group account that is allowed write access, then the Access Token for that logged-on user will contain both SIDs, and the DACL will allow read and write access to the object. Deny ACEs still override any accumulation of permission.

The ACEs in the SACL are formed the same way as the ACEs in the DACL (they are composed of a SID and an access mask), but the access mask, in this case, identifies those services of the object for which the account will be audited.

Not every object has a DACL or a SACL. The FAT file system, for example, does not record security information, so file and directory objects stored on a FAT volume lack DACLs and SACLs. When a DACL is missing, any user account may access any of the object's services. This is not the same as when an object has an empty DACL. In that case, no account may access the object. When there is no SACL for an object, that object may not be audited.

The Security Reference Monitor

Processes do not directly access objects such as files, directories, or printers. The Windows 2000 operating system (specifically, the Win32 portion of it) accesses the objects on behalf of your processes. The primary reason is to make programs simpler. The program doesn't have to know how to directly manipulate every kind of object; it simply asks the operating system to do it. Another important benefit, especially from the security point of view, is that because the operating system is performing the operations for the process, the operating system can enforce object security.

When a process asks the Win32 subsystem to perform an operation on an object (such as reading a file), the Win32 subsystem checks with the Security Reference Monitor to make sure the process has permission to perform the operation on the object. The Security Reference Monitor compares the Access Token of the process with the DACL of the object by checking each SID in the Access Token against the SIDs in the DACL. If there is an ACE with a matching SID that contains an access mask that allows the operation and there is no ACE with a matching SID containing a deny mask to the object for the operation, then the Security Reference Monitor allows the Win32 subsystem to perform the operation.

The Security Reference Monitor also checks to see if the object access is audited and should be reported in the Windows 2000 Security Event Log. It checks for auditing the same way it checks for permissions—by comparing each SID in the Access Token with each access control entry's SID. If it finds a match, it checks to see if the operation (or service) being performed is one of those services indicated in the access mask. If it is, and the result of the security check against the SACL matches the kind of auditing being performed (the access failed and failure is being audited, or the access succeeded and the success is being audited, or both), then the audit event is written to the Event Log.

Part II

Rights versus Permissions

Some activities do not apply to any specific object but instead apply to a group of objects or to the operating system as a whole. Shutting down the operating system, for example, affects every object in the system. The user must have *user rights* to perform such operations.

Earlier in this chapter, I mentioned that the Local Security Authority includes a Locally Unique Identifier when it creates an Access Token. The LUID describes which of the user rights that particular user account has. The LSA creates the LUID from security information in the SAM database (local computer account) or the Active Directory (domain account). The LUID is a combination of the rights of that specific user account and the rights of all the groups of which that account is a member.

Rights take precedence over *permissions*. That's why the Administrator account can take ownership of a file whose owner has removed all access permissions; the Administrator has the Take Ownership of Files or Other Objects right. The Windows 2000 operating system checks the user rights first, and then (if there is no user right specifically allowing the operation) the operating system checks the ACEs stored in the DACL against the SIDs in the Access Token.

User accounts have the right to read or write to an object the user account owns even in the case of a deny ACE permission. A user account may also change the permissions to an object owned by that user account.

NTFS File System Permissions

The NTFS file system is the bastion of Windows 2000 security. Being the platform upon which a secure Windows 2000 computer runs, NTFS is the gatekeeper of persistent security.

The LSA makes sure that running programs cannot violate each other's memory space and that all calls into the kernel are properly authorized. But what keeps a program from replacing the files the make up the LSA with an equivalent service that doesn't work? The answer to that question is NTFS, and that example highlights why a secure file system is mandatory for a secure operating system. Without the ability to trust the file system that stores system files, you can't trust the system that executes from those files.

Consider the case of virus strike on a Windows 95 machine. The user executes a program containing a virus. The virus identifies which program started the current program and infects it, thus propagating itself back one level. The next time that program starts, the virus does the same thing, as well as infect every program spawned from that program. Within a few cycles, the virus has propagated back to the core operating system, thereby infecting every file run from it.

In Windows 2000, the user runs a program containing a virus. That program tries to rewrite `explorer.exe` with the virus header, but it is blocked by NTFS file system security because the user doesn't have write permission to `explorer.exe`. Thanks to NTFS, this type of virus is stopped cold by Windows 2000. Granted, some viruses are content to hang out in user mode (such as Word macro viruses and Outlook worms), but those viruses still can't infect the operating system itself—unless the virus was launched by a user account with administrative access to the machine, which is why you should never run non–operating system software from an administrative account.

TIP

Instead of logging on as Administrator, use the Run As feature of Windows 2000 to launch administrative tasks. To easily set this up in the `Administrative Tools` folder, simply right-click the icon in the Start menu, select Properties, and check Run As Different User. Then you can log on using a normal user account and provide your administrative credentials only when performing an administrative task.

NTFS works by comparing a user's Access Token to the ACL associated with each requested file before allowing access to the file. This simple mechanism keeps unauthorized users from modifying the operating system or anything else they're not given specific access to.

Unfortunately, the default state of Windows 2000 is to provide full control to the "everyone" group at the root of all drives, so that all permissions inherited by files created therein are accessible by everyone. To receive any real benefit from NTFS file system security for applications and user-stored files, you must remove the permission granting full control to everyone and replace it with appropriate security for each folder in your computer.

Managing NTFS File System Permissions

Managing NTFS file system permissions in Windows 2000 is simple, and it works like permissions settings did in earlier versions of Windows NT.

To change security permissions on a file or folder, browse to the file or folder object using the Windows Explorer, right-click the file or folder, select the Security tab, select the appropriate group or user account, and make the appropriate settings in the ACE list.

Inheritance is handled differently in Windows 2000 than it was in Windows NT. In Windows NT, inherited permissions were simply the same as the parent objects and could be immediately modified. In Windows 2000, if the object is inheriting permissions from a containing folder object, you'll have to clear the Allow Inheritable Permissions check box to create a copy of the inherited permissions and then modify the existing permissions. You can create new ACE entries without overriding the inheritance setting.

Encrypting File System

The Encrypting File System is a file system driver that provides the ability to encrypt and decrypt files on the fly. The service is very simple to use: Users check the encrypted attribute on a file or directory. The EFS service generates an encryption certificate in the background and uses it to encrypt the affected files. When those files are requested from the NTFS file system driver, the EFS service automatically decrypts the file for delivery.

File encryption sounds like a really cool feature, but the current implementation in Windows 2000 is so flawed that EFS is mostly worthless, except perhaps on laptops.

The biggest problem with EFS is that it only works for individual users, making it useful only on client computers. Encryption certificates for files are created based on a user identity, so encrypted files can only be used by the account that created them. Encryption certificates cannot be assigned to group objects, so encryption can't protect general files stored on a server. This architecture would require the exchange of private keys over the network, so an encrypted channel would have to be established to exchange keys.

EFS will not allow encrypted files to be shared because it decrypts them before it delivers them. This too is shortsighted. If encryption certificates were held by a group, the encrypted file could be delivered over the network to the client in its encrypted state, and the client computer could use its participation in the group having the decryption certificate to decrypt the file. Kerberos could create session keys to encrypt the certificates to keep them secure while they're transported to members of the group. File-sharing could be secure enough to use over the Internet without a private tunnel.

Furthermore, loss of the encryption certificate—the Achilles' heel of encryption—would not be such a big deal. As long as any member of the group having the certificate still existed, that user would still have a copy of the certificate to decrypt the files. In its current incarnation, EFS always makes a key for the recovery agent (the local administrator by default) whether or not the user wants the recovery agent to be able to decrypt the file.

Alas, EFS (like file replication) is another example of a service that would have been great if Microsoft had done it right. As it is, Microsoft did just enough to say it had file system encryption.

Aside from the fact that it only works for individuals, there are a number of other problems with EFS:

▶ Encryption certificates are stored by default in the Registry of the local machine, where they can be recovered and used to decrypt the files on the machine. For EFS to function correctly as a secure encryption service, certificates must be moved from the local machine to a physically secure certificate server or exported to removable media that isn't left with the machine. Because the vast majority of users don't know or do this, the file system should be more accurately called the Obfuscating File Service.

▶ The only way to secure local EFS certificates is to use smart card authentication or to use SysKey (select Start ➢ Run ➢ SysKey) to move the System Key (a hash used to encrypt the local SAM accounts database that contains the EFS decryption certificate) to a floppy or use it as a password at boot time—and that password or floppy must be available to everyone who needs to boot the computer.

▶ Drag-and-drop Copy operations into an encrypted folder will not automatically encrypt the file, because move operations do not change the attributes of a file. Cut and Paste operations do, because you're effectively deleting the old file and creating a new one. This is a major problem with the Explorer interface because most people don't know any better and move files using drag and drop, believing their files are secure when in fact they're stored as plain-text files.

▶ Encrypted files will be decrypted if they are moved to non-NTFS volumes, which do not support encryption. Be certain you know what file system type you're copying encrypted files to. In my opinion, EFS should copy the file in its encrypted state to the non-NTFS store, where it would be useless until it was moved back to an NTFS store. No crypto service should ever automatically decrypt anything without the consent of the user.

▶ Encrypted files cannot be shared by being located in a shared folder. This restriction is designed to keep them encrypted; shared files are sent as plain text over the wire, so anyone with a network sniffer could decrypt them. A more robust encrypting file system would simply transmit the encrypted file over the wire and trust that the receiver had the appropriate certificate to decrypt it.

▶ Many programs (most Microsoft Office programs) create temporary files either in the local directory or in a temp directory when a file is being edited. Encryption for temp files follows the normal rule: If the file is created in a folder that has the encryption flag set, the temp file will be encrypted. Otherwise, it will not be encrypted and will foil your encryption security. To solve this problem, simply set the encryption flag on the temp directory to ensure that all temporary files are encrypted. You also need to know exactly where temp files are being created—just because the temp directory exists doesn't mean that every program uses it. Many third-party applications create their own temp directories.

▶ Printing is another vector for accidental decryption: When you print a document that is encrypted, the file is decrypted by the source application and sent via plain text to the print spooler. If the spooler is configured to spool documents (as most are), then the printed data is written to a file that could be undeleted to recover your encrypted data. To avoid this situation, you must either configure printing to avoid spooling documents throughout your network or set the encryption flag on the folder that the spooler uses to create spooled documents.

TIP

EFS requires a data recovery agents policy, so you can disable EFS throughout a domain by creating a group policy object for the domain that specifies an empty policy for encrypted data recovery agents. The policy must exist and it must be empty, because a no policy setting will allow the local workstation's policy to override the domain policy.

I don't recommend using EFS except on single-user computers that can't otherwise be physically secured. Its ease of use is a security blanket rather than real security. There are so many holes in EFS and so many accidental decryption vectors that it would be hard for a security expert to remember them all, much less a typical user. EFS is valuable for high-theft computers such as laptops that are configured to encrypt the print spool directory, temp folders, and the My Documents directory. For everyone else, it's worse than nothing because it makes you feel secure when you probably aren't.

WINDOWS 2000 NETWORK SECURITY

Windows 2000 network security is based on a few principal services:

- ▶ Active Directory
- ▶ Kerberos
- ▶ Group Policy
- ▶ Share Security
- ▶ Network Layer Encryption

These services work together to form a coherent whole: IPSec is defined by group policies that are stored in the Active Directory and can be configured to use Kerberos for automatic private key exchange. Share Security is based on user identity as proven by Kerberos based on password hashes stored in the Active Directory. Managing security policy through the Active Directory allows administrators to create policies that can be automatically applied throughout the organization.

Part II

Active Directory

Active Directory is not a security service, but nearly all the security mechanisms built into Windows 2000 rely upon Active Directory as a storage mechanism for security information like the domain hierarchy, trust relationships, crypto keys, certificates, policies, and security principal accounts.

Because nearly all of Windows 2000's security mechanisms are integrated with Active Directory, you'll use it to manage and apply security. Most of the subjects covered in the following sections could be considered components of Active Directory because they're so tightly integrated with it.

Although Active Directory is not a security service, it can be secured: Active Directory containers and objects have ACLs just like NTFS files do. In Active Directory, permissions can be applied in much the same way as they can in NTFS.

Unlike NTFS file system permissions, you can set permissions for the fields inside specific objects so that different users or security groups are responsible for portions of an object's data. For example, although you wouldn't give a user the ability to change anything about their own user account, you can allow them to update their contact information. This is possible using Active Directory permissions.

Kerberos Authentication and Domain Security

Kerberos authentication was developed by the Massachusetts Institute of Technology (MIT) to provide an intercomputer trust system capable of verifying the identity of security principals (such as a user or a computer) over an open, unsecured network. Kerberos does not rely on authentication by the computers involved or the privacy of the network communications. For this reason, Kerberos is ideal for authentication over the Internet and on large networks.

Kerberos operates as a trusted third-party authentication service by using shared secret keys. Essentially, a computer implicitly trusts the Kerberos Key Distribution Center (KDC) because they both know the same secret, which has been placed there as part of a trusted administrative process. In Windows 2000, the shared secret is generated when the computer joins the domain. Because both parties to a Kerberos session trust the KDC, they trust each other. In practice, this trust is implemented as a secure exchange of encryption keys that prove the identities of the parties involved to one another.

Kerberos authentication works like this:

1. A client requests a valid set of credentials for a given server from the KDC by sending a plain-text request containing the client's name (identifier).

2. The KDC looks up the secret keys of both the client and the server in its database (the Active Directory) and creates a *ticket* containing a random session key, the current time on the KDC, an expiration time determined by policy, and optionally any other information stored in the database. In the case of Windows 2000, SIDs are contained in the ticket.

3. The ticket is encrypted using the client's secret key.

4. A second ticket called the *session ticket* is created, which contains the session key and optional authentication data that is encrypted using the server's secret key.

5. The combined tickets are transmitted back to the client. Note that the authenticating server does not need to authenticate the client explicitly because only a valid client can decrypt the ticket.

6. Once the client is in possession of a valid ticket and session key for a server, it initiates communications directly with the server. To do so, the client constructs an *authenticator* consisting of the current time, the client's name, an application-specific checksum if desired, and a randomly generated initial sequence number and/or a session subkey used to retrieve a unique session identifier specific to the service in question. Authenticators are only valid for a single attempt and cannot be reused or exploited through a replay attack because they are dependent upon the current time. The authenticator is encrypted using the session key and transmitted along with the session ticket to the server from which service is requested.

7. When the server receives the ticket from the client, it decrypts the session ticket using the server's shared secret (which secret, if more than one exist, is indicated in the plain-text portion of the ticket).

8. The server then retrieves the session key from the ticket and uses it to decrypt the authenticator. The server's ability to decrypt the ticket proves that it was encrypted using the

server's secret key known only to the KDC and the server itself, so the client's identity is trusted. The authenticator is used to ensure that the communication is recent and is not a replay attack.

Figure 5.1 shows the entire Kerberos authentication process.

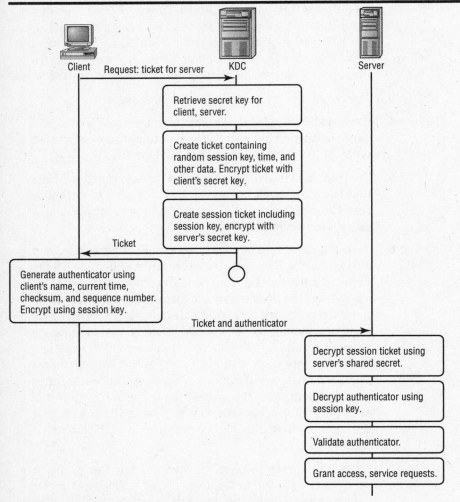

FIGURE 5.1:   Kerberos authentication uses a mutually trusted third party to communicate trust between two security principals.

Tickets can be reused for a duration specified by domain security policy, not to exceed eight hours. This reduces the burden on the KDC by requiring ticket requests as infrequently as once per workday. Clients cache their session tickets in a secure store located in RAM and destroy them when they expire.

Kerberos shortcuts the granting of tickets by granting a session ticket for itself as well as the requested target server the first time a client makes contact. The KDC responds to this initial request first with a session ticket for further ticket requests, called a *Ticket-Granting Ticket (TGT)*, and then with a session ticket for the requested server. The TGT obviates further Active Directory lookups of the client by pre-authenticating subsequent ticket requests in exactly the same manner that Kerberos authenticates all other requests. Like any session ticket, the TGT is valid until it expires, which depends upon domain security policy.

Kerberos is technically divided into two services: the TGT service (the only service that actually authenticates against the Active Directory) and the Ticket-Granting service, which issues session tickets when presented with a valid TGT.

Trust Relationships between Domains

Kerberos works across domain boundaries (domains are called *realms* in Kerberos terminology; the terms are equivalent).

The name of the domain that a security principal belongs to is part of the security principal's name (for example, `titanium.sandiego.connetic.net`). Membership in the same Active Directory tree automatically creates interdomain keys for Kerberos between a parent domain and its child domains.

The exchange of interdomain keys registers the domain controllers of one domain as security principals in the trusted domain. This simple concept makes it possible for any security principal in the domain to get a session ticket on the foreign KDC.

What actually happens is a bit more complex:

1. When a security principal in one domain wants to access a security principal in an adjacent domain (one domain is the parent; one is the child), it sends a session ticket request to its local KDC.

2. The KDC determines that the target is not in the local domain and replies to the client with a *referral ticket*, which is a session ticket encrypted using the interdomain key.

3. The client uses the referral ticket to request a session ticket directly from the foreign KDC.

4. The foreign KDC decrypts the referral ticket because it has the interdomain key, which proves that the trusted domain controller trusts the client (or it would not have granted the referral key).

5. The foreign KDC grants a session ticket valid for the foreign target server.

The process simply reiterates for domains that are farther away. To access a security principal in a domain that is two hops away in the Active Directory domain hierarchy, the client requests a session ticket for the target server against its KDC, which responds with a referral ticket to the next domain away. The client then requests the session ticket using the referral ticket just granted. That server will reply with a referral ticket valid on the next server in line. This process continues until the local domain for the target security principal is reached. At that point, a session key (technically, a TGT and a session key) is granted to the requesting client, which can then authenticate against the target security principal directly. Figure 5.2 shows the Kerberos exchange involved in a complex domain trust transit.

The TGT authentication service is especially important in interdomain ticket requests. After a computer has walked down the referral path once, it receives a TGT from the final KDC in the foreign domain. This ensures that subsequent requests in that domain (which are highly likely) won't require the referral walk again. The TGT can simply be used against the foreign KDC to request whatever session tickets are necessary in the foreign domain.

The final important concept in Kerberos authentication is that of delegation of authentication. Essentially, *delegation of authentication* is a mechanism whereby a security principal allows another security principal with which it has established a session to request authentication on its behalf from a third security principal. This mechanism is important in multitier applications, such as a database-driven website. Using delegation of authentication, the web browser client can authenticate with the web server and then provide the web server with a special TGT that it can

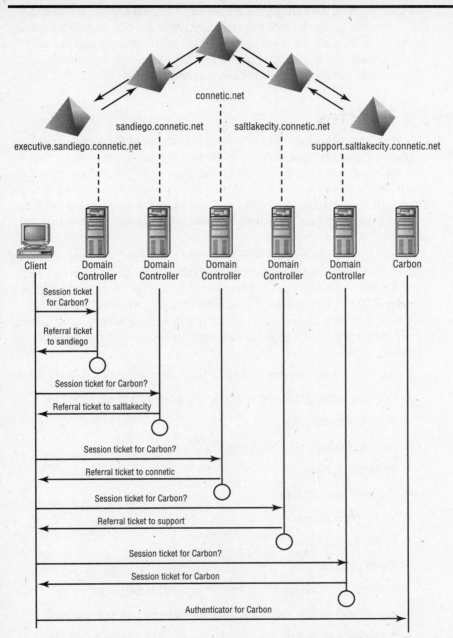

FIGURE 5.2:   The Kerberos-based transitive trust mechanism is simple in Kerberos terms.

use to request session tickets on its behalf. The web server can then use the forwarded credentials of the web client to authenticate with the database server. This allows the database server to use appropriate security for the actual web client, rather than use the web server's credentials, which would have completely different access than the actual client.

Group Policies

Group Policy is Windows 2000's primary mechanism for controlling the configuration of client workstations for security as well as administration. *Policies* in general are simply a set of changes to the default settings of a computer. Policies are usually organized so that individual policies contain changes that implement a specific goal—for example, disabling or enabling file system encryption or controlling which programs a user is allowed to run.

Group policies are applied to members of an Active Directory container (such as a domain or Organizational Unit). Security groups can be used to filter group policies, but policies cannot be applied to security groups. Windows 2000's Group Policy is not strictly a security mechanism—its primary purpose is change and configuration management—but it allows administrators to create more secure systems by limiting the users' range of actions.

Group policies can be used to control the following for computer policies:

- ▶ Registry settings related to security configuration and control
- ▶ Software installation
- ▶ Startup/shutdown and logon/logoff scripts
- ▶ Services startup
- ▶ Registry permissions
- ▶ NTFS permissions
- ▶ Public key policies
- ▶ IPSec policies
- ▶ System, network, and Windows components settings

Group policies can be used to control the following for *user policies*:

- ▶ Software installation
- ▶ Internet Explorer settings

- ▶ Logon/logoff scripts

- ▶ Security settings

- ▶ Remote Installation Service

- ▶ Folder redirection

- ▶ Windows components

- ▶ Start menu, Taskbar, Desktop, and Control Panel settings

- ▶ Network settings

- ▶ System settings

Mechanics of Group Policy

Group Policy Objects are essentially custom Registry files (and supporting files such as .msi packages and scripts) defined by policy settings that are downloaded and applied to domain member client computers when the computer is booted (computer configuration) and when a user logs in (user configuration). Group Policy Objects and any supporting files required for a group policy are stored on domain controllers in the SysVol share. Multiple group policies can be applied to the same computer; each policy overwrites the previous policy's settings in a "last application wins" scenario—unless a specific policy is configured not to be overwritten.

Each Group Policy Object has two parts: computer configuration and user configuration. You can configure both user and computer settings in a single Group Policy Object, and you can disable the computer or user portion of a Group Policy Object in the policy's Properties window. I recommend splitting all policies to apply either to users or computers, because the policies are downloaded at different times and because the configuration requirements for the two types of security principals are highly likely to diverge over time, requiring the application of different policy anyway.

Computer policies are applied at system initialization before a user logs in (and during periodic refreshes). Computer policies control the operating system, applications (including Windows Explorer), and startup and shutdown scripts. Think of computer policies as applying to the HKEY_Local _Machine portion of the Registry. Computer policies usually take precedence over user policies in the event of a conflict. Use computer policies whenever a configuration is required that does not depend on who logs in to the computer. You can apply company-wide policy easily to computer policies.

User policies are applied after a user logs in but before they're able to work on the computer, as well as during the periodic refresh cycle. User policies control operating system behavior, Desktop settings, application settings, folder redirection, and user logon/logoff scripts. Think of user policies as applying to the HKEY_Current_User portion of the Registry. Use user policies whenever a configuration is specific to a user or group of users, even if those users always use the same computers. By applying security-related settings to users rather than to computers, you can ensure that those settings travel with the user in the event that they use someone else's computer—and that those policies don't apply to administrative or support personnel who may need to log on to the computer (of course, security group membership could be used to filter settings for support personnel as well).

Group policies are called group policies because they're applied to groups of users; specifically, membership in Active Directory containers like domains or Organizational Units. Group policies are also hierarchical in nature: Many policies can be applied to a single computer or user, and they are applied in hierarchical order. Furthermore, later policies can override the settings of earlier policies. This means that individual elements of policy can be refined from the broad policies applied to large groups such as domains to narrowly focused policies applied to smaller groups such as Organizational Units.

Group polices are configured at the following levels in the following order:

Local Machine   Group policy is applied first so that it can be overridden by domain policy. Every computer has one local group policy that it is subject to. Beyond the local group policy, group policies are downloaded from the Active Directory depending upon the user and computer's location in the Active Directory.

Site   Group policies are unique in that they are managed from the Active Directory Sites and Services snap-in. Site policies apply to sites, so they should be used for issues relating to the physical location of users and computers rather than for domain security participation. Physical location issues are rare, so you won't use site policy very often. If your organization has only one site, which policies apply to the site may not be obvious, but you should still apply policies by location if the policy truly relates to location because your organization may some day have multiple physical sites.

Domain   Group policies apply to all users and computers in the domain, and this should be the primary place where you implement global policies in your organization. For example, if your company has a security policy document that requires specific configuration of logon passwords for all users, apply that policy to the domain.

Organizational Unit (OU)   Group policies apply to their member users and computers. Group policies are applied from top to bottom (parent, then child) in the OU hierarchy.

Security Group   These work differently than the actual domain containers. Rather than having group policies that can be applied to a security group, group policies that are applied to the user are filtered (allowed or disallowed) by a user's association with security groups. For example, you cannot apply a specific group policy to members of a Sales security group, but you can apply the policy to the Sales and Marketing OU and then set security group filters so that the policy would only apply to members of the Sales group. A more coherent (and more easily documented) method, however, would be to create subordinate OUs within the Sales and Marketing OU. You should use security group filtering when policies should be applied based on some criterion other than a user's position within the company, such as temporary members of "new employees"—a security status that will quickly change. Use security group filtering only when creating a new OU doesn't make sense.

You cannot link a group policy to generic folders or containers other than those listed here. If you need to create a container for Group Policy, use an OU.

Group policies are either all or nothing in their application; you cannot specify that only part of a policy be applied. If you need to implement variations on a policy theme for different users, simply create one policy for each variation and apply the variants to the appropriate Active Directory container or filter by security group.

A single group policy can be applied to more than one container in the Active Directory because group policies are not stored in the Active

Directory at the location where you apply them. Only a link to the Group Policy Object is stored; the objects themselves are actually stored in the replicated SysVol share of the domain controllers in the domain.

Creating Effective Group Policy

Group policies give administrators a tremendous amount of flexibility in the application of configuration information on a client computer. This flexibility makes it easy to create group policies that will be difficult to manage in the future because they were applied at the wrong level in the Active Directory domain hierarchy, or were made local when they should have been nonlocal, or were applied too broadly.

Rather than sitting down in front of the Group Policy Manager and clicking away to create policies that seem like a good idea, use requirements planning techniques to create effective policies. To create your requirements, write down the goals you want to achieve. For example:

▶ Only administrative users should be able to install software. (Applies to the domain, filtered by the Administrator security group.)

▶ New users should not be able to access the Internet. (Applies to the domain, filtered by the New Users security group.)

▶ Members of the Sales department should only be able to run the Sales Tracking application. (Applies to the Sales OU or domain.)

▶ Everything transmitted by members of the San Diego Finance group to the UK domain should be encrypted. (Applies to site policy, filtered by the Finance group. Why site policy? Because it's geographic in nature; this wouldn't apply to Finance members working in other locations.)

▶ No desktop users except administrators and people who work in Research and Development should have access to removable media drives. (Applies to the domain, overridden in the R&D OU by another policy, and filtered by the Administrators security group.)

▶ People should change their password at least once per month. (Applies to the domain.)

Notice how these requirements make both the purpose and scope of an individual policy easy to determine? Each of these bulleted items should constitute a group policy, and their applicability should be obvious from the statement:

To Whom Does This Policy Apply?   If the answer is "Everyone" or "Anyone who uses this computer," then your configuration should probably be implemented as a computer policy. If the answer is anything else, then it's a user policy.

Is This Policy Specific to Certain Locations?   If so, it's a site policy—not a domain policy—even if the two happen to be coincidental. Don't get into the habit of using domain policy for everything, because when your company grows, you'll find yourself deleting links and moving policies around quite a bit.

Is This Policy Unique to One Computer?   Sometimes elements of Group Policy are unique to a single computer—for example, to a computer that operates on the Internet as a public server, or the endpoint to an encrypted tunnel. Also, you may need to use a local policy to control the configuration of laptop computers that aren't always connected to the network. In these cases, local group policy makes sense. It's extremely rare for a local policy to make sense for constantly connected client computers, however, and it's exceptionally rare for user policy to be correctly applied to a local computer in a domain environment. Consider the reasons why you would use a local policy carefully and be sure that the policy wouldn't be more effectively managed as a nonlocal group policy.

Is This Policy Specific to a Group of Users?   If so, ask yourself if that group represents an OU. If it does, create the OU and then apply the security policy to it rather than using a security group to filter the policy. This approach will allow for easier management of future policies that would apply to the same group and is more easily managed and documented. If the group doesn't represent an OU (for example, New Users), then use security groups to filter the application of Group Policy.

Is This Configuration One Policy or Is It Multiple Policies?
Policies are all or nothing in their application, so you should get in the habit of making many small policies that are created for

specific purposes, rather than creating sweeping policies for people or computers. For example, rather than creating a policy for Sales, create policies that affect certain configurations (such as "Lotus Notes User Application Policy") and apply those many specific configurations to groups. Doing so makes it far more likely that the work you've done to create a policy can be applied to various users and allows you to see at a glance what the effects of policy are when applied to various containers in the Active Directory.

Once you've answered these questions, it should be pretty obvious which container in the Active Directory should be linked to each group policy.

There is a downside to using many small, purpose-specific policies: It takes more time at boot time and logon to apply multiple policies. You can optimize the process by combining requirements that are always applied the same way into a single policy. For example, numerous requirements apply to everyone, so it's perfectly fine to combine those into a single policy. I don't recommend optimizing beyond combining policies that apply to the same Active Directory container and security groups, however, because you'll wind up creating confusion as to which combined policies apply to which situations.

Managing Group Policy

Domain group policy is managed through the Active Directory Sites and Services snap-in (for site group policy) or the Active Directory Users and Computers snap-in (for all other nonlocal group policy).

To manage group policy, open the Active Directory Users and Computers snap-in (or the Sites and Services snap-in if you want to apply a policy to a site), right-click the container to which you want to apply the policy (domain or OU), and select Properties. Then select the Group Policy tab. Figure 5.3 shows the Group Policy page for the domain controller's OU.

From this page, you can create new Group Policy Objects, add a link to an existing object, edit and delete objects, change the application order, and change the override polices of objects. Creating a new group policy is easy—just click the New button and select the point in the Active

Directory where you want the policy to be applied. Once you've created and named the policy, click Edit to modify it.

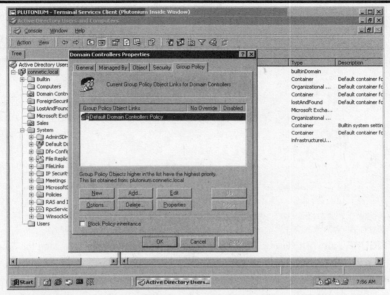

FIGURE 5.3:   Manage the order and application of group policies using the Properties window of the Active Directory container.

To change which security groups a policy is applied to (to use security group filtering), right-click the group policy you want to filter, select Properties, and then select the Security tab. You'll see an Apply Group Policy Access Control Entry in the ACE list. Simply select the group you want to filter on, select the Apply Group Policy ACE, and check Allow or Deny as appropriate to create the filter.

Editing policies is simple. Click the Edit button to open the Group Policy Editor (shown in Figure 5.4) and expand the hierarchy tree to expose the element of policy you want to change. Select the element in the list view you want to change, and double-click it.

Every policy element must be defined in order to be included the in Group Policy Object. Check Define This Policy Setting to enable the input field for the setting. The input field will vary by setting to allow the correct type of data to be entered.

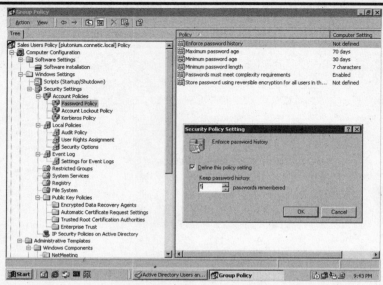

FIGURE 5.4: The Group Policy Editor provides a convenient interface for defining Group Policy Objects.

The same policy can be applied to multiple Active Directory containers, although it is not necessary to apply a policy explicitly to the children of a container to which the policy is already applied because the policy will already have been applied to the security principal. To apply an existing policy to a security container, right-click the container in the Active Directory Users and Computers snap-in and select Properties. Select the Group Policy tab, click Add, select the appropriate tab to display the group policy, select the group policy, and click OK to confirm.

Share Security

Shares are directories or volumes on a workstation or server that can be accessed by other computers in the network. Shares can be publicly available, or their access can be controlled with permissions. Shares use *share-level security*, which controls permissions for shared directories but not for anything specific within the directory. File-level security is superior to share-level security but can only be used on NTFS volumes.

Although you can set up a reasonably secure small network with shares, share security techniques don't really scale well for larger networks and environments where security is required. A new share must be created whenever security requirements change, and multiple shares with different security levels can be applied to the same directories.

Using and Securing Shares

The main reason to set up a network is to share files. Any directory on any workstation or server in the network can be set up as a shared directory. Although shares don't have the same level of security as NTFS directories on a dedicated server, Windows 2000 does provide a simple set of security features for shared directories.

NOTE

Although it's often associated with the workgroup model, you can also share files from workstations within a domain. In order to do this, the Server service must be running.

Creating a Share   You can create a share with any volume or any directory within a volume. You can create shares in either NTFS or FAT partitions, although shares in NTFS partitions can be made more secure. To create a share, right-click a drive or directory in an Explorer window and select the Sharing option. The Sharing Properties dialog box is displayed.

From this dialog box you can specify these options:

Not Shared/Shared As   Specify whether the volume or directory should be shared.

Share Name   Choose a name for the share. This name will appear as a directory name when users view a directory listing for the server. If the share will be accessed by users running Windows 3.x, or if your users use DOS applications, be sure to use a DOS-compatible name for the share.

Comment   Enter a description of the share's purpose or other information. (This is optional.) The contents of this field are displayed in the Explorer window to the right of the share name in Details view.

User Limit   If Maximum Allowed is selected, the number of users accessing the share is limited only by the Windows 2000 license. If a number is specified, only that many concurrent users can access the share.

Permissions   Clicking this button displays a dialog box that allows you to change permissions for the share, as described later in this chapter in the "Share Permissions" section.

Caching   Click this button to configure caching options for this share. Offline caching allows users to store the file locally on their hard disk so it's available if they're not online or if the server is unavailable.

When a directory or drive is shared, it is listed in the Explorer with a special icon that shows a hand underneath the drive or folder icon.

Accessing Shares   Although a server might have several shares configured—some entire volumes, some directories several levels deep—they all appear to users as a single listing under the server's name. Users can navigate to the server name using the My Network Places icon, and then open it to display a list of shares. Unfortunately, share names are not shown automatically in the Active Directory when you double-click a computer; they must be manually added in the Active Directory hierarchy.

As an example, suppose you created several shares, including VOL_F for an entire NTFS volume, and IE4 for the \Program Files\Plus!\ Microsoft Internet directory. A user who navigated to the server through Network Neighborhood would see a flat list of shares.

To make access to shares more convenient for users in the workgroup, you can create Desktop shortcuts to particular directories. You can also map a drive letter on the workstation to the share. This method has the benefit of fooling not only users into thinking it's a local drive, but also DOS and older Windows applications that otherwise might not support network access. To map a drive to a share, right-click the My Network Places icon, and then select Map Network Drive. Mapping drives is not normally necessary to access files from Windows Explorer or from Win32 applications.

To use this dialog box, choose a local drive letter, and then choose a server name and path to map the drive to. The window at the bottom of the dialog box displays a list of servers and shares. Select the Reconnect at Logon option to have the drive mapped each time the user logs on.

As an administrator, you have another option for displaying a list of shares on a server. The Computer Management snap-in's Shared Folders extension allows you to list shares on the local machine, add or remove shares, and monitor users who are currently accessing shares. The tool is available in the `Administrative Tools` folder and works just like every other MMC snap-in.

Default Shares   When you look at the Shared Folder Manager, you'll notice several shares with names ending in a dollar sign: C$, ADMIN$, and so forth. These are *administrative shares*—shares automatically configured by Windows 2000 and accessible only to administrators and the operating system itself. These shares are used for remote administration and communication between systems.

Each drive is automatically given an administrative share, with the share name being the drive letter followed by a dollar sign. The ADMIN$ share is connected to the \WINNT directory on each server. There is also an IPC$ share, used for interprocess communication between Windows 2000 servers, and a PRINT$ share, which shares printer information between servers. Domain controllers have a SYSVOL$ share used to distribute group policies, scripts, and installation packages.

As you've probably noticed, these shares don't appear in the browse lists that you can view from the Explorer. The only way to list them is with the Computer Management snap-in, which was described in the previous section.

TIP

You can create your own "administrative" shares. Any share name ending with a dollar sign ($) will be hidden from browse lists. Users (administrators or not) can access the share if they know its exact name.

Administrative shares present a potential security risk. A hacker who has gained access to the Administrator account on a single workstation in the workgroup can access the system drives of other workstations, effectively allowing administrator-level access to the entire workgroup.

You can improve security by disabling the automatic administrative shares created for the roots of hard disk drives (C$, D$, and so on). You can remove the shares from each drive's Properties window, or use the Shared Folder extension's Stop Sharing option. It's best to disable all of these, and then add a share for any specific drives or directories that need to be available across the network. Don't disable the other administrative shares or you will have problems with your machines.

Share versus File Security   Share-level security is similar to file system security, but not nearly as sophisticated (or as secure) because share

Part II

access control entries can be applied only to the share as a whole. Security cannot be customized within a share.

There is one significant advantage of share-level security: It works with any shared directory, whether it's on an NTFS or FAT volume. Share-level security is the only way to secure FAT directories. However, the share permissions you set only affect remote users. Users logged on to the machine locally can access anything on a FAT volume, shared or not. Share-level security also does not apply to users logged on locally or to Terminal Services clients.

Share Permissions   To set permissions for a share, click the Permissions button from the Sharing Properties dialog box. By default, the Everyone built-in group is given Full Control access to the share—in other words, share security is not implemented by default. The first thing you should do to secure a share is remove Everyone from the list. You can then add any number of users or groups and give them specific permissions. The following are the permissions available for shares, and each can be allowed or denied:

Read   Allows users to list contents of the directory, open and read files, and execute programs.

Change   Allows all Read permissions. In addition, users can create, delete, and modify files.

Full Control   Allows all Read and Change permissions. In addition, users can change permissions and change file ownerships.

Network Layer Encryption

Virtual private networks (VPNs) are a cost-effective way to extend your LAN over the Internet to remote networks and remote client computers. VPNs use the Internet to route LAN traffic from one private network to another by encapsulating the LAN traffic in IP packets. The encrypted packets are unreadable by intermediary Internet computers and can contain any kind of LAN communications, including file and print access, LAN e-mail, Remote Procedure Calls, and client/server database access.

VPNs between LANs can be established using server computers, firewalls, or routers. Client access to the VPNs can be made using VPN software on the client computers, or by dialing in to ISPs that support the VPN protocol. Using this second method, however, makes the ISP a partner in your network security in the same way that relying on an ISP for your firewall does.

Pure VPN systems do not provide adequate network protection. You also need a firewall and other Internet security services to keep your network safe. PPTP in particular has security problems, and you should take steps to correct them in your own network.

Using the Internet to link LANs and give remote computers LAN access causes security, performance, reliability, and management problems. Your LAN is a protected environment that only members of your organization are allowed to use. The LAN clients and servers should be protected from the Internet by a network-address-translating firewall and/or proxy servers so that (ideally) network intruders can't even identify their existence, much less target them for individual attack. In order to make it more difficult for hackers to capture private company information, most firewalls are configured not to pass typical LAN service protocols such as SMB, NetBIOS, the NetWare Core Protocol, or NFS.

SMB works particularly well in the clear over the Internet. Given a high-speed link, you can simply use file sharing without firewalls over the Internet, or you could configure your firewall to pass SMB and Kerberos or NetBIOS traffic and allow your employees to have remote access to file and print services. This would allow hackers to attempt to access your data simply by providing a valid account name and password or by attacking the protocol to exploit a bug that would allow access.

Exposing your LAN's file-sharing traffic in this manner effectively makes the whole Internet your LAN. It is virtual, but not private. Not only can your sales force print to your engineering department's printers or log on to your accounting department's file server, anyone on the Internet can print to the printer or log on to the file server. An intruder would have to guess a password, of course, but hackers have a lot of experience in guessing passwords. Automated password-guessing tools can crack most user account passwords in less than a day over the Internet.

WARNING

You should never leave SMB open to the Internet. Use firewalls to restrict the SMB ports on your corporate network and disable the file and print-sharing service on computers directly connected to the Internet.

Part II

VPN Technologies

Virtual private networks solve the problem of direct Internet access to servers through a combination of the following fundamental security components:

▶ IP encapsulation

▶ Cryptographic authentication

▶ Data payload encryption

All three components must exist in a true VPN. Although cryptographic authentication and data payload encryption may seem like the same thing at first, they are actually entirely different functions and may exist independently of each other. For example, the Secure Socket Layer performs data payload encryption without cryptographic authentication of the remote user, and Kerberos performs cryptographic authentication without performing data payload encryption.

IP Encapsulation   You need to protect the data traffic that travels between your LANs over the Internet. Ideally, the computers in each LAN should be unaware that there is anything special about communicating with the computers in the other LANs. Computers outside your virtual network should not be able to snoop on the traffic exchanged between the LANs or be able to insert their own data into the communications stream. Essentially, what you need is a private and protected tunnel through the public Internet.

An IP packet can contain any kind of information: program files, spreadsheet data, audio streams, or even other IP packets. When an IP packet contains another IP packet, it is called *IP encapsulation*, *IP on IP*, or *IP/IP*. You can encapsulate one IP packet in another in several ways; Microsoft does it in two different but related ways as specified in PPTP and L2TP. Microsoft also supports IPSec, which does not necessarily use encapsulation.

Why encapsulate IP within IP? Because doing so makes it possible to refer to a host within another network when a routed connection may not exist. IP encapsulation can make it appear to network computers that two distant networks are actually adjacent, separated from each other by a single router, when in fact they are separated by many Internet routers and gateways that may not even use the same address space because both internal networks are using address translation.

The tunnel endpoint, be it a router, a VPN appliance, or a server running a tunneling protocol, will remove the internal packet, decrypt it, and then apply its routing rules to send the embedded packet on its way in the internal network.

As an example, consider two IP networks linked by a router. Both are Class C–sized IP subnets—one with the network address of 10.1.1.0/24 and the other with the network address of 10.1.2.0/24. In this example, the fourth number in each network is reserved for the station address and can be from 1 to 254. The router must have a network interface adapter on each network so that it can move IP traffic between the two LANs. The .1 and .127 station addresses are typical addresses reserved for routers and gateways, so in this network, the router has one adapter with the IP address of 10.1.1.1 and another with the IP address of 10.1.2.1. All of the computers in both networks have a net mask of 255.255.255.0.

When a computer in the 10.1.1.0 network (for example, 10.1.1.23) needs to send an IP packet to a computer in the 10.1.2.0 network (such as 10.1.2.99), the communication proceeds as follows:

1. The originating computer first notices that the network portion of the destination address (10.1.2.99) does not match its own network address.

2. Instead of attempting to send the packet directly to the destination, the originating computer sends the packet to the default gateway address for its subnet (10.1.1.1).

3. The router at that address reads the packet.

4. The router determines that the packet should be placed on the 10.1.2.0 network.

5. The router sends the packet from its adapter (10.1.2.1) to the destination address (10.1.2.99) on that network.

6. The destination computer reads the packet.

In comparison with the preceding example, consider two IP networks linked by RRAS servers using PPTP. One LAN has the network address 10.1.1.0, and the other has the network address 10.1.2.0. In this example, the RRAS servers on each network provide the network connection to the Internet. One RRAS server has a LAN IP address of 10.1.1.1 and an Internet address of 250.121.13.12 assigned by the ISP it is connected to, while

Part II

the other has a LAN IP address of 10.1.2.1 and an Internet address of 110.121.112.34 assigned by its ISP.

Communication in the PPTP-connected LANs starts and ends the same way it does in router-connected LANs. The IP packets have further to go, though, so more work is done in the middle. Compare the following example to the previous one:

1. The originating computer (10.1.1.23) first notices that the destination address (10.1.2.99) is not in the same network as itself.

2. Instead of attempting to send the packet directly to the destination, the originating computer sends the packet to the default gateway address for its subnet (10.1.1.1).

3. The RRAS server on the 10.1.1.0 network reads the packet.

4. The RRAS server on the 10.1.1.0 network determines that the packet should be placed on the 10.1.2.0 network subnet, for which it has a PPTP connection established over the Internet.

5. The RRAS server encrypts the packet and encapsulates it in another IP packet.

6. The router sends the encapsulated packet from its network interface connected to the Internet (250.121.13.12) to the Internet address (110.121.112.34) of the RRAS server of the 10.1.2.0 network.

7. The RRAS server of the 10.1.2.0 network reads the encapsulated and encrypted packet from its Internet interface.

8. The RRAS server of the 10.1.2.0 network unpackages and decrypts the IP packet, verifying that it is a valid packet that has not been tampered with and that it comes from a trusted source (another RRAS server).

9. The RRAS server of the 10.1.2.0 network sends the packet from its adapter (10.1.2.1) to the destination address (10.1.2.99) on that network subnet.

10. The destination computer reads the packet.

Note that from the point of view of the two network client computers, it doesn't matter how the packet got from one IP subnet to the other. As far as the network client computers are concerned, a router is the same thing as two RRAS servers and a PPTP connection.

Cryptographic Authentication   *Cryptographic authentication* is used to securely validate the identity of the remote user so the system can determine what level of security is appropriate for that user. VPNs use cryptographic authentication to determine whether the user can participate in the encrypted tunnel and may also use the authentication to exchange the secret or public key used for payload encryption.

Many different forms of cryptographic authentication exist, in two general categories:

> **Secret Key Encryption**   Also called *shared secret* or *symmetric encryption*, relies upon a secret value known to both parties. Simply knowing the value proves to the provider that the requester is to be trusted. Challenge and response can be used to make sure that only hashes of the secret, not the secret itself, are transmitted on the network, and one-time-password variations can be used to ensure that the secret changes each time it's used.

> **Public Key Encryption**   Relies on the exchange of *unidirectional keys*—keys that can only be used to encrypt data. This means that the decryption key is held on the receiver and never transmitted over a public network, which makes the encrypted data secure during transmission because it can't be decrypted. Tunnel end-systems may exchange pairs of public keys to form a bidirectional channel, or the public key receiver may encrypt a shared secret key and transmit it to the public key transmitter to use for future communications (because secret key encryption is faster than public key encryption).

If a hacker intercepted the public or encrypting key, they could only encrypt data and transmit it to the receiver; they could not decrypt the contents of data they intercept.

Data Payload Encryption   *Data payload encryption* is used to obfuscate the contents of the encapsulated data. By encrypting the encapsulated IP packets, both the data and the internal nature of the private networks is kept secret. Data payload encryption can be accomplished using any one of a number of secure cryptographic methods, which differ based on your VPN solution.

Part II

IPSec

IPSec is the IETF standards suite for secure IP communications that relies on encryption to ensure the authenticity and privacy of IP communications. IPSec provides mechanisms that can accomplish the following:

▶ Authenticate individual IP packets and guarantee that they are unmodified

▶ Encrypt the payload of individual IP packets between two end-systems

▶ Encapsulate a TCP or UDP socket between two end-systems (hosts) inside an encrypted IP link (tunnel) established between intermediate systems (routers) to provide virtual private networking

IPSec performs these three functions using two independent mechanisms: *Authentication Headers (AH)* to provide authenticity and *Encapsulating Security Payload (ESP)* to encrypt the data portion of an IP packet. These two mechanisms may be used together or independently.

The AH mechanism works by computing a checksum of all the TCP/IP header information and encrypting the checksum with the secret key of the receiver. The receiver then decrypts the checksum using its secret key and then checks the header against the decrypted checksum. If the computed checksum is different than the header checksum, then either the decryption failed because the key was wrong or the header was modified in transit. In either case, the packet is dropped.

NOTE

Because NAT changes header information, IPSec Authentication Headers cannot pass through a network address translator. ESP can still be used to encrypt the payload, but support for ESP without AH varies among implementations of IPSec. Unfortunately, Windows 2000 only supports tunnel mode between gateways with fixed IP addresses and uses transport mode for L2TP connections, so they cannot be network address translated.

With ESP, the transmitter encrypts the payload of an IP packet using the public key of the receiver. The receiver then decrypts the payload upon receipt and acts accordingly.

IPSec can operate in one of two modes: *transport mode*, which works exactly like regular IP except that the headers are authenticated (AH) and the contents are encrypted (ESP), or *tunnel mode*, where complete IP packets are encapsulated inside AH or ESP packets to provide a secure tunnel. Transport mode is used for providing secure or authenticated communication over public IP ranges between any Internet-connected hosts for any purpose, whereas tunnel mode is used to create secure links between routers or other network endpoints for the purpose of linking two private networks.

Microsoft recommends IPSec for use in gateway-to-gateway communications and does not consider IPSec suitable for client-to-gateway communications because the protocol itself does not include user authentication.

TIP

Download step-by-step instructions for implementing a gateway-to-gateway VPN using Windows 2000 IPSec from Microsoft at www.microsoft.com/ TechNet/win2000/win2ksrv/technote/ispstep.asp.

The root of the problem is that client and machine authentication are handled separately; use of the correct machine gains access to the network, and then a separate authentication protocol gains access to private network resources. A hacker could exploit the window between machine authentication and user authentication to run probes against the network without logging in or to run automated password attacks against the network.

Consider the following example: A legitimate network user uses an IPSec-configured laptop to gain access to the local network and then simply logs in to the domain over the connection. While the user is traveling, the laptop is stolen at the airport and winds up in the hands of an opportunistic hacker. The hacker uses commonly available password-patching tools to gain local access to the laptop and discovers that it is automatically connecting to a remote network via IPSec. This provides the hacker remote access to the private network, so he uses network-scanning tools to "sniff out" the structure of the network. He then finds a client computer and runs a network-based password-guessing program over the course of a few days to guess the password of the user who lost the laptop.

When user authentication is combined with machine authentication at the security gateway, this attack is not possible because access to the private network is not granted unless both the machine and the user are authenticated.

The bias against IPSec as a client-to-gateway technology is somewhat esoteric, because it can encapsulate secure authentication methods like Kerberos to provide user authentication. When an IPSec tunnel is established between a client system and an IPSec gateway, and then a secure authentication protocol like Kerberos is used for secure authentication of the user at the client station, security remains intact. Although a gap between machine authentication and user authentication exists that could technically be exploited, this level of security is sufficient for most business purposes. I've used IPSec for client-to-gateway authentication since shortly after its availability in this mode, and I've found it to be both more reliable and more secure than PPTP.

Microsoft recommends using L2TP/IPSec for client-to-gateway authentication.

Tunnel Mode   In a normal routed connection, a host transmits an IP packet to its default gateway, which forwards the packet until it reaches the default gateway of the receiver, which then transmits it to the end host. All computers in the connection must be in the same public address space.

In IP over IP, or IP/IP, the default gateway (or another router down the line) receives the packet and notices that its route for that packet specifies an IP/IP tunnel, so it establishes a TCP/IP connection to the remote gateway. Using that connection, the gateway transmits all of the originating host's IP traffic inside that connection rather than forwarding it. IP/IP is useful for virtual networking, so that private IP addresses (in the 192.168.0.0 range, for example) can be passed over the public Internet.

IPSec implements both IP/IP and IPSec/IP. IP/IP provides a non-encrypted virtual tunnel between two end-systems (which can use AH to guarantee authenticity), and IPSec/IP uses ESP to encrypt the payload of the carrier IP, thus encrypting the entire encapsulated IP packet.

Internet Key Exchange   IPSec uses public key cryptography to encrypt data between end-systems. In order to establish an IPSec connection to a receiving host, the transmitting host must know that host's public key. Technically, the transmitter could simply ask the host for a public key, but that doesn't provide authentication—any host could ask for the key and get it. This is how SSL works; the identity of the machine is not important, and SSL relies upon some other protocol to authenticate the user once the tunnel is established. That's fine for public websites, but IPSec was designed from the outset to perform host authentication through knowledge of appropriate keys.

NOTE

IPSec is defined by RFCs 2401 through 2409, along with numerous other RFCs that describe supporting protocols.

IPSec uses the concept of *Security Associations (SA)* to create named combinations of keys and policy use to protect information for a specific function. The policy may indicate a specific user, host IP address, or network address to be authenticated or to specify the route for information to take.

In early IPSec systems, public keys for each SA were manually installed via file transfer or by actually typing them in. For each SA, each machine's public key had to be installed on the reciprocal machine. As the number of SAs a host required increased, the burden of manually keying in SA machines keys became seriously problematic; because of this, IPSec was used primarily only for point-to-point systems.

Internet Key Exchange (IKE) eliminates the necessity to manually key systems. IKE uses secret key security to validate its authority to create an IPSec connection and to securely exchange public keys. IKE is also capable of negotiating a compatible set of encryption protocols with the foreign host, so that administrators don't have to know exactly which encryption protocols are supported on the opposite host. Once the public keys are exchanged and the encryption protocols are negotiated, an SA is automatically created on both hosts, and normal IPSec communications can be established. With IKE, each computer that needs to communicate via IPSec needs only to be keyed with a single secret key. That key can be used to create an IPSec connection to any other IPSec host that has the same secret key.

TIP

In Windows 2000, you can configure IPSec policies to use Kerberos to automatically exchange secret keys for IKE. Doing so eliminates the need for manual keying and allows for completely automatic secure encryption between members of the same Active Directory in Windows 2000 networks.

The IKE initiator begins an IKE request by sending a plain-text connection request to the remote host. The remote host generates a random number, keeps a copy, and sends a copy back to the initiator. The initiator encrypts its secret key using the random number and sends it to the remote host. The remote host decrypts the secret key using its kept random number and compares the private key to its secret key (or list of keys, called a *keyring*). If the secret key does not match, the remote host will drop the connection. If it does match, the remote host will encrypt its public key using the secret key and transmit it back to the initiator. The initiator then uses the public key to establish an IPSec session with the remote host. Figure 5.5 illustrates this process.

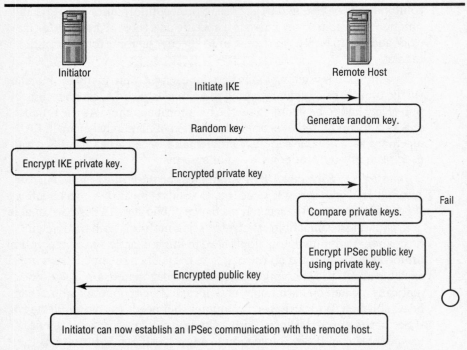

FIGURE 5.5:   Internet Key Exchange uses private key security to simplify IPSec keying.

Like nearly everything in Windows 2000, IPSec configurations are managed by creating a policy. For IPSec, you create a different policy for each receiving computer that has unique IPSec requirements. Destination networks, computers, and tunnel endpoints are specified by IP address. For each IPSec policy, you can define the exact encryption protocols used by the policy and the keying method used for IKE.

In Windows 2000, you manage IPSec through the Security Manager snap-in, which is embedded in the Active Directory Users and Computers snap-in (see Figure 5.6) or through the IP Security Policies snap-in.

TIP

Use the ipsecmon utility to monitor IPSec traffic to and from your server. From the Start menu, select Run and type **ipsecmon** to start this utility.

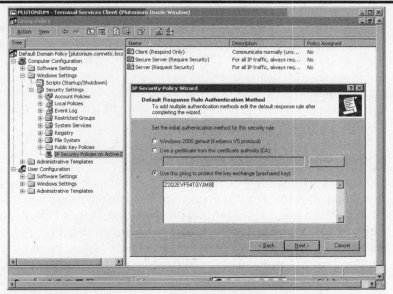

FIGURE 5.6:   Manage IPSec policy using the Security Manager.

Problems with Windows 2000's IPSec Implementation   Microsoft's implementation of IPSec is incomplete because IPSec standards are still emerging. The practical implication is that Windows 2000's implementation of IPSec is not compatible with the implementations of most firewall vendors by default. In every case I've tested, I can't configure IPSec in Windows 2000 to connect to an IPSec-compatible firewall without installing some sort of IPSec client software.

Although Windows 2000 IPSec supports tunnel mode, it disables that support when a dynamic IP address is detected, thus forcing users to use L2TP for remote access to corporate VPNs. If you want to connect a Windows 2000 computer to a third-party firewall IPSec implementation that does not support L2P2, the computer must have a fixed IP address.

TIP

Microsoft Knowledge Base article Q252735 describes the mechanism for establishing an IPSec tunnel-mode connection between gateways. Knowledge Base article Q259335 describes basic L2TP/IPSec troubleshooting tactics and has links to numerous other IPSec-related articles.

Windows 2000 automatically disables IPSec communications when transmitting data to Windows 9x or NT computers—even when an administrator may think there's an IPSec communication in place and that the communication is secure. It would be far more secure to disallow communication unless an express policy allowing the unencrypted communication was in place. Security features should never be automatically, invisibly disabled by the operating system.

L2TP

The Layer 2 Tunneling Protocol is an extension to PPP that allows the separation of the data-link endpoint and the network access point. In traditional PPP, a user (typically a dial-up user) establishes a PPP connection with a remote access server. That server answers the data-link layer connection (modem call) and also serves as a network access point by removing the data encapsulated in the PPP message and forwarding it on the destination network. The encapsulated data might be an AppleTalk frame, IP packet, IPX packet, NetBIOS packet, or any other network layer packet.

NOTE

In this section, I use the generic term *remote access server* to refer to any L2TP-compatible remote access server, which could be a Unix computer, a Windows 2000 computer, or a dedicated remote access appliance. In Windows 2000, this service is called RRAS.

L2TP separates the call-answering from the network access routing. With L2TP, a caller can call a modem bank (or DSL Access Module, or whatever), and that equipment can simply encapsulate the received L2TP packets into Frame Relay, ATM, or TCP/IP packets for further transport to a remote access server. Upon reaching the remote access server, the LT2P packets are unwrapped and their payload is forwarded onto the local network.

L2TP is designed to allow for less-expensive ISP equipment by separating the remote access server functions into a hardware function (physically receiving the connection) and a software function (gating the encapsulated PPP data) that can be performed on separate machines. This separation has a number of important benefits:

▶ Users can dial a local modem bank that will forward L2TP to a distant remote access server, thus avoiding long distance charges for direct-dial remote access.

▶ L2TP payloads can be encrypted using IPSec to provide secure authenticated remote access.

▶ Multilink L2TP sessions can be physically answered by different receivers and correctly bonded on a single remote access server. With current PPP multilinks, all the channels must be connected to the same remote access server.

L2TP can use IPSec to encrypt PPP frames, thus providing what amounts to a secure PPP session for remote users. L2TP was specifically designed to provide remote user authentication and connection to remote networks. Because L2TP is an extension of PPP, any network layer protocol (such as IPX, NetBEUI, or AppleTalk) can be embedded inside L2TP. In contrast, PPTP and IPSec are both specific to IP networks and do not function with other protocols. The use of PPP also provides support for all of the standard user authentication protocols, including CHAP, MS-CHAP, and EAP.

L2TP uses UDP rather than TCP/IP as its data transport because the embedded PPP protocol can provide the necessary guarantee of reliability for the stream. L2TP operates over UDP port 1701.

Microsoft considers L2TP to be the ideal user authentication mechanism for completing the strong security requirements of remote access users. Because L2TP provides secure user authentication and then uses IPSec to provide machine authentication, it allows remote users to connect without the authentication gap that would occur if user authentication were separated from secure tunnel establishment.

PPTP

PPTP was Microsoft's first attempt at secure remote access for network users. Essentially, PPTP creates an encrypted PPP session between TCP/IP hosts. Unlike L2TP, PPTP operates only over TCP/IP; L2TP can operate over any packet transport, including Frame Relay and ATM. PPTP does not use IPSec to encrypt packets; rather, it uses a hash of the user's

Windows 2000 password to create a private key between the client and the remote server that (in the 128-bit encrypted version) is salted with a random number to increase the encryption strength.

L2TP is the successor to PPTP—it is more generalized in that it works over any packet transport, and its encryption strength is far stronger thanks to IPSec encryption. PPTP should be used for legacy compatibility, but new installations should favor L2TP for secure remote access.

SUMMARY

Security is the effort taken to prevent the loss or disclosure of information in a network. Because you can't absolutely eliminate the possibility of loss in useful systems, a certain amount of risk is necessary, and your system's security is fundamentally based on providing access only to trusted security principals (users or computers).

To control security, any system must

▶ Control access

▶ Identify users

▶ Restrict or permit access

▶ Record user activity

▶ Communicate privately between systems

▶ Minimize the risk of misconfiguration

Encryption, the process of obfuscating a message using a mathematical algorithm (cipher) and a secret value (key) known only to the legitimate participants, is the foundation of all modern computer security. Encryption can be used to prove the identity of a user or computer, to validate data, or to hide the contents of a data store or communication stream.

Windows 2000 security is based on user authentication. By logging in to Windows 2000, users prove their identity in order to gain access to files, programs, and shared data on servers. Windows 2000 uses a pervasive security model that attaches the user's identity to every action they perform on the computer, rather than providing wide access to the computer once a successful logon has occurred.

For an operating system to be trusted, it must be able to ensure that it has not become compromised and that information can be kept secure from users. Windows 2000 uses NTFS file system permissions to control access to files, including the files Windows 2000 boots from. Permission can be granted to users and to groups of users for each file system function. Files can also be encrypted on disk to ensure that they cannot be accessed, even when the computer is not running.

Windows 2000 network security is managed using the Active Directory as a repository for Kerberos password hashes, Group Policy, and IPSec policy. Active Directory defines the relationship among security principals as well.

Windows 2000 uses Kerberos to validate user identity over the network. Kerberos is a trusted third-party security system. Because both endpoints in a communication trust and are trusted by the Kerberos server, they trust one another. Kerberos servers can trust other Kerberos servers, so transitive trust relationships can be created allowing endpoints from widely separated networks to establish authenticated communication sessions. Kerberos is integrated with Active Directory (all domain controllers are Kerberos Key Distribution Centers), and participation in the same domain tree automatically creates transitive two-way trust relationships.

Group policies are used to define the security requirements and configuration of computers and user accounts in the domain, site, or Organizational Unit. You can use group policies to control nearly every element of user and computer security. You manage group policies through the Active Directory Users and Computers snap-in or through the Active Directory Sites and Services snap-in.

IPSec is the Internet standard for proving the authenticity of IP packets and for encrypting the data payload of IP packets. IPSec works with many different security algorithms and can operate in the normal transport mode or tunnel mode to simulate a private circuit over a public network like the Internet.

WHAT'S NEXT

In Chapter 6, you will learn about Microsoft's latest incarnation of the Windows operating system: Windows XP. Windows XP builds on the Windows NT kernel, taking the best security features of Windows 2000 and adding an updated, visually stunning user interface.

Chapter 6

LIVING WITH WINDOWS XP PROFESSIONAL STRICT SECURITY

F rom its inception, the NT family of operating systems was designed with security as a primary feature, and, of course, this architectural element is omnipresent in the Windows XP Professional.

Unlike some other operating systems, Windows XP Professional requires you to create a user account for yourself right on your PC before you can do anything on that PC. Yes, the idea that you must create your own user account on your personal PC before you can do anything with the PC is unusual—after all, most of us are accustomed to requiring network accounts, but not particular accounts on a workstation. But—as your father might say when you complain that something you don't like isn't fair—get used to it!

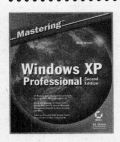

Adapted from *Mastering™ Windows® XP Professional*, Second Edition by Mark Minasi
ISBN 0-7821-4114-5 $39.99

The user account is an integral part of Windows XP Professional and has some great benefits. For example, suppose you and Sue share a computer. You can set up the computer so that you own a folder on the hard disk and Sue owns another folder on the hard disk, and *it is completely impossible for Sue to access your data* (and vice versa) unless you give her permission.

In addition, you can restrict access to files and folders by setting permissions. As you may recall, in Windows XP Professional you can use the FAT, FAT32, or NTFS file system. If you use either FAT system, you can exercise only a limited amount of control over file and folder access, but if you use the NTFS system, you can exercise a great deal of control—whether the files are on your local computer or on your network.

In this chapter, we'll first look at how to set up user accounts, and then we'll look in detail at establishing permissions for shares, files, and folders.

In this chapter:

▶ Understanding and creating accounts in Windows XP Professional

▶ Setting permissions

▶ Understanding ownership

UNDERSTANDING USER ACCOUNTS IN WINDOWS XP PROFESSIONAL

As you have just read, you must create separate user accounts on a Windows XP Professional machine before any user can log on to the workstation—and, unlike Windows 9*x*, Windows XP Professional won't let you get anywhere until you log on.

If your computer is part of a Windows XP Professional client-server network, two types of user accounts are available: domain accounts and local accounts. A domain account gives you access to the network and to the network resources for which you have permission. The manager of the server normally sets up domain accounts, which are stored in a directory on the server. The directory can either be Active Directory or a Windows NT domain directory.

A local user account is valid only on your local computer; local user accounts sit in a database called the *Security Accounts Manager* (SAM).

You create user accounts with the Users and Passwords applet, which you'll meet later in this chapter.

In this chapter, I'm going to talk about local user accounts only. If you happen to be the administrator of a domain on a network and you need help creating domain user accounts, take a look at *Mastering Windows 2000 Server, 4th ed.* (Sybex, 2002).

Before I get into how you change or create an account, we need to look at the types of accounts in Windows XP Professional. The two broad categories are users and groups. A user account identifies a user on the basis of their username and password. A group account contains other accounts, and these accounts share common privileges.

User accounts are of three types:

Computer Administrator   This account has full and complete rights to the computer and can do just about anything to the computer. The Computer Administrator account is created during installation and setup of Windows XP Professional. The Computer Administrator account cannot be deleted. You'll need to log on as Computer Administrator when you want to create new accounts, take ownership of files or other objects, install software that will be available to all users, and so on.

Limited   This account is intended for use by regular old users, those who should not be allowed to install software or hardware or change their username. Someone with a limited account can change their password and logon picture.

Guest   This built-in account allows a user to log on to the computer even though the user does not have an account. No password is associated with the Guest account. It is disabled by default, and you should leave it that way. If you want to give a visitor or an occasional user access to the system, create an account for that person, and then delete the account when it is no longer needed.

As I said earlier, a group is an account that contains other accounts, and a group is defined by function. Using groups, an administrator can easily create collections of users who all have identical privileges. By default, every Windows XP Professional system contains the following built-in groups:

Administrators   Can do just about anything to the computer. The things that they can do that no other type of user can do include loading and unloading device drivers, managing security audit functions, and taking ownership of files and other objects.

Backup Operators   Can log on to the computer and run backups or perform restores. You might put someone in this group if you wanted them to be able to get on your system and run backups but not to have complete administrative control. Backup operators can also shut down the system but cannot change security settings.

Guests   Have minimal access to network resources. As I mentioned earlier, creating user accounts for occasional users is a much safer bet than using Guest accounts.

Network Configuration Operators   Can manage network configuration with administrative-type access. Although they do not have administrative access to your system, these users can modify network and dial-up connections.

Power Users   Can create new printer and file shares, change the system time, force the system to shut down from another system, and change priorities of processes in the system. They can't run backups, load or unload device drivers, or take ownership.

Remote Desktop Users   Have the right to log on remotely.

Replicator   Enables your computer to receive replicated files from a server machine.

Users   Can run programs and access data on a computer, shut it down, and access data on the computer from over the network. Users cannot share folders or create local printers.

HelpServicesGroup   A group of users for the Help and Support Center.

IIS_WPG   The Internet Information Services Worker Process Group; available only if you have installed IIS. A member of this group can manage the IIS Web server (not content, just service).

Understanding User Rights

But what's this about shutting down the machine or loading and unloading drivers? Well, actually, the notion of a *user right* is an integral part of how Windows XP Professional security works. Basically, the difference between regular old users and administrators lies in the kinds of actions that they can perform; for example, administrators can create new user accounts but regular old users cannot. In Windows XP Professional terminology, the ability to perform a particular function is a user right. To take a look at the user rights in Windows XP Professional and the types of users to whom they are assigned, follow these steps:

1. In Control Panel, click Performance and Maintenance, click Administrative Tools, and then click Local Security Policy to open the Local Security Settings window:

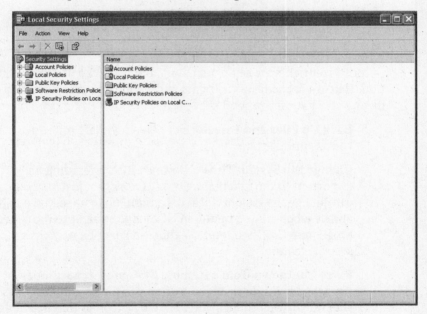

2. In the Security Settings pane, expand Local Policies, and then click User Rights Assignment to display a list of user rights in the pane on the right:

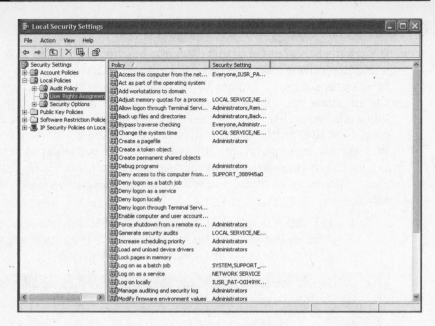

Most user rights are self-explanatory, but a few can use some clarification. Here's a list some of the rights and, where necessary, what they mean and what they're good for:

Back Up Files and Directories   This right lets you run backup utilities.

Change the System Time   Because the system time is important to the functioning of a network, not just anybody can change the system clock; it's a right. (Of course, you could always reboot the computer in DOS or go straight to the setup program in CMOS to reset the time, so it's not a very airtight security feature.)

Force Shutdown from a Remote System   Some utilities let you select a Windows XP Professional machine and force it to shut down, even though you're not logged on to that machine. (One such utility comes with the Resource Kit.) Because you wouldn't want just anybody doing a forced shutdown, Microsoft made this a right.

Load and Unload Device Drivers   A device driver is not only a video driver or SCSI driver; a device driver may be part of a software application or operating system subsystem. Without this right, you'll often be unable to install new software, and you'll usually be unable to change drivers or add and remove parts of the operating system.

Log on Locally   You can sit down at the computer and log on.

Manage Auditing and Security Log   You can optionally turn on a Windows XP Security Log, which will report every single action that woke up any part of the security subsystems in Windows XP Professional. In general, I don't recommend using the Security Log unless you have a specific reason to do so, because the output is quite cryptic and can be *huge*; logging all security events can fill up your hard disk quickly, and the CPU overhead of keeping track of the log will slow down your computer. You can't enable any security logging unless you have this right.

Restore Files and Directories   This right lets you do what the name states.

Take Ownership of Files or Other Objects   If you have this right, you can seize control of any file, folder, or other object even if you're not *supposed* to have access to it. This right is obviously quite powerful, which is why only administrators have it.

NOTE

The user right to Take Ownership of Files or Other Objects is the secret to the administrator's power. You can do whatever you like to keep an administrator out of your data, but remember that the Computer Administrator can always take ownership of the file, and as owner, do whatever they want to the file including changing permissions. You cannot keep an administrator out; you can only make it difficult to get in.

Creating a User Account

OK, now that you understand about the types of accounts and the concept of rights, let's create a new user account. You can do so in a couple of ways: using the Users and Passwords applet and using Computer

Management. I'll start with the steps for creating a new user account with the Users Accounts applet:

1. Log on as Computer Administrator.

2. Choose Start ➤ Control Panel to open Control Panel, and then click User Accounts to open User Accounts.

3. Click the Create a New Account link to open the Name the New Account screen:

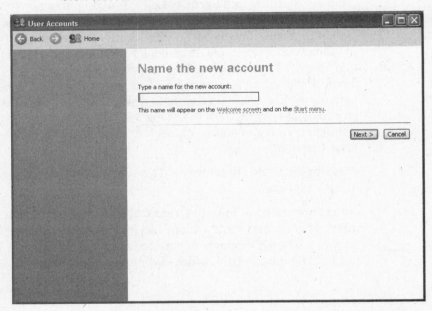

4. Enter a username for the person, and then click Next.

NOTE

In Windows XP Professional, a username can be a maximum of 20 characters and is not case sensitive.

5. Specify the type of account you want this user to have, and then click Create Account.

6. Back in User Accounts, click Change an Account, click the account you just created, and then click Create Password to open the screen on which you can create a password for the account.

NOTE

In Windows XP Professional, a password can be a maximum of 127 characters if you are in a pure Windows XP Professional environment. If you have Windows 9*x* machines on your network, keep the password to a maximum of 14 characters. Passwords are case sensitive.

7. In the Type a New Password box, enter a password, and then enter it again in the Type the New Password Again to Confirm box. If you want, you can then type a hint (which can be seen by anyone using this computer) to trigger your remembrance of the password if you forget it.

8. Click Create Password to establish the password for the new user account.

To gain more control over the process of managing user accounts on Windows XP Professional, you will need to use the Local User Manager. In Control Panel, click Performance and Maintenance, click Administrative Tools, and then click Computer Management to open the Computer Management window. In the Computer Management (Local) pane, expand System Tools, expand Local Users and Groups, and then select Users to display a list of users in the right pane. Choose Action ➤ New User to open the New User dialog box, as shown in Figure 6.1.

Part II

New User   [?] [X]

User name:	
Full name:	
Description:	

| Password: | |
| Confirm password: | |

☑ User must change password at next logon
☐ User cannot change password
☐ Password never expires
☐ Account is disabled

[Create]   [Close]

FIGURE 6.1:   Use the New User dialog box to add a new user to your system.

Now follow these steps:

1. Enter a username for this new account.

2. Enter the person's full name.

3. Enter a description.

4. Enter and confirm a password.

5. Set the password options. The default option is User Must Change Password at Next Logon. This option means that only that user will know the password, which means better security. If you uncheck this option, the other two options become available. Select User Cannot Change Password if this account will be used for a service or for someone you do not want to give the ability to change their own password. Select Password Never Expires if this password should be considered "permanent" and not have an automatic expiration.

6. The final option is to specify whether the account should be disabled. This is often a good idea if you want to change other properties of the account before it can be used, such as setting permissions on files and folders that this user will use. If this is the case, check the Account Is Disabled box.

7. When all options are selected, click Create to complete the process of making the new user account.

NOTE

To enable a disabled account, in the Local Users and Groups window, right-click the account and choose Properties from the shortcut menu to open the Properties dialog box for that account. Clear the Account Is Disabled check box.

Creating a Group Account

The process of creating a new group account is similar to creating a new user account. Local groups are useful for assigning permissions to resources. To create a new group account, follow these steps:

1. In Control Panel, click Performance and Maintenance, click Administrative Tools, and then click Computer Management to open the Computer Management window.

2. Expand System Tools, expand Local User and Groups, right-click Groups, and choose New Group from the shortcut menu to open the New Group dialog box:

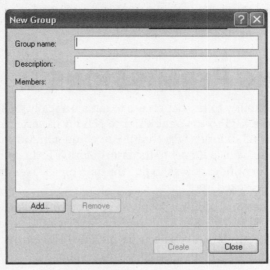

3. Type a name for the group in the space provided. The name can contain any numbers or letters and can be a maximum of 256 characters. The name must be unique in the local database.

4. Enter some text in the Description field that will describe the membership and purpose of this group.

5. Click the Add button to open the Select Users dialog box:

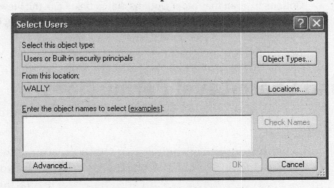

Part II

6. In the Enter the Object Names to Select box, enter the name of the user you want to add to the group, and then click OK. Repeat step 5 and this step to add more users to the group.

7. Back in the New Group dialog box, click Close, and then close Computer Management.

SETTING PERMISSIONS

The capability to restrict access to data is a really great feature of NT and Windows XP Professional. Prior to NT, my experience with operating systems of all kinds was that if you could gain physical access to a computer, you could get to its data; before NT, the only way to secure data with any confidence was to put the data on a server and put the server behind a locked door.

But network security is only as good as you make it. If a person can gain physical access to your machine, they can remove your hard disk and have all your data. Data security includes educating users to protect passwords and to apply permissions responsibly.

In this section, I'm going to show you how to set permissions at the share level and at the file and folder level. Remember, however, that you can establish file and folder security only if you are using the NTFS file system.

NOTE

To set permissions on a shared resource, you need to disable simple file sharing, which is enabled by default. In an Explorer window, choose Tools ➤ Folder Options to open the Folder Options dialog box. Click the View tab, and then in the Advanced Settings list, clear the Use Simple File Sharing (Recommended) check box.

Setting Share-Level Permissions

To give access to shared resources, you will need to set permissions as follows:

1. In Explorer, right-click the shared resource and choose Sharing and Security from the shortcut menu to open the Properties dialog box for the share at the Sharing tab.

2. Click the Permissions button to open the Permissions dialog box:

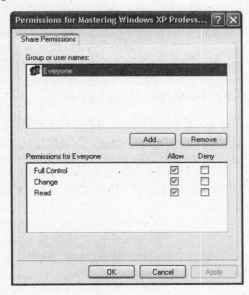

NOTE

The default shared permission in Windows XP Professional is for the Everyone group to have Full Control. In a secure environment, be sure to remove this permission before assigning specific permissions to users and groups.

3. Click Add to open the Select Users or Groups dialog box, in which you can select which groups have access to a shared file or folder:

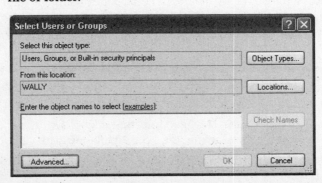

Part II

4. In the Enter the Object Names to Select box, enter the name of the user or group to whom you are granting permission, and click OK.

5. Back in the Permissions dialog box, you'll see that the user or group has been added to the Group or User Names list. In the Permissions section, click Allow or Deny to specify the type of permission you want to grant this user or group. Table 6.1 explains the choices.

6. When you've granted the permissions, click OK.

TABLE 6.1:   File Permissions

PERMISSION	DESCRIPTION
Full Control	The assigned group can perform any and all functions on all files and folders through the share.
Change	The assigned group can read and execute, as well as change and delete, files and folders through the share.
Read	The assigned group can read and execute files and folders but cannot modify or delete anything through the share.

Types of File and Folder Permissions

Share-level permissions determine who can access resources across the network and the type of access they will have. However, you can still assign more detailed permissions to the folders and files that can be accessed through the share. In addition, by using file- and folder-level permissions, you can restrict access to resources even if someone logs on to the system.

MULTIPLE GROUPS ACCUMULATE PERMISSIONS

You might have one group in your network called Accountants and another called Managers, and they might have different permission levels—for example, the Accountants might be able to only read

CONTINUED ➡

files, and the Managers might have Change access, which in NT was called Read and Write access. What about the manager of the Accounting department, who belongs to both the Managers and the Accountants groups—does he have Read access or does he have Change access?

In general, your permissions to a network resource *add up*—so if you have Read access from one group and Change from another group, you end up with Read *and* Change access. However, because Change access *includes* all the things that you can do with Read access, there's no practical difference between having Read and Change and having only Change access.

You've already seen that network shares have three types of permission levels: Read, Change, and Full Control. The permission types for files and folders are much more extensive, and each primary type includes still other types. Here are the primary types:

Read   Allows you to view the contents, permissions, and attributes associated with a resource. If the resource is a file, you can view the file. If the resource is an executable file, you can run it. If the resource is a folder, you can view the contents of the folder.

Write   Allows you to create a new file or subfolder within a folder if the resource is a folder. To change a file, you must also have Read permission, although you can append data to a file without opening the file if you have only Write permission.

Read & Execute   Allows you the permissions associated with Read and with Write and also allows you to *traverse* a folder, which means you can pass through a folder for which you have no access to get to a file or folder for which you do have access.

Modify   Allows you the permissions associated with Read & Execute and with Write, but also gives you Delete permission.

Full Control   Allows you the permissions associated with all the other permissions I've listed so far and lets you change permissions and take ownership of resources. In addition, you can delete subfolders and files even if you don't specifically have permission to do so.

List Folder Contents   Allows you to view the contents of folders.

If these levels of access are a bit coarse for your needs, you can fine-tune someone's access with what Microsoft calls *special access*. To modify the special access permissions for a file or folder, follow these steps:

1. In Explorer, right-click the resource whose permissions you want to modify and choose Properties from the shortcut menu to open the Properties dialog box for that resource.

2. Click the Security tab, and then click Advanced to open the Advanced Security Settings dialog box:

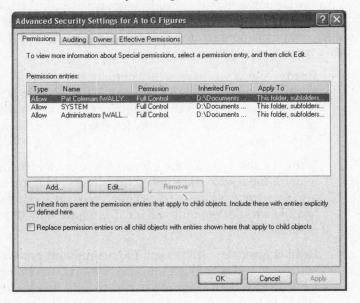

NOTE

If you don't see the Security tab in the Advanced Security Settings dialog box, in the Explorer view of My Computer choose Tools ➢ Folder Options to open the Folder Options dialog box. Click the View tab, and in the Advanced Settings list, clear the Use Simple File Sharing (Recommended) check box and click OK.

3. Click Edit to open the Permission Entry dialog box:

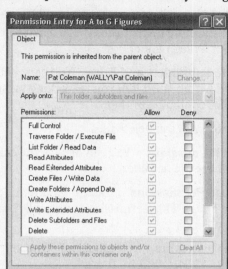

Here's a description of each of these permissions:

Full Control   This permission works as its name indicates and as discussed earlier in this chapter.

Traverse Folder/Execute File   You can change folders through this folder, and you can run this file.

List Folder/Read Data   You can read the contents of a file and display the contents of a folder.

Read Attributes   You can display the current attributes of a file or folder.

Read Extended Attributes   You can display the extended attributes of a file or folder, if there are any.

Create Files/Write Data   You can write data to a new file. When applied to a folder, this permission means you can write files into the folder, but you can't view what's already in the folder.

Create Folders/Append Data   You can create new folders in this location, and you can append data to existing files.

Write Attributes   You can modify the attributes of a file or folder.

Write Extended Attributes   You can create extended attributes for a file or folder.

Delete Subfolders and Files   You can remove folders contained within the folder you're working in, and you can remove the files contained in them.

Delete   You can delete files.

Read Permissions   You can display the current permissions list for the file or folder.

Change Permissions   You can modify the permissions for the file or folder. This permission is normally only included in Full Control.

Take Ownership   You can claim ownership of a file or folder.

These levels of granularity make security considerations more difficult to grasp initially, but they give a skilled administrator much finer control over how files and folders will be accessed.

To prevent someone from accessing a file or folder, you have two choices. The first, and usually the best, is simply to not grant the person access to the file or folder. That means, don't add their account to the list of permissions. The second method is to add the person's account to the permissions list, but check Deny for each permission. Doing so creates an explicit No Access–type permission.

NOTE

The special access items are all check boxes, not radio boxes, so you can mix and match as you like.

Assigning File and Folder Permissions

Now that you know something about the types of permissions you can place on files and folders, let's walk though the steps to assign them:

1. In Explorer, right-click the file or folder for which you want to establish permissions and choose Properties from the shortcut menu to open the Properties dialog box for that file or folder.

2. Click the Security tab:

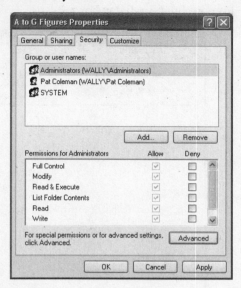

3. Click Add to open the Select Users or Groups dialog box.

4. In the Enter the Object Names to Select box, enter the name of the user or group to whom you are granting permission and click OK.

5. Back in the Properties dialog box, you'll see that those groups or users have been added to the Group or User Names list. Click OK.

Auditing Files and Folders

In addition to assigning file and folder permissions, Windows XP Professional lets you keep track of who accessed a file and when. You can audit everyone or only specific users or groups. To enable, set up, and view auditing, you need to be logged on as an administrator. Enabling auditing is a bit of a pain, but you have to do it before you can set up auditing. Bear with me, and follow these steps:

1. At a command prompt, type **mmc/a** and press Enter to open the Microsoft Management Console.

Part II

2. Choose File ➤ Add/Remove Snap-In to open the Add/Remove Snap-In dialog box:

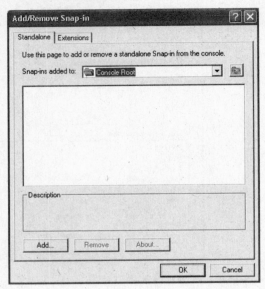

3. Click Add to open the Add Standalone Snap-In dialog box:

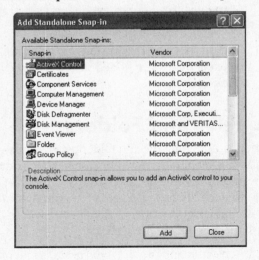

4. In the Snap-In list, select Group Policy, and then click Add to start the Group Policy Wizard:

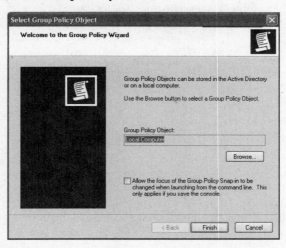

5. If Local Computer is not selected in the Group Policy Object box, browse for it, and then click Finish.

6. Back in the Add Standalone Snap-In dialog box, click Close.

7. Back in the Add/Remove Snap-In dialog box, click OK.

8. Back in the MMC, expand Local Computer Policy, expand Computer Configuration, expand Windows Settings, expand Security Settings, expand Local Policies, and then click Audit Policy. You'll see the following:

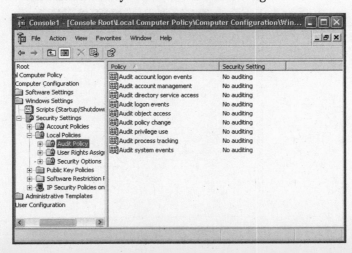

9. In the pane on the right, right-click Audit Object Access and choose Properties from the shortcut menu to open the Audit Object Access Properties dialog box:

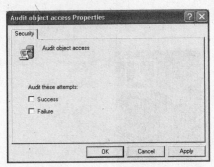

10. Click the check boxes to audit for success and failure, and then click OK.

11. Close the MMC.

Whew! Now you're ready to set up auditing. Follow these steps:

1. In Explorer, right-click the share you want to audit and choose Properties from the shortcut menu to open the Properties dialog box for that share.

2. Click the Security tab, click the Advanced button to open the Advanced Security Settings dialog box, and click the Auditing tab:

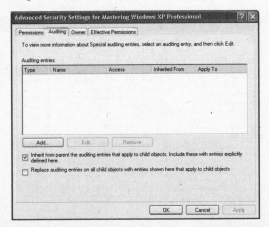

3. Click Add to open the Select User or Group dialog box.

4. In the Enter the Object Names to Select box, enter the name of a user or a group to audit, and then click OK to open the Auditing Entry dialog box:

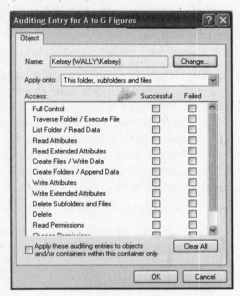

5. Select the entries that you want to audit, and then click OK three times.

To take a look at the events you've selected to audit, follow these steps:

1. In Control Panel, click Performance and Maintenance, click Administrative Tools, and then click Event Viewer to open the Event Viewer window.

2. In the pane on the left, select Security Log to display a list of audited events in the right pane.

UNDERSTANDING OWNERSHIP

Ownership—what a confusing concept. *Ownership* is a process by which you can take exclusive control over a file or a folder; and you can do all of this with a click of a button. But before you get power drunk with the possibilities, let's take a closer look at what being the owner of a file really means.

Defining Ownership

Now, having worked with NT since its inception, I don't mind telling you that the whole idea of a folder or file's "owner" seemed a bit confusing until I finally figured out the definition. Here's a definition—and from this point on, let me shorten the term *file* or *folder* to *object*:

Minasi's Definition of an Owner An object's owner is a user who can *always* modify that object's permissions.

Ordinarily, only an administrator can control settings such as an object's permissions. But you want your users to be able to control objects in their own area, their own home folder, without having to involve you at every turn. For example, suppose you want to give another user access to a folder in your home folder. Rather than having to seek out an administrator and ask the administrator to extend access permissions to another user, you as the owner can change the permissions directly. Ownership lets users become mini-administrators, rulers of their small fiefdoms.

To find out who owns an object, follow these steps:

1. In Explorer, right-click an object and choose Properties from the shortcut menu to open the Properties dialog box for that object.

2. Select the Security tab, and then click Advanced to open the Advanced Security Settings dialog box.

3. Select the Owner tab:

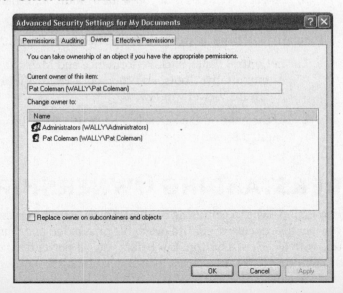

Taking Ownership

Users can't force themselves onto the permissions list for an object; but if they have the Take Ownership permission they *can* become the owner, and once they are the owner, *then* they can add themselves to the permissions list.

If you highlight your name in the Change Owner To list and click OK, you can become the owner of the object, but you can't see what's in the object because you are still not on the permissions list.

NOTE

Owners of files can't necessarily access those files. All that the owners of files can do is change the permissions on those files.

Okay, then, how do you get to the object? Well, because you are an owner, you can change permissions. So you will add yourself to the permissions list and *then* gain access to the object.

Why are you able to do that? Because of a user right that all administrators have by default: Take Ownership. Perhaps if you were a more user-oriented than administrator-oriented company, you could remove the Administrators group from that right. By doing so, however, an administrator would be unable to poke around a user's area.

Further, users can always shore up their security just a bit by taking control of their home folder from the administrators. Recall that users have Full Control of their home folder, and Full Control includes the ability to take ownership of an object.

And if you're concerned about an administrator being able to take control at any time—where's the security in that?—consider that an administrator must *take* ownership in order to add themselves to the object's permissions list. In doing that, they leave fingerprints behind; if you log on one day and find that you're no longer the owner of something that you owned yesterday, you know that an administrator has been snooping—and if file auditing is in place, you can even find out who snooped.

NOTE

You can't *give* ownership; you can only exercise the permission to take ownership. If an administrator were to take ownership of a file, they could not edit the file and then give ownership back to the original owner.

To summarize permissions and ownership:

▶ By default, new files and new subfolders inherit permissions from the folder in which they are created.

▶ A user who creates a file or a folder is the owner of that file or folder, and the owner can always control access to the file or folder by changing the permissions on it.

▶ When you change the permissions on an existing folder, you can choose whether those changes will apply to all files and subfolders within the folder.

▶ Users and groups can be denied access to a file or a folder simply by not granting the user or group any permissions for it.

WARNING

It is possible to lock out everyone including the operating system itself if you do not apply permissions correctly.

WHAT'S NEXT

In this chapter, we've looked at creating user and group accounts and at the rights that the various kinds of users and groups can have. I've also walked you through the steps involved in setting permissions for shares, files, and folders. Understanding and following these procedures is essential if you want the information on your Windows XP Professional system to be secure. And presumably that's one of the main reasons you're working with Windows XP Professional, right?

In Chapter 7, we will move from Microsoft operating systems to an operating system with a long history of security on PC-based networks: Novell NetWare

Chapter 7

SECURING YOUR NETWARE 6 NETWORK

N ovell Netware is one of the most robust network operating systems available for PC networking today. Since its introduction, Netware has constantly improved its security mechanisms, and Netware 6 is no exception. Netware 6 builds on the mature strength of Novell Directory Services (now eDirectory), adding improved auditing features and new management tools.

This chapter begins with a brief introduction to firewall technologies and then discusses file security. Once you have learned the basics of file security, you will move into NDS security, which is at the heart of Netware's security system. We'll discuss ConsoleOne, the new management tool of choice, and finally, you will learn how to protect your network from virus threats.

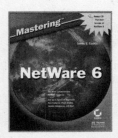

Adapted from *Mastering™ NetWare® 6*
by James E. Gaskin
ISBN 0-7821-4023-8 $69.99

THE INTERNET AND FIREWALLS

No intelligent network manager will connect to the Internet without some type of firewall in place to provide security. If your company already has an Internet connection and you are adding your own NetWare network to the list of Internet-aware networks, a firewall is in place already. Talk to the network administrator in charge of your TCP/IP network, and get the details you need to feel good about network security.

Firewall is an unusually descriptive term, even for the term-spewing computer industry. In construction, a firewall stands against disasters by forming an impenetrable shield around the protected area (I got the impenetrable shield slogan from my deodorant). Most disasters in buildings revolve around fires; hence, the term firewall.

NOTE

For more information on various network firewalls see Part III: "Firewalls," comprising Chapters 11–16.

The goal of a firewall is simple: to control access to a protected network. Firewall managers use two philosophies during configuration:

► Allow everything except designated packets

► Block everything except designated packets

Today, the proper attitude is to block everything except designated packets. Novell's products come this way straight from the box. When you enable filtering, everything is blocked, and you must designate what is allowed to pass through the firewall and/or filtering software.

There are four types of firewalls. Table 7.1 shows each type of firewall matched up with where it functions in the OSI seven-layer model.

TABLE 7.1: Matching Security Filters and Network Layers

OSI MODEL LAYER	INTERNET PROTOCOLS	FIREWALLS
Application	HTTP, FTP, DNS, NFS, Ping, SMTP, Telnet	Application-level gateway, stateful inspection firewall

TABLE 7.1 continued: Matching Security Filters and Network Layers

OSI MODEL LAYER	INTERNET PROTOCOLS	FIREWALLS
Presentation		
Session	TCP	Circuit-level gateway
Transport	TCP	
Network	IP	Packet-filtering firewall
Data Link		
Physical		

Let's see what each of these firewalls can do for you:

Packet Filters (FILTCFG)   The lowest level, packet filters, was once enough to protect your network, but that is no longer true. IP addresses are used to allow or deny packets, and IP address spoofing (disguised packets) has ruined the idea of this level of protection being enough to protect your network.

Circuit-Level Gateways   Circuit-level gateways do more to control internal traffic leaving your protected network than to keep outsiders at bay. Rules for users, such as allowable hosts to visit and time limits, are handled at this level.

Application-Level Gateways   Application-level gateways are specific to network services, such as FTP or e-mail. These are most common today with web browsers, used by software meant to monitor or block web access to certain sites.

Stateful Inspection Firewalls   Finally, the most critical area is the stateful inspection firewall, used by Novell and a few others. This software examines incoming packets to match them to appropriate outgoing packets and is able to examine packet contents to maintain control. The more options you have, the better your security, and NetWare gives you plenty of options. Of course, you'll need more time to configure more settings, but NetWare utilities will help with that chore.

Part II

PROTECT YOUR CORPORATE NETWORK

If your network is the corporate network, check out Novell's BorderManager software. You aren't familiar with this product? It adds a complete security- and performance-enhancing software server to any NetWare 4, 5, or 6 server.

You can run both the NetWare 6 server and BorderManager on the same hardware. Larger networks will want to separate the Border-Manager software on its own server for performance reasons. One BorderManager server protects your entire network when configured correctly. Feel free to look up my *IntranetWare BorderManager* book, also from Sybex, at your local bookstore or favorite online shopping destination.

KEEPING UP WITH SECURITY THREATS

Can one person, namely you, keep up with all the network miscreants out there? No, but there are more people on your side than you might imagine.

Enlist the resources of your firewall vendor, whether Novell for Border-Manager or another vendor. Keep up-to-date on all bug fixes, patches, and upgrades for your firewall software. Maintain proper security for the physical firewall system (lock it up in the server room or equivalent).

Also, watch the trade magazines and websites pertaining to security. Security information is all over the place if you keep your eyes open. Please don't be one of those who become paranoid *after* you get burned. Go ahead and start being paranoid, or at least well informed, before something serious happens to your network.

Here's a regularly repeated warning: *Watch your users carefully*. Some companies are using "internal" firewalls to keep employees out of sensitive areas. A serious security breach, where valuable information is stolen or compromised, almost always includes help from the inside. Every user is a potential thief. Always provide new services with tighter rather than looser security, and then loosen the leash as you and your management feel more comfortable with the security situation on your network. Most data thieves walk out rather than break in.

When the network is new, or a security problem has occurred, everyone is conscientious. After a time, however, human nature takes over and everyone gets sloppy.

Your network changes constantly, and each change is a potential security disaster. Add a new user? Did you take care to match the new user to an existing group with well-defined security and access controls? How about new files created by the users themselves? Do you have a plan for watching the access level of those files? Do users have the ability to allow other users access into a home directory? If so, no private file will be safe. Don't allow file sharing within each person's private directory. Send the file by e-mail or have a common directory in which users can place files to share. Do not allow them more file rights to the \PUBLIC directory, even though some users will ask for it.

Watch new applications. Many vendors have modified NetWare rights for files and directories for years, especially during installation. Are these loopholes closed in the new application directories you created just last week? Take the time to check.

Part II

PASSWORDS AND LOGIN RESTRICTIONS

Password and login security is essential. Let's take a look at each: Passwords   Each user must have a password. Here are some tips for your passwords:

▶ The longer the password, the better. Novell's default minimum is five characters; try for six or lucky seven.

▶ Encourage the use of mixed alpha and numeric characters in the password.

▶ Set passwords to expire (the default is 40 days).

▶ Let the system keep track of passwords to force unique ones. The limit is 20.

▶ Limit the grace logins; two is enough.

Login Restrictions   Using login restrictions, you can limit users' network access and track the resources they use. Here are some tips for setting login restrictions:

▶ Limit concurrent connections for all users.

- ▶ Set an account expiration date for all temporary workers.
- ▶ Disable accounts for users away from the office who don't communicate remotely to your network.

THE ADMIN USER, ADMIN RIGHTS, AND SUPERVISOR RIGHT

The only user created with NetWare 6 is named Admin, short for Administrator. If you just climbed up the version tree from NetWare 3.1x, don't bother looking for SUPERVISOR, because Admin replaced SUPERVISOR.

Make the mental note that the Admin user is separate from the Admin rights over the network operating system and included objects. As you'll see later, the more advanced management techniques that arrived with object management and the Admin user are a way to block this SUPERVISOR equivalent from managing parts of the network. Oops.

The Admin user is a supervisor's supervisor, able to control the network completely as the old SUPERVISOR did in earlier NetWare versions. The Supervisor right, however, may be granted to any user for particular NDS eDirectory objects or containers. Being able to set up subadministrators for specific tasks can be a great help.

This flexibility of supervision is an important feature of NetWare 6—one of the many features that place NetWare ahead of the competition. With global enterprise networking the norm for many companies today, the job of supervision is far beyond the abilities of any one person. NetWare 6 allows the supervision chores to be distributed in whatever method you prefer.

You can have different administrators for different parts of the tree, as well as different volumes, directories, or files. Admin may control the NDS design and overall setup but have no control over the files. Filesystem supervisors in each container will handle those chores. Admin in Chicago may share duties with Admin in Cleveland, with each responsible primarily for his or her own city but able to support the other network across the WAN if necessary.

UNDERSTANDING FILESYSTEM SECURITY

There are two main security areas for NetWare 6: filesystem and NDS security. If you are familiar with NetWare 3.x, you will be familiar with filesystem security. NetWare 4.1x added some attributes to support data compression and data migration features and changed a bit of the terminology, but most of the details and the security goals remain the same, even in NetWare 6. The main goal is to provide users access to and control of the proper files and directories.

NetWare files are protected in two ways:

▶ Users must be granted the right to use files and directories.

▶ File and directory attributes provide hidden protection.

What is hidden protection? Suppose that Doug has the right to create and delete files in the \LETTERS directory. If he writes a letter named SLS_GOAL.OCT and decides he doesn't like that file, he can delete it. Files can be deleted from within applications or from the DOS prompt. He can use Windows Explorer.

What if Doug's mouse slips a fraction within Explorer, and he tries to delete the SLS_GOAL.PLN file, the template for all the sales goal letters? Is the file doomed?

Not necessarily. If the network administrator (probably you) has set the attribute to SLS_GOAL.PLN as Read Only or Delete Inhibit, Doug can't delete the file. However, if Doug also has the right to modify the file attributes (a bad idea, knowing Doug), he could change the Read Only or Delete Inhibit designation and delete the file anyway. But he would need to work at deleting the file; he couldn't do it by accident.

When granting Doug rights to use the \LETTERS directory, we call him a *trustee* of the directory, given to him by way of a *trustee assignment*. He has been trusted to use the directory and files properly. The trustee concept works with objects and NDS items, as you'll soon see.

Someone in authority must grant Doug, or a group or container Doug is a member of, the rights to use the file, directory, or object in question. The administrator is the person who places trust in Doug, making him a trustee of the rights of the object. This is referred to as making trustee assignments to a directory, file, or object. The trustee assignments are stored in the object's ACL (Access Control List) property inside NDS eDirectory.

The rights granted to users flow downhill (kind of like *stuff* on a bad day). This means that the rights Doug has in one directory apply to all subdirectories. This idea works well, and the official name is *inheritance*. If your system is set up with \LETTERS as the main directory, and Doug has rights to use that directory, he will automatically have the same rights in the \LETTERS\SALES and \LETTERS\PROSPECT subdirectories. He will inherit the same rights in \LETTERS\SALES as he has in \LETTERS.

One way to stop Doug from having full access to a subdirectory is to use the IRF (Inherited Rights Filter). The IRF filters the rights a user may have in subdirectories and will be covered later in this chapter. The other way is to explicitly make a new trustee assignment to this subdirectory. A new assignment always overrides the inherited settings.

NOTE

NetWare 3.*x* had Inherited Rights Masks (IRMs). NetWare 4.1 and later have Inherited Rights Filters (IRFs). The name has changed, but the actions are the same.

[Public] is a special trustee for use by all the users on the network, and it can always be specified as a trustee of a file, directory, or object. Although it sounds similar to the group EVERYONE in earlier NetWare versions, containers act more like the EVERYONE group than [Public] does.

File and Directory Rights

The rights to use directories and files are similar, so we'll take a look at the directory situation first. Users' rights in dealing with files and directories are also similar, making explanations fairly simple.

Directory Rights for Users and Groups

There are reasons to grant rights to directories rather than files, not the least of which is the time savings. Even with wildcards available, I would rather set the rights of users to use a directory and all subdirectories than set their rights to the files in each directory.

What are these rights that users can have over a directory? And did that last sentence in the previous paragraph mean subdirectories? Yes it did. The directory rights available to users are summarized in Table 7.2.

TABLE 7.2:   Directory Rights in NetWare 6

RIGHT	DESCRIPTION
Supervisor (S)	Grants all rights to the directory, its files, and all subdirectories, overriding any restrictions placed on subdirectories or files with an IRF. Users with this right in a directory can grant other users Supervisor rights to the same directory, its files, and its subdirectories.
Read (R)	Allows the user to open and read the directory. Earlier NetWare versions needed an Open right; Read now includes Open.
Write (W)	Allows the user to open and write files, but existing files are not displayed without Read authorization.
Create (C)	Allows the user to create directories and files. With Create authorization, a user can create a file and write data into the file (authority for Write is included with Create). Read and File Scan authority are not part of the Create right.
Modify (M)	Allows the user to change directory and file attributes, including the right to rename the directory, its files, and its subdirectories. Modify does not refer to the file contents.
File Scan (F)	Allows the user to see filenames in a directory listing. Without this right, the user will be told the directory is empty.
Access Control (A)	Allows the user to change directory trustee assignments and the IRFs for directories. This right should be granted to supervisory personnel only, because users with Access Control rights can grant all rights except Supervisor to another user, including rights the Access Control user doesn't have. The user can also modify file trustee assignments within the directory.

Part II

Let's see how these directory rights appear in ConsoleOne. Figure 7.1 shows the group Techies and the file and directory rights the members have. (Why use ConsoleOne rather than NetWare Administrator? To get ready for the future, because ConsoleOne gets the Novell developer's attention today, while NetWare Administrator remains static. Like it or not, ConsoleOne is the future.)

The Effective Rights dialog box in Figure 7.1 appears when you click the Effective Rights command button in the Rights to Files and Folders tab of the Techies property page. The odd arrangement here helps show all the pieces without blocking the parent window. Unlike NetWare Administrator, ConsoleOne requires you to drill down through the volume to the directory in the Select Object dialog box (not shown here).

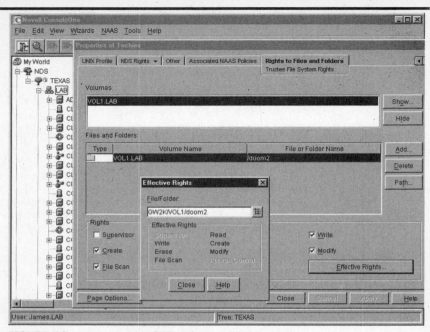

FIGURE 7.1: An example of the rights a group can have

The Supervisor and Access Control check boxes are clear in the Rights area. This means that the group Techies does not have those two rights. Giving a group of users (especially a group of techs) the Supervisor right could be dangerous. Giving a person or group the Access Control right is equally dangerous. With the Access Control right, the user or group member can change his or her own rights and add more rights without your knowledge or consent.

These rights apply to the directory where they are granted and to all subdirectories. Rights are inherited from the top directory levels through all the existing subdirectory levels.

The rights are displayed (in DOS with the RIGHTS command) as a string of the initials within brackets: [SRWCEMFA]. If some are missing, a space is put in their place. For instance, the most rights nonadministrative users generally have are [_RWCEMF_]. As you can see, underscores were put in place of the S (Supervisor) and A (Access Control) rights. If the generic user listed previously didn't have the rights to Erase in a particular directory, the listing would appear as [_RWC_MF_].

File Rights for Users and Groups

In contrast to directory rights, file rights address only specified files. Sometimes the files are identified individually, and sometimes they are specified by a wildcard group (*.EXE, for example). There are minor differences between how the rights are applied to a directory and to a file. Table 7.3 summarizes the file rights.

TABLE 7.3: File Rights in NetWare 6

RIGHT	DESCRIPTION
Supervisor (S)	Grants all rights to the file, and users with this right may grant any file right to another user. This right also allows modification of all the rights in the file's IRF.
Read (R)	Allows the user to open and read the file.
Write (W)	Allows the user to open and write to the file.
Create (C)	Allows the user to create new files and salvage a file after it has been deleted. Perhaps the latter should be called the Re-create right.
Erase (E)	Allows the user to delete the file.
Modify (M)	Allows the user to modify the file attributes, including renaming the file. This does not apply to the contents of the file.
File Scan (F)	Allows the user to see the file when viewing the contents of the directory.
Access Control (A)	Allows the user to change the file's trustee assignments and IRF. Users with this right can grant any right (except Supervisor) for this file to any other user, including rights that they themselves have not been granted.

Part II

    You might notice that the Create right is a bit different, and the Supervisor and Access Control rights apply to individual files. Why do we have the differences between directory and file rights?

The IRF and File and Directory Rights

Let's pretend that your filesystem is set up so that all the accounting data is parceled into subdirectories under the main \DATA directory in the volume ACCOUNTING. Many people on your network will need access to the information in these accounting files. Some will need to use the accounting programs, some will need to gather the information into reports, and others may need to write applications that use those data files.

Directory rights flow downhill, so this will be easy: Give the group ACCOUNTING rights to use the \DATA directory, and the information in \DATA\AR, \DATA\AP, \DATA\GL, and \DATA\PAYROLL is available to everyone. But suddenly your boss realizes that giving everyone rights to see the information in \DATA\PAYROLL is not smart (your boss must be slow, because salary information paranoia runs pretty high in most bosses).

This is what the IRF was made for. The IRF controls the rights passed between a higher-level directory and a lower-level directory. In our example, that would be \DATA to \DATA\PAYROLL. The IRF does not grant rights; it strictly revokes them. The IRF default is to let all rights flow down unless otherwise instructed.

Figure 7.2 shows a simple look at our example. Everyone has access to all directories except \DATA\PAYROLL. The IRF is blocking the rights for everyone in that directory.

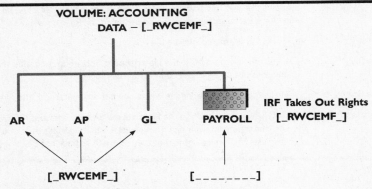

FIGURE 7.2:   Keeping prying eyes out of PAYROLL

There's a problem here: How does anyone see the \DATA\PAYROLL directory? The network administrator must specifically grant rights to the \DATA\PAYROLL directory for those users who belong there. The IRF filters between the parent directory and subdirectory. It does not dictate the rights assigned specifically to the subdirectory.

When you type **RIGHTS** from the DOS command line, you see your rights in the current directory listed with an explanation. If you have all rights in a directory, such as your home directory, the RIGHTS command will show something like the display for user Alex in Figure 7.3.

NOTE

Do you like Figure 7.3's old screenshot using Novell DOS? Yes, they had it for a while until they sold it to Caldera—the Linux people.

```
[Novell DOS] I:\HOME\ALEX>rights
GATEWAY2000\PROJECTS:\HOME\ALEX
Your rights for this directory:   [SRWCEMFA]
    Supervisor rights to directory.        (S)
    Read from a file in a directory.       (R)
    Write to a file in a directory.        (W)
    Create subdirectories and files.       (C)
    Erase directory and files.             (E)
    Modify directory and files.            (M)
    Scan for files and directories.        (F)
    Change access control.                 (A)

[Novell DOS] I:\HOME\ALEX>
```

FIGURE 7.3: Results of the RIGHTS command

If you have no rights in a directory, such as if our friend Alex typed the RIGHTS command in the HOME directory above his own, the result would look something like this:

```
GATEWAY2000\PROJECTS:\HOME
Your rights for this directory: [   ]
```

You can approach the IRF in two ways: Ignore it and set up your filesystem so that inheritance is never a problem, or take a minute to figure out how it works. The problem with the first option is that reality always rises up and bites you when you try to ignore problems, such as the previous example with the \DATA\PAYROLL directory. Inheritance is always going to be with us, and the IRF makes good sense in certain situations, so let's look at another view of the IRF.

First, let's add a complication: group rights. Users can be assigned rights directly, or they can get them through group memberships. The individual and group rights are additive. If you have one right granted individually and another granted through group membership, you effectively have both rights.

The IRF works against both the individual and group rights. The results of the individual plus group rights minus those taken away by the IRF are called the *effective rights*. Figure 7.4 stacks up the individual and group rights, subtracts the IRF, and shows the effective rights.

Part II

Individual Rights	[_RWCE_F_]	[_RWCEMFA]	[_RW_E_F_]
plus Group Rights +	[_____M_A]		[_R___MF_]
minus IRF −		[_____M_A]	[__W_EM__]
Effective Rights	[_RWCEMFA]	[_RWCE_F_]	[_R____F_]

FIGURE 7.4:   Stacking and subtracting rights

Notice that the Supervisor (S) rights aren't mentioned anywhere. The IRF does not block the Supervisor rights, whether granted to the individual or a group. This is true only of the directory and file rights IRF. Later, you'll see that the object rights are a different story.

Directory and File Security Guidelines

No two networks are alike or use the same security profile. However, some general guidelines are applicable:

▶ Design your network top-down, from tighter security at the higher directories to looser security in the lower directories.

▶ Fight the urge to grant trustee rights to individuals. Always look for groups first, second, and third before you work with the individual user.

▶ Plan for inheritance. Grant Read and File Scan rights high, and Create, Erase, and Modify rights lower in the NDS eDirectory tree.

▶ Avoid granting any destructive rights high in the directory structure.

▶ Remember that the Supervisor right for the filesystem cannot be blocked by the IRF. Grant that right carefully, if at all.

File Attributes as a Security Enhancement

File attributes in NetWare, as in DOS, detail the characteristics of a file or directory. NetWare administrators often call these attributes *flags*. The NetWare DOS command-line utility FLAG.EXE displays and modifies these attributes.

Because we've decided that security includes making sure all network resources are available, the safety of files on the file server is important. Someone besides you deleting or renaming files is a security problem.

File and directory attributes are not a defense for cases of willful destruction and sabotage. They are a defense against mistakes and typos by innocent users. Haven't you ever had a user type **DEL** *.* in a directory on drive G: instead of drive C:? Having some of the files set as Read Only or Delete Inhibit may lessen the damage from a confused user.

Attributes control what can and can't be done with files and directories. They are also a limited form of virus protection. Most viruses work by modifying executable files, so keeping those executables Ro (Read Only) will stop viruses from trying to rewrite files and save them back with the same name.

WARNING

Ro flags won't help with the new genre of Word macro viruses or with many of the other multitude of viruses out there. Flagging files Ro is never enough virus protection; it just helps a little.

Filesystem: Directory Attributes

As is the case with much of NetWare, there are attributes for directories as well as files. Again, this makes sense. Unlike the rights to use an object, most directory rights don't directly affect the files in the directory. The attributes dealing with compression and data migration obviously do impact individual files. Compression may be set by volume, so the Immediate Compress attribute may be used more often than the Don't Compress attribute. Table 7.4 lists the directory attributes with their abbreviations and descriptions.

TABLE 7.4: Directory Attributes in NetWare 6

ATTRIBUTE	DESCRIPTION
All (All)	Sets all available directory attributes.
Don't Compress (Dc)	Stops compression on any files in the directory. This attribute overrides the compression setting for the volume.
Delete Inhibit (Di)	Stops users from erasing the directory, even if the user has the Erase trustee right. This attribute can be reset by a user with the Modify right.
Don't Migrate (Dm)	Stops files within the directory from being migrated to secondary storage.
Hidden (H)	Hides directories from DOS DIR scans. NDIR will display these directories if the user has appropriate File Scan rights.
Immediate Compress (Ic)	Forces the filesystem to compress files as soon as the operating system can handle the action.

TABLE 7.4 continued: Directory Attributes in NetWare 6

ATTRIBUTE	DESCRIPTION
Normal (N)	Flags a directory as Read/Write and nonshareable. It removes most other flags. This is the standard setting for user directories on the server handling DOS programs.
Purge (P)	Forces NetWare to completely delete files as the user deletes them, rather than tracking the deletions for the SALVAGE command to use later.
Rename Inhibit (Ri)	Stops users from renaming directories, even those users who have been granted the Modify trustee right. However, if the user has the Modify trustee right, that user can remove this attribute from the directory and then rename the directory.
System (Sy)	Hides directories from DOS DIR scans and prevents them from being deleted or copied. The NDIR program will display these directories if the user has appropriate File Scan rights.

NOTE

The Don't Compress, Immediate Compress, and Don't Migrate attributes for files and directories were added when NetWare 4 introduced compression and advanced storage features.

Most of these directory attributes are seldom used to protect a directory from confused users. The options you will probably use the most are those that concern the operating system, such as Don't Compress and Immediate Compress. The Normal attribute will be used most often, if your network follows true to form.

Filesystem: File Attributes

Most flagging happens at the file level and doesn't get changed all that often. After all, once you set the files in a directory the way you want (all the .EXE and .COM files Read Only and Shareable, for instance), few occasions require you to change them.

The time to worry about file attributes is during and immediately after installation of a new software product. Many product vendors today advertise, "Yes, it runs with NetWare," and they normally set the flags for you during installation. However, it's good practice to check newly installed applications, just in case the developers forgot to set a flag or three. The available file attributes are listed in Table 7.5, with their abbreviations and meanings.

TABLE 7.5:   File Attributes in NetWare 6

ATTRIBUTE	DESCRIPTION
All (All)	Sets all available file attributes.
Archive Needed (A)	DOS's Archive bit that identifies files modified after the last backup. NetWare assigns this bit automatically.
Copy Inhibit (Ci)	Prevents Macintosh clients from copying the file, even those clients with Read and File Scan trustee rights. This attribute can be changed by users with the Modify right.
Don't Compress (Dc)	Prevents the file from being compressed. This attribute overrides settings for automatic compression of files.
Delete Inhibit (Di)	Prevents clients from deleting the file, even those clients with the Erase trustee right. This attribute can be changed by users with the Modify right.
Don't Migrate (Dm)	Prevents files from being migrated from the server's hard disk to another storage medium.
Hidden (H)	Hides files from the DOS DIR command. The NDIR program will display these files if the user has appropriate File Scan rights.
Immediate Compress (Ic)	Forces files to be compressed as soon as the file is closed.
Normal (N)	Shorthand for Read/Write, because there is no N attribute bit for file attributes. This is the default setting for files.
Purge (P)	Forces NetWare to automatically purge the file after it has been deleted.
Rename Inhibit (Ri)	Prevents the filename from being modified. Users with the Modify trustee right may change this attribute and then rename the file.
Read Only (Ro)	Prevents a file from being modified. This attribute automatically sets Delete Inhibit and Rename Inhibit. It's extremely useful for keeping .COM and .EXE files from being deleted by users, and it helps stop a virus from mutating the file.
Read Write (Rw)	The default attribute for all files. Allows users to read and write to the file.
Shareable (Sh)	Allows more than one user to access a file simultaneously. Normally used with the Read Only attribute so that a file being used by multiple users cannot be modified. All the utility files in the \PUBLIC directory are flagged Sh (and Ro, Di, and Ri).
System File (Sy)	Prevents a file from being deleted or copied and hides it from the DOS DIR command. NetWare's NDIR program will display these directories as System if the user has appropriate File Scan rights.
Transactional (T)	Forces the file to be tracked and protected by the Transaction Tracking System (TTS).

Part II

File attributes are normally assigned to the files using a wildcard with the FLAG command, as in this example:

```
FLAG *.EXE RO Sh
```

This command says, "Change the file attributes of all files with the .EXE extension to be readable, but not writable, and to share the file by allowing multiple clients to use the program file concurrently."

 TIP

When a user has a problem with a file, the first two things to check are the user's rights in that directory and the flags set on the problem file. One of these two settings, mismatched in some way, accounts for 80 percent or more of user file problems.

Let's look at how to type an exploratory FLAG command and examine the results. Figure 7.5 shows the command and result.

```
MS-DOS Prompt                                                    _ □ ×
  8 x 12 ▼
J:\PUBLIC>flag m*.*
Files           = The name of the files found
Directories     = The name of the directories found
DOS Attr        = The DOS attributes for the specified file
NetWare Attr    = The NetWare attributes for the specified file or directory
Status          = The current status of migration and compression for a file
                  or directory
Owner           = The current owner of the file or directory
Mode            = The search mode set for the current file

Files                   DOS Attr NetWare Attr          Status Owner        Mode

MAP.EXE                 [Ro----] [------Di--Ri------]          .[Supervisor] 0
MFC42.DLL               [Ro----] [------Di--Ri------]          .[Supervisor] N/A
MODIFY.BAT              [Rw---A] [------------------]          .James.LAB    N/A
MSVCP50.DLL             [Ro----] [------Di--Ri------]          .[Supervisor] N/A
MSVCRT.DLL              [Ro----] [------Di--Ri------]          .[Supervisor] N/A
MSVCRT40.DLL            [Ro----] [------Di--Ri------]          .[Supervisor] N/A

Directories             NetWare Attr    Owner

MGMT                    [------------] .[Supervisor]

J:\PUBLIC>
```

FIGURE 7.5:   Checking the FLAG setting in the \PUBLIC directory

In this example, you can see the file attributes for a few of the NetWare utility files. Most are Ro (Read Only), meaning they have the NetWare attributes of Di (Delete Inhibit) and Ri (Rename Inhibit) set as well. Looking at the second set of attributes, you see this is true.

The MODIFY.BAT file was created by me (James). You can tell because the flag is set to Rw (Read Write) and the Archive attribute is set, meaning the file changed since the last backup. The rest of the files in the example are owned by the Supervisor. The ownership for these files was set during installation.

To check for all the various FLAG command-line switches, from the DOS command line, type:

```
FLAG /? ALL
```

You'll see six screens' worth of information.

NOTE

Don't think that FLAG is the only way to change file attributes. The FILER, ConsoleOne, and NetWare Administrator utilities allow these same functions, just not as quickly and easily (in my opinion).

ConsoleOne's new beefy manifestation, like the weakling working out after being embarrassed, impresses me with its progress. Early versions of ConsoleOne couldn't get to the file level, but Novell engineers whipped that problem in NetWare 5.1. See Figure 7.6 for ConsoleOne's new file-control features.

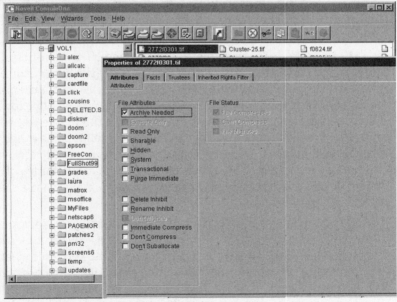

FIGURE 7.6:   ConsoleOne now displays file attributes.

Notice the strange icons on the ConsoleOne toolbar? The red X means delete, the scissors mean cut, the pages mean copy, and the A with a strikeout and a B means rename. Not the best iconography for rename, I grant you, but new and impressive overall.

UNDERSTANDING NDS SECURITY

Because NDS was new to NetWare 4, the idea of NDS security was new to old NetWare hands at the time, and it may still be new to those just jumping up from good old NetWare 3. NDS security is concerned with the management and protection of the NDS database and its objects.

The SUPERVISOR user in NetWare 3 was concerned about both file security (as we just discussed) and network resources security. The second part of the job included creating and managing users, setting network access privileges for all network users, and creating and managing network resources, such as printers and volumes.

The Admin user has, by default, all the rights and power of the SUPERVISOR user. In NetWare 6, however, the management can easily be split between NDS security and filesystem security. It's entirely possible to have one administrator with no control over file and user trustee rights and another administrator with no control over containers, Organizations, or Organizational Units. You can also set up subadministrators with complete control over their containers, having both file and property rights.

Let's be quite clear about this: Filesystem and NDS security systems are (almost) completely separate from each other (the Supervisor right crosses the line). Just as filesystem security controls which users can control which files, NDS security controls the same functions for the NDS objects. Having the rights to control a container gives you no authority over a file kept on a volume in that container, unless rights are granted to that volume. The two security systems are not in any way related. Let me repeat: Having control over the NDS attributes of an object (let's say a disk volume) does not grant the rights to the files contained in that volume.

The NDS database allows multiple management layers. You can create as many Organizations and Organizational Units as you want, nesting the Organizational Units as many levels as you want. As you'll see when I talk about how the IRF works on object and property rights, it's possible for the Admin of a network to have full control over the Organization and the first Organizational Unit, but no control over the final Organizational Unit. Make sure this is what you have in mind before setting up such a system, however. If you can't trust your Admin with access to everything, you have more problems than can be solved by NetWare.

Object Rights versus Property Rights

There are two types of rights in NDS: object rights and property rights. *Object rights* determine what a trustee (a user with the proper rights) can do to an object, such as creating, deleting, or renaming the object. *Property rights* determine whether a trustee can examine, use, or change the values of the various properties of an object.

Only in one case does an object right intrude into the property rights arena: the Supervisor right. A trustee with the Supervisor right to an object also has full rights to all properties of that object. But unlike with file and directory rights, the Supervisor right can be blocked on object and property rights by the IRF.

The opposite of the Supervisor right is the Browse right. This is the default right for users in the network. It allows users to see, but not modify, objects in the NDS eDirectory tree.

Object rights concern the object as a whole in the Browser. Actions taken on an object in the Browser, such as moving a User object from one context to another, exemplify object rights.

Property rights concern the values of all the properties of an object. The User object that was moved in the last paragraph has hundreds of properties. The ability to change a property value, such as Minimum Account Balance or Telephone Number, requires property rights.

Objects have inheritance rights, meaning a trustee of one object has the same rights over a subsidiary object. If a trustee has rights over one container, that trustee has the same rights over any container objects inside the main container.

Let's play "Pick Your Analogy." Object rights are like moving boxes, and the box contents are properties. The movers have authority over the boxes (object rights) but not over the contents of the boxes (property rights). A mover supervisor, however, has the rights to the boxes and to the contents (property rights) of those boxes for management situations.

When you turn your car over to a parking lot attendant, you give that attendant object rights: Your car can be placed anywhere in the parking lot. The attendant has full control over where your car is and if it needs to be moved while you're gone. You probably exclude the Delete right from the attendant, however. The property rights to your car, such as the items in your trunk, glove compartment, and backseat, do not belong to the parking lot attendant. You have granted the attendant some object rights to your car, but no property rights. Do you think armored car drivers have object rights or property rights to the money bags? Which would you prefer if you were a driver? Which if you owned the bag contents?

To keep things consistent, object rights and property rights overlap only in the Supervisor right. The trick is to remember that sometimes a C means Create and sometimes it means Compare. Take a look at the official list of object rights in Table 7.6.

TABLE 7.6:   Object Rights in NetWare 6

RIGHT	DESCRIPTION
Supervisor (S)	Grants all access privileges, including unrestricted access to all properties. The Supervisor right can be blocked by an IRF, unlike with file and directory rights.
Browse (B)	Grants the right to see this object in the eDirectory tree. The name of the object is returned when a search is made, if the search criteria match the object.
Create (C)	Grants the right to create a new object below this object in the eDirectory tree. No rights are defined for the new object. This right applies only to container objects, because only container objects can have subordinates.
Delete (D)	Grants the right to delete the object from the eDirectory tree. Objects that have subordinates can't be deleted unless the subordinates are deleted first, just like a DOS directory can't be deleted if it still contains files or subdirectories.
Rename (R)	Grants the right to change the name of the object. This action officially modifies the Name property of the object, changing the object's complete name.

The object rights tend to be used by managers, not by users. Create, Delete, and Rename rights are not the type of things normally given to users. The Browse object right is granted automatically to [Root], meaning everyone can browse the NDS eDirectory tree. Remember that the Supervisor object right automatically allows full access to all property rights. The property rights are listed in Table 7.7.

TABLE 7.7:   Property Rights in NetWare 6

Right	Description
Supervisor (S)	Grants all rights to the property. The Supervisor right can be blocked by an IRF, unlike with file and directory rights.
Compare (C)	Grants the right to compare any value with a value of the property for search purposes. With the Compare right, a search operation can return True or False, but you can't see the value of the property. The Read right includes the Compare right.
Read (R)	Grants the right to read all the values of the property. Compare is a subset of Read. If the Read right is given, Compare operations are also allowed.
Write (W)	Grants the right to add, change, or remove any values of the property. Write also includes the Add or Delete Self right.
Add or Delete Self (A)	Grants a trustee the right to add or remove itself as a value of the property, but no other values of the property may be changed. This right is meaningful only for properties that contain object names as values, such as group membership lists or mailing lists. The Write right includes the Add or Delete Self right.

The Access Control List (ACL)

The ACL is the object property that stores the information about who may access the object. Just as Joe is a value of the Name property, the ACL contains trustee assignments for both object and property rights. The ACL also includes the IRF.

To change the ACL, you must have a property right that allows you to modify that ACL value for that object. Write will allow this, as will the Supervisor object right. Add or Delete Self is for users to add or remove themselves from a Members List property of a Group object.

Do you want to grant object or property rights to another object? You must have the Write, Add or Delete Self, or Supervisor right to the ACL property of the object in question.

Although it sounds as if the ACL is a list somewhere, it's really just one of many properties held by an object. Each object has an ACL. If a user is not listed in the ACL for an object, that user cannot change the properties of that object.

How Rights Inheritance Works

As I said before, rights flow downhill (ask a plumber what else flows downhill). Directory rights pass down to subdirectories, and container rights flow down to subcontainers. The only way to stop rights from flowing to a subcontainer is to use the IRF in the subcontainer. This forces users with rights to the parent container to also get the trustee rights to the subcontainer in a separate operation. That means the network supervisor (probably you) must go back and grant trustee rights to those users who need access to the subcontainer.

The system works well, with one exception: Selected property rights are not inherited. If a user is granted trustee rights to an object for selected property rights only, those rights do not move down to the subcontainer or other objects. Figure 7.7 shows an example of the process of granting a user selected property rights.

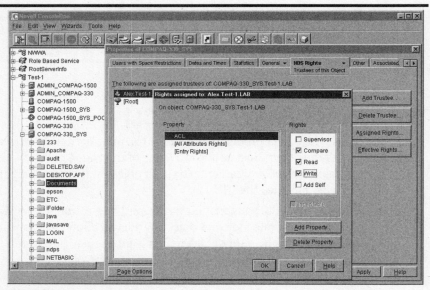

FIGURE 7.7: Granting limited rights that cannot be inherited

Selected property rights always take precedence over inherited rights. Even without an IRF, setting particular trustee rights in one container puts those rights in effect, no matter which rights are assigned to the container above. ConsoleOne shows these rights assignments in a different way than we're used to, but you can see in Figure 7.7 that we just added property rights to the ACL property for the Documents volume for Alex. I clicked the Add Property button in the foreground dialog box to pop up the long list of rights to choose for Alex.

The IRF and Object and Property Rights

The IRF works the same with object and property rights as it does with file and directory rights. The IRF doesn't give rights to anyone; it only takes rights away.

You, as network manager, set the level of rights users should have to an object. If a particular user has more rights than that, the IRF will filter that particular user to the level of access you set.

The big difference in the IRF when dealing with the NDS object and property rights is the ability to block the Supervisor object right. This gives some departments a warm fuzzy feeling, because no one except their administrator can control their part of the eDirectory tree. But care must be taken in organizing your system.

NetWare helps safeguard against accidentally eliminating all supervision for part of your tree by not allowing you to block the Supervisor object right to an object unless at least one other object has already been granted the Supervisor right to that object. The problem comes if the other Supervisor object is deleted. Deleting the sole Supervisor for part of your NDS eDirectory tree leaves part of the system without management, which is not a good thing.

This is a good reason to never delete the Admin user, even if you have one or two Admin-equivalent users. Over time, something will happen to both equivalent users, and suddenly your network will not have anyone able to perform supervisory functions over the entire tree. Some paranoid people have both Admin-equivalent users and users not set as Admin-equivalent but granted the full set of rights. Why? If Admin is deleted or the properties are garbled, the Admin equivalency may be worthless as well.

So, when you grant someone the Supervisor trustee right to a section of the eDirectory tree, also grant them all other trustee rights. This precaution allows that person to maintain the ability to create, delete, rename, and modify objects, even if the Supervisor right is blocked by the IRF.

Part II

NDS Security Guidelines

Security management is not the most exciting stuff in the world, 99 percent of the time. The goal of this section is to help you ensure that the one percent of security management that is exciting—a security breach—happens only in the mildest way possible. (Maybe only a bad joke breach.)

Realize that few users need to create, delete, or modify objects (users, printers, and so on) during their normal workday. Those users who have occasion to need these trustee rights should be made an official or un-official helper. The designation of "Power User for Marketing" will help that person feel better about spending extra time helping other users without getting paid for it. At least recognize those power users, because recognized helpers will help keep security strong, not tear it down. The big problems come when someone accidentally gets too many rights, not when the department's power user has defined a new printer.

A CNI (Certified NetWare Instructor) friend of mine offers these guidelines for granting rights:

▶ Start with the default assignments. Defaults are in place to give users access to the resources they need without giving them access to resources or information they do not need.

▶ Avoid assigning rights through the All Properties option. Avoiding All Properties will protect private information about users and other resources on the network.

▶ Use Selected Properties to assign property rights. This will allow you to assign more specific rights and avoid future security problems.

▶ Use caution when assigning the Write property right to the ACL property of any object. This right effectively gives the trustee the ability to grant anyone, including himself or herself, all rights, including the Supervisor right. This is another reason to use extreme care when making rights assignments with All Properties.

▶ Use caution when granting the Supervisor object right to a Server object. This gives Supervisor filesystem rights to all volumes linked to that server. This object rights assignment should be made only after considering the implication of a network admin-istrator having access to all files on all volumes linked to a particular server. Furthermore, granting the Write property right to the ACL property of the Server object will also give Supervisor filesystem rights to all volumes linked to that particular server.

▶ Granting the Supervisor object right implies granting the Supervisor right to all properties. For some container administrators, you might want to grant all object rights except the Supervisor right and then grant property rights through the Selected Properties option.

▶ Use caution when filtering Supervisor rights with an IRF. For example, a container administrator uses an IRF to filter the network administrator's rights to a particular branch of the NDS eDirectory tree. If the network administrator (who has the Supervisor right to the container administrator's User object) deletes the User object of the container administrator, that particular branch of the NDS eDirectory tree can no longer be managed.

Here's my security slogan: Grant to containers or groups; ignore the individuals. The more individual users you administer, the more time and trouble it will take. I've known some NetWare managers to make groups holding only one person. That sounds stupid, but consider the alternative: When a second person comes, and then a third person, you'll find yourself handling each one by hand. If a group is in place, each new person who arrives takes only a few seconds to install and give all the necessary trustee rights and network resource mappings.

Whenever possible, handle security (access to network resources) through the container. If not a container, then through a group. If not a group, look harder to make the need fit an existing group or develop a new group. The more adamant you are about securing your network by groups rather than by individual users, the lighter your network management burden. The more you use the container to grant rights, the neater things are.

MANAGING SECURITY WITH CONSOLEONE

When NDS first installs, there are two objects: Admin and [Public]. By default, the Admin object has Supervisor object rights to [Root], which allows Admin to create and administer all other network objects.

The [Public] object has the following object and property rights by default:

▶ Browse object rights to [Root], which allows all users to see the NDS eDirectory tree and all objects on the tree

▶ Read property right to the Default Server property, which determines the default server for the User object

When you create User objects, each has a certain set of default rights. These rights include what the User object can do to manage itself, such as Read and Write the user's login script and print job configuration. To get around in the eDirectory tree, users are also granted limited rights to [Root] and [Public]. Here's a summary of the default User object trustee, default rights, and what these rights allow a user to do:

▶ Read right to all property rights, which allows the reading of properties stored in the User object

▶ Read and Write property rights to the user's own Login Script property, which allows users to execute and modify their own login scripts

▶ Read and Write property rights to the user's own Print Configuration property, which allows users to create print jobs and send them to the printer

The [Root] object has one default property right: the Read property right to Network Address and Group Membership, which identifies the network address and any group memberships.

As you can see, the default NDS rights are fairly limited. A new user can see the network, change his or her own login script and printer configuration, and wait for help.

If that's too much—perhaps you don't want users to have the ability to change (and mess up) their own login scripts—change it. Merely revoke the User object's Login Script property right. Figure 7.8 shows the User object details, with the Write capability for the Login Script property revoked. The Read capability is necessary so that the user can log in.

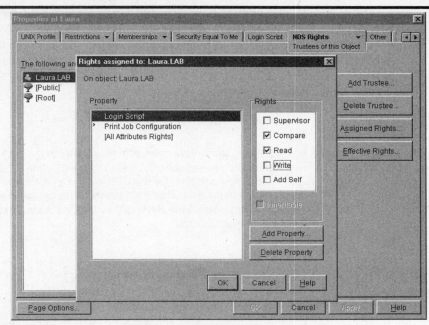

FIGURE 7.8: Preventing Laura from changing her login script

Revoking a Property Right

Think of this process as a prelude to the other security-management tasks we're going to do in the following sections. First, you must start ConsoleOne from some Java Virtual Machine (JVM)–enabled system and highlight the User object that you want to modify. You must either right-click and choose Properties or use the File ➢ Properties menu choice.

When we get to the property page for the User object (as you can see in Figure 7.8 in the previous section), we want to change the Property Rights setting. It may sound odd, or at least different, but with ConsoleOne, we need to check the Trustees of This Object right under NDS Rights. Drill down to Laura.LAB.TEXAS. Then click the Assigned Rights command button, which opens the Rights Assigned To dialog box. Scroll through the list, find Login Script, highlight it, and review the rights.

The default is to have both Read and Write capabilities. By clicking the Write check box, that right is cleared from our user. The change will become active after the dialog box is saved with the new setting and the NDS database has a second to digest the change.

In Figure 7.8, I also opened the Rights Assigned to: Laura.LAB dialog box by clicking the Effective Rights button from the NDS Rights page. When I highlighted Login Script, the rights for user Laura to her own login script were shown: Compare and Read appeared in the Rights box. So now we know user Laura has the capability to read, and therefore execute, the login script, but not to change it.

TIP

The other way to prevent users from playing with their login scripts is to bypass them entirely. Remember the sequence of login script execution? The User object's login script comes last. Just use the EXIT command in the container login script, and the personal login script for everyone in the container will be bypassed. Users can then make all the changes they want in their login scripts, but it won't make a bit of difference.

Setting or Modifying Directory and File Rights

You can allow a user or group of users access to a directory in two ways:

▶ You can go through the user side and use the rights-to-files-and-directories approach.

▶ You can go to the directory to be accessed and use the trustees-of-this-directory angle.

Which method you use depends on whether you're making one directory available to many users or granting trustee rights to one set of users to a lot of other network objects. We'll take a look at both approaches.

From the Group or User's Point of View

You can easily grant trustee rights for a single object to multiple volumes, directories, or files. The object gaining the rights should be a group of some kind, such as an Organization, an Organizational Unit, or a Group object, but it works for single User objects as well.

Start ConsoleOne as either the Admin user or another user with the Supervisor right to both the user side and the network resource side of this equation. Drill down until the group appears on the right side of Console One. We'll work with our Techies group in this example. Right-click that group, choose Properties, click the Rights to Files and Folders tab, and you'll see most of what appears in Figure 7.9.

First, click the Show command button to find and select the correct volume (COMPAQ-330_SYS: in this case). Then click the Add command button, select down to the directory level, and choose the Apache directory. Techs demand access to web pages and source code, so let them have it.

Notice that all rights are being granted to Techies. If you don't give them all rights, they'll just whine and complain until you change your mind and upgrade their rights. Give them all rights the first time, and then let them worry about what happens if they screw up. They're programmers, so if they do screw up, they'll never admit a thing. That's what I'm doing in Figure 7.9—giving them all rights to the Apache directory.

Unlike in NetWare Administrator or other Windows utilities, Console-One won't allow you to select multiple files or directories on the Rights to Files and Folders tab of the group's property page. You could use another utility, but I would rather you take the hint: Don't change one file at a time, but focus on the directory.

The default rights to any new volume, directory, or file are Read and File Scan. Figure 7.10 shows that this is the case for the Techies group's effective rights to the Documents directory.

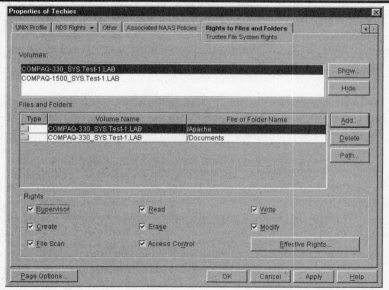

FIGURE 7.9:   Granting Techies access to the Apache directory

Contrast the limited array of rights (the default rights) in Figure 7.10 to the full platter of rights available in Figure 7.9. Although we all agree Techies can make good use of their full access to the web server directory,

Part II

giving them access to corporate documents may prove less useful. This is why they have almost no rights to the Documents folder. Trust me, writers hate to let techs attempt to write or edit their work.

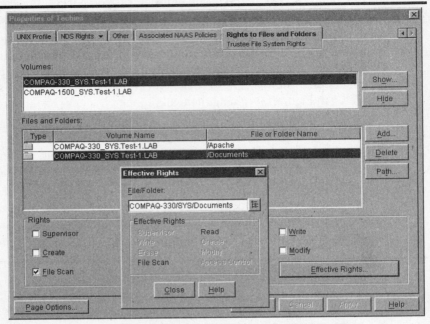

FIGURE 7.10:   Granted rights are bold; excluded rights are gray.

Granting rights to a directory in another container is not a problem, but one more step may be needed. If the users want to map a drive to another container in their login script, they can't get there from here. You must create an Alias object for the remote volume and then map the groups and users to the Alias.

You can grant trustee rights to a Volume object rather than to a directory or file. If you do, the object with those rights has complete access to the root directory, meaning the entire volume. If you have enough volumes to parcel them out in that manner, that's great, but many networks grant rights to a directory. That allows plenty of accessibility for the users, because they can build a full directory structure while still maintaining an easy method of control.

From the Directory or File's Point of View

Approaching rights from the directory's (or file's) point of view is the best method to use when granting several users or groups trustee rights to the same volume, directory, or file. One screen allows you to choose multiple trustees at once and yet assign different rights to each of them. Although this technique can work with volumes and files, let's use a common scenario: making a group of users trustees to a directory.

Start the ConsoleOne program. Browse through the NDS eDirectory tree as necessary to locate and highlight the object that you want to make available to the new user or users. In our example, the Documents directory is the one to be shared with Sandi and now the Writers Organizational Unit (yes, an OU can have trustee rights, as we discussed earlier).

Once the volume is highlighted in the left pane, the directories will appear in the right pane. Pressing Enter will display the directories in the left pane, leaving the right pane still empty. Right-click the directory name (in either pane you prefer) and choose Properties.

We added Sandi and the Techies earlier, so she and that group appear as trustees of the directory. Click the Add Trustee command button to open the Select Objects dialog box, and then select the Writers OU, as shown in Figure 7.11. Once you've found it, click OK to add the Writers OU to the list of trustees for the Documents directory.

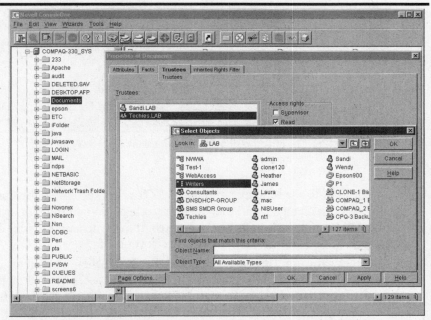

FIGURE 7.11:   Adding the Writers OU to the Documents directory's Trustees list

Once the new trustees are copied to the list, checking the Access Rights boxes for each group will set the level of control the group has over the directory. Few groups should ever have Supervisor rights, so leave that box unchecked.

In ConsoleOne, the Access Rights check boxes do an excellent job of showing the Effective Rights. In Figure 7.12, you can see that the Writers OU has all rights to the directory except Supervisor.

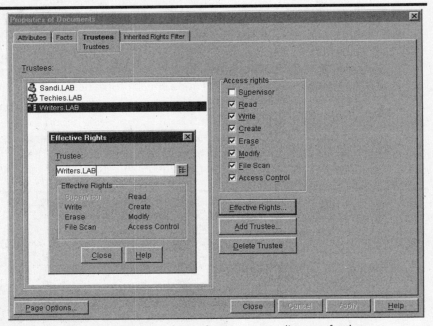

FIGURE 7.12:   The effective rights to the Documents directory for the Writers OU

Click OK to save and exit, or just click Close because the rights have already been changed, and then reenter to check that all the rights you planned to grant have in fact been granted. It's easy to skip a mouse-click here and there, so make it a habit to check yourself.

Once again, granting rights to a directory in another container is not a problem, but one more step may be needed. If the users want to map a drive to another container in their login script, they can't get there from here. You must create an Alias object for the remote volume and then map the groups and users to the Alias.

Setting or Modifying Object and Property Rights

Sometimes, one network resource must be managed, controlled, or modified by multiple other objects. That's what we did in the previous section. And sometimes, one object must manage or control multiple other objects.

The network administrator does this, of course, for the entire network. But many users need some control over more than just their home directory. Even medium-power users can help by controlling a department printer or volume. Real power users can become de facto subadministrators with the proper cooperation with your department.

Do you want to give an object trustee rights to more than one other object at a time? Here's the place. This procedure allows you to grant trustee rights to multiple objects from one screen.

As the Admin user or equivalent, start ConsoleOne. Highlight the object, such as a user, a group, or a container, that you want to make a trustee of one or more other objects, right-click, and choose Properties. Then click the NDS Rights tab and select Trustees of This Object from its menu.

The first step is to discover what the object already has rights to. This requires your first real search operation. Figure 7.13 shows the Select Objects dialog box open, with the user Laura's NDS Rights property page in the background. The Select Objects dialog box offers two ways to cruise the NDS eDirectory tree, and Figure 7.13 shows one of them.

When the dialog box opens, the current context displays. Use the down arrow at the end of the Look In box to display the full eDirectory tree down to your current context. If you need to go up only one context level, you can click the up-arrow icon to the right of the down arrow instead. Drill down, or slide up, the eDirectory tree until you find what you need. Because you're going to let Laura control some servers in a minute, you need to move up to the Test-1 Organization level.

Your goal is to Add Trustee. Browse through the NDS eDirectory tree and highlight the object or objects to gain trustee rights over, as shown in Figure 7.14. In our example, Laura now gains some control over the COMPAQ-1500 and COMPAQ-330 servers.

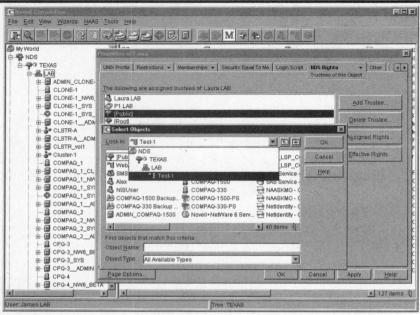

FIGURE 7.13: Searching for other objects for Laura to control

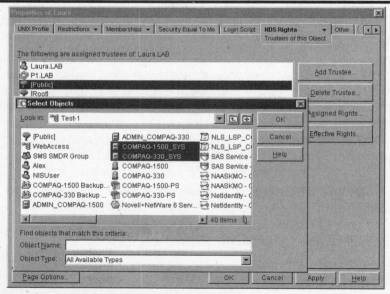

FIGURE 7.14: Laura selects volumes to control.

Notice that you may once again tag several objects in one screen by using either the Ctrl-key-and-multiple-click or the Shift-key-and-inclusive-click technique. You can see the current context of the items you're choosing, not the context of the objects gaining the trustee rights. Click OK to save your choices and move them to the Trustees of This Object property page for final configuration.

Figure 7.15 shows the final step in this process. You can configure both of your chosen objects concurrently. As long as one or more items in the Rights Assigned To list is highlighted, the check boxes will apply to all of the objects. Click the Assigned Rights button, and then click the rights you want the object to have over the target object (in our example, the rights of Laura over COMPAQ-1500_SYS and COMPAQ-330_SYS). When you're finished, click OK to save and exit the object's property page.

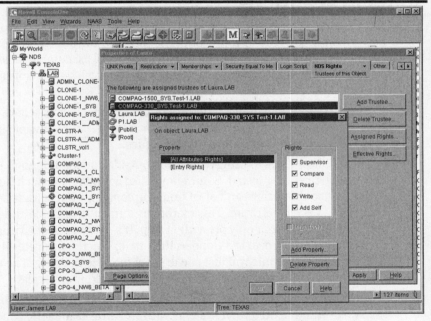

FIGURE 7.15:   Granting trustee rights to more than one object at a time

The same process works for modifying existing rights to objects. In that case, making sure you search the entire network for all objects is even more important. If you want to delete the assignment, highlight the previously Assigned Rights and click the Delete Property command button. The rights assignment, not the object itself, will be deleted.

PROTECTING YOUR NETWORK FROM VIRUSES

Viruses are always a concern, even if they are statistically insignificant. People worrying about viruses waste more time than viruses waste, although the proliferation of operating systems with Swiss cheese security (the initials are Microsoft) makes virus protection more critical than in years past. Knowing that a virus attack is rare doesn't make you feel any better or get your network back to normal any faster if it does happen. Time spent preventing viruses is much more fun than time spent cleaning up after one.

Some Precautions

You can take some precautions without adding optional software to your network or much time to your workday. Mark all .EXE and .COM files as Read Only. Viruses generally function by modifying executable files. If all your executable files are read-only, viruses have a much harder time getting started.

Keep a tight watch on users' access rights to system areas—there shouldn't be any. Only managers, with a proper understanding of virus prevention, should have access to system files.

Do not allow users to bring disks from outside and load them to the network before being tested. Some companies go so far as to lock floppy drives, not so that users can't steal from the company, but so that users can't load infected software. This method is difficult to enforce and not good enough to be your only prevention step. It's better to offer a virus-free check station for users to test floppies than try to ban floppies altogether. If you ban them, people will just sneak them into the building. The same goes for CDs, the preferred method of program distribution today.

The days when users regularly downloaded unknown files from bulletin boards and booted their systems with those disks are long gone. That's good. Commercially sponsored download sites now pride themselves on running a clean site. That's also good. But the number of files copied from unknown sources across the Internet is growing tremendously, and that's bad. Unix administrators often don't know which DOS and Windows files are on their systems, and they don't have the time or tools to test them for viruses. That's also bad.

Feel free to restrict or eliminate FTP (File Transfer Protocol) programs from your Internet suite of applications, except for those trustworthy users who understand the need for virus protection. Although you can't always stop users from downloading files with a web browser such as Netscape, keeping the FTP programs away from the general user population may help a little, even though few "regular" users ever attempt using FTP.

Virus-Protection Software

Special virus-protection software is available for networks, often in conjunction with software metering or network user management. If your company is overly concerned with a virus attack, the software may give some peace of mind. However, antivirus software used inconsistently is worse than none at all. When you have none, people are more careful. When you have antivirus software used poorly, people develop a false sense of protection.

Here are some of the virus-protection features the optional programs provide:

▶ Install and configure easily. NetWare versions are run as NLMs (new Java versions have yet to appear).

▶ Block unprotected clients from logging in to a protected server.

▶ Distribute protection to multiple servers and clients.

▶ Include an administration program for Windows as well as DOS.

▶ Send alerts to specified users when a questionable event occurs.

▶ Schedule when and how security sweeps are made.

▶ Report on status and other statistics.

There are two major camps regarding the primary means of protection against the virus-developer community. One idea is to track the signature of all viruses. The *signature* is a piece of code inside the virus that identifies that virus, usually included by the virus criminal as an ego enhancer. As more viruses are discovered, the signature database must grow. Those systems that scan for known virus signatures should receive regular database updates.

The other option is to register a *CRC* (cyclical redundancy check) of every executable file on the server when the file is installed. The CRC is checked each time the file is read from the server. If the CRC value changes, this means that the file has been tampered with. The alert sounds, and the software shuts down the use of that file.

I lean toward the CRC method, for several reasons. First, a new virus obviously can cause you problems, and this threat is eliminated with a CRC. Second, the overhead of checking a large virus database with every file-read request will only get heavier. As the demands on servers grow, this overhead will become burdensome. Finally, my friend John McCann was one of the first programmers to make quality add-on NetWare utilities, and he says the CRC method is better. He knows more about NetWare programming than anyone else I know, so I'll take his word for it. (It's especially easy when I agree with his conclusion anyway.)

Do you have a favorite antivirus program? Do I? Not really. Be sure to check several major brands if you don't have virus protection already (and why don't you have protection already?). Those readers with multivendor networks (which usually means some Windows NT or 2000 servers) will find that many of the companies in this market make virus products for both NetWare and NT/2000.

Some people ask about the values of server-based versus client-based virus protection. We could even have separate sections extolling the virtues of both types of protection. But we won't, because I feel strongly that you can't trust users to do your job for you. Yes, the users will suffer if they have a virus attack on their personal system, but they will demand that you fix things for them. So, asking them to protect against virus attacks on the client is asking them to do your job for you. Even if they were willing, they don't have the mental discipline to do a good job. They'll trust a file from a friend, assuming their friend knows the file's history. That's usually a bad move, as recent virus writers have demonstrated by forwarding viruses through every contact in an infected system's Outlook address book (thanks again, Windows).

A critical part of virus protection is regular updates. Server-based products need a single update session to protect hundreds of clients. This is much more efficient (and reliable) than upgrading hundreds of clients individually.

Verify that your virus protection works on the client when the user logs in. Kicking off a check of the client during the login process catches most of the viruses introduced by careless users. You won't catch them all, unfortunately, because if you make the process idiot-proof, your company will hire a better idiot. Just make sure the virus doesn't spread.

TIP

If your manager is particularly scared of a virus attack, use that fear to your advantage. Clip an article about a virus attack and the resulting damage to the company. Nearly every single report includes a line about how the company had an inadequate backup procedure in place, meaning extra loss. If you've been angling for a bigger tape backup system or an upgrade, play the cards you're dealt, and hit your manager with the tape backup request in one hand while waving the virus attack article in the other hand. Is this dishonest? Not at all. Some people need to be pushed into doing the right thing. You should take care to push your manager when he or she is already staggering. This way, you don't need to push noticeably hard, but you still get what your network needs. Our world will never be virus-free again, so you must keep upgrading your protection systems. Nudge and/or blackmail your management as necessary.

NetWare 6 Security Improvements

Ever-evolving features required Novell to add some bang to the security section of NetWare 4.1x and NetWare 5. Novell could have done this by adding a few extra security screens everyone ignores, marked the security matrix as "improved," and gone on with its business.

Security became much more prominent than that. Novell hired one of the original developers of the U.S. government's "Red Book" security project. That developer, and other work done by Novell deep inside the operating system, helped certify NetWare 4.11 as a "C2 Red Book" network. This is a big deal. NetWare 6 must also be certified, but Novell officials declared this rating important and will submit NetWare 6 soon.

Part II

WHY IS C2 SECURITY CERTIFICATION A BIG DEAL?

First of all, it's a big deal because Microsoft made so much noise about Windows NT getting C2 security. The Novell folks can't stand for Microsoft to beat them in any purchase order check-off category, and that's what was happening. The fact that Windows NT was only C2 secure in stand-alone mode left the door open for Novell to top Microsoft, at least in the PR war. Not that the government followed its own regulations; departments regularly ignored the security guidelines and bought NT.

Second, it's a big deal for customers who support and use such security systems already, such as the government, the armed forces, and paranoid corporations. It's true that the government has a sizable NetWare installed base, and huge areas of some departments can't run computer equipment rated lower than C2.

Does C2 security do much for you? Probably not. Realistically, C2-level security is a giant hassle, and few companies go to that much trouble. If your company is one of the C2 adherents, you know of what I speak.

I will be amazed if your company increases your NetWare security profile up to the C2 level, unless you work for one of the aforementioned groups such as the military. For one thing, only C2-authorized software can run on a NetWare NTCB (Network Trusted Computing Base). All those NLMs you have will be gone, unless they've been certified.

Are you and the other administrators certified? Gone. Do you have NetWare 3.x networks still running on your corporate network? Gone. Only secure systems can run on a secure network. Do you have your server under lock and key? Gone until that's done. Have you limited access to remote console programs, such as RCONSOLE? Gone. See what I mean? It's more trouble than it's worth, at least for the majority of corporations.

Adding the JVM will make your NetWare 6 server more popular for all types of utilities for the server, including security. Distributed applications are all the rage today, and security is becoming a consideration in the design phase. This falls under the heading of "a good thing," as Martha Stewart would say.

NetWare 6 includes a certificate authority for added security, but don't confuse that with C2 security certification. Those certificates guarantee that traffic across the Internet came from whom you think it came from and have nothing to do with normal, intracompany network business. We won't go into much depth with the Internet security options, because that topic deserves a book or two or 10 devoted to ways to secure Internet traffic.

WHEN SECURITY STINKS, MANAGEMENT SMELLS THE WORST

A "rock and a hard place" describes security. The tougher the security, the more people will hate the network. Looser security makes for happier users but more virus problems and file mishaps.

Remember, here we're speaking about NetWare security, not complete Internet security for all your web and e-mail servers. That subject has its own bookshelf.

Your company routinely allows access to every room of your building to the lowest paid, and least monitored, employees: cleaning crews. The biggest risk is crews employed by the building management, especially those who use temporary helpers. Do you have any idea what these people are doing? Does your management? Probably not.

This is one of the areas where hard choices must be made, and your management must make them. If your bosses won't do their jobs, push a little. If they still refuse, document the security measures in place and the reasons for those measures, and apply them absolutely. When users complain to their bosses, and their bosses complain to your boss, let your boss modify the procedure. Then get your boss to sign any changes. Accountability is shared; blame is yours alone.

Don't let management overcompensate for lousy security elsewhere by tightening the screws on the network. That's like a bank that has a vault full of cash, while the bearer bonds, cashier checks, and negotiable securities are lying out in the open, ready to be picked up and carried away.

Force management to define a consistent security profile. It makes no sense to restrict network users to the bone while leaving the president's file cabinet unlocked. People looking to steal information, both from the inside and outside, will happily take paper or computer disks. Although it isn't legal to steal a report off your computer system, it is legal to grab a printout of that same report out of the dumpster.

Inconsistent security control runs both ways. I once had a customer so worried about security that he refused to have a fax server on the network. The owner was afraid of dial-in hackers going through the fax modem into the computer system. We finally convinced the owner that this was impossible.

The flip side was a major oil company in the mid-1980s that had the typical tight security on its mainframe. Terminal and user IDs were tracked, users were monitored, and passwords were everywhere—the whole bit. Then someone noticed it was possible to copy information from the mainframe to a PC connected with an IRMA board (an adapter in the PC that connected via coax to an SNA cluster controller, effectively making the PC a 3270 terminal). A management committee studied the matter and verified that yes, anyone could copy any information from the mainframe to disks and paper. The information could then be dropped in the trash, carried home, or sold to a competitor. All these options obviously violated the company's security guidelines.

What did the managers do? They decided to ignore the problem and placed no security on PCs with IRMA boards beyond what they had on the terminals the PCs replaced. It may be noble to trust the employees, but it was inconsistent security. Those users with PCs deserved security training and a warning about the severity of potential security leaks. They got nothing, because corporate management was too lazy to do its job. If a problem developed, who would be blamed? You know—the computer managers who had no control over the decision.

If you thought your managers were paranoid before, wait until they come to you waving copies of the *Wall Street Journal* predicting doom and gloom because hackers stopped another website for a few minutes. Is this a realistic threat to your servers? Probably not, especially when running your web servers on NetWare. Is this a realistic threat to your schedule because of paranoid managers? Probably—your whole day will be wasted chasing nonexistent loopholes and manager security blankets.

WHAT'S NEXT

In this chapter, you learned about securing a Novell Netware 6 network. As with the other chapters in this part of the book, you learned how to use login security and directory permissions, and we offered general guidelines for creating a secure network. In Chapter 8 you will learn about another operating system gaining popularity—Linux—and how to create a secure system install.

Chapter 8

Linux System Installation and Setup

T his chapter discusses the security implications of the following Linux server administration tasks:

- ▶ Choosing a Linux distribution
- ▶ Building a secure kernel
- ▶ User account security
- ▶ File and directory permissions
- ▶ `syslog` security
- ▶ Filesystem encryption

Note that you will be taking on these tasks before you even connect your server to the network. Although most of us associate security with network layer services, a number of important security issues must be decided during the setup and configuration of the system itself. This chapter guides you through the

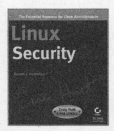

Adapted from *Linux Security* by Ramón J. Hontañón
ISBN 0-7821-2741-X $49.99

process of choosing the distribution that is best suited for your security needs and goes on to offer specific advice on how to configure your kernel to maximize system and network security. Finally, this chapter gives you practical advice on securing the accounts and the filesystem to ensure that you can offer your users an adequate level of protection against attacks from other legitimate, or seemingly legitimate, system users. You'll learn how to minimize the exposure of your root user, and you'll learn about the tools available to implement filesystem encryption on your Linux server.

Let's start by taking a look at the process of selecting a Linux distribution that's right for you.

Choosing a Linux Distribution

A crucial step in building a secure Linux server is selecting the distribution that best fits the needs outlined in your security policy. This decision is going to determine much of your success in installing and maintaining a secure Linux server. But what exactly makes a distribution "secure"? Here is a set of criteria to consider before making that decision:

- ▶ Does the vendor have a well-known mechanism to report security vulnerabilities found in its distribution?

- ▶ Does the vendor issue periodic security advisories that warn users of vulnerabilities found in its distribution?

- ▶ How often are security issues resolved? Does the vendor devote a well-delineated portion of its web or FTP site to security information (patches, security updates, and so on)?

- ▶ How often does the vendor release general distribution upgrades? A slow-moving release schedule is likely to prolong the exposure of known vulnerabilities.

- ▶ Does the vendor offer an intuitive, easy-to-use tool for installing and updating software packages?

- ▶ Does the vendor support open source efforts to improve Linux security or to create vendor-neutral security scripts and tools?

- ▶ How long has the vendor has been in existence?

- ▶ Have the previous versions been secure and well maintained?

As with any other choice of Linux software, there is no clear winner here, but you can make a more educated decision by finding out the vendor's general stance in these areas. The following sections look at the most prominent Linux distributions and examine the security features of each one.

Red Hat

As the most successful Linux vendor to date, Red Hat has been able to devote considerable resources to the tracking, dissemination, and resolution of security flaws in the packages that it distributes. Its RPM package management system is the industry standard, and its release schedule calls for a major revision every six months or so, which ensures that you're always running recent (and often more secure) software packages. This schedule is a good compromise between having up-to-date software and avoiding the "bleeding edge" of the latest (and often unstable) versions of most tools.

Red Hat's numbering scheme seems to use the .0 minor number for an initial major release (for example, 7.0) and .1 and .2 for the subsequent maintenance updates. If you opt for Red Hat, you should try to upgrade up from a .0 release as soon as the update is available. You may want to wait until the company releases the 7.1 or later version to make sure that any critical bugs have been fixed in the previous version.

Caldera

Rivaling Red Hat's success, Caldera's OpenLinux has grown into a major player in the Linux distribution market. Unlike Red Hat, Caldera maintains two separate release lines for clients (eDesktop) and servers (eServer). Both of these packages are now in a stable release line, although new versions are usually not available as often as Red Hat's.

Like Red Hat, Caldera offers a well-laid-out mechanism for updating releases by downloading the appropriate packages (also in RPM format) from its FTP site. Caldera seems to be increasingly committed to offering a security-minded distribution, and most vulnerabilities are addressed by software updates within one or two days of being identified.

Security advisories for OpenLinux can be found at www.calderasystems .com/support/security/ (see Figure 8.1). This is the longest running resource of its kind, and it includes a chronological list of advisories for all OpenLinux packages and all the available patches or solutions.

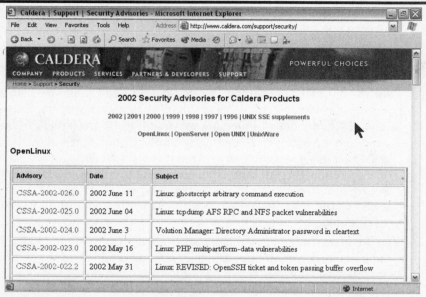

FIGURE 8.1: OpenLinux security advisories

SuSE

An extremely popular distribution in the European market, SuSE offers a full-featured set of supported packages (six CDs worth of them!) and also uses the RPM package management system. Its release schedule is similar to Red Hat's with the .0 minor numbers signaling the initial offering of a major release. However, SuSE typically offers up to four minor releases (such as 6.4) before moving on to another major version. Red Hat, on the other hand, generally has only two minor releases with each version.

One of SuSE's distinguishing characteristics is the inclusion of the seccheckscript that can be periodically invoked from cron, to test the overall security of the system in a number of areas. The vendor also includes a utility that you can use to "harden" your server installation (harden_suse). This is a sign that this vendor is concerned with security and is willing to spend development and maintenance resources to prove it.

You can find this vendor's security clearinghouse at www.suse.com/ us/support/security/index.html (see Figure 8.2), including a comprehensive list of advisories and pointers to their two security-related mailing lists.

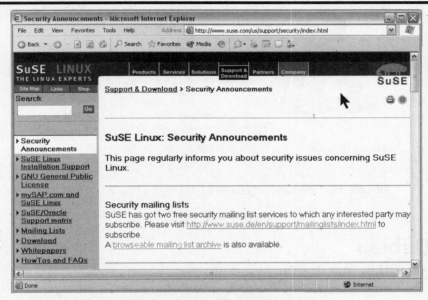

FIGURE 8.2: SuSE security page on the World Wide Web

Turbolinux

This vendor has been in the Linux market since 1992 and has had a great deal of success in the Asian and European markets. Even though it has not been embraced as widely as Red Hat and Caldera in the U.S., it has gained a lot of momentum in recent months, especially in the high-end server application market.

The Turbolinux release schedule is significantly longer than Red Hat's and Caldera's, but this vendor maintains a list of security updates for each release at www.turbolinux.com/security (see Figure 8.3). It also includes a separate security subdirectory for each release update section in its FTP site.

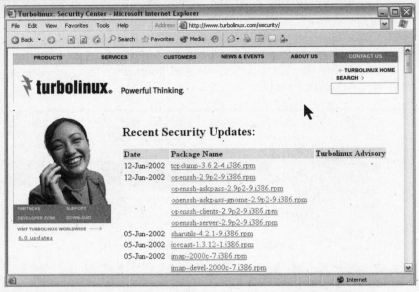

FIGURE 8.3: Turbolinux Security Center page on the World Wide Web

Debian

This Linux distribution is maintained by a group of about 500 volunteer developers around the world. Due to its nonprofit nature, the release schedule for Debian's Linux distribution is different from most commercial vendors', focusing on small interim minor releases rather than major updates. These small releases are often driven by a number of security fixes, and are usually about 100 days apart.

Unlike most commercial vendors, Debian has a clearinghouse for security information at www.debian.org/security/ that you can use for this purpose (see Figure 8.4). This is one of the most straightforward vendor security sites available. The content is well organized, and the security advisories are easier to find than those of the other vendors. In addition, the page includes links to the archives of the Debian-specific security mailing list, going back at least two years.

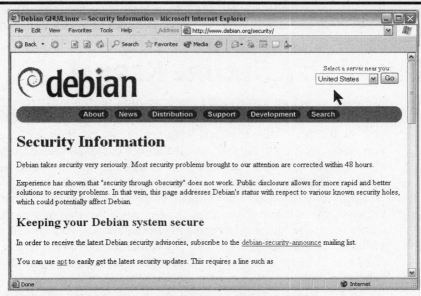

FIGURE 8.4:   Debian's security page on the World Wide Web

And the Winner Is...

All Linux distributions can be made secure, and all vendors are making an effort to keep users informed of vulnerabilities and patch availability. Although each vendor seems to excel in a different aspect of security, there are no clear winners or losers here.

Your choice of a Linux distribution should depend on your administrative style. If you're willing to spend some time every few days catching up with the latest vulnerabilities, and you're willing to install incremental patches as needed, Debian is a good choice for you. If instead you prefer to bundle security updates with vendor releases, you should opt for a more actively updated distribution, such as Red Hat, Caldera, SuSE, or Turbolinux.

In either case, you should plan to make use of the security resources of your vendor of choice, including a daily scan through its web page and a subscription to its security mailing list. In addition, you should monitor

the BugTraq mailing list (online.securityfocus.com/cgi-bin/
sfonline/forums.pl) for vulnerabilities common to all Linux vendors.

BUILDING A SECURE KERNEL

Although most Linux users are content to run the standard kernel provided in the latest distribution, you'll need to become familiar with the
process of downloading the kernel sources, modifying their configuration, and building a custom kernel. Building a custom kernel has its
advantages: You're specifying the security options that you want, and
you're also building a lean kernel, compiling only the driver support
that you need. Another benefit to compiling your own kernel is that you
know what is in it and you can see any security holes that may need to be
addressed in the future or immediately (if the holes are big enough). In
addition, the solution to many security vulnerabilities comes in the form
of a patch to be applied to the Linux kernel, which requires you to recompile the kernel.

The first step in building a custom kernel is to obtain the kernel sources.
If you're using Red Hat, you need both the kernel-headers and kernel-
source RPM packages. To install either of these packages, use one of the
following commands:

```
[root]# rpm -q kernel-headers
kernel-headers-2.2.12-20
[root]# rpm -q kernel-source
kernel-source-2.2.12-20
```

These two packages populate the /usr/src/linux directory, which
should contain all the source and configuration files necessary to compile
the Linux kernel from scratch.

TIP

Before you install your new kernel, create an emergency boot disk in case
the new kernel has problems booting. On Red Hat, use the command:
mkbootdisk –device /dev/fd0 2.2.12-20 (assuming that your system
modules directory is /lib/modules/2.2.12-20).

Logged on as root, go to the Linux source directory and clean up any lingering configurations from previous kernel builds using the following commands:

```
[root]# cd /usr/local/linux
[root]# make mrproper
```

At this point, you're ready to specify the options that you'd like to build into the kernel using this command:

```
[root]# make config
```

This command prompts you for a series of options that you can choose to add to your kernel (Y), leave out (N), or add as a dynamically loaded module (M). Table 8.1 shows the 2.2.X kernel options that have security implications and should be set to the appropriate value during the make config step.

TABLE 8.1:   Kernel Configuration: Recommended Security Options

CONFIGURE OPTION	RECOMMENDATION	DESCRIPTION
CONFIG_PACKET	Y	Protocol used by applications to communicate with network devices without a need for an intermediate kernel protocol
CONFIG_NETLINK	Y	Two-way communication between the kernel and user processes
CONFIG_FIREWALL	Y	Firewalling support
CONFIG_INET	Y	Internet (TCP/IP) protocols
CONFIG_IP_FIREWALL	Y	IP packet-filtering support
CONFIG_SYN_COOKIES	Y	Protection against synflooding denial of service attacks
CONFIG_NET_IPIP	N	IP inside IP encapsulation
CONFIG_IP_ROUTER	N	IP routing
CONFIG_IP_FORWARD	N	IP packet forwarding (routing)
CONFIG_IP_MULTICAST	N	IP Multicast (transmission of one data stream for multiple destinations)

Part II

The CONFIG_SYN_COOKIES option prevents the kernel from entering a deadlock state whenever its incoming connection buffers are filled with half-open TCP connections. Note that in the 2.2.X kernels, setting CONFIG_SYN_COOKIES simply enables the option, but does not actually activate it. You must enter the following to activate SYN_COOKIES support:

```
[root]# echo 1 > /proc/sys/net/ipv4/tcp_syncookies
```

The CONFIG_IP_ROUTER and CONFIG_IP_FORWARD options allow a multi-homed Linux server to forward packets from one interface to another. This option should be disabled because there is a possibility that an intruder could use your Linux server as a router, circumventing the normal path of entry into your network (the one you are policing).

The final step before actually compiling the kernel sources is to build a list of dependencies using this command:

```
[root]# make dep
```

Now you're ready to compile your new kernel. Execute the following command to compile and link a compressed kernel image:

```
[root]# make zImage
```

If you have chosen loadable module support during the previous make config step, you'll also need to execute the following commands:

```
[root]# make modules
```

```
[root]# make modules_install
```

To boot the new kernel, you must first move it from the source directory to its final destination. Make a backup of the old image first using these commands:

```
[root]# cp /zImage /zImage.BACKUP
```

```
[root]# mv /usr/src/linux/arch/i386/boot/zImage /zImage
```

```
[root]# /sbin/lilo
```

Rerun lilo every time you update the kernel image on your hard drive. In addition, it is a good idea to create a separate lilo.conf entry for your backup kernel (/zImage.BACKUP), even though you have an emergency boot diskette, because planning for disasters is an important part of security. When you are updating your version of Linux, it is always good to be able to go back to the old version if the newer one does not work as it should. See *Linux Network Servers 24seven* by Craig Hunt (Sybex, 1999) if you need more information about lilo and lilo.conf.

You should now restart your system to make sure that you can boot the new kernel. Don't forget to have your emergency boot disk close by in case there are problems.

WARNING

Be prepared for the worst, because if you aren't prepared, the worst is going to happen to you.

USER ACCOUNT SECURITY

The CSI/FBI Computer Crime and Security Survey (www.gocsi.com/press/20020407.html) shows, year after year, that the overwhelming majority of successful system attacks come from insiders—that is, disgruntled (or just bored) nonprivileged users who manage to gain root authority through subversive means. Even when the attack comes from the outside, seizing a misconfigured or stagnant user account is one of the easiest ways to crack access to root. It's also important to protect against your own mistakes, because root access can be a powerful and dangerous tool, even in the proper hands.

You should pay special attention to the part of your security policy that regulates the creation and maintenance of user accounts. Here is my recommended set of considerations for managing your Linux server accounts:

> **Disable Inactive Accounts.**   Attackers look for accounts that have not been accessed for a while in order to seize them for their nefarious ends. This gives attackers the luxury of being able to "squat" the account and hide their exploits without being noticed or reported. Most Linux distributions allow you to specify the conditions under which an account should be disabled. I recommend that you disable all accounts as soon as the password expires (more on password expiration later), while allowing users a week to change their passwords before they expire. Red Hat's linuxconf provides a graphical interface to specify this policy (see Figure 8.5).
>
> I usually set passwords to expire every four months (120 days) and allow users seven days to change their passwords. The 0 value under Account Expire After # Days simply directs the system to disable the account if the password expires. The default value

of −1 directs the system never to cause the account to expire, so make sure you change this default.

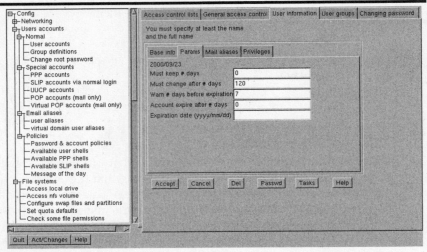

FIGURE 8.5:   Setting user account expiration parameters with `linuxconf`

Disable Root Access Across NFS Mounts.   Pay special attention to the /etc/exports file, where you declare the local filesystems that you'd like to share via Network File System (NFS). By default, the NFS server on most Linux distributions maps user ID 0 (root) to a nonprivileged user, like nobody. This behavior, however, can be overridden by the no_root_squash option in the NFS server's /etc/exports file. Avoid this option at all costs. It leaves your entire NFS server at the mercy of a root user on any of your clients.

See *Linux NFS and Automounter Administration* by Erez Zadok (Sybex, 2001) if you have set up your Linux clients to mount remote NFS shares automatically.

Restrict the Use of Your Root User to When It's Absolutely Necessary.   You should resist the temptation to log on to root to execute an administration command and stay logged on to execute other user-level commands. The longer you're logged on as root, the longer you're exposed to a number of vulnerabilities, such as Trojan horses and session hijacking.

Use a Descriptive Root Prompt.   Sometimes you are your worst enemy. When you have several terminals active on your

X-display, it's important to be able to tell at a glance which ones are root terminals. This helps you avoid executing a user-level command on a root window by mistake. Make sure the root prompt is distinctive enough and that it includes a root-specific character, such as a sharp sign (#).

Use a Minimal *$PATH* for Your Root Account.   A common attack on the root account is to place Trojan horse versions of frequently used utilities in a directory that is included in the root $PATH. This is a very subtle attack, and the only way to protect against it is to ensure that you know the contents of your $PATH variable and the contents of the directories included in the variable. To minimize the chance of running a Trojan horse, avoid having directories in your $PATH that are writeable by any user other than root.

Use Special-Purpose System Accounts.   An operator who simply needs to shut down the system does not need full root privileges. That's the purpose of default Linux accounts such as operator and shutdown. In addition, I recommend that you install and use sudo, which is described in detail in the section "The sudo Utility" later in this chapter.

Use Group Memberships.   As a Linux administrator, you'll often be asked to make a file or directory available for reading and writing to several users who are collaborating on a single task. Although it is easy to simply make these resources world-writeable, don't do it. Take the time to add a new group, make each of the users a member of this group, and make the resources accessible only to members of the group. Think of files with wide-open permissions as vulnerabilities waiting to be exploited.

Restrict Root Logins to the System Console.   To monitor who is logging in as root, configure the /etc/securetty file to allow direct root access only from the console. This action forces authorized root users to use su or sudo to gain root privileges, thus allowing you to easily log these events. The standard Linux default is to allow root logins only from the eight virtual system consoles (function keys on the keyboard):

```
[root]# more /etc/securetty
tty1
tty2
tty3
```

```
tty4
tty5
tty6
tty7
tty8
```

Aside from the logging advantage, this is an extra hurdle in the event that the root password becomes compromised. Intruders would have to first gain access to a regular user's account (or to the physical console) to exploit their finding.

Using good user account practices is paramount to ensuring the security of your system, but by choosing a poor password, users can undermine all the work you have done to protect their accounts. The next section offers some practical advice on choosing strong passwords and enforcing their use.

Good Passwords

Although stronger modes of authentication are becoming increasingly commonplace, using a username and password remains the most widely used method of authentication for Linux servers. Much has been said and written about the importance of password security, so I'll keep this discussion brief and to the point. There are some very simple rules to follow that can go a long way toward locking down your password policy:

Don't Set Your System to Cause Passwords to Expire Too Quickly.   If the period between password expirations is too short, users are more likely to feel that they'll forget their passwords, so they will write them down. In addition, users will use cyclic, predictable password patterns. When it comes to password expiration, anything less than three months should be considered too short.

Don't Allow Your Passwords to Get Stale.   Conversely, if you allow your users to have the same password for a year, they're exposing it for a longer time than is safe. Four months is a good compromise, but six months is not an unreasonably long expiration period.

Avoid Short Passwords.   Force your users to pick passwords that are at least six characters in length. Anything shorter than that is too easy to guess using brute force attacks, even if random characters are chosen. Figure 8.6 illustrates how you can enforce a password length minimum using a systems administration tool like Red Hat's linuxconf. Note that in addition to enforcing the six-character limit, this page forces the user to use a minimum of two nonalphanumeric characters.

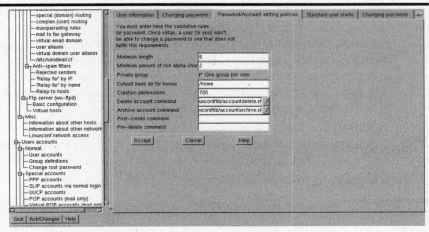

FIGURE 8.6: Setting password length parameters with linuxconf

Crack Your Own Passwords. As part of your periodic system security audit, use password-guessing tools to look for weak passwords in your /etc/passwd file. Contact the guilty users directly and suggest to them that they use longer passwords, with more nonalphanumeric characters and a mix of uppercase and lowercase characters.

Delete Unused Accounts. Most Linux servers don't offer Unix-to-Unix Copy (UUCP), Point-to-Point Protocol (PPP), Network News Transfer Protocol (NNTP), Gopher, or Postgres services, yet most Linux distributions ship with these accounts. Completely remove these accounts and any others that don't make sense in your environment.

Avoid Empty Password Fields. Never set up users with no password, even if their shell is highly restricted. Gaining access to any user on your system gets intruders halfway to their destination.

An effective way to minimize the risk associated with user passwords is to configure support for shadow password and group files. This is the topic of the next section.

Shadow Passwords

One of the easiest system vulnerabilities to overlook is the ability by any user to *crack* another user's password. This can be done quickly and easily, using tools readily available on the Internet. To prevent this, enable *shadow passwords*. Shadow passwords split the password files into two: the /etc/passwd file, which contains a placeholder in the actual password field entries, and the /etc/shadow file, which contains the encrypted password. The /etc/shadow file does not need to be readable by anyone except root, which makes it more difficult for a regular user to attempt to crack another user's password (including root).

Most Linux distributions also support the concept of *shadow groups*, where the actual members of each group are not listed in the main /etc/group file, but rather in the /etc/gshadow file, which, like the /etc/shadow file, is readable only by root.

TIP

Some Linux distributions do not have shadow passwords enabled by default. If your distribution is one of these, enable this feature right away.

Listing 8.1 shows how you should look for the existence of the /etc/shadow file. If it does not exist, simply create it with the pwconv command. Note the change in the /etc/passwd file after the conversion:

Listing 8.1: Creating a Shadow Password File

```
[root]# ls -1 /etc/shadow
ls: /etc/shadow: No such file or directory
[root]# more /etc/passwd
root:PV/67t9IGeTjU:0:0:root:/root:/bin/bash
bin:*:1:1:bin:/bin:
daemon:*:2:2:daemon:/sbin:
adm:*:3:4:adm:/var/adm:
lp:*:4:7:lp:/var/spool/lpd:
sync:*:5:0:sync:/sbin:/bin/sync
shutdown:*:6:0:shutdown:/sbin:/sbin/shutdown
halt:*:7:0:halt:/sbin:/sbin/halt
mail:*:8:12:mail:/var/spool/mail:
operator:*:11:0:operator:/root:
ftp:*:14:50:FTP User:/home/ftp:
```

```
nobody:*:99:99:Nobody:/:
ramon:aalg0.pAVx2uA:501:100:Ramon J. Hontanon:/home/ramon:
   /bin/bash
[root]# pwconv
[root]# ls -l /etc/shadow
-r-----   1 root     root            563 Sep 23 15:27 /etc/shadow
[root]# more /etc/passwd
root:x:0:0:root:/root:/bin/bash
bin:x:1:1:bin:/bin:
daemon:x:2:2:daemon:/sbin:
adm:x:3:4:adm:/var/adm:
lp:x:4:7:lp:/var/spool/lpd:
sync:x:5:0:sync:/sbin:/bin/sync
shutdown:x:6:0:shutdown:/sbin:/sbin/shutdown
halt:x:7:0:halt:/sbin:/sbin/halt
mail:x:8:12:mail:/var/spool/mail:
operator:x:11:0:operator:/root:
ftp:x:14:50:FTP User:/home/ftp:
nobody:x:99:99:Nobody:/:
ramon:x:501:100:Ramon J. Hontanon:/home/ramon:/bin/bash
[root]# more /etc/shadow
root:PV/67t9IGeTjU:11223:0:99999:7:::
bin:*:11223:0:99999:7:::
daemon:*:11223:0:99999:7:::
adm:*:11223:0:99999:7:::
lp:*:11223:0:99999:7:::
sync:*:11223:0:99999:7:::
shutdown:*:11223:0:99999:7:::
halt:*:11223:0:99999:7:::
mail:*:11223:0:99999:7:::
operator:*:11223:0:99999:7:::
ftp:*:11223:0:99999:7:::
nobody:*:11223:0:99999:7:::
ramon:aalg0.pAVx2uA:11223:0:99999:7
```

The next section of this chapter discusses the sudo utility, a useful tool to minimize the exposure of the root password to your Linux server.

The sudo Utility

During the normal course of administering my Linux systems, I often go several weeks before actually logging on as the root user. In fact, there have been times when I have come close to forgetting the root password.

The sudo utility affords me this luxury, and I recommend that you install this tool on every system that you administer. By allowing the system administrator to predefine root access for regular users, sudo can be used to execute commands with root privileges in lieu of actually logging in as root and exposing the root password on the network. In general, the less often the root password is actually typed, the more secure it will be.

Installing *sudo*

You can download sudo in both RPM and source format. I recommend that you use the RPM package system to install it, because the default compilation parameters are typically rational, and there is very little need for customization.

Let's start the installation by ensuring that sudo is not already present:

```
[root]# rpm -q sudo
sudo-1.5.9p4-1
```

In this case, you do have a previous installation of sudo, but it's out of date, so delete it and install a more current version using the following commands:

```
[root]# rpm -e sudo
[root]# rpm -i ./sudo-1.6.3p5-1rh62.i386.rpm
[root]# rpm -q sudo
sudo-1.6.3p5-1
```

You now have installed the sudo utility. Make sure you take a look through /usr/doc for the documentation that comes with the source package before you start using the tool.

The *sudoers* file

As with any Linux utility, sudo comes with a configuration file where you can customize its operation. This file is in /etc/sudoers by default, and contains, among other things, the list of users who should be allowed to run the sudo command, along with the set of commands that each sudo user is allowed to execute.

The general format used to add users to this file is as follows:

```
user    host(s)=command(s)[run_as_user(s)]
```

For example, if you'd like to grant user alice permission to run the shutdown command, you specify the following:

```
alice ALL = /etc/shutdown
```

Note that the ALL directive can be used as a wildcard for any fields in the sudoers file. Let's consider another example where user bob is given access to all root commands, as any user:

```
bob ALL = ALL
```

And finally, let's consider the case where you'd like user charlie to be allowed to run su to become user operator:

```
charlie ALL = /bin/su operator
```

WARNING

If you're using sudo to grant a user root access to a limited set of commands, make sure that none of these commands allow an "escape" to a Linux shell, because that would give the user unrestricted root access to *all* system commands. Note that some Linux editors (such as vi) include this shell escape feature.

Using ⌊udo

The basic usage of the sudo command is as follows:

```
sudo [command line options] [username] [command]
```

Table 8.2 contains a summary of the most important sudo command-line options.

TABLE 8.2: sudo Command-Line Options

OPTION	PARAMETER	PURPOSE
-u	username	Runs the command as the specified username (default is root)
-v	N/A	Prints out the current version
-l	N/A	Lists the allowed and forbidden commands for this user
-h	N/A	Prints a usage message
-b	N/A	Runs the command in the background

For example, to show the contents of the shadow password directory, simply use:

```
sudo cat /etc/shadow
```

To edit a file in a user's directory preserving his or her permissions, use the following:

```
sudo -u fred vi /export/home/fred/.forward
```

I recommend that you use the sudo command strictly to log the root activity of users who are fully trusted to execute any root command on your Linux server (including yourself), rather than using it to allow certain users to execute a small set of system utilities. It is relatively easy for a user to maliciously extend the privilege of a given command by executing an escape command to the root shell.

The following section describes sudo's logging features, as well as the format of the sudo log file.

The *sudo.log* file

By default, sudo logs all its activity to the file /var/log/sudo.log. The format of entries into this file is as follows:

```
date:user:HOST=hostname:TTY=terminal:PWD=dir:USER=user:
    COMMAND=cmd
```

Each of these fields has the following meaning:

▶ *date*: Timestamp of the log entry

▶ *user*: Username that executed sudo

▶ *hostname*: Host address on which the sudo command was executed

▶ *terminal*: Controlling terminal from which sudo was invoked

▶ *dir*: Current directory from which the command was invoked

▶ *user*: Username that the command was run as

▶ *command*: Command that was executed through sudo

For example, Listing 8.2 illustrates a typical sudo.log file showing six entries, all executed by username ramon, invoking commands to be run as root.

Listing 8.2: Contents of the sudo.log File

```
Sep 23 14:41:37 : ramon : HOST=redhat : TTY=pts/0 ;
➡PWD=/home/ramon USER=root ; COMMAND=/bin/more /etc/shadow
Sep 23 14:43:42 : ramon : HOST=redhat : TTY=pts/0 ;
➡PWD=/home/ramon USER=root ; COMMAND=/usr/sbin/pwconv
Sep 23 14:43:51 : ramon : HOST=redhat : TTY=pts/0 ;
➡PWD=/home/ramon USER=root ; COMMAND=/bin/more /etc/shadow
Sep 23 14:55:30 : ramon : HOST=redhat : TTY=pts/0 ;
➡PWD=/home/ramon USER=root ; COMMAND=/bin/cat /etc/securetty
Sep 23 15:12:27 : ramon : HOST=redhat : TTY=pts/1 ;
➡PWD=/home/ramon USER=root ; COMMAND=/bin/linuxconf
Sep 23 15:23:37 : ramon : HOST=redhat : TTY=pts/0 ;
➡PWD=/home/ramon USER=root ; COMMAND=/usr/sbin/pwunconv
```

FILE AND DIRECTORY PERMISSIONS

Perhaps one of the most difficult aspects of Linux administration, file permissions are a vital aspect of system security. Linux (like all Unix variants) treats most resources as files, whether they're directories, disk devices, pipes, or terminals. Although this makes for straightforward software architecture, it also introduces a fundamental challenge to the Linux administrator charged with ensuring the security of these resources.

Permissions on files and directories have a direct effect on the security of your system. Make the permissions too tight and you limit your users' ability to get their work done. Make permissions too lax and you invite unauthorized use of other users' files and general system resources.

The next subsection of this chapter examines the specifics of suid and sgid permissions on the Linux operating system.

ᴀuid and ᴀgid

Linux supports device and file permissions for three distinct groups of users, each of which is represented by three bits of information in the

Part II

permissions mask, in addition to two special-purpose high-order bits, for a total of 12 bits:

AAABBBCCCDDD

Each of these bits has the following meaning:

AAA   setuid, setgid, sticky-bit

BBB   User (read, write, execute)

CCC   Group (read, write, execute)

DDD   Other (read, write, execute)

Therefore, if you have a new executable file called `report` that you want read, written, and executed only by the file's owner, but read and executed by everybody else, you set its permissions to the appropriate bit-mask value as follows:

```
[ramon]$ chmod 0755 report
[ramon]$ ls -l report
-rwxr-xr-x   1 ramon      users       19032 Sep 25 19:48 report
```

Note that 7 is the octal representation of the binary number 111. The permissions displayed include only three bits per portion (user, group, other), but in reality, Linux allows you to specify four bits for each of the groups. This is addressed by overloading the representation of the third bit with the following values:

x   execute

s   execute + [setuid or setgid] (applicable only to the user and group portions)

S   [setuid or setgid] (applicable only to the user and group portions)

t   execute + sticky (applicable only to the other portion)

T   sticky (applicable only to the other portion)

Now consider the case where you'd like this file to be executed with root permissions because it has to read and write to privileged areas of the filesystem, but you would like nonprivileged users to be able to execute it. You can achieve this by setting the very first bit of the permissions mask as follows:

```
[ramon]$ sudo chown root:root report
[ramon]$ sudo chmod 4755 report
```

```
[ramon]$ ls -l report
-rwsr-xr-x   1 root     root          19032 Sep 25 20:30 report
```

As noted earlier, s in the user portion of the permissions mask denotes that the setuid and execute bits are set for the user (file owner). This means that the file will execute with the user permissions of the file owner (root) instead of the executing user (ramon). In addition, you can set the setgid bit in order to have the file execute with the group permissions of root, as follows:

```
[ramon]$ sudo chmod 6755 report
[ramon]$ ls -l report
-rwsr-sr-x   1 root     root          19032 Sep 25 20:30 report
```

The third bit in the permissions mask is often referred to as the *sticky bit*, and it is used in directories to signal the Linux kernel that it should not allow a user to delete another user's files, even if the directory is world-writeable. This is most often used in the /tmp directory, which has wide-open permissions:

```
[ramon]$ ls -ld /tmp
drwxrwxrwt   7 root     root          1024 Sep 25 21:05 /tmp
```

Note the final t in the mask. This prevents you from deleting your fellow user's files in that directory unless they explicitly allow you to do so by setting write permissions for others.

In general, use of setuid and setgid should be restricted to those partitions that are only writeable by root. I recommend that you explicitly disallow use of setuid/setgid on the /home directory, by specifying the nosuid option in the /etc/fstab file, as shown in Listing 8.3.

Listing 8.3: Contents of the /etc/fstab File

```
[ramon]$ cat /etc/fstab
/dev/sda8       /             ext2     defaults              1 1
/dev/sda1       /boot         ext2     defaults              1 2
/dev/sda6       /home         ext2     exec,nodev,nosuid,rw  1 2
/dev/sda5       /usr          ext2     defaults              1 2
/dev/sda7       /var          ext2     defaults              1 2
/dev/sda9       swap          swap     defaults              0 0
/dev/fd0        /mnt/floppy   ext2     noauto                0 0
/dev/cdrom      /mnt/cdrom    iso9660  noauto,ro             0 0
none            /proc         proc     defaults              0 0
none            /dev/pts      devpts   mode=0622             0 0
```

Part II

Figure 8.7 illustrates how this option can be specified from Red Hat's `linuxconf` utility.

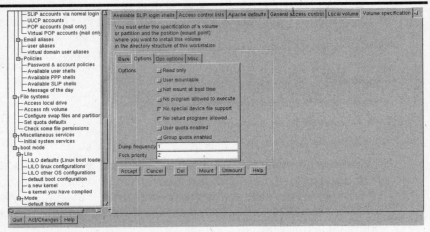

FIGURE 8.7: Setting the `nosuid` option on a local filesystem with `linuxconf`

Also, note that the No Special Device File Support option (option `nodev` in `/etc/fstab`) is selected. This effectively prevents a user from creating a block device in the `/home` filesystem, which would be considered a highly suspect action by a nonprivileged user.

Having taken these precautions, you still need to be vigilant of the `setuid/setgid` present in your Linux server. I suggest that you run this command in `cron`, piping its output to an e-mail report to your mailbox every morning, as follows:

```
find / -type f \( -perm -04000 -o -perm -02000 \) -exec ls -l
{} \;
```

This command should report on all the scripts that have either the `setuid` or the `setgid` bit set in the permissions mask. Compare the current report with the previous day's report, and ensure that any new files have been created by the administration staff. At the very least, you should have the output of this command written to a separate file within `/var/log`.

NOTE

The Linux kernel allows you to use `setuid/setgid` permissions only on binary executables, not on shell scripts. This restriction protects against malicious tampering with shell scripts, a common occurrence that can result in a serious compromise of root.

The *umask* Setting

The default permissions for new files created on your server can have a profound impact on its overall security. Users who create world-writeable files by default are effectively poking tiny holes in your system security. Linux uses the umask configuration setting to control default file permissions. Its usage is

    umask AAA

where AAA is the octal complement of a default permissions mask of 666 (777 for directories). For instance, a umask of 022 would yield a default permission of 644 for files (the result of subtracting 022 from 666). Let's look at the examples in Listing 8.4.

Listing 8.4 umask **Configuration Examples**

```
[ramon]$ umask 000
[ramon]$ touch example1
[ramon]$ ls -l example1
-rw-rw-rw-  1 ramon     users        0 Sep 25 22:08 example1
[ramon]$ umask 022
[ramon]$ touch example2
[ramon]$ ls -l example2
-rw-r-r-  1 ramon     users        0 Sep 25 22:08 example2
[ramon]$ umask 66
[ramon]$ touch example3
[ramon]$ ls -l example3
-rw----  1 ramon     users        0 Sep 25 22:08 example3
```

I recommend that you edit your /etc/profile file to assign a mask of 066 to the root user and assign a mask of 022 to your regular users. This ensures that root-created files have no permissions for group and others, whereas any other files are created with world-read permissions only.

Limiting Core Dump Size

A common means for a local user to gain root privileges is to force a setuid/setgid program to dump a core file (upon crashing) in a specific location within the filesystem. By using this method to overwrite arbitrary files anywhere on the server, including /etc/passwd, /etc/hosts .equiv, or .rhosts, intruders can effectively create for themselves a user with root privileges. With today's servers having gigabytes of physical memory available, these core files could potentially fill an entire disk, which would result in a denial of service (DoS) attack for other users relying on the same filesystem.

There is an effective way to keep core files under control. Using the ulimit command, you can control the resource utilization limits of any user, including the maximum size of a core dump file. You should simply set this size to 0, using the following command:

```
ulimit -c 0
```

You can include this command in the global /etc/profile configuration file also.

SYSLOG SECURITY

One of the most significant skills of sophisticated intruders is their ability to clean up all evidence that an attack has taken place. This is the electronic equivalent of a criminal using gloves at the scene of the crime, and it's a constant source of frustration for those who make a living out of tracking down the actions of these intruders.

You should go to whatever lengths are necessary to make sure that you can safeguard *some* evidence that your system was tampered with. The problem is that it's very difficult to guarantee that your log files are correct when attackers could be modifying them with their root privileges. You should take advantage of the syslog program's ability to send a copy of all log events to a remote server.

For example, in order to send all your kernel, mail, and news messages to a remote syslog server (hostname zurich), add the following line to your /etc/syslog.conf configuration file:

```
kern.*, mail.*, news.*    [TAB]@zurich
```

(Don't forget that the syntax of this file calls for a tab character to be inserted between fields.)

After making this modification, you must send the -HUP (hang-up) signal to the syslog daemon to force it to read its configuration:

```
[ramon]$ sudo killall -HUP syslogd
```

Keep in mind, however, that some services may not be configured or able to log events via syslog. You should use cron to move those services' log files to a remote server several times throughout the day—the more often the better.

FILESYSTEM ENCRYPTION

However strong your physical and system security measures are, you need to be ready for the time when a user gains access to some other user's files. Cryptography is your last line of defense. By encrypting the contents of sensitive directories, users can protect the privacy of their data even after an intrusion has succeeded.

This section describes two different ways to do this, both of which are based on secret-key technology using standard encryption algorithms. Let's take a look at each of them in more detail.

The Cryptographic File System

The Cryptographic File System (CFS) was developed by Unix pioneer Matt Blaze and constitutes the first full-blown integration of secret-key encryption into the Linux filesystem. One of the most important advantages of CFS is its support of both local filesystem types (such as ext2) as well as remote filesystems such as NFS. This support protects your data as it sits in your server and also as it travels through the network whenever you share an NFS mount point. CFS supports several encryption algorithms including Data Encryption Standard (DES), triple-DES (3DES), MacGuffin, SAFER-SK128, and Blowfish.

CFS's main drawback, however, is performance. If you elect to use 3DES encryption (which I recommend because DES is barely adequate nowadays), you will pay a price, and you'll see a noticeable delay in your disk access, especially for large files. This is partly due to the fact that CFS operates in user space (outside of the kernel). However, running in user space can actually be an advantage, because other cryptographic filesystem modules are offered as a patch to particular versions of Linux kernels, and they're often not available for the latest stable kernel.

Let's start by installing the software on your server.

Installing CFS

The package can be obtained in source form, and it's also available from www.zedz.net (or ftp.zedz.net) in RPM format, as shown in Listing 8.5.

Listing 8.5: Downloading the CFS Distribution in RPM Format

```
[ramon]$ ftp ftp.zedz.net
Connected to ftp.zedz.net.
```

Part II

```
220 warez.zedz.net FTP server ready.
Name (ftp.zedz.net:ramon): anonymous
331 Guest login ok, send your complete e-mail address as
    password.
Password: rhontanon@sybex.com
230 Guest login ok, access restrictions apply.
Remote system type is UNIX.
Using binary mode to transfer files.
ftp> cd /pub/crypto/disk/cfs/
250 CWD command successful.
ftp> get cfs-1.3.3bf-1.i386.rpm
local: cfs-1.3.3bf-1.i386.rpm remote: cfs-1.3.3bf-1.i386.rpm
200 PORT command successful.
150 Opening BINARY mode data connection for cfs-1.3.3bf-
    1.i386.rpm (194436 bytes).
226 Transfer complete.
194436 bytes received in 22.7 secs (8.4 Kbytes/sec)
ftp> quit
221-You have transferred 194436 bytes in 1 files.
221-Total traffic for this session was 197280 bytes in 2
    transfers.
221-Thank you for using the FTP service on warez.zedz.net.
221 Goodbye.
[ramon]$ sudo rpm -i cfs-1.3.3bf-1.i386.rpm
```

At this point you have installed CFS on your system (note that there is no need to rebuild the kernel or reboot the server). Let's take a look at configuring CFS in the next step.

Configuring CFS

The first step is to make sure your server is configured to run NFS services (statd, portmapper, and mountd). This is a requirement for CFS to work correctly. CFS actually protects the privacy of NFS shares, so perhaps this is just the tool you were looking for to add NFS back into your security policy. You can verify that NFS is running on your system by looking for the mountd line with the following command:

```
[ramon]$ ps aux | grep mountd
root   5756  0.0  0.7  1132  456 ?  S   19:15  0:00 rpc.mountd
```

Next, create a /null directory. CFS refers to this directory as the *bootstrap mount point*. In addition, you need to create the directory that you want to use as the root for all encrypted data (I chose /crypt for this purpose):

```
[ramon]$ sudo mkdir /null
[ramon]$ sudo chmod 0000 /null
[ramon]$ sudo mkdir /crypt
```

Add the /null directory to the list of exported filesystems using the following command:

```
[ramon]$ echo "/null localhost" >> /etc/exports
```

Add the following commands to the end of /etc/rc.d/rc.local:

```
if [ -x /usr/sbin/cfsd ]; then
        /usr/sbin/cfsd && \
            /bin/mount -o port=3049,intr localhost:/null /crypt
fi
```

That's the end of the installation. You're now ready to try CFS. You can either restart your system or type the commands that you just added in the rc.local file by hand.

Using CFS

There are three commands that support the operation of the CFS package:

```
cmkdir [-1] [private_directory]
cattach [private_directory] [cleartext_directory]
cdetach [private_directory]
```

Start by creating a directory that is going to contain all your confidential information:

```
[ramon]$ cmkdir secret
```

The command prompts you for a passphrase, which is then used to hash out an appropriate secret encrypting key. You'll need this passphrase to be able to get at the data in this directory.

WARNING

Note that by default, CFS uses the 3DES algorithm for encryption. This is noticeably slower than the DES variant that can be specified using the -1 switch (# cmkdir -1 secret). I strongly recommend against this option, because the DES algorithm has been known to be vulnerable to brute force attacks. If you're encrypting data that you expect to keep around for a while, you should make it as resistant as possible to cryptanalysis.

Part II

The next step is to attach this newly created directory to the master CFS tree:

```
[ramon]$ cattach secret decrypted
```

You are then prompted for the same passphrase that you provided when you created the directory. If you authenticate successfully, the secret directory will be available to you as /crypt/decrypted in cleartext form. Once you're done working with the cleartext directory, simply make it unavailable using the following command:

```
[ramon]$ cdetach secret
```

As with any other encryption, CFS is only as strong as your ability to protect the passphrase used to encrypt the data. In addition, you should ensure the integrity of the CFS utilities themselves (cmkdir, cattach, cdetach) to be sure that they have not been replaced with Trojan horse versions. Chapter 9, "Linux System Monitoring and Auditing," shows you how to use file integrity tools to ensure that these and other important system utilities have not been tampered with.

Practical Privacy Disk Driver

A more recent alternative to CFS is Allan Latham's Practical Privacy Disk Driver (PPDD). Unlike CFS, this utility actually creates a disk driver similar to a physical disk device, but its behavior is controlled by the PPDD software. Also unlike CFS, there is built-in support for only one encryption algorithm: Blowfish. This shouldn't be considered a drawback because Blowfish has fared well so far in the many attempts to crack it via both cryptanalysis and brute force.

The goal of this utility is to provide an encryption device that is totally transparent to the user, who can access the PPDD-protected directories without the need for any special procedures. Let's take a closer look at PPDD, starting with its installation.

Installing PPDD

As of this writing, there is no RPM package for PPDD, probably because the installation requires a kernel patch and rebuild. So you need to download the package in source format from ftp.gwdg.de (see Listing 8.6).

Listing 8.6: Downloading the PPDD Distribution

```
[ramon]$ ftp ftp.gwdg.de
Connected to ftp.gwdg.de.
220 ftp.gwdg.de FTP server (Version wu-2.4.2-academ [BETA-18]
➥(1) Mon Jul 31 14:25:08 MET DST 2000) ready.
Name (ftp.gwdg.de:ramon): anonymous
331 Guest login ok, send your complete e-mail address as
    password.
Password:rhontanon@sybex.com
230-Hello User at 204.254.33.77, there are 44 (max 250
230-Local time is: Wed Sep 27 03:00:15 2000
230 Guest login ok, access restrictions apply.
Remote system type is UNIX.
Using binary mode to transfer files.
ftp> cd /pub/linux/misc/ppdd
250 CWD command successful.
ftp> get ppdd-1.2.zip
local: ppdd-1.2.zip remote: ppdd-1.2.zip
200 PORT command successful.
150 Opening BINARY mode data connection for ppdd-1.2.zip
    (198959 bytes).
226 Transfer complete.
198959 bytes received in 28.4 secs (6.9 Kbytes/sec)
ftp>
```

Once you have verified that the file has been successfully downloaded (and it is of the right size), you need to unzip it and extract the tar file, as shown in Listing 8.7.

Listing 8.7 Installing the PPDD Distribution

```
[ramon]$ unzip ppdd-1.2.zip
Archive:  ppdd-1.2.zip
  extracting: tmp/ppdd-1.2.tgz.sig
  inflating: tmp/ppdd-1.2.tgz
[ramon]$ tar zxf tmp/ppdd-1.2.tar
```

At this point you should have a new subdirectory called ppdd-1.2 in your current directory. The PPDD distribution will be applying a patch against the current Linux sources, so make sure that you have a good set of kernel source and header files in /usr/linux and that you have been able to successfully build a working kernel from these files. Don't forget to make a backup copy of the kernel before patching it.

Next, go into the PPDD source directory and apply the kernel patches:

```
[ramon]$ cd ppdd-1.2
[ramon]$ sudo make apply_patch
```

This results in a modification to the Linux sources, so you should rebuild your kernel and install the resulting boot file at this point. Don't forget to reconfigure lilo and have an emergency boot disk handy!

If the new image boots without any errors, you're ready to create the encryption device. The following command assumes that you'll be using /dev/hdc1 as your encrypted disk partition:

```
[ramon]$ sudo ppddinit /dev/ppdd0 /dev/hdc1
```

It is at this stage that you'll be prompted for a passphrase, whose hash will constitute the secret key used in the Blowfish algorithm.

Next, you need to set up the newly created device, and you need to write an ext2 filesystem on it using the following commands:

```
[ramon]$ sudo ppddsetup -s /dev/ppdd0 /dev/hdc1
[ramon]$ sudo mkfs /dev/ppdd0
```

Using PPDD

To use PPDD, simply mount the encrypted device on a real mount point (I'll use /crypt for consistency):

```
[ramon]$ sudo mount /dev/ppdd0 /crypt
```

From this point on, your users can access resources within /crypt transparently, as if it were a regular filesystem.

Before you shut down the server, you should unmount the /crypt filesystem as you would any other partition, and you should also disconnect the ppdd0 driver, as follows:

```
[ramon]$ sudo umount /crypt
[ramon]$ sudo ppddsetup -d /dev/ppdd0
```

PPDD encrypts an entire filesystem with a key derived from a single passphrase and allows users to access the files within the filesystem using the standard Linux permissions model. This makes PPDD a good candidate for protecting a server's disk from being read by an intruder who has physically seized the system, as well as for protecting backup media that have fallen into the wrong hands.

What's Next

This chapter examined the issues involved in system-level Linux security and provides a set of recommended configurations and utilities that can aid in protecting your server from unauthorized access by local users. All the popular Linux distributions are becoming increasingly security conscious, but a staggering number of vulnerabilities are still being reported daily.

It's important to understand the impact of all kernel parameters and recognize which ones can have a direct influence on the security of your server. You should build your own custom kernel for efficiency, but also for security and accountability.

You should protect your server against root exploits. One way to do this is by constantly monitoring the permissions of your system files, and by guarding against the perils of setuid/setgid executables. Setting the correct default umask for your users ensures that they're creating files with a safe set of permissions. Also, limiting the size of core files with the ulimit command can prevent a common type of root compromise attack.

When all else fails, filesystem encryption can protect the data that has been compromised. The Cryptographic File System (CFS) provides good granularity for individual protection of user information, while the Practical Privacy Disk Driver (PPDD) is an efficient, transparent method for encrypting filesystems (and backups) in bulk.

Chapter 9 covers the monitoring and auditing of your system and describes the tools that you can use to ensure the integrity of your system files. This is an essential part of system security and should be used in conjunction with the recommendations in this chapter.

Part II

Chapter 9
Linux System Monitoring and Auditing

Monitoring your system for abnormal behavior is an essential task in both system administration and information security. Most attackers leave their "fingerprints" in the system log files, and examining these logs is a fundamental step in the process of network forensics. More important, examining log files on a regular basis, looking for erratic or suspicious user behavior, can prevent attacks and enhance the overall security of your server.

There are attackers who may be able to penetrate your system without leaving any evidence in the log files. However, even the best attackers will not be able to delete or modify a history file without being noticed. Examining log files is just one critical part of your overall security plan.

You should be looking at the system log files for

► Repeated authentication failures

► Unusual shutdowns

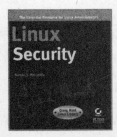

Adapted from *Linux Security* by Ramón J. Hontañón
ISBN 0-7821-2741-X $49.99

- ▶ Attempts to relay messages through your mail server
- ▶ Any events that seem out of the ordinary

A single authentication failure for a single user can be attributed to a mistyped password. Multiple authentication failures for a single user can be attributed to an acute case of "fat-finger" syndrome. Multiple authentication failures for multiple users, however, are a clear sign of an attack in the making, or a sign that one of your internal users may be trying to guess the root password in an effort to gain greater access to your server.

Through the use of the centralized syslog facility, Linux offers a wealth of real-time diagnostics that are often not used to their full extent—not because they don't offer the right kind of information, but because most system administrators don't know exactly how to use them. The problem is that the standard Linux syslog files are too verbose to be of any value. A typical /var/log/messages file on a standard Red Hat or Caldera distribution can grow by 500–600KB in a typical day for a average-load server.

Human inspection of log files has two major shortcomings:

- ▶ The task is tedious and expensive because it has to be performed by a (highly paid) system administrator who is trained to recognize the trouble signs.

- ▶ Humans are prone to error, especially when scanning large text files full of repetitive sequences.

Luckily, the Linux community has responded to the challenge and has developed a number of useful log-monitoring tools that can be run batch style to identify certain keywords or patterns that are known to spell trouble. The section "System Log Monitoring" later in this chapter illustrates the concept of log monitoring using two such tools: swatch and logcheck.

SYSTEM LOGGING WITH *SYSLOG*

The syslog utility allows the system administrator to configure and manage log files generated by heterogeneous system utilities and applications from a central location. Linux comes standard with the syslog utility configured and the syslogd daemon active upon startup. The system administrator specifies in the /etc/syslog.conf file which messages they would like to see logged, and the application directs the messages to the appropriate log file. Most generic messages are directed to the /var/log/messages file, although the system administrator can choose any arbitrary file as the destination. In general, Linux uses the following initial log files:

/var/log/messages   This is the primary Linux log file, used for recording most common system events.

/var/log/secure   Authentication failures for daemons started from /etc/inetd.conf are logged here.

/var/log/maillog   The sendmail daemon is notoriously verbose (and often very busy), so it makes sense to dedicate this separate log file to keep track of mail-delivery messages.

/var/log/spooler   This is the log file where other daemons such as UUCP and News (NNTP) log their messages.

/var/log/boot.log   The boot-up messages displayed when the system is coming up are typically logged in this file.

These five log files are automatically rotated by the system via the /etc/logrotate.d/syslog script. Rotating essentially means renaming the current log file to something like logfile.1 while creating a new (empty) file called logfile to record only those events that took place since the last rotation. At the next rotation, the logfile.1 file is renamed to logfile.2 and the logfile.11 file (if you're only keeping 10 log files) is deleted.

syslog.conf File

Listing 9.1 shows a typical syslog.conf file on a Linux system. It includes references to the five log files described earlier in this section.

Listing 9.1: A Typical Linux /etc/syslog.conf File

```
# Log all kernel messages to the console.
# Logging much else clutters up the screen.
kern.*                                    /dev/console

# Log anything (except mail) of level info or higher.
# Don't log private authentication messages!
*.info;mail.none;authpriv.none            /var/log/messages
```

```
# The authpriv file has restricted access.
authpriv.*                                      /var/log/secure

# Log all the mail messages in one place.
mail.*                                          /var/log/maillog

# Everybody gets emergency messages, plus log them on another
# machine.
*.emerg                                                        *
*.emerg                                               @loghost


# Save mail and news errors of level err and higher in a
# special file.
uucp,news.crit                                  /var/log/spooler

# Save boot messages also to boot.log
local7.*                                        /var/log/boot.log
```

The general format of the entries in the `syslog.conf` file is as follows:

facility.priority[;*facility.priority*] [TAB]*action*

Each field is defined as follows:

> **facility**   The *facility* field is the subsystem that you want to log events from. The current supported subsystems are:
>
> > ▶ `auth`: Secure and authentication messages
> >
> > ▶ `authpriv`: Private secure and authentication messages
> >
> > ▶ `cron`: Clock/scheduler daemon
> >
> > ▶ `daemon`: Other system daemons
> >
> > ▶ `kern`: Linux kernel messages
> >
> > ▶ `lpr`: Line printer system messages
> >
> > ▶ `mail`: Mail system
> >
> > ▶ `news`: Network news subsystem
> >
> > ▶ `sysloguser`: Internal `syslog` messages
> >
> > ▶ `uucp`: Unix-to-Unix copy subsystem
> >
> > ▶ `local0-local7`: Reserved for local use

The special character * can be used to denote any (and all) facilities.

priority   The *priority* field specifies the priority level of the message within a given subsystem. The current priorities are (in ascending order of criticality):

- ▶ debug: Debug-level messages for troubleshooting
- ▶ info: Informational messages
- ▶ notice: Normal messages of special interest
- ▶ warning: Abnormal messages signaling impending failure
- ▶ error: Failure condition messages
- ▶ crit: Critical error-condition messages
- ▶ alert: Condition needing immediate action
- ▶ emerg: Error condition leading to system failure

The special character * can be used to denote any (and all) priorities.

destination   The *destination* field defines the destination for log messages that match the given facility and priority combination. This can be a filename, or a host name when the @ sign precedes the keyword. The * character takes on a special meaning here, denoting all users; in other words, all users who are currently logged on will receive a copy of the message on their active terminals. Needless to say, you should only use this for absolutely critical messages that might impact the user's ability to continue to work on the system.

action   The *action* field can be one of the following:

- ▶ A regular file. In this case, all messages will be appended to the end of the file. The file must be specified with a full path name, starting with the / character.
- ▶ A named pipe. In this case, the messages are used as the standard input to the pipe.
- ▶ A terminal or console. In this case, the messages are displayed over the given device.
- ▶ A remote machine. In this case, the messages are sent to a remote host's syslogd daemon.

Part II

▶ A list of users. In this case, the messages are broadcast to the terminals owned by any active users. The special character * is used to send messages to all users that are currently logged on.

Applying these facility, priority, destination, and action values, you can see that the syslog.conf file in Listing 9.1 is instructing the syslogd daemon to:

▶ Log all kernel messages to the console.

▶ Log authpriv and mail messages to secure and maillog respectively.

▶ Log emergency messages to all the users' terminals and to the remote system loghost.

▶ Log uucp and news messages (critical and above) to spooler.

▶ Log local7 (boot) messages to boot.log.

▶ Log the remaining messages (info and above) to messages.

Some messages are critical enough to the system that they should be stored outside the system itself. This is necessary to make sure that you can continue to log events, even when the local disk is full or is otherwise unavailable. Keeping a set of log files on a separate system also has clear security advantages, because a sophisticated attacker will most likely delete or otherwise tamper with the log files on the attacked system. An attacker would have to repeat all the steps used to get on the first server to get on the second server in order to completely erase their trail.

The next section describes the operation of remote syslog and discusses the security implications of running this service on the remote server.

syslog Server Security

The Linux model is one where services can easily transcend physical servers, and the syslog facility is no exception. When the action @loghost for kernel emergency messages is specified in Listing 9.1, the implication is that there is a system named (or aliased to) loghost that is actively listening on UDP port 514 for incoming syslog requests.

Although this facility makes a more robust logging mechanism, it also introduces a known vulnerability: Attackers can target port 514 UDP by sending very large files to this service to fill up the disks and make the server unavailable. This can then be followed by a stealth attack on the servers that this loghost was logging for in the first place.

If you deploy remote syslogd servers, I recommend that you take at least one of the following precautions:

▶ Protect access to port 514 UDP by ensuring that only authorized servers are allowed to write to that service.

▶ Deploy your remote syslogd server on a separate, dedicated network segment that is exclusive for this use (for example, a 10.0.0/24 management network).

▶ Use a dedicated partition to write remote syslogd messages. This partition could fill up completely without having any other adverse effect on the system. (Note, however, that when the log files fill up, the system is really no longer useful.)

TIP

In order to allow your remote syslogd server to accept messages from other machines, don't forget to use the -r flag when invoking syslog.

SYSTEM LOG MONITORING

The basic idea behind log file monitoring is to define a set of system log files of interest, and a set of *triggers,* or regular expressions, to monitor for. When the tool finds a trigger in the appropriate log file, it executes a specified action (sends an e-mail, executes a command, pages the administrator, and so on). Two full-featured system log monitoring tools are swatch and logcheck.

swatch

The Simple WATCHer (swatch) is a monitoring tool developed by Todd Atkins at University of California, Santa Barbara (UCSB). It is composed of a large Perl script that does all the monitoring and a configuration file where you can specify your triggers and a set of actions for each trigger. The following sections describe the installation, configuration, and use of swatch.

Installing swatch

Although swatch is readily available in RPM format, be aware that most Linux distributions lack three of the Perl packages required by swatch:

- ▶ perl-File-Tail: A Perl module for reading from continuously updated files

- ▶ perl-Time-HiRes: A Perl module for handling high-resolution time variables

- ▶ perl-Date-Calc: A Perl module for Gregorian calendar date calculations

These modules are part of the CPAN Perl archive that is also available in RPM format. Once you have downloaded these three Perl packages, as well as the latest swatch RPM, then install all four packages in the order shown in Listing 9.2.

Listing 9.2: The swatch Installation Process

```
[ramon]$ ls -l *.rpm
-rw-r-r-   1 ramon     users          55922 Sep 30 22:49
➡perl-Date-Calc-4.2-2.i386.rpm
-rw-r-r-   1 ramon     users          12280 Sep 30 22:49
➡perl-File-Tail-0.91-2.i386.rpm
-rw-r-r-   1 ramon     users          12500 Sep 30 22:49
➡perl-Time-HiRes-01.20-2.i386.rpm
-rw-r-r-   1 ramon     users          28279 Sep 30 22:45
➡swatch-3.0b4-1.noarch.rpm
[ramon]$ sudo rpm -i perl-Date-Calc-4.2-2.i386.rpm
[ramon]$ sudo rpm -i perl-File-Tail-0.91-2.i386.rpm
[ramon]$ sudo rpm -i perl-Time-HiRes-01.20-2.i386.rpm
[ramon]$ sudo rpm -i swatch-3.0b4-1.noarch.rpm
```

If there are no errors during these installation steps, you are now ready to configure and use the swatch utility.

Configuring swatch

There is only one swatch configuration file, typically called .swatchrc or swatchrc. This file contains a definition of the triggers that you'd like to monitor, as well as the appropriate action that you would like taken in the presence of each of the triggers. The file should have one keyword per line, with an optional equal sign (=) and an optional value for the keyword.

The following section defines the keywords used in the `swatchrc` configuration file.

Pattern-Matching   There are two options available in `swatchrc` for specifying triggers, or patterns, to watch out for:

Watch for *regex*   Take the appropriate action when the regular expression specified in *regex* is found within the file or command being monitored.

Ignore *regex*   Take the appropriate action when there is any activity within the file or command being monitored, except for events that match the expression specified in *regex*.

Pattern-Matching Action   Once the pattern has been identified, you must specify the action to be taken. Here are the options available:

echo   Write the event that matches the pattern being monitored.

bell   Ring a bell by printing the appropriate ASCII character. This action is appropriate only if you're directing the output of `swatch` to `stdout`.

exec *command*   Execute the specified command as if it were typed in at the command line. You can pass positional variables from the matched line to the command. For example, $1 is the first character in the line, $2 is the second character, and so on. $* is the entire line.

mail[=address:*address*:...][,*subject=your_ subject*]   Send an electronic mail message to the address you specify (*address*), with an optional subject header (*your_ subject*). Note that if the recipient is omitted, the message is sent to the user who owns the `swatch` process on the local server.

Pipe *command*   Pipe the matched lines from the monitored file as input to the specified command.

throttle *hours*:*minutes*:*seconds*   This option is useful for patterns that appear repetitively. Rather than taking action on each appearance of the trigger, `swatch` can signal the event only periodically. However, you will get a report of how many times the event occurred during that time.

when *day:hour* This option is used to restrict the use of an action to a day of the week and an hour of the day. It's useful to configure swatch to page the system administration staff in some instances or to simply e-mail them in other instances, depending on their availability.

swatch Configuration File Examples

The following is a sample swatch configuration file to alert the system administrator of any user authentication failures in the last 30 minutes. This example specifies that you'd like to be notified by pager whenever one of the filesystems has reached capacity. You are instructing swatch to look for the expression "authentication failure," and you are specifying an e-mail message that indicates what action to take. The e-mail message will have the subject "Auth Failure Report." The echo directive instructs swatch to include the offending message in the e-mail. The throttle directive ensures that you are alerted only once every 30 minutes, regardless of the frequency of the message within the 30-minute period:

```
watchfor /authentication failure/
        echo
        bell
        throttle 00:30
        mail=sysadmin@example.com,subject=Auth Failure
        Report
```

If it's after hours, the following configuration file entry indicates that the staff should also be paged. This example looks for occurrences of the string "filesystem full" and sends two separate e-mail messages: one to sysadmin@example.com and another to sysadmin-pager@example.com, but only during the hours of 5 P.M. to 9 A.M.:

```
watchfor /filesystem full/
        echo
        mail=sysadmin@example.com,subject=Filesystem Full
        mail=sysadmin-pager@example.com,when=1-7:17-9
```

Finally, consider the following example of a swatch configuration file that triggers corrective action at the same time that the administration staff is informed of the condition. This example is similar to the previous two, except that it invokes the execution of a script (`cleanup_old_files`) whenever the string "filesystem full" is encountered:

```
watchfor /filesystem full/
        echo
        mail=sysadmin@example.com,subject=Cleaning Files
        exec "cleanup_old_files"
```

Running *swatch*

The `swatch` script accepts several command-line options. Table 9.1 describes the ones that you need to be most interested in.

TABLE 9.1:   swatch Command-Line Options

CONFIGURE OPTION	DESCRIPTION	DEFAULT
`--config-file=filename`	Location of the configuration file.	`$HOME/.swatchrc`
`--help`	Display a short help summary.	N/A
`--version`	Display the swatch script version.	N/A
`--tail-file=filename`	Examine lines of text as they're added to the file.	Note: Only one of these options can be specified at any one time. The default is: `--tail-file=/var/log/messages`.
`--read-pipe=command`	Examine input piped in from the specified command.	
`--examine=filename`	Examine specified filename in a single pass.	

I recommend that you always include the `--config-file` option, and that you place the configuration file in an obvious place, like /etc /swatchrc, where it's easier to track and manage. When no command-line options are specified, the default `swatch` command is

```
swatch --config-file=~/.swatchrc --tail-file=/var/log/messages
```

More typical invocations of the `swatch` command would be

```
swatch --config-file=/etc/swatchrc.messages --tail-
➥file=/var/log/messages
```

```
swatch --config-file=/etc/swatchrc.htmlaccess.log --tail-
➥file=/var/log/htmlaccess.log

swatch --config-file=/etc/swatchrc.authlog --tail-
➥file=/var/log/authlog
```

Note that these commands specify separate configuration files for each system log file to be monitored. I recommend that you invoke each of these `swatch` commands (or whichever commands you find useful) on a separate virtual terminal (or `xterm` in the system console) and review the output periodically. As always, the severity of the alert (`echo`, `mail`, `page`, and so on) should be in accordance with the type of event and its recommended handling as stated in your security policy.

logcheck

Maintained by Craig Rowland of Psionic, `logcheck` is an adaptation of `frequentcheck.sh`, a log-monitoring package that once accompanied the Gauntlet firewall from Trusted Information Systems, although some of the most important components have been totally rewritten. Unlike `swatch`, the `logcheck` design is such that you don't have to have a constantly running process scrutinizing your log files, which should cut down on overhead on the server. In addition, `logcheck` can alert you of unusual events, even if you have not defined them as triggers to look for.

The `logcheck` package contains two executables: `logtail` and `logcheck.sh`. `logtail` keeps track of how much of the log file was monitored last time, and it is written in C for performance reasons. `logcheck.sh` controls all processing and inspects the contents of the log files. It is meant to be invoked from `cron` and should be configured to run at least hourly.

Installing logcheck

Fortunately, the RPM version of the `logcheck` package is ubiquitous. I recommend that you use the following installation method, because there is no need for special configuration of the sources. Once you have obtained the `.rpm` file, simply install it using the `rpm` utility:

```
[ramon]$ ls -l logcheck-1.1.1-1.i386.rpm
-rw-r-r-  1 ramon users  33707 Sep 28 20:04 logcheck-1.1.1-
   i386_rpm
[ramon]$ sudo rpm -i logcheck-1.1.1-1.i386.rpm
```

TIP

Don't forget to erase any previous or outdated versions of `logcheck` **before** running the command that installs `logcheck`.

Configuring *logcheck*

Upon installation, `logcheck` writes a number of reference files in the /etc/logcheck directory, which it uses for default pattern matching. The most interesting of these files is `logcheck.hacking` (shown in Listing 9.3), in which the author has placed a number of regular expressions that are often associated with documented attacks on Linux servers, such as:

- ▶ VRFY root

- ▶ EXPN root

- ▶ A `sendmail` command that is used to obtain more information on legitimate mail users (EXPN, VRFY), as well as login failure attempts from accounts that enjoy system privileges (root)

- ▶ The command `login.*; .*LOGIN FAILURE.* FROM .*root`, which signals a root login with the wrong password

Listing 9.3: The Standard /etc/logcheck/logcheck.hacking **Reference File**

```
"wiz"
"WIZ"
"debug"
"DEBUG"
ATTACK
nested
VRFY bbs
VRFY decode
VRFY uudecode
VRFY lp
VRFY demo
VRFY guest
VRFY root
VRFY uucp
VRFY oracle
VRFY sybase
```

Part II

```
VRFY games
vrfy bbs
vrfy decode
vrfy uudecode
vrfy lp
vrfy demo
vrfy guest
vrfy root
vrfy uucp
vrfy oracle
vrfy sybase
vrfy games
expn decode
expn uudecode
expn wheel
expn root
EXPN decode
EXPN uudecode
EXPN wheel
EXPN root
LOGIN root REFUSED
rlogind.*: Connection from .* on illegal port
rshd.*: Connection from .* on illegal port
sendmail.*: user .* attempted to run daemon
uucico.*: refused connect from .*
tftpd.*: refused connect from .*
login.*: .*LOGIN FAILURE.* FROM .*root
login.*: .*LOGIN FAILURE.* FROM .*guest
login.*: .*LOGIN FAILURE.* FROM .*bin
login.*: .*LOGIN FAILURE.* FROM .*uucp
login.*: .*LOGIN FAILURE.* FROM .*adm
login.*: .*LOGIN FAILURE.* FROM .*bbs
login.*: .*LOGIN FAILURE.* FROM .*games
login.*: .*LOGIN FAILURE.* FROM .*sync
login.*: .*LOGIN FAILURE.* FROM .*oracle
login.*: .*LOGIN FAILURE.* FROM .*sybase
kernel: Oversized packet received from
attackalert
```

In addition, the /etc/logcheck directory includes a file named logcheck.violations containing patterns that, although they should be flagged as suspicious, don't quite constitute evidence of an attack in progress. For example, a line such as

```
RETR passwd
```

indicates that someone tried to retrieve the password file via FTP. This is not an illegal action per se, but you should at least question the motive of the user who performed this transfer.

The `logcheck.violations` file also contains references to failed login attempts and other system access diagnostics, such as file transfers and kernel warnings, that are less critical than the `logcheck.hacking` file but still warrant further investigation.

Listing 9.4 shows the contents of the `logcheck.violations` file.

Listing 9.4: The Standard `/etc/logcheck/logcheck.violations` **Reference File**

```
!=
-ERR Password
ATTACK
BAD
CWD etc
DEBUG
EXPN
FAILURE
ILLEGAL
LOGIN FAILURE
LOGIN REFUSED
PERMITTED
REFUSED
RETR group
RETR passwd
RETR pwd.db
ROOT LOGIN
SITE EXEC
VRFY
"WIZ"
admin
alias database
debug
denied
deny
deny host
expn
failed
illegal
kernel: Oversized packet received from
nested
```

```
permitted
reject
rexec
rshd
securityalert
setsender
shutdown
smrsh
su root
su:
sucked
unapproved
vrfy
attackalert
```

You should update the `logcheck.hacking` and the `logcheck`
`.violations` files regularly with newly discovered log message patterns,
or, better yet, make sure that you always have an up-to-date `logcheck`
installation on all your servers. In addition, take the time to add items
to these files that are specific to your server and your system needs. For
example, add message patterns from Apache if you're running an HTTP
server, or from `sendmail` if you're running a mail server.

Note that by default, the Linux version of `logcheck` scans the `/var/`
`log/messages` file for all events, so make sure that this file is indeed seeing
all application log messages. Your `/etc/syslog.conf` file should have
the following line in it:

```
*.info          /var/log/messages
```

Although there are no real configuration files, the actual `logcheck`
shell script (`/usr/sbin/logcheck`) is very readable, and it has a few
variable definitions toward the front. I recommend that you only change
the line

```
SYSADMIN=root
```

to a username other than root, if you have a special account to which the
logs should be e-mailed instead.

Running *logcheck*

The `logcheck` command uses `cron` to schedule periodic runs. Make
sure that your system is indeed running `crond` (the `cron` daemon) by

issuing the following command:

```
[ramon]$ ps aux | grep cron
root       403  0.0  0.4  1284   304 ?        S    Sep24
0:00 crond
```

Upon installation, the logcheck RPM distribution creates the following file in the /etc directory:

```
/etc/cron.hourly/logcheck
```

This file forces the cron job on your server to execute logcheck at the top of the hour, resulting in hourly e-mail messages to the root account on the server. This e-mail message includes a report on the security violations and any unusual system events recorded during the last hour.

Listing 9.5 shows an example of this hourly report. In this report, logcheck reports that there was a SOCKS5 client that failed to properly authenticate to the local server, as well as a regular user (ramon) who performed a su command to inspect the /var/log/messages file.

Listing 9.5: Sample E-Mail Sent By logcheck to the Local Root User

```
From: root <root@redhat.example.com>
Message-Id: <200010012201.SAA16387@redhat.example.com>
To: root@redhat.example.com
Subject: redhat.example.com 10/01/00:18.01 system check
Status: RO
Content-Length: 222
Lines: 8
Security Violations
=-=-=-=-=-=-=-=-=
Oct 1 17:28:14 redhat Socks5[16296]: Auth Failed: (204.168.33.2:_
1196)
Unusual System Events
=-=-=-=-=-=-=-=-=-=
Oct 1 17:28:14 redhat Socks5[16296]: Auth Failed: (204.168.33.2:_
1196)
Oct 1 18:17:15 redhat sudo:     ramon : TTY=pts/3 ; PWD=/usr/doc/_
logcheck-1.1.1 ; USER=root ; COMMAND=/usr/bin/tail/var/log/messages
```

swatch versus logcheck

Both swatch and logcheck have a place in your system defense. Whereas swatch makes for a better real-time log notification tool, logcheck provides a straightforward, easy-to-install tool that you can use to create custom reports that can be periodically examined by the administration staff.

Whichever tool you choose to implement, it's crucial to choose a recipient who will have enough time and dedicate enough energy to read the reports thoroughly. These tools are meant to help in one of the most tedious aspects of systems security, but ultimately, there is no substitute for human scrutiny and appropriate response.

FILE INTEGRITY AUDITING

Ensuring the integrity of system executables, configuration files, and log files is paramount to a successful security defense. Consider the case where an intruder manages to replace a commonly executed file (like `login`) with a Trojan horse version. If the attacker manages to create a Trojan horse `login` that performs just like the original, this attack could go undetected forever. Because you can't easily "look" inside executables, the only way you can flag such a compromise is by comparing the current *signature* of the current `login` utility to the signature taken when the system was first installed.

These signatures are cryptographic hash functions whose properties ensure that two different files can never yield the same hash. Therefore, the slightest modification in one of these files can cause the signature to be drastically different. This is the fundamental principle behind most file integrity assurance tools. By taking a *signature snapshot* of all the executable files before the system goes on the network, you create a baseline that can be stored in a database, preferably on a write-once, read-many-times medium (to ensure that it cannot be tampered with). You can then periodically compare these signatures to the current state of the files and deal with any changes appropriately.

The following section introduces `tripwire`, the most popular Linux file integrity assurance utility, and explains its installation, configuration, and use as part of a comprehensive system security strategy.

tripwire

Born in 1992 under the auspices of Dr. Gene Spafford at Purdue University, `tripwire` was the first tool to be offered in the field of file integrity assurance. In 1999, the maintenance and development of the tool was taken over by Tripwire, Inc., a commercial endeavor spearheaded by Gene Kim, one of tripwire's original developers, while working for Dr. Spafford back at Purdue.

Installing *tripwire*

Although the company offers a fully supported line of commercial products based on the tripwire concept, Tripwire, Inc. makes the Linux version of its tool available for free download. You can obtain a compressed archive containing the distribution at www.tripwire.com/downloads. Once you have downloaded the archive file, decompress it and extract the contents of the resulting .tar file to the current directory using the following commands:

```
[ramon]$ gunzip Tripwire_221_for_Linux_x86.tar.gz
[ramon]$ tar xf Tripwire_221_for_Linux_x86.tar
[ramon]$ rm Tripwire_221_for_Linux_x86.tar
[ramon]$ ls -l
total 8814
-r--r--r--  1 ramon  users   9825 Jan 11  2000 License.txt
-r--r--r--  1 ramon  users   7060 Jan 11  2000 README
-r--r--r--  1 ramon  users  23065 Jan 11  2000 Release_Notes
-r--r--r--  1 ramon  users   3300 Jan 11  2000 install.cfg
-r-xr-xr-x  1 ramon  users  31919 Jan 11  2000 install.sh
drwxr-xr-x  2 ramon  users   1024 Jan 11  2000 pkg
```

Before proceeding with the installation, take a look at the install.cfg file, which contains a number of environment variables that control the installation process. Table 9.2 shows the options that you should examine, along with their default settings. I recommend that you change the value of TWROOT to the location where you normally install system tools (for example, /usr/local/tripwire) because most other environment variables build on this base directory.

NOTE
Despite my suggestion, I use /usr/TSS in these examples to make the text more compatible with other tripwire documentation.

Part II

TABLE 9.2: `tripwire install.cfg` Environment Variables

VARIABLE	DESCRIPTION	DEFAULT
TWROOT	The root directory	/usr/TSS
TWBIN	Location of the program executables and configuration files	${TWROOT}/bin
TWPOLICY	Location of policy files	${TWROOT}/policy
TWMAN	Location of the man pages	${TWROOT}/man
TWDB	Location of the databases	${TWROOT}/db
TWSITEKEYDIR	Location of key used to secure the configuration and policy files	${TWROOT}/key
TWLOCALKEYDIR	Location of key used to secure database files and reports	${TWROOT}/key
TWREPORT	Location of results of integrity checks	${TWROOT}/report

Next, simply execute the supplied install `.sh` script as the root user:

```
[ramon]$ sudo ./install.sh
```

During the installation process, you are prompted to enter a passphrase to protect the confidentiality and integrity of the configuration and policy files. You are also asked to enter the name of the database that will eventually contain the signatures to the system files that you choose to monitor. Choose a good passphrase composed of at least 16 characters. (`tripwire` accepts passphrases of up to 1,023 characters!)

NOTE

If you choose to accept the installation directory default of /usr/TSS, you should at least include /usr/TSS/bin in your PATH environment variable if you want to execute `tripwire` commands without supplying a fully qualified file path. Do not include this path in root's PATH variable, however. You may also want to include /usr/TSS/man in your MANPATH environment variable so you can display the supplied man pages.

Configuring *tripwire*

Once the package has been installed in the appropriate directory, you must create a configuration file, as well as a default policy, that will also be stored in a text file. After these two files are created, use the twadmin utility to encode and sign both files to ensure that their contents are not modified. The next step is to initialize the signature database, which allows you to run your first integrity check.

The following sections explain in more detail the process of creating a tripwire configuration file and a policy file.

The *tripwire* Configuration File   The tripwire configuration file is typically found at the following location:

```
${ROOT}/bin/twcfg.txt
```

The purpose of this configuration file is to control the location of all the other files in the tripwire distribution after it has been installed. Listing 9.6 contains the default contents of the file.

Listing 9.6: Initial Contents of the tripwire Configuration File (twcfg.txt)

```
ROOT                   =/usr/TSS
POLFILE                =/usr/TSS/policy/tw.pol
DBFILE                 =/usr/TSS/db/$(HOSTNAME).twd
REPORTFILE             =/usr/TSS/report/$(HOSTNAME)-$(DATE).twr
SITEKEYFILE            =/usr/TSS/key/site.key
LOCALKEYFILE           =/usr/TSS/key/redhat.example.com-local.key
EDITOR                 =/bin/vi
LATEPROMPTING =false
LOOSEDIRECTORYCHECKING =false
MAILNOVIOLATIONS =true
EMAILREPORTLEVEL =3
REPORTLEVEL            =3
MAILMETHOD      =SENDMAIL
SYSLOGREPORTING =false
MAILPROGRAM            =/usr/lib/sendmail -oi -t
```

If you specified a custom value for TWROOT before the installation, the paths in this file should reflect that fact. Note that the first six variables in the twcfg.txt file are needed for tripwire operation, and the rest are optional. Table 9.3 contains a description of the environment variables in this file that are different from the ones in the installation configuration (see Table 9.2 for those). Unless you have a very specific need to do so, I recommend that you do *not* change the default contents of this configuration file.

Part II

TABLE 9.3: `tripwire twcfg.txt` Environment Variables

VARIABLE	DESCRIPTION
EDITOR	Editor for interactive reports.
LATEPROMPTING	Delay the prompting of the passphrase to minimize exposure.
LOOSEDIRECTORYCHECKING	Don't check files for properties that are likely to change often.
MAILNOVIOLATIONS	Send an e-mail report even if no violations occurred.
EMAILREPORTINGLEVEL	Default verbosity level of the e-mail report (0 through 4).
REPORTLEVEL	Default verbosity level of the printed report (0 through 4).
MAILMETHOD	Choice of mail transport (SMTP or Sendmail).
SYSLOGREPORTING	Send `user.notice` reports through `syslog`.
MAILPROGRAM	Program invoked for mailing `tripwire` violation reports.

The next section describes the syntax and maintenance of the policy file and the last steps needed to get `tripwire` up and running.

The *tripwire* Policy File   Now that you have defined the operational parameters of `tripwire`, you're ready to tell it which files to watch. This is done in the policy file, which is located by default in `/usr/TSS/policy/twpol.txt`.

A typical `tripwire` policy file has three distinct sections:

▶ Global definitions of variables whose scope includes the entire policy file

▶ File severity levels that allow you to prioritize the execution of policies

▶ Rules or group of properties to be checked for each file or object

Consider the sample (partial) policy of the `tripwire` policy file (`twpol.txt`) in the examples in this section. This example contains the global variables that determine the location of the `tripwire` root directory (TWROOT), binary directory (TWBIN), policy (TWPOL), database (TWDB), key files (TWSKEY, TWLKEY), and report (TWREPORT):

```
@@section GLOBAL
TWROOT="/usr/TSS";
```

```
TWBIN="/usr/TSS/bin";
TWPOL="/usr/TSS/policy";
TWDB="/usr/TSS/db";
TWSKEY="/usr/TSS/key";
TWLKEY="/usr/TSS/key";
TWREPORT="/usr/TSS/report";
HOSTNAME=redhat.example.com;
```

The next example shows the file severity level section of the tripwire policy file. This example defines a number of macros to be used later in the policy. It uses several built-in property masks that tell the policy which events to examine or ignore (IgnoreNone, ReadOnly, Dynamic, Growing), as well as some user-defined property masks (+pug, 33, 66, 100). These masks direct tripwire to look for certain types of changes in a given file or directory (see Table 9.4 for a complete list of the characters used in tripwire's property masks):

```
@@section FS
SEC_CRIT = $(IgnoreNone)-SHa;  # Critical files - we can't
                               # afford to miss any changes.

SEC_SUID = $(IgnoreNone)-SHa;  # Binaries with the SUID or SGID
                               # flags set.

SEC_TCB  = $(ReadOnly);        # Members of the Trusted
                               # Computing Base.

SEC_BIN  = $(ReadOnly);        # Binaries that shouldn't change.
SEC_CONFIG  = $(Dynamic);      # Config files that are changed
                               # infrequently but accessed
                               # often.

SEC_LOG   = $(Growing);        # Files that grow, but that
                               # should never change ownership.

SEC_INVARIANT = +pug;          # Directories that should
                               # never change permission or
                               # ownership.

SIG_LOW    = 33;               # Non-critical files that are
                               # of minimal security impact.

SIG_MED    = 66;               # Non-critical files that are
                               # of significant security impact.
```

```
SIG_HI        = 100;            # Critical files that are
                               # significant points of
                               # vulnerability.
```

TABLE 9.4: `tripwire` Policy File Property Mask Characters

PROPERTY	DESCRIPTION
–	Ignore properties
+	Record and check properties
p	File permissions
I	Inode number
n	Number of links
u	User id of file owner
g	Group id of file owner
t	File type
s	File size
d	Device number of disk
I	Device number to which inode points
b	Number of blocks allocated
a	Access timestamp
m	Modification timestamp
c	Inode creation/modification time stamp
c	Cyclic redundancy check

The Tripwire Binaries rule instructs `tripwire` to watch the binaries themselves and tag any violation with the highest severity value:

```
# Tripwire Binaries
(rulename = "Tripwire Binaries", severity = $(SIG_HI))
{
    $(TWBIN)/siggen   -> $(ReadOnly);
    $(TWBIN)/tripwire -> $(ReadOnly);
    $(TWBIN)/twadmin  -> $(ReadOnly);
    $(TWBIN)/twprint  -> $(ReadOnly);
}
```

The Tripwire Data Files rule also instructs tripwire to watch the policy configuration and key files. Note that in the file severity section earlier, SEC_BIN was defined to be ReadOnly, so you're telling tripwire that the policy, configuration, and key files should not change at all. Here's an example of the Tripwire Date Files rule:

```
# Tripwire Data Files - Configuration Files, Policy Files,
  Keys,_
  Reports, Databases
(rulename = "Tripwire Data Files", severity = $(SIG_HI))
{
$(TWDB)                          -> $(Dynamic) -i;
$(TWPOL)/tw.pol                  -> $(SEC_BIN) -i;
  $(TWBIN)/tw.cfg                -> $(SEC_BIN) -i;
  $(TWLKEY)/$(HOSTNAME)-local.key  -> $(SEC_BIN) ;
  $(TWSKEY)/site.key             -> $(SEC_BIN) ;


  #don't scan the individual reports
  $(TWREPORT)                    -> $(Dynamic)
                                    (recurse=0);

}
```

Make sure to define rules to monitor the integrity of the policy directory, the key files, and the reports, as in the previous example. Note that the content of the report files is considered to be dynamic, and the recurse=0 directive instructs tripwire not to go into any of the report subdirectories.

The following is an example of a medium severity rule that defines a set of files that can change on a regular basis, but must retain their user and group ownership:

```
# Commonly accessed directories that should remain static
  with_
  regards to owner and group
(rulename = "Invariant Directories", severity = $(SIG_MED))
{
  /      -> $(SEC_INVARIANT) (recurse = 0);
  /home  -> $(SEC_INVARIANT) (recurse = 0);
  /etc   -> $(SEC_INVARIANT) (recurse = 0);
}
```

Part II

After you have edited the textual policy file to make any necessary additions or modifications, encrypt it and sign it with the following command:

```
[ramon]$ sudo /usr/TSS/bin/twadmin --create-polfile
➥/usr/TSS/policy/twpol.txt
```

This results in the creation of a binary file called /usr/TSS/policy/ tw.pol. At this point, you have a valid configuration file and an initial policy file in place.

The next section explains how to initialize the tripwire database and how to start using the application.

Running *tripwire*

You're almost ready, but before you start comparing file signatures to look for tampering, you need to snap a baseline of what the signatures should look like on all the files in your policy. This takes place when you first initialize the signature database using the following command:

```
[ramon]$ /usr/TSS/bin/tripwire --init
```

Whenever you want to check the integrity of the current state of the files, simply issue the command

```
[ramon]$ /usr/TSS/bin/tripwire --check
```

which results in a report being written to stdout and saved to the file location specified in the REPORTFILE environment variable (see Listing 9.6).

If you would like the report to be e-mailed to you instead, use the following variant of the previous command:

```
[ramon]$ /usr/TSS/bin/tripwire --check --email-report
```

Once you have reviewed the report, you can confirm that any integrity differences have been acknowledged by writing the new integrity results to the database. Do this by using the following command:

```
[ramon]$ /usr/TSS/bin/tripwire --update
```

Finally, as you make changes to the policy file, you need to force tripwire to reload its policy definitions using the following command:

```
[ramon]$ /usr/TSS/bin/tripwire --update-policy
```

TIP

I recommend that you run tripwire at least twice a day and examine the integrity reports carefully before updating the signature database. Ideally, you should simply add the tripwire --check --email-report command to a cron job. This command should be executed first thing in the morning and shortly before the system administration staff goes home for the day.

Password Auditing

Keeping track of logs and ensuring the integrity of your files can significantly strengthen your server, but it's easy to fall prey to the "crunchy on the outside, chewy on the inside" syndrome. The weakest links in most of today's Linux servers are the users and, more specifically, their choices of passwords. Your security policy should always include a section outlining the properties of good passwords, and you should also take a proactive approach to password security and conduct periodic audits of all your users' passwords.

As with any other Unix system, the Linux passwords are stored as the result of a one-way Data Encryption Standard (DES) encryption operation on the original cleartext password. (Some Linux systems also support MD5 hashing for password protection.) This means that the actual password is never stored in the clear. Whenever a user attempts to log on to the system, the login program encrypts the password entered and compares the result to the one found in /etc/passwd (or /etc/shadow). The user is allowed access to the system only if the two passwords match.

There are several password-auditing tools available for Linux. These tools take as input the encrypted password file, and they attempt to guess each user's password by staging a *dictionary attack*, where a collection of commonly used words is DES-encrypted one by one and the results are compared to the /etc/passwd entries. If a match is found, the username is recorded and included in the output report for the security administrator.

This section describes one of these tools, John the Ripper, developed as part of the Openwall project (www.openwall.com).

John the Ripper

An alternative to the original crack program, John the Ripper is a robust password-guessing tool that uses its own routines to attempt to crack passwords, rather than using the Linux crypt(3) system call. This results in a noticeable performance advantage over the earlier version of the crack tool. Another advantage is that John the Ripper runs on a variety of platforms (most Unix, DOS, and Windows systems), so you can use other machines in your network to try to crack your Linux servers' passwords.

By using John the Ripper to try to guess your own users' passwords, you can alert them that they have chosen too short or too weak a password and exhort them to change it before an attacker with the same tool guesses it and breaks into their account.

Installing *john*

The john installation is trivial. Download it from www.openwall.com/ john (it's not available in RPM form), decompress it, and expand the archive (see the steps in Listing 9.7). Once you have expanded the sources into their own directory, go to the src directory and run the make command. Note that you have several options for the target executables (type make with no arguments to see the options). Listing 9.7 shows a build for an ELF format executable on the i386 architecture.

Listing 9.7: *Installing and Compiling* **john**

```
[ramon]$ ls -l john-1.6.tar.gz
-rw-r--r-- 1 ramon     users        497354 Oct  3 19:27 john-_
1.6.tar.gz
[ramon]$ gunzip john-1.6.tar.gz
[ramon]$ tar xf john-1.6.tar
[ramon]$ cd john-1.6
[ramon]$ ls
README  doc  run  src
[ramon]$ cd src
[ramon]$ make
To build John the Ripper, type:
        make SYSTEM
where SYSTEM can be one of the following:
linux-x86-any-elf        Linux, x86, ELF binaries
linux-x86-mmx-elf        Linux, x86 with MMX, ELF binaries
linux-x86-k6-elf         Linux, AMD K6, ELF binaries
linux-x86-any-a.out      Linux, x86, a.out binaries
linux-alpha              Linux, Alpha
linux-sparc              Linux, SPARC
generic                  Any other UNIX system with gcc
[ramon]$ make linux-x86-any-elf
```

```
ln -sf x86-any.h arch.h
make ../run/john ../run/unshadow ../run/unafs ../run/unique \
JOHN_OBJS="DES_fmt.o DES_std.o BSDI_fmt.o MD5_fmt.o
MD5_std.o_
    BF_fmt.o BF_std.o AFS_fmt.o LM_fmt.o batch.o bench.o
    charset.o_
    common.o compiler.o config.o cracker.o external.o
    formats.o_
    getopt.o idle.o inc.o john.o list.o loader.o logger.o
    math.o_
    memory.o misc.o options.o params.o path.o recovery.o rpp.o_
    rules.o signals.o single.o status.o tty.o wordlist.o
    unshadow.o_
    unafs.o unique.o x86.o" \
        CFLAGS="-c -Wall -O2 -fomit-frame-pointer -m486"
make[1]: Entering directory `/home/ramon/john-1.6/src'
gcc -c -Wall -O2 -fomit-frame-pointer -m486 -funroll-loops
DES_fmt.c
gcc -s DES_fmt.o DES_std.o BSDI_fmt.o MD5_fmt.o MD5_std.o
BF_fmt.o BF_std.o AFS_fmt.o LM_fmt.o batch.o bench.o
    charset.o_
    common.o compiler.o config.o cracker.o external.o
    formats.o_
    getopt.o idle.o inc.o john.o list.o loader.o logger.o
    math.o_
    memory.o misc.o options.o params.o path.o recovery.o
    rpp.o_
    rules.o signals.o single.o status.o tty.o wordlist.o
    unshadow.o_
    unafs.o unique.o x86.o -o ../run/john
ln -s john ../run/unshadow
ln -s john ../run/unafs
ln -s john ../run/unique
make[1]: Leaving directory `/home/ramon/john-1.6/src'
[ramon]$ ls -l ../run/john
-rwxr-xr-x    1 ramon    users       148428 Oct  3 19:59
../run/john
```

There is no make installation step, so simply copy the executable to the appropriate place in your filesystem using the following command:

```
[ramon]$ sudo cp ../run/john /usr/local/bin
```

Configuring *john*

All configuration parameters are kept in the file ~\john.ini, which must be present in the current directory when john is invoked. There are four environment variables that can be configured in this file:

wordfile   The wordfile variable is the file that contains the word list to be used to crack passwords in batch style.

idle   When set to Y, the idle variable forces john to use only idle CPU cycles. I recommend this setting if you need to run john on a production server. The default value is N.

save   The save variable is the delay (in seconds) of the crash recovery file. This file contains checkpoints of the work done so far in case of an interruption. The default value is 600.

beep   When the beep variable set to Y, john beeps every time a password is successfully cracked. The default value is N.

The following is the [options] portion of a sample john.ini file containing these environment variables:

```
[ramon]$ more john.ini
#
# This file is part of John the Ripper password cracker,
# Copyright (c) 1996-98 by Solar Designer
#
[Options]
# Wordlist file name, to be used in batch mode
Wordfile = ~/password.lst
# Use idle cycles only
Idle = N
# Crash recovery file saving delay in seconds
Save = 600
# Beep when a password is found (who needs this anyway?)
Beep = N
```

Running *john*

By invoking john with no options, you can allow john to come up with enough random tries to crack the passwords:

```
[ramon]$ john /etc/passwd
```

Alternatively, you can supply a list of commonly used words for john to try. The word list can be a file; the following example uses the file my_guesses:

[ramon]$ **john -wordfile:my_guesses /etc/passwd**

As a third option, the word list can be piped in via stdin, as in the following command:

[ramon]$ **cat my_guesses | john -stdin /etc/passwd**

Note that in general, john runs for a long time, and it writes its findings as it goes along into the ~/john.pot file. If you wish to see the passwords that john has cracked so far, issue the following command:

[ramon]$ **john -show /etc/passwd**

Also, if you are using shadow passwords, you need to merge /etc/passwd and /etc/shadow into a single file for john to work properly. The john executable can do this conversion when invoked as unshadow. Start by creating a symbolic link using the command

[ramon]: **sudo ln -s /usr/local/bin/john /usr/local/bin/unshadow**

and then invoke the unshadow script with both files using the command

[ramon]$ **unshadow /etc/passwd /etc/shadow > mypasswd**

You now have a file (mypasswd) that you can try to crack through john:

[ramon]$ **john mypasswd**

Although it's very stable in its current form, the john utility is still being actively developed, and new versions often introduce a dramatic increase in performance. Check the website www.openwall.com periodically to look for updates.

WHAT'S NEXT

Security is a process, and putting up a strong defense is virtually useless unless you're willing to monitor your system for intrusions and stay vigilant. The syslog facility is a powerful system security tool, especially when the resulting log files are periodically monitored for abnormal behavior. This chapter describes two such tools: swatch and logcheck.

The value of examining log files, however, is greatly diminished if you can't be sure that their contents haven't been modified by an intruder in order to cover his/her tracks. Part of your security-monitoring procedures should include an integrity check on both log files and important system executables. This serves to assure you that the log files haven't been tampered with and that the executables haven't been replaced by Trojan horse versions.

Finally, it's easy to underestimate the importance of using good passwords that can stand up to simple intrusion attempts. Among the password-auditing tools currently available for Linux, John the Ripper stands out as a clear winner because of its performance and its ease of use.

In Chapter 10, "Samba Security Considerations," you will learn how to protect one of the most popular services running on a Linux server: Samba.

Chapter 10

SAMBA SECURITY CONSIDERATIONS

Part II

S amba is an extremely powerful server and, therefore, can be an extremely useful network tool. Unfortunately, Samba's power also makes it a potentially dangerous tool, particularly if an unwanted outsider (or even an unauthorized insider) gains access to the server. A miscreant who breaks into a computer through a Samba logon may be able to do anything from no damage to substantial damage, depending upon Samba's configuration and the configuration of other servers on the computer. This chapter describes Samba's security features and presents information to help you design a Samba security system that can help keep out those who should remain out.

We begin with an overview of Samba's first lines of defense: by-system access control, passwords, and password encryption. The chapter then describes Samba's interactions with Linux's file security features—ownership and permissions. In particularly high security environments, you may want to use the *Secure Sockets Layer (SSL)* to encrypt all the data passing between the

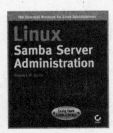

Samba server and its clients, so we'll discuss this option. Finally, the chapter covers an assortment of Samba characteristics and methods you can use to help secure Samba by using other programs and network features.

CONTROLLING INITIAL ACCESS TO SAMBA

Samba provides a wide range of access control options. You can configure a Samba server with extremely lax security, so that anybody can access the server without even sending a password; or you can configure Samba to be very fussy about the systems and individuals it allows to connect. There are two main types of access control: restrictions based on the client computer, and those based on usernames and passwords sent by the calling system. Microsoft Windows employs the latter method. The by-system access methods can be extremely powerful and useful, however, and if you want to run a secure server, it's generally a good idea to set up by-system access controls in addition to password-based access controls.

No matter what security methods you opt for, they'll have implications and uses that are both more and less appropriate for particular situations. It's important that you understand these access restrictions and how they interact, so that you can design an appropriate security system for your network.

Binding Samba to Specific Network Interfaces

Some servers host more than one network interface—one that links to a network from which Samba must be accessible, and another that doesn't. This might be the case if your Samba server runs on a network of Windows computers as well as a network of Unix or Macintosh systems. You can run appropriate servers for both networks, serving the same files to a wide variety of computers. In such situations, it's ideal to bind servers only to the interfaces that require them. Fortunately, Samba includes two global parameters to allow just such a configuration:

interfaces   This parameter allows you to specify interfaces to which Samba will bind itself. Remember that it's important to add the local host address (127.0.0.1) to this line, if you use it.

Failure to do so may cause the Samba Web Administration Tool (SWAT) and smbpasswd to work improperly, because they use this interface internally. You can list interfaces in any of several formats:

- ▶ An interface name, such as eth0. You can also use wildcards, as in eth*, to bind to all Ethernet interfaces.

- ▶ The IP address by which the server is known on a network, as in 192.168.56.9. Samba then locates the interface associated with that address.

- ▶ The network address with netmask, as in 192.168.56 .0/24 or 192.168.56.0/255.255.255.0.

bind interfaces only   By itself, the interfaces parameter has little effect. You must also set bind interfaces only = Yes to limit access to the server. This parameter has a slightly different effect on the nmbd name server daemon than on the smbd file server daemon. To be precise, nmbd uses the interface information to reject accesses from clients based on their claimed IP addresses, whereas smbd rejects accesses based on the network interface. This fact means that nmbd may be susceptible to IP spoofing attacks even when bind interfaces only = Yes is in use; smbd, on the other hand, is only vulnerable to such attacks if the real and spoofed addresses both arrive over the same physical interface.

Part II

If you want to provide Samba services to only one physical interface, using the interfaces and bind interfaces only parameters is a very good idea. When Samba isn't listening to packets coming from a less-trusted network, no amount of password theft or similar actions will gain an intruder access to your system.

There are other ways to erect similar barriers, using external utilities such as ipchains and xinetd. As a general rule, I recommend using several layers of defense; if one fails, another may succeed in keeping intruders out. A few external tools that can help secure Samba are mentioned later in this chapter, in "Samba in the Broader Security World."

Restricting Access by Computer

Whenever a client connects to a Samba server, the client must provide a way for the server to return information, such as files to be read. When using TCP/IP networking, as is normally the case with Samba, this return information comes in the form of an IP address. This fact provides an opportunity for restricting access to the server: The server can be programmed to ignore access attempts from unauthorized IP addresses.

Access restrictions based on IP addresses can take one of two forms: absolute restrictions, which replace the more traditional Server Message Block / Common Internet File System (SMB/CIFS) usernames and passwords; or initial screens, which block access from unauthorized sources but leave the username/password requirements intact. When you configure Samba to use absolute restrictions, the system operates much like an NFS server; Samba effectively passes all responsibility for authentication to the client. An initial screen configuration is usually more secure, because any would-be client must pass multiple tests before gaining access.

Samba options for per-computer accesses include the following:

allow trusted domains   This global parameter works only with Server or Domain security (described shortly, in "Authenticating Users by Username and Password"). When set to Yes (the default), Samba accepts logons from clients in all the domains that are trusted by the domain controller. When set to No, Samba accepts logons only from computers belonging to its own domain.

hosts equiv   If you want Samba to trust certain computers or users without asking for passwords, you can list the names of those computers and users in a file, and pass the name of the file with the global hosts equiv parameter. The file format used is the same as in the /etc/hosts.equiv file, if it's present on your computer. Specifically, each line of the file contains an optional plus sign (+) to allow access, or a minus sign (-) to deny access, followed by a hostname and optional username. (The username is ineffective with most Samba clients.) Activating this option can create a major gap in security.

use rhosts   If you set use rhosts = Yes, individual users can create files called .rhosts in their home directories, and Samba allows connections from any computer listed in these files without further authentication. These .rhosts files are the same as those used for rlogin and similar protocols, and they take the same form as the file used by hosts equiv. Just like rlogin and the hosts equiv parameter, the global use rhosts is potentially very dangerous, so it defaults to No.

NOTE

The hosts equiv parameter can point to a file other than /etc/hosts.equiv, so you don't need to activate host equivalency in other utilities that use this file, such as rlogin and rsh. The use rhosts parameter, by contrast, uses the ~/.rhosts file and no other. Therefore, any utility that looks for this file is affected if you set use rhosts = Yes and your users create ~/.rhosts files for Samba use only.

hosts allow   This parameter can be used either globally or on individual shares. You can specify one or more computers or networks with this parameter. Samba allows access from computers listed on the hosts allow line, but disallows access from all others. The default is to allow access to all computers. This parameter does not bypass Samba's normal password authentication features. Even if you list computers, 127.0.0.1 (the local computer) is given access, unless explicitly denied via the hosts deny parameter. A synonym for this parameter is allow hosts.

hosts deny   This parameter is the opposite of hosts allow—it specifies a "blacklist" of computers that aren't allowed access to the server. The default value is a null string—no computers are denied access to the server. A synonym for this parameter is deny hosts.

The hosts allow and hosts deny parameters can both take fairly complex lists of hosts. You can specify individual computers, networks, and exceptions. You can also use either IP addresses or DNS hostnames. The rules Samba allows are very similar to those used by the /etc/hosts.allow and /etc/hosts.deny configuration files of TCP Wrappers. Specifically, you can designate the following:

▶ An individual computer by IP address, as in hosts deny = 192.168.66.6.

▶ An individual computer by its DNS name, as in hosts allow = dreyfus.panther.edu. You can omit the network name if the Samba server is in the same network.

▶ A network of computers by IP address, by listing only the numbers for the network address, followed by a period; hosts allow = 192.168.65. is an example of this usage.

Part II

▶ A network of computers by IP address, by using an IP address/netmask pair, as in hosts allow=192.168.65.0/ 255.255.255.0.

▶ A network of computers by its DNS name, preceded by a period, as in hosts deny = .panther.edu. This example matches dreyfus .panther.edu, clouseau.panther.edu, olga.diamond.panther .edu, and so on.

▶ A network of computers by its NIS name, preceded by an ampersand, as in hosts deny = @panther. For this option to work, your computer must have access to an NIS server.

▶ Any combination of options, separated by spaces. For instance, hosts allow = clouseau.panther.edu 192.168.34. allows access to all computers on the 192.168.34.0/24 network and the computer clouseau.panther.edu.

▶ An exception, which can be any pattern preceded by the keyword EXCEPT. In hosts deny = 10.34. EXCEPT .diamond.panther.edu, access is denied to all computers in the 10.34.0.0/16 network, except for computers in the diamond.panther.edu subdomain.

TIP

As a general rule, I recommend you set hosts allow to a value that grants access only to computers in your network. This greatly reduces the risk of your Samba server's being accessed and damaged by someone outside your environment.

You can use hosts allow and hosts deny together, or in conjunction with other security-related parameters. If a computer is listed on both the hosts allow and hosts deny lists, hosts allow takes precedence. Therefore, if you want to grant access to all but a few computers on a network, use the EXCEPT clause to hosts allow to block the exception computers; do not rely on hosts deny to override hosts allow!

Authenticating Users by Username and Password

The usual method of authentication for Samba is to accept a username and password from the client, and to authenticate the user based on this information. Samba includes several parameters that influence the way it goes about this task. It's important that you understand these parameters, so that you can design an authentication system that's appropriate for your network.

NOTE

One set of user authentication features—the use or nonuse of encrypted passwords—is of critical practical importance. Details about this essential feature are provided later in this chapter, in "Encrypted versus Cleartext Passwords."

The Security Model

The security global parameter determines the *security model* used by the server. There are two basic security models: *share* and *user*. In share-level security, Samba attempts to protect each share independently of the others, and Samba doesn't explicitly require a username before it allows a connection. In user-level security, Samba uses a more traditional username/ password pair to grant users entry to all shares. Samba supports three variants of user-level security: one for local authentication and two that defer to a domain controller for authentication. Altogether, then, the security parameter has four possible values: Share, User, Server, and Domain.

NOTE

Samba's security model does not affect SWAT. To use SWAT, you must enter a valid Linux username and password, and SWAT authentication is never passed on to a domain controller.

Share-Level Security   When security = Share, Samba attempts to validate users much as a Windows 9x computer does. By default, Windows 9x associates a password with each share and allows a client access to those shares if the client sends the correct password. Windows 9x does not, by default, use usernames, and each share can have a different password. Adapting this security model to Samba is tricky, because in Linux every action by a server program such as Samba must be associated with a user. Therefore, it's not possible to create a password that's directly linked to a share. Rather, Samba tries to associate the password against several different usernames. The process works like this:

1.   If the share specifies guest only = Yes, then Samba tries to match the password against the username specified by the

guest account parameter. If this test fails, then Samba rejects the authentication request.

2. If the client sent a username along with the password, then Samba tries to authenticate the password against that username.

3. If the client has successfully logged on to another share, then Samba tries authenticating the current password against the username that worked on the previous share.

4. Samba tries using the share name as a username. For example, if the share is [bigdrive], then Samba tries authenticating against the user bigdrive.

5. Samba tries the client's NetBIOS name as the username.

6. If a share specifies an explicit username parameter, then Samba uses the usernames listed on that parameter.

To best mimic the security operation of a Windows 9x computer, you should set the guest only = Yes parameter for each share, and set the guest account parameter to a "dummy" account (possibly a different account for each share). Samba then skips the subsequent authentication steps. (No other steps bypass subsequent attempts.)

It's seldom advantageous to use security = Share authentication. Unless you set guest only = Yes, share-level security opens several opportunities for matching passwords, which creates greater exposure to security risks than are present with other security models. The other three security models (user, server, and domain) are much closer matches to Linux's native security model, and all modern SMB/CIFS clients work quite happily with these more Linux-friendly security arrangements. Share-level security makes sense only when you must replace an existing Windows 9x server with minimal disruption to users, or if you're using very old clients that don't pass usernames to the server.

User-Level Security   When you set security = User, Samba requires that the client send a username along with a password. Without the username, the user cannot gain access to the computer. Unless the share includes a force user parameter, Samba uses the username passed with the password (or a derivative based on the username map parameter, described in "Other Authentication Parameters") to determine the user's permissions. If jacques connects to a share to which he has read-only permissions based on the Linux permissions on the server, then `jacques` cannot create or modify files on the share, even if the share is read/write for other users.

One implication of user-level security is that every Samba user must have an account on the server, unless you enable guest access. With share-level security, a user can potentially access the server even without a Linux account. Depending on the password encryption options, Samba run with user-level security may use the user's normal logon password or a special Samba-only encrypted password to determine whether to allow access to the server.

Server-Level Security   If `security` = `Server`, Samba operates much as it does in user-level security, except that Samba passes authentication requests along to the domain controller. You must specify the domain controller in the `password server` parameter, which takes a NetBIOS name or IP address as its value (for example, `password server` = `DREYFUS`). The password server computer can be another Samba computer that's configured to accept such requests via the `domain logons` = `Yes` parameter. Alternatively, the password server can be a Windows NT or 2000 domain controller.

WARNING

No matter what you use as the password server, be sure that system can be trusted! If your chosen password server has been compromised, then the individual who's broken into the password server can gain access to any user's shares. Also, be sure you *do not* set `password server` to point to the Samba server you're configuring. You can set this value to point to *another* Samba server, but if it points to itself, the result is an endless loop of password lookups that causes nothing but problems and possibly even a server crash.

Using `security` = `Server` does not by itself obviate the need for local accounts associated with each user. Your Samba server must still have these accounts—it's just that, for purposes of Samba access, another computer handles the authentication. You can use the `add user script` parameter in conjunction with `security` = `Server`, however, to bypass the need to maintain user accounts. Give the complete path to a script that accepts as its only parameter a username. This script should add a Linux user to the system. If Samba doesn't find a user of a given name, but the password server does authenticate the username and password, Samba calls the script indicated by `add user script`.

TIP

The add user script parameter is a convenient way to add user accounts to a Linux computer that's been added to an existing network of Windows computers.

WARNING

When you create a user-adding script, be sure it doesn't set the password on new accounts to anything constant or obvious. Ideally, the account should be disabled for Linux shell access. If you want to automatically provide Linux logon access, be sure the script generates random passwords and delivers them to the user in some secure way.

If you use a Windows NT system as the password server, the Samba server must have a trust account on that system. This is not a requirement, however, if you use a Samba server as the password server.

Domain-Level Security   Server-level security can be a useful way to centralize authentication. Instead of having to store and, potentially, change passwords on several servers, one domain controller handles the task. A Samba system running with server-level security does not, however, participate fully in the domain. A NetBIOS domain is a workgroup that includes several special features. One of these features is that the password server issues tokens to clients. These tokens help provide speedy logons to all the servers in the domain. When you set security = Domain, Samba participates more fully in the domain than when you set security = Server. In both server- and domain-level security, you must specify the domain controller with the password server parameter. Domain-level security also requires that you use encrypted passwords, which is not a requirement for server-level security.

When a server uses domain-level security, it must have a trust account on the domain controller. The Samba server must also join the domain. You can accomplish this with the smbpasswd command, as in

```
# smbpasswd -j PANTHER -r DREYFUS
```

This command joins the Samba server to the PANTHER domain, using the domain controller DREYFUS. The domain controller listed in this command is normally the same one you list with the password server parameter in smb.conf, although you can mix and match if your domain uses both primary and secondary domain controllers.

In the end, domain- and server-level security operate very similarly as far as a Samba server is concerned. Both of these, in turn, look the same as user-level security from the client's point of view. Which model you use, therefore, depends on whether you want to centralize your authentication.

At present, the extent of Samba's participation in a domain is limited, even with domain-level security specified. The experimental Samba TNG branch of Samba development includes additional domain support. Future versions of Samba will no doubt further Samba's domain participation, to allow remote administration of Samba servers from Windows systems using Windows tools rather than only local administration or administration through Samba-specific tools such as SWAT (which work equally well no matter what security model you use).

Other Authentication Parameters

In addition to the security parameter, Samba includes a number of other parameters that affect how it performs authentication:

min password length This parameter sets the minimum number of characters Samba accepts in a cleartext password. The default value is 5. There is no way to set a minimum number of characters for an encrypted password.

null passwords This parameter defaults to No, which disallows access to accounts that have no set passwords. When it's set to Yes, users can log on to Samba using no password when an account has no password set—a potentially huge hole in security.

password level SMB/CIFS uses case-insensitive passwords, so m1nkey and M1NKEY are equivalent. Linux, on the other hand, uses case-sensitive passwords—and Samba uses the password level parameter to bridge the gap. No matter how this parameter is set, Samba first tries to use the password as it's sent by the client, and then converted to all lowercase. If password level is set to a value higher than the default 0, Samba then tries all possible passwords with some characters converted to uppercase (from 1 to the value of password level). For example, if the client sent m1nkey as the password and if password level = 2, Samba tries M1nkey, m1Nkey, and so on through m1nkeY, then M1Nkey, M1nKey, and so on through m1nkEY.

Part II

The `password level` parameter is critical when your users have mixed-case passwords and a client converts passwords to all uppercase or all lowercase before sending them. This sometimes happens with Windows for Workgroups. The parameter is useful only when Samba uses unencrypted passwords; encrypted passwords aren't afflicted by the password case differences between Samba and Linux.

username level   This parameter works much like `password level`, but applied to usernames rather than passwords. Initially, Samba tries the username as sent but converted to all lowercase, then with the first letter capitalized. For example, if the client sends JACQUES as the username, Samba tries `jacques` and then `Jacques`. When `username level` is set higher than the default 0, Samba tries converting some letters to uppercase, as described for `password level`.

The `username level` parameter is particularly likely to be useful with DOS clients, which convert usernames to uppercase. Unlike `password level`, this parameter works with both encrypted and unencrypted passwords.

restrict anonymous   If set to Yes, this parameter causes Samba to refuse all anonymous connections to the server. Normally, some clients (such as Windows NT 4.0) rely on anonymous access for some tasks—renewing browse lists, for example. The default value is, therefore, No because Yes can cause browsing problems, particularly after a user has logged off a Windows NT client.

revalidate   This parameter works only when `security = User`. Normally, `revalidate` is set to No, which allows a client to connect to new shares on a server without going through the authentication procedure a second time. Setting the parameter to Yes can improve security by a small amount, but at the cost of marginally increased network traffic. Also, if the client doesn't cache passwords, users may have to enter passwords several times.

All of these parameters are global and affect access to the server. Samba includes many additional parameters that affect access within specific shares, many of which are described in "File Ownership and Permissions" later in this chapter.

ENCRYPTED VERSUS CLEARTEXT PASSWORDS

One point mentioned repeatedly earlier in this chapter is the distinction between *cleartext* and *encrypted* passwords. This is a critically important aspect of Samba's password handling and, in fact, is perhaps the most common challenge for new Samba administrators. That's because Samba's default encryption policies don't work with the most recent versions of Windows, as described shortly, in "Default Encryption for Versions of Windows."

When something is transmitted as ordinary text, it's said to be sent as *cleartext*. A *cleartext password* is, therefore, a password that's sent as plain (ASCII) text. If a client sends m1nkey as a cleartext password, the string m1nkey appears somewhere in the packets that travel from the client to the server.

Encrypted information, on the other hand, is scrambled in some way. The goal of a typical encryption algorithm is to allow only the desired recipient to use the encrypted information. Typically, two *keys* are used— one to encode the text and another to decode it. In transferring a password, the server can send an encryption (or public) key to the client and retain a matched decryption (or private) key locally or store pre-encrypted passwords locally. When the client sends the password using the encryption key, nobody else can decode the password, because only the server has the matching decryption key. When the client sends the password m1nkey in an encrypted form, that string doesn't appear in any packet; instead, it traverses the wire as ciphertext or encrypted text.

Advantages and Drawbacks of Encrypted and Cleartext Passwords

Both cleartext and encrypted passwords have their advantages and disadvantages. Before reviewing these, you should understand that TCP/IP networking is inherently insecure. Consider the network depicted in Figure 10.1. If CLOUSEAU is a server, and DALA connects to CLOUSEAU, then several different types of computer may be able to inspect every packet that travels between the two computers, including packets containing sensitive passwords. Specifically:

▶ LITTON, on DALA's home network, can inspect all traffic from and to DALA if the local network uses coaxial Ethernet, twisted-pair

Part II

Ethernet with a hub, or various other types of networking hardware. Chances are, a switch will keep LITTON from examining DALA's traffic, though.

▶ DREYFUS, on CLOUSEAU's home network, can inspect all traffic from and to CLOUSEAU, under the same circumstances applying on the other side of the connection.

▶ Figure 10.1 depicts the Internet as a blob. In fact, the Internet is a mass of computers. Although the vast majority of these computers cannot inspect packets that pass between systems, many can. In particular, routers that lie between the two end-point networks, and possibly other computers on these routers' local networks, can inspect packets that traverse the network.

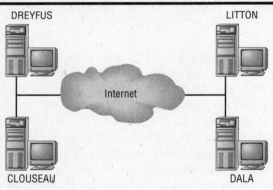

FIGURE 10.1: Network traffic from one computer to another passes through a potentially large number of intermediary computers.

The key point to remember is that, on most network accesses that involve routing from one network to another, a large number of computers over which you have no control may be able to access your data, including passwords. Even on local networks, passwords can often be "sniffed" from computers on those local networks. If one of your network's computers has been compromised by an outsider, that outsider may be able to obtain passwords by using a packet sniffer utility on your own computer.

Considering Samba specifically, password encryption has several advantages and disadvantages. On the plus side, encryption provides these important benefits:

Improved Security When you use encrypted passwords, you make it harder for an outsider to sniff passwords. This benefit is particularly important if you must allow access to Samba from outside your local network.

No password level Hassles   The password level parameter, described in "Other Authentication Parameters," applies to unencrypted passwords, not encrypted passwords. This fact makes the handling of encrypted Samba passwords simpler in some ways than the handling of unencrypted passwords, because you need not be concerned with configuring Samba to try matching variants of the password provided by the client.

Separate Linux and Samba Passwords   When you use encrypted passwords, you maintain separate Linux and Samba passwords. Your users can therefore use different passwords for shell access and Samba access. Alternatively, you can disable password-based access to Linux except through Samba, if you want users to be able to use a server only through Samba.

Defaults for Recent Versions of Windows   As described in greater detail in "Default Encryption for Versions of Windows," all currently available versions of Windows use encrypted passwords by default. If you do not enable encrypted password use in Samba, these clients will not be able to access shares on a Samba server, at least not without being modified themselves to send cleartext passwords.

Required for Domains   Domains function on encrypted passwords. This is a rule that cannot be broken; so if you use a domain, you must use encrypted passwords.

The advantages of encrypted passwords create a very powerful argument in their favor. There are, however, drawbacks to their use, including the following:

Separate Linux and Samba Passwords   This feature is both an advantage and a disadvantage to encrypted passwords. Maintaining a separate encrypted password database for Samba requires extra administrative work on your part. Fortunately, Samba includes some tools that can help you keep your Linux and Samba password databases synchronized, if that is your desire. Unfortunately, setting up encrypted passwords initially can be a major nuisance, particularly if your server hosts many users.

Older Client Expectations Older clients use cleartext passwords. Although Samba can fall back on cleartext passwords when it's configured for encrypted passwords, doing so can result in verification of cleartext passwords against Linux's normal password database, and of encrypted passwords against Samba's encrypted password database. This can cause user confusion if the two don't match.

NOTE

Linux's passwords, stored in /etc/passwd or /etc/shadow, are encrypted. Linux uses a different encryption scheme for its own passwords than NetBIOS uses for its passwords, and the two can't be converted from one to another. When Linux receives a cleartext password (whether from Samba or for any other purpose), it encrypts the password and checks the result against the encrypted form stored in its database.

On the whole, the advantages of encrypted passwords outweigh the advantages of cleartext passwords for most networks. If you have an isolated network that's already configured to use cleartext passwords, however, converting it to encrypted passwords may be more trouble than it's worth. You may be planning to add new Windows 98, Windows Me, or Windows 2000 computers, and so can prepare to convert to encrypted passwords. You should also give serious consideration to doing so if your network is accessible from the Internet at large. If a cracker breaks into one of your computers (even a client system), cleartext passwords can often be easily sniffed, opening a door into your Samba server.

Default Encryption for Versions of Windows

As installed, the versions of Windows use different default encryption policies:

▶ Cleartext is used by Windows for Workgroups, Windows 95, and Windows NT 3.1–4.0.

▶ Encryption is used by Windows 95 OEM Service Release 2 (OSR2), Windows 98, Windows Me, Windows NT 4.0 Service Pack 3 and higher, and Windows 2000.

It's virtually certain that future versions of Windows will use encrypted passwords by default. Samba's default encryption policy is to expect cleartext passwords. When configured to send encrypted passwords, Windows computers don't fall back to using cleartext passwords. Therefore, if both Samba and Windows clients are set for their defaults, Samba cannot authenticate recent versions of Windows clients. You must change either Samba's configuration or the Windows configuration to use Samba with recent Windows clients. The next two sections describe how to do this.

Using Samba's Encryption Policy

Samba includes a large number of features that control its handling of password encryption. Many of these are parameters in the smb.conf file. Others are support programs that allow you to change encrypted passwords or prepare the system to use encrypted passwords.

Encryption Parameters in *smb.conf*

A handful of global smb.conf parameters control Samba's password encryption policies:

encrypt passwords   This Boolean parameter defaults to No, which causes Samba to use normal Linux authentication methods and cleartext passwords. If you change it to Yes, Samba uses encrypted passwords stored in the smbpasswd file or an external password server in lieu of Linux's normal authentication methods. The security parameter controls whether Samba uses an smbpasswd file or an external password server.

smb passwd file   This parameter sets the name of the smbpasswd file, including a complete path. The default value is a compile-time option, but it's normally a file called smbpasswd located in the same directory as the smb.conf file, or in a subdirectory with tighter security settings.

WARNING

The smbpasswd file is extremely sensitive. Although the passwords stored in smbpasswd are encrypted, crackers can attack the encryption of these passwords in various ways (such as by encrypting every word in a dictionary and comparing the results against smbpasswd's contents, to locate weak passwords). You should, therefore, ensure that smbpasswd has very restrictive permissions—0600 with root ownership works well in most cases. To prevent ordinary users from even finding the file, you may also want to store it in a directory with 0700 permissions and root ownership.

update encrypted   This parameter is intended as a tool when migrating a network from cleartext to encrypted passwords. It defaults to No; but when set to Yes, Samba runs smbpasswd to update the Samba encrypted password file whenever a user logs on using a cleartext password. The idea behind use of this parameter is that you create an encrypted password file with null passwords for all users, and then set update encrypted = Yes and leave encrypt passwords = No for a time. Users can then use the server normally and, after a few days, most or all of the encrypted passwords will be set to the same values as the normal Linux passwords. You can then set update encrypted = No and encrypt passwords = Yes and add clients that require encrypted passwords, or convert clients to use encrypted passwords. The transition is smooth from your users' point of view. The alternative is to require all users to run smbpasswd from a Linux shell prompt, or you can assign passwords randomly and require users to use these assigned passwords. "Samba's Password Support Programs" describes migrating from cleartext to encrypted passwords in more detail.

unix password sync   This parameter controls whether Samba tries to change the Linux password for a user whenever the Samba encrypted password is changed. The default value is No, which leaves the user or administrator to synchronize passwords manually, if desired.

passwd program   This parameter specifies the complete path to the program that Linux uses to change users' passwords. On most systems, this value defaults to /bin/passwd, but you can change it if necessary. Samba uses this value only when changing the encrypted password and if unix password sync = Yes.

passwd chat   A typical Linux passwd program displays information, accepts a response, displays more information, and so on until the password is changed. Samba uses the passwd chat parameter to control its responses to the passwd program's output, in order to change the password. The default value of this parameter varies from one installation to another, but probably resembles the following:

```
*new*password* %n\n *new*password* %n\n *changed*
```

Components of this parameter include the following:

Asterisks (*)	These represent any received character or set of characters.
Ordinary text	Plain text represents itself. It's most likely to be used in the expect portion of the string—that is, what Samba expects to see from the passwd program.
Variables (%o and %n)	These may be used in the send string to represent the old and new passwords. Depending on how the program is called, however, Samba may not know the old password. Specifically, if you call the smbpassword program as root, smbpassword doesn't ask for the old password; and because the encryption used to store the password isn't reversible, Samba can't provide the old password in this situation.
Escape characters	You can use the standard two-character escape sequences for carriage return, line feed, tab, or space: \r, \n, \t, or \s, respectively.
Double quotes (")	Use double quotes to enclose strings that contain spaces, to ensure that they're interpreted correctly.
Full stops (.)	In the passwd chat parameter, full stops (a.k.a. periods) are interpreted as meaning no input or no output.

Many Linux distributions come with smb.conf files set with passwd chat and related parameters that are appropriate for the distribution's version of the passwd program. If this isn't the case and you want to use automatic password updates, try using the default values; just set unix password sync = Yes to enable password synchronization. When you change a Samba password, as described in "Samba's Password Support Programs," check to see if the matching Linux password also changed. If it didn't, try using passwd directly and compare its output and what it expects against the default passwd chat parameter's contents, and

Part II

adjust it as necessary. Attention to detail is critical when setting this feature, because chat scripts like this are notoriously picky about things that humans easily overlook, such as the case of strings and the presence or absence of spaces or tabs.

One critical point to consider when you create a password-change script is that Samba runs passwd as root. When run in this way, passwd doesn't normally ask for the original password.

Samba's Password Support Programs

Samba includes several support programs that allow you to create and maintain an encrypted password file. The smbpasswd program is the most important in day-to-day use, but additional tools are critical when it comes to setting up your server or migrating it from using cleartext to encrypted passwords.

Using *smbpasswd*

The most important password support tool is smbpasswd, which is the Samba equivalent of the passwd program—it lets you change encrypted Samba passwords. The smbpasswd program uses the following syntax:

```
smbpasswd [-a] [-d] [-e] [-D debuglevel] [-n] [-r
➥ machinename] [-U username] [-h] [-s] [username]
```

NOTE

Don't confuse the smbpasswd *program* with the smbpasswd *file*. Both bear the same name, but they're very different things. Because they're so different, you'll be able to see from context which one is meant in any given discussion in this chapter. When necessary, the word *program* or *file* is used to distinguish the two.

The various optional parameters to smbpasswd include the following:

-a This parameter adds a user to the smbpasswd file. This option is honored only when root runs smbpasswd.

-d This parameter disables the specified username. Subsequent attempts to log on using the specified username fail. Only root can use this option.

-e The opposite of -d, this parameter enables the specified username. Only root can use this option.

-D *debuglevel*   This parameter sets the debug level to a value between 0 and 10 (the default is 0). Higher values write additional information to the Samba log files. Try -D 1 if you have a problem. Levels above 3 are likely to be useful only to Samba developers.

-n   Only available to root, this parameter sets a null password for the specified user. If you use null passwords = Yes, as described in "Other Authentication Parameters," anybody is allowed to log on to the share. Otherwise, the result is effectively the same as disabling the username with -d.

-r *machinename*   This parameter lets you adjust the password on a remote computer, which can be either another Samba server or a Windows NT or 2000 system.

-U *username*   Use this parameter in conjunction with the -r parameter to specify the user whose password you want to change.

-h   Use this parameter to display a summary of options available from smbpasswd.

-s   This parameter causes smbpasswd to use standard input and output, rather than /dev/tty. If you want to write a script that calls smbpasswd, this option may be necessary. You can use it along with redirection operators (such as < and >) to get smbpasswd to accept input from and send output to files or other programs.

username   When root runs smbpasswd, you have to specify the user whose password should be changed.

The two most common uses of smbpasswd are by a user who changes his or her own password, and by the administrator to change a user's password. In the first case, the exchange resembles the following:

```
$ smbpasswd
Old SMB password:
New SMB password:
Retype new SMB password:
Password changed for user jacques
```

When run this way, smbpasswd doesn't require that a username be specified, but the program does need the user's old password. Neither the old nor the new password echoes to the screen, as a security measure.

When root runs smbpasswd, the behavior is slightly different:

```
# smbpasswd jacques
New SMB password:
Retype new SMB password:
Password changed for user jacques.
```

In this case, root must specify the username but does not need to provide the old password.

Setting Up Encrypted Passwords

When you first configure a Samba server to use encrypted passwords, you must do several things:

1. Create an smbpasswd file. There are a couple of options for doing this, as described shortly.

2. Populate the smbpasswd file with valid passwords. You can do this a couple of different ways, as described shortly.

3. Reconfigure Samba to use smbpasswd. This is a matter of setting encrypt passwords = Yes in smb.conf.

4. Add clients that use encrypted passwords to your network, or convert existing clients to use encrypted passwords.

One way of creating an smbpasswd file is to run smbpasswd as root with the -a parameter. Although smbpasswd complains about not being able to open a file, it creates a new one and adds the user you specify. You can then rerun smbpasswd -a to add more users to its list. This procedure may be useful if you have few users or want to assign passwords, rather than let users choose their own. If you have many users, however, creating them all this way can be awkward. Although you can automate the process by using a script, the issue of password assignment can impose difficulties.

Another way to create an smbpasswd file is to run the helper program mksmbpasswd—a script that comes with most Linux Samba distributions. (On some distributions, it's called mksmbpasswd.sh.) This program accepts as input the /etc/passwd file and creates as output a model smbpasswd file with null passwords. You can use it as follows:

```
# cat /etc/passwd | mksmbpasswd > smbpasswd
```

Once you've created the smbpasswd file, you should edit it to remove users who have no need to access Samba. Chances are, the file created by mksmbpasswd will have several such users at the top—these are users that Linux uses internally, such as ftp and daemon. Be sure to remove root from this list, as well. When you're done editing the file, move it to /etc, /etc/samba.d, or wherever Samba expects to find the smbpasswd file. You then have three choices for how to proceed:

▶ Use smbpasswd as root to assign passwords to all users. If you intend to do this, though, there's no reason to use mksmbpasswd; you could simply call smbpasswd with the -a parameter to do the job in one step.

▶ Have users set their Samba passwords. This could be accomplished several ways, including the following:

  ▶ Have users log on using shell accounts and issue the smbpasswd command. This may be a viable option if users have shell access.

  ▶ Set smbpasswd to be the users' logon shells. When users use Telnet or Secure Shell (SSH) to try to log on, they get the smbpasswd program and can set their passwords; then the system ends the connection. This can be a good option if users don't have or need shell access to the server. It can also be useful for future Samba password changes.

  ▶ Use SWAT to enable users to change their passwords.

  ▶ Have users approach you individually to run smbpasswd. This approach allows you to supervise the process, but may be very time-consuming if you have many users.

▶ Set the update encrypted = Yes parameter in smb.conf, which lets Samba automatically update the encrypted passwords based on the cleartext passwords used by Linux. This option is useful if your network currently uses cleartext passwords but you want to migrate over to encrypted passwords. It's not useful if your network already uses encrypted passwords. This option is described earlier, in "Encryption Parameters in smb.conf." After running for a time with this option set, most or all of the users' smbpasswd entries will be set to match their Linux passwords.

As you can see, setting up encrypted passwords on a new server can involve a substantial amount of work, particularly if you're trying to migrate an existing large user base from another platform. By planning carefully, though, you can minimize your troubles by letting your users do the bulk of the work of entering passwords, either through `smbpasswd` or the `update encrypted` parameter. Another option is to use an existing password server. If your network already contains such a server, it's likely to be much easier to set up Samba to use that server than to duplicate its user and password list locally.

Setting the Windows Encryption Policy

As described in "Default Encryption for Versions of Windows," Microsoft in the late 1990s shifted its default encryption policy for Windows from using cleartext passwords by default to using encrypted passwords. If you're running an older network that still employs cleartext passwords, it's often easier to reconfigure new clients to use cleartext passwords than it is to enable encrypted passwords on your Samba server—at least in the short term.

To continue to use cleartext passwords, you can enable them on Windows clients by following these steps:

1. On the Samba server, locate the `WinVer_PlainPassword` `.reg` files (where `WinVer` is a version of Windows, such as `Win98`). These files should be in your Samba documentation directory, such as `/usr/doc/samba-2.0.7` or `/usr/doc/packages/samba`.

2. Copy the `WinVer_PlainPassword.reg` files to a floppy disk that uses the FAT filesystem. You only need to copy the files that correspond to the clients you have on your network.

3. Remove the floppy disk you created in step 2 from the Linux server and insert it in the floppy drive of a client you want to reconfigure to use cleartext passwords.

4. On the client, open the floppy disk and double-click the appropriate `WinVer_PlainPassword.reg` file. This action creates a new Windows Registry entry that disables the use of encrypted passwords. (On Windows NT and 2000 clients, you must perform this step as the Administrator.)

5. Reboot the client computer. It should now use cleartext passwords.

NOTE

You can use a method other than a floppy disk to transport these files, if you like—FTP, for instance. You can't use Samba, however (at least not directly), because Windows clients configured to use encrypted passwords can't access a cleartext-only Samba server.

To reverse this process, you'll have to edit the *WinVer_PlainPassword* .*reg* file. This file should have a line that reads

```
"EnablePlainTextPassword"=dword:00000001
```

Change this line so that it reads

```
"EnablePlainTextPassword"=dword:00000000
```

You can then perform steps 2 through 5 with the modified file to re-enable encrypted passwords.

FILE OWNERSHIP AND PERMISSIONS

One important aspect of security on a Samba server is in configuring ownership and permissions on individual shares and files. Samba includes a number of parameters, including force user, create mask, and directory mask, that affect who can access a share, what Linux permissions Samba gives to files it creates, and so on. This section describes some of the consequences of using these file-sharing parameters.

Evaluating Per-Share Ownership and Permissions

Each share has associated with it certain security characteristics. For example, you can make a share read-only or read/write (via the writeable parameter), you can set the permissions Samba uses to create files in a share (via create mask, force create mode, and similar parameters), and you can set the ownership of files created in a share (via force user).

It's worth reiterating, however, that you should give considerable thought to the security consequences of any configuration you might produce. Here are some questions to ask yourself:

▶ When a user accesses the computer from a shell prompt, does that user have any sort of special access to a share? Can the user create links that lead outside the share from a shell prompt? Can the user create or delete files in a read-only share from a shell prompt? Can the user change permissions in ways that might cause problems?

▶ When a user accesses a share using Samba, what privileges are granted? If a link exists in a share pointing to an area outside the share, can a user do any damage using that link? Can a user overwrite other users' files? If so, is this desirable?

▶ If you use force user, with what Linux privileges will Samba users be accessing the computer? Does that account have unusual rights? Does it correspond with a real user (which is usually not a good idea)? Do you use the same "dummy" account for multiple shares? (Again, this may be a step toward problems in some cases.)

▶ Do you rely on specific ownership or permissions in a share? If so, is there any way, short of intervention from root, that files with differing ownership or permissions might appear in the share? This might happen because of users with shell access or other servers, for example, and might cause files to be undeletable or inaccessible from Samba.

The answers to many of these questions can be good, bad, or indifferent, depending on your uses for the shares and your server's configuration. For example, the ability of users to create files with assorted ownership within a share can cause problems in some cases, but this ability may be desirable or even necessary in others. You should, therefore, think about the answers to these questions with respect to *your environment's specific* requirements.

If you carefully consider the security consequences of share-level access controls when you configure your Samba server, you should have no problems as a result of these features. Failure to consider the consequences of a configuration, however, may entangle your server in a web of file-access difficulties. When you first deal with a Samba server, it's probably best to stick to simple configurations, if at all possible. Providing access to users' home shares and perhaps one or two read-only shared areas is usually not too demanding. On the other hand, juggling multiple groups of users with complex needs for cross-group sharing and security can turn into a brain-teasing logical puzzle.

Evaluating Per-User Access Controls

Many of Samba's access control mechanisms operate on the level of individual users. These parameters are normally share parameters, so you can set one share's security features to be quite different from another share on the same server. Here is a brief rundown:

read list   With this parameter you can specify a list of users who are to be given read-only access to an otherwise read/write share. For example, read list = jacques, simone prevents these two users from writing to a share.

write list   This parameter functions as the opposite of read list; users included on the write list can write to a share that is read-only to other users. If a share includes both a read list and a write list and a user appears on both lists, the write list entry takes precedence.

valid users   When you want to restrict access to a share to just a few users, this parameter lets you do so. For example, valid users = jacques, simone configures Samba to allow only jacques and simone to access a share. Other users can see the share in browse lists, but they aren't allowed in.

invalid users   This parameter is the opposite of valid users; users listed in this parameter are not allowed access to the share, whereas other users can access it. If a share has both valid users and invalid users lists and a user appears on both lists, then invalid users takes precedence; the user is not granted access.

Per-user access controls can be extremely useful in tightening security on a Samba server. Considered only within the Samba security model, these parameters give you fine and arbitrary control over user access to shares. You can restrict access such that simone, for instance, cannot read a share, or can read it but not write to it, even when simone belongs to all the same Linux groups as other users who can access the share. This arbitrary control can be extremely useful if you want to restrict access. It can also be employed when you want to *loosen* restrictions for some reason. For example, you might have a read-only share that contains program files. In the event you need to update those files, however, it's necessary that somebody have write access to the share. Using write list provides a wedge into the share; you can use one account as a designated maintenance account for otherwise read-only shares.

Be aware that the utility of these per-user access parameters is reduced when you add Linux shell account access to the mix. When a user has access to a directory from a shell account, Samba access restrictions suddenly become meaningless—at least, if serious security is your goal. If you only want to protect against accidents, the Samba-only features may be adequate. When your users have Linux shell accounts, you must consider how permissions on the directories in question interact with standard Linux security to bypass Samba's features.

Integrating ACLs with Samba

Windows NT and 2000 support a security model built around access control lists (ACLs). ACLs use users, groups, and both read and write permissions to files, just as does Linux's native security model. ACLs go further, however, in that they use *lists* of users and groups to control access. You can, therefore, specify an arbitrary list of users or groups who have particular types of access to a file or directory. Although it's often possible to mimic the effects of ACLs in Linux by using a large number of groups, one for each arbitrary group of users, this practice can be tedious to implement.

Because ACLs are more flexible than Linux's native file ownership and security model, Samba doesn't completely implement ACLs. However, Samba does provide Windows NT and 2000 clients with access to Linux file security options through Windows's ACL mechanisms. Samba includes several parameters that influence ACL support:

nt acl support   This global parameter determines whether Samba gives Windows NT clients access to Linux security information. The default value is Yes.

security mask   This parameter sets the permission bits that a Windows NT client may access. The default value is the same as the create mask parameter. To give Windows NT clients full access to Linux permission bits, set security mask = 0777.

directory security mask   This parameter works much like the security mask parameter, but it applies to directories rather than files. The default value is the same as the directory mask parameter.

force security mode   The security mask option sets permission bits that a Windows NT client *may* set. The force security mode parameter, in contrast, sets the permission bits that will automatically be set when clients try to change permissions. It defaults to the value of the force create mode parameter, which has a default of 0000.

force directory security mode   This parameter works like force security mode, but it applies to directories rather than files. It defaults to the value of the force directory mode parameter.

NOTE

Windows NT's permission controls provide access to the Linux execute bit. Samba uses this bit to double for the FAT-style archive, system, and hidden bits. Therefore, if you change the execute bits on any file, you'll also find that the file's archive, system, or hidden status changes.

On most networks, the default values for these ACL-integration parameters produce reasonable results. Windows NT clients can adjust permissions on files and directories on the Linux server up to the limits imposed by the create mask and directory mask parameters.

From Windows NT 4.0, you can access the Linux permission information as follows:

1. Open a window on the directory that contains a file or directory you want to modify.

2. Right-click the file or directory you want to modify. In the pop-up menu, select Properties. Windows displays a Properties dialog box.

3. In the Properties dialog box, click the Security tab. The Properties dialog box should now resemble the one shown in Figure 10.2. Windows provides three security features: Permissions, Auditing, and Ownership. Auditing does not work with a Samba server. Ownership allows you to see who the owner of the file is, but the Take Ownership button in the Owner dialog box doesn't work. Permissions works within the limits of the Linux permissions model, as described in the next steps.

2

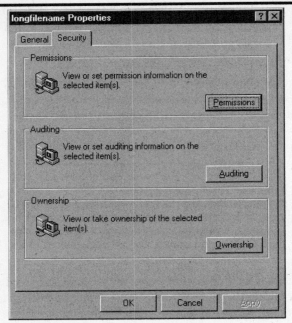

FIGURE 10.2: Of the three security features, only Permissions can be changed on files stored on a Samba server.

4. Click the Permissions button. Windows displays the File Permissions dialog box shown in Figure 10.3. There are three access groups in this case: Everyone (Linux's world permissions), the owner (rodsmith), and the group (users).

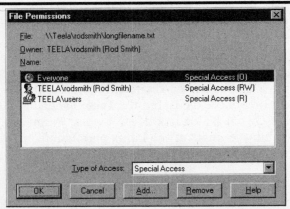

FIGURE 10.3: Files stored on a Samba server always have three sets of permissions: Everyone, the owner, and the users group.

5. Click one of the three permissions groups, and then click Special Access... in the Type of Access field. Windows displays the Special Access dialog box shown in Figure 10.4.

NOTE

Windows displays two entries called Special Access in the Type of Access field. One is followed by an ellipsis (...), and the other isn't. Select the one that includes the ellipsis. The one without the ellipsis doesn't allow you to modify the settings.

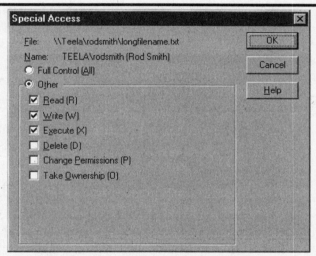

FIGURE 10.4: You can set Linux permission bits in the Special Access dialog box, but not all of the box's features are useful.

6. In the Special Access dialog box, you can check Read (R), Write (W), or Execute (X) to set the appropriate bits on the Samba server, assuming the `security mask` or `directory security mask` parameters allow you to do so. If you enable other options, or options that are disallowed by your `smb.conf` configuration, Samba ignores them.

Part II

7. Click OK in the Special Access dialog box. Windows shows your changed permissions in parentheses following the words "Special Access" in the File Permissions dialog box (Figure 10.3). If you've removed all permissions, Windows displays an "O" in parentheses (you can see this in the Everyone line in Figure 10.3). At this point, Windows displays your changed permissions as you've entered them, even if you've selected options that Samba doesn't support or allow.

8. Click OK in the File Permissions dialog box and again in the Properties dialog box.

The result of all this activity is a change in permissions on the Samba server. Because Samba maps Linux user, group, and world permissions onto constructs that Windows can deal with, access to those permissions from Windows is fairly straightforward.

As an alternative to steps 5 through 7, you might try selecting a preconfigured set of permissions from the Type of Access list. Samba will accept such a selection, but if the option you choose includes permissions that are meaningless under Linux, Samba ignores these settings just as if you selected them from the Special Access dialog box (Figure 10.4).

Setting permissions in Windows 2000 is somewhat easier than in Windows NT 4.0. In Windows 2000, you have direct control over the permissions from the Security tab of the Properties dialog box (see Figure 10.5). There's no need to click a Permissions button in the Properties dialog box or open a Special Access dialog box to change permissions.

NOTE

If the server runs Samba 2.0.6 or earlier, Windows 2000 doesn't display the owner or group name correctly; instead, it displays a long numeric code. With Samba 2.0.7 and later versions, Windows 2000 displays the file's owner and group names accurately.

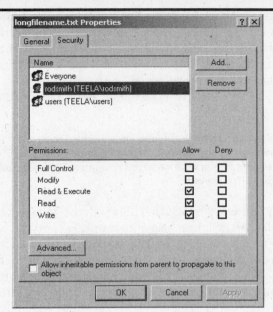

FIGURE 10.5: Windows 2000 provides more-direct access to Linux permissions than does Windows NT 4.0.

When you manipulate files on an NTFS partition on a Windows computer, you can use the Add button in the File Permissions dialog box (shown earlier in Figure 10.3) to add permissions for an arbitrary number of users or groups. You cannot do this with files stored on a Samba server. If you try, you'll get an error message, either when you select the group or when you click the OK button in the Add Users and Groups dialog box.

SAMBA OVER SSL

SMB/CIFS was designed at a time when network security concerns were, by today's standards, simple. Aside from encrypted passwords, SMB/CIFS doesn't encrypt any other data passing over the network. As a result, all the files you transfer with SMB/CIFS might be read by somebody using a packet sniffer on the source, the destination, or an intervening network. This fact can be a major drawback to the protocol in certain situations— for example, if you want to pass data across the Internet, or if you're using SMB/CIFS in a *very* high-security environment that requires encryption even on your local network connections. In these cases, it's useful to be able to add another package to encrypt SMB/CIFS connections. Samba includes support for one such protocol, the *Secure Sockets Layer (SSL)*, which is also used on many secure websites. Unfortunately, configuring Samba and its clients to use SSL is a bit tedious, but it can be done, and it greatly enhances security if you need to use clients and servers that are separated by networks you don't trust.

NOTE

Another option is to use Samba in conjunction with the *Secure Shell (SSH)*, which is most commonly used as a replacement for Telnet. Like SSL, SSH can be used to encrypt data from a wide variety of programs. Samba includes no explicit support for SSH, however.

The type of security addressed by SSL and SSH is that of the readability of the *files* you transfer. An SSL link also automatically encrypts your passwords, but if you're only concerned with password security, `encrypt passwords = Yes` is a much simpler (although also somewhat less effective) option than SSL. You should consider SSL only if your shared files contain extremely sensitive data, such as trade secrets or confidential medical information.

WARNING

Before proceeding further, check to be sure that running SSL in your environment is legal. Russia and some other countries restrict the use of cryptographic software such as SSL and SSH. In the past, the United States restricted the export of cryptographic software, even when it was readily available outside the U.S. For these reasons, SSL hasn't been integrated more closely into Samba or Linux. The U.S. has loosened its export restrictions, however, leading to easier availability of SSL and similar packages.

Configuring SSL

The first step to using SSL with Samba is to install and configure an SSL package. This process can be intimidating if you're not used to dealing with cryptographic software, certificates, and so on, but it's not too difficult if you follow the steps described here.

Installing SSL on Linux

Two major SSL implementations are available for Linux:

▶ SSLeay (http://www2.psy.uq.edu.au/~ftp/Crypto/ssleay/)

▶ OpenSSL (http://www.openssl.org/)

In addition, you can find links to many mirror sites that host OpenSSL RPMs at www.openssh.com/portable.html, and the Debian website (www.debian.org/) lists SSL packages for Debian-based distributions.

NOTE

Red Hat 7 ships with both OpenSSL and an SSL-enabled version of Samba. Future versions of other distributions may follow suit. Chances are you won't need to install SSL on such a system, but you will still need to create SSL certificates.

The following sections discuss the configuration of OpenSSL, but the configuration of SSLeay is quite similar; only the locations of a few configuration files differ.

Assuming you have an RPM-based Linux distribution, you can install the OpenSSL RPMs just as you would any other RPM files, by entering this:

```
# rpm -Uvh openssl-0.9.5a-1.i386.rpm
openssl-devel-0.9.5a-1.i386.rpm
```

If you need to compile SSL from source, follow the instructions that come with the package. Typically, you must run a configure script and then run make and make install.

TIP

In preparing this chapter, I ran across an SSLeay binary package that didn't work well with Samba. During the Samba configuration phase, the configure script complained that it could not create a summary. Replacing this binary with an OpenSSL binary or a version of SSLeay compiled from source code on the same system solved this problem. If you encounter difficulties compiling Samba with SSL, try replacing the SSL package with another one.

Basic SSL Configuration

Basic SSL configuration involves telling SSL where it will find certain key files and setting up the program so it can be run easily. Perform the following configuration steps as root:

1. Set up the SSL binary so that it's accessible on your path. If you installed the program from an RPM or Debian package, this has probably already been done. If you compiled the

program yourself, you may need to add the SSL binary path to your PATH environment variable. You can adjust this variable system-wide by editing it in /etc/profile.

Alternatively, you can create a link called ssleay in a directory that's on your path (such as /usr/local/bin) to the SSL binary (ssleay or openssh) in its particular directory.

2. SSL relies on random numbers for part of its security. To prime SSL's random number generator, you'll need to create a file with random characters. To do so, enter the command

    ```
    # cat > /tmp/private.txt
    ```

    and then type characters randomly for a minute or more. When you're done, press Ctrl+D to stop input. The result will be a file called /tmp/private.txt that contains gibberish.

3. Convert the /tmp/private.txt file you just created into a form that's usable by SSL. To do this, enter the command

    ```
    # ssleay genrsa -rand /tmp/private.txt > /dev/null
    ```

    The result is a 1,024-byte file called /root/.rnd based on /tmp/private.txt. You can and should then delete /tmp/private.txt.

4. Create a directory in which SSL will store certificates. A good choice for this duty is /etc/certificates. Be sure to use chmod to restrict access to this directory once you've created it, as in **chmod 0700 /etc/certificates**.

5. Edit the /var/ssl/misc/CA.sh file (which may reside in some other directory if you built SSH yourself or used SSLeay rather than OpenSSH). Locate the line that defines CATOP; it probably reads CATOP=./demoCA. Change this line to read CATOP=/etc/certificates.

6. Edit the /var/ssl/openssl.cnf file. This file may reside elsewhere if you built SSL yourself, and it's called ssleay.cnf in SSLeay. Find the entry that reads dir = ./demoCA and change it to read dir = /etc/certificates.

These steps lay the groundwork for creating certificates, as described next. These certificates help to authenticate one computer to another, but they don't replace the usual SMB/CIFS password mechanisms.

Creating Certificates

Ordinarily, SSL is used in conjunction with a *certificate* issued by a *certification authority (CA)*. The CA's "stamp of approval" guarantees that a web-based retailer, for example, is the organization it claims to be and not an imposter. In most Samba SSL configurations, you don't need an external CA to provide this sort of guarantee; you can generate your own certificates, thereby serving as your own CA. This arrangement is certainly good enough for in-house use of Samba and SSL. If you run a secure website, however, you'll probably want to register with a CA. You can use these registrations with Samba over SSL.

Web servers typically don't require certificates on their clients, because the primary concern in web commerce is that the server be trustworthy. In file sharing, however, the identity of the client is at least as important as the identity of the server; you don't want unauthorized computers accessing your server. Generating certificates for your clients can help verify that your clients are who they claim to be.

Creating a CA Configuration

The first step to creating a certificate is to run the certificate authority setup script, CA.sh. If you installed SSL from the OpenSSL RPM files, this script is in the /var/ssl/misc directory. Listing 10.1 shows the results of running this script. You'll be asked to enter information identifying yourself and your organization. The passphrase you enter early on is like a password but should be substantially longer than a typical password. The script doesn't echo the passphrase you type, for security reasons.

Listing 10.1: Results of Running the Certificate Authority Setup Script

```
# /var/ssl/misc/CA.sh -newca
mkdir: cannot make directory '/etc/certificates': File exists
CA certificate filename (or enter to create)

Making CA certificate ...
Using configuration from /var/ssl/openssl.cnf
Generating a 1024 bit RSA private key
..........................................++++++
........++++++
writing new private key to
   '/etc/certificates/private/./cakey.pem'
```

```
Enter PEM pass phrase:
Verifying password - Enter PEM pass phrase:
---
You are about to be asked to enter information that will be
    incorporated
into your certificate request.
What you are about to enter is what is called a Distinguished
    Name or a DN.
There are quite a few fields but you can leave some blank
For some fields there will be a default value,
If you enter '.', the field will be left blank.
---
Country Name (2 letter code) [AU]:US
State or Province Name (full name) [Some-State]:Massachusetts
Locality Name (eg, city) []:Malden
Organization Name (eg, company) [Internet Widgits Pty
    Ltd]:The Panther School
Organizational Unit Name (eg, section) []:None
Common Name (eg, YOUR name) []:clouseau.panther.edu
Email Address []:jacques@panther.edu
```

Most of the details you enter, such as the organization's name, are unimportant. By default, however, the client and server must contain the same information for the country code, state, and organization name. (The upcoming section "Creating Client Certificates" describes entry of this information for the client certificates.)

As indicated early in the CA.sh output, the script creates a file called /etc/certificates/private/cakey.pem. This is a highly sensitive key file, so do not copy it onto other systems.

Creating Client Certificates

The next step is to create certificate files for use by clients. You can skip this step if you don't intend to use client certificates; however, because client certificates can provide an added component of security, I recommend you use them. Suppose the client you want to link to the server using SSL is called SIMONE. To avoid confusion, you can create certificates whose filenames are based on the client's name. First, you create a file called simone.key, by using the ssleay program:

```
# ssleay genrsa -des3 1024 >simone.key
Generating RSA private key, 1024 bit long modulus
...............++++++
...................++++++
```

```
e is 65537 (0x10001)
Enter PEM pass phrase:
Verifying password - Enter PEM pass phrase:
```

Note that creating the simone.key file requires that you enter a passphrase, just as you did when creating the cakey.pem file. This passphrase should not be the same as the passphrase used for the server.

You must now create a temporary client file:

```
# ssleay req -new -key simone.key -out simone-csr
Using configuration from /var/ssl/openssl.cnf
Enter PEM pass phrase:
```

The passphrase you enter here is the one for the client, not for the server. You only need to enter it once, because it's being used for authentication purposes, not to change or create the passphrase to begin with. At this point, you must enter the organization information from Listing 10.1 again, but this time, you should respond in a way that's appropriate for the client.

You must now use your CA configuration to "sign" the client's certificate. Doing so will allow the server to verify that the client has been approved to connect to the server. To do this, you use ssleay again:

```
# ssleay ca -days 1000 -infiles simone-csr >simone.pem
Using configuration from /var/ssl/openssl.cnf
Enter PEM pass phrase:
Check that the request matches the signature
Signature ok
```

To sign the client certificate, you enter the passphrase for the server. As with other passphrase entries, this information is not echoed to the screen. The program proceeds to display the information you've entered about the client's certificate. If all goes well, the program asks if you want to sign the certificate. Respond by typing **y**. Before committing changes to the server's certificate database (in /etc/certificates), the program asks once more for confirmation. Again, respond with **y**. The program finishes by confirming that it's written the changes.

If, rather than asking for these confirmations, the program complains that data did not match (for instance, if the states for the client and server don't match), then you should check your client and server configurations and make changes as appropriate.

Part II

NOTE

You specify the number of days for which a certificate is valid when you create it. This is the -days 1000 parameter in the preceding example. At the end of this time, you'll need to generate a new certificate.

The result of this certification creation process is as follows:

▶ An entry is made in the SSL certificates database on the server, in the /etc/certificates directory. You don't need to concern yourself with the details of this entry, except to be sure it's protected from harm, tampering, or unauthorized access.

▶ Two files (simone.key and simone.pem in the examples) are created; you will ultimately transport them to the client. These files are very sensitive; with them and the client passphrase, an unscrupulous individual could gain access to your server. Therefore, you should transport these files in the most secure manner possible—hand-delivered by floppy disk, for example.

I recommend that you generate client certificates for the server. Doing so will allow you to test the server configuration using smbclient to connect to the local computer.

With these certifications in hand, you'll now configure Samba to use SSL and set up SSL on your client system.

Configuring Samba to Use SSL

Before you can use SSL with Samba, you must compile an SSL-enabled version of the server. Unfortunately, Samba servers in most Linux distributions do not come with SSL support enabled. (Red Hat 7 is an exception to this rule, and there may be more exceptions in the future.) Once you've recompiled Samba with SSL support (and installed an SSL package), basic SSL functionality is a matter of setting a few parameters in smb.conf. You can then test for basic functionality by using smbclient to connect the server to itself.

Creating an SSL-Enabled Samba

Chances are good that you'll need to compile a copy of Samba with SSL support enabled. If you're uncertain about this requirement, skip ahead to "Setting Samba's SSL Parameters." Create an smb.conf file that contains

SSL support, and then type **testparm**. If testparm complains that it doesn't recognize the SSL parameters, you need to remove your current Samba installation and create a new one with SSL support.

Of critical importance is the –with-ssl parameter to configure. You *must* include this parameter to compile Samba with SSL support. In order for this option to work, SSL *and* the SSL development libraries must be installed on your system. These libraries often come in a separate package from the main SSL package, with a name similar to openssl-devel-0.9.5a-1.i386.rpm.

Note that Samba's SSL support assumes that certain SSL development files, most importantly ssl.h, are in typical locations. This arrangement isn't true of some SSL packages, including OpenSSL. In theory, using the –with-sslinc=*/path/to/ssl/libraries* parameter should fix this problem. In practice, you may need to create a symbolic link from a directory on your include path to the ssl.h file, wherever it might be. Alternatively, try creating a directory called /usr/local/ssl; then create in that directory a symbolic link called include to wherever your SSL include files are, and *do not* use the –with-sslinc parameter to configure.

Setting Samba's SSL Parameters

Samba includes a fairly large number of global SSL-related parameters. You can configure a basic SSL-enabled Samba server with just a handful of these parameters, including the following:

ssl   This Boolean parameter enables or disables SSL support. The default value is No, so you must set this parameter to Yes to allow SSL connections.

ssl server cert   This parameter accepts the full path to the SSL server certification file. If you've used /etc/certificates as the SSL certificates directory, you should use ssl server cert = /etc/certificates/cacert.pem. There is no default value.

ssl server key   You designate the location of the server's own key file in this parameter. If you've configured your server as specified in this chapter, then an appropriate setting is ssl server key = /etc/certificates/private/cakey.pem. This parameter has no default value.

The foregoing three parameters are enough to enable a basic SSL server configuration, but this configuration supports only encryption and not certificates. To use certificates, you must set the following additional options:

ssl ca certfile This parameter specifies the location of the certificates of all the trusted CAs. On a small server, this file may contain information on just one CA. To use certificates, you *must* use either this parameter or the ssl ca certdir parameter (but not both). If you've configured SSL as described earlier in "Basic SSL Configuration," you should point this parameter to /etc/certificates/cacert.pem. There is no default value.

ssl ca certdir This parameter specifies the location of the SSL CA certificates directory. The directory works like an SSL certification file, but each CA has its own file in the directory. This configuration, although it involves more work to set up if you have just a few CAs, may be preferable if you use a large number of CAs. There is no default value.

ssl client cert This parameter specifies an SSL client certificate file's location, such as the simone.pem file described earlier in "Creating Client Certificates." The smbclient parameter uses this client file when connecting to an SSL-enabled server. This file must be located in a directory that's readable by anybody who uses smbclient. If you want to use certificates as a client, you must set this option.

WARNING

Even though the SSL client certification file must be readable by anyone using an SSL-enabled connection, the file is still sensitive, so you should protect it as best you can given its required availability. You may want to create an SSL user group that can read the file, while restricting access to other users.

ssl client key This parameter specifies the location of an SSL client key file, such as simone.key, described in "Creating Client Certificates." This option is required if you want to use the computer as a client with a certificate. This key should be protected by placing it in a directory that's readable only by root.

ssl require clientcert This Boolean parameter determines whether Samba as a server will accept a connection from a client that lacks a certificate. The default value is No, which means that the server does not require a client certificate. Such connections are encrypted, but there's still a chance that one will come from an unauthorized source.

ssl require servercert This Boolean parameter determines whether smbclient will connect to a server that has no certification. As with ssl require clientcert, the default value is No, which enables encryption of connections but does little to guarantee the identity of the server.

Samba supports a number of additional SSL features, some of which require configuration options. You may want to use one or more of the following options to expand or fine-tune your configuration:

ssl hosts This parameter allows you to specify clients that *must* use SSL to connect to the server. It takes a list of computer names or IP addresses as a value, using the same syntax as the hosts allow and hosts deny parameters described in "Restricting Access by Computer" at the beginning of in this chapter. If neither this parameter nor the ssl hosts resign parameter is used, and if ssl = Yes, Samba requires *all* connections to be made through SSL.

ssl hosts resign This parameter is the opposite of ssl hosts; it specifies a list of clients that need not use SSL to connect to an SSL-enabled server. You might set up this parameter if you require only connections that arrive through routers to be SSL-enabled. You can specify your local network's IP addresses on ssl hosts resign, to exempt them from using SSL.

ssl ciphers You can specify which *ciphers* (that is, encryption schemes) Samba will use when negotiating a connection. Possible values are DEFAULT, DES-CFB-M1, NULL-MD5, RC4-MD5, EXP-RC4-MD5, RC2-CBC-MD5, EXP-RC2-CBC-MD5, IDEA-CBC-MD5, DES-CBC-MD5, DES-CBC-SHA, DES-CBC3-MD5, DES-CBC3-SHA, RC4-64-MD5, and NULL. Unless you're an SSL expert, I recommend you not adjust this parameter.

ssl version This parameter specifies which versions of the SSL protocol Samba will attempt to use. The default value is ssl2or3, which indicates that versions 2 and 3 will both be accepted. If necessary, you can set this parameter to tls1, ssl2, or ssl3.

ssl compatibility This parameter configures Samba to use some older SSL implementations. The default value is No, and chances are you won't need to change this.

If your server accepts both SSL-encrypted and unencrypted connections, you may need to use the ssl hosts or ssl hosts resign parameters. The latter is generally more secure because it sets up an exception to the SSL requirement rather than requiring SSL for only some connections. The rest of these parameters are advanced features that you probably won't need to adjust.

Testing Samba's SSL Functionality

The easiest way to test Samba's SSL functionality is to configure SSL with the three necessary SSL parameters (described in "Setting Samba's SSL Parameters") plus any certificate parameters necessary for your SSL configuration. You must then restart the Samba daemons. When you start smbd, you must enter your server's passphrase. If you're *not* asked for a passphrase, you're not using an SSL-enabled version of Samba with SSL features turned on.

Once Samba is running, use the smbclient program from the SSL-enabled Samba package to connect to the local computer. For example, if Samba is running on clouseau, you might type **smbclient //clouseau/ shares**. If all goes well, smbclient prompts you for the client's passphrase. After that, smbclient prompts for the normal Samba password for your user. During this process, the SSL component reports what SSL encryption method (or *cipher*) has been negotiated, such as DES-CBC3-SHA.

WARNING

If SSL reports that it's using NULL for a cipher, it means your data is not being encrypted. You should review your settings, particularly the ssl ciphers parameter.

If SSL reports an error, such as unknown error 18, check your certification settings. Although you can connect without certification and ignore this error message, any attempt to use either client or server certificates with incorrect certification parameters will cause the system to fail.

Configuring a Client to Use SSL

Some of the Samba configuration options discussed in "Setting Samba's SSL Parameters" govern client configuration. You can use these options to configure smbclient as an SSL-enabled client. As of Samba 2.0.7, smbmount does not support SSL functionality, but you can use smbmount through an SSL proxy. Windows doesn't natively support SSL. Therefore, the only way to use Windows systems as SSL-enabled Samba clients is to use them through a proxy. There are two ways to do this: by running a separate proxy server computer or by running an SSL proxy on the client itself. Both options are explained in the next two sections.

Using an SSL Proxy Server Computer

If you're using Windows clients, SSL functionality is much more difficult to implement than it is when using smbclient. The usual way to use SSL with Windows clients is to use an SSL *proxy server*: a computer that stands in for another one. In the case of an SSL connection to a Samba server, it works as shown in Figure 10.6. The client computer connects to the proxy server, which then encrypts the communications that pass over an untrusted network to reach the server.

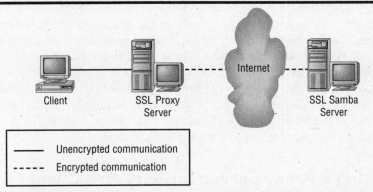

Client   SSL Proxy Server   Internet   SSL Samba Server

——— Unencrypted communication
- - - - - Encrypted communication

FIGURE 10.6: An SSL proxy server uses unencrypted communication with the client but encrypted communication with the server.

Several SSL proxy servers support SMB/CIFS networking. Two popular choices are SSL Proxy (http://obdev.at/Products/sslproxy.html) and Stunnel (www.stunnel.org/). Both of these packages are available for both Windows and Unix. For Linux, you can compile the Unix source code. You'll need the same SSL libraries that are required to compile an SSL-enabled version of Samba.

WARNING

The Windows binary versions of SSL Proxy available from the SSL Proxy website include separate .EXE and .DLL files. Unfortunately, Netscape for Windows corrupts .DLL files when downloading them. You can download the files with Internet Explorer or the Linux version of Netscape to work around this problem.

As an example, let's consider SSL Proxy. Once you have a binary version and client certificate files, you can run it as follows:

```
# sslproxy -1 139 -R server -r 139 -n -c certif.pem -k
   certif.key
```

You can run the program precisely the same way on either a Windows or Linux proxy server. The program asks for the client passphrase. It should then display the following information:

```
SSL: No verify locations, trying default

proxy ready, listening for connections
```

The first line is merely information to the effect that the program is reading some data from default files. The second line indicates that the program is running correctly. You can then try using an unencrypted connection from a client on the proxy server's local network to the proxy server. The proxy server should allow connections to shares on the SSL-enabled Samba server.

One drawback to using SSL Proxy as just described is that the program only forwards TCP port traffic. This means the proxy server (and hence the remote system) won't show up in Network Neighborhood. However, you can directly address the server by entering the proxy server's name in a Windows file browser's Address field, as in \\PROXY. Doing so should produce a list of the shares available through the proxy server. If the proxy server is a Linux system, you can run nmbd *without* smbd on the proxy server to work around the problem.

Using a Proxy Server Directly on a Client

As I've just described it, the proxy server usurps TCP port 139, which is normally used by smbd or the Windows implementation of SMB/CIFS. This fact means you can't use normal SMB/CIFS tools on the proxy server. If you must run Samba on a Linux SSL proxy, you can use the -p option to the Samba daemons to bind them to nonstandard ports—but doing so will mean that only clients supporting similar options, such as smbclient, can use the Samba server. On either Linux or Windows, one alternative is to bind the proxy server only to the localhost (127.0.0.1) address. You can accomplish this task by using a command like the following:

```
# sslproxy -L 127.0.0.1 -1 139 -R server -r 139 -n -c
   certif.pem -k certif.key
```

When you use this technique, it helps to add an entry to the lmhosts file (this is C:\WINDOWS\LMHOSTS on Windows 9*x*, C:\WINNT\SYSTEM32\

DRIVERS\ETC\LMHOSTS on Windows NT, or lmhosts in your Samba configuration directory on Linux). The entry in lmhosts should link the
127.0.0.1 IP address to some useful name, like localhost. Such an entry
looks like this:

```
127.0.0.1    localhost
```

When you run SSL Proxy in this way, you can access the SSL-enabled
Samba server by connecting to the computer called LOCALHOST. For
instance, you can mount a share in Windows with this command:

```
C:> NET USE G: \\LOCALHOST\JACQUES
```

If the server you specified in the sslproxy command hosts the JACQUES
share, this command mounts that share as G:. From the point of view of
Windows's SMB/CIFS networking, Windows is making an unencrypted
connection to itself. Because this connection is entirely internal, no unencrypted data leaks onto the network. SSL Proxy encrypts the data and sends
it out over the network. This sort of configuration can be extremely useful if
you want the highest level of security even on your local network wires.

Windows normally binds its SMB/CIFS servers only to real network
interfaces, not the localhost interface. Samba, however, binds to the
localhost interface as well as others. You can use the interfaces and
bind interfaces only parameters, described earlier in "Binding Samba
to Specific Network Interfaces," to keep Samba from using these interfaces so that SSL Proxy can use them. Unfortunately, doing so causes
SWAT and smbpasswd to malfunction because they use the localhost
interface internally.

SAMBA IN THE BROADER SECURITY WORLD

As discussed in this chapter, Samba includes many features that can
enhance your server's security. The capability of blocking accesses based
on port or IP address can present a high initial hurdle to troublemakers.
Appropriate use of password policies and password encryption can help
more. Encrypting entire sessions with SSL contributes still more.

All these features are built into Samba, however, or they at least use
Samba in conjunction with SSL or another tool. In principle, a critical
flaw at a low enough level of Samba could make many of these security
features moot. Therefore, it's wise to use external mechanisms to block

access to Samba from at least some potentially undesirable sources. This section covers a few such tools: external firewalls, the Linux ipchains program, and xinetd.

Ports Used by SMB/CIFS

External security tools usually work by blocking access to specific ports on a computer. In this context, a port is a means of reaching a particular program that's running on the server. A port is analogous to a telephone number. When a client contacts a server, it does so by contacting the port number associated with the server, just as you can contact a person by dialing that individual's telephone number. In some cases, including Windows SMB/CIFS clients, the client calls from a fixed port number itself; but in most cases, including Samba clients, the client's originating port number is variable.

The TCP/IP stack supports several different types of ports. The two that are important for this discussion are the User Datagram Protocol (UDP) and Transmission Control Protocol (TCP). UDP ports are used for quick and possibly unreliable transmissions, whereas TCP is used for extended and reliable connections. A specific port number may be used by one protocol for UDP and another for TCP, although in most cases a single protocol claims both UDP and TCP ports, even if it doesn't use both.

SMB/CIFS uses port numbers 137 and 138 as UDP ports and 139 as a TCP port, but the entire range 137–139 is reserved for SMB/CIFS on both UDP and TCP. You can use this arrangement to block access to Samba from clients that should not be accessing the server—you need only block both TCP and UDP ports from 137–139.

Using *ipchains* or a Firewall to Block Samba Access

A *firewall* is a computer that sits between a protected network of computers and an untrusted network (such as the Internet) to block undesirable access from the outside, and sometimes to block unauthorized access to the outside from the inside. Figure 10.7 illustrates this arrangement. As illustrated in this figure, the only way for traffic to pass between the internal network and the Internet is for it to pass through the firewall computer.

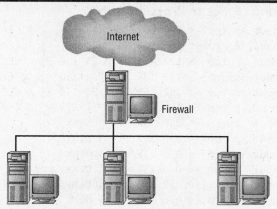

FIGURE 10.7: A firewall computer, like a physical firewall in a car or building, serves as a barrier between unsecured computers and the Internet.

Firewalls can be specialized pieces of equipment or ordinary computers running an ordinary OS and configured with minimal but specialized tools. If you have a stand-alone firewall, you should consult its documentation to learn how to block ports 137–139. Assuming the firewall works properly, this configuration will protect your network from attack via SMB/CIFS.

NOTE

For more information on firewalls and ipchains on a Linux computer, see Chapter 16, "Linux Network-Layer Firewalls."

Linux computers can function as firewalls. At the core of Linux's firewall capabilities is the ipchains tool. With ipchains, you can configure Linux to accept or reject packets based on characteristics such as the network interface, the source address, the destination address, the source port, and the destination port. You can use ipchains either to create a simple stand-alone firewall, similar to the one in Figure 10.7, or to protect a single computer. Although the details of ipchains configuration are well beyond the scope of this chapter, an example set of ipchains rules that can run on a Samba server is shown in Listing 10.2.

Part II

Listing 10.2: ipchains Rules to Protect Samba

```
ipchains -A input -p tcp -s 192.168.34.0/24 137 -j ACCEPT
ipchains -A input -p udp -s 192.168.34.0/24 137 -j ACCEPT
ipchains -A input -p tcp -s 192.168.34.0/24 138 -j ACCEPT
ipchains -A input -p udp -s 192.168.34.0/24 138 -j ACCEPT
ipchains -A input -p tcp -s 192.168.34.0/24 139 -j ACCEPT
ipchains -A input -p udp -s 192.168.34.0/24 139 -j ACCEPT
ipchains -A input -p tcp -s 0/0 137 -l -j DENY
ipchains -A input -p udp -s 0/0 137 -l -j DENY
ipchains -A input -p tcp -s 0/0 138 -l -j DENY
ipchains -A input -p udp -s 0/0 138 -l -j DENY
ipchains -A input -p tcp -s 0/0 139 -l -j DENY
ipchains -A input -p udp -s 0/0 139 -l -j DENY
ipchains -A output -p tcp -d 192.168.34.0/24 137 -j ACCEPT
ipchains -A output -p udp -d 192.168.34.0/24 137 -j ACCEPT
ipchains -A output -p tcp -d 192.168.34.0/24 138 -j ACCEPT
ipchains -A output -p udp -d 192.168.34.0/24 138 -j ACCEPT
ipchains -A output -p tcp -d 192.168.34.0/24 139 -j ACCEPT
ipchains -A output -p udp -d 192.168.34.0/24 139 -j ACCEPT
ipchains -A output -p tcp -d 0/0 137 -l -j DENY
ipchains -A output -p udp -d 0/0 137 -l -j DENY
ipchains -A output -p tcp -d 0/0 138 -l -j DENY
ipchains -A output -p udp -d 0/0 138 -l -j DENY
ipchains -A output -p tcp -d 0/0 139 -l -j DENY
ipchains -A output -p udp -d 0/0 139 -l -j DENY
```

Although it contains 24 lines and 24 rules, Listing 10.2 is actually fairly simple. It's constructed of four sections, each of which has six variant commands: one for each of the three UDP ports and three TCP ports. The four major sections control the following accesses:

▶ Input to the Samba ports from the 192.168.34.0/24 network is explicitly allowed. This set of rules allows computers on the local network to use the server. (Naturally, you must change this address to fit your network.)

▶ Input to the Samba ports from all other IP addresses is explicitly denied. Foreign computers, therefore, can't use the server.

▶ Output directed at the SMB/CIFS ports on the 192.168.34.0/24 network is explicitly allowed. This set of rules allows Samba to reply to requests that originate from the SMB/CIFS ports, which is how most Windows systems operate. It also lets the computer run as a client.

▶ Output directed at the SMB/CIFS ports on all other IP addresses is explicitly denied. This set of rules blocks output directed at foreign SMB/CIFS servers, or replies to foreign Windows SMB/CIFS clients. These rules can prevent local users from abusing others' computers.

Although ipchains is often thought of as a firewall tool, it can be very useful for restricting access to server programs on individual server computers. In fact, the rules in Listing 10.2 are designed for such a configuration. If Listing 10.2 were used as the basis for a Samba policy on a stand-alone firewall, you'd need to add options to restrict the rules' application to particular network interfaces.

NOTE

ipchains is the tool used for packet filtering on the 2.2.x kernel series. The older 2.0.x kernels used a similar tool called ipfwadm, and the newer 2.4.x kernels (not yet released at this writing) will use a newer utility called iptables. Configuration details for these packages differ, but the basics as I've described them here are the same: You can block access to Samba's ports based on IP addresses, network interface, and so on.

Whether you use a stand-alone firewall computer or a set of ipchains rules on your Samba servers, blocking access to Samba with something other than Samba is a good idea. In fact, it wouldn't hurt to use *both* an external firewall *and* a set of ipchains rules on your Samba servers.

Running Samba through TCP Wrappers or *xinetd*

Most serious Samba servers run the Samba daemons directly. It is possible, however, to run Samba through inetd, the so-called *super server*. Doing this can result in a reduced memory load on the server, but at the cost of slowed responses to access attempts and seriously hindered capacity as a domain controller, NBNS server, or master browser. These drawbacks make running Samba through inetd a poor choice for most servers. You might want to consider using this option if your server is seldom used (for instance, if your computer is principally a client to which others connect only rarely).

If the drawbacks of running Samba through inetd aren't overwhelming, you can use assorted access control features to help improve Samba's security. One of these is to use TCP Wrappers to block access to Samba based on the client's IP address or assorted other features. This functionality is similar to that provided by the Samba hosts allow and hosts deny parameters. Because it's implemented in a separate program, however, there may be some modest security benefits if a flaw is discovered in Samba's implementation of these features.

One alternative to inetd and TCP Wrappers is a package called xinetd (www.xinetd.org). This program improves on inetd with TCP Wrappers because xinetd allows you to bind a server to a specific network interface. This fact can reduce the susceptibility of the servers to IP spoofing attacks. Unfortunately, Samba's nmbd doesn't run properly from xinetd, although smbd does. If your Samba server has two or more network interfaces and you don't need access to Samba from all of them, you might want to consider running nmbd separately and running smbd via xinetd.

Non-Samba Servers

As a general rule, you should run as few servers as possible on any one computer. Many Linux distributions ship with a distressingly large number of servers active by default. This fact leaves the system vulnerable to outside attack. Bugs or misconfiguration of any of these servers could allow outsiders access to the server or make it possible for a malicious local user to abuse the system. Ideally, a Samba server should run only Samba. In practice, this is often impossible; you may require SSH or Telnet to gain access to the system to administer it; or you may need to run NFS, Netatalk, or some other file server to make the system a useful cross-platform server. Nevertheless, it's wise to examine your server's configuration for opportunities to remove unnecessary servers.

The /etc/inetd.conf file is a good place to start tracking down unnecessary servers. In this file, a typical Linux computer includes many lines like the following:

```
ftp     stream tcp  nowait  root  /usr/sbin/tcpd  proftpd
telnet  stream tcp  nowait  root  /usr/sbin/tcpd  in.telnetd
# nntp  stream tcp  nowait  news  /usr/sbin/tcpd
/usr/sbin/leafnode
pop3    stream tcp  nowait  root  /usr/sbin/tcpd
/usr/sbin/popper -s
```

These four lines enable three servers—FTP, Telnet, and POP3. The NNTP server line is commented out and, therefore, disabled.

TIP

As a general rule, if you don't know what a server does, you should disable it. A better policy is to learn what a server does and disable it once you've determined you don't need it. Adding a pound sign (#) to the start of the server's line in /etc/inetd.conf disables it.

Some servers run apart from inetd. Typically, these servers are started through startup scripts located in the /etc/rc.d directory tree. You can disable these servers by moving their startup scripts from /etc/rc.d or /etc/rc.d/init.d to some other directory.

For added safety, you should remove unused servers entirely from your system. If you're using an RPM- or Debian-based Linux distribution, you can accomplish this removal quite easily using the rpm or dpkg tool. For example, rpm -e proftpd removes the proftpd FTP server package.

Once you've removed unnecessary servers from your system, Samba will be more secure because it's that much more protected from compromise via an intermediary network server.

What's Next

Samba is a powerful, yet dangerous network access tool. With its diverse options, almost any network can benefit from Samba, yet still maintain security. In this chapter you have learned some of the specifics for implementing Samba security.

In the next chapter, you will move from Samba server–specific security to an introduction of network-border security using firewalls.

Part II

Part III

FIREWALLS

Chapter 11

UNDERSTANDING FIREWALLS

N ations without controlled borders cannot ensure the security and safety of their citizens, nor can they prevent piracy and theft. Networks without controlled access cannot ensure the security or privacy of stored data, nor can they keep network resources from being exploited by hackers.

The communication efficiency provided by the Internet has caused a rush to attach private networks directly to it. Direct Internet connections make it easy for hackers to exploit private network resources. Prior to the Internet, the only widely available way for a hacker to connect from home to a private network was by direct dialing with modems and the public telephony network. Remote access security was a relatively small issue.

When you connect your private network to the Internet, you are actually connecting your network directly to every other network that's attached to the Internet directly. There's no inherent central point of security control—in fact, there's no inherent security at all.

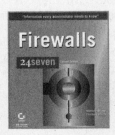

Adapted from *Firewalls 24seven™*, Second Edition
by Matthew Strebe and Charles Perkins
ISBN 0-7821-4054-8 $49.99

Part III

Firewalls are used to create security checkpoints at the boundaries of private networks. At these checkpoints, firewalls inspect all packets passing between the private network and the Internet and determine whether to pass or drop the packets depending on how they match the policy rules programmed into the firewall. If your firewall is properly configured, is capable of inspecting every protocol you allow to pass, and contains no serious exploitable bugs, your network will be as free from risk as possible.

There are literally hundreds of firewall products available, and different security experts have different theories about how firewalls should be used to secure your network. This chapter will explore the operation of a generic firewall in detail, outline the important features you need in a firewall, and discuss how firewalls should be deployed in networks of any size.

FIREWALL ELEMENTS

Firewalls keep your Internet connection as secure as possible by inspecting and then approving or rejecting each connection attempt made between your internal network and external networks like the Internet. Strong firewalls protect your network at all software layers—from the Data Link layer up through the Application layer.

Firewalls sit on the borders of your network, connected directly to the circuits that provide access to other networks. For that reason, firewalls are frequently referred to as *border security*. The concept of border security is important—without it, every host on your network would have to perform the functions of a firewall themselves, needlessly consuming computer resources and increasing the amount of time required to connect, authenticate, and encrypt data in local area, high-speed networks. Firewalls allow you to centralize all external security services in machines that are optimized for and dedicated to the task. Inspecting traffic at the border gateways also has the benefit of preventing hacking traffic from consuming the bandwidth on your internal network.

By their nature, firewalls create bottlenecks between the internal and external networks, because all traffic transiting between the internal network and the external must pass through a single point of control. This is a small price to pay for security. Because external leased-line connections are relatively slow compared to the speed of modern computers, the latency caused by firewalls can be completely transparent. For most users, relatively inexpensive firewall devices are more than sufficient to keep up with a standard T1 connection to the Internet. For businesses and ISPs whose Internet traffic is far higher, a new breed of extremely high-speed (and high-cost) firewalls has been developed, which can keep up with even the most demanding private networks. Some countries actually censor the Internet using high-speed firewalls.

Firewalls function primarily by using three fundamental methods:

Packet Filtering   Rejects TCP/IP packets from unauthorized hosts and rejects connection attempts to unauthorized services.

Network Address Translation (NAT)   Translates the IP addresses of internal hosts to hide them from outside monitoring. You may hear NAT referred to as *IP masquerading*.

Proxy Services   Makes high-level application connections on behalf of internal hosts in order to completely break the Network layer connection between internal and external hosts.

You can use devices or servers that perform only one of these functions; for instance, you could have a router that performs packet filtering, and then a proxy server in a separate machine. This way, either the packet filter must pass traffic through to the proxy server, or the proxy server must sit outside your network without the protection of packet filtering. Both arrangements are more dangerous than using a single firewall product that performs all the security functions in one place. Most firewalls also perform two other important security services:

Encrypted Authentication   Allows users on the public network to prove their identity to the firewall, in order to gain access to the private network from external locations.

Virtual Private Networking   Establishes a secure connection between two private networks over a public medium like the Internet. It allows physically separated networks to use the Internet rather than leased-line connections to communicate. VPNs are also called *encrypted tunnels*.

Some firewalls also provide additional subscription-based services that are not strictly related to security, but which many users will find useful:

Virus Scanning   Searches inbound data streams for the signatures of viruses. Keeping up with current virus signatures

requires a subscription to the virus update service provided by
the firewall vendor.

Content Filtering   Allows you to block internal users from
accessing certain types of content by category, such as hate-
group propaganda, hacking information, and pornography.
Keeping up with the current list of blocked sites for a specific
category also requires a subscription.

Nearly all firewalls use these basic methods to provide a security service. Hundreds of firewall products are on the market, all vying for your
security dollar. Most are very strong products that vary only in superficial
details. The remainder of this section covers the five primary functions
that most firewalls support.

Packet Filters

The first Internet firewalls were simply packet filters, and packet filtering
remains one of the key functions of today's firewalls. Filters compare network protocols (such as IP) and transport protocol packets (such as TCP)
to a database of rules and forward only those packets that conform to the
criteria specified in the database of rules. Filters can be implemented
either in routers or in the TCP/IP stacks of servers (see Figure 11.1).

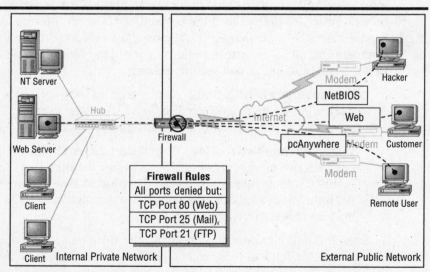

FIGURE 11.1:   Filtered Internet connections block undesired traffic.

Filters implemented inside routers prevent suspicious traffic from reaching the destination network, whereas TCP/IP filter modules in servers merely prevent that specific machine from responding to suspicious traffic. The traffic still reaches the network and could target any machine on it. Filtered routers protect all the machines on the destination network from suspicious traffic. For that reason, filtering in the TCP/IP stacks of servers (such as that provided by Windows NT) should only be used in addition to router filtering, not instead of it.

Filters typically follow these rules:

- ► Drop inbound connection attempts but allow outbound connection attempts to pass.

- ► Eliminate TCP packets bound for those ports that shouldn't be available to the Internet (such as the NetBIOS session port) but allow packets that should be available (such as Simple Mail Transfer Protocol [SMTP]) to pass. Most filters can specify exactly which server a specific sort of traffic should go to—for instance, SMTP traffic on port 25 should only go to the IP address of a mail server.

- ► Restrict inbound access to certain IP ranges.

WARNING

Simple packet filters or routers with a packet filtering function that requires opening ports above 1023 for return channels are not effective security devices. These packet filters do not prevent internal users or Trojan horses from setting up a service on a client station in the port range above 1024 and simply listening for connection attempts from the outside. Firewalls (stateful inspection filters and security proxies) only open channels for servers that have been invited back in by a connection attempt from inside the security perimeter; choose them over simple packet filters that can't maintain the state of a connection.

Sophisticated filters examine the states of all connections that flow through them, looking for the telltale signs of hacking, such as source routing, Internet Control Message Protocol (ICMP) redirection, and IP spoofing. Connections that exhibit these characteristics are dropped.

Internal clients are generally allowed to create connections to outside hosts, and external hosts are usually prevented from initiating connection attempts. When an internal host decides to initiate a TCP connection, it sends a TCP message to the IP address and port number of the public server (for example, www.microsoft.com:80 to connect to

Microsoft's website). In the connection initiation message, it tells the remote server what its IP address is and on which port it is listening for a response (for example, localhost:2050).

The external server sends data back by transmitting it to the port given by the internal client. Because your firewall inspects all the traffic exchanged between both hosts, it knows that the connection was initiated by an internal host attached to its internal interface, what that host's IP address is, and on what port that host expects to receive return traffic. The firewall then remembers to allow the host addressed in the connection message to return traffic to the internal host's IP address only at the port specified.

When the hosts involved in the connection close down the TCP connection, the firewall removes the entry in its state table (its connection memory) that allows the remote host to return traffic to the internal host. If the internal host stops responding before closing the TCP connection (because, for example, it has crashed), or if the protocol in question does not support sessions (for example, User Datagram Protocol [UDP]), the firewall will remove the entry in its state table after a programmed time-out of a few minutes.

Operating System Filtering

You might not be aware that most versions of Unix and Windows include packet filtering in the TCP/IP protocol interface. You can use this filtering in addition to a strong firewall to control access to individual servers; you can also use this filtering to provide an additional measure of internal security inside your organization without the cost of a firewall. Just as filtering alone is not sufficient to protect your network entirely, your operating system's internal filtering is not sufficient to create a completely secure environment.

Security Limitations of Packet Filtering

Filtering does not completely solve the Internet security problem. First, the IP addresses of computers inside the filter are present in outbound traffic, which makes it somewhat easy to determine the type and number of Internet hosts inside a filter and to target attacks against those addresses. Filtering does not hide the identity of hosts inside the filter.

Additionally, filters cannot check all the fragments of an IP message based on higher-level protocols like TCP headers because the header exists only in the first fragment. Subsequent fragments have no header information and can only be compared to IP level rules, which are usually relaxed to allow some traffic through the filter. This situation allows bugs in the destination IP stacks of computers on the network to be exploited, and could allow communications with a Trojan horse installed inside the network. More modern true firewalls support rebuilding fragmented packets and then applying firewall rules to them.

Finally, filters are not complex enough to check the legitimacy of the protocols inside the Network layer packets. For example, filters don't inspect the HTTP packets contained in TCP packets to determine if they contain exploits that target the web browser or web server on your end of the connection. Most modern hacking attempts are based on exploiting these higher-level services, because firewalls have nearly eliminated successful Network layer–hacking beyond the nuisance of denial-of-service attacks.

VARIANTS OF WINDOWS

There are three major versions of Windows:

- ▶ 16-bit versions of Windows that run on top of MS-DOS, including Windows 3.0, 3.1, and 3.11

- ▶ 32-bit versions of Windows that run on MS-DOS, including Windows 95, 98, and ME

- ▶ 32-bit versions of Windows that run on the NT Kernel, including NT 3.1, NT 3.5, NT 3.51, NT 4, 2000, and XP

Part III

Do not rely on your operating system's built-in filtering alone to protect your network. You should use your operating system's filtering functions inside your network to establish filters to pass only those protocols you explicitly intend to serve. Doing so prevents software from working in ways you don't expect and keeps Trojan horses from functioning even if they manage to get installed.

Basic OS filtering allows you to define acceptance criteria for each network adapter in your computer for incoming connections based on the following:

- ▶ IP protocol number
- ▶ TCP port number
- ▶ UDP port number

The filtering usually does not apply to outbound connections (those originating on your server) and is defined separately for each adapter in your system.

NOTE
Windows 2000 supports outbound filtering; Windows NT 4 does not.

A typical server sets up services to listen on the following ports. These ports must be open through your filter in order for these services to work correctly.

Simple TCP/IP services usually listen on the following ports:

Port	TCP/IP Service
7	Echo (Ping)
9	Discard
13	Daytime
17	Quote of the Day
19	Character Generator

Internet servers usually listen on the following ports:

Port	Server
21	File Transfer Protocol (FTP)
23	Telnet
70	Gopher
80	World Wide Web (HTTP)
119	Net News (NNTP)
22	Secure Shell
443	Secure HTTP (HTTPS)

File servers usually listen on the following ports:

Port	Service
53	Domain Name Service (DNS service, if installed)
135	RPC Locator Service (Windows NT only)

137	NetBIOS Name Service (WINS servers only)
139	NetBIOS Session Service (Windows network and SMB/CIFS servers only)
515	LPR (used by the TCP/IP print service, if installed)
530	Remote Procedure Call (RPC connections are used by the Windows NT WinLogon service as well as many other high-level network applications)
3389	Windows Terminal Services (accepts connections on this port using the RDP protocol)

Mail servers are usually configured to listen on the following ports:

Port	Mail Server
25	Simple Mail Transfer Protocol (mail server-to-server exchanges)
110	Post Office Protocol version 3 (server-to-client mail exchanges)
143	Internet Mail Access Protocol (client access to mail server)

If you install other service software, you must make sure your server's filter is set up to listen on the ports required by the service—otherwise the service will not work. Find out from the software manufacturer which ports are required for that service. This does not apply to border firewalls, which should only be configured to pass a service if you intend to provide that service to the public.

General Rules for Packet Filtering

You can take two basic approaches to security: Pessimistic, where you disable all access except that which you know is necessary, and optimistic, where you allow all traffic except that which you know is harmful. For security purposes, you should always take a pessimistic approach, because the optimistic approach presumes that you know every possible threat in advance, which is not possible. Consider the following general guidelines when you use packet filtering:

▶ Disallow all protocols and addresses by default, and then explicitly allow services and hosts you wish to support.

▶ Disallow all connection attempts to hosts inside your network. By allowing any inbound connections, you allow hackers to

Part III

establish connections to Trojan horses or exploit bugs in service software.

► Filter out and do not respond to ICMP redirect and echo (ping) messages. Drop all packets that are TCP source routed. Source routing is rarely used for legitimate purposes.

► Drop all external routing protocol (Router Information Protocol [RIP], Open Shortest Path First [OSPF]) updates bound for internal routers. No one outside your network should be transmitting RIP updates.

► Consider disallowing fragments beyond number zero, because this functionality is largely obsolete and often exploited.

► Place public service hosts like web servers and SMTP servers outside your packet filters rather than opening holes through your packet filters.

► Do not rely on packet filtering alone to protect your network.

Network Address Translation

Network Address Translation (NAT) solves the problem of hiding internal hosts. NAT is actually a Network layer proxy: A single host makes requests on behalf of all internal hosts, thus hiding their identity from the public network. Windows 2000 and XP, Linux, and many modern Unix operating systems provide this functionality as part of the operating system distribution; Windows NT does not.

NAT hides internal IP addresses by converting all internal host addresses to the address of the firewall. The firewall then retransmits the data payload of the internal host from its own address using the TCP port number to keep track of which connections on the public side map to which hosts on the private side. To the Internet, all the traffic on your network appears to be coming from one extremely busy computer.

NAT effectively hides all TCP/IP-level information about your internal hosts from prying eyes on the Internet. Address translation also allows you to use any IP address range you want on your internal network, even if those addresses are already in use elsewhere on the Internet. This means you don't have to request a large block of IP addresses from the American Registry for Internet Numbers (ARIN) or reassign network numbers from those you simply plugged in before you connected your network to the Internet.

WARNING

Although you can use any block of IP addresses behind a firewall with NAT, be aware that you may encounter strange problems accessing Internet hosts that have the same public IP address as a computer inside your network. For that reason, use the reserved 192.168.0.0 network or the 10.0.0.0 network inside your firewall to avoid these problems.

Finally, NAT allows you to multiplex a single public IP address across an entire network. Many small companies rely on the services of an upstream Internet service provider that may be reluctant to provide large blocks of addresses because their own range is relatively restricted. You may want to share a single dial-up or cable modem address without telling your ISP. These options are all possible using NAT.

On the downside, NAT is implemented only at the TCP/IP level. As a result, information hidden in the data payload of TCP/IP traffic could be transmitted to a higher-level service and used to exploit weaknesses in higher-level traffic or to communicate with a Trojan horse. You'll still have to use a higher-level service like a proxy to prevent higher-level service security breaches.

Additionally, many protocols include the host's IP address in the data payload, so when the address is rewritten while passing through the NAT, the address in the payload becomes invalid. This occurs with active-mode FTP, H.323, IP Security (IPSec), and nearly every other protocol that relies upon establishing a secondary communication stream between the client and the server.

NAT is also a problem for network administrators who may want to connect to clients behind the NAT for administrative purposes. Because the NAT has only one IP address, there's no way to specify which internal client you want to reach. This restriction keeps hackers from connecting to internal clients, but it also keeps legitimate users at bay. Fortunately, most modern NAT implementations allow you to create port-forwarding rules that allow internal hosts to be reached.

Proxies

NAT solves many of the problems associated with direct Internet connections, but it still doesn't completely restrict the flow of packets through your firewall. It's possible for someone with a network monitor to watch traffic coming out of your firewall and determine that the firewall is translating addresses for other machines. It is then possible for a hacker to hijack TCP connections or to spoof connections back through the firewall.

Part III

Application-level proxies prevent this. They allow you to completely disconnect the flow of network-level protocols through your firewall and restrict traffic only to higher-level protocols like HTTP, FTP, and SMTP. Application-level proxies are a combination of a server and a client for the specific protocol in question. For example, a web proxy is a combination of a web server and a web client. The protocol server side of the proxy accepts connections from clients on the internal network, and the proto-col client side of the proxy connects to the public server. When the client side of the proxy receives data from the public server, the server side of the proxy application sends it to the ultimate inside client. Figure 11.2 shows exactly how this works.

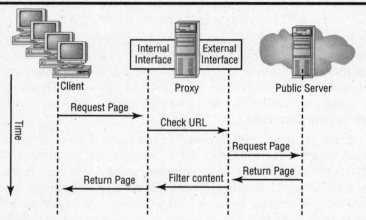

FIGURE 11.2: Proxy servers receive requests on the private network and regenerate them on the public network.

Proxies straddle two networks that are not connected by routers. When a client on the protected network makes a connection to a server on the public side, the proxy receives the connection request and then makes the connection on behalf of the protected client. The proxy then forwards the response from the public server onto the internal network. Proxies essentially perform a benign man-in-the-middle attack, and they provide a good example of how any intermediate system between you and another end system could potentially perform a more malicious sort of processing without your permission.

Application proxies (like Microsoft Proxy Server) are unlike Network Address Translators and filters in that the Internet client application is (usually) set up to talk to the proxy. For instance, you tell Internet

Explorer the address of your web proxy, and Internet Explorer sends all web requests to that server rather than resolving the IP address and establishing a connection directly.

Application proxies don't have to run on firewalls; any server, either inside or outside your network, can perform the role of a proxy. Without a firewall, you still don't have any real security, so you need both. At least some sort of packet filter must be in place to protect the proxy server from Network layer denial-of-service attacks (like the infamous "ping of death"). And, if the proxy doesn't run on the firewall, you'll have to open a channel through your firewall one way or another. Ideally, your firewall should perform the proxy function. Doing so keeps packets from the public side from being forwarded through your firewall.

Some firewall proxies are more sophisticated than others. Some have the functionality of an IP filter and masquerade, so they can simply block outbound connection attempts (on port 80 in the case of HTTP) to remote hosts rather than having the client software configured to address the proxy service specifically. The firewall proxy then connects to the remote server and requests data on behalf of the blocked client. The retrieved data is returned to the requesting client using the firewall's NAT functionality in order to look just like the actual remote server. Proxies that operate in this manner are said to be *transparent*.

Security proxies are even capable of performing application-level filtering for specific content. For instance, some firewall HTTP proxies look for tags in HTML pages that refer to Java or ActiveX embedded applets and then strip out that content from them. This process prevents the applet from executing on your client computers and eliminates the risk that a user will accidentally download a Trojan horse. This sort of filtering is extremely important because filtering, proxying, and masquerading can't prevent your network from being compromised if your users are lured into downloading a Trojan horse embedded in an ActiveX applet.

You may have noticed that as we climb through the networking layers, the security services have gotten more specific. For instance, filtering is specific to IP and then to TCP and UDP. Applications that use IP with other protocols like Banyan Vines must use special high-cost or unusually robust firewalls.

Proxies are extremely specific because they can only work for a specific application. For instance, you must have a proxy software module for HTTP, another proxy module for FTP, and another module for Telnet. As these protocols evolve (HTTP is particularly fast moving), the proxy module for that protocol will have to be updated.

Many protocols are either proprietary or rare enough that no security proxies exist. Proxies don't exist for proprietary application protocols like Lotus Notes, so those protocols must either be sent through a Network layer filter or be proxied by a generic TCP proxy that regenerates the packet but simply transfers the payload. SOCKS is a specific form of generic proxy, sometimes called a *circuit-level gateway*. Although generic proxying cannot prevent attacks from the content of a protocol, it is still more secure than filtered routing because the Network layer packets are completely regenerated and thus scrubbed of malformations that might not be detected by the firewall.

In many cases, you "roll your own" proxy by using a combination of the protocol server and the protocol's client on the same machine. For example, say you've got a network that is disconnected from the Internet, but a Windows server has two network interfaces, one on the Internet and one on the private network. If you use the Terminal Services functionality of Windows 2000 to attach to the server on its public side, you can then run a Terminal Services client on that machine to reach a machine on the interior of the network. In practice, this process works a lot better than you might presume, although it's not a particularly good security practice.

Whenever possible, use proxy servers for all application protocols. Consider disallowing services for which you do not have proxy servers. Use high-level proxies capable of stripping executable content, like ActiveX and Java, from web pages.

Virtual Private Networks

Virtual Private Networks (VPNs), also called *encrypted tunnels*, allow you to securely connect two physically separated networks over the Internet without exposing your data to viewing by unauthorized intermediate parties. VPNs by themselves could be subject to redirection attempts, spoofed connection initiation, and all manner of hacking indignity while the tunnel is being established. But when implemented as an integral part of a firewall, the firewall authentication and security services can be used to prevent exploitation while the tunnel is being established.

Once established, VPNs are impervious to exploitation so long as the encryption remains secure. And, because firewalls sit at the Internet borders, they exist at the perfect terminal points for each end of the tunnel. Essentially, your private networks can pass traffic as if they were two subnets in the same domain.

VPNs also allow users to address remote internal hosts directly by their hidden IP addresses; Network Address Translators and packet filters would prevent this if the connection attempt came directly from the Internet.

TIP

The Point-to-Point Tunneling Protocol (PPTP) for Windows NT provides an encrypted tunnel using the security services of the Remote Access Server. Windows 2000 provides support for the more modern Layer-2 Tunneling Protocol (L2TP) and IP Security (IPSec) in transport mode. Most distributions of Linux include support for encrypted tunnels, such as the Point-to-Point Protocol (PPP) over Secure Sockets Layer (SSL).

Use leased lines rather than VPNs whenever doing so is cost effective. Use VPNs for all communications over the Internet between organizational units when leased lines are not available or are cost prohibitive. If you are using VPNs as your primary connection method between organizational units, you'll have far better performance if you use the same ISP at every site, because the VPN traffic won't have to be routed through the congested commercial Internet exchanges. Never communicate private information between organizational units over the Internet without using some form of encryption. Unencrypted packet headers contain valuable nuggets of information about the structure of your internal network.

NOTE

Technically, leased lines are not guaranteed to be secure either, but they are free of Internet hackers. If you need to secure your data from the possibility of government wiretaps or serious corporate espionage, you should use a VPN over leased lines as well.

Encrypted Authentication

Encrypted authentication allows external users on the Internet to prove to a firewall that they are authorized users and thereby authorized to open a connection through the firewall to the internal network. The encrypted authentication might use any number of secure authentication protocols. Once the connection is established, it may or may not be encrypted, depending on the firewall product in use and whether additional software has been installed on the client to support tunneling.

Using encryption authentication is convenient because it occurs at the transport level between a client software package and the firewall. Once the connection is open, all normal application software and operating system logon software will run without hindrance—so you don't have to use special software packages that support your specific firewall.

Unfortunately, encrypted authentication reduces the security of your firewall. By its nature, it causes the following problems:

▶ The firewall must respond on some port because it listens for connection attempts. This action can show hackers that the firewall exists.

▶ The connection could be redirected using ICMP after establishment, especially if it's not encrypted.

▶ A hacker who monitored the establishment might be able to spoof the address of the authorized client to gain access inside the network without redirecting any existing connections.

▶ A stolen laptop computer with the appropriate keys could be used to gain access to the network.

▶ Work-at-home employees could become a target for breaking and entering because their computers are able to access the private network.

▶ The authentication procedure could be buggy or less than completely secure, thus allowing anyone on the Internet to open holes through the firewall.

Each of these risks is less than likely to actually occur. Administrators of medium- to low-risk environments should not feel uncomfortable using encrypted authentication as long as the connection is encrypted for the duration.

CREATING EFFECTIVE BORDER SECURITY

To maintain the absolute minimum level of effective Internet security, you must control your border security using firewalls that perform all three of the basic firewall functions (packet filtering, Network Address Translation, and high-level service proxying). Your firewalls must also be dedicated primarily to the performance of firewall functions; avoid the temptation to run mail, web, or other public services on the firewall unless the service software comes from the firewall software vendor. Even in this case, be aware that you are increasing your risk, because a bug in any of the high-level services running on your firewall might be exploited to bypass the firewall completely. This recommendation is not as theoretical as it sounds: Unix Sendmail is notorious for the number of buffer-overrun attacks it has been susceptible to, as is Internet Information Services (IIS), the Windows web server. If these services run on your firewall, it can be compromised easily.

Again, simply minimize the services running on the firewalls. Doing so reduces the complexity of the software running on the machine, thereby reducing the probability that a bug in the operating system or security software will allow a security breach. In the case of Windows, very few of the services in the service Control Panel are needed for a computer running only as a firewall. Turn off all services that the server will allow you to shut off, and set them to start manually. In the case of Linux, install only those packages necessary for the operation of the firewall, or select the "firewall" installation option if the distribution has one. Normally, you won't have to deal with this issue because the firewall software installation program will shut down all unnecessary services for you. If it doesn't, look elsewhere for firewall software.

It's always tempting to pile services like HTTP, FTP, Telnet, Gopher, and mail onto the same machine you use as an Internet router and firewall because doing so is cheaper and because that machine probably has a lot of spare compute time and disk space. Unfortunately, few operating systems are both secure enough and bug-free enough to guarantee that services won't interfere with each other or that a service won't crash the firewall. It's also quite probable that a high-level service running on the firewall, even if it doesn't affect other security services, could provide a way to circumvent the security services of the firewall. And finally, many services contain logon banners or automatically generated error pages that identify the firewall product you are using. These features could be dangerous if hackers have found a weakness in your specific firewall. You want to make it difficult to determine which operating system your firewall is running.

You must also enforce a single point of control in your firewall policy. If you have more than one firewall in your company (perhaps one firewall attaching each remote office to the Internet), you need to make absolutely certain they are all configured the same way. Enterprise firewall management software features aid in this endeavor.

Part III

WARNING

A lapse on any of your firewalls can compromise your entire network, especially if you use secure tunneling or private leased lines to connect offices. Hackers can be relied on to use the path of least resistance.

Comparing Firewall Functionality

There is a common misconception among network administrators that a firewall has to be based on the same operating system as the network file servers—Unix firewalls for Unix-based networks and NT firewalls for Windows NT–based networks. In fact, there's no functional reason why the operating system used by a firewall should be the same as that used by the network, because (and only in very special circumstances) you'll never run any other software on the firewall computer. In fact, these days, most firewalls come as preconfigured computers running a completely proprietary operating system.

All firewalls filter TCP/IP traffic, and in most cases you'll set them up once and leave them to do their job, with minor tweaks as security policies and work habits change in the organization. Some firewalls run proprietary operating systems that aren't related to Unix or Windows at all; they are just as appropriate on any network.

The second most important factor in choosing a firewall operating system (after security, of course) is familiarity—the administrator should be familiar with the user interface and know how to configure the firewall correctly. Most Windows-based firewalls are easier to set up than Unix-based firewalls, but many Unix-based firewalls are catching up by using Java or web-based graphical interfaces that run remotely on the administrator's PC.

Some firewall vendors claim that their products are superior to firewalls based on Windows or standard versions of Unix because the products are based on a "hardened" implementation of the TCP/IP protocol stack or a theoretically more secure operating system. They also claim that bugs in Windows NT or Unix releases can be exploited to get past the firewall software of their competitors. Although this may be true, those vendors can't prove that similar bugs don't exist in their own software. In fact, there's no practical way to prove that complex code is bug free, and firewall vendors are no more likely to get it absolutely right than are large vendors like Microsoft or Sun.

One major advantage of using a widely available operating system as the foundation of a firewall is that the code is put through its paces by millions of users. Bugs are more likely to be found and corrected, and patches are available far sooner and with greater regularity than is true for proprietary products provided by smaller vendors that usually don't have the programming resources to throw at problems as they arise. On the downside, common operating systems are subject to far more hacking attempts than uncommon ones; Windows bears the brunt of hacking attempts because it's the most common operating system and because many hackers hate Microsoft. For this reason, it's the most often compromised operating system, although Unix (including Linux) isn't theoretically any more secure.

Many firewall products that are based on a standard operating system don't rely on the standard TCP/IP stack or higher-level services that ship with the operating system; they implement their own TCP/IP stack so that they can have absolute control over its operation. The base operating system serves only as a platform for the firewall software, providing functions like booting, multitasking, and user interface.

Firewall products vary in the following ways:

Security   Some firewall products are fundamentally flawed because they rely too heavily on the host operating system, because they contain bugs that can be exploited, or because there is a flaw in the authentication protocol used for remote authentication.

Interface   Some firewalls are very difficult to configure because you must administer them via Telnet or an attached console and learn a cryptic command-line interface. Others use intuitive graphical interfaces that make configuration easy and obvious (well, obvious to us geeks, anyway).

Enterprise Functionality   Some firewalls are fortresses unto themselves, whereas others use a centrally maintained security policy that is replicated among all firewalls in the enterprise.

Security Features   Many firewalls offer important security features such as VPN and encrypted authentication to allow remote office networking with a high degree of security. In many firewalls, VPN is an extra-cost feature that must be enabled by purchasing an additional license.

Service Features   Some firewalls include services such as FTP, Telnet, HTTP, and so forth, so that you don't have to dedicate a machine to those functions. These features can be convenient, but they're often somewhat obsolete in functionality and can reduce the security of the firewall if they aren't properly implemented. Also, many services reveal a copyright that tells hackers exactly which firewall product you are using and allows them to target any weaknesses it may have.

Your primary criterion for firewalls should be security. The next most important feature is ease of use for you; you must be able to correctly configure a firewall for it to work correctly. Flashy features, performance, and services galore are tertiary considerations after the key issues of security and ease of use.

Problems Firewalls Can't Solve

No network attached to the Internet can be made completely secure. Firewalls are extremely effective and they will keep the hacking masses at bay, but there are so many different ways to exploit network connections that no method is entirely secure. Many administrators mistakenly assume that once their firewall is online and shown to be effective, their security problem is gone. That's simply not the case.

For example, let's say that the only thing you allow through your firewall is e-mail. An employee gets a message from a branch office asking him to e-mail a CAD file to them. So, the employee looks at the From address, verifies that it's correct, clicks Reply, attaches the file, and unknowingly sends the CAD file to the hackers who forged the e-mail request because the Reply-to address isn't the same as the From address. Your firewall can't realistically do anything about this type of exploitation because many typical users have different From and Reply-to addresses for valid reasons (for example, they send mail from multiple e-mail addresses but only want to receive mail at one).

Another problem firewalls can't solve is protection against protocols you decide to allow. For example, if you have a Windows-based IIS public web server on your network, your firewall must forward port 80 to it. Hackers can then attach to the web server as if they were typical web browsers and exploit the hundreds of known bugs in IIS to gain remote administrative access to it. Once they have control of your web server, they're "inside" your network and can use that web server to proxy an attack to the interior of your network, unless you have additional firewall policy preventing it.

There is another serious threat to the security of your network: hidden border crossings. Modems provide the ability for any user on your network to dial out to their own Internet service provider and completely circumvent your firewall. Modems are cheap, and they come in most computers sold these days. All modern client operating systems come with the software required for setting up modems to connect to a dial-up Internet service provider. And it's a good bet that most of your computer-savvy employees have their own dial-up networking accounts they could use from work.

Most users don't understand that all IP connections are a security risk. Modem PPP connections to the Internet are bidirectional just like leased lines. There's a good chance that a user's client has file sharing turned on, so their computer can be exploited directly from the Internet.

WARNING

It's quite common for businesses with firewalls to allow unrestricted file and print sharing among peers because it's an easy and efficient way for users to transfer files. If one of those users is dialed into the Net, it's also an easy and efficient way for hackers to transfer your files. Remember that the AOL dialer provides PPP service, so it's not any more secure than any other dial-up ISP.

Why would a user choose a dial-up modem connection when they have a fast and secure Internet connection? Reasons might include the following:

- Your firewall doesn't pass Internet Relay Chat, and they want to talk to their friends.

- They want to use NetPhone to talk to their mother for free.

- They want to work from home using pcAnywhere.

- AOL uses a port your firewall doesn't pass, and they want to check their personal e-mail.

- You filter FTP, and they want to download a file.

- Your network is configured to block pornography sites.

Users dial out so they can circumvent your security policy without your knowledge. To control border security, you must control all the border crossings; it must be impossible to establish a new border crossing without your permission. Exceptions to this rule endanger the security of your entire network.

Reinforcing the Borders

Here are some tips for taking control of your border crossings:

▶ Reduce the number of connections to the Internet to the minimum number possible: one per campus. Many large organizations allow only a single link to the Internet at headquarters and then route all remote offices to that point using the same Frame Relay lines used to connect internal networks. Even if you use VPN to connect your remote offices, consider requiring them to route through your central firewall to reach the Internet—this way, you can control firewall policy on a single machine.

▶ Don't allow dial-up connections to the Internet. Remove modems and all other uncontrolled network access devices. Disable free COM ports in the BIOS settings of client computers and password-protect the BIOS to prevent users from overriding your security settings.

▶ Don't allow unrestricted file sharing. Use file sharing with user-based authentication or, at the very least, with passwords. Don't install file and print sharing on client computers unless absolutely necessary. Encourage users to store all files on network file servers, and create server pools of resources like CD-ROMs or modems that can be centrally controlled.

▶ Configure internal client computers with IP addresses in the 192.168.0.0 or the 10.0.0.0 domains, which are not routed over the Internet. Use NAT to translate these internal addresses to routable external addresses on your firewall. Doing so may prevent hackers from exploiting modem connections into your network beyond the computer that established the connection.

Border Security Options

Once you've got your firewall running on the border between your private network and the Internet, you're going to run into a problem: How do you provide the public services your customers need while securing your internal network from attack? There is more than one answer to this question, and which one is right depends entirely upon your security posture and the level of service you need to provide.

Methods used by companies to protect their networks range from the simple to the complex, and from the risky to the very secure. Such methods include the following (in order of security risk from highest to lowest):

1. Filtered packet services
2. Single firewall with internal public servers
3. Single firewall with external public servers
4. Dual firewalls or demilitarized zone (DMZ) firewalls
5. Enterprise firewalls
6. Disconnection

The following sections discuss each method in detail, along with relative risks and issues.

Filtered Packet Services

Most Internet service providers provide packet filtering as a value-added service for leased-line customers. For a small monthly charge (generally about $100), your ISP will set up its firewall to filter traffic into and out of your network. Some ISPs also offer proxy servers and NAT, but you may still be at risk from security attacks by other customers served by that ISP. Remember that all hackers have ISPs too. Figure 11.3 illustrates how filtered packet services work.

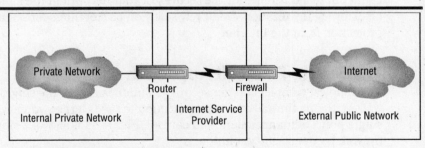

FIGURE 11.3:   Filtered packet service

There are a number of problems with filtered firewall services:

▶ Packet filters can be exploited more easily than complete firewalls.

▶ Your security is in the hands of a third party. Their motivations may not always coincide with yours, especially if a legal dispute arises between your company and theirs.

▶ The responsibility for reliability isn't controllable.

▶ It's not in the best interest of the ISP to alert you that there has been a compromise.

▶ There's rarely any provision for alarming and alerting.

▶ Configuration is a difficult and error-prone administrative hassle. Reconfiguration is also a pain in the neck if the ISP doesn't have a strong customer support ethic.

▶ You are probably vulnerable to the ISP's other subscribers, who are usually inside the same firewall.

ISP-provided packet filters have the following advantage:

▶ No up-front capital expenditure is required.

Even if the firewall service provided by an ISP were complete, it would still never be a good idea to put the security of your network in the hands of another organization. You don't know anything about your ISP's employees, and you don't know what measures your ISP might take if for some reason a dispute arose between your company and theirs. Add to that these simple facts: Most people who can hack do so at least occasionally, and many good hackers work for the people who can get them closest to the action.

Locally control and administer all security services for your network. Don't put responsibility for the security of your network in the hands of an external organization. Don't rely solely on packet filters for security protection from the Internet.

The Single-Firewall Approach

The simplest complete border security solution is that of the single firewall. With one firewall and one connection to the Internet, you have a single point of management and control. Figure 11.4 shows a single firewall border security solution.

You have a problem if you intend to provide public services like an FTP site or website, or if you want to operate a mail server. You must either open a connection through your firewall to an internal host, or you must expose your public server to the Internet without the protection of a firewall. Both methods are risky.

The problem with putting public servers, like mail servers, outside your firewall is that they are at risk for unrestricted hacking. You can set up these computers so that they don't contain much useful information, but hacking attempts could easily cause denial of service if your servers are crashed, or at least cause embarrassment if hackers modify your web pages. Figure 11.5 shows public servers inside the firewall.

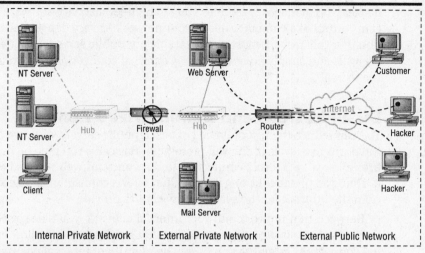

FIGURE 11.4: A single firewall with public servers exposed to the Internet

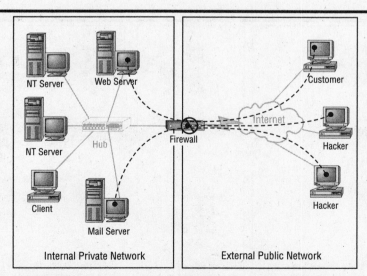

FIGURE 11.5: A single firewall with public servers protected but allowing external traffic in through the firewall

The problem with opening a path through your firewall for externally sourced connection attempts is that inappropriate packets could potentially make their way onto your internal network if they look like packets that conform to the rules used by your packet filter. It also means that a hacker who manages to exploit a bug in high-level service software might gain control of a computer inside your network—a very dangerous situation. For this reason, most organizations put public servers outside their firewalls and simply do not allow any external connections in through the firewall.

Dual Firewalls and Demilitarized Zones

You can reduce the risk of having exposed public servers with two firewalls and two levels of firewall protection. Basically, you put the first firewall at your Internet connection and secure your web servers behind it. Doing so provides strong security, but allows connection attempts from the Internet for the services you want to provide.

Between that network and your internal network, you place a second firewall with a stronger security policy that simply does not allow external connection attempts and hides the identity of internal clients. Figure 11.6 shows a network with two firewalls providing two levels of security.

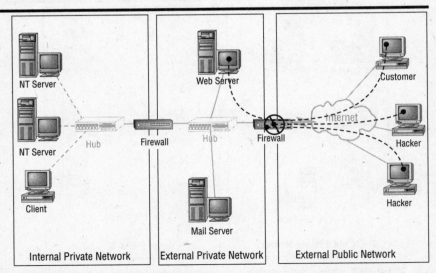

FIGURE 11.6:   Two firewalls acting in concert to completely protect a network

Most modern firewall products allow the use of demilitarized zones (DMZ), which provide the functionality of having two firewalls by having different security policies for each attached interface in the firewall. With three interfaces—external network, internal network, and public server network—you can customize your security policy to block connection attempts to your internal network but pass certain protocols to your public servers. This allows you the functionality of two firewalls using a single product. This approach is sometimes referred to as a *trihomed firewall.* Figure 11.7 shows a trihomed firewall with different security settings for each network.

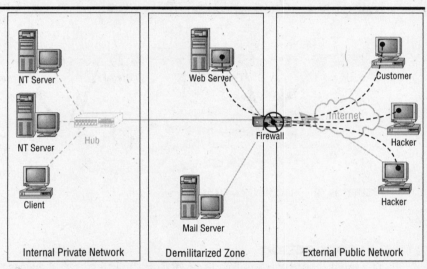

FIGURE 11.7:   A DMZ firewall provides different security for different needs.

NOTE

Always use a DMZ firewall or dual firewalls if you need to provide public services *and* protect an interior network. Every different security policy requires its own firewall or network interface.

Enterprise Firewalls

Enterprise firewalls are those products that share a single, centralized firewall policy among multiple firewalls. Enterprise firewalls allow you to retain central control of security policy without having to worry about whether the policy is correctly implemented on each of the firewalls in your organization. The firewall policy is usually defined on a security workstation and then replicated to each firewall in your organization using some means of secure authentication. Figure 11.8 shows an enterprise with multiple firewalls, one at each Internet connection.

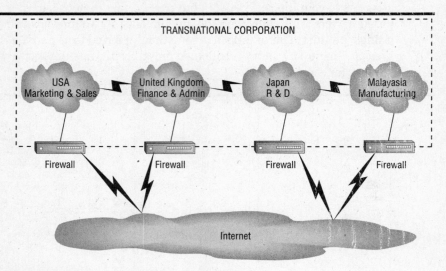

FIGURE 11.8: Multiple firewalls in an enterprise

Disconnection

The most secure way to provide service on the Internet and access for internal users is not to connect your internal network to the Internet at all, but to have a separate network used only for Internet-related services. Figure 11.9 shows an internal network that is disconnected from the Internet.

This method is absolutely impenetrable from the Internet because no connection exists between the internal and the external networks. The public-access servers for web, FTP, and mail are located on a small network segment that is attached to the Internet along with a few clients. The client stations contain e-mail, news, and web browsers but no sensitive information. Employees travel to the external clients to check their e-mail, browse the web, or perform any other Internet-related tasks.

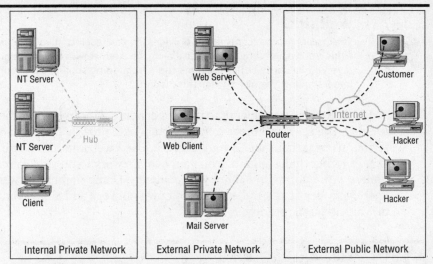

FIGURE 11.9: The disconnected security model provides the most protection from Internet intrusion.

This model has three very important benefits:

▶ The private network is absolutely secure. Data can't flow freely between the external and internal networks. You may consider putting a high-capacity removable media drive on one of the clients to facilitate large file transfers when necessary—but this can be a security problem!

▶ It's free. It doesn't require esoteric software or sophisticated hardware, and you can use outdated computers for the client stations.

▶ It provides a natural disincentive for employees to waste time surfing the Web randomly or downloading content that could cause legal liability problems.

And of course, there is one very important detractor: Employees hate it. They have to travel to access stations, which are typically located in one central area. Transferring files becomes problematic. It can cause a work bottleneck if there aren't enough access stations. Many employees simply won't use it, which reduces the efficiency of e-mail and other such important business tools.

In a nutshell, disconnection is the most secure and the least efficient way to connect your employees to the Internet.

WARNING

The disconnected security model provides the greatest incentive for employees to blow off your security policy and dial up the Internet with their modem. Make sure your security policy prevents them from doing so, and that your users understand why you've chosen this model.

Don't attach your network to public networks if it can possibly be avoided. Use the disconnected network model to provide Internet access to your users rather than to your network. Use a web and FTP hosting service rather than computers on your own network to provide your customers with information about your company. Doing so puts the web hosting agency at risk rather than your own network and allows you to provide no public services.

FIREWALL OPTIONS

Recently, we were hired to perform ethical hacking against the network of a "famous name" company that used another large multinational to provide third-party security services. The security service involved placing a strong Unix-based firewall at the client's site and performing remote administration and monitoring of the firewall and of hacking attempts

When we began our attack, we used the traditional method of port scanning to determine what we could see in the client's network. Port scanning is easy to detect and was supposed to be part of the monitored services the client received from its security vendor. The scan revealed a potential vulnerability (port 139 was open to one of the internal servers). We used another traditional method to try to exploit the vulnerability: automated password guessing over the Internet using a common password list. This technique is also very easy to detect and was specifically listed as one of the hacking techniques the service provider monitored and provided protection against.

The password list we used was specially created by hackers from an analysis of hundreds of thousands of exploited user accounts. The hackers created a statistical ranking of the commonality of passwords and created this list that order.

Using this list, our automated password scanner guessed the local administrative password so quickly that we were still in the process of explaining to the client that we probably would not be able to

CONTINUED ➡

exploit the machine using this technique unless the passwords were really simple. In this specific case, it hit using the eleventh most commonly used password.

After we screenshot the contents of the web server's hard disk and completed our report, our client waited for notification from the monitored security service. Notification never came. In fact, our client finally gave up waiting for a call after two weeks and fired the service provider.

In a separate incident, another customer of ours relied on a filtered packet service from its Internet service provider for security. Because the client runs a very small startup business and is strapped for cash, we didn't put up too much resistance to this arrangement initially.

As part of our services for the client, we made periodic light hacking attempts against its server to make sure no easily exploitable methods could be used to gain access. After having verified the service a number of times, one scan showed that the service had suddenly failed, exposing the NetBIOS session ports of the NT server to the Internet. We mapped a drive connection right to the server over the Internet!

A panicked call to the client's ISP verified that for some reason the filter had been turned off. The ISP could not explain why or how this had happened and did not know how long the filter had been down. It simply turned the filter service back on and apologized.

Our client decided that it needed to administer security itself, because the ISP could not be trusted to maintain filtering. To keep costs as low as possible, we suggested using a Linux-based firewall product or perhaps Linux alone. Our client was not comfortable with the user interface, however, and decided to go with a Windows NT–based firewall solution. We acquired a machine running Windows NT Workstation and installed Checkpoint Firewall-1. Although Firewall-1 is a more expensive solution, its interface is fairly intuitive. We were able to train the client to administer policy without the help of a consultant, which served to lower the total cost of ownership. The client now has a reliable and secure connection to the Internet.

Part III

What's Next

In this chapter, you have learned the basic concepts that are part of any firewall system. Throughout the next few chapters, you will learn more about some of the specific firewall methods mentioned in this chapter.

Chapter 12

PACKET FILTERING

P acket filters were the original firewalls. The first attempts to make TCP/IP secure were based on the idea that it's pretty easy for a router to inspect the header of TCP/IP packets and simply drop packets that don't conform to the specifications you want to accept.

However, packet filters have problems that make them insufficient to provide total security for an internal network. They are now combined with proxy servers and Network Address Translators to solve those problems.

Proxy servers were originally designed to make the World Wide Web faster. Network Address Translators were originally designed to increase the address space available to private organizations and to solve IP address numbering problems associated with attaching existing private TCP/IP networks to the Internet. The serendipitous security benefits of both of these functions were integrated with packet filtering and encryption technology to create the modern effective firewalls in use today.

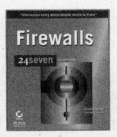

Adapted from *Firewalls 24seven™*, Second Edition by Matthew Strebe and Charles Perkins

ISBN 0-7821-4054-8 $49.99

Part III

Neither proxy servers nor Network Address Translators can be properly secured without a packet filter, and a packet filter cannot provide total security without the services of a proxy server or a Network Address Translator. Because these services must be combined into a single coherent security function to be effective, you should use firewalls that make effective use of all three methods to truly secure your network.

There are two primary types of packet filtering:

▶ Original, or *stateless* packet filtering, often used by routers and operating systems

▶ *Stateful* inspection packet filtering, used in all modern firewalls

This chapter discusses "pure" packet filtering: packet filtering not combined with proxy or Network Address Translation functions. Pure packet filters are still in use all over the place, so this discussion remains very current.

How Stateless Packet Filters Work

Packet filters are border routers that increase security by determining whether to forward a packet based on information contained in the header of every individual packet. Filters can theoretically be configured to determine this based on any part of the protocol header, but most filters can be configured only to filter on the most useful data fields:

▶ Protocol type

▶ IP address

▶ TCP/UDP port

▶ Source routing information

▶ Fragment number

The following sections detail each of these fields.

Protocol Filtering

Protocol filtering filters packets based on the content of the IP protocol field. The protocol field can be used to discriminate against entire suites of services, such as:

▶ User Datagram Protocol (UDP)

▶ Transmission Control Protocol (TCP)

▶ Internet Control Message Protocol (ICMP)

▶ Internet Group Management Protocol (IGMP)

For example, if you have a single-purpose server serving a TCP-based service like HTTP, you could filter out all UDP services. Unfortunately, the protocol field is so general (only four common protocols are available to filter on) that most servers and routers will have to leave all of them open.

IP Address Filtering

IP address filtering allows you to limit connections to (or from) specific hosts and networks based on their IP address. Most filters allow you to either deny access to all hosts except an accepted list or allow access to all hosts except a denied list.

Specific denial of certain hosts is almost worthless, because you'd have to keep track of every hacker who had ever attacked your network and assume that they have no way to gain information from a different IP address, which they always will. Relying on specific denial is not a strong security policy.

Specific acceptance of certain host addresses provides particularly strong security, however; it is the strongest form of security that a stateless packet filter can provide. By denying access to all hosts except a list of known IP addresses, you can ensure that your routers can only be reached by the IP addresses of machines or networks you know about. This list could be other networks in your organization, the networks of your customers, or the networks of work-at-home users. By denying access to all other IP addresses, you make it nearly impossible for a hacker to exploit your network. To hack into your network, a hacker would have to have access to your list of allowed IP addresses.

It is possible for hackers to use source routing (explained in detail in the next section) to "spoof" IP addresses. Source routing would allow a hacker to put an allowed address into a packet and then capture the return by specifying that responses be routed back to his computer. For this reason, packet filters should always be configured to drop source-routed packets.

Part III

Good packet filters will allow you to specify hosts on a per-protocol basis, so (for example) you could allow all hosts to access TCP port 80 for HTTP service but only hosts from your company network to access TCP port 23 (Telnet). Most simple filters don't have allowed lists per protocol, so you can only assign a single list of hosts allowed for all protocols.

It's important to remember that a filter can only limit addresses based on the IP address field's contents, which could be different than the actual source host. It's easy for hackers to forge the IP address field of a packet, so it's certainly possible for them to get a packet past a packet filter if they know an address that the filter will pass. This would be useful in instances where a round-trip is not necessary, such as in a denial-of-service attack or where the return address for the protocol is contained in the payload of the packet as well as the header (as in FTP).

TCP/UDP Ports

TCP or UDP port information is the most commonly used information to filter on because this data field indicates most specifically what the packet is for. Port filtering is also commonly referred to as *protocol filtering* because the TCP or UDP port number identifies higher-level protocols. Figure 12.1 shows how a stateless packet filter discriminates based on the TCP or UDP port number.

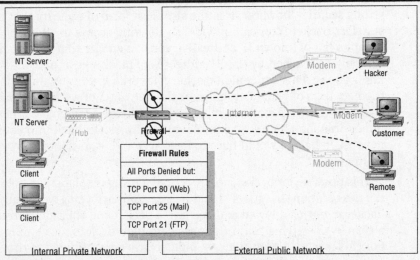

FIGURE 12.1: A packet filter rejects undesired traffic.

Common protocols that can be filtered based on the TCP or UDP port field are:

Daytime	DNS	NetBIOS Session
Echo	HTTP	IMAP
Quote	Gopher	NFS
FTP	POP	Whois
Telnet	SNMP	RSH
SMTP	NNTP	

As with IP addresses, most packet filters allow you to either pass all protocols except a denied list or pass no protocols except an allowed list; and as with IP addresses, passing no protocols except an allowed list is more secure. Unlike IP address filtering, blocking only certain ports is still useful because most hacking exploits target only a few specific protocols. The most important protocols to block are listed here:

Telnet   Leaving this port open on a host will allow hackers to open a command prompt with a large amount of access to your machine.

NetBIOS Session   Leaving this port open to the Internet on Windows or Server Message Block (SMB) serving hosts will allow hackers to attach to your file servers as if they were local clients.

POP   You should implement a virtual private network (VPN) connection for remote clients who need to check their mail, because POP uses plaintext passwords to allow access. The use of plaintext will allow hackers to sniff user's passwords off the network.

NFS   Unix clients should not leave open access to Network File System (NFS) ports for the same reason Windows clients should not leave open access to the NetBIOS ports.

X Windows   Running X client software (the terms *client* and *server* in X environments have the opposite of their usual meanings) will leave your server vulnerable to attack.

Windows Terminal Services   Exposing Windows Terminal Services to the Internet means your terminal server is protected by just a username and password. There are numerous ways to extract that information from clients on your network.

Part III

These ports are especially sensitive to attack because of the high level of functional control they give the attacker. Other ports, like DNS, could be used to damage some specific information, but the services themselves are not rich enough to control the machine directly and are therefore of less value to attackers (of course, all listening services are potentially vulnerable to buffer overrun and related exploits).

Other ports you should block include any sort of remote access or remote control software such as pcAnywhere or VNC.

Filtering on Other Information

In addition to the standard fields, headers contain other information that can be used to determine whether a packet should be passed.

Source routing and fragmentation are two techniques supported by the IP protocol that are largely obsolete and frequently exploited by hackers. Most packet filters will allow you to simply drop any packets that are source routed or fragmented.

Source Routing

Source routing is the process of defining the exact route a packet must take between hosts in an IP connection. Source routing was originally used for debugging and testing purposes, but it is now frequently used by hackers who can put any address in the source field and still ensure the packet will return by specifying their own machine in the source route.

Two types of source routing exist:

▶ *Loose source routing* indicates one or more hosts the packet must flow through, but not a complete list.

▶ *Strict source routing* indicates the exact route a packet must follow between hosts.

Of the two types, loose source routing is most often used by hackers because they can simply plug in the IP address of their machine to make sure the packet comes back to them by any means.

Unless you use source routing in your network, configure your filters to drop any source-routed packets. No protocol or ISP requires source routing.

Fragmentation

Fragmentation was developed to support the passage of large IP packets through routers that could not forward them due to the frame size constraints encountered in some early networks. Fragmentation gave any router in the path between two hosts the ability to chop up an inbound IP packet into multiple smaller packets and then forward them on size-constrained networks. The receiving system simply waited for all fragments of the packet to reassemble it to its original form.

The problem with fragmentation comes from the fact that the most useful filter data—the TCP or UDP port number—is provided only in the beginning of an IP packet, so it will only be contained in fragment 0. Fragments 1 and higher cannot be filtered based on port information because they don't contain any port information. So, most early filters simply forwarded all subsequent fragments with the assumption that if the 0th fragment had been dropped, the subsequent fragments would be worthless.

But that's not always the case. Many flawed versions of TCP/IP running on internal hosts might reassemble the packet anyway, and if the first through nth packets contained a valid TCP packet, they'd go ahead and use it. This meant that hackers could modify their IP stack to start all fragment numbers at 1 and effectively bypass the filter altogether.

Problems with Stateless Packet Filters

Packet filters suffer from two problems that prevent them from being completely effective:

▶ They cannot check the payload of packets.

▶ They do not retain the state of connections.

These problems make packet filters alone insufficient to secure your network.

No Service-Specific Security

Packet filters make pass/drop decisions based solely on header information; they do not inspect content for the presence of dangerous or malformed data to determine whether that data should be passed. For this reason, packet filters alone do not constitute effective security.

For example, HTTP content flowing back into your network could contain Trojan horses embedded in ActiveX controls. Your packet filter cannot determine this, so it simply passes the content through. Or you may allow Simple Mail Transfer Protocol (SMTP) port 25 through to your mail server to receive e-mail, but the filter can't determine that a malformed e-mail passing through it will crash your e-mail server.

Service-specific security can be implemented only by the service-specific filters used by proxy servers and true firewalls.

Part III

No Connection State Security

Most packet filters are stateless—that is, they do not retain information about connections in use. They simply make pass/drop determinations packet by packet and based only on the information contained within that packet. Stateless packet filters cannot determine whether to drop fragments, because they retain no information about the fragment's service port. Stateless packet filters also cannot determine when a return socket connection applies to a connection established from inside the network, so they must be configured to simply pass all TCP ports in the range of a normal return socket. For this reason, many early packet filters simply pass all TCP ports above 1024.

Modern port filters and all modern firewalls use state information to keep track of connection status and thereby more positively control the routing of packets through your network.

If you can't use proxy servers to eliminate routing at your border, use state-based packet filtering and Network Address Translation.

OS Packet Filtering

Most modern operating systems, Unix and Windows included, include packet filtering as part of the TCP/IP stack. This means that you can configure unique packet filtering rules for each server based on its individual function. This is called *end-system packet filtering* because the final computer in the route (the host to which the packet is actually addressed) performs the filtration.

Intermediate systems like packet-filtering routers and firewalls can be configured to drop or pass packets based on the ultimate address, so end-system packet filtering may seem unnecessary. But no border system can protect your server from an internal attack or from an attack that somehow sidesteps your border security by exploiting an improperly secured VPN or dial-up connection.

By including backup packet filtering directly on servers, you can provide an extra level of security that will still be in place if your border security fails or if the attack comes from inside your network.

You should use the packet-filtering functionality of your server's operating systems to guarantee that you are serving only those protocols you intend to serve publicly. Host-based packet filtering allows you to ensure that each server exposes only those services you intend.

How Stateful Inspection Packet Filters Work

Standard packet filters have a number of flaws, all of which stem from the fact that a single packet in a communication does not contain enough information to determine whether it should be dropped, because it is part of a larger communication. Stateful inspection packet filters solve this problem by retaining the state of all the communication flowing through the firewall in memory, and using that remembered state to determine whether individual packets should be dropped. Stateful inspectors filter entire communication streams, not just packets.

Stateful packet filters remember the state of connections at the network and session layers by recording the session establishment information that passes through the filter gateway. The filters then use that information to discriminate valid return packets from invalid connection attempts or hacking.

Most stateless packet filters simply allow all ports above 1024 to pass through the firewall because those ports are used for the return sockets of connections initiated inside the firewall. This is extremely poor security—nothing prevents Trojan horses from waiting inside your network on a service port above 1024, so stateless packet filters cannot prevent this sort of intrusion.

Stateful packet filters, on the other hand, do not allow any services through the firewall except those services they're programmed to allow and connections that they already maintain in their state tables.

When a trusted internal host connects to a TCP socket on an external untrusted host, it transmits with the connection synchronization packet the socket (IP address and port) on which it expects to receive a response. When that SYN packet is routed through the stateful inspection filter, the filter makes an entry in its state table containing the destination socket and the response socket, and then forwards the packet on to the untrusted network. When the response comes back, the filter can simply look up the packet's source and destination sockets in its state table, see that they match an expected response, and pass the packet. If no table entry exists, the packet is dropped because it was not requested from inside the network. Figure 12.2 shows the establishment phase of a stateful filter.

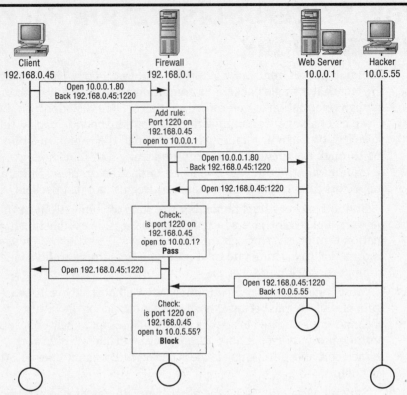

FIGURE 12.2:   A stateful inspection packet filter allows return data.

The filter removes state table entries when the TCP close session negotiation packets are routed through, or after some period of delay, usually a few minutes. This action ensures that dropped connections don't leave state table "holes" open. Figure 12.3 shows a filter removing the table entry that allows return data from a connection.

Stateful filters are then programmed with rules (usually called *policies*) that modify that basic behavior. Policies usually include rules for packets that are always dropped, packets that are never dropped, services that are allowed to pass from the outside to specific hosts inside, and so forth. On multifunction firewalls, the policies also control network address translation and proxying; they usually abstract IP addresses, networks, and ports into objects, areas, and services so that rather than blocking port 80 from network 192.168.12.0, you're blocking "web service" from "accounting."

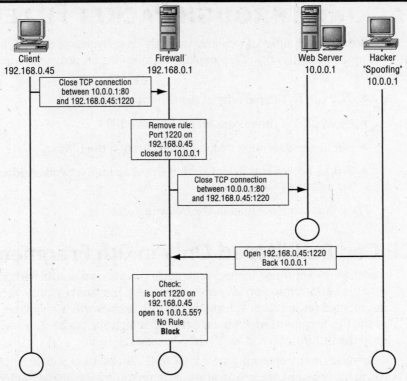

FIGURE 12.3: A stateful inspection filter leaves holes open only as long as they're necessary.

Because stateful filters can filter on all the same information that stateless filters can, and can additionally filter fragments, which side of the firewall a connection is initiated from, and other more complex information, stateful filters are considerably more secure.

Stateless packet filters still don't solve the problem of internal protocol analysis for higher-level protocols like HTTP and FTP, but higher-end firewalls like Firewall-1 do provide a proxy-like higher-layer filtration service for common protocols like HTTP, FTP, and SMTP. Although far more secure than not having higher-level inspection at all, the packets are not regenerated the way they are on a proxy server, so there's still a chance that malformed original data could pass through the filter to a target inside your network.

Part III

HACKING THROUGH PACKET FILTERS

Hackers use a number of well-known methods to bypass packet filters and get inside your network. They exploit the following security problems with packet filters:

► TCP can be filtered only in the 0th fragments.

► Older packet filters pass all ports above 1024.

► Public services must be forwarded through the filter.

► Trojan horses can defeat packet filters using Network Address Translation (NAT).

These hacks are detailed in the following sections.

TCP Can Be Filtered Only in 0th Fragments

Stateless packet filters inspect each packet on its own merits without retaining information about previous packets. For this reason, when a fragmented packet comes through, the TCP header will be available only in the 0th fragment, which means that although the packet filter will drop the 0th fragment, it won't drop fragments past 0.

Because many operating system TCP/IP stacks don't pay attention to fragment ordering, these operating systems will reassemble a fragmented packet until they get a packet with the final fragment flag set. If the data in their IP buffer constitutes a valid packet, they'll pass it along to the operating system.

Hackers exploit this to pass data right through a packet filter to a specific host inside your network. By transmitting all packets with the fragment number set to 1, but containing the entire TCP packet, the filter will ignore the TCP payload and allow it to pass to the internal network. The addressed end system sees that the final fragment message is set and passes the TCP packet along to the operating system. In this way, hackers can connect directly to hosts inside your network as if the packet filter didn't even exist.

The two solutions to this problem are to use only hardened TCP/IP stacks on your internal hosts and to use state-based packet filters like true firewalls. Windows NT 4 Service Pack 3 hardens the TCP/IP stack against this vulnerability, but earlier editions of NT are vulnerable. Many

Unix implementations are hardened against this attack, but many are not—even some firewalls are vulnerable to this attack. Search the Web for your specific version and variation to determine if this exploit will work against your operating system.

Low Pass Blocking Filters Don't Catch High Port Connections

Stateless packet filters and the packet-filtering services provided by ISPs usually open ports above 1024 so that the return socket of a connection can be established back to a host. As a result, any protocol running with a TCP port higher than 1024 cannot be protected by these packet filters.

Make sure your packet filter is state-based and blocks all inbound connection attempts except those you want to allow and those that were initiated from inside your network.

Public Services Must Be Forwarded

These days, hackers don't usually bother with TCP-level exploits because they know you have to open your web and e-mail servers to the public anyway. They just use protocol exploits to reach these servers, and then try to initiate connections to the interior of your network from those servers. If you've set up additional rules in your firewall to allow connections to and from your web server—for example, to publish changes to the website— then hackers can use that way in to gain access to the interior of the network.

Internal NATs Can Defeat Filtering

If a user inside your network sets up a Network Address Translator on a machine (a Linux computer, for example), then that machine can be used to perform port and address translation to change a protocol inbound on a high, unfiltered port (say 8080) back down to a protocol on a filtered port (80) and then pass it to an internal server. Internal proxy servers could also be used to cause this vulnerability. This exploit would allow uncontrolled access to your internal services.

Trojan horses perform exactly this sort of protocol translation for the purpose of allowing hackers to access your internal network directly. Unsuspecting users might get e-mail from your e-mail address with instructions to click the setup file of the attached program, which would then install the Trojan horse. Hackers could then exploit the Network Address Translator in the Trojan horse to bypass your filter.

BEST PACKET FILTERING PRACTICES

Pure packet filters are subject to a few glaring security problems. Use these recommendations to keep your packet filtering secure:

- ▶ Use at least a stateful filter if you can't use a proxy.
- ▶ Disable all ports by default.
- ▶ Secure the base operating system.

These practices are detailed in the following sections.

Use a Real Firewall

Do not rely on simple packet filters or the packet filtering functionality of your operating system to keep your network secure. Pure packet filters cannot adequately secure a network.

Disable All Ports By Default

Do not pass all protocols by default and then block those you consider dangerous. Although doing so is convenient, it opens you up for attack by Trojan horses and unintended user mode services like pcAnywhere.

Block all ports by default, and pass only the ports you intend to serve and the return channels from connections initiated from inside your network.

Secure the Base OS

Make sure the base operating system is secure. As with all security software, the security of a packet filter is based on the security of the device on which it's run. Most packet filter appliances (routers) can be configured via Telnet, meaning that a hacker could telnet into your packet filter and reconfigure it to allow more useful ports to be opened.

LEAKY FILTERS

When a customer of mine attached its network to the Internet in 1994, we put a "firewall" in place on the routed connection. In those days, a firewall was a router with a packet filter. We used Telnet to block all inbound ports below 1024 except ports 80 (the customer ran a web server on a SPARC machine), 21 (FTP), and 25 (SMTP). We felt perfectly secure.

Then a scientist downloaded a Trojan horse embedded in a freeware utility without knowing about it. It wasn't a virus, so the virus scanning software didn't pick it up.

One day a few months later, the scientist was working at his desk when an MS-DOS command prompt popped up on the screen. At the C:\> prompt, the letters format c: slowly appeared one at a time, as if they were being typed by someone directly—except he wasn't typing them.

The hacker apparently paused for some reason before hitting the Enter key, and during that pause, the scientist wisely unplugged his network connection. He immediately got on the phone to me, and I came in to take a look.

I had never seen such a brazen intrusion before. Until then, Trojan horses to me were a theoretical possibility that were too esoteric to bother thinking about. I knew how difficult it would be to write a useful one, so I didn't worry about them.

This specific Trojan horse set itself up as a server on port 12345 and waited for connections. Upon receiving a connection, it would open a command prompt and vector the I/O to that command prompt over the TCP connection. This action effectively gave hackers a remote command prompt on infected machines. Hackers could simply scan wide ranges of IP addresses, browsing for open connections on port 12345 to find running instances of the Trojan horse.

Of course, I was called to the mat to explain how the firewall had failed. It hadn't, I explained; it just wasn't designed to prevent that sort of intrusion because this specific firewall could only block ports below 1024, like many early packet filters. The budget for security went up considerably, and we used it to install a Firewall-1–based stateful inspection gateway. We also bought port-scanning tools to search for other instances of unknown services running inside the network.

What's Next

In this chapter, you have learned how packet filters can be used to analyze information traveling in and out of your firewall. In Chapter 13, you will learn how NAT can be combined with packet filtering to increase the security of your network.

Chapter 13

NETWORK ADDRESS TRANSLATION

N etwork Address Translation (NAT) converts private IP
addresses in your private network to globally unique public
IP addresses for use on the Internet. Although NAT was originally
implemented as a hack to make more IP addresses available to
private networks, it has a serendipitous security aspect that has
proven at least as important—internal host hiding.

Network Address Translation effectively hides all TCP/IP-
level information about your internal hosts from hackers on the
Internet by making all your traffic appear to come from a single
IP address. NAT also allows you to use any IP address range
you want on your internal network (even if those addresses are
already in use elsewhere on the Internet, although you won't
be able to reach public servers on the public Internet that are
within the range of addresses you use on your private Internet).
This means you don't have to register a large, expensive block
from the American Registry for Internet Numbers (ARIN) or
your ISP or reassign network numbers from those you simply
plugged in before you connected your network to the Internet.

Part III

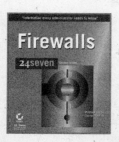

Adapted from *Firewalls 24seven*™, Second Edition
by Matthew Strebe and Charles Perkins
ISBN 0-7821-4054-8 $49.99

NAT hides internal IP addresses by converting all internal host addresses to the address of the firewall (or an address responded to by the firewall) as packets are routed through the firewall. The firewall then retransmits the data payload of the internal host from its own address using a translation table to keep track of which sockets on the exterior interface equate to which sockets on the interior interface. To the Internet, all the traffic on your network appears to be coming from one extremely busy computer.

NOTE

RFC 1631 describes Network Address Translation.

NAT is actually a fundamental proxy: A single host makes requests on behalf of all internal hosts, thus hiding their identity from the public network. Windows NT did not provide this function; however, Windows 2000 and subsequent Microsoft operating systems can provide NAT for computers connecting through them to outside networks (and the Internet). Many versions of Unix provide or can use publicly available IP masquerade software. All modern firewalls provide NAT.

NAT is implemented only at the transport layer. This means that information hidden in the data payload of TCP/IP traffic could be transmitted to a higher-level service and used to exploit weaknesses in higher-level traffic or to communicate with a Trojan horse. You'll still have to use a higher-level service like a proxy to prevent higher-level service security breaches.

TIP

NAT is so effective at IP address re-use that the implementation of IP version 6 has been practically stalled due to lack of interest, and the threat of IP address scarcity has been eliminated for the foreseeable future. NAT allows an entire Class A–sized network to hide behind a single IP address.

NAT Explained

To perform Network Address Translation, firewalls maintain a table of interior sockets matched to exterior sockets. When an interior client establishes a connection to an exterior host, the firewall changes the source socket to one of the firewall's exterior sockets and makes a new entry in the translation table indicating the actual interior source socket, the destination socket, and the mated firewall socket.

When an exterior host sends data back to the interior host's socket, the firewall performs the reverse translation. If no entry exists in the translation table for the socket address or if the IP address of the source is different than the address the firewall expects to see, then the packet is dropped.

This process is easiest to explain with an example. Let's say that interior host 192.168.1.9 wants to establish a web session with exterior host 10.50.23.11. Using the next available port, 192.168.1.9:1234 transmits a TCP packet to 10.50.23.11:80.

The router/firewall (192.168.1.1 interior address, 10.0.30.2 exterior address) receives the packet and makes the following record in its translation table:

Source	192.168.1.9:1234
Public Host	10.50.23.11:80
Translation	10.0.30.2:15465

It then transmits the packet on the Internet using the translated IP address and port number, so 10.50.23.11:80 (the public host) receives a connection attempt coming from 10.0.30.2:15465 (the firewall's exterior address). When the public host transmits back, it responds to the source that it thinks originated the request: 10.0.30.2:15465.

Upon receiving the packet, the firewall searches its translation table for a matching socket and finds it. It then verifies that the source of the packet is the same as the public host recorded in the translation table when the entry was made. The presence of a table entry confirms that the packet was requested by an internal host—had the packet not been requested, no translation entry would be present matching both the translated socket and the recorded public host socket. If no matching entry is found, the packet is dropped and logged.

The firewall then modifies the packet with the internal source client's socket number and passes it to the interior network for transmission to the ultimate client.

On the public host side, NAT is also used in "port forwarding" mode—the web server in this case is protected by another NAT, which is configured to receive connections on its public IP address and translate them to the interior of the network. Unlike the NAT on the browser's connection,

Part III

this configuration is not automatic; the administrator must specifically configure the NAT device for this translation.

In this example, the NAT receives an HTTP connection on 10.50.23.11: 80. It examines its port forwarding tables and sees that port 80 is mapped to the interior host 192.168.0.5:80. So the NAT rewrites the IP address from 10.50.23.11:80 to 192.168.0.5:80 and forwards the packet. On the return stream, it performs the inverse translation, so the packet sent to 10.0.30.2:1234 (the browser's NAT's public IP address) from 192.168.0.5:80 is rewritten to come from 10.50.23.11:80 by the NAT device. Figure 13.1 illustrates this process.

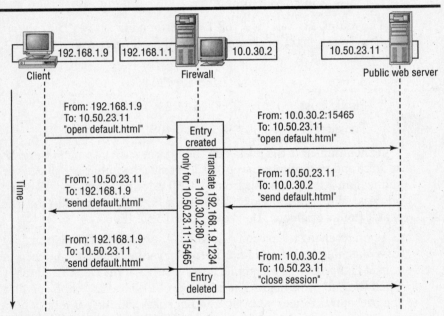

FIGURE 13.1: Network Address Translation

Because NAT changes the IP address in the packet, it is almost always necessary to make entries in your routing tables to ensure that translated packets reach their proper destination inside your network.

In the case of port forwarding, no "dynamic" entry needs to be made or remembered—the IP address rewriting is the same coming and going for every host. Port forwarding is therefore slightly simpler and doesn't require a substantial amount of RAM on the NAT device.

WARNING

Because NAT performs only simple substitutions at the packet layer, it does not need to perform complex analyses on the contained data, as application proxies must. This means that most implementations of NAT are nearly as fast as straight routing. NAT requires far less processor overhead than higher-level application proxying. Firewalls performing Network Address Translation must have at least one valid public IP address, and that address cannot be concealed.

Because NAT changes the contents of the IP header, systems that rely on that data remaining unchanged (such as Header Authentication in IPSec, the Internet Protocol Security suite of protocols) will not work through NAT. Another difficulty with IPSec is that NAT has a difficult time differentiating IPSec traffic coming from multiple interior clients, so firewalls that perform IPSec passthrough typically allow only one interior client at a time to establish IPSec tunnels to exterior locations.

WARNING

NAT and IPSec don't mix well. Either have your firewall be the end point of your virtual private network (VPN) connection (in the ideal situation) or expect only one interior client at a time to use the IPSec passthrough feature of your firewall—and kiss header authentication good-bye while you're at it.

Translation Modes

Many firewalls support various types of Network Address Translation. The four primary functions of a NAT firewall are defined here in order of their popularity and availability:

Dynamic Translation (or NAPT, or IP Masquerade)   A large group of internal clients shares a single or small group of internal IP addresses for the purpose of hiding their identities or expanding the internal network address space. Ports on the single public IP address can be forwarded to specified private IP addresses.

Static Translation   A specific block of public addresses is statically translated to a same-sized block of private addresses. In this mode, an internal network resource (usually a server) has a fixed translation that never changes.

Part III

Load Balancing Translation A single IP address and port are translated to a pool of identically configured servers, so that a single public address can be served by a number of servers.

Network Redundancy Translation Multiple Internet connections are attached to a single NAT firewall. The firewall chooses and uses a network based on bandwidth, congestion, and availability.

WARNING

Not every firewall supports each type of NAT. Read the firewall's documentation carefully before you purchase it to make sure its form of NAT is the type you need.

Dynamic Translation

Dynamic translation, also referred to as IP Masquerade or just *masking*, protects internal hosts by replacing their IP address with an address that routes to the firewall. Individual hosts inside the firewall are identified based on the port number in each connection flowing through the firewall.

NOTE

RFC 1631 does not describe the use of port addresses to extend the applicability of a single IP address, but every existing NAT implementation I know of uses this method. Purists call this method NAPT, for Network Address and Port Translation.

Because a translation entry does not exist until an interior client establishes a connection out through the firewall, external computers have no method to address an internal host that is protected using a dynamically translated IP address. And because most firewalls create translations that are valid only for the addressed host and port, there's no way for any computer except the computer addressed to attack the host—no other route exists back to it.

Technically, it is possible to use the Internet Protocol's source-routing feature to route through a NAT device. Source routing allows you to specify intermediate routers through which a packet must travel. By specifying the NAT device as an intermediate router between a public machine and an interior private address, you can route packets through a NAT device. But because any NAT device sold as a security device is configured to drop any packets that are source-routed, this routing can be accomplished only through simple or improperly configured NAT devices. You should test any NAT devices you deploy to ensure that they do drop source-routed packets for this reason.

It's important to note that NAT does nothing to protect the client other than to keep external hosts from connecting to it. If the client is seduced into connecting to a malicious external host, or if a Trojan horse is somehow installed on the computer that connects to a specific external host, the client can be compromised just as easily as if there were no firewall. For this reason, NAT alone is not sufficient to protect your network.

Seducing a client into connecting to a malicious site is surprisingly easy. For example, if your boss sent you e-mail saying, "Check out this site. It's remarkably close to what we want to do," you'd probably click on the hyperlink included in the e-mail without a second thought. That's all it takes, and forging e-mail is child's play for a hacker.

REALITY CHECK: FORGING E-MAIL TO GAIN CONTROL

Forging e-mail to gain control of a computer is easy if the intended victim views their e-mail in HTML format and has JavaScript enabled (which is the default configuration for both Outlook and Outlook Express). In this case, the e-mail can contain JavaScript event triggers that will automatically start your web browser and pull up the page of the attacker's choice, which would subsequently allow the malicious website operator to perform every heinous act listed on Microsoft's support site when you search on "malicious website operator."

Worse, if you've ever selected the option to automatically open executable downloads, and the attacker points your web browser at an executable file, your web browser will automatically download file and then execute it—all without asking you anything. To show how simple this exploit is to perpetrate, import the following HTML/JavaScript code into an Outlook Express e-mail using the import text feature (the import is a bit tricky and doesn't just work by cutting and pasting); then, send the e-mail to yourself. If you have JavaScript enabled and view your e-mail as HTML, Outlook

CONTINUED →

Express will open Google's search page automatically when you close the e-mail message:

```
<html>
<head>
<title>This is funny!</title>
</head>
<body onunload="Leave()">
<script language="JavaScript">
var leave=true;
function Leave()
{if (leave)
open("http://google.com");}
</script>
Hi Folks, This is funny.<p>
</Body>
</html>
```

Some protocols do not function correctly when the port is changed. These protocols will not work through a dynamically translated connection. Any protocol that relies on the ability to establish a separate reverse connection to the source client will work correctly only if the firewall is designed to make exceptions for that specific protocol.

When you use dynamic translation, you must establish an IP address to which to translate the internal addresses. This address will be visible to the outside world for outbound connections. Most firewalls allow you to use the firewall's own address or another address that routes to the firewall and for which the firewall will answer using Address Resolution Protocol (ARP).

Each IP address can support a theoretical maximum of 65,536 (or 2^{16}) connections, because the port address pool used for multiplexing the client connections is only 16 bits wide. Most firewalls are further limited to about 50,000 connections because many ports are reserved for other uses. Linux's default IP Masquerade settings make only 4,096 ports available for translation, but that number can be modified easily.

In any case, the number of ports is large and shouldn't cause a problem unless your users maintain hundreds of simultaneous Internet connections while they work. If you do find yourself running out of ports, you'll have to have more than one IP address behind which to hide hosts.

Static Translation

Static translation is used when you have resources inside your firewall that you want to be publicly available or (in rare cases) when you use a protocol that must have certain port or IP addresses to operate.

You can use static translation to map a range of public IP addresses to the same-sized block of internal private addresses. For example, you could translate 128.110.121.0–128.110.121.255 to the internal range 10.1.2.0–10.1.2.255. The firewall performs a simple static translation for each of the IP addresses in the range.

Port forwarding is a type of static translation that refers to the process of forwarding just a specific port, rather than an entire IP address or block of addresses. Let's say your e-mail server's IP address is 10.1.1.21, and your firewall's external IP address is 10.0.30.2. You can statically map socket 10.0.30.2:25 to address 10.1.1.21:25. This static connection will cause the firewall to translate any connections to its Simple Mail Transfer Protocol (SMTP) port to the e-mail server inside your firewall.

You can use port forwarding to establish a number of different complex services on a single IP address. For example, you could have an e-mail server statically translated on the SMTP and POP ports, a web server statically translated on the HTTP port, and a news server on the Network News Transfer Protocol (NNTP) port. Because the translations can specify any IP address, these services can be split among many machines inside your firewall.

Load Balancing

Some firewalls support IP load balancing using the static NAT facility. This support allows you to spread the load of one very popular website across a number of different servers by using the firewall to choose which internal server each external client should connect to on either a round-robin or balanced load basis. Load balancing is somewhat similar to dynamic translation in reverse—the firewall chooses which server each connection attempt should go to from among a pool of clones.

To choose based on load, the servers in the pool must have some facility to transmit their load levels to the firewall. Because there is no standard way to do this, your firewall must implement a proprietary method. For that reason, many simpler firewalls assume that each connection creates about the same amount of load and assign connections to the next server in the list. Other more sophisticated load-balancing firewalls attempt to average the number of simultaneous connections to each interior host or attempt to average the amount of network bandwidth exchanged with each interior host.

Part III

IP load balancing only works with protocols that are stateless or that maintain their state on the client. For websites, IP load balancing is perfect because the server does not maintain any information about the client between page transmittals—it doesn't matter if a specific client gets the same server each time it loads a page. Consider the problem with mail, though. If a firewall provides load balancing for a number of e-mail servers, each of a user's e-mail messages will arrive on any of the servers depending on which server the firewall selects for the SMTP connection. When the user connects to a server, the firewall will again select one server for the POP connection, so the only messages that user will see are those that happen to have been received by that server—the user will not see all of her received messages.

IP load balancing is particularly important for e-commerce sites that have a heavy processing load because they make heavy use of Active Server Pages, CGI or Perl scripts, or Java servlets. These technologies all put a significant compute burden on a web server, which reduces the maximum number of clients the server can support. Figure 13.2 shows a complex e-commerce website being load balanced by a firewall.

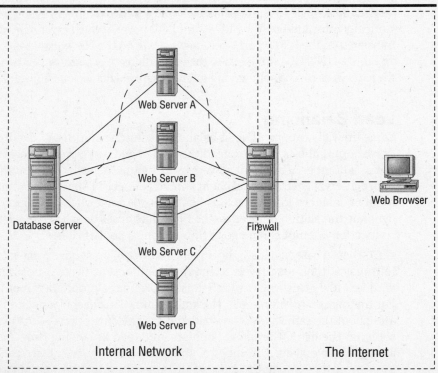

FIGURE 13.2: Using firewalls to perform load balancing

Network Redundancy

It is possible to use a NAT-based firewall to perform Internet network redundancy, either to balance the load of clients across multiple low-cost Internet connections or to compensate automatically for the failure of any given link.

Network redundancy works with dynamic translation in much the same way that IP load balancing works with static translation. In network redundancy, the firewall is connected to multiple ISPs through multiple interfaces and has a public masquerade address for each ISP. Each time an internal host makes a connection through the firewall, the firewall chooses on a least-loaded basis the network on which to establish the translated connection. In this way, the firewall is able to spread the internal client load across multiple networks.

The failure of any network is then treated as if that network is completely loaded; the firewall simply will not route new clients through it. Although session-based protocols will have to be reestablished from the client hosts, stateless protocols like HTTP can survive a link failure without the client knowing anything has occurred. Figure 13.3 shows network redundancy. Notice that because the IP address is translated, it does not matter which ISP the firewall uses to connect to the public website.

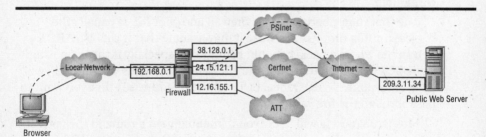

FIGURE 13.3: Network redundancy

Router Configuration for NAT

When you use Network Address Translation with IP addresses other than the IP address of the firewall, you'll have to configure the routing in your network to make sure packets reach the firewall. You also may have to configure routing on the firewall to make sure packets are relayed to the correct interfaces.

Whether you have to configure routing separately from the firewall's configuration depends on whether the firewall routes packets itself or whether it relies on the host system for routing. If the firewall relies on the host operating system to perform the routing function, you then need to know whether the firewall translates addresses before or after the routing function has occurred.

You can tell whether the firewall relies on the host system for routing in Unix by checking whether the firewall requires the use of the routed daemon. If the firewall requires the routed daemon, then it relies on that daemon to perform the routing function.

In Windows, you can tell if the firewall relies on the operating system to route if the firewall enables the Enable IP Forwarding setting in the network Control Panel, or if it instructs you to enable it manually.

If the firewall relies on the operating system for routing, you must ensure that the internal routing tables are correct for the various translation modes you establish. Some firewalls configure the routing tables for you; others do not. If the firewall performs the routing function, you can assume that the firewall will correctly route packets without intervention. In either case, you should thoroughly read the firewall documentation on routing and test the routing through your firewall once it's completely configured.

The first router between your firewall and your ISP is usually the biggest routing problem, because it may assume that it can use ARP to determine where a packet should be routed—especially if there's no static route between the router and your firewall. This means your firewall will have to respond to ARP requests for all the IP addresses that you want to pass through the firewall.

Most true routers will allow you to manually set a route to the correct interface on the firewall, so this isn't an issue. But many new high-speed data link devices like cable modems and DSL interfaces aren't actually routers—they're just bridges, and they assume that every device they talk to will be connected to the same collision domain as their Ethernet adapter.

In Unix, this is no problem. Just use the ARP command to set the IP addresses for which the external interface will use ARP (or respond as the correct interface for said IP address), and add routing entries to make sure the packets will be routed to their correct location as shown in Table 13.1.

In Windows NT, this is a serious problem. Windows NT includes an ARP command, but it does not properly implement the ARP protocol for proxy ARP (when an interface responds to ARP requests for multiple IP addresses). Manual ARP entries remain cached for only about an hour, after which time your routing will fail.

The only way to handle this problem is for the firewall software to implement some method to properly implement proxy ARP for the IP addresses the firewall uses for translation.

Adding IP addresses to the external adapter will not solve the problem because these addresses are automatically used to create the routing tables for NT. These tables will then be incorrect for further routing to the interior of the network.

An example will explain why this is the case. If the firewall has two interfaces, 10.0.0.1 and 10.0.30.2, then the default entries in the routing table will look like those in Table 13.1.

TABLE 13.1: Firewall Routing Table Entries

NETWORK	MASK	GATEWAY
10.0.0.0	10.0.0.255	10.0.0.1
128.110.121.0	128.110.121.255	10.0.30.2

Suppose host 10.0.0.12 has its address translated to 128.110.121.44 as it goes through firewall 10.0.30.2. A return packet will be addressed to 128.110.121.44. When that packet reaches the firewall router, the packet will be routed to interface 10.0.30.2 by default, because the address translation will have occurred after the routing function has already happened. The firewall will then translate the address to 10.0.0.12, but it will be too late—the packet already will have been routed to the incorrect interface, so it will be transmitted on the 128.110.121.0 network.

If you try to solve the problem by adding IP address 128.110.121.44 to the 128.110.121.1 interface or the 10.0.0.1 interface, Windows NT will automatically generate routing rules for that interface that unfortunately stipulate incorrect routing—and these automatically generated rules cannot be removed.

To solve the problem, use the firewall's ARP facility and make a routing entry on the firewall that specifies a route for each IP address that the firewall proxy ARPs:

```
Route add 128.110.121.44 10.0.0.1 1
```

Part III

This will ensure that packets coming in on the proxy ARP address will be routed to interface 10.0.0.1. They will be transmitted on the correct interface once the address is translated.

IANA Private Use Network Numbers

The Internet Assigned Numbers Authority (IANA) has designated three blocks of addresses for private use without coordination:

- ▶ 10.0.0.0 to 10.255.255.255

- ▶ 172.16.0.0 to 172.31.255.255

- ▶ 192.168.0.0 to 192.168.255.255

NOTE

The IANA function is now operated by the Internet Corporation for Assigned Names and Numbers (ICANN). The term now officially refers to the function provided by the former IANA organization, as now operated by ICANN.

Internet routers are configured not to route these addresses on the Internet backbone. You can use these addresses in your own network with a certain amount of impunity, unless your ISP also uses them. Most ISPs use portions of the 10.0.0.0 domain for their own internal routing, with NAT into and out of the range.

For that reason, I generally recommend that clients use the 192.168.0.0 network range for their own private networking. Doing so prevents conflicts with ISPs that use the 10 domain for internal routing, and you don't have to remember which block of addresses is valid inside the 192.168.0.0 domain. You can use all 16 bits of address space with impunity.

PROBLEMS WITH NAT

A few protocols cannot be used with NAT because they require the ability to open a back channel to the client, embed TCP/IP address information inside the higher-level protocol, encrypt TCP header information, or use the original IP address for some security purpose:

- ▶ Back channels will not work because no separate route back to the internal hosts exists. This situation occurs with H.323 video teleconferencing.

▶ Software that embeds TCP/IP address information inside TCP/IP packets and then relies on that information will not work because the interior TCP/IP address information will be incorrect. This problem occurs with FTP and some other protocols.

▶ Software that encrypts the TCP header information will not work correctly with NAT because the TCP information must be accessible to the firewall. You can solve these problems by making the firewall the encryption end point. This situation occurs with Point-to-Point Tunneling Protocol (PPTP) and IPSec Header Authentication.

▶ Software that relies on TCP/IP address information for security checking will fail because the IP address information has changed. This problem occurs with Sqlnet2.

More advanced firewall software can inspect outgoing connections for these protocols and establish a translation entry to wait for the destination public host to respond with the back-channel open request. Most firewalls do not support service-specific NAT; rather, they use service-specific proxy software in combination with the NAT mechanism to perform these functions.

NAT cannot be used with the following services without some form of higher-level proxying or a patch to the basic NAT code:

H.323, CUSeeMe, and VDO Live   These video teleconferencing software programs cannot be used because they rely on the ability to establish a back channel to the host. Some firewalls may make special entries in their translation tables to allow a specific host to create the back channel.

Xing   This software fails for the same reason video teleconferencing programs do.

Rshell   This software fails for the same reason video teleconferencing programs do.

IRC   This software fails for the same reason video teleconferencing programs do.

PPTP   This software fails because it relies on encrypted IP information inside its stream, but other non-TCP/IP protocols can be tunneled inside PPTP with an end point on the firewall to get around this problem.

Part III

Sqlnet2   This software requires the numerical difference between the host and client IP addresses to be the same as if both IP addresses were not translated. Thus the protocol will nearly always fail unless you design your network around this strange restriction.

FTP   This software must be RFC 1631–compliant to work with NAT. FTP embeds IP address information in ASCII text inside the TCP packets, the length of which is likely to change through an address translation.

ICMP (Internet Control Message Protocol)   This software sometimes embeds the first part of the original packet in ICMP messages. This first portion will contain the untranslated address. The secure solution is simply not to pass ICMP traffic through your firewall.

IPSec   IPSec-authenticated headers cannot pass through a NAT device because the Authentication Header (AH) uses a hash to determine if any part of the packet has been changed in transit. The purpose of NAT is to change the IP address, so the AH hash will no longer be correct, and the end systems will drop the AH packets because they fail authentication.

Encapsulating Security Payload (ESP) in transport mode cannot transit a NAT for the same reason AH can't—checksums won't match if the IP addresses have changed. However, some VPN clients allow the administrator to ignore checksums, so these implementations may be able to get ESP transport mode through a NAT.

ESP in tunnel mode (wherein the original packet is encrypted and becomes the payload of a non-encrypted packet) can traverse static NAT mappings. However, when using dynamic (NAPT) translation, there's no way to differentiate which interior host different inbound IPSec connections should go to; so, only one IPSec connection will work through the dynamic NAT.

Finally, most implementations of Internet Key Exchange (IKE) use pre-shared keys to prove their identity and bind the original IP address as part of the key. Again, because the original IP addresses change, the key changes, and the IKE negotiation fails. The solution in this case is to configure your firewall and

VPN clients to use X.509 certificates or some proprietary key-ing mechanism to transit the NAT.

Basically, configuring IPSec to transit a NAT device is much harder than simply end-pointing the VPN on the firewall. That's the logical and most secure place to do it anyway.

HACKING THROUGH NAT

If Network Address Translation makes clients invisible, it's impossible to hack, right? Wrong. Here's where NAT can fail:

► Static translation does not protect the internal host.

► If the client establishes the connection, a return connection exists.

► If the connection can be intercepted or subjected to a man-in-the-middle attack, the man-in-the-middle is the end point.

► If the firewall's NAT implementation is flawed, it could be subject to exploitation.

► Source routing can specify the NAT device as an intermediate system and then route through it.

These hacks are further explained in the following sections.

Static Translation = No Security

Static translation merely replaces port information on a one-to-one basis. It affords no protection to statically translated hosts—hacking attacks will be translated just as efficiently as any valid connection attempt.

The solution to security for statically translated hosts that must provide public services is to reduce the number of attack vectors to one, and then to use (if necessary) application proxy software or other application-based security measures to further protect the internal host.

For example, to protect e-mail servers inside a firewall, Checkpoint's Firewall-1 software has a simple SMTP store-and-forward mechanism that eliminates the nasty problem of e-mail buffer overflows. Firewall-1's e-mail proxy receives all e-mail inbound on its port 25 (SMTP) and writes each message to the hard disk. A separate service running in a different process reads the e-mail messages and transmits them to the internal

Part III

e-mail server. This mechanism eliminates the possibility that a buffer overflow from a malformed e-mail message will affect anything but the firewall—and in that case, it will only shut down the e-mail receiver. The firewall's internal consistency checker can then simply restart the e-mail receiver afresh.

Internal Host Seduction

Even if hackers can't get inside your network, you can't prevent your users from going to the hackers. Forged e-mail with a website link, a Trojan horse, or a seductive content website can entice your users to attach to a machine whose purpose is to glean information about your network. HTTP is a reasonably robust protocol, and extensions to it by the major browser vendors have made it a potent source for exploitation. Because nearly any type of content can be downloaded through an HTTP connection, your users can easily be compromised once they connect to a hacker's machine.

Higher-level, application-specific proxies are once again the solution. By inspecting the contents of those protocols for what will most likely be exploited (like HTTP), your firewall can sniff for suspicious content like Java applets, ActiveX controls, downloadable executables, malformed URLs, and other tools hackers use to perform their mischief. By filtering out or at least logging and alerting on the presence of this content, you can keep your users from being exploited through seductive means.

The State Table Timeout Problem

NAT has one hackable aspect to its function. When a client connects to the outside world, the firewall must remember which internal host has connected to which external host so that it can route the return portion of the TCP connection back to the source host. Without this functionality, only unidirectional (and therefore worthless) transmissions can be made.

But how does the firewall know when the client is finished with the connection? If the firewall relies only on TCP information, it can sniff for close session information. But many protocols don't have an obvious ending negotiation, and there's always the possibility that a connection may be dropped without proper closing negotiation. In those cases, to remain as protocol-generic as possible, most firewalls implement a timeout value.

The length of this timeout varies greatly, and firewall publishers never tell you how long it is.

Before the timeout occurs, a connection through the firewall to the originating internal host exists. This connection could potentially be exploited by a hacker, although the hacker would have to know exactly which IP address and port to use, and would probably have to know the IP address of the original destination in order to get through the firewall. This information would be known only if the hacker had been snooping on the connection.

The theoretical possibility of this exploitation exists, but it would require a lot of information to execute. Even if the client had not closed the connection, it wouldn't be listening on the high number port it had opened to initiate the connection. This attack could be most effectively used to send malformed packets to a host in a denial-of-service attack.

Source Routing through NAT

Dynamic NAT naturally protects clients by eliminating a direct route to them from the Internet. Because no forward route exists, there's simply no way to get to an internal client from the Internet. Any attack stops at the NAT device—unless the hacker uses source routing and knows an internal IP address. Source routing is a feature of IP that was originally used for testing, but is now most often exploited by hackers to hijack TCP connections by specifying routes back to themselves rather than to legitimate hosts.

In a normal IP packet transmission, the header contains just the source and destination addresses, and relies on a series of default gateways and routers to know how to get it from one router to the next. With source routing, the source host of the packet can specify a list of routers that the packet must be transmitted to other than the default route. The mechanism is simple—rather than transmitting the packet to the final destination, the packet is forwarded to the next router in the source router list. Once it arrives at that router, the router sends it to the next address in line—either another router or the final system. There are two flavors of source routing: *strict*, where the entire router list is specified and the packets will be dropped if they can't make it using that route; and *loose*, where one or more intermediate systems are listed, but where any number of other intermediate systems can be transited between the listed systems.

Part III

So, to get through NAT, the hacker need only specify the final internal IP address of the host but include the NAT as an intermediate system in a loose source-routed packet. The original host will then transmit the packet to the NAT device, which will then transmit the packet to the interior of the network because it does know the identity of the final destination.

Of course, the hacker would have to know the network numbering scheme inside your network. But that's easy: By simply scanning the standard private ranges (10, 192.168., and so on) using source-routed ICMP packets, he'll see ping responses from whatever computers exist and quickly be able to build a map of the internal portion of your network.

The solution is to configure your firewall to drop source-routed packets, because the few legitimate purposes for them are easily accomplished using other means and because no standard operating system or router generates them by default.

WARNING

Be sure you test simple NAT devices for the source-routing vulnerability before you deploy them as security on home or small office networks.

TRIAL BY FIREWALL

A few years ago, a customer of mine wanted to implement Network Address Translation in its network for security reasons and because it used a DSL adapter that provided only 16 public IP addresses. Because the customer was an all-Microsoft shop and a small business, we decided to use Checkpoint Firewall-1, which has good automatic support for NAT.

After setting up the firewall for standard use and creating the appropriate policies, I set up NAT for the internal client computers to use the firewall's IP address. I then created a static translation for the mail server, which was internal.

The client access worked fine, but I realized that I'd have to set a route in the DSL adapter to route the static IP address for the mail server. Because the DSL adapter was owned by the ISP, I called its technical support number and asked to have a route programmed into the adapter.

Much to my surprise, the support technician had no idea what I was talking about. He'd never heard of adding a route to anything.

CONTINUED ➡

I asked to speak with his supervisor, who then informed me that the DSL adapter was not a router at all—it was merely a Data Link–layer bridge. Any devices it talked to would have to be present on the same Ethernet collision domain.

This was problematic because we needed to protect the e-mail server (and because I didn't want to buy a hub to put between the firewall and the DSL adapter). So I decided to use proxy ARP, which I was familiar with from the Unix world, but which I'd never used in Windows NT.

I sat down to the NT server and typed **ARP**. The command existed and worked as expected. I typed in the ARP command to bind the static translation address to the MAC address of the external adapter. The server accepted the command, and voilà! Traffic began to flow. I verified that I could connect from the outside world to the e-mail server and that mail could flow from the ISP. Everything seemed fine.

After chatting with my contact at the client site, I packed up my laptop and tools and began to leave. At that point, one of the employees said that the e-mail service seemed to have gone down. I checked for connectivity again, and found that, indeed, the static mapping no longer worked.

I was stumped. I checked the firewall—no difference. I re-issued the ARP command with the parameter to indicate a static mapping. That worked as it had the first time, and traffic flowed again.

This time I was wary. I left my laptop in place, running a constant ping from the Internet (through a dial-up account) to the mail server's static address mapping. Sure enough, about an hour later the ping began to fail.

For some reason, Windows NT would not retain the ARP mapping. I fired up Internet Explorer and searched Microsoft's tech support site to no avail—almost no information existed about the default ARP command. So I went to Alta Vista and did a net-wide search. Surprisingly few pages matched, but I did find one that specifically mentioned that NT's ARP command could not retain address resolutions—exactly the problem I was having.

I figured Firewall-1 must have some sort of solution to the problem. I pulled up the documentation on the CD-ROM (which is normally very complete) and dug around. I found a description of the proxy

CONTINUED ➡

Part III

ARP problem, but the solution said to manually enter a proxy ARP command—which I'd already done.

Next, I added the statically mapped IP address to the protocol stack of the NT machine as a second IP address on the external adapter. Unfortunately, Firewall-1 performs late translation, which means the IP addresses are translated after the operating system has routed the packet. Thus the packets bound for the statically translated address were being "bounced" back out the external adapter by the default routing NT adds for each adapter, which I could not defeat. Only true proxy ARP, which NT didn't support, would solve my problem.

I couldn't imagine that I was the first person to have this problem, so I called Checkpoint's tech support. They told me they could open a support incident for $500, which frosted me, but I gladly would have paid if they had guaranteed me a solution. They would not, so I decided not to pay them.

As I sat and stewed about the problem, my phone suddenly rang. It was the Checkpoint support technician, who said he'd send me e-mail with a URL to click on. I checked my mail, read the message, and clicked into a private area in Checkpoint's support website that described the exact problem and how to solve it.

It seems that Firewall-1's firewalling engine for NT is designed to support proxy ARP because NT doesn't, but there's no user interface for doing it or documentation about how to do it. Firewall-1 will support ARP via entries to a `config.arp` file in Firewall-1's configuration directory. The file is a simple list of Ethernet MAC addresses for the adapter and the IP address to respond to.

I added the entry for the static mapping and restarted the firewall. Everything worked fine after that.

This situation highlights my basic problem with the fee-for-support arrangements that nearly all firewall vendors set up. Vendors are naturally inclined to hold out until users pay for support and to provide minimal documentation so as to increase the number of paid support calls. Vendors claim that they have to pay their support costs, but making effective user interfaces and completely documenting software can nearly eliminate support calls. Be sure to do a thorough search for your issue on the Internet and at Google Groups (`groups.google.com`) before you pay for technical support.

WHAT'S NEXT

In this chapter, you learned how to use Network Address Translation to hide the internal addresses on your network. In Chapter 14, you will learn about firewall products based on the Windows platform that use many of the security features already discussed.

Chapter 14

WINDOWS FIREWALLS

There are now so many firewall products available that it's difficult to determine what you should use. This chapter will familiarize you with the firewall market, applying the theoretical information we've discussed in the last few chapters to the practical selection of a real firewall. This chapter is specific to Windows firewalls, although most of them also have versions that run under other operating systems.

This chapter details the following firewalls:

► Checkpoint Firewall-1

► Symantec Enterprise Firewall

► Microsoft Internet Security and Acceleration (ISA) Server

These firewalls represent the high-end firewall market for firewalls that run on the Windows NT kernel–based operating systems. These firewalls make use of the user interface, services

Part III

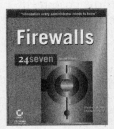

Adapted from *Firewalls 24seven™*, Second Edition by Matthew Strebe and Charles Perkins
ISBN 0-7821-4054-8 $49.99

architecture, and in some cases the network interface functionality of Windows, and add only those components related directly to security of the operating system. Basing the firewall on an existing operating system is a double-edged sword: It allows the security systems vendor to concentrate on writing security software rather than operating system software, but it can also make the resulting product vulnerable to flaws in the operating system if the vendor hasn't taken special preventative precautions.

With the exception of Microsoft ISA Server, the firewalls profiled in this chapter support a remarkably similar set of technologies. They all cost about the same amount of money and are ICSA-certified.

The group is divided into two types based on their primary security posture:

Stateful Inspection Filters   Use complex filters based on retained information about connection state and protocols to either block or pass traffic. Firewall-1 falls into this group.

Proxy Servers   Receive and then completely regenerate allowed services through the gateway, and ignore protocols for which there is no established proxy. Gauntlet, Symantec Enterprise Firewall, and ISA Server fall into this group.

The primary security posture of a firewall doesn't tell the whole story; most stateful inspectors include proxy or proxy-like services, and most proxy servers include stateful packet filters. The division in this case depends on the philosophy on which the architecture of the firewall is based, and which services are added on to shore up deficiencies in the basic architecture.

There are two things you will not find in this chapter:

► Performance ratings

► Hacking tests

We decided not to include performance information because we believe performance should not be a deciding factor in your security posture. It would be something like comparing the top speeds of tractors—performance isn't the point. The essential problem is that more inspection and rigor takes more time, so the better a firewall is, the slower it will perform. If you are in the rare circumstance that must use a high-performing firewall, use a stateful inspector. Otherwise, proxy servers provide more security, albeit at considerably reduced performance rates.

We performed a number of hacking tests against these products once they were properly secured, using publicly available hacking tools. We were not able to find any case in which a firewall was susceptible to intrusion or denial of service except when we knew architectural flaws existed in the software. So, we decided not to write about our lack of results. Psychological attacks using forged e-mail or rogue websites remain the only ways we know of to penetrate these firewalls.

NOTE

This chapter contains discussions of various firewall products based on evaluation software and hardware provided by the vendors, their documentation, and our installation and testing of the evaluation software or device (except where noted). We were not able to review the product source code for dormant flaws and cannot ensure that these products will remain secure in a continually changing security environment.

Each firewall is detailed in its own section throughout the remainder of this chapter.

CHECKPOINT FIREWALL-1

Checkpoint Firewall-1 is a policy-based stateful inspection filter with an integrated Network Address Translator and a small set of nonintegrated protocol-specific security filters for common Internet protocols. Checkpoint Firewall-1 was the best-selling firewall in the world until about two years ago, when the firewall device market overtook it.

The most recent version of Firewall-1 (included as part of the Checkpoint NG Enterprise Suite or available as a separate product) is an incremental improvement that removes most of the most annoying configuration problems with Firewall-1: the need for routing rules on the host OS to support Network Address Translation (NAT), the requirement for proxy-ARP, and so forth. By addressing these issues, Firewall-1 is now substantially easier to successfully install and configure than prior versions were.

Checkpoint developed the concept of stateful inspection to improve the security of packet filters without requiring the overhead of proxy servers. Once a packet passes the suite of tests applied by the inspector module, the original packet is forwarded into the network. This means that any deformations not detected by the inspector module are passed through without modification by the firewall module.

Stateful inspection is a middle ground between simple packet filters and application proxies. Because stateful inspectors maintain state information about each connection, they can make more rigorous pass/fail checks on packets. But they do not usually have the ability to monitor the internal content of the various protocols, so they are more closely related to packet filters than to proxy servers.

Firewall-1 solves this problem to some degree by allowing plug-in protocol filters that are similar to actual proxies. These protocol filters understand the content of popular protocols like HTTP, Simple Mail Transfer Protocol (SMTP), and FTP (the three provided with Firewall-1), so they can inspect and make pass/fail decisions on those protocols. These filters are able to perform high-level filtering functions like Java blocking and attachment stripping. Filters remain less secure than proxies because the packets are routed through the firewall, rather than being re-created as they are in proxies. The Firewall-1 SMTP filter is a true proxy: It writes e-mail to its disk and then has a separate service forward the e-mail through the gateway. This method is designed to prevent the buffer overflow problems that plague e-mail systems.

Don't confuse content filters with simple protocol support. Firewall-1's documentation claims to support more than 120 protocols out of the box. By "support," Checkpoint means it has defined an object that encapsulates a protocol's protocol header number, not a content filter. Firewall-1 provides content filters for just three common protocols: HTTP, FTP, and SMTP.

The management console requires a Win32 or Sun Solaris host. The firewall modules can run on Unix, Linux, or Windows computers or on numerous commercial routers from Cisco, Bay Networks, and others. Perhaps the coolest design feature of Firewall-1 is that with it, you can convert your existing inventory of border routers into strong firewalls.

Firewall-1's documentation assumes you have a working knowledge of TCP/IP and the platform on which you are installing the software.

Major Feature Set

Firewall-1 supports the following major features:

► Stateful packet filter

► Protocol-specific transparent proxies (HTTP, SMTP, and FTP)

► Reverse proxies (HTTP, SMTP, FTP)

► Network Address Translation

► Port redirection

- DMZ (demilitarized zone) support

- VPN firewall-to-firewall and firewall-to-remote client add-on components (available at additional cost)

- VPN client software (Windows 98/NT/2000/XP, Macintosh, Unix, Linux)

- Logging and e-mail notification (including SNMP trap)

VPN Features

The VPN-1 component of the Checkpoint NG Suite is actually a separate product from Firewall-1, but they are closely integrated. The VPN-1 product supports a wide range of remote client authentication schemes, including Checkpoint's proprietary authentication, NT Challenge/Response, SecureID, RADIUS, Azent Pathways Defender, TACACS/+, and X.509 certificates.

For encryption, VPN-1 supports Advanced Encryption Standard (AES), Data Encryption Standard (DES), and triple-DES (3DES) using IPSec/IKE (Internet Key Exchange) and supports IP Compression (IPCOMP). VPN-1 can be integrated into a Public Key Infrastructure (PKI) system.

The SecuRemote VPN client for VPN-1 is available for Windows 98, NT, 2000, and XP, as well as for the Macintosh, Linux, and most major variants of Unix.

Additional Optional Features

Checkpoint NG Enterprise Suite includes the FloodGate Quality-of-Service traffic shaper, the ConnectControl module for load balancing and high availability, and separate firewall high-availability features.

Minor Feature Set

Firewall-1 supports the following minor features:

- Content filtering (Java, ActiveX, virus scanning, URL blocking)

- Scan detection, spoofing detection, and automatic blocking

- SYN flood protection

- Security server (proxy authentication)

- Real-time monitoring

Part III

- Centralized administration

- Policy-based configuration and management

- Highly configurable alerting

- Execution of arbitrary programs upon event detection

- Diagnostic tools

- Dynamic Host Configuration Protocol (DHCP) and Simple Network Management Protocol (SNMP)

- LDAP (Lightweight Directory Access Protocol) integration

- Demand dialing of PPP connections

- Split DNS

- Support for third-party content scanners

- SQL proxying

- Online help

- Host OS boot security

- Process watchdog

Policy-Based Configuration and Management

Policy-based configuration and management makes it easy to view, manage, and understand the configuration of the firewall. Like most GUI-based firewalls, Firewall-1 lets you create protocol definitions called *objects* that associate a friendly name with a collection of protocol identifiers like the port number and IP protocol type. This way, you can work with objects like FTP instead of TCP Port 21, so you won't get confused during the configuration process. Because the abstraction allowed by identifying protocols, addresses, users, and time ranges as named objects is easy to understand, management is simple. This tends to reduce the number of mistakes made when configuring the firewall.

Centralized Client/Server Management

What separates Firewall-1 from the majority of policy-based firewalls is its support for a single enterprise-wide policy interface that can automatically generate custom-compiled firewall policies for each firewall in your enterprise. So, rather than managing firewalls separately and mapping your security needs to each firewall's specific place in your network, you can maintain and configure a singe policy that is automatically customized for each of your firewalled devices.

Content Vectoring Protocol

The Content Vectoring Protocol (CVP) allows you to plug in filters to handle very specific protocols like HTTP, mail, and FTP. CVP-compatible filters can strip attachments and executable content, and can perform virus checking, URL blocking, or any other protocol-specific filtration. NAI and Symantec both make CVP-compatible virus scanners that work with Firewall-1 and are available at additional cost.

Automatic Address Translation

Automatic address translation handles objects on an individual basis. Once an object is defined and an address translation mode is assigned to it, address translation rules are automatically generated for every case where the object is used in the rule base. Address translation rules can be manually created for those cases where automatic translation doesn't accomplish your goals.

Firewall Module Synchronization

Module synchronization allows firewalls to trade state with each other. If two firewalls on the same connection are used, one can fail without affecting the connections running through them. This feature can also be used to perform load balancing across a range of firewalls.

Interface

Firewall-1 is a client/server architecture that allows you to centrally control any number of firewall modules from a single management console. The GUI is easy to read and comprehend without being overly busy. The latest version has solved a number of the annoying design problems that plagued earlier versions of Firewall-1; the result is a simple and very usable policy-editing interface.

Firewall-1 abstracts devices, users, and networks as objects defined by IP or network addresses and referred to by a uniquely assigned name identifier. You define pass/drop rules by selecting a source object (including Any to encompass the Internet as well as internal systems), a destination object, one or more protocols, the action to apply, and the logging or

Part III

alerting level. The collection of rules is called a *rule base*; it is synonymous with the strategies used by most firewalls. Figure 14.1 shows the Firewall-1 interface with a complete rule base displayed.

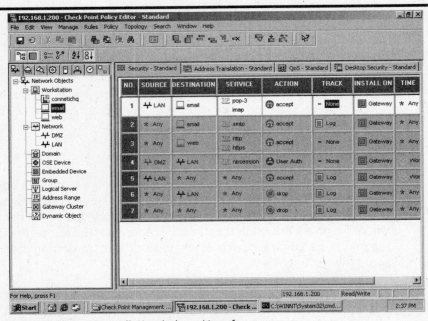

FIGURE 14.1:   Firewall-1's rule-based interface

Rules are interpreted from the top to the bottom of the rule base as it is displayed on the screen. The first rule that applies to a packet is used, so you can add a number of rules pertaining to the same protocol in an intuitive and obvious manner. This process lets you create various levels of security for different groups. The last rule in the rule base is "Any source, any destination, any protocol: drop with no logging." This rule is implicit and is not shown in the rule base, but it guarantees that anything not specifically allowed is specifically denied.

Network address directives are assigned per object; so, once the rule base is complete, a NAT strategy is automatically defined. You can add manual address translation rules, but doing so is usually not necessary.

Once a policy is defined, it must be compiled and applied to the appropriate gateways. This step is easy to complete; but unfortunately it is possible for the GUI to allow you to create policies that won't compile correctly. In that case, you must go through something of a compile/debug cycle to create a working policy. A solid user interface would simply prevent you from creating problem policies in the first place.

Security

Checkpoint devised the idea of the stateful inspection packet filter, which improves on the basic packet filter by more closely examining the packets used to set up connections and store connection information (the *state*). This stored state is used to determine which packets should be passed and which should be dropped based on their participation in a connection. Stateful inspection is very fast because the computation done to examine packets is fairly slim, and once a connection has been established, the filtering of packets through the connection takes little time. Stateful inspection filters are capable of operating nearly as fast as a standard IP router.

But throughput is not the purpose of a firewall; it is merely a feature. Strong security, which can be achieved only through rigorous examination of all possible protocol information, remains paramount. Because stateful inspectors like Firewall-1 perform only cursory examination of TCP-layer information and do not typically filter the contents of packets, they are not as secure as pure proxy servers like NAI Gauntlet or Symantec Enterprise Firewall.

To close that security boundary, Firewall-1 includes a small set of security filters for common services like SMTP and HTTP; however, these filters are not well integrated into the management paradigm. Firewall-1 also includes a protocol filter for HTTP that is capable of stripping out dangerous content like executable files and Java applets.

Documentation

Firewall-1's online documentation is among the best in the business. It teaches about firewall theory, applications, and the user interface, and it is packed with examples. It is professionally written and appropriate for the target audience. Most network administrators will be able to establish a firewall without technical assistance now that most of the major problems in the Firewall-1 configuration set have been eliminated.

If you intend to purchase and install a firewall by yourself without prior experience, you should consider Firewall-1 based on the strength of its documentation. Any Unix Administrator, Microsoft Certified Systems Engineer (MCSE), or equivalent should be able to figure out Firewall-1 from the documentation alone and construct a reasonable, secure firewall policy for it.

Cost and Support

Firewall-1 is sold a number of different ways:

▶ Single gateway products support a specific number of users. The management console and gateway are installed on a single machine. This product is sufficient for small businesses with fewer than that number of IP addresses on their network (which is how the firewall determines how many hosts it will work with).

▶ Enterprise products protect an unlimited number of internal hosts and are sold on a per-module basis. You purchase the number of firewall modules you require (one per border gateway) and the number of encryption modules you require to support the VPN functionality.

Minimum platform requirements for Firewall-1 are easy to meet and should not be expensive:

▶ Pentium processor

▶ At least two network interfaces

▶ 40MB of disk space

▶ 128MB RAM

▶ CD-ROM drive

Checkpoint is stingy with online support and charges an exorbitant $400 per incident for telephone technical support (for which they will not guarantee a solution to your problem). I can understand not wanting to deal with first-time network integrators, but it seems that Checkpoint has decided technical support is a lucrative market. Competition will inevitably change the company's mind. That said, its technicians seem very competent, as far as I could determine without providing my credit card number.

Firewall-1 is sold on a per-module basis, with a simple 5-user Small Office product for $300 and a 250-user module costing $6,000. You can get modules for firewalling, VPN, and Quality-of-Service at various comparable prices, and you need a module for each device in your enterprise that you want to firewall. Operating systems supported are Windows, Linux, and Solaris.

The VPN-1 and remote authentication module are about as expensive, and costs for additional users hover around the $100-per-user point.

SYMANTEC ENTERPRISE FIREWALL

Symantec Enterprise Firewall (formerly Axent Raptor, formerly Raptor Eagle Firewall) is Gauntlet's strongest competitor in the area of security. Like Gauntlet, Symantec Enterprise Firewall is a security proxy. Unlike Gauntlet, Symantec Enterprise Firewall does not include the adaptive proxy filter technology that increases the speed of Gauntlet to near that of a stateful inspector. Symantec Enterprise Firewall is among the fastest proxy firewalls, however, and is capable of handling dedicated circuits up to T3 (45Mbps).

Symantec Enterprise Firewall runs on Windows NT 4 SP 6a, Windows 2000, and Sun Solaris (SPARC), and is multithreaded to take advantage of multiple processors. You can use it with Windows NT Cluster Server and Windows 2000 Advanced or Datacenter Server to create high-availability firewall services. However, Symantec Enterprise Firewall is not compatible with Windows 2000's Advanced Server's Windows Load Balancing service.

Unlike most firewalls we're discussing, Symantec Enterprise Firewall relies on "best-fit" policies that are not order-dependent. This means the firewall applies the policy that most closely applies to each connection, rather than filtering the connection down through a policy rule base until either a pass condition is met or the connection is dropped.

Major Feature Set

Symantec Enterprise Firewall supports the following major features:

- ▶ Packet security filter for the gateway
- ▶ Network Address Translation
- ▶ Security proxy
- ▶ Remote authentication
- ▶ VPN support through the add-on Symantec Enterprise Firewall VPN and Symantec Enterprise Firewall Mobile VPN products

Packet Filtering

Unlike other firewalls, Symantec Enterprise Firewall does not allow network-level routing and therefore does not include a packet filter. All data—even low-level information like Internet Control Message Protocol

Part III

(ICMP) and TCP generic services—is routed through Application-layer proxy services and regenerated on the firewall. This is the most secure method of passing information between interfaces, because it guarantees that no malformed packets can cross through the gateway.

In addition to performing no routing, the firewall automatically drops source-routed packets and packets containing internal addresses that appear on external interfaces. These packets are dropped before any connection proxying can be performed on them.

It is not entirely clear whether the firewall is capable of protecting the operating system's TCP/IP stack from denial-of-service attacks, because it does not appear to include an NDIS-layer adapter driver. Considering that the installation requires updating the operating system to the latest security hotfixes, it's likely that Symantec Enterprise Firewall is indeed susceptible to network-level attacks directed at the operating system. None of these attacks provide access to the system, but they can deny Internet services.

Network Address Translation (NAT)

Symantec Enterprise Firewall relies primarily on its proxy service to perform the standard many-to-one address translation. However, it also uses reverse address translation to support services on interior machines and true NAT through a feature Symantec Enterprise Firewall calls *Virtual Clients*. The Virtual Clients facility also allows support for Illegal Network Address Translation.

Security Proxies

Symantec Enterprise Firewall is primarily a security proxy that uses separate security proxies for every supported protocol. Third-party products must be used to perform virus scanning and Java filtration. Symantec Enterprise Firewall includes security proxies for the following services:

- ▶ SMB/CIFS (Windows/LAN Manager network file and print sharing)
- ▶ SQL*Net (Oracle SQL servers)
- ▶ Telnet
- ▶ FTP
- ▶ SMTP

- HTTP 1.1
- HTTP-FTP
- HTTP-Gopher and Gopher+
- HTTPS
- H.323
- Ping
- NNTP (Network News Transfer Protocol)
- RealAudio and RealVideo
- NDS
- NTP (Network Time Protocol)

Authentication Support

Symantec Enterprise Firewall can be configured to support the following authentication protocols:

- Security Dynamics ACE
- BellCore S/Key
- Defender (by Axent)
- CRYPTOCard
- Gateway password
- Windows NT Challenge/Response
- RADIUS
- TACACs+

Minor Feature Set

Symantec Enterprise Firewall includes support for the following minor features:

MIMEsweeper Virus Scanning   This feature can be used to strip viruses out of downloads and attachments. Symantec Enterprise Firewall is missing support for the standard CVP content-vectoring protocol, however.

URL Blocking   This feature is based on a client/server updated list of sites that have been categorized. There's no real way to keep up with the ever-changing world of the unseemly, however, so I doubt that any simple URL filter would keep people from accessing this sort of content.

Paging and Audible Alerts   This feature can be used if your firewall has a Hayes-compatible modem and/or a sound card. The paging alert is especially useful for administrators who want to maintain a real-time response capability.

Transparency   You won't have to configure client applications or rely on clients that are proxy compatible to use Symantec Enterprise Firewall.

Illegal NAT   This support feature, using the Virtual Clients facility, allows you to perform client address translation through the gateway for networks that use illegal IP addresses.

Dual DNS   This configuration feature allows different DNS names to be served to the public and private sides of the proxy.

Security

Symantec Enterprise Firewall's gateway security architecture is extremely strong; it's highly unlikely that attacks through the firewall will succeed due to the proxy-only architecture. The Application-layer support for NAT is also very strong and transparent.

Symantec Enterprise Firewall's Achilles' heel is its reliance upon a stable operating system and TCP/IP stack. Telling requirements in the Symantec Enterprise Firewall installation documents (like the necessity for the latest service pack) show that everything in the firewall operates above the Network layer. There appears to be no MAC-layer protection (such as a packet filter) for the operating system itself, so there's no support for things like anti-spoofing. This is a fairly common problem for pure proxies. Ultimately, it means hackers could bring down your firewall and cause a denial of service, but they would not be able to penetrate the firewall to access your secured network.

Symantec Enterprise Firewall does not include any native high-availability or load-balancing features and is not compatible with the Windows Load Balancing Service. However, you can use a RadWare plug-in to achieve high availability or load balancing; more information is available from Symantec.

Interface

Symantec Enterprise Firewall version 6 uses the Microsoft Management Console to achieve a highly integrated and very useful user interface—it's the best user interface I've seen on a firewall. Despite the recent purchase and name change, Symantec Enterprise Firewall still calls its MMC snap-in the Raptor Management Console, or RMC. The RMC is client/server based and can support any number of firewalls. The interface is hierarchical, following the architectural requirements of the MMC. Figure 14.2 shows the user interface for Symantec Enterprise Firewall.

Management objects are completely hierarchical and very coherent, although the management interface is more complex than most firewalls. Network administrators familiar with the MMC should have no problems.

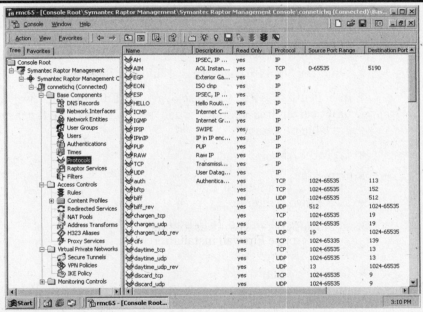

FIGURE 14.2: Raptor Management Console for the Symantec Enterprise Firewall user interface

Documentation

The included documentation is very thorough and is task oriented rather than technology/training oriented, although solid coverage of basic topics is provided. You can easily download a trial version from Symantec's website, but obtaining pricing information is nearly impossible.

Cost and Support

Support is via the website or support agreement only.

Licensing costs for the firewall (with VPN) are as follows:

- ▶ 1–100 users: $4,000
- ▶ 1–250 users: $8,500
- ▶ Unlimited users: $12,500

There is also a "deviceafied" version that comes preinstalled on a Sun Raq 1U Linux server. Oddly, its prices are about the same as the software-only versions, so it's a better deal—considering that you don't have to license an operating system or buy a computer.

System requirements are as follows:

- ▶ Windows NT 4 SP 6a Server or Windows 2000 Server SP-1
- ▶ Intel Pentium II 233 (because Symantec Enterprise Firewall is a proxy server, it is compute bound, so you should use the fastest available processor)
- ▶ 128MB RAM
- ▶ 2GB disk
- ▶ Two network interfaces

Standard support prices are as follows:

- ▶ 25 users: $375
- ▶ 100 users: $600
- ▶ 250 users: $1,275
- ▶ Unlimited: $1,875 per year

You can purchase 24/7 priority support as a single product rather than on a per-incident basis. Prices vary, depending on which product modules you have. Prices without VPN support are:

- ▶ 100 users: $900
- ▶ 250 users: $2,000
- ▶ Unlimited: $2,800

MICROSOFT INTERNET SECURITY AND ACCELERATION SERVER

Microsoft ISA Server replaces Microsoft Proxy Server 2.0 as Microsoft's firewall product. The two products have no similarity whatsoever—if they share any code, it's not apparent. Proxy Server was a simple HTTP proxy server that Microsoft claimed was a firewall. ISA Server is a real ICSA-certified firewall that performs all manner of forward, reverse, and transparent proxying for numerous protocols.

The difference in maturity between the two products is so extreme that it's difficult to believe they came from the same vendor within two years of each other. Unlike most of the other updated firewalls we've discussed, which underwent minor usability updates, name changes, and interface improvements, ISA Server is a completely new product that dramatically improves Microsoft's standing in the firewall market.

That said, ISA Server suffers from some problems. It relies heavily (although not completely) on Windows 2000's built-in security mechanisms—those low-level (Layer 4 and below) problems that affect Windows 2000 are highly likely to affect ISA Server.

ISA Server's tree-browser interface, while easy to figure out and configure initially, does not provide any sort of overview of your security policy the way most policy-based firewalls do. Considering that there is usually more than one way to achieve the same result in ISA Server, it can be excruciatingly difficult to determine what to change down the road when you want to reconfigure your policy.

Major Feature Set

Microsoft Internet Security and Acceleration Server provides the following major features:

- ► Stateful packet inspection
- ► Circuit layer (SOCKS) proxy
- ► Application-layer filtering in- and outbound
- ► IPSec, Point-to-Point Tunneling Protocol (PPTP), and Layer 2 Tunneling Protocol (L2TP) VPN
- ► Numerous authentication methods

Part III

Stateful Packet Inspection

ISA Server builds on the built-in filtering in Windows 2000 by adding a stateful inspection filter. (Windows 2000's packet filtering is stateless.) Stateful inspection ensures that inbound return channels on the firewall are closed when the TCP session had ended or timed out. The stateful inspection facility is also used to provide the SecureNAT feature of the firewall, which improves on Windows 2000's built-in network address translation by providing circuit layer regeneration rather than simple packet address translation.

Circuit Layer Proxy

ISA Server allows you to define circuit layer proxies that are protocol generic and that will work with any Windows SOCKS–based protocol, as well as with most Berkeley sockets–based protocols. A circuit layer proxy is a generic proxy that acts as the end point for TCP sessions and then regenerates them on the other side of the firewall. The effect is much the same as a stateful inspection firewall, except that the original TCP/IP packets themselves are not passed through—they are regenerated on the outbound interface so that no Network- or Session-layer malformations make it through. A circuit layer proxy is essentially the same thing as setting up a Unix redir service to receive and redirect a socket on a Unix machine.

Application-Layer Filtering

ISA Server comes with a number of Application layer security filters that can process rules for a specific application. The default set of filters includes:

▶ SMTP

▶ FTP

▶ HTTP

Numerous third-party content filters, virus scanners, and content blockers are available for ISA server. If you have programming talent available, you can use the SDK to create your own content filters as well.

Virtual Private Networking

ISA Server manages the built-in IPSec, PPTP, and L2TP VPN services of Windows 2000. Although it does not provide these services, it does create a simple, unified management platform; it also provides wizards for setting up such common schemes as a VPN remote access server and firewall-to-firewall VPN connectivity.

Authentication

Authentication is another area where ISA Server gets a free feature from its strong integration with Windows 2000. Because it passes authentication through to the server below, ISA Server can support all Windows 2000–supported authentication schemes, including plain-text passwords, NTLM encrypted passwords, Kerberos, X.509 certificates, smart cards, and third-party biometrics.

But with the good comes the bad—many of these authentication schemes are weak, and using them for the sake of convenience can seriously jeopardize your overall security posture. Although Microsoft considers it a "feature" that ISA Server can be configured to authenticate users based upon their internal account names and passwords, I would never use internal accounts for external security because usernames and passwords are far too easy to obtain from other sources, like malicious websites and Windows 95/98/Me .pwd files. Always use certificate-based authentication at the very minimum when configuring ISA Server as a remote access server.

Minor Feature Set

Microsoft Internet Security and Acceleration Server has the following minor features:

- ▶ Strong intrusion detection
- ▶ OS system hardening
- ▶ Highly configurable logging
- ▶ Ability to send e-mail or run arbitrary programs in response to alerts
- ▶ Transparent proxying
- ▶ Inbound content caching
- ▶ Outbound published content caching
- ▶ Policy-based configuration
- ▶ Secure Sockets Layer (SSL) bridging
- ▶ High availability and load balancing
- ▶ Quality of Service bandwidth allocation
- ▶ Enterprise management

Strong Intrusion Detection

ISA Server's intrusion detection filters are based on Internet Security Systems' ISS intrusion detection suite. I'm not a huge fan of fingerprint-based ID systems running stand-alone, but they're a marvelous addition to a firewall when your only other option would be the simple "someone connected to this blocked port" logging that you get with most firewalls. The intrusion-detection filters in ISA Server work at the Network (packet) layer and at the Application layer. Third-party Application-layer filters can trigger intrusion-detection alerts based on malformations in the protocols they filter.

OS System Hardening

ISA Server performs automatic operating system hardening for three different purposes as part of its setup wizard. This OS hardening feature was sorely lacking in Proxy Server 1 and 2, because Microsoft naively assumed that everyone knew how to make an NT or 2000 box secure. By packaging OS hardening as a "select one" configuration, ISA Server closes the holes that made Proxy Server a mere security placebo.

The OS Hardening Wizard allows you to select "dedicated mode" for servers that are dedicated to firewalling, or "secure mode" for installing on public Internet web and database servers that must protect themselves. There's also a hybrid mode that combines the features of the two.

Strong Logging and Alerting

Like all truly good firewalls, ISA Server gives you plenty of options when an alert comes in. You can send an e-mail, log it to the Windows event log, or stop or start a specific service. Stopping services automatically would be useful, for example, when your web server comes under concerted attack from the Internet and you're more interested in preventing intrusion than in remaining online. Finally, ISA Server can launch and run arbitrary programs in response to specific alerts, which gives you complete flexibility in dealing with intrusion attempts.

Transparent Proxying

ISA Server supports transparent proxying and Application-layer filtering for clients running in SecureNAT mode on the interior of the network. This eliminates machine-by-machine proxy configuration, which was required in MS-Proxy Server and was relatively easy for users to defeat.

Inbound and Outbound Caching

ISA Server's ascent from a simple HTTP proxy leaves it with strong HTTP caching abilities. You can configure the server to cache content for inbound users, and even distribute the cache among ISA Servers in your enterprise. Doing so can dramatically improve performance for websites that are visited frequently (which is becoming more common as businesses begin transacting with one another over the Web) but is ineffective for random surfing.

You can also configure an ISA Server (or an array of machines running ISA Server) to cache outbound content from your web server farm. So, for example, instead of having 10 web servers for which you must maintain identical configurations, you could have a single configured web server and an array of 10 ISA Servers in front of it delivering its cached content. Of course, your mileage will vary depending on the structure and activity of your site, but any site that transmits graphics will make good use of an outbound caching content server like ISA Server.

Policy-Based Configuration

Like all high-end firewalls, ISA Server's rules are based on abstract policies built from objects (called *Policy Elements* in ISA parlance). Objects include destinations, users, timeframes, protocols, and so forth.

There is no single place where you can look at the entire ruleset, however, and it's confusing to determine exactly how ISA Server will apply rules. For example, with protocol-based rules, ISA Server applies a "best fit" methodology with a deny-by-default policy, whereas for user groups it applies a "top-down first wins" methodology with an undeletable bottom rule that forms the default. This situation leads to a somewhat incoherent view of what's really going on that makes it difficult to survey an existing policy on a machine.

SSL Bridging

An unusual feature of ISA server is its SSL bridging capability. An ISA Server can initiate or terminate any SSL connection that flows through it. For example, if for some reason you don't want SSL flowing through the interior of your network, you can create a rule that will cause the ISA Server to respond to interior HTTP requests by creating an HTTPS connection to a secure public server. I can't figure out why this would be a good thing, but there are other purposes for SSL bridging. Another example would be connecting branch office users to an intranet at another site by creating an SSL bridge automatically between the ISA border servers. But, you'd probably just use VPN to do this. You can also have a front-line array of ISA servers terminate SSL in front of a secure web server to reduce its compute load. I suppose you could terminate outbound SSL connections at the firewall, inspect them, and then re-create them on the way out, so that users would have no idea you were able to filter their secure connections—that must be what this feature is really for.

High Availability and Load Balancing

ISA Server is capable of using Windows 2000 Advanced Server's high-availability and load-balancing services to protect against the failure of firewalls. By configuring border ISA Servers in an array and using the built-in load-balancing facility of Windows 2000 Advance Server, you could theoretically withstand the loss of all but one of your servers and still remain online.

Quality of Service Bandwidth Allocation

ISA Server also provides a management interface for the Quality of Service scheduler (QoS) built into all versions of Windows 2000. By abstracting bandwidth into its policy schema, ISA Server makes it easy to manage the bandwidth services of Windows 2000.

Enterprise Management Features

By integrating ISA Server Enterprise Edition with Active Directory, Microsoft has made it possible to publish ISA Server policies to the Active Directory for replication throughout the Enterprise. There's a bit of a chicken-and-egg problem to deal with if you intend to use an ISA Server–based VPN to connect your enterprise, but once you've got data flowing (and assuming you have an Active Directory schema set up and running), further updates are relatively simple.

Security

The security improvements in ISA Server are dramatic when compared to Proxy Server. Proxy Server came with an anemic recommendation to "lock down the host server," without so much as bothering to explain what that process entailed. Proxy Server ran as a service and literally did nothing to secure the base operating system against exploitation. Beyond that, Proxy Server was capable of proxying only HTTP and acting as a generic SOCKS proxy for other applications. Although this did disconnect the direct route through the proxy and eliminate the passage of Layer-3 packets through the proxy, it did nothing to secure against higher-layer attacks.

ISA Server, on the other hand, includes a simple wizard to lock down the server based on your firewalling needs, which configures the built-in security features of Windows 2000 to conform to the level of security required of a firewall. It also automatically configures the NAT and VPN features of the operating system to conform to the policies you set in the ISA Server interface, so that you have a single unified security interface on the firewall.

Basing its firewall on a complete general-purpose operating system like Windows 2000 provides Microsoft with a feature set that is second to none in the firewall market: ISA Server supports a rich set of authentication methods, installable IPSec encryption protocols, NAT, and a host of other minor features. But the foundation on a general-purpose operating system is also the potential Achilles' heel of the firewall. Unlike other firewalls, Windows 2000 is the subject of an enormous hacking effort, and failures of its core TCP/IP networking stack are highly likely to affect ISA Server as well.

But Microsoft has done a very good job of integrating Application-layer security. ISA Server was capable of defending against the Code Red virus the day it came out, assuming your access policies were strict. And although NIMDA made it through the majority of ISA installations, it did so as an e-mail attachment that a strong e-mail stripping policy could have prevented. Few other firewalls were proof against these attacks.

Finally, ISA Server supports third-party content modules and includes an SDK for developing your own in-house security filters and proxies. It provides the ability for those seriously interested in security to take matters into their own hands in a way that only open-source firewalls have allowed until now.

Interface

The user interface in ISA Server is the standard Microsoft Management Console that is used to configure all Windows 2000 administrative tools. As such, it's intuitive and easy to figure out for anyone familiar with Windows 2000 administration. The interface looks a lot like that of Symantec Enterprise Firewall, but the functionality is quite different.

The basic interface shows a tree consisting of all ISA Servers in your enterprise. Below the view of each server are located access policies, object definitions, forwarding rules, and so forth. Unfortunately, because the policy view is force-fit into a tree view, there's no room for viewing all access policies and then viewing which servers have those policies applied. The interface separates the pool of ISA servers rather than joining them into a single coherent policy as Checkpoint Firewall-1 does.

Figure 14.3 shows the Microsoft ISA Server's MMC interface.

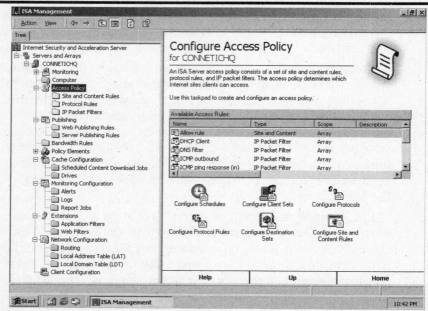

FIGURE 14.3:   Microsoft ISA Server

Cost and Support

ISA Server is sold in two editions: Standard and Enterprise. The only difference between them is that the Standard edition is limited to running on a single machine with up to four processors, so it does not support firewall arrays, policy enforcement on remote machines, or any of the other enterprise-management features. The Enterprise edition has none of these limitations.

Like many of Microsoft's newer BackOffice products, ISA Server is licensed per processor, which means you pay a licensing fee for every processor in the machines you're using. The Standard edition costs $1,500 per processor, and the Enterprise edition costs $6,000 per processor.

Microsoft support is the standard $250 per call, with one free call during the first 90 days. The product is fairly easy to set up and configure, so a support call should not be necessary.

WINDOWS AS A FIREWALL

Device-based firewalls are killing the traditional server-based firewall market because they're easier to buy, configure, install, and operate than the bulkier server-based products — plus, they tend to cost the same as firewall software alone, and the hardware they run on is usually more reliable than a PC-based server. These advantages add up to quick extinction for the server-based firewall market.

Responding to this threat, both NAI Gauntlet and Symantec Enterprise Firewall are available as devices. NAI Gauntlet can be ordered pre-installed on a Sun Netra 1U server, and Symantec Enterprise Firewall is sold as the Symantec VelociRaptor Firewall device on a Sun Raq 1U box running Linux. Although convenient, these devices are more expensive than their true device-based brethren and still contain hard disk drives, which makes them more susceptible to failure.

Two years from now, I expect that the only firewalls you'll be able to buy for Windows will be the venerable Firewall-1 (before its sagging sales make it a takeover target for the voracious appetite of Computer Associates) and Microsoft's ISA Server.

But I don't expect ISA Server to be around as a separate product much longer. Microsoft will probably roll ISA Server's features into the next version of Windows Server in order to shore up Windows' much-publicized security failures. This will allow the company to publicize its server operating system as a strong firewall by itself, and will alleviate the concern that many companies have about deploying .NET XML services on the Windows platform that is directly connected to the Internet.

Once Microsoft rolls ISA Server into the standard version of Windows, there won't be any real reason to use anyone else's Windows-based firewall on that platform. With the strong support for stateful packet inspection built into Linux now, I can think of no reason why anyone would pay for a server-based firewall a few short years from now.

That is how things always should have been.

WHAT'S NEXT

In this chapter, you have learned about several of the most popular firewalls based on the Windows platform. In Chapter 15, you will learn about firewalls based on the Unix operating system; we'll provide a basis to compare the various products.

Chapter 15

UNIX FIREWALLS

A version of Unix exists for every microprocessor being mass-produced today and for nearly every type of computer. Unix is the closest thing to a universal operating system that has ever existed. You can load many kinds of Unix (Solaris, Linux, BSD, and so on) on your PC; you can get OS X, Linux, or BSD for your Macintosh; and you can run Unix on your IBM mainframe, your Cray supercomputer, or your VAX, if you still have a VAX. You can even get Unix for your iPAQ pocket computer.

Most commercial versions of Unix (and all the versions discussed in this chapter) are based on the original AT&T Unix, whereas most open-source Unixes are based on either the Unix derivative developed somewhat independently by the University of California at Berkeley, or on Linux, a completely independent version of the Unix operating system that was designed to be compatible with both AT&T's Unix and Berkeley's Unix. A program written for one version of Unix will probably compile and run on another version of Unix with just a little porting effort; so, if you're looking for a firewall for your specific brand of high-performance workstation, you might find it in this chapter.

Part III

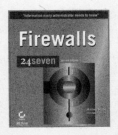

Adapted from *Firewalls 24seven*™, Second Edition by Matthew Strebe and Charles Perkins
ISBN 0-7821-4054-8 • $49.99

COMPUTER ASSOCIATES ETRUST FIREWALL

In really big networks containing hundreds or thousands of computers, the task of administering all those clients and servers can be overwhelming. Computer Associates developed the Unicenter TNG suite of tools to help network administrators centrally administer a large number of network devices, including client workstations, file servers, messaging servers, network devices, routers, and firewalls. The portion that implements a firewall for Unicenter-managed networks is the eTrust firewall, formerly designated the Network Security Option for Unicenter TNG, or GuardIT.

The eTrust firewall runs on various versions of Unix and on Windows NT. Unicenter provides for centralized management of multiple eTrust firewalls distributed throughout your enterprise, providing ease of configuration and use as well as a consistent security policy for your network. Because eTrust ties into the rest of the Unicenter resource management tools, you can combine user authentication and resource access rules with the typical address and port restrictions of packet filtering.

The eTrust firewall provides stateful packet inspection, Network Address Translation (NAT), packet inspection and rewriting for supported protocols, generic proxying for redirectable protocols, and centralized authentication. The sophisticated security event monitoring, logging, and response features of this firewall even allow for automatic reconfiguration of the security policy when suspicious or threatening activity is detected, which allows the system to lock itself down and gives you time to respond to the problem.

Pros and cons of the eTrust firewall are as follows:

Pros	Cons
Runs on Unix and Windows NT	Cost
Integrates with Unicenter	Requires Unicenter TNG
Centralized management	Long learning curve
Strong remote management	
Fast and flexible	

The platform requirements are as follows:

- ▶ Intel Pentium microprocessor or Unix workstation of equivalent power
- ▶ 64MB RAM (128MB recommended)
- ▶ 500MB hard disk drive; additional for caching
- ▶ Unix or Windows NT
- ▶ At least two network interfaces

Major Feature Set

The major features of eTrust include the following:

- ▶ Packet filter (stateful)
- ▶ Network Address Translator (dynamic, static)
- ▶ DMZ (demilitarized zone) support
- ▶ Port redirection
- ▶ Proxies (HTTP, FTP, RealAudio, and so on)
- ▶ Transparent proxies
- ▶ Reverse proxies (HTTP, SMTP [Simple Mail Transfer Protocol], FTP, and so on)
- ▶ Secure authentication (NT Server, RADIUS Server)
- ▶ Logging to databases and e-mail notification

The included stateful inspection filter is very strong and comparable to the stateful inspection services provided by Checkpoint Firewall-1. NAT is built into the stateful inspector.

The proxy functionality of eTrust doesn't really occur at the Application layer; protocol payloads are rewritten directly by the stateful inspector rather than being handed off to a separate Application-layer service, which regenerates the connection in its entirety. Rewriting provides much the same benefit; portions of the protocol that the firewall doesn't know about can't be rewritten, and such parameters as proper buffer length can be checked to prevent buffer overrun conditions.

Part III

Minor Feature Set

Some of the minor features of eTrust include the following:

- Content filtering (Java, virus scanning, URL blocking) through the additional eTrust Content Inspection and eTrust AntiVirus packages
- Scan detection, spoofing detection, and automatic blocking through the additional eTrust Intrusion Detection package
- Graphical administration
- Remote administration
- Centralized administration
- Integration with overall enterprise management tools
- Transparent ARP (Address Resolution Protocol) support
- SYN flood protection
- Anti-spoofing control
- Real-time monitoring and reporting
- Policy-based configuration and management
- Calendar support

A central policy-based management application (Unicenter TNG) provides strong centralized management for the firewall. Policies can easily be created and applied across the enterprise from the Unicenter control application. Unicenter TNG also provides a platform for strong integration with the other IT management options available for the system and provides the foundation for the log, alert, event detection, and response features.

The calendar support of the eTrust firewall is a useful feature that allows you to change the firewall policy based on the time. For example, you could significantly restrict outbound communications from your protected LAN after working hours, when users are not expected to be using the network. Violations can be logged and investigated as potentially compromised computers opening a back channel to outside hosts.

Interface

With eTrust, there is a graphical interface for both Windows NT and Unix. Firewalls appear as resources to be administered from the Unicenter administration suite. Because eTrust uses the same framework as all the other Unicenter options, administrators in a Unicenter shop will find the interface to be friendly and comfortable.

The graphical interface makes it easy to set up rules and enable or disable specific services for particular computers or users. The security objects are integrated with the other components of the Unicenter system (such as the Single Log On option), sparing you the effort of both establishing user account information and recording security restrictions in multiple locations.

Security

The eTrust firewall uses a stateful inspection packet filter, which keeps track of connection information across multiple packets. These include User Datagram Protocol (UDP) packets, which do not retain session information. The packet filter checks all the typical IP packet features such as source and destination addresses, port numbers, options set, SYN bit, Internet Control Message Protocol (ICMP) messages, and so on. The packet filter can also integrate into its rule set additional information obtained from the rest of the Unicenter framework, including user identity, allowed access times, and network resource restrictions. The firewall checks every packet before the IP stack processes it, thereby blocking attacks against the firewall itself using malformed and maliciously constructed IP packets, such as the Ping of Death, teardrop attacks, and so on.

One performance advantage of the firewall is that it can perform the equivalent of protocol proxying for some protocols by directly manipulating the IP packets, rather than handing off the packets to a separate proxy server application. This process provides for much faster proxying and therefore increased throughput and reduced latency between your network and the Internet. The firewall also provides for generic port redirection and integration with the Internet Web Management option to Unicenter TNG.

Documentation, Cost, and Support

Using eTrust requires a Unicenter TNG network infrastructure, which is designed for larger businesses. Because pricing varies widely and depends largely on your Unicenter infrastructure, there's no meaningful way for us to provide pricing information. Contact a Computer Associates sales representative directly to obtain pricing information if you use or want to use Unicenter TNG.

Part III

TIP

You can get more information about Unicenter TNG at www.cai.com.

SECURIT FIREWALL

The SecurIT firewall from SLMsoft (formerly MilkyWay) is available for both Unix and Windows NT. This firewall, like the free TIS FWTK, does not perform any packet filtering. Instead, it provides Application-level proxies for each of the protocols that will pass from the internal network to the Internet. Also like FWTK, the SecurIT firewall uses authentication to provide user-based as well as IP address–based access control. Where SecurIT really shines, however, is in the wide variety of protocols it "scrubs" or provides proxy redirection for. In addition to the proxies, SecurIT has a strong virtual private network (VPN) component that allows you to establish encrypted IP tunnels between your protected LANs over the Internet.

Its pros and cons are as follows:

Pros	Cons
Runs on Unix and Windows NT	No packet filtering
Supports a wide range of protocols	NT version does not harden OS
VPN	Cost
Centralized authentication	Difficult to acquire
High-speed application proxying	

Platform requirements for the SecurIT firewall include the following:

- ▶ SunSparc 5 or any Ultra-SPARC, Intel Pentium
- ▶ 2GB hard disk drive
- ▶ 32MB RAM
- ▶ PCI Quad adapter
- ▶ 2 or more network cards
- ▶ CD-ROM drive

Major Feature Set

SecurIT provides the following major features:

- ▶ Bidirectional transparent proxy services for a wide variety of protocols
- ▶ VPN between SecurIT-protected networks
- ▶ DMZ support
- ▶ Secure authentication (Unix passwords, S/Key software, SecureID, Safeword Enigma Logic)
- ▶ Logging to databases and e-mail notification

SecurIT provides numerous security proxies for common Internet protocols, which makes its protocol security very strong. SecurIT uses its generic TCP proxy functionality to perform client hiding, a function the documentation calls Network Address Translation. The functionality is not equivalent to true Network-layer NAT.

Secure authentication is performed via Bellcore's (now Telcordia's) S/Key one-time password algorithm.

Conspicuously missing from the major feature set are packet filtering and NAT. Neither function is necessary in a strong security proxy as long as the base operating system is sufficiently hardened. However, neither Solaris nor NT is hardened in our opinion, which considerably weakens the ability of firewalls that do not implement their own packet filtering accordingly. SecurIT ships with a version of Solaris that has apparently been hardened, and recommends security patches as additional vulnerabilities are discovered; but the NT version is susceptible to a wide range of denial-of-service attacks.

Minor Feature Set

SecurIT provides the following minor features:

- ▶ SQL proxying
- ▶ Remote administration
- ▶ Content filtering (Java, virus scanning, URL blocking, and so on)

As with most true firewalls, SecurIT is capable of logging to databases and transmitting e-mail to alert on security events. A SQL security proxy is provided to support SQL*Net transactions through the firewall.

Part III

Security

SecurIT does not filter packets before they are delivered to the IP stack for processing. The firewall relies on the underlying operating system to be resistant to IP-level attacks. Both Solaris and Windows NT, at their most current patch or service pack, have finally been made highly resistant to known attacks, but undiscovered vulnerabilities almost certainly exist in both operating systems. SecurIT for Solaris ships with a hardened version of Solaris.

Instead, SecurIT is a proxy server. It examines the data portions of IP packets to ensure that the traffic traversing a particular port conforms to the protocol for that port (that only HTTP requests and replies are going over port 80, for example).

SecurIT is designed with performance in mind. This highly optimized proxy server uses threads and shared memory to minimize the time required to filter the proxied protocols, allowing more traffic to pass through the firewall while still fully examining all the data to ensure that it conforms to protocol specifications.

SecurIT comes with a number of application-specific firewall proxies. In addition to providing content filtering for the specific protocol (guaranteeing that the port is actually used by the appropriate protocol instead of some other program), each protocol can be configured to block certain IP addresses and Internet domains. SecurIT provides proxies for the following protocols:

▶ FTP—A standard FTP service proxy

▶ Generic SOCKS—Allows the administrator to redirect proxied protocols easily by specifying the address and port where TCP and UDP packets should be forwarded

▶ Gopher—Proxies the text-based hypertext protocol that (barely) predates the Web

▶ HTTP++—Allows basic web traffic, but lets the administrator block applets and URLs

▶ HTTP—For basic port 80 proxying or for web traffic on other ports, but using the HTTP protocol

▶ LDAP (Lightweight Directory Access Protocol)—Allows network clients to access directory servers exterior to your firewall

▶ Mail—Stores and forwards e-mail delivered to the firewall for delivery on your local network

- ▶ NNTP (Network News Transfer Protocol)—Forwards Usenet news through the firewall

- ▶ POP—Provides a channel for internal clients to access external e-mail servers

- ▶ Real Media—Channels audio and video conforming to the Real Media standard through the firewall

- ▶ RPC—Provides for secure Remote Procedure Calls through the firewall

- ▶ SSL (Secure Sockets Layer)—Forwards secure socket communication through the firewall

- ▶ Telnet—Proxies command-line control of remote computers

- ▶ VDO Live—Mediates VDO multimedia from internal clients to external multimedia servers

Documentation, Cost, and Support

The SecurIT firewall is sold by the number of open simultaneous connections (sessions) rather than the number of IP addresses inside the network. This means, for example, that a 15-user network could probably get away with a 10-session version of the firewall if only 66 percent of the users were using the Internet at any one time. Prices shown are for the Solaris edition with one year of included support. The U.S. distributor would not quote pricing for the Windows NT version, because it considered the Windows operating system to be nonsecure. The product is sold primarily to military and government channels, because SLM has no significant marketing through commercial channels.

The product ships with a hardened version of Solaris, so there's no need to purchase the operating system. Hardware costs for a Sun Ultra-5 run about $5,000:

- ▶ 10 sessions: $3,600

- ▶ 40 sessions: $7,200

- ▶ 100 sessions: $16,200

- ▶ Unlimited: $23,400

- ▶ VPN: +$1,200

Part III

TIP

You can browse SLMsoft's website at `slmsoft.com`. To purchase SecurIT, contact Neoteric at (212) 625-9300.

NETWALL

Group Bull, a major European manufacturer of electronics and software, has packaged its internal IP security expertise into a firewall product called NetWall. This firewall runs on Sun's Solaris and IBM's AIX versions of Unix as well as Windows. The secure remote control software for the firewall runs on Windows platforms as well as AIX.

NetWall gives you the full range of security options to work with—from stateful packet inspection to Application-level proxies for a wide variety of protocols, NAT, VPN, authentication, load balancing, remote control, and support for third-party content inspectors. Its pros and cons are as follows:

Pros	Cons
High speed	Cost
High reliability	
Centralized authentication	
Versatile proxying	

NetWall suffers from a difficult setup and a lack of integration among software components. Configuring the firewall is not particularly easy compared to the majority of firewall offerings discussed in this book.

Major Feature Set

NetWall offers the following major features:

- ▶ Packet filter (stateful)
- ▶ Network Address Translator (dynamic, static)
- ▶ DMZ support
- ▶ Port redirection

- ▶ Transparent and reverse proxies (SOCKS [IP, IPX], HTTP, Telnet, Gopher, SMTP, FTP, POP, IMAP, RealAudio/Video, H.323)

- ▶ Secure authentication (plain, proprietary, Security Dynamics, Crypto Card, S/Key, RACAL, RADIUS Server)

- ▶ VPN (proprietary)

- ▶ VPN client software (Windows 98/NT/2000/XP)

- ▶ Redirection for load balancing and high availability through add-in package

- ▶ Firewall high availability

- ▶ Logging to databases and e-mail notification

NetWall includes a strong stateful inspection filter and Network Address Translator that supports both static and dynamic address mapping.

NetWall supports a broad range of authentication features, including low security options like ASCII plain-text passwords and higher security options like RADIUS, MD/5 Challenge/Response, Bellcore S/Key one-time passwords, SecurID Cards, and smart cards. NetWall also includes a complete set of APIs to allow third-party vendors or organizations with programming support to create other authentication options.

The remote access VPN is different than the firewall-to-firewall VPN. The remote access VPN is somewhat unique in that it is based on a SOCKS proxy transmitted through an SSL tunnel, rather than IPSec. The remote access VPN supports standard 40-, 56-, and 128-bit key lengths. The firewall-firewall VPN is based on Data Encryption Standard (DES) and triple-DES, and supports key lengths up to 192 bits.

Minor Feature Set

NetWall offers the following minor features:

- ▶ Content filtering (Java, virus scanning, URL blocking) through MimeSweeper and VirusWall plug-ins

- ▶ Graphical administration

- ▶ Remote administration

- ▶ Centralized administration

- ▶ OS hardening

- ▶ SQL proxying

Multiple NetWall firewalls can be used to balance the connection load between them and to continue operating in the event that one of them fails. This feature allows you to provide high availability of Internet services and protects you in the event of a denial-of-service attack.

NetWall supports content vectoring to third-party content scanning applications such as MimeSweeper or VirusWall.

Firewall management can be performed remotely from any Windows or AIX workstation. Communication between the firewall and the management workstation is encrypted.

Interface

NetWall's GUI interface is typical of policy-based firewall managers, providing a look and feel similar to Checkpoint Firewall-1's interface. As with Firewall-1, the interface can be run locally on the firewall or on a remote management workstation.

Security

NetWall's IP filter performs stateful packet inspection, keeping track of the state of TCP and UDP data streams. (The state mechanism allows the firewall to keep track of UDP in spite of the fact that UDP doesn't keep session information in the packets.) The NetWall packet-inspection engine can also inspect the data portion of some IP packets directly, which simplifies and improves the proxying performance of certain protocols. Protocol filters that the IP filter accelerates include HTTP, SMTP, FTP, Telnet, RPC, SQL* Net, and SAP.

The IP filter accelerates the proxies and protects the firewall server from IP-level attacks, and the application proxies make sure that only safe data traffic transits your firewall. NetWall comes with an impressive range of proxies, including the following:

▶ FTP—Filters FTP traffic

▶ Generic—Allows the administrator to redirect easily proxied protocols by specifying the address and port to which TCP and UDP packets should be forwarded

▶ Gopher—Proxies the non-multimedia hypertext protocol that (barely) predates the Web

- ▶ HTTP—Proxies for basic port 80 or for web traffic on other ports, but using the HTTP protocol
- ▶ SHTTP/SSL—Proxies for encrypted web traffic and for Secure Socket Layer communication
- ▶ LDAP—Allows network clients to access directory servers exterior to your firewall
- ▶ SMTP—Stores and forwards e-mail delivered to the firewall for delivery on your local network
- ▶ IMAP4—Mediates mail delivery and mailbox checking through the firewall
- ▶ NNTP—Forwards Usenet news through the firewall
- ▶ POP3—Provides a channel for internal clients to access external e-mail servers
- ▶ Real Audio/Video—Channels audio and video conforming to the Real Media standard through the firewall (AIX version only)
- ▶ H.323—Allows for videoconferencing through the firewall (AIX version only)
- ▶ Telnet—Proxies command-line control of remote computers
- ▶ TN3270—Proxies TCP/IP access to mainframe and minicomputers
- ▶ TNVIP—Allows TNVIP access across the firewall
- ▶ SOCKSV5—Redirects protocols specifically designed to be redirected through the SOCKS proxy service

Documentation, Cost, and Support

Bull has firmed up distribution of its firewall in the U.S. since the first edition of this book. Contact www.evidian.com/accessmaster/netwall for more information and contact information regarding this product.

NETWORK ASSOCIATES GAUNTLET ON THE WEBSHIELD E-PPLIANCE

Network Associates (NAI), the new owner of Gauntlet, is the result of the merger of McAffee (of virus-scanning fame) and Network General (makers of the Sniffer network protocol analyzer). The company then purchased PGP, Phil Zimmerman's encryption technology company, and Trusted Information Systems (TIS), the makers of Gauntlet. TIS developed the first security proxies under contract to the Department of Defense's Advanced Research Projects Agency (DARPA) when DARPA decided that stateless packet filters were not effective security devices. These original TIS security proxies are still available at no charge on the Internet.

NAI has put Gauntlet in the PGP group. The company is in the process of merging all of its security products together through a mechanism it calls *active security*. Active security is an event-driven publish/subscribe mechanism that allows the various software components of a security infrastructure to report exceptional events to other components in the security group. The security components are then able to make adjustments to their security policy to deal with the changed circumstance.

The level of conformance to this new active security infrastructure is low—most products can do little more than report events. But it does show that NAI is serious about integrating its security products, and that it understands how such integration needs to be done. No other security product vendor has shown as much understanding of total security as NAI in this respect. How much of this talk becomes reality, and how useful the product will be when it does, remains to be seen.

Gauntlet is widely regarded in the security industry to be the most secure firewall on the market, because it uses security proxies for all secured services rather than relying on stateful packet inspection. Recent versions include support for adaptive filtering, whereby connections are inspected at the Application layer by a proxy server during initiation and are then dropped down to the Network layer for stateful filtering once the connection is established and authenticated. This process improves the performance of the firewall dramatically.

Gauntlet is available for Windows NT and Unix. The firewall is multi-threaded, which means it provides higher performance on multiprocessor machines. In addition to a software package, you can purchase software that has been pre-installed on a Sun workstation and sold as an *e-ppliance*. This turns the Gauntlet software into a firewall; however, the e-ppliance contains hard drives (therefore it is not solid-state and is more likely to fail eventually), and it contains a feature-rich operating environment that hackers can use in the unlikely event that they penetrate the Gauntlet firewall security.

Gauntlet's pros and cons are as follows:

Pros	Cons
High speed	High cost
High reliability	
VPN support	
Centralized authentication	
Cross-platform and device packaged	

Major Feature Set

Gauntlet provides the basic components required of a modern firewall:

- ▶ Packet filter (stateful)
- ▶ Network Address Translator (dynamic, static)
- ▶ DMZ support
- ▶ Port redirection
- ▶ Transparent and reverse proxies
- ▶ Secure authentication (SecureID, RADIUS S/KEY, CryptoCard, ActiveCard, Microsoft Windows NT Challenge/Response)
- ▶ VPN (IPSec/IKE accelerated)
- ▶ VPN client software (Windows 98/NT/2000/XP, Macintosh, Unix, Linux)
- ▶ Redirection for load balancing and high availability
- ▶ Firewall high availability
- ▶ Bandwidth control and Quality of Service
- ▶ Logging to databases and e-mail notification

The Gauntlet Packet Filter

Gauntlet is now a combination of a security proxy and a stateful inspection filter. Each time a connection is established, the initial connection establishment packets are transmitted through the application proxy.

Part III

Depending on the security settings established by the security administrator, the proxy can continue to proxy all the data in the connection or determine that the connection is trustable and direct the packet filter to simply forward remaining packets in the connection without further inspection through the proxy. This approach lessens the rather serious performance and load problems from which security proxies suffer, but retains most of the security provided by an application proxy.

Proxy Services

Gauntlet provides support for an impressive range of both traditional Internet services and the newer multimedia and database services.

Standard Internet services include:

- FTP
- HTTP
- LDAP
- NNTP
- POP3
- PPTP (Point-to-Point Tunneling Protocol)
- SMTP
- SNMP (Simple Network Management Protocol)
- SSL
- Telnet

H.323 Multimedia services include:

- NetMeeting
- NetShow
- RealAudio
- RealVideo
- VDOLive

SQL services include:

- Microsoft

- Oracle
- Sybase

Network Address Translation (NAT)

Illegal Network Address Translation (INAT) is NAT in an environment where valid IP addresses (those not in the 10, 192.168, or 176 domain) assigned to other owners are in use in your network and must be translated to legal addresses for proper operation on the Internet. INAT can deal with the special problems posed by illegal addresses.

TIP

Reconfigure your entire network to use the legal, non-routable 10 domain for internal addresses. There are illegal address problems that INAT translators can't solve. I've had customers who have tried for years to deal with their illegal address schemes rather than put in the few days of intense, IT organization-wide effort it would take to rebuild the address infrastructure using DHCP and legal addresses. If your network is so encrusted that you don't dare change IP addresses, it's a disaster waiting to happen anyway.

Minor Feature Set

Gauntlet supports the following minor features:

- Content filtering (Java, virus scanning, URL blocking)
- Scan detection, spoofing detection, and automatic blocking
- Graphical administration
- Remote administration
- Centralized administration
- Transparent ARP support
- SYN flood protection
- Anti-spoofing control
- Real-time monitoring and reporting
- Content Vectoring Protocol (CVP)

Part III

- Policy-based configuration and management
- High performance
- OS hardening
- SQL proxying

The Gauntlet CVP allows firewall vendors and third-party providers to create connectable content scanners through which certain types of content must pass before they clear the firewall. Gauntlet's virus protection and Java filtering are performed using CVP technology.

NAI uses the CVP to tie the Gauntlet firewall in to its McAfee content-filtering service, which periodically updates the firewall with new fingerprint files for viruses, Trojan horses, and other malicious content that may attempt to transit your firewall in HTTP, SMTP, FTP, or some other protocol. Gauntlet is an attractive solution for networks that already use the popular McAfee virus-scanning software on their workstations.

Security

Gauntlet secures the firewall with various policies that are accumulations of service proxy rules. You are free to develop as many different policies as you need. These policies are then mapped to network interfaces for implementation. Two default policies are created when the product is installed:

- Trusted policies are mapped to network adapters that you identify as "inside" during the installation process.
- Untrusted policies are mapped to interfaces you identify as "outside" during the installation process.

The trusted policy engages the following proxy services:

- FTP
- H.323
- HTTP
- LDAP
- NetShow
- NNTP
- PPTP

- RAP
- SMTP
- StreamWorks
- Telnet
- VDOLive

The default trusted policy disallows the following proxy services:

- MS-SQL
- POP3
- SNMP
- SQL-GW
- Sybase-SQL

The effect of this policy is to allow most normal consumption content to pass through the firewall, but to block attempts by internal clients to interact directly with foreign untrusted e-mail servers or SQL servers.

The default untrusted policy allows the following services:

- FTP
- NNTP
- POP3
- SMTP
- Telnet

The policy disallows all others. This allows untrusted hosts to make FTP, NNTP, e-mail, and Telnet connections inside the network. Authentication is required for all of these services.

Interface

The Gauntlet interface is clean and simple—it's much less cartoonish than either Guardian or Firewall-1. The firewall manager application uses a tabbed view to switch between the various dialogs used to configure the firewall.

Documentation

All documentation included with the evaluation edition of Gauntlet comes in the form of the help file for the firewall manager. This makes the documentation somewhat difficult to read straight through, but easier to read in a digressional click-through manner. HTML-based documentation would have combined the best of both worlds.

The documentation is light, focusing on simple explanations of broad security concepts and relying on the administrator to figure out the technical nuances of firewall operation.

Cost and Support

Cost information about NAI Gauntlet can only be obtained on a per-configuration basis from a Gauntlet sales representative, so it's very difficult to compare the firewall's price against the competition.

The device we tested for this book—an unlimited e-ppliance with VPN—weighed in at a hefty $17,500, making it by far the most expensive firewall we tested. Only ISP-grade, high-speed firewalls cost more.

Evaluation editions of the Gauntlet firewall can be downloaded at www.nai.com.

SUNSCREEN SECURE NET 3.1

All the big information technology companies have crafted their own firewall software, and Sun is no exception. It has a firewall called (cleverly enough) SunScreen, which runs on Sun SPARC workstations and Intel computers under Solaris and is expertly designed for providing high-throughput protection for large networks.

Its pros and cons are as follows:

Pros	Cons
High speed	High cost
High reliability	No content filtering
VPN support	
Centralized authentication	
Java-based administration	

NOTE

In addition to selling its own firewall software, Sun provides the hardware for the appliance versions of the Gauntlet, Raptor, and SLM firewalls.

Major Feature Set

SunScreen provides the following major features:

- ▶ Packet filter (stateful)
- ▶ Network Address Translator (dynamic, static)
- ▶ DMZ support
- ▶ Port redirection
- ▶ Proxies (HTTP, SMTP, FTP, Telnet)
- ▶ Secure authentication (Plain, SecureID, RADIUS, SKIP [Simple Key Management Protocol for IP])
- ▶ VPN (IPSec/IKE, SKIP)
- ▶ VPN client software (Windows 98/NT/2000/XP, Macintosh, Unix, Linux)
- ▶ Firewall high availability
- ▶ Bandwidth control and Quality of Service
- ▶ Logging and e-mail notification

Sun's firewall provides all the major features you'd want in a network firewall, which is to be expected from the company that coined the phrase "The network is the computer." Also gratifying is the use of industry-standard protocols for VPN support, so you can connect any client for whom you have IPSec software to your LAN. The firewall doesn't give you anything you can't get in other firewalls, though, so the best reason to install SunScreen is if you're already a Sun shop.

Minor Feature Set

SunScreen provides the following minor features:

- ▶ Scan detection, spoofing detection, and automatic blocking
- ▶ Graphical administration

Part III

- ▶ Remote administration

- ▶ Centralized administration

- ▶ Transparent ARP support

- ▶ SYN flood protection

- ▶ Anti-spoofing control

- ▶ Policy-based configuration and management

- ▶ High performance

- ▶ OS hardening

- ▶ Stealth

The interesting feature is SunScreen's support for *stealth* or *drop-in* firewalling, where the firewall interposes itself between the hosts on a network and the outside network. In stealth mode, the firewall does not present any IP addresses to either the LAN or to the WAN connection; instead, it monitors all network traffic on its interfaces and forwards packets or does not forward them as appropriate. The firewall itself is not addressable and therefore is unsusceptible to most firewall subversion methods.

One noticeable lack in the SunScreen software is built-in support for content filtering. The SunScreen proxies ensure that you're using HTTP on the HTTP port, but they do not keep you from downloading a virus. Perhaps this is a reflection of Sun's Unix culture, which is far less suscep-tible to the viruses, malicious ActiveX controls, and Visual Basic scripting worms that plague Windows networks. Nevertheless, if you need to pro-tect Windows computers, you should consider adding a virus scanner to your network in addition to the SunScreen firewall; many virus scanner products that will run on Solaris alongside the firewall.

Interface

Centralized management of multiple bastion hosts is performed via a Java applet running in web browsers. This makes administration very flexible, because you can administer the firewall from any Java-enabled browser with SKIP installed. It's no surprise that Sun would provide this option because Sun developed Java and is Java-enabling all of its enterprise software.

The interface is clean and simple, and it makes good use of Java technology. Management is policy based. Figure 15.1 shows the initial policy page.

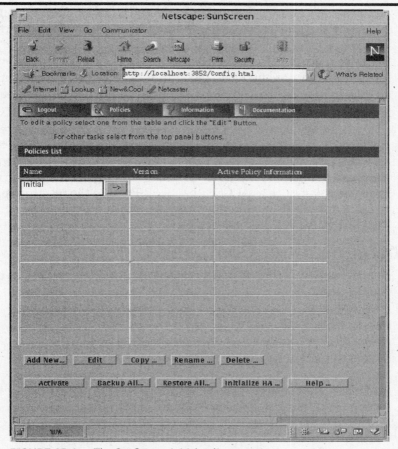

FIGURE 15.1: The SunScreen initial policy page

Security

SunScreen hardens a Sun SPARC or Intel workstation running Solaris to perform as a packet filter and Network Address Translator. All packets are processed by the packet filter before being routed or translated. SunScreen provides the full range of packet filtering options, including the SYN bit, source and destination IP addresses, source and destination ports, packet type, and so on.

Because SunScreen does not inspect the data portions of the packets and locks down the operating system (so naive administrators can't compromise security by running insecure services on the server), you will need a proxy server running on another computer to ensure that the traffic traversing a particular port conforms to the protocol for that port (that only HTTP requests and replies are going over port 80, for example). Many web servers will also act as HTTP proxies, and you can use servers for store-and-forward protocols (such as SMTP and NNTP) unmodified as protocol proxies for their services. Ideally, you should use address translation to redirect the appropriate traffic to and from these servers.

SunScreen evaluates every packet received by the network adapters in the firewall computer according to a set of rules you establish from the Java administration console. The rules are applied in order and one at a time until SunScreen finds a rule that matches the packet and specifies a terminal action, such as ACCEPT or DROP. Because the rules are applied in order, it is vitally important to craft the rules in the right order.

Documentation, Cost, and Support

SunScreen EFS is sold on a per-user basis, with VPN licensing as a separate cost:

- ▶ SunScreen EFS 3.0, unlimited users, single server: $10,000
- ▶ 250 client licenses for SunScreen SKIP: $10,000
- ▶ SSN 3.0 Competitive Upgrade: $3,000
- ▶ SSN 3.0 for Workgroups unlimited + 100 clients for SKIP: $7,000
- ▶ SSN 3.0 Evaluation Kit: $100
- ▶ SSN 3.0/WG with 100 uses + 100 SKIP: $3,000
- ▶ SSN 3.0 Site + 250 SKIP clients: $35,0000
- ▶ SSN 3.0/WG unlimited use + 250 SKIP clients: $70,000
- ▶ SKIP client for Windows 9x/NT (1 server, 1 user): $150
- ▶ SKIP clients, 1,000 pack: $41,000

TIP
Visit Sun's website at www.sun.com/security.

TRY TO BUY

To provide cost and support information for the various firewalls in this book, I went through the same sales channels that any knowledgeable consultant would use. Primarily based on vendor websites, I searched for sales channels for the product, got in touch with the contacts listed, and basically did whatever the company's website told me to do to acquire the firewall. I felt this approach would closely approximate the typical firewall buying experience.

Surprisingly, my survey yielded mixed results. Some firewalls were incredibly easy to buy—their websites went through to an online store willing to take your credit card number and ship you the product the next day. Others went the more traditional route of listing numerous distributors. I also had great success finding firewalls available from online distributors at www.shopper.com, for those firewalls in a traditional distribution channel.

Other firewalls' pricing information was so difficult to obtain that I would have given up had I not been doing research for a book. The companies that sell these firewalls have chosen to work exclusively through value-added reseller agreements, which leads customers down a Byzantine maze of voicemail in an attempt to find product sales information.

For one product, my phone calls to the numbers listed on the company's web pages yielded numerous incorrect and out-of-date phone numbers. Calling their tech support reached a voicemail box, and leaving a message did not generate a return call. When I called the main number and asked for pricing information, I was transferred six times until I reached a voicemail box. I received a call back from a sales representative who directed me to the company's primary U.S. distributor; this company appeared to be a very small operation—it had only one sales person who was qualified to provide pricing information about the firewall.

I found it simply impossible to obtain U.S. pricing information for another product from a major multinational vendor. When I contacted the company the website listed as the U.S. distributor, that company had no idea that it carried the product. I was then transferred to another distributor that had no idea what I was talking about. I finally just gave up.

CONTINUED ➡

Part III

Firewall vendors that can't figure out how to sell their product are likely to be completely unable to support it. Although I hate to make recommendations based on non-technical criteria like sales and marketing, especially when the two firewalls that suffered from these problems are very strong security proxies, I just don't think it's worth the potential support problems you'll have with a completely non-responsive company.

WHAT'S NEXT

In this chapter, you have learned about a wide variety of firewall products for the Unix platform. Many of the firewalls in this chapter work at all seven layers of the OSI model. In Chapter 16, we will discuss firewall products for Linux, focusing on the Network layer.

Chapter 16

LINUX NETWORK-LAYER FIREWALLS

U nlike the bricks-and-mortar version, a network firewall must not only protect the inside network from intrusion, but it must also allow users to reach outside resources while allowing certain connections back to those users. This sounds like a simple concept, but its implementation is often challenging.

The good news, however, is that Linux itself easily serves as an efficient firewall device. The Linux kernel has the native ability to inspect the headers of packets received by the system. The `iptables` tool provides full control of packet filtering, Network Address Translation (NAT), and even *stateful inspection*, where the decision of whether to accept or reject a packet is made in the context of a previously established flow (like an outgoing Telnet request).

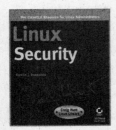

Adapted from *Linux Security* by Ramón J. Hontañón
ISBN 0-7821-2741-X $49.99

The classic example of the stateful inspection capability is what allows a firewall to permit an incoming `ftp-data` connection (TCP port 20) only when a local host has initiated an `ftp-control` connection (TCP port 21). By remembering the *state* of the outgoing connection from a given internal IP address, the firewall allows the incoming `ftp-data` connection only while the outgoing `ftp-control` connection is still in the ESTABLISHED state.

The combination of `iptables/ipnatctl` and kernel support makes Linux a very solid platform on which to protect your network perimeter.

LINUX AS A FIREWALL PLATFORM

So why should you choose the Linux platform over the competing offerings, both open source and commercial? Ultimately, you are seeking the best protection for your network perimeter. So, before jumping into the discussion of *how* you go about setting up a Linux firewall, let's talk briefly about the reason *why* you would want to do this. These are the major advantages of a Linux platform over its competition:

Uniform Administration   There is nothing magical about using a Linux server to act as a firewall device, except for the fact that you'll be running a number of commands that affect kernel packet filtering and perhaps NAT. Your training and experience as a Linux administrator can be applied toward the administration of your firewall. You know Linux and you understand it, which is your best protection when something goes wrong.

Commodity Hardware   Unlike some of the commercial firewall appliances that employ proprietary (in other words, expensive) and sometimes obscure hardware, the Linux firewall can be built with an existing off-the-shelf PC-compatible system, a PowerPC, or a Sparc/Ultra machine. Thus it's much easier to maintain spare parts and repair the system in the event of an outage.

Robust Kernel-Based Filtering   Although Linux uses user-level tools for configuring its firewall feature, the heart of its packet-filtering capability is implemented in the kernel, where it's safer and more efficient.

Tested Platform   Both the kernel and the user tools are widely deployed around the world, where they enjoy the constant enhancement and support of thousands of dedicated developers. Vulnerabilities are discovered and divulged in a timely fashion, and patches are often available within hours.

Performance   With native support for fast Ethernet and even some WAN technologies (ISDN, T1), the Linux operating system can keep up with just about any type of connection that your company uses to reach the Internet. The bottleneck is likely to be that connection, even when you take into account the time it takes the firewall to inspect every packet that reaches its interfaces.

Cost   Using an open-source operating system as well as commodity hardware, a Linux firewall is the overall cost winner, often outperforming much larger commercial offerings. Not surprisingly, the more cost effective of these commercial firewalls are typically the ones based on the Linux operating system, like the Watchguard Firebox (`www.watchguard.com`) and the Xsentry Internet Firewall package (`www.trustix.com`).

There are, however, a few disadvantages to choosing Linux firewall support. Here are two of them:

Support   I'm not going to enter into the age-old argument of open source versus commercial, but the fact remains that many enterprises still feel uneasy about relying on an open-source system for protection. Although there are plenty of support offerings for the Linux operating system, the firewall application support offered by most commercial vendors is bound to be more enticing to your CIO.

Application Bundling   Although some open-source packages offer graphical user interface (GUI) interfaces to the command-line tools used to control packet filtering, the commercial sector is further ahead in offering all-encompassing firewall applications. These applications often include an installation and deinstallation script, a GUI, and a set of monitoring, logging, and reporting tools. These features are of relative value, however, unless your company lacks the expertise necessary to install the more laborious "build-your-own" Linux alternative.

Part III

If you have analyzed these pros and cons, and are still ready to use Linux to protect your network, then read on! The next section introduces the concept of packet filtering, which is central to the way a Linux firewall goes about protecting your perimeter at the Network layer.

PACKET FILTERING

The basic steps of packet filtering are as follows:

1. A packet arrives in one of the interfaces.

2. After the interface strips out the packet's Data Link layer header, it passes the Network layer payload to the kernel.

3. The kernel inspects the packet's header (IP address, port) and decides to drop it or forward it based on a set of rules. This operation can take place in near real time and is totally transparent to the end user.

Packet filtering is not exclusive to firewalls, because any Linux host can be configured to perform it; but it is most useful for building a perimeter control device (such as a firewall). A Linux server can be configured to act as a cost-effective firewall using the latest kernel's packet-filtering support. In fact, even an average machine (an entry-level Pentium with 48MB of RAM and a very small disk) has been shown to be more than adequate to keep up with Ethernet speeds while performing packet filtering and address translation.

The main advantage of packet filtering is that it is an efficient and nonintrusive way of adding security to your network. Users need to be aware of proxy-level firewalls. They don't need to be aware of packet-filtering firewalls, and they don't need to authenticate themselves to use any outgoing services.

One important drawback to packet filtering is its inability to provide secure access to remote users who receive their addresses dynamically (using dial-up accounts via bootp or Dynamic Host Configuration Protocol [DHCP]). A second drawback is the lack of user-level authentication authorization, especially when a remote host houses a number of users.

However, the most successful approach to security is a multilayered one, and packet filtering should play a critical role in the overall defense of your network. The last section of this chapter explains the concept of

Network Address Translation, which is used in conjunction with packet filtering in most Linux firewalls.

THE LEGACY: *IPFWADM* AND *IPCHAINS*

Starting with kernel version 1.2.1, Linux has offered a number of utilities to configure the rules used by the kernel to accept or discard IP packets. The first incarnation of this utility was Alan Cox's and Jos Vos's ipfwadm utility, which was based on BSD's ipfw utility and worked with kernel versions 1.2 through 2.1. The last version of ipfwadm was released in July 1996. Starting with kernel version 2.1.102 and later, ipfwadm was replaced by Paul "Rusty" Russell's and Michael Neuling's ipchains; this utility addresses some of ipfwadm's limitations, namely:

▶ The 32-bit counters, which were previously unable to keep track of packets coming into high-speed network interfaces

▶ Its inability to deal adequately with IP fragmentation

▶ No support for transport layer protocols other than UDP and TCP

▶ No support for inverse rules, where you look for the opposite of a condition (for example, -i !eth0)

If your Linux distribution only supports ipfwadm, you are running an old system and you should upgrade to a newer version. Most recent Linux vendors include the ipchains utility in their standard distribution. The next section explains how to use the ipchains command and includes some real-life examples of how you can use it to build a Network layer firewall.

Using *ipchains*

The name ipchains refers to the fact that the Linux kernel consults three separate *chains*, or sequences of rules, when it receives a Network layer packet. Three chains come built-in with the Linux kernel:

Input Chain   The input chain handles packets that arrive at one of the server's interfaces and are bound for the local host.

Output Chain   The output chain handles packets that are originated by the local system and are bound for a remote host.

Forward Chain   The forward chain handles packets that arrive
at one of the server's interfaces and are bound for a remote host.

Each of these three chains can contain a set of rules that define access
controls based on the source/destination address, the TCP/UDP port, or
the protocol ID. By specifying a set of rules that enforces the provisions
of your security policy, you can build a firewall device using the Linux
kernel as the underlying system and ipchains as your configuration tool.

The ipchains utility uses the following syntax:

```
ipchains command chain rule-specifications [options] -j
➥action
```

The *command* field is used to maintain the list of rules for a given
chain. For example, it defines whether you're adding a rule, deleting a
rule, or simply listing the rules that have already been defined for that
chain. Table 16.1 contains a list of valid commands supported in
ipchains.

TABLE 16.1:   *ipchains* Commands

SWITCH	MEANING
-A	Add a rule to a chain (append to end of the chain).
-D	Delete a rule from a chain.
-C	Create a new chain.
-R	Replace an existing rule in the chain.
-L	List all rules in the chain.
-I	Insert numbered rules in the chain.
-F	Flush all rules from the chain (empty the chain).
-Z	Zero (reset) the packet and byte counters on all chains.
-N	Create a new chain.
-X	Delete the user-defined chain.
-P	Set policy for the chain to the given target.
-E	Rename the chain.
-M	View currently masqueraded connections.
-C	Check a given packet against a selected chain.
-S	Change the timeout values used for masquerading.

The *chain* field can be one of INPUT, OUTPUT, or FORWARD, or it can be a user-created chain (in the case of the -C command). You'll learn more about user-created chains later in this section.

In the *rule-specifications* field, you can specify one or more rules to be applied to each packet. Each incoming packet is compared to the parameters included in each rule, and, if a match is found, the appropriate *action* is taken for that packet. Table 16.2 lists the set of available constructors for the ipchains rules.

TABLE 16.2: *ipchains* Rule Specification Parameters

PARAMETER	MEANING
-p [!]*protocol*	Protocol ID to match. This value can be tcp, udp, icmp, or any numeric or alphabetic representation of a service in /etc/services.
-s [!]*address[/mask]*	Source address to match. This value can be a host name, an IP address, or a network name in network/mask format.
--sport [*port:[port]*]	Source port or source port range.
-d [!]*address[/mask]*	Destination address to match. Follows the same rules as the -s parameter.
--dport [*port:[port]*]	Destination port or destination port range.
-j *target*	Action to take when the rule finds a match (for example, accept, drop). Note that in addition to being the name of an action, *target* can also be a user-specified chain or a built-in chain.
-i [!]*interface*	Interface through which the packet was received, such as eth0.
-o [!]*interface*	Interface through which the packet is to be sent, such as eth0.
[!] -f	Indication that the packet is a second or subsequent fragment of a larger fragmented packet.
-y	Instruction to only match TCP packets with the SYN bit set.

Part III

The parameters listed in Table 16.2 allow you to define any combination of source/destination IP address, port, protocol ID, and interface, along with the inverse of each of these conditions, by simply preceding the parameter with the exclamation mark (!).

Finally, the ipchains command needs to be told what action to take with each packet that matches the given rule. The action field is preceded by the -j option (which literally stands for *jump*) and can be one of the following:

- ▶ *chain*—This value can be a user-defined chain. It allows you to "call" a chain within another chain, similar to the case where a subroutine calls another to perform a defined operation.

- ▶ accept—Let the packet through.

- ▶ deny—Quietly drop the packet on the floor.

- ▶ reject—Drop the packet and inform the sender via an Internet Control Message Protocol (ICMP) message.

- ▶ masq—Modify (*masquerade*) the packet's source IP address as if it had originated from the local host. This action applies only to the forward chain and to any user-defined chains.

- ▶ redirect—Forward the packet to a local socket even if its destination is a remote host. This action applies only to the input chain and to any user-defined chains.

- ▶ return—Exit the present chain and return to the calling chain.

ipchains Examples

Let's look at some examples of the ipchains command. Consider a Linux server called watchtower.example.com with the following interfaces:

- ▶ eth0: 63.54.66.1 (public interface)

- ▶ eth1: 38.110.200.1 (private interface)

Let's start by flushing the three built-in chains from all previously specified rules using the following commands:

```
ipchains -F input
ipchains -F output
ipchains -F forward
```

To set up a policy whereby all packets that are not matched by a specific rule within the chain will be rejected, use the following commands:

```
ipchains -P input REJECT
```

```
ipchains -P output REJECT
ipchains -P forward REJECT
```

The previous three commands set up a restrictive policy where you have to explicitly define the kinds of traffic you want to allow through your firewall. Suppose your security policy allows incoming mail, HTTP, and Telnet connections from any public host. You enforce it by adding the appropriate rule to the `forward` chain:

```
ipchains -A forward -s 0.0.0.0/0 -d 38.110.200.0/24
➥-dport smtp -j  ACCEPT
ipchains -A forward -s 0.0.0.0/0 -d 38.110.200.0/24
➥-dport http -j  ACCEPT
ipchains -A forward -s 0.0.0.0/0 -d 38.110.200.0/24
➥-dport telnet -j  ACCEPT


ipchains -A forward -s 38.110.200. /24  -d 0.0.0.0/0
➥-sport smtp -j  ACCEPT
ipchains -A forward -s 38.110.200. /24  -d 0.0.0.0/0
➥-sport http -j  ACCEPT
ipchains -A forward -s 38.110.200. /24  -d 0.0.0.0/0
➥-sport telnet -j  ACCEPT
```

Note that the first three rules will match incoming connections, whereas the last three rules will match outgoing responses to those connections. Because you have only added rules to the forward chain, you're not yet allowing any connections to the Linux firewall itself. Perhaps you want to be able to telnet to the server for maintenance, but only from a known internal host of IP address 38.110.200.10 (ideally, the system administrator's workstation). The following two rules will allow you to do so:

```
ipchains -A input -s 38.110.200.10 -dport telnet -j ACCEPT
ipchains -A output -d 38.110.200.10 -sport telnet -j ACCEPT
```

As with the previous example, you need to allow incoming access for the Telnet traffic, but also outgoing access for the responses.

Finally, let's say you want to guard against packet spoofing by ensuring that all traffic that leaves the internal network has the proper source address:

```
ipchains -A forward -i eth1 -s !38.110.200.0/24 -j REJECT
```

This command uses an inverse rule by stating that all traffic that enters the server at interface eth1 (the private interface) and does not contain a source IP address in the 38.110.200.0 class-C network should be rejected.

As of Linux kernel 2.4, the functionality once provided by ipwfadm and ipchains is now provided by Netfilter and its iptables user space tool. I recommend that you deploy your Linux firewall on a 2.4 kernel machine and that you use the Netfilter package for packet filtering. This is the topic of discussion of the next section.

THE PRESENT: NETFILTER

Linux kernel 2.4 includes a number of features and stability enhancements that make it a very robust platform to use for your firewall. One of the most noticeable improvements of this kernel version is the packet-filtering subsystem, which is now named *Netfilter*. The development of Netfilter has been largely funded by Watchguard Technologies. This U.S.–based company develops and markets commercial firewalls appliances based on Linux platforms, as well as security services based on its firewall platforms.

The next section explains how to configure your Linux kernel using Netfilter support to build a Network layer firewall using a Linux server.

Configuring Netfilter

In order to configure Netfilter support into the kernel, install the 2.4 kernel sources and enter **Y** to the CONFIG_NETFILTER question during the make config stage of the kernel configuration.

NOTE
The details of kernel configuration are beyond the scope of a security book. See *Linux System Administration* by Vicki Stanfield and Roderick W. Smith (Sybex, 2001) to find out more about Linux kernel configuration.

By default, a Linux system is configured as a network host—not as a router. The RFCs that define Internet standards require that hosts do *not* forward packets. However, for a Linux system to act as a firewall, it must forward packets. In effect, for a Linux system to act as a firewall, it must first act as a router. Therefore, once the kernel is configured to support filtering, you enable IP forwarding by setting the `ip_forward` switch to `true`. You can do so by setting the variable to 1. One way to do this is to set the value of the `ip_forward` switch through the `/proc` filesystem, as in the following example:

```
echo 1 > /proc/sys/net/ipv4/ip_forward
```

Every time the system restarts, the `ip_forward` switch is cleared to 0 and must be explicitly reset to 1. Add the `echo` line to a startup script such as `/etc/rc.d/rc.local` to set the switch back to 1. Some Linux distributions (for example, Red Hat and Caldera) attempt to simplify this process by providing an argument to the `network` startup script that explicitly sets the `ip_forward` switch. For example, on a Red Hat 7 system, setting `net.ipv4.ip_forward` in the `/etc/sysctl.conf` file sets the `ip_forward` switch to a corresponding value. The following example sets `ip_forward` to 1:

```
[ramon]$ head -2 /etc/sysctl.conf
# Enables packet forwarding
net.ipv4.ip_forward = 1
```

On a Caldera system, the `ip_forward` value can be set through the `/etc/sysconfig/network` file by setting a value for `IPFORWARDING`. If `IPFORWARDING` is set to `true` or `yes`, `ip_forward` is set to 1. If it is set to `false` or `no`, `ip_forward` is set to 0. The following example sets `ip_forward` to 1 to enable forwarding:

```
[ramon]$ cat /etc/sysconfig/network
NETWORKING=yes
IPFORWARDING=yes
HOSTNAME=ibis.foobirds.org
```

Personally, I recommend that you use the `echo` command to directly set `/proc/sys/net/ipv4/ip_forward`. The extensions that various vendors add to simplify setting this switch often increase the complexity of the task because the extensions are different. The `echo` command works the same on all Linux distributions.

NOTE
The Netfilter kernel feature provides backward compatibility by allowing you to create packet-filtering rules with both `ipfwadm` and `ipchains`.

Part III

iptables

An integral part of Rusty Russell's Netfilter package, iptables, is the user space utility that you use to affect changes in the three built-in Network-layer kernel-filtering chains (input, output, and forward). An evolution of the ipchains utility, iptables only runs on the 2.3 and 2.4 Linux kernels, and it differs from ipchains in a number of important areas:

▶ The names of the built-in parameters (INPUT, OUTPUT, and FORWARD) have changed from lowercase to uppercase.

▶ The -i (interface descriptor) flag now designates the *incoming* interface and only works in the input and forward chains. If you need an interface descriptor for a rule in the forward or output chain, use the -o flag instead.

▶ The ipchains -y flag (to match IP packets with the SYN bit set) is now --syn.

▶ You can now zero a single chain (with the -Z option) while listing it. (This capability did not work in ipchains.)

▶ Zeroing built-in chains clears policy counters (also a bug fix).

▶ REJECT and LOG chain actions are now extended targets (separate kernel modules).

▶ Chain names can now be up to 31 characters.

▶ The ipchains MASQ chain is now called MASQUERADE and uses a different syntax (see the section "Network Address Translation").

Figure 16.1 shows the flow of packets as they move around the kernel and shows where the three chains fit within the overall process flow.

As discussed in the "Using ipchains" section, *chain* is the term used to describe a set of rules that are checked in sequence. These rules determine what is done with the packets. Consider the following example:

```
[ramon]$ sudo iptables -A INPUT -p tcp –dport smtp -j ACCEPT
[ramon]$ sudo iptables -A INPUT -j DROP
```

This simple example adds two rules to the input built-in chain. The first rule matches all packets whose Transport layer protocol is TCP and whose destination TCP port is 25 (Internet mail or Simple Mail Transfer Protocol [SMTP]). If a packet matches this rule, Netfilter is to accept this packet. The second rule is a *catchall rule* (sometimes called the *stealth rule* because it hides the server from all external systems not explicitly allowed to talk directly to it). The catchall rule instructs Netfilter to drop all other input chain traffic. The two rules in the preceding example might be used to ensure that your mail server is only accepting connections destined for the SMTP port.

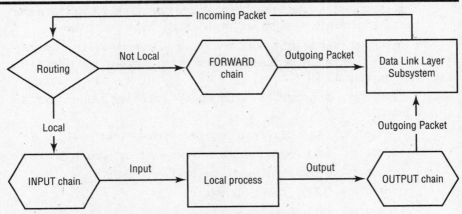

FIGURE 16.1:   Linux kernel packet-filtering built-in chains

NOTE

One of the most important enhancements of the Netfilter framework over the legacy packet-filtering support in pre-2.4 Linux kernels is the handling of both the input and output chains. Before Netfilter, the kernel consulted the input chain for all packets received from the network driver, regardless of whether the packet would eventually be bound for another system (routing) or for the local system (local processing). The same applied to the output chain, with both forwarded and locally originated packets. This situation forced network administrators to apply nonintuitive rules to the input chain to account for both types of packets. With Netfilter, only packets bound for local processing are subject to the input chain, and only packets originated at the local host and bound for another host are subject to the output chain.

Both iptables and its ancestors (ipfwadm, ipchains) fulfill the same need: to reinstate a number of packet-filtering rules to the kernel every time the system reboots. Because the kernel does not have any non-volatile storage, you need to reinitialize your packet-filtering policy using the iptables scripts every time your system comes up. These rules do not survive system reboots, so you must place your iptables commands in a script file and place the script in the /etc/rc.d/init.d directory.

Part III

Using *iptables*

Not all Linux distributions ship with iptables standard. Simply browse on over to your favorite RPM depot (my favorite is www.rpmfind.net) and install the latest version as follows:

```
[ramon]$ sudo rpm -i iptables-1.1.1-2.i386.rpm
```

This command installs a number of shared libraries in /usr/lib; a man page for iptables; and /sbin/iptables, the main executable.

You must operate with root privileges at all times when invoking the iptables command, because it is actually writing the chain rules to the running kernel.

The general command-line syntax of the iptables command is as follows:

```
iptables -[ADC] chain rule-specifications [options]

iptables -[RI] chain rulenum rule-specifications [options]

iptables -D chain rulenum [options]

iptables -[LFZ] [chain] [options]

iptables -[NX] chain

iptables -P chain target [options]

iptables -E old-chain-name new-chain-name
```

The command-line switches and their meanings are listed in Table 16.3.

TABLE 16.3: *iptables* Command-Line Switches

Switch	Meaning
-t *table*	Select the table to act upon. There are currently three of them: filter (the default), nat (Network Address Translation, and mangle (specialized packet translation).
-A	Add a rule to a chain (append to the end of the chain).
-D	Delete a rule from a chain.
-C	Create a new chain.
-R	Replace an existing rule in the chain.
-L	List all rules in the chain.
-I	Insert numbered rules in the chain.
-F	Flush all rules from the chain (empty the chain).
-Z	Zero (reset) the packet and byte counters on all chains.

TABLE 16.3 continued: *iptables* Command-Line Switches

Switch	Meaning
-N	Create a new chain.
-X	Delete the user-defined chain.
-P	Set policy for the chain to the given target.
-E	Rename the chain.

The [*options*] field for the iptables command can take one of values listed in Table 16.4.

TABLE 16.4: *iptables* Command-Line Options

Option	Meaning
--verbose	Display rich (verbose) output.
--numeric	Output IP addresses in numeric format (no DNS lookup).
--exact	Expand numbers in the output.
--line-numbers	Show line numbers when listing the rules.

iptables Rule Specifications

The real power in the iptables command is its ability to match a specific type of traffic using its rich ruleset. Every packet that is forwarded from the server arrives at the server, or is originated by the server, and is compared to the ruleset for the appropriate chain (forward, input, or output). If the packet matches the rule, the specified action (defined by the -j *action* option) is taken. Table 16.5 lists the parameters to be used in the rule-specifications portion of the iptables command.

TABLE 16.5: *iptables* Rule Specification Parameters

Parameter	Meaning
-p [!]*protocol*	Protocol ID to match. This value can be tcp, udp, icmp, or any numeric or alphabetic representation of a service in /etc/services.

TABLE 16.5 continued: *iptables* Rule Specification Parameters

PARAMETER	MEANING
-s [!]*address[/*mask*]*	Source address to match. This value can be a host name, an IP address, or a network name in network/mask format.
--sport [*port:*[*port*]]	Source port or source port range.
-d [!]*address[/*mask*]*	Destination address to match. Follows the same rules as the -s parameter.
--dport [*port:*[*port*]]	Destination port or destination port range.
-i [!]*interface*	Interface through which the packet was received, such as eth0, ppp0, and so on.
-o [!]*interface*	Interface through which the packet is to be sent, such as eth0, ppp0, and so on.
[!] -f	Indication that the packet is a second or subsequent fragment of a larger fragmented packet.

Note that for each of the parameters listed in Table 16.5, a leading exclamation mark (!) instructs iptables to look for packets that do not meet that criterion. The rule specification parameters for iptables are very similar to the parameters available to ipchains, and they include options to match the protocol ID of the incoming packet (-p), the source and destination address (-s and -d), and the source and destination port number (-sport and -dport).

In addition to these basic parameters, you can specify extended matching parameters for packets of certain types (such as tcp, udp, and icmp) by using protocol-specific rules. For example, the following iptables line will match and accept all ICMP packets that carry the echo-request type (the type of packets used by the ping application):

```
iptables -A INPUT -p icmp --icmp-type echo-request -j ACCEPT
```

The converse of the previous command is

```
iptables -A OUTPUT -p icmp --icmp-type echo-reply -j ACCEPT
```

where you allow the local system to reply to the echo-request with an echo-reply, so that your system responds to ping requests properly.

Table 16.6 lists the protocol-specific parameters corresponding to the TCP, UDP, and ICMP traffic types included in iptables.

TABLE 16.6: *iptables* Protocol-Specific Packet-Matching Parameters

PARAMETER	MEANING	PROTOCOL TYPE
`--sport [!]` `[port[:port]]`	Matches packets with a given source port, or from a given *port:port* range.	`tcp, udp`
`--dport [!]` `[port[:port]]`	Matches packets with a given destination port, or from a given *port:port* range.	
`--port [!]` *port*	Matches packets with an equal source and destination port.	
`--tcp-flags [!]` *mask comp*	Matches packets with TCP flags as specified. Flags are SYN, ACK, FIN, RST, URG, PSH, ALL, and NONE.	`tcp`
`[!] --syn`	Matches TCP packets with the SYN bit set and the ACK and FIN bits cleared.	
`--tcp-option [!]` *number*	Matches if the packet has the TCP option set.	
`--icmp-type [!]` *typename*	Matches if the packet has the given ICMP type.	`icmp`

In addition, `iptables` allows you to load so-called *extended packet-matching modules*. These are similar to external plug-ins that can be added to the basic `iptables` package to dynamically extend its ability to match packets. In order to extend the syntax of an `iptables` command with one of these modules, simply use the `-m` *module* option.

The following extended packet-matching modules are included in the standard `iptables` distribution:

- `owner`—Matches packets on the characteristics of the local packet creator. As such, it applies only to the output chain.

- `state`—Allows access to the connection-tracking state for this packet.

- `tos`—Matches the eight bits of the type-of-service field in the IP header.

Part III

▶ limit—Regulates the rate at which the rule should match incoming packets. It is most often used to reduce the rate at which packets are accepted into an interface to avoid denial-of-service attacks.

Table 16.7 lists the parameters that are available for building rules when preceded by the -m *module* switch. The leftmost column includes the module to which the parameter applies.

TABLE 16.7: *iptables* Extended Packet-Matching Parameters

PARAMETER	EXTENDED MODULE	MEANING
--uid-owner *userid*	-m owner	Matches if the packet was created by a process with the given user ID.
--gid-owner *groupid*		Matches if the packet was created by a process with the given group ID.
--pid-owner *processid*		Matches if the packet was created by a process with the given process ID.
--sid-owner *sessionid*		Matches if the packet was created by a process with the given session group.
--state *state*	-m state	Matches one of the following states: INVALID, ESTABLISHED, NEW, or RELATED.
--tos *tos*	-m tos	Matches the 8-bit type-of-service (TOS) field in the standard IPv4 packet.
--limit *rate*	-m limit	Maximum average packet rate. Used to restrict a certain kind of packets to a maximum frequency. The rate must have one of the following suffixes: /second, /minute, /hour, or /day. Default is 5/hour.
--limit-burst *number*		Maximum initial number of packets. Used to restrict the maximum burst of packets of a given type. Default is 5.

For example, let's say your firewall is protecting a private server whose primary mission is to serve web content but that also runs an FTP server for a few of your customers. You would like to allow unrestricted HTTP traffic to this server:

```
iptables -A FORWARD -p tcp -dport 80 -j ACCEPT
```

But, you want to limit FTP connections to one every 30 seconds (or two per minute):

```
iptables -A FORWARD -p tcp --syn -dport 21 -m limit --limit
➡2/minute  -j ACCEPT

iptables -A FORWARD -p tcp -dport 21 -j ACCEPT
```

Note that in addition to the -m limit extended match, you're also matching --syn type connections in the first command in the preceding example. Doing so ensures that you only rate-limit connection requests. The rest of FTP traffic is accepted by the second command.

As you can see, the iptables command has a very complex syntax. The next section presents some examples of how you can use iptables, describes a number of real-world network architecture scenarios, and offers suggested iptables commands that would be used in each case.

SAMPLE FIREWALL SCENARIOS

The following example scenarios should capture the most popular network architectures in place today, from the simple dial-on-demand connection to a complex scenario featuring a dedicated router and a demilitarized zone where you can offer public services without compromising the security of your private network.

Single-Homed Dial-up Server

Most small enterprises or branch offices have a single, non-dedicated connection to the Internet, and they don't want anyone coming back into their network or their firewall. Furthermore, many of these temporary connections are broadband (Internet over cable) connections, where the medium is shared by all the subscribers who are currently connected. This is breeding ground for intrusion and eavesdropping, and firewall protection should always be included in such a scenario.

In addition, most home users who use DSL or cable connections typically have more than one host on their network from which they want to access the public Internet. Linux offers NPAT Network Address Translation through Netfilter's masquerading feature.

Consider the example (illustrated in Figure 16.2) in which your dial-up server has two interfaces:

▶ ppp0, a dial-on-demand Point-to-Point Protocol (PPP) connection to your ISP

▶ eth0, a fast Ethernet connection to your private LAN

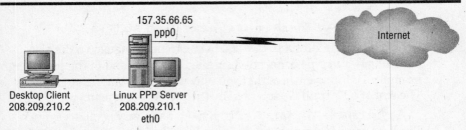

FIGURE 16.2:   Single-homed dial-up server architecture

Let's create an iptables configuration for this scenario. Take a look at Listing 16.1.

Listing 16.1: Single-Homed Dial-Up Server

```
iptables -N protect
iptables -A protect -m state --state ESTABLISHED,RELATED -j
➡ACCEPT
iptables -A protect -m state --state NEW -i ! ppp0 -j ACCEPT
iptables -A protect -j DROP
iptables -A INPUT -j protect
iptables -A FORWARD -j protect
```

The first line defines a new chain called protect, which is where you'll do all your filtering. (This is done for convenience, so you don't have to enter the same filter rules in multiple built-in chains.) The second line instructs iptables to allow any incoming packets to the dial-up server as long as they are in response to a previously open connection (ESTABLISHED, RELATED). The third line allows new connections to be forwarded through the firewall, but only if the connection is not coming from interface ppp0; therefore, it must be coming from eth0, the only other interface on the server. This step ensures that it is an outgoing connection. The fourth line finishes the protect chain with a stealth rule, ensuring that any traffic that does not match a previous rule is dropped by the firewall.

The last two lines in Listing 16.1 are not part of the newly created `protect` chain, as the –A options of those lines clearly indicate. These two lines are the rules that send packets to the new chain by forwarding packets that arrive in the input, forward chains to the `protect` chain. Note that you are not restricting the output chain at all, so you are allowing any outbound connections that originate from the dial-up server itself.

Dual-Homed Firewall: Public and Private Addresses

At a company's central location and at some of its larger branch offices, you'll typically find a dedicated router supporting a full-time connection to the Internet. The most straightforward perimeter security architecture calls for a firewall device *in series* with the LAN connection to the router. Such a device ensures that all traffic coming in and out of the Internet is inspected by the packet-filtering firewall. Consider the sample architecture depicted in Figure 16.3, where the local network is 208.209.210.0/24 and the router's public interface is 157.35.66.65.

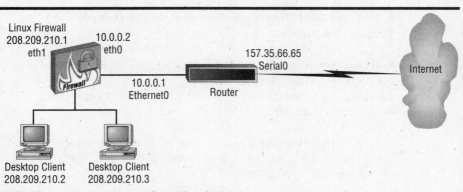

FIGURE 16.3: Dual-homed firewall architecture

NOTE

The firewall's public interface and the router's private interface do not need routable addresses because their connection is in essence point-to-point. You use the 10.0.0.0/24 network for this connection.

Let's consider a policy (in Listing 16.2) that allows for Secure Shell (SSH) inbound access, while blocking all other type of requests. All types of outbound TCP connections are still permitted. ICMP inbound traffic is restricted to echo requests (service 0).

Listing 16.2: Dual-Homed Firewall Architecture: SSH Incoming Services

```
# Flush all the rules out of the the chains
iptables -F INPUT
iptables -F OUTPUT
iptables -F FORWARD

# Set the default policy for the FORWARD chain to deny all
iptables -P FORWARD deny

# Block all incoming traffic coming from public interface
➥(eth0)
iptables -A INPUT -i eth0 -j DROP

# Block all outgoing traffic going out the public interface
➥(eth0)
iptables -A OUTPUT -o eth0 -j DROP

# Instruct Netfilter to accept fragmented packets (-f)
iptables -A FORWARD -f -j ACCEPT

# Accept incoming TCP packets from established connections
# (--state ESTABLISHED,RELATED)
iptables -A FORWARD -m state -p tcp --state ESTABLISHED,
➥RELATED -j ACCEPT

# Accept incoming TCP connections to SSH arriving at eth0
iptables -A FORWARD  -p tcp -i eth0 -d 208.209.210.0/24
➥--dport ssh -j ACCEPT

# Accept all outgoing TCP connections entering the private
# interface (eth1)
iptables -A FORWARD -p tcp -i eth1 -j ACCEPT

# Accept all outgoing UDP connections entering the private
# interface (eth1)
iptables -A FORWARD -p udp -i eth1 -j ACCEPT
```

```
# Accept incoming ICMP packet of "echo reply (=0)" type
➡(ping replies)
iptables -A FORWARD  -p icmp -i eth0 -d 208.209.210.0/24
    --icmp-type 0 -j ACCEPT

# Accept all outgoing ICMP connections entering the private
# interface (eth1)
iptables -A FORWARD -p icmp -i eth1 -j ACCEPT

# Drop all other traffic in the FORWARD chain
iptables -A FORWARD -j DROP
```

Note that the last line is not really needed because you have established a deny policy (where everything is denied by default unless specifically allowed) for the forward chain at the top of the script. However, it's always a good idea to err on the side of caution.

Next, let's restrict the previous policy by only allowing SSH, WWW, SMTP, and DNS outbound services (see Listing 16.3). The lines in **bold-face** are the changes from the previous scenario in Listing 16.2.

Listing 16.3: Dual-Homed Firewall Architecture: SSH Incoming Services; SSH, WWW, SMTP, and DNS Outgoing Services Only

```
# Flush all the rules out of the chains
iptables -F INPUT
iptables -F OUTPUT
iptables -F FORWARD

# Set the default policy for the FORWARD chain to deny all
iptables -P FORWARD deny

# Block all incoming traffic coming from public interface
➡(eth0)
iptables -A INPUT -i eth0 -j DROP

# Block all outgoing traffic going out the public interface
➡(etho)
iptables -A OUTPUT -o eth0 -j DROP

# Instruct Netfilter to accept fragmented packets (-f)
iptables -A FORWARD -f -j ACCEPT
```

Part III

```
# Accept incoming TCP packets from established connections
# (--state ESTABLISHED,RELATED)iptables -A FORWARD -m state -p
➥tcp --state ESTABLISHED,RELATED -j ACCEPT

# Accept incoming TCP connections to SSH arriving at eth0
iptables -A FORWARD  -p tcp -i eth0 -d 208.209.210.0/24
➥--dport ssh -j ACCEPT

# Accept outgoing TCP connections to SSH, WWW, SMTP only
iptables -A FORWARD  -p tcp -i eth1 --dport ssh,www,smtp -j
➥ACCEPT

# Accept incoming UDP packets as response from DNS service
➥(port 53)
iptables -A FORWARD -p udp -i eth0 --sport domain -j ACCEPT

# Accept outgoing UDP connections to port 53 (DNS) only
iptables -A FORWARD -p udp -i eth1 --dport domain -j ACCEPT

# Accept incoming ICMP packet of "echo reply (=0)" type
➥(ping replies)
iptables -A FORWARD  -p icmp -i eth0 -d 208.209.210.0/24
    --icmp-type 0 -j ACCEPT

# Accept all outgoing ICMP connections entering the private
# interface (eth1)
iptables -A FORWARD -p icmp -i eth1 -j ACCEPT

# Drop all other traffic in the FORWARD chain
iptables -A FORWARD -j DROP
```

Note that, unlike TCP services like SSH and Telnet, you cannot effectively restrict return UDP traffic to packets that reflect an established outgoing connection. This means you need to allow your firewall to accept all UDP traffic whose source port is 53 (DNS—domain lookup service).

Trihomed Firewall with a Demilitarized Zone

A more elaborate network architecture features a trihomed firewall, including a public interface, a private interface, and a third interface that services

a demilitarized zone (DMZ). The DMZ allows you to offer public services with some degree of control, and without allowing anonymous
users entry in your private network space. Figure 16.4 illustrates the
trihomed firewall, which adds a new network 64.65.66.0/24 that serves
the DMZ with two servers (web and mail) to the architecture depicted
in Figure 16.3.

To extend the dual-homed firewall example (SSH and Telnet inbound,
all outbound), you add a policy (see Listing 16.4) that allows only your
remote branch users (from network 208.209.210.0/24) access to the
DMZ web server, while granting unrestricted Internet access to the DMZ
mail server. The lines in **boldface** are the changes from the previous scenario (Listing 16.3).

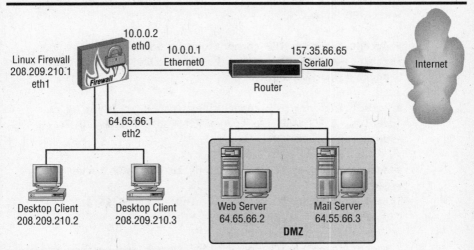

FIGURE 16.4:   Trihomed firewall architecture with DMZ

Listing 16.4: Sample *iptables* Script for Trihomed Firewall Architecture with DMZ

```
# Flush all the rules out of all three default chains
iptables -F INPUT
iptables -F OUTPUT
iptables -F FORWARD

# Set the default policy for the FORWARD chain to deny all
iptables -P FORWARD deny
```

```
# Block all incoming traffic coming from public interface
➥(eth0)
iptables -A INPUT -i eth0 -j DROP

# Block all outgoing traffic going out the public interface
➥(eth0)
iptables -A OUTPUT -o eth0 -j DROP

# Instruct Netfilter to accept fragmented packets (-f)
iptables -A FORWARD -f -j ACCEPT

# Accept incoming TCP packets from established connections
# (--state ESTABLISHED,RELATED)
iptables -A FORWARD -m state -p tcp --state ESTABLISHED,
➥RELATED -j ACCEPT

# Accept incoming TCP connections to SSH arriving at eth0
iptables -A FORWARD  -p tcp -i eth0 -d 208.209.210.0/24
--dport ssh -j ACCEPT

# Accept incoming TCP connections to SSH arriving at eth0
iptables -A FORWARD  -p tcp -i eth0 -d 208.209.210.0/24
--dport ssh -j ACCEPT

# Accept incoming TCP connections to DMZ SMTP server
➥(64.65.66.3)
iptables -A FORWARD  -p tcp -i eth0 -d 64.65.66.3
--dport smtp -j ACCEPT

# Accept incoming TCP connections to web server from remote
➥branch only
iptables -A FORWARD  -p tcp -i eth0 -s 128.129.130.0/24 -d
➥64.65.66.2 --dport  www -j ACCEPT

# Accept all outgoing TCP connections received via both
➥eth1 and eth2
# (the private and the DMZ interfaces respectively)
iptables -A FORWARD -p tcp -i eth1,eth2 -j ACCEPT

# Accept all outgoing UDP connections received via both
➥eth1 and eth2
# (the private and the DMZ interfaces respectively)
iptables -A FORWARD -p udp -i eth1,eth2 -j ACCEPT
```

```
# Accept incoming ICMP packet of "echo reply (=0)" type
➥(ping replies)
iptables -A FORWARD  -p icmp -i eth0 -d 208.209.210.0/24
    --icmp-type 0 -j ACCEPT
iptables -A FORWARD  -p icmp -i eth0 -d 64.65.66.0/24
    --icmp-type 0 -j ACCEPT

# Accept all outoing ICMP connections received from either
➥the
# private interface (eth1) or the DMZ interface (eth2)
iptables -A FORWARD -p icmp -i eth1, eth2 -j ACCEPT

# Drop all other traffic in the FORWARD chain
iptables -A FORWARD -j DROP
```

In Listing 16.4, you have simply added two rules to the forward chain: one to allow all SMTP traffic to the mail server (64.65.66.3) and another to allow traffic source from 208.209.210.0/24 to connect to port 80 of the DMZ web server (64.65.66.3). Note that you must also allow ICMP responses to enter eth0bound for the DMZ and to exit through the DMZ interface, eth2.

Protecting against Well-Known Attacks

In addition to the capability to enforce access control to your internal hosts, Netfilter and iptables can be used to protect against specific types of Internet attacks by filtering traffic that matches the fingerprint of the attack. This section describes sample iptables statements that you can use to address a number of these well-known vulnerabilities.

Address Spoofing

Many firewall configurations allow the packet to be forwarded after verifying that it has an address from the private network in the source field of the header. The problem is that it's trivial for an attacker to synthetically create a "spoofed" packet generated from their network but with your source address. You can protect your site from address spoofing by requiring that packets with the local network's source address be received on the interface connected to the local network using an iptables command like the following:

```
iptables -A FORWARD -s internal_network -i public_interface
➥-j DROP
```

Part III

This command adds a rule to the forward chain that matches traffic sourced from the internal network, but that enters the system at the public interface. By adding this command, you are forcing Netfilter to drop spoofed packets arriving at the public interface of your firewall.

For example, consider the dual-homed firewall architecture depicted back in Figure 16.3, where the local network is 208.209.210.0/24 and the router's public interface is 157.35.66.65. An address-spoofing rule for this firewall would look like the following:

```
iptables -A FORWARD -s 208.209.210.0/24 -i eth0 -j DROP
```

This rule examines packets that arrive in the public interface (eth0) and drops them quietly if they carry a source address in the (private) 208.209.210.0/24 network.

Smurf Attack

A *smurf* attack is staged by sending an ICMP echo request (ping) packet to the broadcast address of your internal network. The packet's source is forged with the address of the target of the smurf attack, which gets flooded by ICMP echo responses from all your internal hosts.

The following iptables command guards against smurf attacks by preventing the forged ICMP echo-request from entering your network:

```
iptables -A FORWARD -p icmp -d
➡internal_network_broadcast_address -j  DENY
```

This command adds a rule to the forward chain that matches any ICMP packets coming into any of the interfaces of the firewall whose destination is the broadcast address of your internal LAN. When this rule is matched, the packet takes the DROP action. For example, in the network depicted back in Figure 16.4, you would use the following command:

```
iptables -A FORWARD -p icmp -d 208.209.210.255 -j DENY
```

In this case, you're looking for ICMP traffic whose destination is 208.209.210.255, the broadcast address of the 208.209.210.0/24 network.

Syn-Flood Attack

A *syn-flood* attack is staged by sending a large number of TCP connection requests (with the SYN flag set) to a host while suppressing the normal SYN–ACK responses, thereby attempting to consume all of the host's available data structures, which are busy keeping track of these half-open connections.

Using the limit external matching module, you can throttle the acceptance of TCP SYN requests to one per second using the following iptables command:

```
iptables -A FORWARD -p tcp --syn -m limit --limit 1/s -j
➥ACCEPT
```

A rate of one TCP SYN request per second should be acceptable for most Internet servers, but it restricts just enough occurrences of incoming SYN requests to ensure that your systems always have enough available resources to handle legitimate connections.

Port-Scanner Attack

Many port-scanner applications try to identify every open TCP and UDP port in your system by sending a SYN or FIN signal to a given port range and expecting an RST signal for those ports not active. You can limit this activity to one incidence per second with the following iptables command:

```
iptables -A FORWARD -p tcp --tcp-flags SYN,ACK,FIN,RST RST
➥-m limit --limit 1/s -j ACCEPT
```

This command adds a rule to the forward chain that matches TCP traffic that arrives at the firewall with the SYN, ACK, and FIN flags unset, and the RST flag set. When packets match this description, they are accepted at a rate of only one per second.

Ping-of-Death Attack

It is possible to kill certain operating systems by sending unusually large and unusually frequent ICMP echo (ping) requests. This is called a *ping-of-death* attack. The following iptables command limits the acceptance of such pings to one per second:

```
iptables -A FORWARD -p icmp --icmp-type echo-request -m limit
➥--limit 1/s -j ACCEPT
```

In fact, I recommend that you block ICMP requests at your firewall altogether using the command

```
iptables -A FORWARD -p icmp --icmp-type echo-request -j DROP
```

unless you have a legitimate need to have your host be reached via ping from the outside.

Part III

NETWORK ADDRESS TRANSLATION

One of the problems facing the current installed base of Internet-connected hosts is the scarcity of network addresses. Although four billion IP addresses may seem like more than enough to go around, a good number of them are not usable because of subnetting and non-contiguous allocation. In addition, many enterprises never felt the need to connect their networks to the public Internet, so they used addresses from the nonroutable blocks (RFC1819), a number of addresses set aside for use in non-Internet-connected networks.

When faced with the task of integrating a privately numbered network with the Internet, you have to make an important choice: renumber or translate. On the one hand, you can request a routable IP block from your Internet service provider and go through the pain of renumbering (and often re-subnetting) your entire network; or, if your connectivity needs are modest, you can use NAT.

The advantages of NAT are twofold:

▶ You are free to use whatever numbering scheme you choose while still allowing your users to connect to the public Internet.

▶ If you use nonroutable internal addresses, intruders can't access your internal hosts as easily as if they were naturally routable, especially when they're hidden behind NAPT, a many-to-one NAT described shortly.

NAT involves modifying the source address of the packet before sending the packet to its destination. This process requires the NAT device to keep track of the modification so that the step can be reversed when a response is received. There are three types of NAT that vary depending on how the NAT device keeps track of the translation:

Network Address Port Translation (NAPT)   Also known as *many-to-one NAT*, NAPT is best suited for network gateways that can only use a single public address. The NAT device accepts outbound connection requests from private clients and keeps track of each connection with two pieces of information:

▶ The private IP address of the internal host

▶ The source port that the NAT device used as the Transport layer port number for the request

This information allows the NAT device to route return traffic properly, even when two internal clients are connecting to the same external server. Deploying NPAT hides your entire private network behind a single public address, thereby reducing your exposure to the Internet and drastically reducing your need for routable address space. The principal disadvantage of NPAT is the fact that you cannot host any services on your internal network because the NPAT device is unable to accept incoming requests from the Internet. Use Static NAT if hosting services on your internal network is a requirement.

Static NAT   Also known as *one-to-one NAT*, Static NAT is the simplest case, where a single public address is mapped to a single private address. The NAT device must be configured to perform this mapping beforehand. Unlike NAPT, for example, where you can have a whole network hiding behind a single address, you must know beforehand which addresses you will be protecting because you need to assign them a public equivalent.

Load-Sharing Network Address Translation (LSNAT)   An extension to plain, Static NAT, LSNAT allows you to advertise a single address to the public Internet while requests made to that address are serviced by a number of internal hosts. Consecutive requests are handed to the pool of internal addresses in a round-robin fashion, which achieves a load-sharing effect for incoming connections. This approach is useful when deploying a web server farm in your DMZ, where all servers can contain exact replicas of your web content. As the demand increases, simply add servers and register the new private address with the binding tables in your NAT device. To the outside world, it still appears as if there is only one web server.

Configuring NAT Using *iptables*

Consider the network architecture depicted in Figure 16.3. If your internal network does not contain routable addresses, and you still want to connect to the Internet from your private hosts, you need to perform NAT. The most popular approach for a small network with a single routable address is NPAT, which is also referred to as *masquerading* or *hiding*. Simply add the line in Listing 16.5 to your iptables configuration.

Part III

Listing 16.5: Sample *iptables* NPAT Configuration

```
iptables -t nat -A POSTROUTING -o ppp0 -j MASQUERADE
```

Notice that the command in Listing 16.5 uses the option -t nat. The majority of iptables commands operate on the *filtering* table (which contains the built-in chains input, output, and forward). NAT relies on a different Netfilter table, appropriately named nat, which contains the built-in chains prerouting, postrouting, and output. These chains have the following characteristics:

▶ The prerouting chain attempts to match the packet as soon as it enters the system.

▶ The postrouting chain attempts to match the packet once the routing decision has been made based on its destination.

▶ The output chain matches locally generated traffic before a routing decision has been made based on its destination.

The -o ppp0 option directs iptables to apply the MASQUERADE rule to the packet just before it goes out the ppp0 interface, so that any other processes on the server itself will see the packet with its original source address. This is an important point because it implies that packet-filtering rules applied to that packet will also see the packet with its original source address. Keep this in mind as you write your iptables rules.

The example in Listing 16.5 performs NPAT on the outgoing packet, using the address assigned to ppp0 as the *masquerade-as address*. What if you want to statically bind a specific routable address (such as 208.209.210.1) to a non-routable, private address (such as 10.10.10.1)? You could use Static NAT by specifying the syntax in Listing 16.6.

Listing 16.6: Sample *iptables* Static NAT Configuration

```
iptables -t nat -A POSTROUTING -s 10.10.10.1 -o eth0 -j
➥SNAT --to 208.209.210.1

iptables -t nat -A PREROUTING -s 208.209.210.1 -i eth0 -j
➥DNAT --to 10.10.10.1
```

The first command in Listing 16.6 makes sure that the source field of packets originating from 192.168.1.1 is changed to 208.209.210.1 just before it leaves interface eth0. The second command performs the opposite destination translation just as the packet arrives in eth0 and before routing takes place.

LSNAT can be accomplished by simply specifying a -j DNAT rule where you perform destination NAT from one incoming address to several destination addresses. For example, consider the case where you are hosting a popular web server on public address 208.209.210.1, but would like to share the incoming load to that server among identical servers 10.10.10.1, 10.10.10.2, and 10.10.10.3. Just modify the commands in the previous example, as shown in Listing 16.7.

Listing 16.7: Sample *iptables* LSNAT Configuration

```
iptables -t nat -A POSTROUTING -s 10.10.10.1 -o eth0 -j
➡SNAT --to 208.209.210.1
iptables -t nat -A PREROUTING -s 208.209.210.1 -i eth0 -j
➡DNAT --to 10.10.10.1-10.10.10.3
```

The only difference between Listing 16.7 and Listing 16.6 is that the second rule is translating the incoming 208.209.201.1 destination into the range 10.10.10.1–10.10.10.3, rather than the single 10.10.10.1 address.

WHAT'S NEXT

Building a Linux firewall is conceptually easy, but the devil is in the details. This chapter walked you through the general concept of packet filtering and its implementation in the Linux kernel. You learned about two user space tools that you can use to define the necessary filtering rules: ipchains (introduced with kernel 2.1) and the newer iptables (introduced with kernel 2.3). You got a chance to look at a number of detailed network scenarios, and you saw several sample iptables configurations that reflected several different security policies.

Although the initial cost of deploying a Linux firewall will be lower than many commercial alternatives, crafting a configuration to reflect your security policy takes some serious attention to detail. Packet filtering is your first level of perimeter defense, but a comprehensive security stance will use protection at the Transport and Application layers as well. In this and preceding chapters, you learned how to establish a firewall to protect and secure your LAN.

In the next part of this book, we will move from firewalls based on network server operating systems to firewalls based on the popular Cisco IOS.

Part III

Part IV
Cisco Security Specialist (CSS1) Highlights

Chapter 17

PIX FIREWALL BASICS

This chapter begins our detailed look at Cisco's firewall solutions, laying the groundwork for all the information you need to know to understand the operation and configuration of a PIX Firewall. (For more information about firewalls in general, see Chapter 11, "Understanding Firewalls.")

Let's begin our discussion with a review of firewall technologies. Then we will introduce the Secure PIX Firewall and Cisco's IOS Firewall feature set. We'll cover the hardware and software components of the PIX Firewall, and explain how they fit together to help protect networks. Finally, we'll discuss the PIX Firewall command-line interface and some of the basic commands used to manage the PIX Firewall.

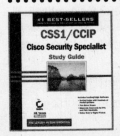

Adapted from *CSS1™/CCIP™: Cisco® Security Specialist Study Guide* by Todd Lammle, Tom Lancaster, Eric Quinn, and Justin Menga

ISBN 0-7821-4049-1 $89.99

Part IV

Reviewing Firewall Technologies

Because there are many types of threats, there are many types of policies to deal with these threats. These policies operate at many different levels, so several different types of firewalls are available. We will concentrate on three common types:

- Application proxy (a type of dual-homed gateway)
- Packet-filtering firewall
- Stateful firewall

Of course, any given "firewall" product may implement one or more of these techniques.

Dual-Homed Gateways

There are several types of dual-homed gateways. *Application proxies* (often called *proxy servers*) and bastion hosts are common examples. All of the dual-homed gateways have one thing in common: Physically and as far as the operating system is concerned, the dual-homed gateway is actually a host on two different networks at the same time. This device is not a router or a switch, whose job it is to forward packets at layer 2 or 3 (the Data Link or Network layer of the OSI model). Rather, the dual-homed gateway acts as a host. Packets are sent to it, and it processes them in the same way as any other host, passing them all the way up to layer 1 (the Application layer), where they are inspected by a proxy application.

The proxy is "application-aware." For example, a web proxy understands the HTTP protocol. It knows what the commands mean and can decide whether users are allowed to access a certain URL or whether specific content returned to the client is allowed inside the network.

Generally speaking, dual-homed gateways are very useful for Application-layer filtering, and they excel at auditing. For instance, if you've used a web proxy server, you may have noticed that the log files are quite detailed and can grow very large.

Unfortunately, dual-homed gateways have several drawbacks:

- They are inherently slow. Their high latency often creates problems with real-time traffic, such as streaming media.

- Because they are application-aware, they must be programmed to understand the application. If the manufacturer does not support the particular service or protocol you need, you will need to find another solution.

- Once it is compromised, the gateway can be used as a launch pad for attacks into the formerly protected network. Typically, this situation is possible on dual-homed gateways because they often run general-purpose operating systems, which makes it easy to develop attack software.

NOTE

Special-purpose operating systems and hardware rarely publish their APIs and other specifications, so developing rogue programs to run on these systems would be an extremely difficult task.

Application gateways are very good at preventing unauthorized access to services or data, both inbound and outbound. They provide some protection against privacy violations on the hosts, but not for data in transit, and they actually become an additional point of failure for denial of service (DoS) attacks.

Packet-Filtering Firewalls

Packet-filtering firewalls operate at a much lower level of the OSI model than dual-homed gateways in the network. In fact, this functionality is often implemented on routers and switches, which only process packets at layers 2 through 4 (Data Link, Network, and Transport).

Packet-filtering firewalls simply match values in the headers of frames and packets and permit or deny packets based on a set of rules. The most commonly used fields are as follows:

- The layer 2 source address and destination address, most often the Media Access Control (MAC) addresses

- The layer 3 source address and destination address, most often the IP or IPX addresses

- The options in the layer 3 header, such as the fragmentation bits

- The layer 4 source address and destination address, most often the TCP or UDP ports

- The options in the layer 4 header, such as the SYN bit

Packet-filtering technology has been around for some time and is often considered an old technology that is no longer useful, but it does have a few advantages:

▶ It is cheap and widely available.

▶ The lower a function is on the OSI model, the faster it is. So, packet-filtering firewalls generally have a tremendous speed advantage compared to application gateways.

▶ Because it is simple, it is fairly reliable and easy to maintain. Its simplicity also makes it easy to implement in hardware.

▶ It is particularly useful in combination with other technologies. In modern security architecture, packet filtering is often used on screening routers.

On the other hand, packet filtering has its share of problems:

▶ The rules are commonly static in nature, so services such as FTP, which use random ports, are often blocked accidentally.

▶ Undesired packets can be fabricated to match the "permit" rules. For instance, a packet could be fabricated to appear as if it was already part of an established TCP connection, and it would be permitted to pass through the firewall.

▶ The order in which the rules are placed is critically important. If you have a large number of rules, it is easy to make mistakes when manually maintaining them.

▶ Older packet-filtering platforms had difficulty with fragmented packets because only the first packet contained the header information. Sending specially formed fragmented packets, or not sending the final fragment, would often crash older host systems.

Despite these shortcomings, packet-filtering technology is still useful. Cisco has implemented this technology in the form of access control lists (ACLs) in all versions of its IOS software. Combining these ACLs with other firewalls, like the PIX Firewall, can create a much more robust security system than either tool by itself.

Stateful Firewalls

Stateful firewalls operate in the same manner as packet-filtering firewalls, but they work on connections instead of packets. Put another way, a stateful firewall has the ability to permit or deny a packet based on other packets. For example, if a TCP packet arrives claiming to be from an established connection (that is, it doesn't have the SYN bit set), the packet-filtering firewall would let it pass; but the stateful firewall can still deny this packet if any of the following conditions are met:

- ▸ It has not seen the three-way handshake of SYN, SYN-ACK, ACK for that connection.

- ▸ The TCP sequence and acknowledgment numbers are not correct (they would be based on the previous packet).

- ▸ The packet contains a response when there wasn't previously a command.

As you can see, when properly implemented, stateful filtering can make forging packets practically impossible.

Stateful firewalls also excel in preventing DoS attacks. For instance, conceivably, you could allow ping traffic into your network. If someone attempted to send you 100,000 Internet Control Message Protocol (ICMP) requests at once, the packet-filtering firewall would let all of them through. However, the stateful firewall could be configured with a reasonable threshold; after this threshold was crossed, it would automatically deny all future requests until the flood subsided.

Generally, stateful firewalls provide the following benefits:

- ▸ Much higher performance than application gateways

- ▸ Stronger security than packet filtering

- ▸ Easy administration

However, because they do not necessarily operate at the Application layer, stateful firewalls do not offer as strong control over applications as do dual-homed gateways. This also means that their auditing will not be as detailed.

Firewall Technology Combinations

Each of the three firewall types mentioned in the previous sections has different strengths and weaknesses. We compare them here academically, but in the real world, they are often used together.

For instance, the application gateway and proxy servers provide some protection for the application, but they themselves are vulnerable to other attacks, such as DoS attacks. To protect the proxy servers, we typically put them in what is called a *screened subnet* or a *DMZ* (demilitarized zone). This is a protected network that sits between a trusted internal network and a totally untrusted external network. From the perspective of a typical company's internal network, the DMZ is trusted less than the internal network, but more than the external network.

Two common screened-subnet designs are used today, as described in the following sections.

Packet-Filtering Router, Stateful Firewall, and Application Proxy Combination

One type of screened subnet employs a packet-filtering router to separate the outside network from the DMZ. Then, a stateful firewall connects the DMZ to the inside network. An application proxy typically resides inside the DMZ, so traffic does not flow directly from the inside network to the outside network or from the outside network directly to the inside network. Instead, all traffic from the inside network to the outside network flows to and from the proxy server. However, traffic from the outside network to the other servers, such as the web and FTP servers, does not pass through the proxy server, but goes directly to the appropriate server. The data flow of this design is shown in Figure 17.1.

The combination of these three firewall technologies provides much more security than any one technology alone. The routers in this network provide high-performance packet filtering, and the application-aware proxy servers make attacks as difficult as possible. The stateful firewall protects the resources on the internal network, without affecting the performance of web servers and other devices in the DMZ.

Another advantage of this design is that the access to the proxy server often requires authentication, based on the user's ID on the internal network (such as an account on a Windows domain). This authentication makes access into the internal network more secure, without requiring the management of an infinite number of accounts on the outside network that are accessing your web and FTP services.

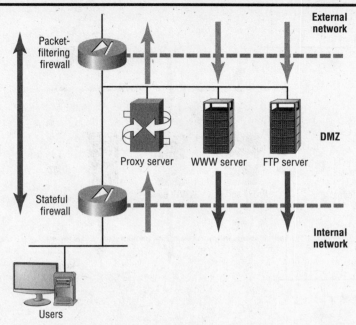

Users

FIGURE 17.1:   Traffic flow in a modern screened subnet

The combination of low-level support by the packet-filtering firewall, application-level support from the dual-homed gateway, and protection from DoS attacks is a classic case of synergy, where the whole is greater than the sum of the parts. This technique is sometimes called *defense-in-depth*.

A Stateful Firewall with Multiple Interfaces

The second type of screened-subnet design is similar to the one just described, but it's a little more efficient and cost-effective. It takes advantage of multiple interfaces on the newer, faster firewalls. However, the traffic flow is fundamentally unchanged. This design is shown in Figure 17.2.

This design has two inherent characteristics, which are both a result of all the data passing through a single firewall. The negative characteristic is that the additional traffic may affect performance. The positive characteristic is that seeing all the traffic may allow the firewall to make more intelligent filtering decisions than a firewall that sees only part of the traffic.

Part IV

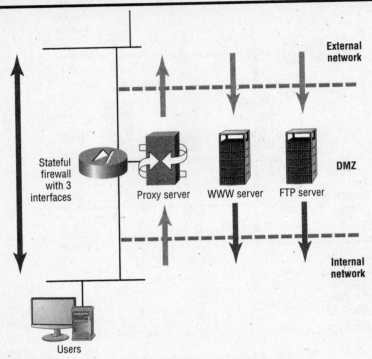

FIGURE 17.2:   A cost-effective alternative DMZ design

INTRODUCING THE CISCO IOS FIREWALL FEATURE SET

Before we move onto our coverage of the PIX Firewall, we will take a quick look at the Cisco IOS Firewall. The IOS Firewall is implemented as a set of features in Cisco's IOS software for use on almost all of Cisco's router platforms. The firewall features were first implemented in version 11.2. The letter *o* in the IOS image's filename designates the presence of the firewall features. For example, the filename c2600-jos56i-mz.120-4.T.bin indicates that the image is version 12.0(4) for the 2600 platform. The j and o indicate it contains the Enterprise and Firewall feature sets, respectively, and the 56 tells you it supports IPSec encryption with a 56-bit key.

WARNING

Although all the features discussed here are in every version of software for the PIX Firewall, do not assume a feature is included in an IOS image. It is possible to buy an IOS Firewall image that does not support IPSec, for instance. The reverse is also true.

The IOS Firewall is designed to be a cost-effective enhancement for the packet filtering that router ACLs have always done. The enhancements specifically include the following:

▶ Stateful inspection

▶ Application-based filtering

▶ Real-time alerts

▶ Defense against network attacks

▶ Per-user authentication and authorization

In addition, full Network Address Translation (NAT) functionality is included in all Cisco IOS Firewall images. NAT is also supported in IP Plus images starting with version 11.2 and IP-only versions 12.0 and higher.

The IOS Firewall is stateful, performs NAT, and does application-based filtering, just like the PIX Firewall. However, it accomplishes these tasks in a much different way internally, even though it may look and act similarly. In fact, the differences are largely transparent to both users and administrators, especially because Cisco has attempted to standardize the command-line syntax as much as possible.

INTRODUCING THE SECURE PIX FIREWALL

Now that you understand the basic firewall technologies and their usefulness, we can describe the basic characteristics of the PIX Firewall. The PIX Firewall is one of the world's premier firewalls because its unique operation provides strong security and very high performance. In this section, we will begin to discuss its operation and various features that contribute to its speed and protection.

Part IV

NOTE

Admittedly, the information in this section is more marketing-related than technical. However, it is important to understand the background and context in which Cisco places the PIX Firewall. This understanding will benefit you immensely when it comes time to select and install a firewall in your network.

The PIX Firewall has its roots in NAT, with the ability to maintain information about the state of each connection that passes through it, and then filter (permit or deny) traffic based on that state. For this reason, it is classified as a stateful firewall.

PIX Firewall Features

The PIX Firewall series uses specially designed hardware and a very small, proprietary, multithreaded kernel. On the lower-end models, the hardware is fixed-configuration, but the higher-end models support modular interface cards for many different types of media, up to gigabit speeds. The advantage is that the extraneous equipment and issues associated with hard drives, CD-ROMs, GUIs, monitors, keyboards, mice, and so on are eliminated, without losing the core functionality of the firewall.

The PIX Firewall features support for IPSec, virtual private networks (VPNs), cut-through proxy switching, inbound and outbound authentication, failover, and more. These features are covered in the following chapters in this section.

Another feature, which administrators will appreciate, is that compared to some firewalls (particularly the ones running on general-purpose operating systems), the PIX Firewall is easy to configure and hard to misconfigure. Unlike many firewalls, the PIX Firewall hardware and software are based on a pessimistic, or restrictive, security model. In other words, by default, everything is denied. To allow network traffic to pass through the PIX Firewall, the PIX must be explicitly configured to accept that traffic.

In contrast, Windows NT and 2000 have a more optimistic model, where practically every service is turned on by default and must be explicitly turned off. Although this is usually done via the firewall's installation scripts, each service still represents an endless supply of vulnerabilities, and the process itself presents the opportunity to misconfigure the firewall.

PIX Firewall Components

In this section, we will explore the parts that make up the PIX Firewall.
Before we get into the nuts and bolts, you should understand that simplicity is an important competitive advantage in the realm of security, because
as components in a system become more complex, there are more opportunities to take advantage of the system. The PIX Firewall has succeeded
in maintaining a very simple, almost minimalist, list of components.

On the PIX Firewall, you can see some of these components by typing
the show version command at the privileged exec prompt (we've boldfaced the sections of interest here for clarity):

```
PIX# show version


Cisco Secure PIX Firewall Version 6.0(1)


Compiled on Thu 17-May-01 20:05 by morlee


PIX up 58 secs


Hardware:  PIX-515, 64 MB RAM, CPU Pentium 200 MHz
Flash i28F640J5 @ 0x300, 16MB
BIOS Flash AT29C257 @ 0xfffd8000, 32KB


0: ethernet0: address is 0050.54ff.076d, irq 10
1: ethernet1: address is 0050.54ff.076e, irq 7
2: ethernet2: address is 00d0.b79d.8856, irq 9


Licensed Features:
Failover:          Enabled
VPN-DES:           Enabled
VPN-3DES:          Disabled
Maximum Interfaces:      6
Cut-through Proxy:     Enabled
Guards:            Enabled
Websense:          Enabled
Throughput:        Unlimited
```

Part IV

```
ISAKMP peers:    Unlimited

Serial Number: 403420127 (0x180bb3df)
Activation Key: 0x9aa99a8d 0xc56166de 0x4ecd338a
  0x5b6d06eb
PIX#
```

As you can see, the components shown by the show version command are the CPU (central processing unit), random access memory (RAM), flash filesystem, BIOS, interfaces, and licensed features. Let's take a closer look at each of these components.

CPU

The PIX Firewall uses the Intel Pentium line of processors as the CPU. This is where the software image is executed and most of the rules are processed. Also, tasks such as encryption using IPSec are performed here (unless an optional VPN accelerator card is installed, which offloads this processing to a dedicated processor).

The show version command shows the type and speed of the processor. The show cpu usage command gives the average processor utilization for the past five seconds, one minute, and five minutes, as in this example:

```
PIX# show cpu usage
CPU utilization for 5 seconds = 0%; 1 minute: 0%;
  5 minutes: 0%
PIX#
```

RAM

RAM is the primary memory used by the PIX Firewall. Instructions being executed by the CPU exist here. Also, RAM is used for packet buffers and the various tables, such as state information, dynamic NAT entries, the translation (xlate) tables (described in the "NAT Mechanisms" section later in this chapter), and more.

The sample show version output shows that this PIX Firewall has 64MB of RAM. You can also use the show memory command to see the available or unused memory:

```
PIX# show memory
67108864 bytes total, 51089408 bytes free
PIX#
```

Flash Filesystem

The physical flash memory used in PIX Firewalls is similar to that used in Cisco's router and switch platforms. However, the filesystem used by the PIX is considerably different.

The filesystem used in Cisco's IOS allows any number of files to be stored, including multiple images, copies of the configuration file, and so on. Each of these can be manipulated by a filename. However, the PIX flash filesystem version 1 divides the flash into four sectors, each of which contains one file. Version 2 of the flash filesystem adds one more sector, for a total of five, to support the GUI configuration software, PIX Device Manager (PDM).

The show flashfs command shows the length of each file, but not its filename:

```
PIX# show flashfs
flash file system:  version:2  magic:0x12345679
  file 0: origin:        0 length:2449464
  file 1: origin: 2490368 length:1463
  file 2: origin:        0 length:0
  file 3: origin:        0 length:0
  file 4: origin: 8257536 length:280
PIX#
```

The files are used as follows:

▶ File 0 is the PIX binary image. This is the BIN file. (See the next section for details on the PIX system image.)

▶ File 1 is the PIX configuration data, viewed with the show config command.

▶ File 2 contains the firewall's IPSec key and certificates.

▶ File 3 contains the PDM software.

▶ File 4 contains downgrade information for previous versions.

Access to these files is much more restricted than access to the IOS flash filesystem. To enhance security, the ability to copy files from flash to FTP, Trivial FTP (TFTP), another file on the flash, or other locations is no longer available. Also gone are flash partitions and the detailed information, such as checksums. Although the lack of these features may not seem like an "enhancement," their exclusion helps prevent your private keys from being stolen. The maintenance of the flash system—such as compacting, formatting, and squeezing—is handled automatically on the PIX Firewall.

System Image

The system image is a binary executable file that resides in file 0 in the flash. Older models store the image on 3.5-inch floppy diskettes. The image contains all the code for the PIX operating system and all the features—NAT, IPSec, filtering, and so on.

Unlike Cisco IOS images, where there are many images for each platform and each image contains only a certain set of features, there is only one image per software version for the PIX Firewall. This image contains all the features Cisco has developed for PIX, but certain features may be enabled and disabled by the licensing keys (see the "Licensed Features" section later in this chapter).

To install or upgrade an image, you must copy it across the network, typically with TFTP, or replace the flash memory with flash containing the new image. For PIX models that use floppy disks, simply swap the floppy with the one containing the new image and reboot.

The PIX operating system itself is non-Unix, real-time, and embedded.

FLASH EXPLOITS

Years ago, it was a trivial (pun intended) exercise to gain unauthorized access to most Cisco routers. The primary reason was that most router administrators would configure TFTP so that they could copy system images to and from the routers and make backup copies of their configuration files. Because TFTP has no authentication and does not even require a password, all intruders needed to know was the name of the configuration file, and they could send a TFTP Get request to the router. The router would promptly return the configuration file, which of course contained the login and enable passwords. Although the password was encrypted in the configuration file, it was just a matter of time before it was cracked. If the password could be found in a dictionary, this "matter of time" was probably a few seconds.

Although it's still possible to configure routers like this, such a configuration would be unusual. Newer versions of IOS have more secure default settings and support more secure protocols, such as FTP (which at least requires a username and password).

CONTINUED ➡

With the PIX Firewall, the security is much tighter. In fact, configuration file theft is exactly the type of attack the PIX Firewall's flash system is designed to thwart. It is immune to this type of attack because you can only send files to the PIX Firewall; you cannot download from it.

BIOS

The BIOS of the PIX Firewall operates in the same way as the BIOS of other Intel processor-based computers. It is responsible for the initial boot sequence and loading the PIX software image located in file 0.

The BIOS is stored in a special chip, separate from flash. Although upgrades to the BIOS are seldom necessary (an example would be date fixes for the Y2K bug), upgrading it is possible.

Interfaces

Most PIX Firewalls have at least three fixed ports: RJ-45 (console connector), DB15 (failover connector), and USB (not currently used).

Depending on the model, PIX Firewalls also have one or two fixed Fast Ethernet interfaces for data traffic and a number of slots for optional interfaces. These interfaces are labeled much like router interfaces: 10/100 Ethernet 0, 10/100 Ethernet 1, and so on.

Internally, the interfaces are numbered and named. For instance, using the command show interface ethernet1, we see that the interface numbered ethernet1 is named inside:

```
PIX# show interface ethernet1
interface ethernet1 "inside" is up, line protocol is up
   Hardware is i82559 ethernet, address is 0050.54ff.076e
   IP address 10.1.1.20, subnet mask 255.255.255.0
   MTU 1500 bytes, BW 100000 Kbit full duplex
      395 packets input, 43128 bytes, 0 no buffer
      Received 395 broadcasts, 0 runts, 0 giants
      0 input errors, 0 CRC, 0 frame, 0 overrun, 0
       ignored, 0 abort
      1 packets output, 64 bytes, 0 underruns
      0 output errors, 0 collisions, 0 interface resets
```

Part IV

```
          0 babbles, 0 late collisions, 0 deferred
          1 lost carrier, 0 no carrier
          input queue (curr/max blocks): hardware (128/128)
            software (0/2)
          output queue (curr/max blocks): hardware (0/2)
            software (0/1)
      PIX#
```

All PIX Firewalls have at least two interfaces, but several models support six or more interfaces. By default, these two interfaces are named
inside and outside. The name inside is reserved for a network that
has a security level of 100 (the maximum). The name outside is reserved
for a network that has a security level of 0 (the minimum). We will discuss the security levels in more depth in the "The Adaptive Security
Algorithm (ASA) and Security Levels" section later in this chapter.

TIP

Some models of the PIX Firewall have more than one internal bus, which
shuttles data from the interfaces to the CPU and RAM. For instance, the PIX 535
has three separate buses: two run at 66MHz or 33MHz, and the third runs only
at 33MHz. Some interface cards, like the Gigabit Ethernet interface card, come
in 33MHz and 66MHz flavors, so the interface you use and the slot you choose
can greatly affect your system's performance.

Licensed Features

Cisco has three basic licenses for the PIX Firewall:

▶ The Restricted license sets a limit on the number of connections
  and interfaces and disables failover.

▶ The Unrestricted license has no limit on connections, enables
  failover, and allows as many interfaces as the hardware supports.

▶ The Failover license (the least expensive) is intended for a backup
  firewall (when using the failover feature) and assumes the license
  characteristics of the primary firewall.

In addition to these licenses, you can purchase special licenses to enable
IPSec at 56 bits and 128 bits. All features, including cut-through proxy,
attack guards, and WebSENSE support are included in the Unrestricted
license. Older models of the PIX Firewall had multiple Restricted versions
that were limited to 128 connections or 1,024 concurrent connections.

Each PIX Firewall has a unique serial number. This serial number and the licenses purchased are used as the inputs to a mathematical formula that generates an activation key. This key is entered as the system image is being installed and determines which features are available on the firewall. When you do a flash upgrade, you also need the serial number of the flash card.

In order to change your license, you must reload the system image. For instance, if you purchase a license-activation key for triple Data Encryption Standard (3DES) encryption and wish to install it on your PIX Firewall, you must copy the system image to the flash (again). During this process, you will be prompted for the activation code.

PIX FIREWALL OPERATION

Now that you understand the components of the PIX Firewall, let's look at how they work together. As we mentioned earlier, the PIX Firewall has its roots in NAT. In fact, when the PIX Firewall was introduced in 1994, it was the first box capable of doing true RFC 1631 NAT.

Although it is possible to configure a PIX Firewall to not translate IP addresses, its switching process is based on NAT, and every packet must use this NAT mechanism. So, in order for you to understand how a PIX forwards packets, we must first define some NAT vocabulary. Then we will discuss the sequence in which packets are processed, and, finally, the Adaptive Security Algorithm.

WARNING
Even if the PIX filtering is configured so that its ACLs will not deny any packets, packets that are not translated will not be forwarded. The PIX Firewall must have a translation slot to switch packets from one interface to another.

NAT Mechanisms

With NAT, a *translation* is a pair of IP addresses: local and global. The local address is on the network connected to the inside, or trusted interface of the PIX Firewall. The global address is part of a network somewhere beyond the *outside interface* that is trusted less than the *inside interface*. The PIX Firewall translates the local address to the global address as the packet passes outbound through the firewall. It translates the global address to the local address as a packet passes inbound through the firewall.

Translations can be either static or dynamic. Static translations must be manually configured. Dynamic translations are created as packets that meet certain criteria arrive.

When the first packet in a series of packets arrives at the PIX Firewall from the inside interface, the PIX Firewall creates a *translation slot*. This "slot" is a software construct that keeps track of translations. Each translation uses one translation slot.

Connection slots are another software construct that the PIX Firewall uses to keep track of stateful information. A given pair of devices, such as a client and server, can multiplex several conversations between their two IP addresses. This is often accomplished via TCP and UDP ports. For instance, a client could connect to a server via Telnet, FTP, and HTTP simultaneously, creating three separate TCP connections between the two devices. If this happened across a PIX Firewall, it would create a single translation slot and three connection slots. Each connection slot is bound to a translation slot.

NOTE

The Restricted licenses used in older PIX models limit the number of connection slots to either 128 or 1,024. As of the time of this writing, "older" means the PIX Classic and those whose model numbers end in zero, such as PIX 520. The current models end in five, such as PIX 515, PIX 525, and PIX 535.

The translation table, which is usually abbreviated *xlate table*, is the actual table in memory that holds all the translation slots and connection slots. It is important to distinguish this table from the configuration file of the PIX Firewall. Just because you have configured a static entry does not mean it will appear in the output of the show xlate command. The PIX places an entry in this table only when a packet arrives. After a certain amount of inactivity (that is, after the PIX does not see any more packets that are part of this conversation), the PIX will remove the entry from the xlate table. Remember that the xlate table shows the current translations and connections.

Packet Processing

Now that you know how NAT works, let's look at how the PIX Firewall processes packets. We'll see how it handles outbound packets, inbound packets, and routing.

Outbound Packets

When a packet arrives on the inside interface, the PIX Firewall first checks the xlate table for a translation slot. Specifically, the PIX checks the source address of the IP header and searches the xlate table for a match. Its next actions depend on whether it finds a match.

Packets with Existing Translation Slots   If the PIX finds a match for the outbound packet's source address, it knows it has seen packets from this address before and already created a dynamic translation slot, or it has a manually configured static translation slot. The PIX then processes the outbound packet as follows:

- ▶ It takes the global address from the translation slot that corresponds to the local address it just looked up in the xlate table and overwrites the source address in the IP header of the packet with the value of the global address.

- ▶ The other attributes, such as the checksums, are recalculated. (Otherwise, the packet would be discarded upon arrival, because the change in the IP header would change the value of the checksum.)

- ▶ Assuming a filter does not block the packet, the packet is then forwarded out the outside interface.

Packets without Existing Translation Slots   If the PIX receives a packet on the inside interface that does not have a current translation slot in the xlate table, it can dynamically create an entry if configured to do so. In this case, when the packet arrives, the PIX checks the source address and finds no match in the xlate table. It then follows these steps to process the outbound packet:

1. The PIX makes sure it has sufficient connections, which are determined by the license.

2. It creates the translation slot by reserving an unused IP address from the global NAT pool and entering this global address along with the source address from the IP header into the translation slot.

3. With the translation slot created, the source address is overwritten with the global address.

4. The checksum and other values are recalculated.

5. The packet is transmitted on the outside interface.

Part IV

Inbound Packets

For packets that arrive on the outside interface, destined for the inside network, the PIX Firewall behaves quite differently than it does for packets that arrive on the inside interface. It does so because the outside network is, by definition, less trusted. By default, packets from the outside do not create translation slots, so they cannot be switched to the inside interface without a static NAT mapping. Thus the PIX is very secure, from an architectural standpoint.

But even before the PIX checks for an existing entry in the xlate table, packets from an outside interface must match criteria specified in an ACL. Only after an incoming packet matches the ACL will it be processed further. The combination of the ACL and translation slot is the primary source of the PIX Firewall's security.

WARNING

Do not confuse the definition of stateful firewalls with this section's description of the operation of the PIX Firewall. There are many brands of stateful firewalls, but the PIX Firewall's operation is unique.

Routing

As you can see from the description of packet processing in the previous sections, the PIX Firewall is not a router. This is an important distinction, because many other brands of firewalls are, in fact, routers, with packet filtering or even stateful capabilities added on. For instance, the IOS Firewall is a full-featured, stateful firewall that runs on a Cisco router; but it processes packets just as it would if it were running a basic IOS image, except that it adds the stateful filtering feature. Although the mode of operation detailed in the previous sections makes the PIX Firewall much more secure, it also has some limitations related to its routing protocol support.

RIP Support   The PIX Firewall's routing information is very limited. For all practical purposes, it acts more like a host on the network than a router. Specifically, it supports the Router Information Protocol (RIP) routing protocol, but this support is limited to three features:

> **Passive Mode**   The PIX operates in a passive mode. This mode is typically used in a network where there are multiple gateways. It allows the PIX to receive RIP routes so that it knows the best path to forward its traffic to, but the PIX cannot

generate nondefault routes. As a passive device, it cannot pass RIP updates received on one interface to a router on another interface. When RIP is being used on both sides, the PIX will always be a boundary, separating the two RIP domains.

Default Route Broadcasts   The PIX is capable of broadcasting a default route using RIP version 1 or 2. This approach is often used because the PIX typically sits on the border of an organization's network, where some security is desired. Also, because most organizations use RFC 1918 private addresses, NAT must be performed at the border. Another reason to use default route broadcasts is that the border represents one of a few points to exit the network, so a default route inside the network, pointing to the egress point of the network, is appropriate.

Static Routes   Although this feature is not specific to RIP, the PIX can be configured with static routes for more security, control, and reliability.

Figure 17.3 illustrates the PIX Firewall's typical role in routing.

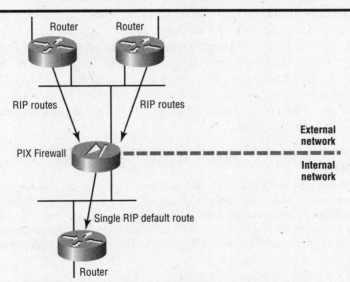

FIGURE 17.3:   Typical routing configuration for a PIX Firewall

Part IV

RIP Information   Although somewhat brief, information about RIP on the PIX Firewall can be displayed via the show rip command. To see the routing information, use the show route command. Here's an example of using these commands:

```
PIX# show rip
rip outside passive version 2
rip inside default version 1
PIX# show route
        outside 0.0.0.0 0.0.0.0 10.2.0.6 1 RIP
        outside 0.0.0.0 0.0.0.0 10.2.0.5 6 RIP
        inside 10.1.1.0 255.255.255.0 10.1.1.20 1
            CONNECT static
        outside 10.2.0.0 255.255.255.0 10.2.0.20 1
            CONNECT static
        DMZ 192.168.1.0 255.255.255.0 192.168.1.20 1
            CONNECT static
PIX#
```

Here, you see that the PIX Firewall is sending a default route out its inside interface and receiving default routes from two different routers, both of which are connected to the outside interface (as shown in Figure 17.3). The default route through 10.2.0.5 has a metric of 6 (which equates to *hops* in RIP), whereas the same route through 10.2.0.6 has a metric of 1. Therefore, the route through 10.2.0.6 will be preferred. It is also possible to broadcast the default route to the outside interface and receive routes from the inside interface, or the PIX can simply receive routes from both interfaces.

NOTE

Although the routing scenarios discussed here are common, you might need a far more complex routing environment. Thus, it is not necessarily appropriate to replace a full-featured Cisco router with a PIX Firewall, just because you need more security. This is particularly true if your network's routing is complex or if you wish to enable quality of service (QoS) or use features such as policy routing.

The Adaptive Security Algorithm (ASA) and Security Levels

Cisco's Adaptive Security Algorithm (ASA) is the basis for the PIX Firewall's security, and it includes much of the information discussed in the previous sections. However, it can be summarized into a few rules that govern how packets are inspected and permitted or denied. These rules are as follows:

- ▶ All packets must have a connection slot to be transmitted.

- ▶ All packets are allowed to travel from a more secure interface to a less secure interface unless specifically denied (for example, by an ACL).

- ▶ All packets from a less secure interface to a more secure interface are denied, unless specifically allowed.

- ▶ All ICMP packets are denied unless you specifically configure the PIX Firewall to accept them.

- ▶ When the PIX Firewall denies a packet, it is *dropped* (received but not transmitted), and the action is noted in the logs.

Like Einstein said, everything is relative. Security on the PIX Firewall is no exception, and it's critical that you understand this fact. Specifically, what is allowed and disallowed by default depends on which interfaces a packet enters and leaves.

Each interface is assigned a value, called the *security level*, from 0 to 100: 100 means the interface is completely trusted, and 0 indicates it's completely untrusted. This system allows a PIX Firewall with several interfaces to be configured securely.

For instance, you might have five interfaces on your PIX Firewall and assign them security levels as follows:

Connection	Security Level	Default Access
Internal network	100	All
Remote-access network	75	Business partner, DMZ, and Internet
Business partner	50	DMZ and Internet
DMZ	25	Internet
Internet	0	None

In this scenario, traffic from your internal network would be, by default, able to access any of the other four networks. Your remote users would be able to get to your business partner, the DMZ, and the Internet; however, you must explicitly configure the PIX Firewall to let them inside your internal network because it has a higher security level. Your business partners would be able to access your shared systems on the DMZ and the Internet by default, although you could restrict this access with an ACL. Your partners would not be able to get to your internal network or the modems on your remote-access network, unless you explicitly granted them permission in the configuration. The systems on the DMZ would be able to access only the Internet. Finally, the Internet would not be able to access any of the other four networks, again, without explicit configuration.

In summary, the PIX Firewall controls access via the translation and connection slots we mentioned earlier. The PIX Firewall simply does not allow a packet from a less trusted interface, destined for a more trusted interface, to create a translation or connection slot, unless you explicitly configure the NAT translation and an ACL.

USING THE PIX COMMAND-LINE INTERFACE

Now that you know what the PIX Firewall is and how it works, it's time to get some hands-on experience with it. In this section, we will discuss the various modes of the command-line interface (CLI), as well as several basic commands. This chapter concentrates on the system and management commands and general navigation between the CLI modes. The bulk of the network and security configuration commands will be discussed in detail in later chapters.

CLI Access Methods

There are a number of ways to access the PIX Firewall's CLI. The most common method is via the console. This is a standard EIA/TIA-232 serial interface that uses an RJ-45 connector and a rolled cable. Typically, the console is connected to the COM port on a PC and accessed via a terminal emulator, such as HyperTerminal or TeraTerm.

Another way to access the CLI is via a Telnet session. However, this option comes with some major caveats. The Telnet protocol itself is almost totally insecure. Although a password is required, it is transmitted in plain text across the network. For this and other reasons, it is possible to telnet to a PIX Firewall from any interface, but sessions connecting to the PIX Firewall from the outside network must be inside an IPSec tunnel.

The preferred method of remotely accessing a PIX Firewall is using the Secure Shell (SSH) protocol. This method is similar to Telnet, but it provides data privacy via encryption.

The actual configuration of these access methods will be discussed in the next chapter. Here, we will continue by explaining what happens once you access and log on to the PIX Firewall.

CLI Modes

The PIX Firewall uses basic modes similar to the IOS-based routers: user mode (called unprivileged mode), privileged mode, and configuration.

Unprivileged Mode

After the initial logon, a user is in unprivileged mode. This is a highly restricted mode that, by default, has only three commands: enable, pager, and quit. The prompt in unprivileged mode is marked by the greater-than symbol (>).

Privileged Mode

To gain access to view and configure the PIX Firewall, a user must type the command enable from the unprivileged-mode prompt. The user will then be prompted for the enable password. After successfully entering this password, the user will be in privileged mode. This mode is marked by the pound symbol (#).

The mode sequence looks like this:

```
PIX> ?
enable      Enter privileged mode or change privileged
            mode password
pager       Control page length for pagination
quit        Disable, end configuration or logout
PIX> enable
Password: *****
PIX#
```

From the privileged mode, the user can manage the flash, view the configuration, use the show commands, view the logs, and more. The command disable returns to unprivileged mode from privileged mode.

Part IV

Configuration Mode

To enter configuration mode on the PIX Firewall, the user types the configure terminal command. Unlike with the IOS, in the PIX operating system, this command can be used only to configure the PIX from the terminal. It cannot be used to configure the PIX from memory.

After entering this command, the prompt will change to include the word config, indicating that the user is in the configuration mode. While in this mode, the user has the ability to modify the current running configuration in the PIX Firewall's memory. Any command the user types will take effect immediately. The user can return to privileged mode by typing the command exit.

Editing in the CLI

The PIX Firewall's CLI uses the same editing conventions as the IOS router software. These conventions are special Ctrl-key combinations or arrow keys that allow you to move the cursor to different places. Table 17.1 lists the key combinations commonly used when editing the PIX Firewall's configuration.

TABLE 17.1: PIX CLI Editing Keys

KEY	FUNCTION
Ctrl+P or up arrow	Causes the previously accepted commands to be displayed. This is handy when you need to enter several similar commands or the same command several times in a row.
Ctrl+N or down arrow	Causes the next accepted command to be displayed. Note that if you make a syntax error and a command is not accepted, it will not be displayed in the history.
Ctrl+W	Deletes the word to the left of the cursor.
Ctrl+U	Deletes the entire line.

Basic Commands

This section presents the basic commands for privileged mode. These commands are organized alphabetically.

The *clear* Command

The clear command resets counters or caches held in the PIX Firewall's memory. It is useful during troubleshooting. You may want to clear the interface statistics, the ARP table, or the xlate table. You can also use this command to clear the PIX Firewall's configuration and clear the contents of the flash before installing a new image.

The *clock set* Command

PIX Firewalls use an internal clock, similar to that on PCs, for a number of purposes. The two primary uses are for generating timestamps on the SYSLOGs and as part of the Public Key Infrastructure (PKI) protocol, to make sure that certificates and other security constructs are removed as they expire. Thus, it is important to set your clock correctly. To do so, use the clock set command. The syntax is as follows:

```
clock set hh:mm:ss month day year
```

The *copy* Command

The copy command is used to copy an image or PDM file from a TFTP server onto the flash. This command uses the URL syntax, as follows:

```
copy tftp[:[[//location][/path]]] flash[:[image | pdm]]
```

After this command is executed, the PIX will prompt you for the IP address of the TFTP server and the source filename that you want to copy.

WARNING

Unlike the copy TFTP operation on Cisco routers using IOS, when upgrading from 5.*x* to 6.*x* images, the PIX does not warn you about erasing all files on the flash, or ask you over and over if you really, really want to copy the file. It just does it. Fortunately, once it has finished verifying that the copy was successful, you have the option of not installing the new image.

The *debug* Commands

The debug commands provide detailed, real-time information about events on the PIX Firewall, including information about packets traversing the firewall, special services like DHCP and failover, the crypto processes of IPSec and ISAKMP (Internet Security Association and Key Management

Part IV

Protocol), and more. Here is an example of the debug output for the RIP routing process:

```
PIX# debug rip
RIP trace on
PIX# 226: RIP: interface outside received v1 update
           from 10.2.0.6
227: RIP: interface outside received v2 update
           from 10.2.0.5
228: RIP: update contains 4 routes
229: RIP: interface inside sending v1 update
           to 255.255.255.255
230: RIP: interface outside received v2 update
           from 10.2.0.5
231: RIP: update contains 4 routes
```

Most debug operations will use the command debug followed by a keyword, such as rip as in the previous example. However, the packet-debugging feature is much more powerful, and the syntax is correspondingly complex:

```
[no] debug packet <if_name> [src <s_ip> [netmask <m>]]
    [dst <d_ip> [netmask <m>]]
    [[proto icmp]|[proto tcp [sport <s_p>] [dport <d_p>]]
    |[proto udp [sport <s_p>] [dport d_p]] [rx|tx|both]
```

As you can see, this feature allows you to explicitly define the types of packets you want to view. Doing so is useful to verify that your filters are operating as you intended.

The *enable password* Command

The enable password command is used to set the password that allows access to the privileged mode. The password is alphanumeric and can be up to 16 characters long. The syntax is as follows:

```
enable password password [encrypted]
```

If you are entering a password that is already encrypted, you must use the encrypted keyword after your password. Also, an encrypted string will always be exactly 16 characters long (so you cannot tell how long the unencrypted password is).

The *passwd* Command

The passwd command sets the password for Telnet access to the PIX Firewall. The syntax is as follows:

```
passwd password [encrypted]
```

The encrypted keyword works just like the enable password command.

The *perfmon* Command

The perfmon command provides a convenient interface for accessing a number of statistics all at once. This command has three parts:

```
perfmon interval seconds
perfmon [verbose | quiet]
perfmon settings
```

The first command tells the PIX how often to report the statistics. The second command turns reporting on and off. The last command shows the current settings. Here is an example of these commands and the perfmon report:

```
PIX# perfmon interval 10
PIX# perfmon verbose
PIX# perfmon settings
interval: 10 (seconds)
verbose
PIX#
```

PERFMON STATS:	Current	Average
Xlates	0/s	0/s
Connections	0/s	0/s
TCP Conns	0/s	0/s
UDP Conns	0/s	0/s
URL Access	0/s	0/s
WebSns Req	0/s	0/s
TCP Fixup	0/s	0/s
TCPIntercept	0/s	0/s
HTTP Fixup	0/s	0/s
FTP Fixup	0/s	0/s
AAA Authen	0/s	0/s
AAA Author	0/s	0/s
AAA Account	0/s	0/s

Part IV

The *reload* Command

The reload command reboots the PIX Firewall after prompting you to confirm that you would like the PIX to reboot itself. Optionally, you can use the keyword noconfirm to bypass confirmation. The syntax is as follows:

```
reload [noconfirm]
show checksum
```

To ensure the integrity of the configuration of the PIX Firewall, the PIX calculates a cryptographic checksum of the configuration. The show checksum command displays this checksum as a series of four 4-byte numbers in hexadecimal. As part of your security procedures, after the PIX is initially configured, you should use the show checksum command and record the checksum. You can then use this checksum as part of your audits, to verify that no one has tampered with the configuration. Here is an example of the output of the show checksum command:

```
PIX# show checksum
Cryptochecksum: eb30f570 92b0f5e6 e29ee8dc 5f0aa42a
```

The *show interface* Command

The show interface command is used often because it provides a great deal of information about the interfaces on the PIX Firewall. The syntax is as follows:

```
show interface [hardware_address]
```

If the optional hardware address is given, the output is limited to information about the address specified; otherwise, information is displayed about all interfaces.

The show interface command is most often used to verify that the interface is "up/up," which refers to the hardware and the line protocol—in this case, Ethernet. In other words, it checks layers 1 and 2 of the OSI model, respectively. The show interface command is also used to show the IP address and the activity on the interface, including packet and byte counts for inbound and outbound traffic, and error statistics. The following shows sample output of this command.

```
PIX# show interface ethernet0
interface ethernet0 "outside" is up, line protocol is up
  Hardware is i82559 ethernet, address is 0050.54ff.076d
  IP address 10.2.0.20, subnet mask 255.255.255.0
```

```
MTU 1500 bytes, BW 100000 Kbit full duplex
      6063 packets input, 608203 bytes, 0 no buffer
      Received 1684 broadcasts, 0 runts, 0 giants
      0 input errors, 0 CRC, 0 frame, 0 overrun,
       0 ignored, 0 abort
      45 packets output, 3530 bytes, 0 underruns
      0 output errors, 0 collisions, 0 interface resets
      0 babbles, 0 late collisions, 0 deferred
      0 lost carrier, 0 no carrier
      input queue (curr/max blocks): hardware (128/128)
       software (0/1)
      output queue (curr/max blocks): hardware (0/1)
       software (0/1)
PIX#
```

The *show tech-support* Command

The show tech-support command is often used at the request of Cisco's Technical Assistance Center (TAC). It is a convenient way to dump the output of several show commands to the screen, so you can cut and paste the output into an e-mail message and forward it to the TAC to help them troubleshoot a problem.

The *shun* Command

The shun command allows an administrator to quickly respond to an incident by deleting the connection information of a given source address and rejecting any future packets from that source without changing the configuration rules of the PIX Firewall. Because the configuration of ACLs and conduits can become quite complex, the shun command can save a great deal of time, which is often critical during an attack.

The syntax of the shun command is as follows:

```
shun src_ip [dst_ip sport dport [prot]]
no shun src_ip
show shun [src_ip|statistics]
clear shun [statistics]
who
```

Part IV

This command shows the TTY ID and IP address of each active Telnet session on the PIX Firewall. The TTY ID is important because it is used with the `kill` command to terminate active Telnet connections.

The *write* Command

The `write` command can be used to copy the current configuration to a number of different locations, as follows:

▶ To copy the current configuration to flash:

```
write memory
```

▶ To display the current configuration on the terminal:

```
write terminal
```

▶ To copy the current configuration to a TFTP server:

```
write network [[server_ip]:[filename]]
```

You can also erase the configuration on the flash by using the following command:

```
write erase
```

WHAT'S NEXT

This chapter began by looking at the three common firewall technologies in use today. Packet-filtering firewalls use rules to deny packets based on the content of the headers. Application proxies are layer 7–aware programs that communicate with systems on untrusted networks on behalf of hosts in the trusted network. Stateful firewalls permit or deny packets based on other packets, typically on a session basis.

We introduced the Cisco IOS Firewall, and then focused on the PIX Firewall. We examined the unique hardware and software components in a PIX Firewall and how they operate together to provide a formidable security solution. Finally, we covered the PIX Firewall CLI (command-line interface) and the common commands used in the day-to-day operation and management of the PIX Firewall.

Now you should have a basic understanding of firewalls in general, and the operation of the PIX Firewall specifically. This knowledge will provide a foundation for the advanced topic of PIX Firewall configuration in the next chapter.

Chapter 18

PIX FIREWALL CONFIGURATION

In this chapter, we will discuss the configuration of the PIX Firewall. We'll begin by discussing the preparatory work you should complete before you configure a PIX Firewall. Then you will learn how to set up a PIX Firewall to allow the traffic of your choice to pass between the inside, outside, and demilitarized zone (DMZ) interfaces. This discussion includes the configuration of interfaces, Network Address Translation (NAT), and Port Address Translation (PAT). This chapter also covers how to configure a PIX Firewall to participate in Router Information Protocol (RIP) domains.

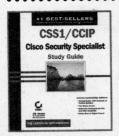

Adapted from *CSS1™/CCIP™: Cisco® Security Specialist Study Guide* by Todd Lammle, Tom Lancaster, Eric Quinn, and Justin Menga

ISBN 0-7821-4049-1 $89.99

Part IV

PREPARING FOR FIREWALL CONFIGURATION

Before you purchase a firewall, you should ask quite a few questions. These typically begin with some touchy-feely, but very important, questions, such as the following:

- ▶ What am I really trying to accomplish?
- ▶ How important is my security?
- ▶ What is my budget?

These questions will help you determine which model of firewall you need, or whether a firewall is appropriate at all.

In order to configure the PIX Firewall, you must answer the following questions at a minimum:

- ▶ What am I trying to protect?
- ▶ What am I trying to protect it from?
- ▶ How many networks will be connected and what are their addresses?
- ▶ Which of these networks do I trust most?
- ▶ Which of these networks do I trust least?
- ▶ Are there any other paths to get from one network to another?
- ▶ What routing protocols are involved and how are they configured?
- ▶ Will address translation be required?
- ▶ If so, how many addresses need to be translated, and how many addresses are available to translate them?
- ▶ What are my application requirements?
- ▶ Which applications will pass through the firewall, and on which interfaces will they arrive and depart?
- ▶ What protocol and/or port number will they use?
- ▶ Who are the users of each application?

- ▶ What are the source and destination IP addresses?

- ▶ What are my organization's security policies?

The answers to these questions will determine much of the configuration. As we go through the configuration procedures in the rest of this chapter, we will point out where the answers to these questions are used.

USING COMMON GLOBAL CONFIGURATION COMMANDS

Before we delve into the important aspects of configuring the PIX Firewall, let's take a brief look at several commands that are largely optional: clock, domain-name, hostnames, names, and logging. Each of these commands plays a part in making the PIX Firewall more secure or more user friendly, and they affect the PIX Firewall as a whole, rather than any one particular interface or rule.

The *clock* Command

The clock command is used to set the system clock. Although the syntax is simple, there are many caveats related to setting the system clock—most of them because the clock is too simple. First, although it may be hard to believe, the PIX Firewall's clock isn't aware of daylight savings time (DST). Thus, it doesn't automatically switch twice per year, although it does compensate for leap years. Second, amazingly, the clock doesn't support time zones.

Both of these problems can cause headaches if you're using the logging timestamp feature, because all log entries are coded with the actual time as opposed to the number of seconds elapsed since the last reboot. Just be careful when analyzing logs. Worse, IPSec's security associations and certificates expiration are tracked via the system clock. All certificates are tracked from Greenwich mean time (GMT). So, in order to use IPSec with other boxes, you need to have the PIX Firewall's clock set to GMT, which is fine if you're in England but can be a pain otherwise. If you're using a centralized SYSLOG server and IPSec certificates at the same time, you could be in for some head-scratching date math.

Part IV

The *domain-name* and *hostname* Commands

The domain-name command accepts a single parameter: the domain name. The domain-name and hostname commands combine to allow the administrator to specify the fully qualified domain name (FQDN). The primary purpose of this command is to facilitate RSA keys, which use the FQDN as an input.

The hostname command also accepts single parameter, which is the name of the host. Although it is also part of the RSA key's input, this command is most often used to set the PIX command-line interface (CLI) prompt.

The *names* Command

A few commands work together to provide aliases for IP addresses, much like the /etc/hosts file in a Unix host. The purpose of the names command is to make the configuration easier to read.

To enable this aliasing, simply type the word **names** from the PIX (config)# prompt. Then create an alias by using the name keyword followed by an IP address and the name (up to 16 characters) that you want to use. For instance, you might type the following:

```
PIX (config)# name 192.168.10.53 proxy1
```

Then you could use the word proxy1 in place of the IP address in all the access-list, nat, and conduit statements. Doing so enhances security by reducing the risk of misconfiguration from typos. It also makes the output from show and other commands much easier to read.

The *logging* Command

Simple Network Management Protocol (SNMP) and SYSLOG logging on the PIX Firewall are controlled by the logging command. This command directs the output of the logging process to several different places, including the console or a SYSLOG daemon on a Unix host (or software that mimics it on a Windows NT or 2000 machine). The logs can also be displayed via Telnet. In all cases, logging must be explicitly enabled by using the following commands:

▶ To turn logging on and off from the config prompt:

```
[no] logging on
```

▶ To display the logs on the console:

```
[no] logging console level
```

▶ To store the logs in a buffer on the PIX that allows them to be displayed with the show logging command:

```
[no] logging console level
```

▶ To send logs to a remote host using the SYSLOG facility:

```
[no] logging host [interface-nam]
     ip_address [protocol/port]
```

▶ To display the logs on Telnet sessions:

```
[no] logging monitor level
```

NOTE

It is possible to send these messages to multiple hosts. You might want to do so for redundancy or to let two different organizations keep tabs on the PIX Firewall, for example. However, you should be aware that sending messages to more than one host entails additional resource usage, so make sure you don't overload the processor.

CONFIGURING PIX FIREWALL INTERFACES

The PIX Firewall must act as a gateway between two networks. As such, it must have, at a minimum, two physical network interfaces.

Actually configuring interfaces on the PIX Firewall is much different than configuring other Cisco devices, such as IOS routers and switches. For starters, you don't enter an interface configuration mode. Instead, you configure the interfaces from the PIX(config)# prompt. Also, you begin by assigning a name and security level to the hardware interface. After you've done so, most configuration commands use the name of the interface instead of its hardware address.

Because IP is the only layer 3 protocol supported by the PIX Firewall, you must gather some specific information before configuring its interfaces:

▶ IP address of each interface

▶ Subnet mask of each interface

▶ Relative security of each interface

Part IV

Of course, each interface must be on a separate IP network because the PIX Firewall does not support subinterfaces or secondary IP addresses (often called *multinetting*). However, if you're using the PIX Firewall's Dynamic Host Configuration Protocol (DHCP) client, you don't actually need the IP address and subnet mask of the interface, but you will need a DHCP server.

Naming an Interface and Assigning a Security Level

To name an interface, use the nameif command. The syntax for this command is as follows:

```
PIX(config)# nameif ?
usage: nameif <hardware_id> <if_name> <security_lvl>
       no nameif
```

Here, *hardware_id* represents the actual name, such as ethernet0, and *security_lvl* is any integer between 0 and 100. The <*if_name*> is a little tricky: It's any string you make up, with the exception that the name inside is reserved for security level 100. The value 100, which indicates the most trusted interface, is always named inside. By convention, an interface with a security value of 0, which indicates the least trusted interface, is usually named outside; however, this name is not required—the interface with security level 0 can be named anything you want.

Here are some examples of using the nameif command:

```
PIX# show nameif
nameif ethernet0 outside security0
nameif ethernet1 inside security100
nameif ethernet2 DMZ security10
PIX# config term
PIX(config)# nameif ethernet1 inside 90
interface name "inside" is reserved for interface with security100
Type help or '?' for a list of available commands.
PIX(config)# nameif ethernet1 cheese 100
security 100 is reserved for the "inside" interface
Type help or '?' for a list of available commands.
```

Notice that when you try to give the same name to two different interfaces, the PIX Firewall's CLI swaps the name, rather than giving you an
error or allowing two interfaces to have the same name.

Also notice that the security value follows the displaced DMZ interface,
but the interface named in your command (in this case, ethernet2)
receives the security level specified in your command.

Next, let's look at some examples that show it is not necessary to have
an inside interface or an outside interface.

```
PIX(config)# nameif ethernet0 cheese 0
PIX(config)# show nameif
nameif ethernet0 cheese security0
nameif ethernet1 inside security100
nameif ethernet2 DMZ security10
PIX(config)# nameif ethernet2 cheese 10
interface 0 name "cheese" swapped with interface 2 name "DMZ"
PIX(config)# show nameif
nameif ethernet0 DMZ security10
nameif ethernet1 inside security100
nameif ethernet2 cheese security10
PIX(config)# nameif ethernet2 cheese 0
PIX(config)# show nameif
nameif ethernet0 DMZ security10
nameif ethernet1 inside security100
nameif ethernet2 cheese security0
PIX(config)# nameif ethernet1 whiz security11
PIX(config)# exit
PIX# show nameif
nameif ethernet0 DMZ security10      ← same security as "cheese"
nameif ethernet1 whiz security11     ← no "inside" or "outside"
nameif ethernet2 cheese security10   ← same security as "DMZ"
PIX#
```

Notice that when we chose the same security level for this interface,
we created two interfaces with the same security level. This poses an
interesting problem for the ASA, because of the method in which NAT

Part IV

translation slots are created: Which interface will be permitted to access the other by default, and which interface will be denied by default? Cisco's answer is that both interfaces are denied by default. In fact, no direct communication is ever possible between two interfaces configured with the same security level!

TIP

Although accidentally configuring two interfaces with the same security level and having to troubleshoot the subsequent "connectivity issue" would be no fun, this "feature" can be not only valid, but very useful. For example, if you wanted an extremely high level of security, you might want to force traffic between two networks through a proxy server or other bastion host. You could configure the two networks with the same security level and put the proxy on a third, higher security network. This approach might also be useful in a B2B scenario, where two customer networks need to communicate with you but definitely not with each other.

To summarize the use of the nameif command with one more example, if you wanted to give the first Ethernet interface of a PIX Firewall the name YellowZone and a security value of 20, you would type the following:

```
PIX(config)# nameif ethernet0 YellowZone 20
```

WARNING

For some reason, the PIX Firewall uses the term *Ethernet* somewhat liberally. Unlike with the IOS, where *Ethernet* refers only to the 10BaseT specification and *Fast Ethernet* refers to 100BaseTX and 100BaseFX, on the PIX Firewall, *Ethernet* refers to both 10 and 100Mbps specifications. This difference is important because many administrators habitually define the auto-negotiation properties of Fast Ethernet, but not Ethernet. If you have hard-coded the speed and duplex values on your Catalyst switch, remember to define them in the PIX Firewall as well, even though the interface says *Ethernet*.

Setting Interface Properties and Shutting Down the Interface

After you enter a nameif statement for each interface on the firewall you wish to use, you continue the configuration by setting the layer 2 properties. To do this, use the interface command.

The syntax of this command is as follows:

```
PIX(config)# interface ?
usage: interface <hardware_id> [<hw_speed> [<shutdown>]]
PIX(config)#
```

For Ethernet interfaces, the `interface` command controls the speed and duplex, and allows the interface to be administratively shut down.

The *hw_speed* parameter is one of the following keywords:

- ▶ `auto` sets the interface to use auto-negotiation.
- ▶ `10BaseT` sets the interface to 10Mbps, half-duplex.
- ▶ `100BaseTX` sets the interface to 100 Mbps, half-duplex.
- ▶ `100full` sets the interface to 100 Mbps, full-duplex.
- ▶ `aui` sets the interface to 10Mbps, half-duplex for an AUI cable.
- ▶ `bnc` sets the interface to 10Mbps, half-duplex for a BNC cable.

On older PIX Firewalls that support Token Ring, the available choices are 4, which sets the ring speed of the interface to 4Mbps, and 16, which sets the ring speed of the interface to 16Mbps.

Using the `shutdown` keyword is intuitively obvious. Just type the hardware address and the word `shutdown`, and the interface is disabled, like so:

```
PIX(config)# interface ethernet0 shutdown
```

However, once the interface is down, how to bring it back up is not so obvious. Unlike with the IOS, you do not type **no interface ethernet0 shutdown** or **interface ethernet0 enable**.

Instead, you enter the `interface` command again, without the shutdown keyword. The tricky part is that when you disable the interface, you do not need to include the *hw_speed* value—but when you enable the interface, you must include this value!

WARNING

If you need to bounce an interface or disable it temporarily, be sure to make a note of the *hw_speed* setting. Otherwise, when you enable it, you could set the speed or duplex incorrectly, which would result in intermittent connectivity or no connectivity at all.

To bring this interface back up, issue the following command:

```
PIX(config)# interface ethernet0 auto
```

Part IV

One last item of interest in this sequence is in the output of the `show interface` command. In the Cisco IOS, when an interface is "administratively down," the line protocol is also down. Here, you see that the interface is administratively down, but the line protocol is still up:

```
PIX(config)# interface ethernet0 shutdown
PIX(config)# exit
PIX# show interface ethernet0
interface ethernet0 "YellowZone" is administratively down,
➡line protocol is up
   Hardware is i82559 ethernet, address is 0050.54ff.076d
   IP address 10.2.0.20, subnet mask 255.255.255.0
   MTU 1500 bytes, BW 100000 Kbit full duplex
        15 packets input, 3153 bytes, 0 no buffer
        Received 15 broadcasts, 0 runts, 0 giants
        0 input errors, 0 CRC, 0 frame, 0 overrun, 0 ignored,
          0 abort
        1 packets output, 64 bytes, 0 underruns
        0 output errors, 0 collisions, 0 interface resets
        0 babbles, 0 late collisions, 0 deferred
        1 lost carrier, 0 no carrier
        input queue (curr/max blocks): hardware (128/128)
          software (0/1)
        output queue (curr/max blocks): hardware (0/2)
          software (0/1)
PIX# conf t
PIX(config)# interface ethernet0 auto
```

From this point on, most of your configuration commands will refer to the interface by name instead of the hardware address. In this case, we'll use YellowZone instead of ethernet0.

Assigning an IP Address

Now, it's time to assign an IP address to the interface. To do so, we use the `ip address` command. The syntax for this command is as follows:

```
PIX(config)# ip address ?
usage: ip address <if_name> <ip_address> [<mask>]
       ip address <if_name> dhcp [setroute] [retry <retry_cnt>]
```

```
ip local pool <poolname> <ip1>[-<ip2>]
ip verify reverse-path interface <if_name>
ip audit [name|signature|interface|attack|info] ...
show|clear ip audit count [global] [interface
    <interface>]
```
PIX(config)#

This command has two options of interest. For most users, all interfaces on the PIX Firewall will have static IP addresses. However, the PIX Firewall also supports dynamic address assignment via DHCP for use in the small office, home office (SOHO) environment, where cable modems and DSL-based Internet connections are common.

NOTE
This dynamic address can also be used for PAT, which will be explained later in this chapter.

In our example, we'll configure the YellowZone interface with an IP address of 10.1.1.1/16:

PIX(config)# **ip address yellowzone 10.1.1.1 255.255.0.0**

Note that if the *mask* is not given, the default classful mask is used. And as you would suspect, this is the mask of the interface. So, all hosts, routers, and other devices on this subnet should be configured with the same mask. Also note that although we entered the name YellowZone as proper case, and it displays in the show commands as proper case, when we enter it in subsequent commands, it is not case sensitive.

If you were connecting the outside address to a cable modem of an ISP that does not use static addresses, you would enter the following command:

PIX(config)# **ip address yellowzone dhcp setroute**

Here, the setroute keyword tells PIX to enter a default route in its routing table. The route points to the "default gateway" address received from the cable modem's DHCP server.

WARNING
PIX Firewall failover features are not compatible with DHCP.

Part IV

Setting the Maximum Transfer Unit

The last interface configuration command we'll cover is the mtu command. This command is used to set the maximum transfer unit (MTU), which is the maximum size of a layer 2 frame. This command is used for both Ethernet and Token Ring. The default for Ethernet is 1500 bytes, and unless you have a good reason for changing it, it should probably be left at the default setting.

The syntax for the mtu command is as follows:

```
PIX(config)# mtu ?
usage: mtu <if_name> <bytes> | (64-65535)
PIX(config)#
```

CONFIGURING NAT AND PAT

After configuring the interfaces on the PIX Firewall, the next step is to configure *Network Address Translation (NAT)* and *Port Address Translation (PAT)*. We will begin this section with a brief introduction to NAT and PAT, and then describe when and how to configure each.

In previous chapters, we introduced the NAT mechanisms used by the PIX Firewall. Here, we will provide a more generic explanation of address translation with NAT and PAT. Although we use Cisco's terminology, these concepts could be applied to any vendor, unless otherwise noted.

Understanding Address Translation

To be perfectly honest, address translation is a hack—a workaround, specified in RFC 1631, to alleviate the problem of IP address depletion. As such, it breaks the rules of IP, which solves an immediate problem, but not without consequences.

In order to solve this problem of more hosts than addresses, RFC 1918 specifies three ranges of addresses (one from each class) that are reserved for private use:

▶ 10.0.0.0 to 10.255.255.255

▶ 172.16.0.0 to 172.31.255.255

▶ 192.168.0.0 to 192.168.255.255

The basic idea is that these addresses are not globally unique. In other words, every organization in the world could use the 10.0.0.0/8 network at the same time, so there is now a theoretically unlimited supply of addresses, because they can be reused. However, these addresses are blocked from the routing tables on the backbone of the Internet. Therefore, in order to get a packet from a private address across the Internet, the address must be translated into a globally unique and registered address. Two common techniques are used to translate addresses: NAT and PAT.

NAT Global and Local Addresses

In theory, NAT is a simple one-to-one mapping of addresses. When a packet with a source IP address such as 10.1.1.100 passes through the NAT process, the IP address in the packet is translated to a single public address, such as 202.199.17.23, and vice versa. These public (or global) addresses are unique and typically advertised on the Internet. If another host on the "ten" network sent a packet through NAT at the same time, it would need to be translated into another public address; for example, 10.1.1.101 might be translated to 202.199.17.24.

In practice, NAT is not so simple. Consider that each packet has two addresses: a source and destination address. Depending on the circumstances, you may want to translate either one or both of these addresses. Thus, it's necessary to distinguish inside and outside addresses, as follows (these terms are consistent across both the PIX and IOS NAT implementations):

Inside Local   The *inside local* address is the IP address that a host on the private network is using. In our example, this address would be 10.1.1.100.

Inside Global   The *inside global* address is the IP address into which the inside address is translated. It is typically a globally unique and routable address, which hosts on the outside network would use to communicate with the inside local address. In our example, this address is 202.199.17.23.

NOTE

Obviously, all IP addresses are *routable* in the usual definition of the term, which is in the context of the OSI model. In this section, by *routable*, we specifically mean that the appropriate hosts on the network have a route to this address. For example, the Internet backbone routers do not know how to get to the "ten" addresses because they don't have a route entry. So, we say that address isn't *routable* on the Internet, although it may be routable inside your network.

Outside Global   Typically, the *outside global* address is a globally unique and routable address of a host that resides on the outside network. Our simple example doesn't use an outside global address.

Outside Local   The *outside local* address is the IP address used to translate the outside global address. This address may or may not be registered, but it must be routable on the inside network. Our simple example doesn't use an outside local address.

The terms *inside* and *outside* are used with respect to NAT, not the names of interfaces on the PIX Firewall. Remember that you may have several interfaces on a PIX Firewall, and you may need to translate addresses between each of them.

The outside global and outside local addresses typically come into play when you want to translate both the source and destination of a packet. We will explore this situation in some of our examples later in this chapter.

Static and Dynamic NAT

To further complicate matters, NAT may be configured statically or dynamically. Static configuration is often used for inbound packets. For instance, you may have a web server on a DMZ, and the DMZ may be configured with private addresses. If a host on the global network wants to access the web server, it cannot, because it has no idea which IP address is being used for translation. To resolve this problem, you can configure a static translation between the outside global and outside local addresses.

In a typical organization, there may be dozens of hosts, such as PCs, and only a couple of registered addresses. When a host sends a packet to the global network, the PIX Firewall will choose the first available registered address from a pool of addresses that you configure. This is the inside global address. If another inside host sends a packet to the global network, the PIX Firewall will again choose the next available address. If no more addresses are available, that host will be unable to communicate with the global network. This behavior is referred to as *dynamic*, because the host does not know (or care) what its inside global address will be, and that address may be different every time it accesses the Internet. The host on the global network always knows what the inside global address is, because it is in the source address field of the IP header.

Although dynamic translation helps solve the address-depletion issue, it still constrains concurrent connections to the total number of registered

IP addresses. For example, if you have 1,000 computers on your network and only 32 registered addresses, only 32 of those 1,000 computers can communicate with the Internet at a time. PAT, often called *overloading*, was created to solve this problem.

PAT

PAT is a method of multiplexing a potentially large number of private addresses through a single registered address. This multiplexing is possible because the PIX Firewall keeps track of the source ports used and translates ports as well as addresses.

For instance, if a couple PCs on the local network request a web page from a server on the global network, the first PC will send a packet addressed as follows:

Source IP	Source Port	Destination IP	Destination Port
10.1.1.100	1026	199.206.253.29	80

For our example, we'll suppose that the firewall's outside interface is 199.206.12.143 and the server's address is 199.206.253.29. When this packet is received on the inside interface, the PIX Firewall will modify only the source IP and port. It will not modify the destination information. The source IP address is changed to make the packet appear as if it originated on the outside interface of the PIX Firewall. In other words, the inside local address is replaced with the inside global address, just as with NAT. However, the source port is also translated to the first unused port above 1024. So, as the packet leaves the PIX Firewall, it looks like this:

Source IP	Source Port	Destination IP	Destination Port
199.206.12.143	1025	199.206.253.29	80

Now, when the next host sent a packet, if dynamic NAT were being used with only one registered address, the packet would be denied. But with PAT, it is just given the next highest port. In this example, we'll suppose the traffic is sent to the same server, although it could be any destination:

Source IP	Source Port	Destination IP	Destination Port
10.1.1.100	1032	199.206.253.29	80

Part IV

When PIX receives this packet, it also translates it using the single registered address, but it uses a different source port, as shown here:

Source IP	Source Port	Destination IP	Destination Port
199.206.12.143	1026	199.206.253.29	80

To the web server, it appears as if the same host is making two requests, but it can distinguish between them via the source port. When the server responds, PIX knows where to send the response, because it knows which destination port maps to which local IP address and port.

Because 65,535 ports are available to TCP and UDP, PAT is capable of supporting a very large number of privately addressed devices.

NOTE

Although NAT and PAT are different things, most networking books and network professionals use the terms interchangeably.

Address Translation Consequences

As we mentioned earlier, address translation comes with a few side effects. Aside from mild reactions like headaches and dizziness as a result of trying to keep the "inside local, outside global" monikers straight, and the increased difficulty during troubleshooting, NAT actually breaks some things.

The most common problem is that many protocols include information about IP addresses in the payload of the packets, instead of taking it only from the headers. The security protocol IPSec is famous for being incompatible with NAT, because it tracks the sender's address for anti-spoofing and nonrepudiation purposes. When the receiver gets the packet, and the value in the IP source address field of the IP header is different from the value in the payload (because the header was translated), the packet is not accepted or decrypted. DHCP, routing protocols, and other protocols are similarly affected.

Cisco's implementation of NAT makes special allowances to enable some protocols, such as DNS A and PTR records and queries, Microsoft's NetMeeting, and FTP. However, it does not support protocols with varying frame formats or frames that are encrypted, such as SNMP and Point-to-Point Tunneling Protocol (PPTP). For this reason, it is possible to have traffic pass through the PIX Firewall without being translated, but the traffic is still handled as if it were being translated. This configuration will be covered later in this chapter.

NAT and Security

In addition to the negative side effects discussed in the previous section, address translation produces a positive side effect: enhanced security. However, popular opinion regards this added security more highly than it deserves. Specifically, many people think that if a host is on the "ten" network and connected to the Internet via NAT, miscreants from the Internet underground will be totally unable to reach this host, because they do not have a route to it. The problem is that this is true only part of the time. The different types of address translation—static NAT, dynamic NAT, and PAT—offer different levels of security.

Static NAT offers no security whatsoever. Although it is true that there isn't a route to the 10.0.0.0/8 network on the Internet backbone, that doesn't matter—the intruders will be using the inside global address instead of the inside local address. In other words, any malicious traffic sent to the inside global address will simply be translated to the inside local address and passed on by NAT.

Dynamic NAT will make it practically impossible to directly communicate with a host on the inside network until that host attempts to communicate with the outside network. In other words, as long as there is no address translation in the firewall (called a *translation slot* in the PIX Firewall, as described in Chapter 17), you're fairly safe. However, the instant you open a browser window or any other application on a client that accesses the Internet, the firewall will dynamically create a translation. Until that translation times out, the host is just as vulnerable as it would be if it had a registered address. So, the only protection dynamic NAT really offers is that the internal hosts are moving targets. Attackers never know which host they will get when attacking an inside global address.

PAT, or overloading, offers a considerable amount of security, because only the port you use is exposed to the Internet. For example, suppose you're running an anonymous FTP service on your host for internal use, and you also open a browser window and initiate a HTTP session to the Internet from the same host that uses a source port of 1026. When an intruder scans the firewall's address, it will find only your 1026 connection (which is fairly safe) and not the TCP port 21. The intruder will continue to be oblivious to the other listening ports on your host, including the anonymous FTP. With static and dynamic NAT, a ping sent to the inside global address will be passed on to the host (inside local), but this is impossible with PAT.

The issue here is that many people assume all versions of NAT provide the same level of protection as PAT, which leaves them with a false sense of security. Fortunately, if you are using a PIX Firewall, by default it won't allow any of those outside connections—such as scans or pings—inbound, even with a static address translation entry. But even though the differences in the levels of security provided by address translation do not necessarily apply to PIX Firewall users, it is important to understand that the ASA of the PIX Firewall provides the protection—not the NAT process itself.

NOTE

Unfortunately, many people have purchased cheap cable-modem routers that have been labeled "firewalls." Many of these "firewalls" perform only NAT. They have the ability to block ports, but ports aren't blocked by default. Without the ASA, the protection offered by NAT on these routers is nearly worthless.

Configuring NAT

Although NAT may appear confusing at first, it's really quite simple if you understand one thing: NAT is always configured between a pair of interfaces. Thus it is easy to focus on only two interfaces at a time, even if you have multiple interfaces to configure. And to make things even easier, there are only two commands to deal with—one per interface.

The address translation on the PIX is always performed between a local and global address, and all you need to do is pick the interfaces. You do not need to define which one is local and which one is global, because the local interface is always the higher security value. This fact will become very important later, when we look at some examples of address translation between four interfaces.

Another important aspect of NAT configuration is the order of operation on the PIX Firewall. Knowing this order will help you understand why NAT is only relevant between pairs of interfaces; and later, it may help you troubleshoot problems.

When the PIX Firewall receives an outbound packet (traveling from a higher security interface to a lower security interface), the first thing it does is determine the outgoing interface based on routing information. At this point, it knows the incoming and outgoing interfaces, and which one is local and global, because it knows their relative security levels. Then it searches for a translation slot. Once it finds or creates one, it checks for security rules, such as ACLs, and then translates the packet and sends it on its way.

For an inbound packet (traveling from a lower security interface to a higher security interface), the operation is a little different. First, the PIX Firewall checks ACLs, and then it determines the outgoing interface, based again on routing information. Last, it checks for a translation slot.

NOTE

Of course, the PIX Firewall performs dozens more tasks. We have simplified the operation greatly to make it easier to understand. For more detailed information, visit the PIX Firewall documentation pages at www.cisco.com.

Now, let's look at the commands used to configure NAT and PAT. We'll begin with simple examples and work progressively up to complex configurations, as we add interfaces and rules to deal with common, real-life situations.

The *nat* and *global* Commands

Two commands are used to configure NAT and PAT on the PIX Firewall: nat and global.

The nat command configures the local interface: It defines the networks to be translated. This command has the following syntax:

```
PIX(config)# nat ?
usage: [no] nat [(<if_name>)] <nat_id> <local_ip> [<mask>
                [<max_conns> [emb_limit] [<norandomseq>]]]]
 [no] nat [(if_name)] 0 [access-list [<acl-name>]]
PIX(config)#
```

The global command configures the global interface: It defines what the translated network will be. The global command has the following syntax:

```
PIX(config)# global ?
usage: [no] global [(<ext_if_name>)] <nat_id>
➡{<global_ip>[-<global_ip>] [netmask <global_mask>]} |
  interface
PIX(config)#
```

Notice that the nat command uses the *if_name* and *local_ip* parameters, whereas the global command uses the *ext_if_name* and *global_ip* parameters. A host with address *local_ip* sending a packet to the PIX Firewall's *if_name* will appear as *global_ip* to devices beyond the PIX Firewall's *ext_if_name*.

For a simple example of using the nat and global commands to configure NAT, consider the two networks separated by a PIX Firewall, shown in Figure 18.1. One host is on the RFC 1918 private network 10.1.1.0/24, and the other is on the public network 65.24.200.0/24. Here, we want any packet that is sent from the inside network 65.24.200.0 to the outside network 10.1.1.0 to be translated.

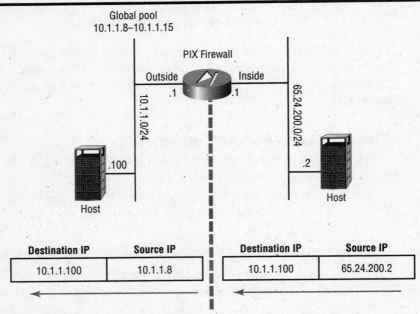

FIGURE 18.1: Simple NAT translation example

WARNING

The local and global interfaces are determined only by the security values. It does not matter which address is private or public! Of course, in the real world, your most trusted inside network will almost always use private addresses, whereas your untrusted outside network will use public addresses. We have configured this example backwards, just to demonstrate the point.

In this case, the *if_name* would be inside, and the *ext_if_name* would be outside. The *local_ip* would be 65.24.200.0 with a mask of 255.255.255.0.

The *global_ip* could be many different values, depending on your environment and how you want the PIX Firewall to behave. In this case, we'll assign the addresses 10.1.1.8 through 10.1.1.15 to the pool. This means up to eight hosts on the inside network could have translations at a time, and these eight hosts will appear to the outside world as .8 through .15.

The last required parameter for the nat and global commands is the *nat_id*. The NAT ID is an arbitrary number between 0 and 2 billion, which allows you to tell the PIX Firewall which global addresses you want to use to translate internal addresses. This may make more sense when we begin configuring multiple interfaces. For now, we can pick any number we want, as long as we use the same number in both the nat and global commands.

NOTE

Using a NAT ID of o tells the PIX not to do any translation. We'll discuss this concept in more detail later in the chapter, in the "Identity NAT" section.

Now we're ready to configure NAT on the PIX Firewall shown in Figure 18.1. We'll begin by verifying that our interfaces are named and addressed correctly, using the show nameif and show ip commands:

```
PIX# show nameif
nameif ethernet0 outside security0
nameif ethernet1 inside security100
nameif ethernet2 intf2 security10
PIX# show ip
System IP Addresses:
        ip address outside 10.1.1.1 255.255.255.0
        ip address inside 65.24.200.1 255.255.255.0
        ip address intf2 127.0.0.1 255.255.255.255
Current IP Addresses:
        ip address outside 10.1.1.1 255.255.255.0
        ip address inside 65.25.200.1 255.255.255.0
        ip address intf2 0.0.0.0 0.0.0.0
PIX#
```

Now, we're ready to tell PIX which addresses we want translated, using the nat command:

```
PIX(config)# nat (inside) 1 65.24.200.0 255.255.255.0
```

WARNING

Don't forget the parentheses around the *if_name* and *ext_if_name*!

The unusual thing about this command is the *mask* field. Unlike the ip address command, where you use the mask of the interface, here the mask is used similarly to the wildcard bits of the IOS. The mask tells the PIX Firewall how many addresses to include in the range. For instance, even though the actual interface 65.24.200.1 has a 24-bit mask, we could use the following command:

```
PIX(config)# nat (inside) 1 65.24.200.0 255.255.255.128
```

This command tells the PIX Firewall that we want only the first half of the address range (65.24.200.1 through 65.24.200.127) to be translated.

Similarly, we could use the following command:

```
PIX(config)# nat (inside) 1 65.24.200.14 255.255.255.255
```

By using the full 32-bit mask, we tell PIX that we want only the host 64.24.200.14 to be translated. In this case, none of the other clients on that network would be translated.

Next, we'll tell PIX which addresses we want these translated into, using the global command:

```
PIX(config)# global (outside) 1 10.1.1.8-10.1.1.15
```

NOTE

Remember that the NAT ID (in this case 1) can be anything you want, as long as it's the same in both the nat and global commands.

This is all that is required to allow hosts on the inside network to access the outside network. Once this command is in place, the default behavior of the PIX Firewall is to let all hosts included in the nat command (in this case, 65.24.200.1 through 65.24.200.254) out, but hosts that want to initiate connections back in are still restricted. In order to allow a host on the outside network to initiate a connection, we use a third command: static.

TIP

Optionally, you can allow all hosts on the inside to be translated by typing the command nat (inside) 1 0 0. As you can imagine, doing so can make configuration a lot less difficult, especially if you have many subnets on your internal network that don't lend themselves to address summarization. However, it is a good idea to explicitly declare the IP addresses that are allowed out, because doing so will make spoofing almost impossible. Nobody wants the embarrassment or liability of having their network used as a DDoS launchpad because they haven't implemented anti-spoofing filters.

The *static* Command

The static command lets a host on the outside network initiate a connection. The static command is different from the nat and global commands because it operates by itself. You enter all the information in one command, rather than two. Here is the syntax of the static command:

```
PIX(config)# static ?
usage: [no] static [(internal_if_name, external_if_name)]
               {<global_ip>|interface} <local_ip> [netmask
                  <mask>]
               [<max_conns>] [<emb_limit>] [<norandomseq>]]]
        [no] static [(internal_if_name, external_if_name)]
           {tcp|udp}
               {<global_ip>|interface} <global_port>
               <local_ip> <local_port> [netmask <mask>]
               [<max_conns>] [<emb_limit>] [<norandomseq>]]]
PIX(config)#
```

For example, let's say we have a web server on our inside network with an IP address of 65.24.200.22. We want all hosts on the outside network to be able to reach this service via the global address 10.1.1.16. To configure this arrangement, we would enter the following command:

```
PIX(config)# static (inside, outside) 10.1.1.16 65.24.200.22
```

Identity NAT

Occasionally, you will want the protection of a PIX Firewall but do not need or desire address translation. This might be the case for several reasons:

▶ Your entire network is using registered addresses.

Part IV

► The firewall's job is to protect some critical area of the internal network from the rest of the internal network, where both are using private addresses. An example is a large company's cluster of accounting or human resource systems that should be accessed only by people in certain departments.

► NAT breaks some protocols, such as SNMP, PPTP, and a lot of streaming media protocols.

The problem is that without a translation slot, nothing gets through the PIX Firewall, and translation slots are only created by the NAT process (as described in the previous chapter). The solution to this problem is to still send packets through the NAT process, but not actually translate them. In other words, the source and destination fields in the IP headers are not modified as they pass through the PIX Firewall. This process is often called *identity NAT*.

You configure identity NAT by using the nat 0 command. For example, if the inside interface of the PIX Firewall is 10.1.1.1/24, and we do not want this network to be translated, we can use the following command:

```
PIX(config)# nat (inside) 0 10.1.1.0 255.255.255.0
```

Note that a corresponding global command is not required for identity NAT.

When we enter this command, the PIX Firewall politely confirms our instruction:

```
PIX(config)# nat (inside) 0 10.1.1.0 255.255.255.0
nat 0 10.1.1.0 will be non-translated
PIX(config)#
```

WARNING
The operation of the nat 0 command, both syntactically and under the hood, has changed dramatically over the last several versions of the PIX operating system. This chapter deals with only the current implementation as of version 6.0(1). If you are using a different version, read the Command Reference documentation on Cisco's website before using the nat 0 command.

Now, let's suppose we want the 10.1.1.0 subnet on the inside interface translated as usual, but we have one host with IP address 10.1.1.15 that frequently establishes IPSec-encrypted tunnels across the PIX Firewall; so, we want every host on this network to be translated except 10.1.1.15. To configure this, we use two commands (not including the corresponding global commands on the outgoing interfaces):

```
PIX(config)# nat (inside) 1 10.1.1.0 255.255.255.0
PIX(config)# nat (inside) 0 10.1.1.15 255.255.255.255
```

Here is the output of the show nat command after these statements have been entered on the PIX Firewall:

```
PIX(config)# nat (inside) 1 10.1.1.0 255.255.255.0
PIX(config)# nat (inside) 0 10.1.1.15 255.255.255.255
nat 0 10.1.1.15 will be non-translated
PIX(config)# show nat
nat (inside) 0 10.1.1.15 255.255.255.255 0 0
nat (inside) 1 10.1.1.0 255.255.255.0 0 0
PIX(config)#
```

Notice that even though the commands were typed out of order, PIX sorted the longest subnet mask to the top of the list.

In these examples, using a zero in the *nat_id* field tells the PIX Firewall to allow packets from the specified hosts to pass through the firewall without being translated. However, there is another use for this command that can be quite confusing. We will explain it in the next section, because it is important that it not be confused with identity NAT.

Access Blocking with ACLs

When many internal networks need to be translated, it can be easy to make data-entry errors. To reduce this possibility, recent versions of the PIX operating system have made the nat command more powerful, but somewhat confusing. In this section we will attempt to explain the proper way to tell the PIX Firewall which networks to translate.

As an example, let's say we have the 10.1.0.0/20 subnet further broken into sixteen 24-bit subnets, from 10.1.0.0/24 to 10.1.15.0/24. All of them access the Internet through the inside interface of our PIX Firewall. Let's further suppose that we want all these networks to be translated except the hosts between 10.1.9.128 and 10.1.9.191. However, in this case, we're not talking about identity NAT, because we don't want these hosts to have any access at all. In other words, PIX should not create a translation slot for hosts in the range 10.1.9.128/26.

You can accomplish this task two ways. The first is shown here, including the commands and the output of the show nat command.

```
PIX(config)# nat (inside) 1 10.1.0.0 255.255.255.0
PIX(config)# nat (inside) 1 10.1.1.0 255.255.255.0
```

```
PIX(config)# nat (inside) 1 10.1.2.0 255.255.255.0
PIX(config)# nat (inside) 1 10.1.3.0 255.255.255.0
PIX(config)# nat (inside) 1 10.1.4.0 255.255.255.0
PIX(config)# nat (inside) 1 10.1.5.0 255.255.255.0
PIX(config)# nat (inside) 1 10.1.6.0 255.255.255.0
PIX(config)# nat (inside) 1 10.1.7.0 255.255.255.0
PIX(config)# nat (inside) 1 10.1.8.0 255.255.255.0
PIX(config)# nat (inside) 1 10.1.9.0 255.255.255.128
PIX(config)# nat (inside) 1 10.1.9.192 255.255.255.192
PIX(config)# nat (inside) 1 10.1.10.0 255.255.255.0
PIX(config)# nat (inside) 1 10.1.11.0 255.255.255.0
PIX(config)# nat (inside) 1 10.1.12.0 255.255.255.0
PIX(config)# nat (inside) 1 10.1.13.0 255.255.255.0
PIX(config)# nat (inside) 1 10.1.14.0 255.255.255.0
PIX(config)# nat (inside) 1 10.1.15.0 255.255.255.0
PIX(config)# exit
PIX# show nat
nat (inside) 1 10.1.9.192 255.255.255.192 0 0
nat (inside) 1 10.1.9.0 255.255.255.128 0 0
nat (inside) 1 10.1.1.0 255.255.255.0 0 0
nat (inside) 1 10.1.2.0 255.255.255.0 0 0
nat (inside) 1 10.1.3.0 255.255.255.0 0 0
nat (inside) 1 10.1.4.0 255.255.255.0 0 0
nat (inside) 1 10.1.5.0 255.255.255.0 0 0
nat (inside) 1 10.1.6.0 255.255.255.0 0 0
nat (inside) 1 10.1.7.0 255.255.255.0 0 0
nat (inside) 1 10.1.8.0 255.255.255.0 0 0
nat (inside) 1 10.1.10.0 255.255.255.0 0 0
nat (inside) 1 10.1.11.0 255.255.255.0 0 0
nat (inside) 1 10.1.12.0 255.255.255.0 0 0
nat (inside) 1 10.1.13.0 255.255.255.0 0 0
nat (inside) 1 10.1.14.0 255.255.255.0 0 0
nat (inside) 1 10.1.15.0 255.255.255.0 0 0
PIX#
```

Here, we type one nat statement for each 24-bit network except the 10.1.9.0 subnet—for it we type two statements, so as not to include the addresses that we do not want translated. In other words, we explicitly define all the networks we want translated.

It's easy to see how you could make mistakes by issuing so many commands. In fact, it's so easy that while I was writing this chapter, I left out the statement for the 10.1.0.0/24 network, and it was more than a week before I noticed my omission! To make matters worse, the PIX Firewall again sorts our longest subnet masks to the top of the list. Although this sorting made things easier to read and understand earlier, it now makes it very difficult, because the subnets are no longer in numerical order. In large organizations where there are often hundreds of networks, variable-length subnet masking (VLSM) is in use, and subnets often aren't contiguous, this situation could quickly get out of hand!

Now compare that method with the access-list feature implemented as of version 5.3:

```
PIX(config)# access-list block permit ip 10.1.9.128
    255.255.255.192 any
PIX(config)# nat (inside) 1 10.1.0.0 255.255.240.0
PIX(config)# nat (inside) 0 access-list block
PIX(config)# exit
PIX# show nat
nat (inside) 0 access-list block
nat (inside) 1 10.1.0.0 255.255.240.0 0 0
PIX# show access-list block
access-list block permit ip 10.1.9.128 255.255.255.192 any
    (hitcnt=0)
PIX#
```

Again, although the corresponding global command has been omitted, we accomplished in three commands what previously took 17! Not only is the input far easier and, by extension, less error-prone, but the output is much simpler and easier to comprehend. The difference is that the entire 10.1.0.0/20 network is covered in one easy-to-read statement, and the address ranges you don't want are defined in an ACL and then applied with the nat 0 statement.

Part IV

TIP

When you are troubleshooting a network problem or responding to an attack, time is critical. Any steps you can take to shorten the time required to understand your configuration will directly affect the time it takes to respond to the situation.

In this section and the previous section, you have seen not only the value of both identity NAT and the ability to block address translation using ACLs, but also that these commands are easily confused. Let's review their use:

- Use nat (*<interface>*) 0 *<network>* *<subnet-mask>* when you want certain hosts to be known outside the PIX Firewall by their actual address.

- Use nat (*<interface>*) 0 access-list *<access-list>* when you want to keep certain hosts from ever sending traffic through the PIX Firewall by preventing them from creating a translation slot.

Configuring PAT

The configuration of PAT is even easier than NAT. We use the same nat command:

```
PIX(config)# nat (inside) 1 65.24.200.0 255.255.255.0
```

However, for the global command, we make one slight modification:

```
PIX(config)# global (outside) 1 10.1.1.8
```

By listing only a single address in the *global pool* (in this case, 10.1.1.8), all the hosts from 65.24.200.1 to 65.24.200.254 will be seen on the outside network as 10.1.1.8. In other words, we've configured PAT.

Here's an example of this command in action:

```
PIX(config)# global (outside) 1 10.1.1.8
Start and end addresses overlap with existing range
Type help or '?' for a list of available commands.
PIX(config)# no global (outside) 1 10.1.1.8-10.1.1.15
PIX(config)# global (outside) 1 10.1.1.8
Global 10.1.1.8 will be Port Address Translated
PIX(config)#
```

We begin by attempting to configure a PAT address that is currently part of an existing global pool. As you can see, PIX won't allow that: You cannot have overlapping address ranges (although you can use NAT and PAT at the same time, as you'll see in the next example). You must remove the first range before assigning the second. Another point of interest is that PIX lets you know what you've done. This helps the PIX Firewall be more secure by preventing a lot of accidental misconfiguration.

Static PAT

Let's take a look at using static PAT for inbound traffic. A common situation for a small to medium business is to use PAT but have a few servers publicly available. Consider the example shown in Figure 18.2.

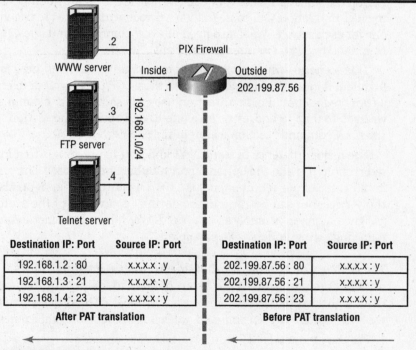

Destination IP: Port	Source IP: Port
192.168.1.2 : 80	x.x.x.x : y
192.168.1.3 : 21	x.x.x.x : y
192.168.1.4 : 23	x.x.x.x : y
After PAT translation	

Destination IP: Port	Source IP: Port
202.199.87.56 : 80	x.x.x.x : y
202.199.87.56 : 21	x.x.x.x : y
202.199.87.56 : 23	x.x.x.x : y
Before PAT translation	

FIGURE 18.2:   Static PAT example

Here we have a web server, an FTP server, and a Unix-based server that is accessed via Telnet. Our fictitious business wants all three of these services to be available to the outside network, but it has only a single global address.

Part IV

We'll readdress our networks so the inside network is 192.168.1.0/24, with the three servers using .2, .3, and .4 respectively. The PIX Firewall will be .1, of course. The ISP has assigned us the single registered address 202.199.87.56 for our outside interface.

This scenario presents a few challenges. We will need to use the PIX Firewall's outside interface address as the global PAT address. Also, we need to direct inbound traffic as follows:

- ▶ Inbound HTTP traffic destined for TCP port 80 to 192.168.1.2
- ▶ Inbound FTP traffic destined for TCP port 21 to 192.168.1.3
- ▶ Inbound Telnet traffic destined for TCP port 23 to 192.168.1.4

No traffic to any other port will be allowed to pass inbound, but all the PCs on the 192.168.1.0 network must be able to access the Internet through the PAT translation. Our configuration will require three static commands: one for each service. We'll also need one nat command and one global command to allow our internal users out.

This scenario—where packets sent to a single global IP address are sent to different local IP addresses based on their TCP port—is often referred to as *port redirection*. Port redirection uses the same static command we used to map IP addresses on a one-to-one basis in the section "The static Command" section earlier in the chapter.

The major difference in static NAT and port redirection is that in port redirection, you add the optional port number and protocol. The protocol for all three of our requirements is TCP. The port number depends on the service, but can be given in the decimal equivalent of the protocol's assigned number or simply as a keyword. We will use both methods in the following configuration as an example.

The *static* Commands for Outside to Inside Requirements   Three static commands take care of our outside to inside requirements. (Although a few of these parameters are optional, such as the two zeros on the end of each static command, we included them for completeness.)

For the inbound HTTP traffic, we use this command:

```
PIX(config)# static (inside, outside) tcp interface
➥80 192.168.1.2 80 netmask 255.255.255.255 0 0
```

This command tells the PIX Firewall that any traffic that arrives on the outside interface, destined for TCP port 80 of the outside interface, should be transmitted out the inside interface to 192.168.1.2, TCP port 80. It also tells the PIX Firewall to change the destination IP address field in the IP header to 192.168.1.2.

Notice the keyword `interface`. This keyword is used to indicate the external or lower security interface so that the actual IP address of the PIX Firewall's outside interface can be used, instead of dedicating a global pool of IP addresses as in the previous examples. Using this interface can occasionally be complicated, but it definitely saves IP addresses.

For the inbound FTP traffic, we use this command:

```
PIX(config)# static (inside, outside) tcp interface
➡21 192.168.1.3 21 netmask 255.255.255.255 0 0
```

This command tells the PIX Firewall that any traffic that arrives on the outside interface, destined for TCP port 21 of the outside interface, should be transmitted out the inside interface to 192.168.1.3, TCP port 21. It also tells the PIX Firewall to change the destination IP address field in the IP header to 192.168.1.3.

For the inbound Telnet traffic, we use this command:

```
PIX(config)# static (inside, outside) tcp interface telnet
➡192.168.1.4 telnet netmask 255.255.255.255 0 0
```

This command is just like the previous two, except that it sends the traffic destined for TCP port 23 to 192.168.1.4. Notice that we used the keyword `telnet` in this example instead of the port number in decimal, to illustrate the command's flexibility. Note that in the `show` commands, and also in configuration mode, PIX will replace these port numbers with its keywords automatically.

The *nat* and *global* Commands for Inside to Outside Requirements

For internal hosts to also access the external network, you need a `nat` and `global` statement. The `nat` statement is identical to the ones used previously, but in the `global` statement, you see the same `interface` keyword. This allows our internal hosts to use the same address as the outside interface as well, again saving IP addresses:

```
PIX(config)# nat (inside) 1 192.168.1.0 255.255.255.0
PIX(config)# global (outside) 1 interface
```

These two commands tell the PIX Firewall to allow all traffic from the 192.168.1.0 network on the inside interface to access resources on the outside interface after being translated with PAT.

Part IV

Checking the Configuration   After entering these commands, we exit
the configuration mode and type a few show commands to see how it looks.

```
PIX# show global
global (outside) 1 interface
PIX# show nat
nat (inside) 1 192.168.1.0 255.255.255.0 0 0
PIX# show static
static (inside,outside) tcp interface www 192.168.1.2
➥www netmask 255.255.255.255 0 0
static (inside,outside) tcp interface ftp 192.168.1.3
➥ftp netmask 255.255.255.255 0 0
static (inside,outside) tcp interface telnet 192.168.1.4
➥telnet netmask 255.255.255.255 0 0
PIX#
```

The show commands indicate that our commands were accepted as
expected. Notice that the port numbers we typed have been converted to
the recognized keywords for easy reading.

Now let's test it. I set up hosts on either side of the firewall and attempted
to telnet to 202.199.87.56; then, I pointed my web browser to the same
address. The show xlate command should prove the configuration is
working. The output is as follows:

```
PIX# show xlate
2 in use, 2 most used
PAT Global 202.199.87.56(23) Local 192.168.1.4(23)
PAT Global 202.199.87.56(80) Local 192.168.1.2(80)
PIX#
```

As you can see, requests to port 23 were forwarded to 192.168.1.4 TCP
port 23, whereas requests to port 80 were sent to 192.168.1.2 TCP port 80.
FTP command sessions would work similarly, but without the fixup
protocol command, our data sessions would be denied.

Configuring NAT on Multiple Interfaces

In practice, networks often start out simply, much like the configurations
we've shown in the previous sections; but they almost always grow in both

size and complexity, as new segments and services are added and the amount of traffic increases. In this section, we'll explain the relationships between interfaces when there are more than just two.

TIP

The configuration of multiple interfaces may seem complicated because of the way packets are translated as they go from one network to another. But as long as you remember that translations always go between pairs of interfaces, and you focus on just the pair in question, configuring multiple interfaces on the PIX Firewall will be much easier to comprehend and troubleshoot.

Configuring Three Interfaces

We'll begin with a simple scenario that has three interfaces: the Internet on the outside interface, a DMZ network containing proxy and web servers, and two private networks on the inside interface. For the ASA, we'll assign 100 to the inside interface, 0 to the outside interface, and 10 to the DMZ interface. Here's a summary:

Interface	Security Level
Inside (two private networks)	100
DMZ (proxy and web servers)	10
Outside (Internet)	0

NOTE

Changing the DMZ interface to a security value of 50 wouldn't alter the PIX Firewall's behavior. That is, increasing or decreasing the value won't automatically make the interface more or less secure. What's important is the value relative to the other interfaces. In this case, as long as the DMZ interface's value is more than that of the outside interface and less than that of the inside interface (that is, between 1 and 99), any number will have the same effect.

This scenario, shown in Figure 18.3, is quite common. We will assume our ISP is allowing us to use the 12 unused, registered addresses on the outside network for our NAT global pool. However, we have 100 user PCs on our 10.1.1.0/24 subnet and another 100 user PCs on the 10.1.2.0/24 subnet. Because 200 is much larger than 12, we'll obviously need to make some allowances.

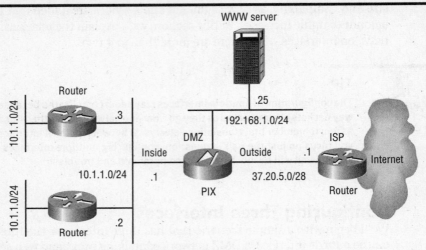

FIGURE 18.3:   A simple multiple interface scenario

Further, let's suppose the users on the 10.1.1.0 subnet are allowed unrestricted access directly to the Internet, but users on the 10.1.2.0 subnet must use a proxy server in the DMZ to access the Internet. These users will be translated from the inside to the DMZ using the global pool 192.168.1.101 to 192.168.1.199. If more than 99 simultaneous connections are needed, the .200 address should be used for PAT. If there are more than 99 simultaneous connections from the 10.1.1.0 subnet to the Internet, the 37.20.5.14 address should be used for PAT.

The proxy server (IP address 192.168.1.25) on the DMZ is allowed to initiate connections to the Internet using NAT but may not initiate connections to the inside network. The web server (IP address 192.168.1.75) is allowed to talk to a database (IP address 10.1.1.50) on the inside network.

Of course, hosts on the Internet are not allowed to initiate any connections to the inside network, and they may only initiate requests to the web server on the DMZ network.

Configuring NAT between the Inside and Outside Interfaces

Now that you understand the requirements, let's begin by configuring NAT between the inside and outside networks. According to our requirements, the only connectivity allowed between the inside and outside interfaces is from the 10.1.1.0 network, and these addresses are supposed to be translated using the addresses 37.20.5.5 through 37.20.5.13. After those addresses are used, any subsequent connections should be translated via PAT using the 37.20.5.14 address. No connections are required from the outside to the inside, so no static commands are necessary. The commands required for this configuration are as follows:

```
PIX(config)# nat (inside) 1 10.1.1.0 255.255.255.0
PIX(config)# global (outside) 1 37.20.5.5-27.20.5.13
PIX(config)# global (outside) 1 37.20.5.14
```

Configuring NAT between the Inside and DMZ Interfaces   Next, we'll configure NAT between the inside and DMZ interfaces. Our primary requirement here is to allow 10.1.2.0 devices access to the proxy server so they can access the Internet. However, any internal device is allowed to access the DMZ. These devices should be translated into 192.168.1.101 to 192.168.1.199. As with the outside interface, we'll use the 192.168.1.200 address for PAT, just in case more than 99 people are accessing it at once. So, our commands here are similar, except that we also have a requirement for the web server to initiate connections into the inside network. This requirement necessitates an additional static command:

```
PIX(config)# nat (inside) 2 0 0
PIX(config)# global (dmz) 2 192.168.1.101-192.168.1.199
PIX(config)# global (dmz) 2 192.168.1.200
PIX(config)# static (inside,dmz) 192.168.1.2 10.1.1.50
➡netmask 255.255.255.255
```

Now you can now see the importance of having a NAT ID. This arbitrary number lets us tell the PIX Firewall exactly which addresses we want to translate when there are multiple outbound interfaces. As you will see in the next pair of interfaces, it also lets us tell PIX which global addresses we want to use when there are multiple inbound interfaces.

Notice in the previous code that the nat statement still uses the inside interface, but the corresponding global statements use the DMZ interface. In all these cases, the nat statement is used on the higher security interface, and the global statements are used on lower security interfaces.

Configuring NAT between the DMZ and Outside Interfaces
Next, we'll configure NAT between the DMZ and the outside interface. To fulfill the requirement that the proxy server be the only device allowed to initiate connections out, we'll choose yet another arbitrary NAT ID and use another pair of nat and global statements. To allow any external

Part IV

device to initiate connections to the web server, we'll need another `static` command. The commands are as follows:

```
PIX(config)# nat (dmz) 3 192.168.1.25 255.255.255.255
PIX(config)# global (outside) 3 37.20.5.4
PIX(config)# static (dmz, outside) 37.20.5.3 192.168.1.75
➥netmask 255.255.255.255
```

Again, the interface with the highest security level is now the DMZ interface, so the `nat` statement is on the DMZ interface and the `global` statement is on the outside interface. Also, by specifying just the proxy server and using a 32-bit mask (255.255.255.255), we have prevented any other host on that network from creating a translation slot in the PIX Firewall.

OUTBOUND CONNECTIONS FROM THE DMZ

Although it may seem safe to allow any device on your DMZ to initiate outbound connections to the Internet, doing so isn't necessarily a good idea. Despite the fact that the network is more trusted than the Internet, it's not totally trusted. As an example of what can go wrong, consider the NIMDA virus and variants from September 2001. This outbreak was particularly annoying because the virus had several delivery mechanisms. Aside from the often-used Outlook e-mail macros, it could also spread from IIS web server to IIS web server.

The moral of the story is that a web server initiating a connection to the Internet is highly suspicious. Unless there is an well-documented need for this privilege, turn it off.

Reviewing the Configuration We'll wrap up this example by showing the relevant part of the configuration. To save space, we've snipped the extraneous stuff:

```
PIX# wr t
Building configuration...
: Saved
:
PIX Version 6.0(1)
nameif ethernet0 outside security0
```

```
nameif ethernet1 inside security100
nameif ethernet2 dmz security10
enable password 8Ry2YjIyt7RRXU24 encrypted
passwd 2KFQnbNIdI.2KYOU encrypted
hostname PIX
<snip>
interface ethernet0 auto
interface ethernet1 auto
interface ethernet2 auto
mtu outside 1500
mtu inside 1500
mtu dmz 1500
ip address outside 37.20.5.2 255.255.255.240
ip address inside 10.1.0.1 255.255.255.0
ip address dmz 192.168.1.1 255.255.255.0
<snip>
global (outside) 1 37.20.5.5-37.20.5.13
global (outside) 1 37.20.5.14
global (outside) 3 37.20.5.4
global (dmz) 2 192.168.1.101-192.168.1.199
global (dmz) 2 192.168.1.200
nat (inside) 1 10.1.1.0 255.255.255.0 0 0
nat (inside) 2 0.0.0.0 0.0.0.0 0 0
nat (dmz) 3 192.168.1.25 255.255.255.255 0 0
static (dmz,outside) 37.20.5.3 192.168.1.75 netmask
   255.255.255.255 0 0
static (inside,dmz) 192.168.1.2 10.1.1.50 netmask
   255.255.255.255 0 0
route inside 10.1.1.0 255.255.255.0 10.1.0.3 1
route inside 10.1.2.0 255.255.255.0 10.1.0.2 1
<snip>
Cryptochecksum:5454bf941e2c2180e5975704c712fe7a
: end
[OK]
PIX#
```

Notice the routing statements required to make the connectivity work. Also notice that we have configured two different PAT addresses on the outside interface. This functionality was implemented in version 5.3; it works great, but it can be confusing. Be careful that you don't try to assign two PAT addresses to the same NAT ID.

Configuring Six Interfaces

Figure 18.4 shows the setup for our next example, which is much more complex than the one described in the previous section. Here we have an organization with an internal network that is connected to the Internet and two partners. We also have a DMZ, which hosts servers that our business partners use, and we have a dedicated remote-access network, where users can dial in from home and access services such as their e-mail.

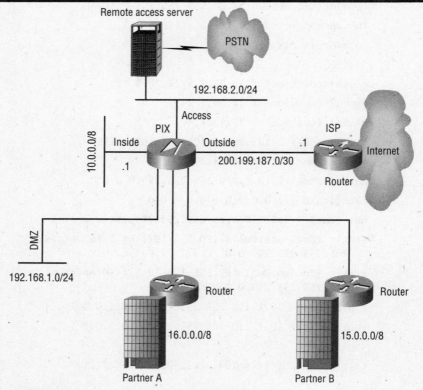

FIGURE 18.4:   Complex six-interface NAT scenario

We want to implement the following basic rules:

▶ Hosts on the inside interface can access anything (we assume our partners have firewalls of their own that prevent us from arbitrarily accessing their equipment).

▶ Only a small group of hosts on the 10.6.98.0/24 inside interface needs to access the remote-access segment, so these hosts can use a shared bank of 32 modems to dial out.

▶ Hosts on the partner networks can access the DMZ.

▶ Hosts on the partner networks cannot access each other or use our Internet connection. We assume they have their own ISP.

▶ Mobile users on the access segment can access anything except the inside interface. That is restricted to the e-mail server on 10.1.1.100.

▶ Hosts on the Internet cannot initiate connections into any other network.

To implement this scenario, we will assign our interfaces the following security level values:

Interface	Security Level
Inside	100
Access	80
Partner A	40
Partner B	40
DMZ	20
Outside	0

Although we assigned all these values (except the inside network) arbitrarily, the relative numbers are important. They immediately accomplish several of the goals. By assigning the same security value to both customer networks, we make it impossible for those two interfaces to communicate directly with one another. In addition, the order of interfaces from highest to lowest allows us to configure the nat and global statements appropriately.

We'll begin our configuration by addressing access to the interfaces in order of security value, from lowest to highest. It is critical to remember that NAT is always between a pair of interfaces.

With six interfaces, the potential exists for many pairs of interfaces, but each pair does not require its own NAT ID. In fact, giving each its own NAT ID would create problems (although it's possible), because the global ranges cannot overlap and the nat ranges cannot be identical. Having several smaller ranges is much less efficient. So, in the sections that follow, we will combine the statements into groups based on the appropriate NAT IDs for efficiency and ease of understanding—but doing so does not change the fact that NAT operates only between a given pair of interfaces.

As an example, if a host on the inside network were translated to 192.168.2.50 for traffic to the DMZ interface, that same host could be translated to a completely different IP address when it conversed with devices through another PIX interface. In this case, that single host would have multiple translation slots.

Configuring the Outside Interface   The outside interface, of course, has the lowest security value. For this interface, we will use one PAT address for all clients coming from the access and inside networks, as follows:

```
PIX(config)# nat (inside) 1 10.0.0.0 255.0.0.0
PIX(config)# nat (access) 1 192.168.2.0 255.255.255.0
PIX(config)# global (outside) 1 interface
```

Here we demonstrate multiple nat statements paired with a single global statement, which is the opposite of the three-interface scenario described in the previous section. Neither of our partners or the DMZ hosts are allowed to use our Internet connection, but if access were allowed, we could easily add three more nat statements. (Note that it is impossible to combine these into one statement by aggregating addresses—you still must specify the interface, and there are three different interfaces.)

Configuring the DMZ Interface   The next highest interface is the DMZ. Because everyone except the outside interface is allowed to access these hosts, we would normally have four nat commands that explicitly define their respective networks and one global command. However, the nat commands for the inside and access segments are already assigned explicitly with a NAT ID of 1. The problem is that you cannot specify the same network in another nat command, because PIX will return a "duplicate NAT entry" error. Our solution is to shorten the subnet mask to include all networks for the inside and access segments, as shown here:

```
PIX(config)# nat (inside) 2 0 0
PIX(config)# nat (access) 2 0 0
PIX(config)# nat (partnera) 2 16.0.0.0 255.0.0.0
PIX(config)# nat (partnerb) 2 15.0.0.0 255.0.0.0
PIX(config)# global (dmz) 2 192.168.1.64-192.168.1.254
```

This interface would normally be nominally less secure because it is theoretically possible to do spoofing. But because this is a DMZ segment, we will accept that small risk and leave our explicit (and correct) statement for use in the NAT ID 1 group that allows access to the Internet.

That takes care of our nat statements. For the global command, we reserve the first 62 addresses for servers on the DMZ segment, and we use the rest for our global NAT pool. It is also important to note that each of these four interfaces with a nat statement must have a higher security value than the interface with the global statement.

Configuring the Partner Interfaces   The next interfaces are our partner interfaces. Here, it is appropriate to reuse the nat statements from NAT ID 1 (which permit only the inside and access segments) and to use the interface addresses to do PAT. Thus, our statements are as follows:

```
PIX(config)# global (partnera) 1 interface
PIX(config)# global (partnerb) 1 interface
```

Configuring the Access Interface   Access to the access segment is next. Here we will use another NAT ID to distinguish between the two we are already using on the inside interface. And, because there are only 32 modems, there's no point to using more than 32 addresses in the global pool—we can have only 32 simultaneous users:

```
PIX(config)# nat (inside) 3 10.6.98.0 255.255.255.0
PIX(config)# global (access) 3 192.168.2.64-192.168.2.95
```

Configuring the Inside Interface   Finally, we need to allow access to the inside network. The only connectivity permitted here is from the access segment to an e-mail server, which requires only a single static statement. This statement allows hosts to access the server using a global address of 192.168.2.63. Therefore, it is important that this address be in the remote user's DNS or in a static hosts file:

```
PIX(config)# static (inside,access) 192.168.2.63 10.1.1.100
➥netmask 255.255.255.255
```

Part IV

NOTE

The `static` command doesn't actually allow access. It only allows the specified host to create a translation slot from a lower security interface to a higher
one. To allow access, you must combine this statement with an `access-list`
or `conduit` command.

Configuring Routing

In most cases, your network is made up of a number of subnetworks. There
may be one or more at each branch office, or you may have the network
configured so that each floor or each closet gets its own IP subnet. In any
case, there are probably several internal routers. The hosts on most, if not
all, of these subnets will need access to external networks, such as business
partners or the Internet.

These internal and external networks are separated by the PIX Firewall,
so routing on the firewall becomes an issue. Typically, the internal routers
use an internal routing protocol, such as Open Shortest Path First (OSPF)
or Enhanced Interior Gateway Routing Protocol (EIGRP), to communicate
Network layer reachability information (NLRI). Presumably, in such a case,
each internal network knows about all the other internal networks. They
also typically use a default route for destinations they don't know about.
In most of your internal networks, this default route points to the PIX
Firewall, which means all traffic leaving the network goes through the
PIX Firewall. The PIX Firewall, in turn, generally needs a default route to
which it can deliver the packets that pass inspection. Recall from the
previous chapter that if the traffic doesn't pass through the firewall, it
can't possibly offer any protection.

In this section, we will cover the commands used to configure IP routing on the PIX Firewall. Our goals are as follows:

► Configure the PIX Firewall to generate a default route so that
   internal routers know where to send packets destined for the
   external networks.

► Configure the PIX Firewall so that it knows where to send packets.

Unfortunately, the only way for the PIX Firewall to communicate with
other routers is via the RIP routing protocol, and even then, all it can do
is generate a single default route and listen for other routes. So, in most

circumstances, you may be better off configuring static default routes on your internal Cisco routers that point to the PIX Firewall's inside interface. Another option is to allow the PIX Firewall to generate the default route via RIP and then redistribute it into a more useful, stable, and secure routing protocol on the Cisco routers before the default route is passed to the rest of the network.

Generating a Default Route

To generate a default route using RIP, you use the `rip` command. The syntax of the `rip` command is as follows:

```
PIX(config)# rip ?
usage: [no] rip <if_name> default|passive [version <1|2>]
➥[authentication <text|md5> <key> <key id>]
PIX(config)#
```

Here's an example of a `rip` command:

```
PIX(config)# rip inside default version 2
```

This command sends the route 0.0.0.0 mask 0.0.0.0 to the multicast address 224.0.0.9 on the inside interface. It will be received and processed by all RIPv2-speaking routers.

Specifying version 1 of RIP will cause the same route to be sent to the broadcast address 255.255.255.255. This process is illustrated here, using the output of the debug `rip` command:

```
PIX# debug rip
RIP trace on
PIX# configure terminal
PIX(config)# rip inside default version 1
PIX(config)# exit
PIX# 8: RIP: interface inside sending v1 update to
    255.255.255.255
PIX# configure terminal
PIX(config)# rip inside default version 2
PIX(config)# exit
PIX# 9: RIP: interface inside sending v2 update to 224.0.0.9
```

Part IV

```
PIX# no debug rip
RIP trace off
PIX#
```

NOTE

Although using RIP to broadcast the default route automates the route-learning process and is extremely easy to configure, it is less secure than using static routes. Distance-vector protocols like RIP are also more susceptible to routing loops than their link-state cousins.

Configuring the PIX Firewall to Route Packets

The next issue to consider is configuring the PIX Firewall so that it knows where to send its packets.

If either the inside or outside networks are using the RIP protocol, you can configure the PIX Firewall to listen to those updates so that it learns its routes dynamically. You do so with the `rip` command, using the `passive` keyword instead of the `default` keyword. For instance, to tell the PIX Firewall to listen for RIP updates on the inside interface, you would use this command:

```
PIX(config)# rip inside passive
```

You can also specify the version and enable authentication with this command.

The alternative to using dynamically learned routes is to manually configure static routes. These routes are configured using the `route` command, which has the following syntax:

```
PIX(config)# route ?
usage: [no] route <if_name> <foreign_ip> <mask> <gateway>
    [<metric>]
PIX(config)#
```

As an example, consider the network shown in Figure 18.5. This network has three internal networks: the directly connected user segment, a remote-user segment, and the WAN link that connects them. The outside interface is connected to our ISP's router, which leads to the Internet, and the DMZ interface has a handful of servers.

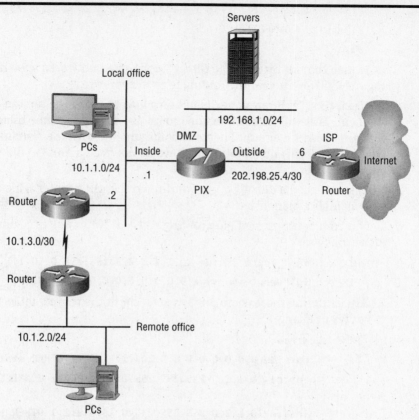

FIGURE 18.5: PIX Firewall routing example

Before we begin entering commands, let's discuss what routes are needed. First, the PIX Firewall automatically enters directly connected networks in its routing table, so no manual entry is needed for the local-user segment, the DMZ, or the network attached to the outside interface. We can use the `show route` command to see the routing table, as follows:

```
PIX# show route
    inside 10.1.1.0 255.255.255.0 10.1.1.1 1 CONNECT
        static
    DMZ 192.168.1.0 255.255.255.0 192.168.1.1 1 CONNECT
        static
```

```
                outside 202.198.25.4 255.255.255.252 202.198.25.5 1
                  CONNECT static
      PIX#
```

Notice that all three of the directly connected networks shown in Figure 18.5 are listed in the routing table shown here.

Next, the PIX Firewall needs to know how to get to the remote-user segment. This will require a manual route. Because we assume there is no business need for external hosts to communicate with the routers that connect the local and remote offices, we do not need a route to the WAN subnet.

Last, we need a default route pointing to the ISP's router. This route also requires a manual entry.

Our commands to configure routing on the PIX Firewall in Figure 18.5 are as follows:

```
      PIX(config)# route inside 10.1.2.0 255.255.255.0 10.1.1.2
      PIX(config)# route outside 0.0.0.0 0.0.0.0 202.198.25.
```

After entering these commands, we can check the routing table again to verify our changes:

```
      PIX# show route
              outside 0.0.0.0 0.0.0.0 202.198.25. 1 OTHER static
              inside 10.1.1.0 255.255.255.0 10.1.1.1 1 CONNECT
                static
              inside 10.1.2.0 255.255.255.0 10.1.1.2 1 OTHER static
              DMZ 192.168.1.0 255.255.255.0 192.168.1.1 1 CONNECT
                static
              outside 202.198.25.4 255.255.255.252 202.198.25.5 1
                ➥CONNECT static
      PIX#
```

The two routes have been added as expected. Also notice that although the routes are all static, the "static" routes are designated by the keyword OTHER, and the directly connected networks are designated by the keyword CONNECT.

One other point of interest in the output of the show route command is that the directly connected interfaces have the same metric (1) as the static routes. This may seem a little unusual if you're used to working with the IOS, where directly connected interfaces always have a metric of 0 and static routes typically have a metric of 1. This curious situation might lead you to believe that it's possible to create all sorts of bizarre routing situations on the PIX Firewall, where traffic destined for directly connected interfaces could take a nonoptimal path. To illustrate that this isn't the case, let's see what happens when we attempt to misconfigure the PIX Firewall shown in Figure 18.5:

```
PIX# configure terminal
PIX(config)# route dmz 10.1.1.0 255.255.255.0 192.168.1.2 1
Route already exists
PIX(config)# route dmz 10.1.1.0 255.255.255.0 192.168.1.2 2
Route already exists
PIX(config)# route inside 10.1.2.0 255.255.255.0 10.1.1.3 1
cannot add route entry
Type help or '?' for a list of available commands.
PIX(config)# route inside 10.1.2.0 255.255.255.0 10.1.1.3 2
PIX(config)# exit
PIX# show route
        outside 0.0.0.0 0.0.0.0 202.198.25.4 1 OTHER static
        inside 10.1.1.0 255.255.255.0 10.1.1.1 1 CONNECT
            static
        inside 10.1.2.0 255.255.255.0 10.1.1.2 1 OTHER static
        inside 10.1.2.0 255.255.255.0 10.1.1.3 2 OTHER static
        DMZ 192.168.1.0 255.255.255.0 192.168.1.1 1 CONNECT
            static
        outside 202.198.25.4 255.255.255.252 202.198.25.5 1
        ➡CONNECT static
    PIX#
```

First, we attempt to reroute traffic destined for the local network on the inside interface out through the DMZ interface, with the same metric as the inside interface. PIX points out our mistake and rejects our command. Next, we try the same command, but with a higher metric. A higher metric on an IOS-based router would tell the router to use this route only if the first route fails. However, PIX doesn't like this either. Although these are unusual but potentially useful configurations, keep in mind that the PIX Firewall consistently foregoes features in favor of security.

Next, we try to tell the PIX Firewall about an alternate route to the remote-user network, which is not directly connected. By assigning an

Part IV

equal-cost route (both routes have a metric of 1), we might expect PIX to load-balance the traffic destined for 10.1.2.0/24 between both the 10.1.1.2 and 10.1.1.3 (not pictured in Figure 18.5) routers. But alas, PIX isn't keen on load balancing either, although the error message it returns is somewhat less precise.

Finally, we try the same route again, but with a higher metric. The PIX Firewall adds this route to its table, as shown by the show route command.

The following are important points to remember about PIX Firewall routing:

▶ The PIX Firewall is not a router.

▶ You can't achieve load balancing by manipulating route metrics.

▶ Static routes are more secure than those learned via RIP.

WHAT'S NEXT

In this chapter, we began by explaining what information you need to gather before configuring a PIX Firewall. Then we discussed the common global commands used to configure services like DNS and logging, and how to set the system clock.

Next, we discussed basic interface configuration, as well as advanced, multiple-interface configuration. Following that, we covered NAT (Network Address Translation) and PAT (Port Address Translation) in detail. Finally, we described how to configure the PIX Firewall to share a default route with other routers and how to receive information from other routers.

In Chapter 19 you will learn about Virtual Private Networks, their basic terminology, and how to establish a VPN tunnel. This chapter is a general introduction, followed by several chapters on specific Cisco devices and configurations.

Chapter 19

Introduction to Virtual Private Networks

This chapter introduces virtual private network (VPN) concepts and explains how virtual private network tunnels are created. The information presented here provides the foundation for the detailed, device-specific material in the following chapter.

We'll begin with some basics, including discussions of the types of VPNs and devices. The remainder of this chapter covers IPSec, which is a standards-based method of negotiating a secure connection between peers, and Internet Key Exchange (IKE), which is a protocol used to provide authentication between peers. We'll discuss the various authentication types, the different ways a VPN tunnel can be built, the steps involved in the process, and the order of events. Finally, we'll address potential problems associated with tunnels and how to troubleshoot them.

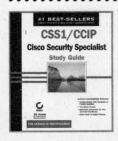

Adapted from *CSS1™/CCIP™: Cisco® Security Specialist Study Guide* by Todd Lammle, Tom Lancaster, Eric Quinn, and Justin Menga

ISBN 0-7821-4049-1 $89.99

VPN Basics

A *virtual private network (VPN)* is an extension of a network. It is *virtual* because it does not use reserved circuits. A VPN may pass over a circuit that is used only for VPN traffic, but this is not a requirement. It is *private* because it is a tunnel. This tunnel does not need to be encrypted or have any sort of protection for the data, although it can use encryption and other security measures. A device can be configured to allow only certain types of traffic to access the tunnel. It is a *network* because it extends an existing network past its natural boundaries.

Major Types of VPNs

There are many types of VPNs, but they are usually defined by how they are created and what purpose they serve. (This is similar to how two pickup trucks may be categorized differently by the Department of Motor Vehicles because one is for commercial use and one is for residential.) The following are three major types of VPNs:

Access VPN   A VPN used to connect to the network over a shared medium like the Internet. People dialing the modem on their PC and connecting to a modem at work are crossing the shared medium of the public telephone system. People connecting to their ISP to use the Internet to transport VPN traffic are connecting to two shared mediums. They first use DSL, cable, or dial-up connections to access their ISP, and then use the Internet to go the rest of the way.

Intranet VPN   A VPN used to connect two trusted locations to each other over a dedicated connection. An example would be a VPN between the corporate headquarters in Maine and a manufacturing facility in Thailand. The key elements are the trusted locations and connection dedicated to VPN traffic.

Extranet VPN   A VPN used to connect untrusted locations to each other over a dedicated connection. An example would be the headquarters office in Maine using a VPN to connect to the ordering system of a supplier in Ohio. There is a certain amount of trust, but not as much as there would be if both sides were part of the same corporate infrastructure.

VPN Devices

A VPN is a *tunnel*, and each tunnel must begin and end somewhere. Cisco has many devices that can act as one end of a VPN tunnel or manage it, including Cisco routers, the PIX Firewall, Cisco VPN Concentrators, and the Cisco Secure VPN client software.

NOTE

Cisco Secure is the name of the product line for Cisco's security products. Cisco Secure Policy Manager (CSPM), a component of Cisco Works, can be used to manage VPNs.

Cisco devices don't need to talk to just other Cisco devices. A Cisco router can talk VPN to a Windows 2000 server, a non-Cisco router, or another IPSec device. IPSec is a standard, and as long as both vendors follow the instructions in the standard and both devices are set up with the correct configuration, they should be able to form a tunnel. (IPSec will be discussed in detail later in this chapter, beginning with the "Introducing IPSec" section.)

Let's take a closer look at each type of Cisco VPN device and its capabilities.

Cisco Routers

Cisco routers come in various flavors and have the ability to do different tasks based on the available hardware and software. Different IOS feature sets will give more or fewer options for creating a VPN tunnel. Cisco routers began supporting IPSec with IOS 11.3(T). Prior to this, they used Cisco Encryption Technology (CET), which should not be used if IPSec is available.

Cisco IOS software is capable of forming many different types of tunnels. Along with IPSec tunnels, Cisco routers can build Layer 2 Forwarding (L2F), Layer 2 Tunneling Protocol (L2TP), Point-to-Point Tunneling Protocol (PPTP), and Generic Routing Encapsulation (GRE) tunnels.

Even low-end routers can do encryption, but what type of encryption depends on the type of router, the version of IOS, and the amount of memory. Newer routers with enough flash and NVRAM can use an IOS image that allows for triple Data Encryption Standard (3DES) encryption. A 1600-series router or a 2500-series router doesn't have the processing ability and is limited to basic DES encryption. Some 800-series routers are capable of using 3DES. (DES and 3DES encryption are discussed in the "Encryption" section later in this chapter.)

It is normally not a good idea to terminate many VPN connections at even a robust router because of the amount of processing that goes on in the encryption and decryption process. The exception to this rule is when your router is outfitted with a VPN module. This module offloads the processing from the CPU, keeping valuable CPU cycles free for other tasks. (For more information about the VPN module, visit www.cisco .com/univercd/cc/td/doc/pcat/vpnnm.htm.)

The PIX Firewall

Cisco has a number of PIX Firewall models available, from the low-end 501 to the high-end 535. The PIX Firewall has supported IPSec since version 5.0. This firewall can form a tunnel with other devices that speak IPSec, including Cisco routers, firewalls, and VPN Concentrators.

All PIX Firewalls are capable of using DES and 3DES encryption, but the device must be licensed for it. If you currently have a PIX Firewall that is not licensed for encryption, you can get a free key for DES by registering at www.cisco.com/kobayashi/sw-center/ciscosecure/pix .shtml. A 3DES license can be purchased through a Cisco reseller.

The Cisco VPN Concentrator

The Cisco VPN Concentrator, formerly the Altiga VPN concentrator, is designed to terminate many client VPN connections. It can also form a tunnel with a router, firewall, or another concentrator.

You should use the VPN Concentrator if you have more than a few users who want to access a network via a VPN tunnel. The concentrator is a stand-alone network device that offloads the task of processing VPN tunnels from routers and firewalls. The VPN Concentrator can be managed via the command-line interface (CLI) or an HTML-based graphical user interface (GUI).

The 3000-series VPN Concentrators can terminate up to 10,000 user tunnels. The 5000-series VPN Concentrators can terminate up to 50,000 tunnels.

VPN Client Software

VPN client software is used on PCs and servers in order for those devices to serve as one end of a tunnel. When users create a VPN from their home PC, it terminates at a router, firewall, or concentrator.

The Cisco Secure VPN client comes in two flavors. The older one is the SafeNet client that Cisco used to connect client PCs to routers and firewalls. There are two versions: 1.0 (which cannot use a certificate from a Windows 2000 certificate authority) and version 1.1 (which can use a certificate from a Windows 2000 certificate authority).

The other type of client is the concentrator client, often referred to as the Altiga client. It is used to connect client PCs to the VPN Concentrator. There are two major versions of this client: 2.5 and 3.0. Use whichever version of the client matches the software version on the concentrator; for example, use a 2.5 client if you have version 2.5 software on the concentrator.

Cisco realized that requiring two different clients when only one can be installed at a time was problematic. The company has merged the two into the Unified Client. The latest version of the Unified Client as of this writing is 3.5, which allows for VPNs to general Cisco devices. This version even comes with a transparent stateful firewall for the client. If you are using Windows XP, you must use version 3.1 or higher.

INTRODUCING IPSEC

IPSec is a standards-based way of creating a tunnel that data will travel along to get to its destination. An example of an IPSec tunnel is shown in Figure 19.1.

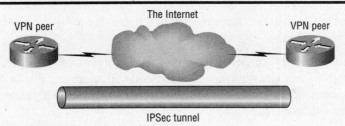

FIGURE 19.1:   An IPSec tunnel

IPSec has the option of using several other standards in order to get the tunnel set up. One of these is Internet Key Exchange (IKE), which is a protocol that works with IPSec. IKE, RSA signatures, and certificate authorities are discussed in the "Introducing IKE" section later in this

Part IV

chapter. Here, we will cover the IPSec components that provide authentication, encryption, and other services. These include the following:

▶ The Authentication Header (AH) and Encapsulating Security Payload (ESP) protocols

▶ Hashing

▶ Transform sets

▶ Data Encryption Standard (DES) and 3DES

▶ Diffie-Hellman

▶ Security Associations (SAs)

However, before we discuss the individual components of IPSec, let's see what services it can provide.

IPSec Services

IPSec can accomplish several tasks, if you wish to configure them. They include the following:

▶ Data confidentiality can be ensured by encrypting traffic as the packets leave the router.

▶ Data integrity can be ensured by verifying that packets have not changed after they were sent. Hashing is used to verify that there have not been any changes to transferred data.

▶ Data-origin authentication verifies the identity of the originator of the packet.

▶ *Anti-replay* is a process by which the receiver can detect that a packet has already been received and will reject any duplicate packets. (This process does not interfere with the TCP retransmission function.)

IPSec Building Blocks: AH and ESP

In order to establish an IPSec tunnel between two devices, those devices must negotiate how the tunnel will be built. IPSec operates at layer 3 (the Network layer) of the OSI model and uses two protocols to build tunnels and protect the data traveling across the tunnel:

> ► *Authentication Header (AH)* uses protocol 51.

> ► *Encapsulating Security Payload (ESP)* uses protocol 50.

Knowing what AH and ESP do is essential to creating a good tunnel blueprint.

Authentication Header

AH, defined in RFC 2402, does not perform any sort of data encryption. Its purpose is to provide data integrity and authentication. It ensures that a packet that crosses the tunnel is the same packet that left the peer device and that no changes have been made. It uses a keyed hash to accomplish this task. Figure 19.2 illustrates the hash creation. (Hashing is discussed in more detail a little later in this chapter.)

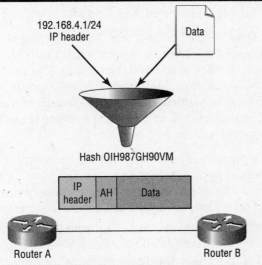

FIGURE 19.2:   The Authentication Header (AH) process

NOTE

Encryption is a very processor-intensive task, so in some situations you might want to use just AH. For example, you might not want to bother to encrypt routing updates, but you will want to make sure the data inside the packets has not changed.

Part IV

The AH information sits in the packet between the spots reserved for layer 3 and layer 4. The AH header consists of six fields:

Next Header This 8-bit field identifies the type of the payload after the AH.

Payload Length This 8-bit field indicates how long the AH header is.

Reserved These 16 bits are reserved and consist of zeros.

Security Parameter Index (SPI) This 32-bit field holds a pseudo-random, arbitrarily assigned number that is paired with other information to identify a particular tunnel. The SPI identifies AH information and links it to an appropriate peer IP address and SA.

Sequence Number This 32-bit field can be used to enable anti-replay, helping prevent old packets from being captured and reused. If anti-replay is not used, this field still exists.

Authentication Data This field is where the data is stored to ensure that the packet hasn't been tampered with. The field size depends on the method used to do the hashing. The two methods used for Cisco devices, MD5 and SHA, will truncate at 96 bits of information. Implementations in IPv4 require blocks of 32 bits, and IPv6 requires blocks of 64 bits. Padding is used to fill any spaces to reach the appropriate block size.

The AH process runs on the entire packet, with the exception of fields in layer 3 that are designed to change. For example, the Time To Live (TTL) field is designed to decrement as the packet goes from one network to the next. It would be rather silly to include this field in a static value.

AH takes the output from the process, encrypts it, and then truncates it so the result will fit in the Authentication Data field. When the packet arrives at the other end of the tunnel, the device performs the same calculation on the packet it received and compares the output it got with the one that was sent by the originator. If they match, the data is authenticated.

WARNING
The IP address is a field that is not designed to be changed. However, many network implementations use Network Address Translation (NAT), which changes the IP address. Creating a tunnel that uses AH across a device using NAT will result in a broken tunnel.

Encapsulating Security Payload

ESP, defined in RFC 2406, can provide for data integrity and authentication, but its primary purpose is to encrypt the data crossing the tunnel. When using the hash to provide for authentication and integrity, ESP does not protect as much of the packet as AH does, but this can be a benefit in some situations.

There are two reasons why ESP is the preferred building block of IPSec tunnels:

▶ The authentication component of ESP does not include any layer 3 information. Thus it can work in conjunction with a network using NAT.

▶ On Cisco devices, ESP supports encryption using DES or 3DES.

Figure 19.3 shows the ESP header and its placement in the packet, depending on whether IPSec is configured in transport mode or tunnel mode. These modes are discussed in detail in the next section.

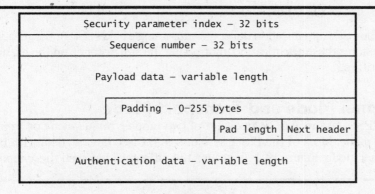

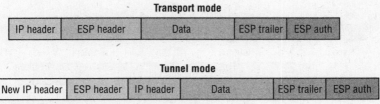

FIGURE 19.3:   The ESP header and packet

Because ESP offers both authentication and encryption, it is possible to do both without needing to use AH. When using both ESP and AH, it is important to remember that encryption comes first. Everything from layer 4 through the end of the data is encrypted. Once the packet has been encrypted, the authentication process is applied.

In addition to the ESP header, which sits right after the layer 3 information, ESP also has a trailer for encryption and a trailer for authentication. There are two 32-bit fields within the ESP header: The Security Parameter Index (SPI) and Sequence Number fields. They work the same way they do in the AH header (described in the previous section). The ESP trailer contains three fields:

Pad Length This 8-bit field indicates how many bytes have been used for padding for encryption.

New Header This 8-bit field identifies the type of data found in the Payload Data field.

Padding This field indicates how much padding has been used to get the encrypted packet to a fixed size. The size used depends on the encryption protocol, but it can be up to a block size of 2,040 bits.

The ESP authentication trailer contains a single field—ESP Authentication—that stores the authentication information. Its size depends on the hashing algorithm.

Tunnel Mode and Transport Mode

An IPSec tunnel can be in either of two modes: *tunnel mode* or *transport mode*. Most of the IPSec sessions that Cisco devices deal with use tunnel mode. Figure 19.4 illustrates the difference between these modes.

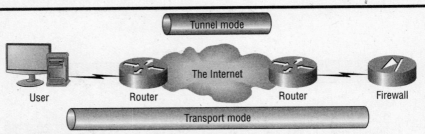

FIGURE 19.4: Tunnel mode versus transport mode

A transport-mode tunnel encrypts from the device that originally created the packet all the way to the device that is receiving the packet. At no time does the packet leave the IPSec tunnel. If users wish to protect their e-mail as they send it to the server, they can encrypt it on their end, and the server will decrypt it. The message is protected from one end all the way to the other. Transport mode might be used if an administrator wanted to be able to administer the router from home via a VPN tunnel, for example.

If the IPSec tunnel does not protect the packet from end to end, then it is a tunnel-mode tunnel. For example, if a company's headquarters has a router and the company's remote site has a router, there could be a tunnel-mode tunnel between them. When users at the remote site check their e-mail, the traffic goes across the tunnel, but it is not protected from end (user) to end (server).

The VPN concept deals with tunnel-mode tunnels. A virtual network is created that spans some other network. A tunnel-mode tunnel actually takes the packet and places it inside another packet. You end up with two IP addresses: one for the tunnel endpoint and one for the origination.

In the example shown in Figure 19.5, a packet with an IP header and payload is depicted at the top. If the packet needs to cross a transport-mode tunnel, the AH process will run on the packet, and the AH header will be inserted. A transport-mode tunnel does nothing to the IP header.

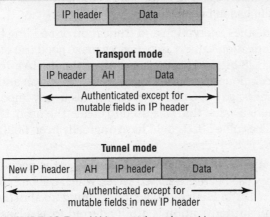

FIGURE 19.5:   AH in tunnel mode and in transport mode

If the packet needs to cross a tunnel-mode tunnel, the IPSec device takes the original packet and places it inside a new packet. The old IP address is now considered to be part of the data field. The new packet has a source IP address of the interface at one end of the tunnel and a destination IP address of the interface at the other end of the tunnel. ESP will work in the same way, except that if both encryption and authentication are used, encryption happens first.

Hashing

Hashing is used to verify that data hasn't changed or to hide data crossing the network. For example, CHAP (Challenge Handshake Authentication Protocol) uses hashing to disguise passwords. In the world of VPNs, hashing is used to verify that there haven't been any changes to data.

A *hash* is a simple thing to create. For example, suppose you want to send the number 12345 across the network and use hashing to make sure there were no changes to this transmission. If the chosen algorithm says to multiply the data by 56,789, invert the result, and chop off all but the first four characters, here is what will happen:

Multiply	$12345 \times 56789 = 701060205$
Invert	$701060205 = 502060107$
Truncate	$502060107 = 5020$

When you send the number 12345, the value 5020 will also be included. In order to make sure the data has not changed, the device on the other end of the tunnel will perform the same computation on the value 12345. Once it comes up with its own four-digit hash, it compares the hashes. If they match, the data has not changed.

A typical hash combines encryption and truncation or padding to get to a fixed-size authentication value. Cisco devices make good use of Message Digest 5 (MD5), 128-bit, and Secure Hash Algorithm (SHA), 160-bit, for hashing. These techniques perform the requisite encryption and then truncate or pad the message to 96 bits. As a result, it is nearly impossible to regenerate the original value that was used to create the hash, if it is not already known. The value 5020 could have originally been 50201, or it could have been 5020983478.

Part of the negotiation of IPSec to set up the tunnel is the negotiation of various keys. The key used here is a shared secret, which will be explained in more detail in the "Diffie-Hellman" section, coming up shortly. The process of hashing an authentication is often referred to as a Hashed Message Authentication Code (HMAC).

Encryption

Encryption is commonly associated with VPN tunnels, but it is not a required component. Encryption involves a message, a key, and a way of combining the two. One type of encryption takes a message and a key and mixes them together in a blender on the "chop" setting; another will combine them using the "puree" setting. The result is a string of seemingly random characters that can be reversed at the other end into its cleartext form.

The tunnel endpoints must use the same type of encryption, which is verified before the tunnel comes up and data can be sent. If a message were encrypted in one form but the other side tried to decrypt it in another form, the output would be undecipherable.

Cisco devices currently support DES and 3DES. DES uses 56-bit encryption, and so does 3DES, but 3DES uses it three times. Whereas DES negotiates a key, 3DES negotiates a key and then breaks it into three parts. The first part is 56-bit encryption, the second process is to decrypt the message with the second key, and then the third key is used to encrypt again. Because the first and second keys are not identical, the second process is just another way of doing 56-bit encryption. 3DES yields encryption that is about twice as strong as regular DES.

NOTE

The U.S. government has approved a new standard called Advanced Encryption Standard (AES) based around an algorithm called Rijndael. Cisco has indicated support for AES and has begun integrating it into some products, such as the Content Accelerator.

Diffie-Hellman Key Exchange

Diffie-Hellman (DH) key exchange is used to create something called a *shared secret*. A shared secret is made when two networking devices create a key and then share part of it with the peer. Diffie-Hellman is defined in RFC 2631.

The first task is for each network device to create a key pair. One mathematical expression is generated and from it, two keys are formed: a private key and a public key, as shown here:

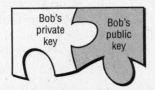

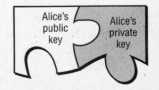

The private key is never shared with any other device, but it is linked mathematically with the public key. Each network device will send its public key to its peer:

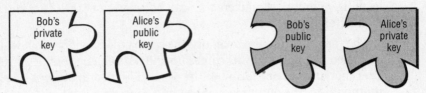

This results in each device having a copy of its private key, its public key, and the peer device's public key. Nothing more will be done with its own public key, but the other two keys are very important. Each device will mathematically combine its own private key with the peer device's public key. This process results in the shared secret:

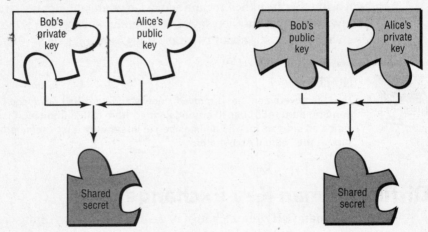

Because the keys are all linked together, each side ends up with the same key. Encrypting and decrypting data using the same key is called *symmetric key* encryption. (The other form is asymmetric key encryption, which will encrypt using one key and decrypt using a different but mathematically related key.)

Diffie-Hellman is used to protect the IPSec tunnel setup process. The Diffie-Hellman tunnel is used to encrypt the IPSec negotiations that are required before the tunnel can come up. The Diffie-Hellman tunnel will not be used to encrypt conventional traffic—for that, you need the IPSec tunnel.

Several strengths of Diffie-Hellman are available, but most Cisco devices support only the two weakest types, called Group 1 and Group 2. Group 1 is 768-bit encryption; Group 2 is 1024-bit encryption.

NOTE

With the approval of the new AES encryption standard, the IETF is working on increasing Diffie-Hellman to 8192 bits.

Transform Sets

In order to build the IPSec tunnel, you need to tell the network device how to use AH and/or ESP. A *transform* is an option that describes how to build the tunnel. For example, a transform may tell a router to use ESP with DES encryption or tell a firewall to use AH with MD5 hashing, or it may say to use several items. An IPSec blueprint, or *transform set*, can have up to three instructions in it: one AH transform and two ESP transforms (one for encryption and one for authentication). Figure 19.6 illustrates the options for transform sets.

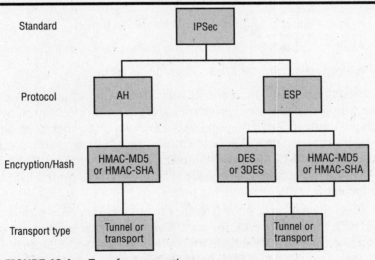

FIGURE 19.6:   Transform set options

Another part of the configuration involves telling the network device if the IPSec tunnel will use tunnel mode or transport mode. The default on the Cisco router is for tunnel mode.

Part IV

NOTE

Other types of transforms are available for odd purposes. For example, the ah-null transform is used to create a tunnel without authentication or encryption.

IPSec Security Associations

A Security Association (SA) contains instructions for how to build a tunnel to a given destination. When two peers decide they will use ESP-DES and AH-MD5 for the IPSec tunnel, this information is stored somewhere along with items like the SA lifetime and appropriate keys. All the properties of the blocks used to build an IPSec tunnel are placed in this database. The SA tells the router the recipe to use when sending traffic through the tunnel to a given destination.

An IPSec SA has several components:

- ▶ The peer IP address (the IP address of the other end of the IPSec tunnel)

- ▶ The Security Parameter Index (SPI), which is a pointer used to identify the characteristics of a tunnel

- ▶ The transform set used to build the IPSec tunnel

- ▶ Keys used to hash or encrypt the traffic that crosses the tunnel

- ▶ Optional attributes, such as the tunnel lifetime

Each tunnel has at least one SA associated with it. An IKE SA is bidirectional; the referenced properties apply in both directions. IPSec tunnels are unidirectional; they apply on a one-way basis only. Because the peers must negotiate and have identical ways of setting up the tunnel, the question, "Why are they unidirectional?" is often raised. The answer is that the router needs to be able to invert the access control list (ACL) for incoming traffic.

When the ACL is created, it applies to outgoing traffic, which is associated with the outgoing SA. In order to make sure that traffic coming in is protected the way it should be, the router makes a mirror image of the ACL and associates it with incoming traffic for the incoming SA.

Each network device is responsible for setting up its outgoing SA. When router A receives traffic that wants to be encrypted, it sends the SA policy information to router B. This becomes router B's incoming SA.

Router B will compile all the information it needs to determine appropriate characteristics for its outgoing SA and send that to router A. The numbers identifying a particular SA (the SPI) will be identical on both sides of the tunnel.

Figure 19.7 shows that there are two separate connections, based on the connection IDs in use (`conn id`). The SPIs are unique on a per-SA basis; each side uses the same SPI when referring to the same SA. Because there are two different SAs, there are two different SPIs. The other information must match across both SAs and on both sides.

Router 1

Router 2

```
outbound esp sas:
  spi: 0x1B781456(460854358)
  transform: esp-des,
  in use settings = {Tunnel, }
  slot: 0, conn id: 18,
   crypto map: mymap
  sa timing: (k/sec)
  replay detection support: N
```

```
inbound esp sas:
  spi: 0x1B781456(460854358)
  transform: esp-des,
  in use settings = {Tunnel, }
  slot: 0, conn id: 18,
   crypto map: mymap
  sa timing: (k/sec)
  replay detection support: N
```

```
inbound esp sas:
  spi: 0x8AE1C9C(145628316)
  transform: esp-des,
  in use settings = {Tunnel, }
  slot: 0, conn id: 17,
   crypto map: mymap
  sa timing: (k/sec)
  replay detection support: N
```

```
outbound esp sas:
  spi: 0x8AE1C9C(145628316)
  transform: esp-des,
  in use settings = {Tunnel, }
  slot: 0, conn id: 17,
   crypto map: mymap
  sa timing: (k/sec)
  replay detection support: N
```

FIGURE 19.7:   IPSec Security Associations (SAs)

NOTE

The `crypto map: mymap` shown in Figure 19.7 defines the crypto map used for IPSec configuration. The crypto map name (such as `mymap` in this example) does not need to match between the peers; it is a locally significant value.

IPSec SAs are traditionally negotiated through IKE (discussed in the next section). It is possible to create an SA manually, but doing so is not

Part IV

advisable for most environments, because it can require additional record keeping and increase the possibility of errors.

INTRODUCING IKE

The Internet Key Exchange (IKE) works hand in hand with IPSec and is defined in RFC 2409. IPSec sets up the tunnel for the traffic to cross in a protected fashion. IKE handles all the administration and gets everything ready so that the IPSec tunnel can form. If there is no connection with IKE, IPSec has no chance of forming a tunnel. Just as a foundation must be laid before a house can be built, an IKE tunnel must exist before IPSec information can be exchanged. The term *IKE* is used synonymously with *ISAKMP* (Internet Security Association Key Management Protocol).

IKE is configured manually on network devices and has several components that must match on both sides of the potential tunnel. Authentication is required to ensure that each device is talking to the correct peer. Cisco devices that support IPSec will support two or three methods of authentication: pre-shared keys, RSA signatures, or RSA encrypted nonces.

In addition to determining how the devices will authenticate, the devices also need to be configured with a peer identifier. Acceptable methods of identifying a peer are via IP address or a fully qualified domain name. The chosen method will apply to the router or firewall as a whole. You may not point to one peer via IP address and another via domain name.

Pre-Shared Keys

A *pre-shared key* can be manually configured on each network device. When you're using pre-shared keys, it is vitally important that the two peers be given the same key. When the process starts, device A sends a packet to device B. This packet includes, among other things, a keyed hash and the data that made the hash. Device B creates a hash using its key and the data that was sent by device A. If the hashes match, then the two devices are using the same key and have authenticated.

Because pre-shared keys must be manually entered, this method of authentication is not recommended for systems with many devices. However, it is a simple way of establishing authentication and works well when only a few devices are involved.

RSA Signatures

An *RSA signature* can be used if the devices have access to a certificate authority (CA). RSA signatures are keys that are generated on network devices and are used to authenticate the peer device. RSA signatures are the primary component when two network devices need to create a shared secret key (as explained in the "Diffie-Hellman Key Exchange" section earlier in this chapter). The peers use a public key and a private key to accomplish this, and they often use a CA to exchange keys.

Each device registers with the CA and gets a device-specific identity certificate. When attempting to authenticate, the devices exchange certificates. The authentication is actually the process of being able to understand the certificate that was received. This method is not efficient if only a few devices are involved, but it can save quite a bit of time if many devices are using IPSec tunnels. CAs are discussed in more detail in the "Certificate Authorities (CAs)" section, after the discussion of RSA encrypted nonces.

NOTE

RSA is a term that occurs frequently in encryption and security white papers and manuals. It stands for Rivest, Shamir, and Adleman, three doctors who invented the RSA Public Key Cryptosystem.

RSA Encrypted Nonces

The RSA encrypted nonce method employs everything that is not desirable in the pre-shared key and RSA signature methods. It is manually configured on each device, so it increases the potential for making mistakes when you're entering data. It also depends on generated keys, so there is a risk that the keys will be compromised.

RSA encrypted nonces start the same way RSA signatures do: Each network device must generate a large number, which is split into public and private keys. The public key must be copied over to the peer device, where the nonce is encrypted in it. When the IPSec session needs to start and IKE needs to be authenticated, the devices exchange nonces. At this point, each side generates a shared secret in the same fashion that Diffie-Hellman key exchange operates.

RSA encrypted nonces do have one advantage: They provide for a deniable transaction. A pre-shared key transaction can happen only with the peer that has the key. Because you have the IP address and the key, it's easy to prove. RSA signatures are difficult to deny because a trusted third party, the CA, maintains records of certificate serial numbers and can identify the device that registered. RSA encrypted nonces have neither of these ways of proving the identity of the other device. After all, it is not hard to spoof an address or hijack an IP address. If deniability is required, go with encrypted nonces.

Certificate Authorities (CAs)

A certificate authority (CA) is a trusted, third-party device that may or may not be under your administrative control. CAs are used to simplify administration of a large number of IPSec devices. Each device needs to register with the CA, rather than have a separate configuration for every peer with which it may wish to create a tunnel. A CA is normally not recommended for small networks because of the initial cost in money and time to set one up.

It doesn't take long to set up four routers to do authentication via pre-shared keys for each of the other three routers in the group; this arrangement uses a total of 12 keys. Expand the model from 4 routers to 400, and then add a new router. Not only will someone need to configure the new router for 400 pre-shared keys—one for each of the existing routers—but someone will need to log in to every one of the existing routers to add a single new key. Adding 800 keys will take quite a while, and troubleshooting the typos will take even longer. With a CA, you can avoid all this work by simply registering the new router with the CA.

In order to enroll to a CA, a device needs to generate an RSA key. As explained earlier, part of the RSA key is a public key and part of it is a private key. During the certificate-enrollment procedure, the network device gets a copy of the CA's public key. The network device also sends its public key to the CA. The CA encrypts the client's public key in a certificate and sends it to the enrolling client.

When two devices wish to form a tunnel and are authenticating via certificates, they need to exchange the certificates. Because the certificates are nothing more than an encrypted packet, the peers must have the necessary information to decrypt them. Because they were encrypted using the CA's private key, a device needs the same CA's public key in order to decrypt the certificate. Once the certificate is decrypted, device A has a copy of device B's public key and vice versa.

It doesn't matter which CA you use; several are available to serve your needs. All CA applications that want to be compatible follow the format specified in the X.509 standards. The CA application gaining the most widespread usage is the one Microsoft includes with Windows 2000 Server. There is no extra cost to use the CA supplied with Windows 2000, unlike other CA applications.

How IPSec Works

In the previous section, we explained that IKE must exist before IPSec can be set up. But before IKE or IPSec can perform their tasks, there must be some traffic that needs to cross the tunnel. Once that occurs, the router can communicate with the tunnel peer to set up the tunnel. IKE tasks are broken into two phases: setting up the IKE tunnel and performing quite a bit of setup for IPSec. Figure 19.8 illustrates these tasks, which are described in more detail in this section.

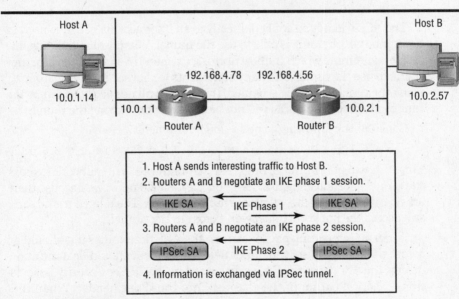

FIGURE 19.8:   The steps of IPSec

Defining Interesting Traffic

Without interesting traffic, there is nothing to trigger the tunnel creation. The tunnel must have a reason to exist, and traffic that wants to cross is that reason. In the network pictured in Figure 19.9, routers A and B are configured to create a tunnel if traffic wants to go from the network host

A resides on to the network that host B resides on. In order to do this, you must configure an ACL.

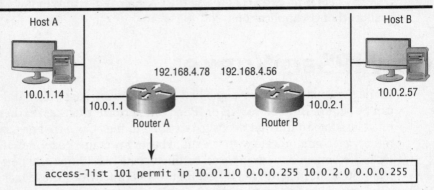

FIGURE 19.9:   Interesting traffic triggers tunnel creation.

The ACL will not be applied directly to an interface; instead, it is used to determine which traffic is able to use the tunnel. When you're building an ACL to determine which traffic will cross, use permit statements to permit traffic to use the tunnel and deny statements to prevent the traffic from using the tunnel. If traffic is denied, that traffic will not be protected by the tunnel. However, the traffic will not be blocked from leaving the router.

Consider the following access-list statement:

```
access-list 101 permit ip 10.0.1.0 0.0.0.255 10.0.2.0 0.0.0.255
```

This ACL will permit traffic originating from the 10.0.1.0 network to cross the tunnel if it is heading to a device on the 10.0.2.0 network. Because there are no other statements, all other traffic is denied. The denied traffic can still access the network; it just won't cross in the tunnel.

When an interesting packet arrives, the ACL determines if it should go across the tunnel. If so, the router determines what should be done and inserts the SPI (from the SA, as discussed in the "IPSec Security Associations" section earlier in the chapter) into the IPSec header. When the packet arrives at the destination peer, the device looks up the IPSec information based on the SPI in the packet.

IKE Phase 1

Once the router has received the interesting traffic and determined that the traffic needs to cross the tunnel, the router buffers the packet and starts the process to bring up the IPSec tunnel.

NOTE
It is not unusual to create an ACL that uses pings for interesting traffic, ping the far side, and watch three to five pings fail. If this happens, test the ACL by pinging again.

In order to bring up the tunnel, the two ends must negotiate what the IKE settings are supposed to be. The following items need to be negotiated:

► IKE SA

► Encryption

► Hash method

► Authentication method

► Diffie-Hellman group

► Tunnel lifetime

Each of these items must match on both sides of the tunnel, with the exception of the tunnel lifetime. A tunnel will not form if one side is using MD5 hashing and the other side is using SHA, or if one side is using Diffie-Hellman Group 1 and the other side is using Group 2. However, if one side leaves the lifetime at the default of one day and the other changes it to half a day, the tunnel will form, and it will expire in half a day.

Each Cisco network device has a default policy that is used for IKE phase one negotiations. This means an administrator needs to make only the desired changes in the configuration; all other settings will use the defaults. For example, if you only need to change the default setting of using a CA for authentication, just change it to pre-shared keys in the profile. The rest of the profile settings will use the built-in defaults.

IKE phase 1 has two different methods of communicating: main mode and aggressive mode.

Main Mode Communication

Main mode involves three, two-way exchanges between the peers:

► In the first exchange, the devices agree on the algorithms and hashing that will be used.

► The second exchange implements Diffie-Hellman to generate the shared secret key information and pass it back and forth.

Part IV

▶ The third exchange involves verifying the identity of the peer device. This process is protected by the Diffie-Hellman tunnel created in the second step.

Once everything is set up, an SA defines the tunnel. As explained in the "IPSec Security Associations" section earlier in the chapter, an SA is nothing more than a pointer to a database entry that defines how the IKE tunnel is formed. The appropriate information includes the hash method used, Diffie-Hellman information, how long the tunnel will stay up, and so on. It is important to remember that the IKE SA is bi-directional: The information the SA provides applies to both incoming and outgoing traffic.

Aggressive Mode Communication

Aggressive mode is great for reducing the latency involved with setting up the IKE tunnel, because only half of the communication is used. The downside is that there is not enough communication to protect the identity information when it is being passed, because it is sent along with the Diffie-Hellman information. The following aggressive mode steps are one-way communications:

▶ Router A sends all the information it can to router B, including policy information like the hash type and Diffie-Hellman group, the Diffie-Hellman public key information, and device identity information.

▶ Router B sends back a similar packet, essentially saying what is being used so that router A knows the tunnel is valid.

▶ Router A acknowledges receipt of the packet router B sent.

It is possible for someone to sniff the wire while an aggressive mode transaction occurs and find out the identity information, because it is not protected like a main-mode transaction.

IKE Phase 2

The purpose of the second phase of IKE is to negotiate the IPSec tunnel parameters. These negotiations are protected by the IKE tunnel created in phase 1. Most of the items the two peers are negotiating are the items configured in the transform sets. If the transform sets do not match, a tunnel will not be set up.

Phase 2 negotiation is also responsible for renegotiating the tunnel when the tunnel lifetime expires. There are two ways to do this: fully renegotiate the keys or partially renegotiate the keys. When the keys are only partially regenerated, it saves computational power because not as much is being redone. It also isn't quite as secure. If you want the keys to be regenerated fully and to have a new Diffie-Hellman tunnel to protect the negotiation, you need to ensure that you are using Perfect Forward Secrecy (PFS).

NOTE

PFS is a switch that tells the VPN device to go through the entire process of generating keys when the IPSec tunnel is about to expire. If PFS is not used, part of the old key may be reused; if the IKE tunnel is still up, it also can be reused. If PFS is enabled, the old IKE tunnel is torn down and rebuilt, and a totally new IPSec key is generated.

Once the IPSec tunnel has come up, packets move along it in both directions. ACLs are used to determine not only which packets need to exit through the tunnel, but also which packets should be arriving via the tunnel.

In the previous example, packets that originated on the 10.0.1.0 network and destined for the 10.0.2.0 network were to be encrypted. If the router received a packet from a 10.0.2.0 course heading for a 10.0.1.0 destination and the packet was not encrypted, the router would know something was wrong and would discard the packet. ACLs determine both which packets should be encrypted as they leave and which packets should be decrypted as they arrive.

The IPSec tunnel stays up for a certain duration. The choices for tunnel duration are a finite time limit in seconds or a number of kilobytes of traffic. The IPSec tunnel collapses once the timeout has been exceeded. More recent versions of code, like IOS 12.1 and PIX software 6.0, let you use both ways. For example, a router can be configured to have an IPSec tunnel that will expire in 12 hours or after 1GB of data has passed through it, whichever comes first.

The peers automatically renegotiate the tunnel 30 seconds or 250KB before the tunnel would expire. On a high-bandwidth link, the possibility exists for the tunnel to expire in the middle of negotiations for a new tunnel, leaving a small gap in communications.

Part IV

IPSec Task Flow

As traffic arrives and leaves and is encrypted and decrypted, decisions need to be made. Now that we've looked at the phases of IPSec tunnel creation, let's examine how the decisions are made in the process. Figure 19.10 shows a flowchart of the decision-making process.

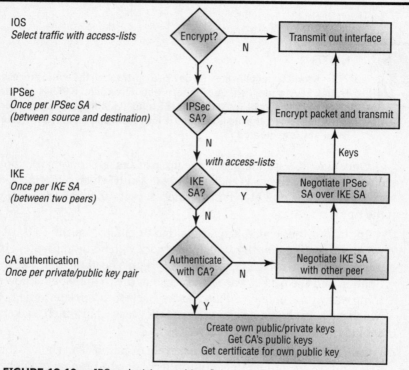

FIGURE 19.10:   IPSec decision-making flow

Let's review each of the decisions in the process:

Does the Traffic Need to Be Encrypted?   The IOS on the router needs to determine what it can do with traffic that arrives. The router compares the packet to the ACL and determines if the traffic should be encrypted. If the ACL says no, the traffic is forwarded out the interface. If the ACL says yes, the traffic goes through the tunnel before leaving the interface.

Does the IPSec SA Need to Be Negotiated?   Before the traffic enters the tunnel, the router needs to make sure the tunnel is up. If the IPSec tunnel already exists, the packet has the appropriate manipulations performed on it before it goes on its way. If the tunnel is not up, the router needs to do some more work.

Does the IKE SA Need to Be Negotiated?   The IPSec and IKE tunnels are two distinct entities. If the IPSec tunnel drops, it doesn't mean the IKE tunnel has dropped as well. If the IPSec tunnel is down, the characteristics need to be negotiated in order for it to come up. This cannot happen if the IKE tunnel is down. If both the IPSec tunnel and the IKE tunnel are down, the IKE tunnel needs to be negotiated in order to protect the negotiations that go on to bring up the IPSec tunnel.

Does the Traffic Need to Be Authenticated with CA?   A decision must be made to use either a CA or pre-shared keys. If a CA is used, the configuration, key creation, and certificate enrollment will all take place before the IKE tunnel negotiation can begin.

IPSEC TROUBLESHOOTING

IPSec is often a good choice for VPNs, but you must be aware of how changes will affect your network. Traffic that is crossing the network through an IPSec tunnel is still IP traffic. So, you need to deal with standard IP issues when passing traffic through the tunnels. The issues you may need to troubleshoot involve traffic delay, filtering, NAT, and ACLs.

Traffic Delay Problems

A certain amount of delay is associated with IP traffic. How much delay depends on several factors. There is propagation delay of about one microsecond per kilometer the packet needs to travel. Packet travel isn't necessarily "as the crow flies," either. Do a traceroute to your destination to see the path being used.

Interfaces also have a delay associated with them. The slower the interface, the more time it takes to place the packet on the network. It also takes time to do the computations and processing to place a packet into the IPSec tunnel. Tests with three 2600 series routers connected via

Part IV

10Mbps Ethernet showed about a 15-millisecond delay to place a ping packet into the IPSec tunnel using only DES encryption.

Encrypting Voice over IP (VoIP) traffic can be unnoticeable, or it can cause enough jitter (delay-triggered jerkiness) to make using VoIP connections undesirable. Test such applications as much as possible before implementing them on a wide-scale basis.

Filtering Problems

If the packets can leave the network device but never reach the far side, it is possible that some filtering is occurring somewhere in the network. If an intermediate router is filtering UDP port 500, then the IKE session will not complete. If the IPSec tunnel comes up but the intermediate router is filtering protocols 51 or 50, then packets with AH or ESP headers will be filtered.

The key to detecting filtering is to debug the setup of both IKE and IPSec and see how far the tasks complete. If the IPSec tunnel comes up, try to ping the far device without encryption. Then try to ping it with the ping configured as interesting traffic.

NOTE
With increasing numbers of high-speed cable Internet connections, filtering is becoming more common. At least one cable provider is filtering IPSec packets generated by subscribers of their low-end residential service in order to force them to upgrade to the more expensive business package.

NAT Problems

Detecting a problem caused by NAT isn't surefire, but it is fairly easy. The main thing to look for are errors on encapsulated packets. If the packets are arriving and being discarded, and the device is configured to use AH, this is a good indication of NAT problems. An appropriate test would be to create a second tunnel from the same two devices using only ESP, and then ping the far end across the tunnel.

ACL Problems

When an ACL is created on a router, the router uses that list to determine which traffic is privileged enough to cross the tunnel. The router also exchanges the source and destination information when examining incoming traffic to see what should have come in via the tunnel. If a packet should have come through the IPSec tunnel but did not, the router drops it.

It is very important that the ACLs on the peer devices be mirror images of each other. If router A permits traffic from 10.1.2.3 to destination 99.5.6.7, then router B should have a line permitting 99.5.6.7 to 10.1.2.3.

What's Next

This chapter serves as an introduction to the rest of the chapters dealing with VPNs. First, you learned about the major types of VPNs and the Cisco VPN devices. The rest of the chapter dealt with IPSec and IKE (Internet Key Exchange). You learned that IKE is the base; IPSec couldn't exist without an IKE foundation. Authentication is a critical component of IKE, and one of the options supported is the CA (certificate authority).

As you learned, IPSec is largely a self-negotiating process. IKE tunnels can be manipulated in many ways, but IPSec configurations usually specify the broad building blocks that will be used and let the two network devices negotiate the details. IPSec's AH (Authentication Header) and EPS (Encapsulating Security Payload) protocols are used to build tunnels. IPSec can use encryption (DES or 3DES) and hashing techniques (MD5 or SHA) to enhance security. Transform sets define a device's IPSec requirements. Actual tunnel creation is triggered by traffic that needs to use a tunnel, as defined by ACLs.

Chapter 20 is an introduction to Cisco VPN devices and how they operate. The chapter also provides basic configuration information.

Chapter 20

INTRODUCTION TO CISCO VPN DEVICES

Although a router or firewall can be used to terminate a VPN, that is not the best use of those devices' CPU cycles. If you have VPNs that need to be terminated, it is better to use a device optimized for VPNs. Cisco has two types of dedicated physical devices that can terminate VPNs: the VPN Concentrator and the VPN Hardware Client. Cisco also offers a software client, which is loaded on a computer so a PC can terminate a VPN tunnel.

This chapter begins with an overview of the Cisco VPN Concentrator models, including their main features. Next, we'll discuss the VPN Hardware Client and how to configure it using the Quick Configuration utility. Finally, we'll cover the VPN software clients, including how to configure them.

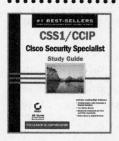

Adapted from *CSS1™/CCIP™: Cisco® Security Specialist Study Guide* by Todd Lammle, Tom Lancaster, Eric Quinn, and Justin Menga

ISBN 0-7821-4049-1 $89.99

Part IV

INTRODUCING THE VPN 3000 CONCENTRATORS

As VPNs gained popularity, Cisco realized that although being able to *terminate* a VPN on a router was a good selling point, terminating more than a few VPNs on a 2500 series router resulted in unacceptable performance degradation. Using a router for VPN termination might be acceptable for an office where one or two people at a time would be using a VPN. However, if an office decided to allow 50 users to telecommute, they often experienced performance problems.

The solution was to develop a hardware device dedicated to terminating VPNs, called a *VPN Concentrator*. Cisco offers two classes of VPN Concentrators: the 3000 series and the 5000 series. The 3000 series is designed for corporate use, and the 5000 series is designed for use by service providers (and handles more connections than the 3000 models). The two series operate in a similar fashion, but they are not configured the same way. This chapter covers only the 3000 series.

NOTE
Cisco's VPN Concentrator is often still referred to as the Altiga concentrator, because Altiga developed it.

In the following sections, we will introduce the VPN 3000 Concentrator series models and summarize their features.

VPN 3005 Concentrator

The 3005 is the low-end VPN Concentrator designed for small to medium-sized offices. This model is a good choice if your organization is not growing very quickly. For example, if a 500-user company has anywhere from 30 to 50 salespeople on the road at any one time and 15 to 20 other employees, this concentrator will handle the job. If the company is expanding at a rapid pace, the 3005 is not the device to choose.

The 3005 can support up to 100 simultaneous tunnels via software-based encryption and is not upgradable. Like the other 3000 series models, it offers the option of using 40-bit or 128-bit Data Encryption Standard (DES), triple-DES (3DES), or Microsoft Point-to-Point Encryption (MPPE).

It can also use Message Digest 5 (MD5) and Secure Hash Algorithm (SHA) for hashing and Diffie-Hellman for key exchanges. (Encryption, hashing, and Diffie-Hellman are discussed in Chapter 19, "Introduction to Virtual Private Networks.")

NOTE

MPPE is an encrypted form of a Point-to-Point Protocol (PPP) packet. For more information about MPPE, refer to RFC 3078.

The 3005 is a 1U device. A *U* is a measurement of height for placement in a rack and is equal to 1.75 inches (4.45 centimeters). For comparison, other 1U devices include the Cisco 2500 and 2600 series routers and the thin Catalyst 1900, 2900, and 3500 series switches.

Table 20.1 summarizes the characteristics of the VPN 3005 Concentrator.

TABLE 20.1:   Characteristics of the VPN 3005 Concentrator

FEATURE	DESCRIPTION
Memory	32MB
Simultaneous users	Up to 100
Power supply	Single
Height	1U
Encryption throughput	4MB
Encryption	Software based
Upgradability	None

Figure 20.1 shows the front and back of a 3005. The front is fairly nondescript, but the 3005 comes with two interfaces on the back. One interface is for the outside connection and is labeled *public*. The other interface is for the inside connection and is labeled *private*. A default configuration comes with each VPN Concentrator, so it is important that these interfaces be attached to the correct connection. In addition to the LAN connections, there is a DB-9 interface for the console port. A standard DB-9 to RJ-45 adapter and a rollover cable can be used for console access.

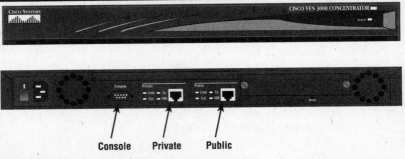

Console   Private   Public

FIGURE 20.1:   The VPN 3005 Concentrator

Each of the LAN interfaces supports 10/100 Ethernet. There is no provision for other types of LAN media (Token Ring, Fiber Distributed Data Interface [FDDI], or Copper Distributed Data Interface [CDDI]) at this time. The interfaces also have LEDs to indicate link, collision, transmit, and receive status.

VPN 3015 through 3080 Concentrators

Models 3015 through 3080 are 2U VPN Concentrators that are more flexible than the 3005. If your organization is growing rapidly or already needs more than 100 tunnels terminated at a time, these are the models to consider.

The 3015 has the same tunnel capacity as the 3005, but it is upgradable to add support for more tunnels. The 3030, 3060, and 3080 models use hardware-based encryption and decryption. Because these tasks are offloaded from the CPU, these devices can terminate more tunnels. All of these models can use 40-bit or 128-bit DES, 3DES, or MPPE encryption; MD5 or SHA for hashing; and Diffie-Hellman for key exchanges.

Table 20.2 summarizes the capabilities of the 3015, 3030, 3060, and 3080 models.

TABLE 20.2:   Base Characteristics of the VPN 3015, 3030, 3060, and 3080 Concentrators

VPN CONCENTRATOR	3015	3030	3060	3080
Simultaneous users	100	1,500	5,000	10,000
Encryption throughput	4Mbps	50Mbps	100Mbps	100Mbps
Encryption method	Software	Hardware	Hardware	Hardware

TABLE 20.2 continued: Base Characteristics of the VPN 3015, 3030, 3060, and 3080 Concentrators

VPN CONCENTRATOR	3015	3030	3060	3080
Encryption (SEP) modules	0	1	2	4
Available expansion slots	4	3	2	N/A
System memory	64MB	128MB	256MB	256MB
Dual-power supply (hot swap)	Optional	Optional	Optional	Default

Figure 20.2 shows the back of a 3015. Just as on the 3005, the console port is a DB-9. The concentrator has both public and private Ethernet ports, as well as a third port that can be used to connect to another LAN segment, like a demilitarized zone (DMZ) or extranet. The 3015 also has an option for a redundant power supply and up to four Scalable Encryption Processing (SEP) modules. The SEP does the hardware-based encryption. Overall, the more memory and the more SEPs, the higher the number of tunnels the concentrator can handle.

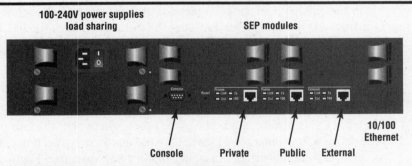

FIGURE 20.2:   The rear of the VPN 3015 Concentrator

NOTE

Cisco used to sell T1/E1 modules for VPN 3015 through 3080 Concentrator models, and Altiga sold a 3005 that had a T1/E1 port. These devices have been discontinued, and support for them in CiscoView is nonexistent after version 5.3. Customers using these products should see "Field Remediation Efforts" at http://www.cisco.com/warp/public/cc/pd/hb/vp3000/prodlit/eoswm_pb.htm.

Part IV

Unlike the 3005, the front of the 3015 actually shows some information. There are quite a few LEDs on the front panel that show the status of the concentrator, as illustrated in Figure 20.3.

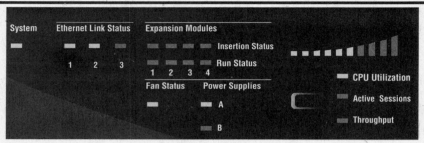

FIGURE 20.3:   The front panel of the VPN 3015 Concentrator

NOTE

On the VPN Concentrator, a blinking green LED for link status does not mean data is passing through the interface. Instead, it means the link is connected but disabled.

On the right side of the LED panel is an LED meter. Below that are a button and three categories. Pressing the button migrates the lit LED through three choices: CPU Utilization, Active Sessions, and Throughput. The meter displays whichever of these three is active.

VPN Concentrator Client Support

The VPN Concentrator should be placed somewhere near the entrance to your network. It is not a good idea to have too many encrypted tunnels going too far into your network because they present a security risk. Figure 20.4 illustrates the concept of a VPN crossing a shared network.

Figure 20.4 shows the client connection coming across the Internet, passing through the router, and terminating at the concentrator. If the router were set to block a certain type of traffic, that router would not be able to check the traffic inside the tunnel as it passed through. This risk becomes more serious when a firewall allows encrypted traffic through. Of course, it may not be possible or desirable to eliminate all VPNs passing beyond a firewall or concentrator, but with good design planning, you can minimize the number of VPNs that do this.

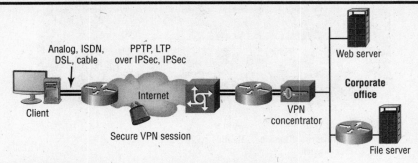

FIGURE 20.4:   Client support for a VPN Concentrator

INTRODUCING THE VPN HARDWARE CLIENT

The VPN Hardware Client is a great tool if your network has several users who need to communicate via a tunnel, but it is impractical to purchase a piece of hardware for every user. Unlike the VPN Concentrator, which was developed by Altiga and picked up by Cisco, the hardware client was developed by Cisco.

The hardware client is nothing more than a basic router whose strong point is creating a tunnel to another location that is serviced by a VPN Concentrator. The purpose of using the VPN Hardware Client is to offload the client-processing requirements when several clients on the same network are creating VPNs to the same destination. This device is most appropriate for use in a small network with fewer than 50 users.

Figure 20.5 is an illustration of the VPN 3002 Hardware Client. There is an RJ-45 console connection if one is required, but unlike the VPN Concentrator, the hardware client comes with an IP address preset on the active private interface. This makes it easy for someone to use a web browser to surf to the administration page to set up the device.

NOTE
In addition to accessing the hardware client via a web browser, using HTTP or HTTPS, the device also supports administrative connections via Telnet and Secure Shell (SSH).

Part IV

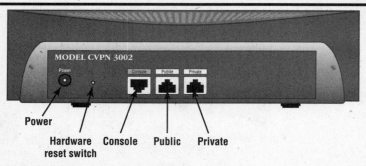

FIGURE 20.5:   The VPN 3002 Hardware Client

The client is configured for the IP address 192.168.10.1 on the private interface. It uses Port Address Translation (PAT), which can be disabled, to provide address translation out to the Internet. The public interface can be configured to use Dynamic Host Configuration Protocol (DHCP) to request an IP address from the service provider.

Once the client is up and running, anyone with the proper credentials can log in and make changes. The client needs to be configured, and then the tunnel needs to be brought up manually. Until this happens, secure communication between the sites does not exist.

Configuring the Hardware Client with the Quick Configuration Utility

The hardware client is easy to set up through its Quick Configuration utility. It is possible to walk a user through setup over the phone.

Although you have the option to configure the client via the command-line interface (CLI) through the console port, most people choose to configure it via the web browser. The first step is to log in to the device. Once the browser is pointed to the correct IP address, the login screen appears, as shown in Figure 20.6. No matter how the client is configured, the default username is admin and the default password is admin.

Anyone who is familiar with setup mode on a router will understand the concept of Quick Configuration. This utility's opening screen is shown in Figure 20.7. As you can see, it takes you through each configuration step:

1. Set the system time, date, and time zone.

2. Configure the Ethernet interface to your private interface.

3. Optionally, upload an existing configuration file.

4. Configure the public interface to a public network.

5. Specify a method for assigning IP addresses.

6. Configure the IPSec tunneling protocol.

7. Set the hardware client to use either PAT or LAN Extension mode.

8. Configure Domain Name System (DNS).

9. Configure static routes.

10. Change the admin password.

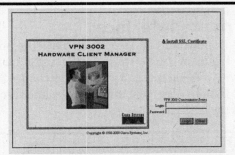

FIGURE 20.6:   Logging in to the hardware client

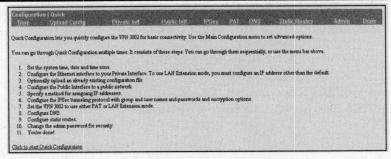

FIGURE 20.7:   The opening Quick Configuration screen

Let's take a look at some of the Quick Configuration details.

Setting the System Time

It is always advisable to ensure that the clock is set to the correct time. If the client will be using a digital certificate, it is also advisable to set the time and time zone to reflect Greenwich mean time (GMT). Setting the time on the client involves entering the time, date, and time zone and specifying whether daylight savings time (DST) is used.

Using an Existing Configuration File

The next section allows the administrator to upload a configuration file. No TFTP server is needed, nor is one supported, but the file does need to reside on a drive that the administrator can access. If the file is on a mapped network drive, you can access it by clicking the Browse button.

Configuring the Private Interface

The Private Interface screen, shown in Figure 20.8, displays the properties of the interface for the inside of the network. By default, it has an IP address of 192.168.10.1 with a 24-bit mask. If you want to change the IP address, select the Yes radio button. Also make sure that the interface has a DHCP server for client addressing.

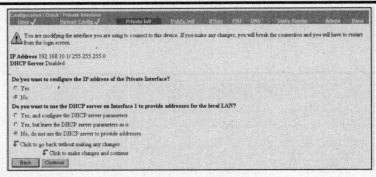

FIGURE 20.8:   Configuring the private interface

Configuring the Public Interface

The Public Interface screen, shown in Figure 20.9, contains properties for the interface going out to the Internet. The IP address may be statically configured or it may be set up via DHCP. Because many DHCP servers require the use of a valid hostname, this is an option on the Public Interface screen.

The public interface also has routing information associated with it. You can configure a default gateway. You can configure other routes later, but most networks that use the hardware client will not have a router further inside the network.

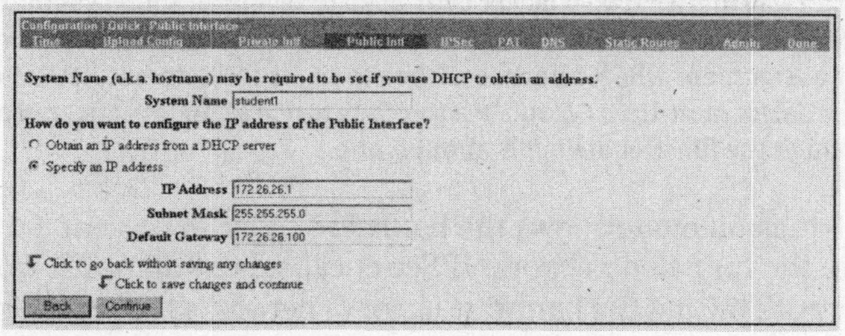

FIGURE 20.9:   Configuring the public interface

Configuring IPSec

All VPNs consist of a tunnel with two endpoints. Because the hardware client is one end of the tunnel, it needs to be told where the other end is. You configure this information on the IPSec screen, shown in Figure 20.10.

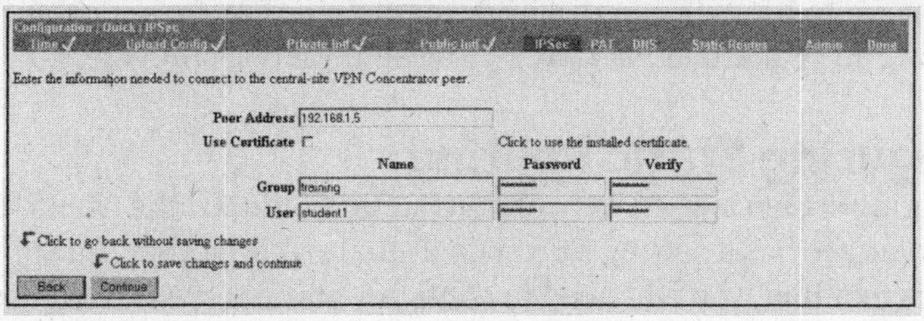

FIGURE 20.10:   Configuring the IPSec peer

You can set up IPSec to use a group name and password, as well as a username and password for remote authentication via a database (such as a Windows NT domain database). Alternatively, IPSec can be set up to use digital certificates. These settings must match on both sides of the tunnel.

Configuring PAT or LAN Extension Mode

PAT is used to translate from one IP address to another. If the default IP address of 192.168.10.1 remains on the private interface, PAT will remain enabled and cannot be disabled. If you do not want to use PAT, you will need to use some other IP address; if the packets will be seen by Internet

Part IV

devices, the IP address must be routable. Also, PAT must be disabled (and a different IP address used) if you want to use LAN Extension mode.

NOTE

PAT is a way that a network device can translate several IP addresses into a single IP address. Each IP address and port assignment equals a like IP address and port assignment when a packet wishes to enter the Internet. PAT allows the potential for more than 64,000 IP addresses to use a single registered address, although the functional limit is about 4,000.

LAN Extension mode allows the hardware client to present a routable network to the tunneled network. IPSec encapsulates all traffic from the private network behind the hardware client to networks behind the central-site concentrator. PAT does not apply. Therefore, devices behind the concentrator have direct access to devices on the hardware client private network through the tunnel.

Configuring DNS

The DNS screen of the Quick Configuration utility contains settings that allow the hardware client to communicate with a DNS server and for a local domain to be configured. The domain name can be important when requesting an IP address via DHCP from some service providers.

Configuring Static Routing

The Routing screen is used to configure static routes for the client. The public interface has a setting for a default route, but if other routing information is required, you will need to configure static routes. Select Add to add a new route. If you need to remove a route, select it and choose Delete.

Changing the Admin Password and Enabling Users

The Admin screen allows you to change the admin password. After you set a new admin password (for security), the Quick Configuration utility displays a screen that lists two other users who are disabled by default:

► The config user is used for quick configuration and monitoring.

► The monitor user works in read-only mode.

You can enable one or both of these users by selecting the Enabled check box above the appropriate user.

TIP

The config and monitor users can be useful additions. If you enable them, you can have one class of administrator to configure the device (the config user) and another class that is able to monitor the device but not make any changes (the monitor user).

Managing the Hardware Client

After you've completed the Quick Configuration utility's steps, the Hardware Client Manager screen appears, as shown in Figure 20.11. This screen has links to three broad areas:

▶ The Configuration option is for configuring device properties such as IP addressing.

▶ The Administration option allows you to change user passwords.

▶ The Monitoring option shows system statistics and allows you to create the tunnel.

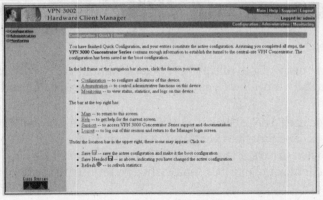

FIGURE 20.11:   The Hardware Client Manager opening screen

To see the status of a tunnel, click Monitoring from the main Hardware Client Manager screen, and then click System Status. If a tunnel exists, it can be disabled. If a tunnel doesn't exist, you can activate one, as shown in Figure 20.12. This screen also shows how long the client has been up and the type of software running.

Part IV

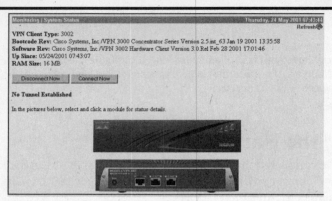

FIGURE 20.12:   Bringing up the tunnel

If a tunnel currently exists, the Monitoring screen will show other information, including how long the tunnel has been up, the Internet Key Exchange (IKE) and IPSec building blocks used to create the tunnel, and how much traffic has passed through the tunnel.

INTRODUCING THE VPN SOFTWARE CLIENTS

Another alternative Cisco offers for VPN termination is the VPN software client. This software allows a single PC or server to act as one end of an IPSec tunnel.

Cisco used the SafeNet client to create tunnels that terminated at routers and firewalls. The SafeNet client cannot communicate with a VPN Concentrator. When Cisco started selling VPN Concentrators, it also included the Altiga client for client PCs that wished to terminate tunnels at a concentrator.

Some users want their PCs to terminate tunnels and don't care which device is handling the termination at the other end. Because users can have only one VPN client installed at a time, they can have only one type of tunnel. To address this problem, Cisco combined the two clients (SafeNet and Altiga) together into what is known as the *Unified Client*.

Configuring the Unified Client

The Altiga client and the software Unified Client look alike, and they are configured in much the same way. Currently, the software Unified Client can communicate with only a VPN Concentrator or a PIX Firewall running version 6.0 software or higher. IOS support will be here shortly.

NOTE

Cisco began supporting tunnels from the Unified Client to an IOS router with IOS version 12.2(8)T in late March 2002.

When the Unified Client starts, nothing is configured by default, as shown in Figure 20.13. To configure the client, you need to set up the connection and set properties.

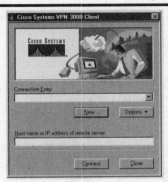

FIGURE 20.13: The Unified Client at initial startup

NOTE

Unified Client versions 3.0 and lower do not support Windows XP. If you install version 3.1 or later, and then upgrade your system to XP, it's possible XP will report that the client is not supported, even though it is. The solution is to uninstall and reinstall the same client.

Configuring the Connection

In order to configure the connection, click the New button to start the process. On the first screen that appears, set the name of the connection along with a description. On the following screen, specify the IP address or hostname of the terminating device.

After you've set the connection name and destination, they will appear in the first window (Figure 20.13). It is possible to configure multiple connections and select among them from a pull-down menu. To create another connection, just select New again.

Part IV

Setting General Properties

To set connection properties, click the Options button and select Properties. (The Options drop-down menu also offers options for duplicating, deleting, or renaming an entry.)

The General tab of the Properties dialog box appears first. Here, you can enter an optional description. There is also a check box to allow IPSec via Network Address Translation (NAT). This does not change the fact that NAT breaks Authentication Headers (AH), as explained in Chapter 19. The Windows 95/98/Me version also includes a section on logging in to a remote system. If you check the Logon to Microsoft Network box, two options become available:

- ▶ Use Default System Logon Credentials
- ▶ Prompt for Network Logon Credentials

Setting Authentication Properties

Authentication can take place via either a digital certificate or a pre-shared key. The Authentication tab of the Properties dialog box, shown in Figure 20.14, allows you to set either group parameters or certificate information. If the system the software client is loaded on does not have any personal digital certificates, the option for using certificates will be grayed out (as it is in Figure 20.14). If a certificate is loaded, the radio button will be available, and the certificate name will appear in the adjacent box.

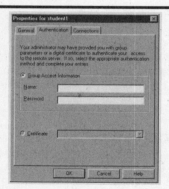

FIGURE 20.14:   The Authentication tab of the Properties dialog box

The group name and password used for the pre-shared key method of authentication must match the ones set up on the destination device.

The newer version of the client includes another text box for password verification.

Setting Connection Properties

The Connections tab of the Properties dialog box, shown in Figure 20.15, allows you to define the other end of the tunnel for this particular configuration. Entries can be added with the Add button and deleted with the Remove button.

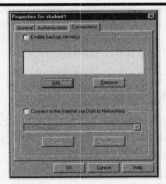

FIGURE 20.15: The Connections tab of the Properties dialog box

Multiple IP addresses are supported when the Enable Backup Servers check box is checked. If the device with the first IP address is unavailable, the second IP address will be tried. Thus an organization can use multiple concentrators for failover purposes.

Preconfiguring Clients

The software client needs to be loaded on each machine that is expected to form the end of a tunnel. In many cases, it is not practical for a member of the IT department to visit the home of a salesperson just to install a single piece of software. Some people who work remotely can be talked through the setup via the phone, but others may find setup difficult.

Cisco has attempted to make it easier to talk users through installations. In addition to the installation being "wizardized," the client uses a configuration file that offers the opportunity to preconfigure the client. You can edit this .ini file and then simply e-mail it to the remote user. Users can copy the .ini file into the directory where the client is installed, and the client will have the necessary settings.

Part IV

In version 2.*x* of the Unified Client, the configuration file is named IPSecdlr.ini. In version 3.*x*, the file is named vpnclient.ini.

TIP

You can find more information about preconfiguring the client, as well as rebranding the client with your own corporate information, at http://www.cisco.com/univercd/cc/td/doc/product/vpn/client/rel_3_5/admn_gd/index.htm.

When a tunnel created via the Unified Client is active, you cannot pull up the IP address information on the tunnel with standard Windows commands. To access that information, double-click the VPN icon in the system tray.

Configuring the SafeNet Client

The SafeNet client will eventually be replaced with the newer software Unified Client. Currently, the only reason to use the SafeNet client is if the VPN is being terminated at an IOS router.

Version 1.0 of the SafeNet client does not support certificates generated by a Windows 2000 CA, but version 1.1 does.

Configuring the Connection

To configure the properties of the other end of the tunnel, you need to define a new connection. In the left pane of the SafeNet client window, shown in Figure 20.16, select Other Connections. Then select the File menu and choose the New Connection option.

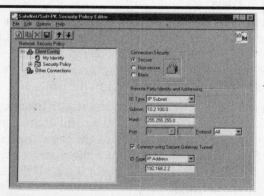

FIGURE 20.16: The SafeNet client

You can configure a number of items:

Connection Security   Choose the Secure option to create the tunnel. Non-secure, the default, allows unencrypted communications. The Block option prevents communication with the IPSec peer.

Remote Party Identity   This section allows the user to identify the remote peer in a number of different ways. Methods include straight IP address, hostname, e-mail address, and others. (This section is usually configured by an administrator.)

Port and Protocol   These sections determine what type of traffic is protected. The default is all ports and all protocols.

Configuring Authentication

To configure authentication, choose My Identity in the left pane of the SafeNet client window, as shown in Figure 20.17. The choices are a digital certificate, if installed, or pre-shared keys. If a computer has multiple interfaces, the tunnel endpoint can be pegged to a particular physical interface by selecting the appropriate name in the Local Network Interface section and entering the correct IP address. The default of Any in these two boxes means that any interface can be the tunnel endpoint.

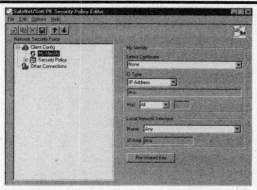

FIGURE 20.17:   SafeNet client authentication options

To use pre-shared keys, click the Pre-Shared Key button at the bottom of the window. A small window will pop up, asking you to enter the pre-shared key in ACSII format.

Part IV

What's Next

Each VPN tunnel has two ends, and each end is a client of the tunnel. The VPN Concentrator, hardware client, and software client are able to offload the VPN process from other network equipment to some dedicated device or service. In this chapter, we introduced these three VPN components.

The software client is portable but requires user intervention in order to run. At the least, the user must start the application and log in. The hardware client and concentrator don't require user intervention, but they aren't portable.

The hardware client is totally GUI-driven and is simple enough to set up that users can be talked through the configuration over the phone. Even better, there is the option of using a preconfiguration file that can be loaded into the client to provide the configuration.

The Altiga and Unified software clients are also fairly easy to set up, and they also come with the option of providing a preconfiguration file. The SafeNet client is a bit more complex, and that is one of the reasons its use is waning.

In Chapter 21, you will learn about the Cisco Intrusion Detection System (IDS), which combines many of the aspects of a firewall and a VPN solution into a comprehensive intrusion warning and detection system.

Chapter 21

INSTALLING CISCO SECURE IDS SENSORS AND IDSMS

In this chapter, you will learn about the Cisco Secure IDS sensor platforms. The sensor is the actual device that monitors traffic, generating alarms if intrusive network activity is detected. The Cisco Secure IDS sensors include the Cisco Secure IDS 4200 series sensors and the Cisco Catalyst 6000 Intrusion Detection System Module (IDSM).

This chapter will initially look at the topic of sensor deployment, which is the process of planning where you should place your sensors on the network. Then you will learn how to install and configure the sensor to a state where it is ready to be managed by your Director platform. You will also learn how to configure your Director platform (Cisco Secure Policy Manager [CSPM]) so that you can define configuration parameters from CSPM and allow CSPM to manage the sensor. Finally, you will learn how to maintain the IDSM, updating its files and troubleshooting problems.

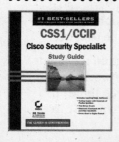

Adapted from *CSS1™/CCIP™: Cisco® Security Specialist Study Guide* by Todd Lammle, Tom Lancaster, Eric Quinn, and Justin Menga

ISBN 0-7821-4049-1 $89.99

Part IV

DEPLOYING SENSORS

Before you install a Cisco Secure IDS sensor or Catalyst IDS module, you must understand the various locations in the network where you can place the sensor. Each location option has pros and cons, and your security, management, and cost requirements will ultimately dictate the optimal location where you should place your sensor. You also must understand the interfaces that each sensor possesses, because the interfaces define the monitoring and management capabilities of the sensor. Once you understand the issues around sensor deployment, you can then decide exactly where you will deploy your sensor(s). We will cover the considerations and procedures for sensor deployment in this section.

General Sensor Placement Considerations

Network IDS systems are generally expensive pieces of equipment, so choosing the appropriate parts of the network to monitor is of critical importance. You must determine the exact number of IDS sensors that your network requires, as well as the optimal locations for each of these sensors. You should consider the following aspects of your network when evaluating IDS sensor deployment:

Connections to Untrusted Networks   You must understand all possible entry points into your network from untrusted networks (such as the Internet and extranets) and remote-access connections (such as dial-up and VPN client connections). Ideally, each entry point should be secured and monitored for traffic violations. You might also consider your internal trusted networks as monitoring points, especially on internal networks that host critical systems.

Critical Resources   Identifying the critical resources in your network often determines where you place your sensors. Critical resources may include servers, mainframes, routers, and firewalls. By placing a sensor in front of these resources, you can detect and react to intrusive activity against the resource.

Performance Requirements   You must understand the bandwidth requirements of key connections in the network. For example, you may wish to monitor a link that uses 100Mbps bandwidth, so your IDS sensor must be able to handle it. You should also understand the different protocols in use on the network (such as TCP, UDP, and HTTP), because each type of traffic has a different performance hit on an IDS system. If the network segment you wish to monitor will exceed a single sensor's capabilities, you can deploy multiple sensors.

Size and Complexity   Normally, the bigger the network, the more entry points to it. This generally means you need to monitor more points in the network, which ultimately means you need to purchase more sensors. Also, some networks have added complexity, such as legacy Fiber Distributed Data Interface (FDDI) networks that your organization may not wish to replace, so the IDS sensors need to be able to support non-Ethernet media.

Common Sensor Locations

Once you have determined and resolved the issues that you must consider before deploying sensors, you can then determine where you want to place sensors. Sensors are commonly placed on entry points into the network. The most common sensor placement locations can be summarized as follows:

Internet Connection   The most common placement is on the Internet demilitarized zone (DMZ) network (the network between a perimeter router and firewall), where you can capture intrusive activity that originates from the Internet before it reaches the firewall. This way, you can understand exactly what threats are out there.

Intranet Connection   You can also place a sensor on your trusted network (also known as intranet connections), where you can detect internal intrusive activity. Doing so is useful to detect any intrusive traffic that manages to pass through the firewall.

Remote-Access and Extranet Connections   Other common locations for IDS sensors are on remote-access networks and connections that terminate an extranet link.

Figure 21.1 illustrates the various points in the network where you can place a sensor. Notice that each sensor is effectively monitoring an entry point into the network or a specific portion of the network.

Part IV

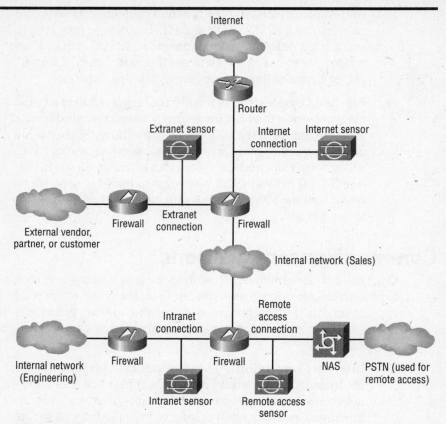

FIGURE 21.1: Common sensor placement locations

Sensor Interfaces

Both the Cisco Secure IDS 4200 series sensors and the Catalyst IDSM sensor use two network interfaces—the monitoring interface and the command-and-control interface—which are key considerations in selecting the location of your sensor. Both of these interfaces must be connected and operational to ensure that your sensor functions correctly.

The *monitoring interface* (operating in promiscuous mode) captures all traffic received on the interface, passing it to the sensor application for analysis. The monitoring interface does not have an IP address, making it totally transparent to the rest of the network. You must connect the sensor-monitoring interface to the network segment that you wish to monitor.

NOTE

The monitoring interface only receives traffic and does not send any traffic except for a single situation. If a sensor is configured to reset a TCP connection that is part of an attack, the monitoring interface (not the command-and-control interface) will send TCP reset packets to the target system.

The *command-and-control interface* provides the management interface to the IDS sensor. Management comprises communications (IDS configuration, alarm notification, and so on) with a Director, and also includes remote Telnet, FTP, or Trivial FTP (TFTP) access (such as upgrading a signature file) to the sensor. The command-and-control interface is also used to provide IP-blocking configuration on a perimeter router, where the sensor essentially opens a Telnet session with the router and applies a blocking access control list (ACL) to an interface. The command-and-control interface must be connected to a network segment that allows IP communications with your Director platform.

The Cisco Secure IDS 4200 series sensor interfaces are located externally on the sensor and plug into either a shared (hub) or a switched-network infrastructure, much like any router or gateway with multiple interfaces. The Catalyst IDSM interfaces are located internally, connected directly to the Catalyst switch backplane. These differences mean the deployment methods for each platform are different, as explained in the following sections.

Cisco Secure IDS 4200 Series Sensor Deployment

Because the Cisco Secure IDS 4200 series sensors do not have trunking support (the ability to support multiple VLANs over a single LAN connection), each network interface on the sensor can exist only in a single network segment or VLAN. This means you must view your network from a physical point of view, selecting a single segment to monitor and a single segment to provide the command-and-control management interface.

When using the 4200 series sensors, you must consider the LAN infrastructure device that provides connectivity for the monitoring interface. If

Part IV

you are using a hub to connect all devices on the segment, all traffic is propagated to every device on the segment, including the monitoring interface, so all traffic transiting the segment can be captured.

If you are using a switch to connect all traffic, this poses a problem because a switch forwards unicast traffic only out the required egress ports. The monitoring interface will not see all traffic on the segment, meaning intrusive activity could be missed. In a switched environment, your switch must be able to mirror all traffic on the segment out the port connected to the sensor-monitoring interface, to ensure all traffic on the segment can be inspected. The mirroring feature is known as Switch Port Analyzer (SPAN).

NOTE

SPAN is required in switched environments for all 4200 series sensors. On the IDSM, another option is available that removes the need for SPAN, but it requires some extra hardware (called a Policy Feature Card [PFC]) on the Catalyst 6000/6500 switch. If you do not have a PFC, you must use SPAN on the switch and mirror VLAN or port traffic to the monitoring interface on the IDSM.

The following common scenarios are used to deploy the 4200 series sensor:

▶ Basic installation

▶ Device management installation

▶ Firewall sandwich installation

▶ Remote installation

These deployment methods are discussed in detail in the following sections.

Basic Installation

The simplest deployment method is the *basic installation*. With the basic installation, the monitoring interface of the sensor is attached to the network segment that you wish to monitor, and the command-and-control interface is attached to an isolated management (out-of-band) network, as illustrated in Figure 21.2. The management network provides a connection to the Director, allowing for configuration and alarm notification for the sensor.

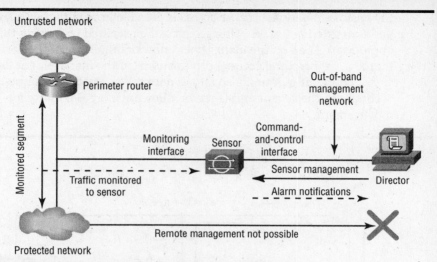

Untrusted network

Perimeter router

Monitored segment

Out-of-band management network

Monitoring interface   Sensor   Command-and-control interface

Traffic monitored to sensor

Sensor management

Alarm notifications

Director

Remote management not possible

Protected network

FIGURE 21.2:   Basic installation sensor deployment

This configuration is secure because both the sensor and Director management interfaces are not accessible from remote networks. However, this configuration is not very flexible. Network operators must physically access the Director console to gain management access. The basic installation also does not allow the sensor to communicate with a perimeter router and apply an IP-blocking ACL, because this function can be performed only via the command-and-control interface.

Device Management Installation

With the *device management installation*, the monitoring interface of the sensor is attached to the network segment that you wish to monitor (just like the basic installation); however, the command-and-control interface of the sensor and the Director management interface are attached to a nonisolated management network, as illustrated in Figure 21.3. The management network provides connectivity between the sensor and Director, but also provides connectivity between the sensor command-and-control interface and a perimeter router.

This configuration allows IP blocking to be implemented, because the sensor can communicate with the perimeter router and download the appropriate blocking ACL. The configuration is less secure than

Part IV

the basic installation, because access is possible from both the trusted and untrusted networks. This access can be secured by placing the appropriate ACLs on the management network interface of the perimeter router, controlling access both to and from the management network. This configuration also allows network operators to remotely access both the sensor and Director, allowing more flexibility for management.

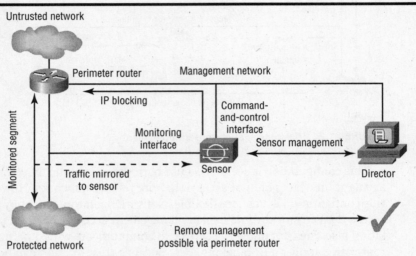

FIGURE 21.3:   Device management installation sensor deployment

Firewall Sandwich Installation

The *firewall sandwich installation* deployment method (no, this is not from a lunch bar menu) is illustrated in Figure 21.4. This deployment method is common when monitoring a segment that provides access to an untrusted network (also known as an Internet DMZ). The Internet DMZ is the segment between the external perimeter router and a firewall device, with the segment normally containing coarsely filtered (by the perimeter router) or unfiltered traffic (no filtering on the perimeter router) from untrusted networks.

The firewall device protects the trusted network from unauthorized access from the outside. The monitoring interface is attached to the Internet DMZ segment, where it monitors traffic coming in from the untrusted network (and also traffic coming out from the trusted network). Most commonly, the command-and-control interface is then attached to the trusted network, where the Director is also attached.

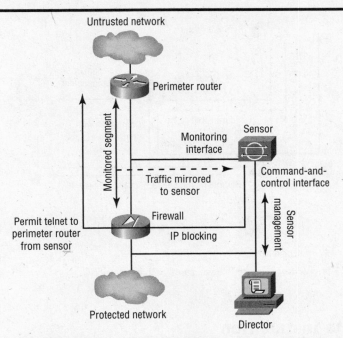

FIGURE 21.4:   Firewall sandwich installation sensor deployment

This deployment method allows for network operators to access the sensor and Director management interfaces remotely, while protecting the management interfaces from the untrusted network (by virtue of the firewall). The sensor can also apply an IP-blocking configuration at the perimeter router; however, the appropriate access (telnet from the sensor to the perimeter router) must be allowed through the firewall for this to occur.

In Figure 21.4, although the sensor and Director management interfaces are protected from the untrusted network, they are not protected from the trusted network (remember, attacks can occur from a trusted network). Figure 21.5 shows a more secure firewall sandwich installation, where the management network is separated from all other networks by the firewall, allowing access controls to be implemented to permit only authorized management access to the sensor and Director.

Part IV

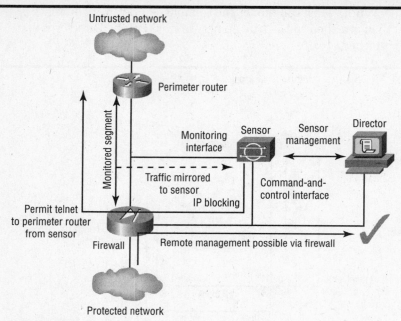

FIGURE 21.5:   A more secure firewall sandwich installation

Remote Installation

The *remote installation* deployment method is not really related to the placement of the sensor, but instead involves the placement of the Director in relation to the sensor, as illustrated in Figure 21.6. The sensor could be placed in either the device management or firewall sandwich deployment configuration at a remote network, with the Director located on a remote management network rather than the same management network.

In this configuration, one or more transit networks between the sensor and Director could be untrusted, so it is recommended that communications between the sensor and Director be encrypted over the untrusted networks. In Figure 21.6, a router-to-router IPSec VPN is used to secure the IDS communications, and the firewalls at each network are configured to allow PostOffice communications (UDP port 45000) between the sensor and Director (and vice versa).

The remote installation method is useful for managing multiple sensors in remote locations, either at an enterprise level or service-provider level. A Director does not need to be physically located along with each sensor; instead, the Director is housed at a central management facility.

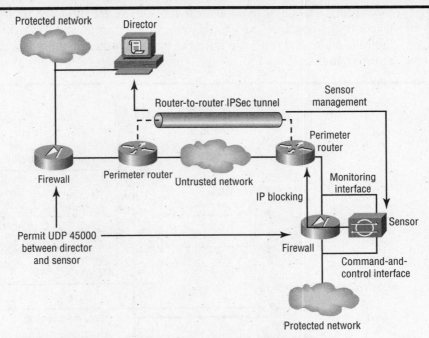

FIGURE 21.6:   Remote installation sensor deployment method

Cisco Catalyst IDSM Sensor Deployment

The Catalyst IDSM provides a monitoring interface that can monitor traffic from multiple VLANs; that is, the monitoring interface is a trunk. The command-and-control interface exists on a single VLAN only.

The trunking capabilities of the IDSM monitoring interface mean that your Catalyst IDSM location is independent of the actual logical segments it is monitoring. For example, you could physically place your IDSM on a trusted network, yet simultaneously monitor traffic from other segments such as a remote-access or extranet segment. Figure 21.7 illustrates this concept.

In Figure 21.7, the Catalyst 6000 switch provides segregated (via a separate VLAN per segment) network connectivity for the trusted VLAN, an extranet entry point VLAN, and a remote-access entry point VLAN. If you're wondering about the security of this scenario, don't worry—traffic cannot pass directly between each VLAN on the switch; it must be passed to a routing device (the firewall in this example) for forwarding. The Catalyst 6000 switching engine is configured to mirror traffic from specific VLANs to the monitoring port on the IDSM, so the IDSM can monitor traffic on both the extranet and remote-access entry point segments.

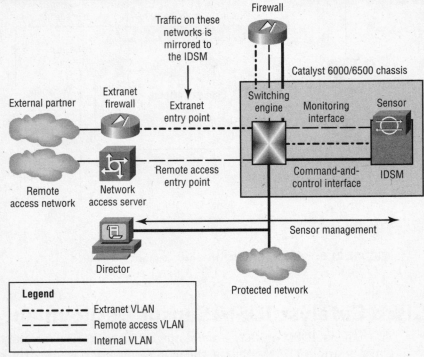

FIGURE 21.7:   Catalyst IDSM sensor deployment

The common scenarios of sensor deployment for the 4200 series sensors, described in the previous sections, also apply to the IDSM. The only real difference is that the IDSM can perform the work of one or more sensors by monitoring traffic from multiple VLANs at the same time.

NOTE

The Cisco Secure IDS sensor software version determines both features and the number of signatures supported by the sensor. An important limitation of the Catalyst IDSM is that it *does not support* IP blocking. IP blocking is supported on the IDSM in version 3.0 of the Cisco Secure IDS sensor software.

INSTALLING AND CONFIGURING CISCO SECURE IDS 4200 SERIES SENSORS

Before performing initial software configuration of a Cisco Secure IDS 4200 series sensor, you must physically install the sensor. After you have installed and powered on the sensor for the first time, you then need to understand how to gain access to the sensor to perform initial configuration and basic sensor setup.

Physically Installing the Sensor

To correctly install an IDS sensor (for example, in a rack with appropriate space), you need to understand the physical characteristics of the sensor and the functions that each physical network interface performs.

4210 Sensor Physical Layout

The Cisco Secure IDS 4210 sensor (Cisco product number IDS-4210) is the entry-level IDS sensor offering from Cisco. The IDS 4210 is a compact, slim-line appliance that includes all the software features of the more expensive IDS 4230, but has lower hardware specifications that reduce the performance capacity of the sensor.

The IDS 4210 is capable of monitoring up to 45Mbps of traffic. Thus it is well suited for external connection segments, which typically use WAN connections to limit the amount of bandwidth to be processed. For example, the IDS 4210 is an ideal sensor to place on the Internet DMZ segment that connects an Internet connection of up to T3 (45Mbps) speed. The IDS 4210 is not well suited to monitor segments that have LAN speed (100Mbps) connections present (such as on an internal network segment).

If you are tasked with the installation of the IDS 4210, you need to understand its physical layout. Figure 21.8 shows the front panel layout for this sensor. As you can see, the only visible slot, or port, is a front-mounted console port, which provides quick console access when required. The removable front panel hides devices such as the floppy drive and CD-ROM that you would normally see on a standard Intel server, in order to give the sensor the look and feel of a network appliance.

Part IV

IDS-4210 front view with panel closed

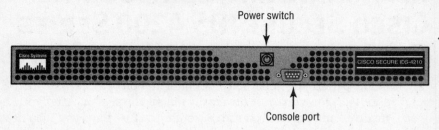

Power switch

Console port

IDS-4210 front view with panel open

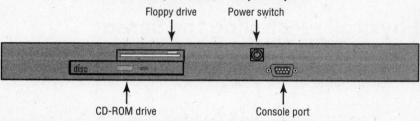

Floppy drive   Power switch

CD-ROM drive   Console port

FIGURE 21.8:   Cisco Secure IDS 4210 sensor front panel

NOTE

The Cisco Secure IDS 4210 and 4230 sensors are actually manufactured by Dell, and they are Intel-based server platforms.

Figure 21.9 shows the rear panel layout for the IDS 4210. The rear panel features the same interfaces and ports as any standard Intel server. Notice the rear panel includes two onboard NICs, with the top interface acting as the command-and-control interface and the bottom interface acting as the monitoring interface. The monitoring interface on the IDS 4210 has a device name of /dev/iprb0, which you need to know when you specify the monitoring interface of a sensor on CSPM (the Director).

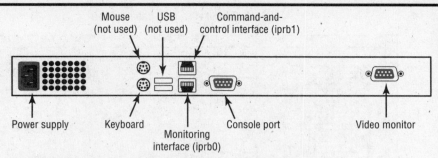

FIGURE 21.9:   Cisco Secure IDS 4210 sensor rear panel

4230 Sensor Physical Layout

The Cisco Secure IDS 4230 sensor (Cisco product number IDS-4230) is a high-performance sensor that can monitor up to 100Mbps of traffic. The IDS 4230 comes in a larger chassis (4U) than the IDS 4210 chassis (1U), which allows for richer expansion options. The IDS 4230 can monitor FDDI networks with the installation of an FDDI-monitoring NIC. The IDS 4230 is well suited for monitoring internal network segments that run at LAN speeds of up to 100Mbps.

NOTE

The 4230 FDDI sensor is no longer available (as of the end of 2000). However, existing networks may have 4230 sensors with FDDI support. Historically, the 4220 sensor (similar to the 4230) provided Token Ring support.

Figure 21.10 shows the front panel layout for the IDS 4230. The IDS 4230 does not have a front-mounted console port like the IDS 4210, and it appears very much like a standard Intel server. The front access panel is lockable, which prevents unauthorized tampering. The front access panel must be opened to gain access to the CD-ROM and floppy drives.

Figure 21.11 shows the rear panel layout for the IDS 4230. The rear panel features standard PC/server interfaces and includes an onboard network interface that acts as the command-and-control interface. The monitoring interface is installed in a PCI slot, and the Ethernet version of the monitoring interface has a device name of /dev/spwr0.

Part IV

IDS-4230 front view with panel closed

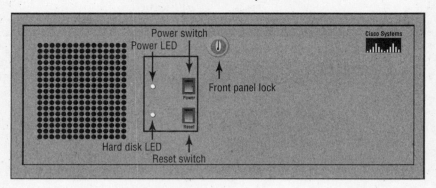

IDS-4230 front view with panel open

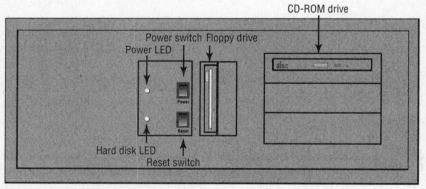

FIGURE 21.10: Cisco Secure IDS 4230 sensor front panel

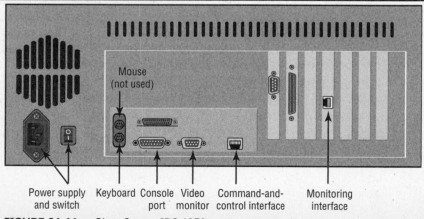

FIGURE 21.11: Cisco Secure IDS 4230 sensor rear panel

The various interface device names for all media (including Token Ring and FDDI) are as follows:

Media	Device Name
Ethernet/Fast Ethernet	/dev/spwr0
Token Ring	/dev/mtok0
Single/Dual FDDI	/dev/ptpci

Gaining Management Access

Once you have physically installed and cabled a sensor appropriately, you need to obtain some form of management access to begin configuration of the box. There are four methods of management access, which are identical for the 4210 and 4230 sensors:

- ▶ Keyboard and monitor
- ▶ Console port
- ▶ Telnet
- ▶ Via a Director platform

When you start up a 4200 series sensor for the first time, by default, you can access the sensor only via the keyboard and monitor or console port. All other options require some initial configuration to enable management access. For example, Telnet access requires an IP address, subnet mask, and default gateway (for remote connections) to be configured. Director management access requires both IP and PostOffice communication parameters to be configured.

NOTE

The console port does not use the standard Cisco console cable. A custom console cable and connector are supplied with the sensor, and they must be used to gain console access. Use a connection with the following settings: 9600bps, 8 data bits, no parity, 1 stop bit, and hardware (or RTS/CTS) flow control.

Logging in to the 4200 Series Sensor

Once you have powered up the sensor for the first time with a keyboard and monitor attached, the next step is to log in to the sensor. The 4200 series runs a preinstalled, custom-built Sun Solaris Unix (Intel 32-bit version) operating system, so it will take a short time to load. After booting is complete, you will be prompted for a Unix-style username and password. Two management accounts are configured that will provide you with access to the sensor:

> ***root***   The root account is an administrative Unix account that is used for performing initial configuration (using the sysconfig-sensor utility, as explained in the next section), service pack or signature updates, and operating system management.
>
> ***netrangr***   The netrangr account is a user account designed to be used with Cisco Secure IDS management commands. This account can execute all Cisco Secure IDS commands and utilities, except the sysconfig-sensor utility.

TIP
The Cisco Secure IDS commands all start with an nr prefix. For example, the nrstop command stops the Cisco Secure IDS application.

The default password for both accounts is attack, and you will automatically be prompted to change this password the first time you log in using the account.

NOTE
Both the username and password on a Unix system are case sensitive, unlike on Windows systems, where the username is not case-sensitive.

When configuring the sensor for the first time, you must log in as root so that you can perform the initial configuration of the sensor. The following example demonstrates logging in to the 4200 series sensor for the first time using the root account:

```
...
The system is ready.

Sensor console login: root
Password: ******
Choose a new password.
New password: *******
Re-enter new password: *******
```

```
login (SYSTEM): passwd successfully changed for root
Mar 12 20:36:58 sensor login: ROOT LOGIN /dev/console
Last login: Fri Sep 22 17:02:05 on console
Sun Microsystems Inc.  SunOS 5.8  Generic February 2000
#
```

Configuring the Sensor for the First Time

After you've logged on as root, you're ready to begin sensor configuration. First, you need to configure initial parameters that will allow the sensor to communicate and be managed by a Cisco Secure IDS Director platform. This initial configuration is performed using the *sysconfig-sensor* utility. To execute this utility, from the command line, type **sysconfig-sensor**, and then press the Enter key.

The sysconfig-sensor utility presents an easy-to-use, menu-style interface. Figure 21.12 shows the sysconfig-sensor configuration menu, from which you can configure the following parameters:

- ▶ IP configuration (options 1 through 5)

- ▶ PostOffice communication (option 6)

- ▶ System management (options 7 through 9)

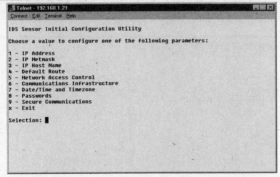

FIGURE 21.12: The sysconfig-sensor main menu

To configure a parameter, simply type in the option number at the Selection prompt and press Enter. At the very least, you must configure IP configuration and PostOffice communication settings.

Part IV

IP Configuration Parameters

A Cisco Secure IDS sensor uses a monitoring interface to detect intrusive activity, and that interface does not have an IP protocol stack associated with it. The command-and-control interface has an IP protocol stack for communication with a Director platform, to allow remote configuration, management, and alarm notification. The sysconfig-sensor utility allows you to configure the appropriate IP addressing and routing information for the command-and-control interface.

IP Addressing   The Cisco Secure IDS sensor is an IP device that requires all the normal IP configuration parameters, such as IP address, subnet mask, and default gateway. The following sysconfig-sensor menu options are used to configure IP addressing and naming parameters:

> ► 1 – IP Address (such as 192.168.1.20)

> ► 2 – IP Netmask (such as 255.255.255.0)

> ► 3 – IP Host Name (such as sensor1)

> ► 4 – Default Route (the default gateway of the sensor, such as 192.168.1.1)

Each of these parameters applies to the command-and-control interface and is required to allow remote IP connectivity for a Director platform and to provide remote Telnet, FTP, or TFTP access. Figure 21.13 shows an example of setting the IP address of the sensor.

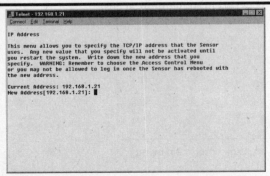

FIGURE 21.13:   Configuring the sensor IP address

Restricting Management Access   The Cisco Secure IDS sensor is a device that needs to be secured in order to ensure that the sensor itself is not compromised and possibly sabotaged. The 4200 series allows you to restrict management access via Telnet, FTP, and TFTP by using a list of hosts that are allowed to attempt to establish management connections. If network administrators require access to the sensor, they must know which hosts can access the sensor remotely, and also know the root or netrangr account and password.

You can specify a list of IP hosts that should be granted management access by choosing Network Access Control (option 5) from the sysconfig-sensor menu. Figure 21.14 shows an example of restricting access to the sensor.

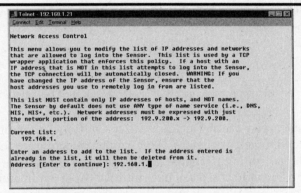

FIGURE 21.14:   Restricting management access

Notice in Figure 21.14 the use of a wildcard to specify a range of addresses that are permitted management access. You specify the required matching octet(s) and terminate the wildcard with a dot. The dot means that any value is allowed in that octet. For example, 192.168.1. means any IP address within the 192.168.1.*x* range (192.168.1.1–192.168.1.254).

NOTE

If you choose options 1 through 5 on the sysconfig-sensor menu and modify any of the parameters, you will need to reboot the sensor for the changes to take effect.

PostOffice Communication Parameters

To allow your Director platform to communicate with and manage your sensor, you must configure the appropriate PostOffice parameters. To configure these parameters, choose Communications Infrastructure

Part IV

(option 6) from the sysconfig-sensor main menu. When you choose this option, you will be able to configure various sensor and Director parameters, as shown in Figure 21.15.

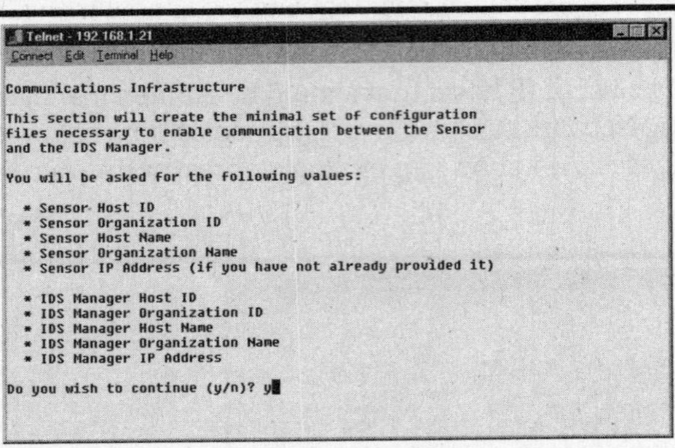

FIGURE 21.15:   Choosing to configure PostOffice communication parameters

First, you must type **y** at the Do You Wish to Continue? prompt to configure the PostOffice parameters. Next, you must configure the host ID/name, organization ID/name, and IP address of both the sensor itself and the Director. Once you have entered these parameters, you are prompted to accept the changes and create or modify a configuration file.

Figure 21.16 shows the Communications Infrastructure screen with configured sensor and Director PostOffice parameters. Type **y** at the OK to Create the Configuration Files? prompt to save the configuration.

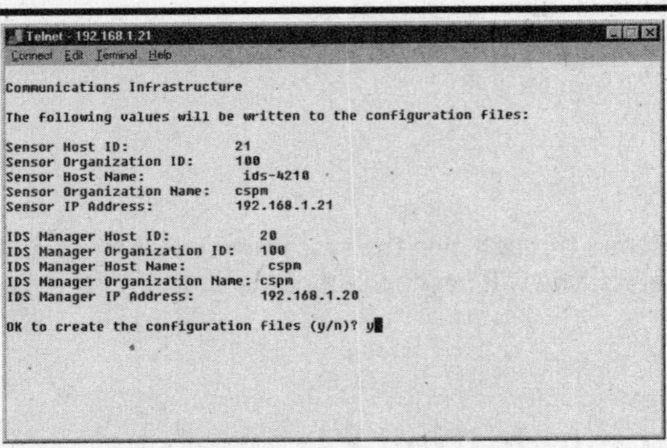

FIGURE 21.16:   Configuring PostOffice communication parameters

System Management Parameters

The following options on the sysconfig-sensor utility main menu allow you to configure system management parameters:

- ▶ 7 – Date/Time and Timezone
- ▶ 8 – Passwords
- ▶ 9 – Secure Communications

System Date and Time   It is important that you set the correct date and time, so that the Director platform knows the accurate date and time an intrusive activity occurred. You can configure the time, date, and local time zone of the sensor by choosing Date/Time and Timezone (option 7) from the sysconfig-sensor main menu. You will see the Date/Time and Timezone menu, as shown in Figure 21.17.

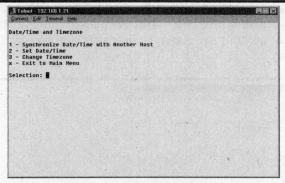

FIGURE 21.17:   Configuring the date, time, and time zone

You can choose Synchronize Date/Time with Another Host (option 1) to synchronize the local sensor time with another host. This option uses the Unix rdate command. You can also manually configure the date and time by choosing Set Date/Time (option 2).

NOTE

The custom Solaris operating system build includes an NTP (Network Time Protocol) client, which is a popular date/time synchronization protocol used on the Internet. To use this NTP client, you must configure it manually via the Solaris operating system. However, be aware that you are not supposed to change the operating system configuration of a Cisco Secure IDS sensor in any way, except via the sysconfig-sensor utility.

Part IV

Changing Passwords   As mentioned earlier, the Cisco Secure IDS 4200 series sensors ship with two accounts (root and netrangr), with the default passwords for each set as attack. These passwords are altered the first time you log in using each account, so the chances are you have already changed the root password if you are using the sysconfig-sensor utility. When you run sysconfig-sensor for the first time, it is highly recommended that you change the password for the netrangr account to protect the sensor from being compromised by the use of default passwords.

When configuring passwords, you should use a long string (eight or more characters) of alphanumeric characters and symbols, so that the password is difficult to guess. The root password should be well protected and provided only to those who need to use the account. The netrangr password should be known only to network administrators who manage the sensors on an ongoing basis.

To change the sensor account passwords, choose Passwords (option 8) from the sysconfig-sensor utility main menu. As shown in Figure 21.18, you must specify the account name and the new password you wish to use for the account.

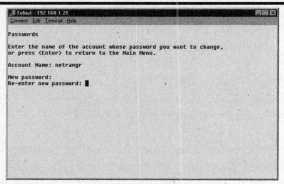

FIGURE 21.18:   Changing passwords

PROTECTING THE *ROOT* PASSWORD

The root account is extremely dangerous because it has full access to the sensor operating system. Although the Solaris operating system has been locked down by Cisco, it still is a general-purpose operating system that is well known.

CONTINUED ➡

Ideally, the root password should be placed in a locked vault and accessed only when required. If the root password is used, it should then be changed, and the new password should be stored in the locked vault once again. In each case, the root password should be known only to the most trusted individuals in the organization (such as the director, CEO, or CIO). In fact, the most secure method is for nobody to know the password—to get the password, the vault must be opened. (Of course, somebody needs to generate the password initially.)

Secure Communications   The Secure Communications option allows you to enable IPSec communications between the sensor and the Director. The CSPM Director requires the installation of the Cisco VPN 1.1 client *before* installation of the CSPM software for this feature to be enabled. The IPSec implementation used is manual, meaning encryption keys used must be manually (and identically) configured on both the sensor and the Director. You can selectively enable or disable secure communications as required.

Completing Initial Sensor Configuration

After you have completed the appropriate initial configuration using the sysconfig-sensor utility, choose Exit (option x) to exit the sysconfig-sensor utility. Because this it the first time you have configured the IDS sensor, you will have configured at least options 1 through 3, which means you must reboot the sensor.

NOTE

Any subsequent modifications to options 1 through 5 of the sysconfig-sensor utility main menu will require a reboot of the sensor. If you modify the Time-zone setting in option 7 of the sysconfig-sensor utility main menu, you must also reboot the sensor.

After reboot, your Cisco Secure IDS 4200 series sensor is ready to communicate with a Director platform, such as CSPM or Cisco Secure IDS Director for Unix. At this stage, your sensor does not need any further configuration and can be fully managed from a Director. The next section discusses the initial configuration required on CSPM to allow CSPM to manage the 4200 series sensor.

Part IV

Configuring CSPM for 4200 Series Sensor Management

Thus far, you have learned how to prepare the 4200 series sensor for communications with a Director platform, such as CSPM. Before the Director can successfully configure, manage, and receive alarm notifications from a sensor, you must add an object to the CSPM database that represents the actual sensor. This section covers the first-time, basic configuration of the sensor and also discusses how to "push" a configuration file to the sensor.

To successfully begin managing a Cisco Secure IDS sensor, you must perform the following actions:

▸ Configure CSPM using the Add Sensor Wizard

▸ Add an object to CSPM to represent the CSPM host

▸ Save and upload the configuration to the sensor

Configuring CSPM Using the Add Sensor Wizard

The CSPM Policy Administrator application includes a wizard that guides you through adding an object in the CSPM database to represent the sensor. To add a new sensor, ensure you are logged in to Policy Administrator with full rights, and select the Wizards ➤ Add Sensor menu item to begin the Add Sensor Wizard.

The Add Sensor Wizard consists of four configuration screens:

▸ Sensor Identification

▸ Default Gateway Address

▸ Sensor Configuration

▸ Sensor Configuration Verification

We will examine the parameters on each of these screens. As you would expect, after you complete the configuration on a wizard screen, click Next to continue to the next screen.

Sensor Identification   Figure 21.19 shows the first screen of the Add Sensor Wizard, which is called the Sensor Identification page. This page allows you to configure the following options:

Sensor Name   Enter a friendly name that identifies the sensor.

Organization Name   Enter a friendly name that identifies the organization to which the sensor belongs.

IP Address   Specify the IP address assigned to the command-and-control interface of the sensor.

Host ID   Enter a numeric value (from 1 to 65535) that uniquely represents the host ID of the sensor within an organization. This value must match the sensor host ID configured on the sensor (under the 6 – Communications Infrastructure option of the sysconfig-sensor utility; see Figure 21.16, shown earlier in the chapter).

Org. ID   Enter a numeric organization identifier value (from 1 to 65535) that uniquely represents the organization to which the sensor belongs. This value must match the sensor organization ID configured on the sensor (under option 6 of the sysconfig-sensor utility; see Figure 21.16).

Associated Network Service   This option defines the network service of CSPM that manages the policy associated with the sensor. Because the Cisco Secure IDS architecture uses the PostOffice protocol to do this, choose the Cisco Post Office service.

Postoffice Heartbeat Interval   This value defines the interval between heartbeat messages (keepalives). It determines how quickly CSPM responds to a sensor failing; nd the default value of 5 seconds is suitable for most networks.

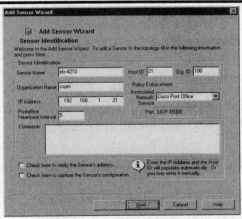

FIGURE 21.19:   The Sensor Identification page of the Add Sensor Wizard

In Figure 21.19, notice the values for each field match the sensor configuration that was defined on the sensor using the sysconfig-sensor utility (see Figure 21.16, shown earlier in the chapter).

Part IV

Default Gateway Address   Next, you see the Default Gateway Address page, as shown in Figure 21.20. As the name suggests, this page allows you to configure the default gateway of the sensor. The default gateway is required because CSPM represents each managed object in a network topology tree (NTT). Because CSPM manages gateway devices such as firewalls, CSPM understands the concepts of perimeter interfaces that allow the gateway to connect to different networks.

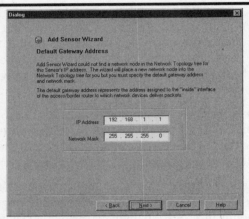

FIGURE 21.20:   The Default Gateway Address page of the Add Sensor Wizard

The default gateway of a subnet is represented as a perimeter interface of the subnet, and CSPM requires each subnet to have at least one perimeter interface configured. Enter the IP address and network mask of the default gateway, and then click the Next button to continue.

Sensor Configuration   The next page of the Add Sensor Wizard is called the Sensor Configuration page, as shown in Figure 21.21. This page allows you to configure the following options:

Distribution Host   This defines the CSPM host object in the NTT that will manage the sensor. In this example, because you have not created an object for the CSPM, the wizard places the CSPM hostname with the (?) suffix in the Host box.

Sensor Version   This defines the sensor Cisco Secure IDS software version installed on the Cisco Secure IDS sensor. Choose from the various versions (Catalyst IDSM versions have an IDSM suffix). It is important that you configure the correct version of sensor software, because it determines what

signatures are known to the sensor (for example, if you configured a higher software version in CSPM, CSPM would think
the sensor understood some signatures that might not be supported in the lower software version running on the sensor).

TIP

If you are unsure of the sensor software version, you can determine it by gaining management access to the sensor (via the console, keyboard/monitor, or
Telnet). Log in to the sensor using the netrangr account, and then execute the
nrvers command, which displays the current sensor software version
installed.

Signature Template   A signature template defines which signatures the sensor monitors for and how the sensor reacts to a
detected signature. In this example, you have not previously
created any templates, so you can choose only the Default
option. Signature templates are covered in detail in Chapter 22,
"Signatures and Alarm Management."

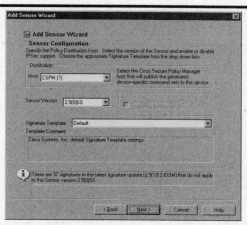

FIGURE 21.21:   The Sensor Configuration page of the Add Sensor Wizard

Sensor Configuration Verification   The final page shown in the
Add Sensor Wizard displays a summary of the configuration parameters of
the sensor object you are about to add to the CSPM database. Once you have
verified that the sensor configuration is correct, click the Finish button to
complete the wizard and add the object to the CSPM database.

Part IV

Adding an Object to the CSPM Database

To allow CSPM to manage sensors, you must ensure that the NTT contains an object that represents the CSPM host itself. Once you have created the CSPM object, you must update the sensor object configuration to ensure that CSPM can distribute the policy to the sensor.

Creating the CSPM Host Object This chapter assumes that your CSPM host resides on the same subnet as the command-and-control interface of your sensor. When you created the sensor object, CSPM automatically created a network object that represents the network on which the sensor resides. The CSPM NTT requires each object to reside in a parent network container. Thus, if your CSPM host resides on that same network, you do not need to create a new network object, because you can add the CSPM host to the previously created network object. If your CSPM host resides on a different network (subnet), you must create a network object in the NTT to allow a CSPM host object to be created.

Creating the CSPM object is extremely simple. Right-click the network object that the CSPM host resides in and select the New ➤ Host option, as shown in Figure 21.22.

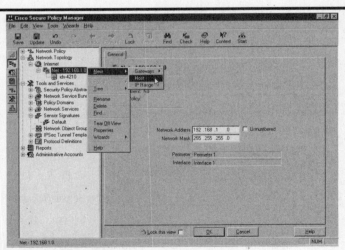

FIGURE 21.22: Configuring the CSPM host object

CSPM will automatically detect itself and prompt you to create an object for itself in the NTT:

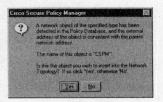

Click the Yes button to complete creation of the object.

Updating the Sensor Object   Each sensor object contains a configuration parameter called a PDP (policy distribution point), which identifies a CSPM host object that manages the sensor. Because you created the sensor object before the CSPM host object was created, this parameter is blank and must be updated with the CSPM host object. To access the sensor object properties, click the sensor object. The object parameters should appear, as shown in Figure 21.23.

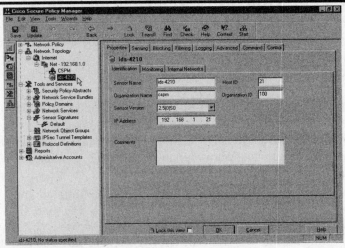

FIGURE 21.23:   Accessing the sensor object properties

Click the Control tab and configure the Policy Distribution Point option by selecting the newly created CSPM host object, as shown in Figure 21.24. Then click the OK button to apply the configuration.

Part IV

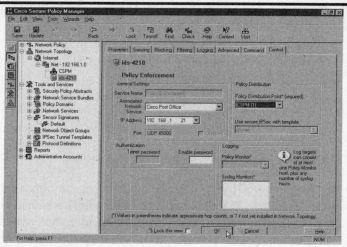

FIGURE 21.24: Configuring the PDP

Saving and Uploading the Configuration to the Sensor

You have now created objects that represent the sensor and CSPM host, and are ready to save the new configuration and upload an initial configuration to the sensor.

Saving and Updating the Configuration CSPM does not automatically save additions, moves, or changes to the CSPM database as you make them. You must manually save and update the CSPM database after any configuration changes to ensure your new configuration is saved.

CSPM has the concept of *saving* and the concept of *updating*. When you save the configuration, the CSPM database is updated and any changes you have made since the last save are applied to the CSPM database. When you update the configuration, CSPM generates new device-specific configuration files from each device's object parameters in the database. This process allows CSPM to be able to apply your configured policy to specific devices.

To save your configuration, click the Save button on the CSPM toolbar (the first button on the left). You will be prompted with an information box that explains the behavior of the File ➤ Save and File ➤ Update command. Click OK, and the new CSPM objects and configuration will be saved to the database.

Once you have saved your configuration, click the Update button on the CSPM toolbar (to the right of the Save button) to generate the device-specific configuration files needed for the sensor.

Uploading the Configuration to the Sensor   Now that your CSPM database is up to date and the appropriate sensor configuration file has been created, you can apply your first configuration to the sensor. To upload the configuration file to the sensor, click the sensor object in the NTT to display the sensor object configuration parameters. Click the Command tab, and then click the Approve Now button to begin the process of uploading a configuration file to the sensor, as shown in Figure 21.25.

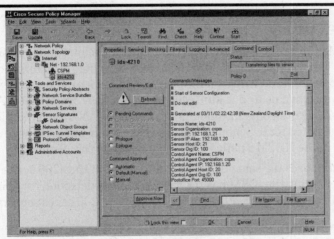

FIGURE 21.25:   Pushing the configuration to the sensor

In Figure 21.25, the Status field shows that the CSPM is currently transferring files to the sensor, in response to the execution of the Approve Now button. Once the upload is completed, the Status field indicates the upload is complete. The Commands/Messages screen shows the commands that are applied to the sensor and messages that appear during upload to the sensor. You can click the Poll button at any time to verify the upload status.

TIP

By default, you must save, update, and push a configuration to a sensor in separate, manual actions. In the Command tab of CSPM, you can select the Automatic option under the Command Approval selection to automatically push a configuration to a sensor after the update process has occurred (by clicking the Update button on the CSPM toolbar).

INTRODUCING THE CISCO CATALYST 6000 IDSM

The Catalyst 6000 IDSM sensor is a line card that is designed for use with the Catalyst 6000 and 6500 family of switches. The IDSM differs from traditional IDS sensors (like the 4200 series) in that it can monitor traffic from multiple LAN segments (VLANs) over a single monitoring interface. The IDSM adds value and functionality to an organization's investment in Catalyst 6000/6500 switches and allows the organization to monitor traffic from a VLAN connected to the switch.

IDSM Features

The IDSM is an exciting product that integrates switching and intrusion detection into a single chassis. The IDSM allows flexible monitoring on traffic of one or more VLANs on the switch, and it does not impact switch performance when using a feature called VLAN access control list (VACL) capture. VACLs overcome the limitations of using SPAN, which traditionally has been required for IDS monitoring in switched networks. (Using VACLs is discussed in the "IDSM Traffic Flow" section later in this chapter.)

The IDSM uses the same IDS sensor software that the 4200 series sensors use, ensuring the IDSM has the same signature-detection capabilities. Table 21.1 compares the features of the IDSM and 4200 series sensors.

TABLE 21.1:   IDSM and 4200 Sensor Feature Comparison

FEATURE	4200 SENSORS	IDSM
Multi-VLAN capture	No	Yes
IP blocking	Yes	No
IP logging	Yes	No
Secure communications (using IPSec)	Yes	No
Signature tuning	No	Yes
Signature port mapping	No	Yes

The information in Table 21.1 assumes Cisco Secure IDS software version 2.5. Notice that the IDSM does not support IP blocking, IP logging, or secure communications (IP blocking is supported in version 3.0).

Also notice that the IDSM is uniquely capable of multi-VLAN capture, signature tuning, and signature port mapping. Signature tuning allows you to fine-tune alarm notifications to ensure your IDS Director is not flooded with alarms. Signature port mapping allows you to apply TCP application/service signatures to TCP ports other than the well-known port for the service. For example, you can configure the IDSM to apply HTTP signature analysis to port 8080 (commonly used for proxy services) as well as well-known port 80.

IDSM Architecture

Before you install, configure, and use the IDSM, you must understand the IDSM architecture and how it interoperates with the Catalyst 6000/6500 switch. The IDSM line card may not look like much, but that is because the IDSM network interfaces are internal and connect to the backplane of the switch. Understanding this internal architecture is crucial to understanding the capabilities of the IDSM. In this section, you will learn about the IDSM physical layout, IDSM traffic capture, and IDSM traffic flow.

IDSM Physical Layout

The IDSM is a standard Catalyst 6000/6500 line card that can be placed in any spare slot on a Catalyst 6000/6500 switch (as long as the switch meets the minimum software and hardware requirements, as described in the "Physically Installing the IDSM" section later in this chapter). Figure 21.26 shows the IDSM line card front panel.

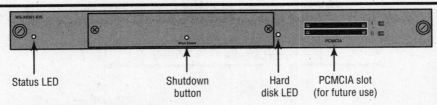

Status LED   Shutdown   Hard   PCMCIA slot
                    button   disk LED   (for future use)

FIGURE 21.26:   IDSM front panel

The front panel of the line card includes a status LED to indicate the state of the IDSM (see Table 21.2), a shutdown button, a hard drive activity LED, and a PCMCIA slot that allows for two PCMCIA cards (reserved for future use).

Part IV

TABLE 21.2: IDSM Status LEDs

COLOR	DESCRIPTION
Green	IDSM is operational; all diagnostics tests passed okay
Red	Diagnostic failed (other than an individual port test)
Amber	IDSM is running self-tests or booting, or IDSM is administratively disabled
Off	IDSM is not powered on

NOTE

The IDSM must be shut down properly to prevent corruption of the IDSM operating system. You normally would shut down the IDSM via a command-line interface (CLI) session to the IDSM using the shutdown command. However, if you cannot do this for some reason, you can push the shutdown button to shut down the IDSM properly.

IDSM Traffic Capture

In order for the IDSM to capture traffic for analysis, it must possess a network interface that allows capture of traffic. Figure 21.27 shows the internal architecture of the IDSM.

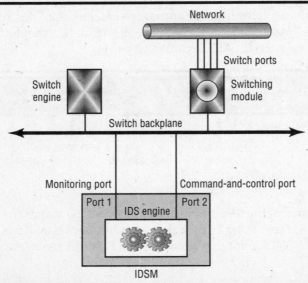

FIGURE 21.27: IDSM internal architecture

Figure 21.27 shows that the network interfaces of the IDSM are internal and connect directly to the Catalyst 6000/6500 backplane. On the IDSM, each network interface is referred to as a *port*, and the IDSM includes the following ports:

Monitoring Port   This is referred to as *port 1* on the IDSM. It captures traffic that is passed to the IDSM sensor application for analysis. The monitoring port is a *trunking* port, which allows it to receive traffic from multiple VLANs.

Command-and-Control Port   This is referred to as *port 2* on the IDSM. It provides the management interface (and is hence assigned an IP address) for the sensor application, allowing communications with a Director platform such as CSPM.

When you install the IDSM module, you place it into a free slot that has a module number. For example, you might install the IDSM into module 2. The switch accesses each IDSM port using the same module/port designation used by the Catalyst 6000 switch. For example, if your IDSM is installed in module 2, the monitoring port is identified as port 2/1 to the switch, and the command-and-control port is identified as port 2/2 to the switch.

IDSM Traffic Flow

As you can see in Figure 21.28, the IDSM has the same types of ports (interfaces) as the 4200 series sensors; however, the ports are not visible and are internally connected to the Catalyst 6000/6500 switch backplane. All traffic is captured off the switch backplane, and the IDSM can monitor up to 100Mbps of traffic. Figure 21.28 illustrates how traffic is captured with the IDSM.

In Figure 21.28, a couple of hosts attached to a Catalyst 6000 switch are communicating. The data is switched over the switch backplane, and that data is mirrored to the IDSM for analysis.

As you learned earlier in the chapter, when the 4200 series sensor is connected to a switched environment, you must use the SPAN feature on the switch connected to the sensor monitoring interface to mirror VLAN traffic to the sensor. Because the IDSM is internally connected to a switch, you would expect that SPAN would also be used to mirror traffic to the IDSM monitoring port. The IDSM can use SPAN for traffic capture, but alternatively it can use VACL capture to monitor traffic. These traffic-capture methods are discussed in the following sections.

Part IV

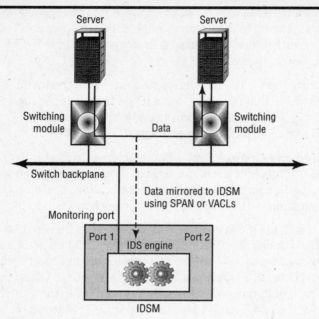

FIGURE 21.28:   IDSM traffic flow

Capturing Traffic Using SPAN   SPAN is the traditional method of capturing some or all traffic from a LAN segment and mirroring that traffic out a destination port. SPAN is useful not only for IDS traffic analysis, but also for any network traffic analysis in general. If you connect a traditional IDS appliance sensor to a switch, you must configure SPAN on the switch to mirror traffic to the sensor monitoring interface. The same applies for the IDSM (although this is not the only method you can use), because the IDSM has a monitoring port just like a traditional IDS appliance sensor.

SPAN is a function of a switch (rather than an IDS sensor). On the Catalyst 6000/6500 switch, there are three different methods of using SPAN:

▶ Ingress SPAN, where network traffic received by one or more source ports is mirrored to a destination port

▶ Egress SPAN, where network traffic sent out one or more source ports is mirrored to a destination port

▶ VLAN SPAN (VSPAN), where network traffic sent and/or received in one or more VLANs is mirrored to a destination port

In SPAN terminology, the monitoring port on the IDSM is the *destination* port, and the network administrator configures one of the methods of SPAN we just listed to define *source* ports from which traffic is mirrored.

Each method just described defines a type of SPAN *session*. A SPAN session is an association of a set of source ports with a single destination port. Only one SPAN session is allowed per destination port, and the Catalyst 6000/6500 has limitations on how many SPAN sessions can operate simultaneously. An ingress SPAN session uses *receive* or *rx* source ports, so a maximum of two ingress SPAN sessions are possible. An egress SPAN session uses *transmit* or *tx* source ports, so up to four egress SPAN sessions are possible. A VSPAN session can use rx, tx, or both rx and tx source ports. A single SPAN session is used to service the IDSM monitoring port. Keep the limitations in mind if you are using other SPAN sessions.

Capturing Traffic Using VACLs   VACLs allow layer 3 and 4 access controls to be applied to traffic on an entire VLAN basis. You can restrict IP traffic that flows within a VLAN based on the following:

- ▶ IP protocol type
- ▶ Source and destination IP addresses
- ▶ Source and destination TCP or UDP ports
- ▶ Combinations of these factors

VACLs require the Catalyst 6000/6500 to have a Policy Feature Card (PFC) installed. The PFC allows VACLs to be stored in ternary content addressable memory (TCAM), which is a specialized memory structure that allows traffic to be inspected in hardware (at wire-speed), rather than in software. Thus a Catalyst 6000/6500 with a PFC installed can apply access control via VACLs with no performance degradation.

VACLs also include a feature that allows you to capture permitted traffic, where the permitted traffic is forwarded normally but is also mirrored to a capture port. If you set the IDSM monitoring port to be the capture port, you can analyze the traffic for intrusive activity. Only a single VACL per protocol (for example, IP or IPX) can be applied to a single VLAN. For the IDSM, this means that only a single IP VACL can be applied per VLAN. However, you can apply the same IP VACL to multiple VLANs. Figure 21.29 illustrates using VACLs to capture traffic for IDSM analysis.

Part IV

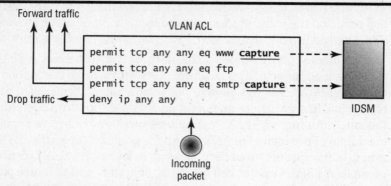

FIGURE 21.29: Using VACLs to capture traffic

In Figure 21.29, incoming traffic into a particular VLAN is inspected using the shown VACL. If the packet matches the first statement (which permits web traffic), then the packet is forwarded *and* mirrored to the IDSM. This happens because the first statement specifies the capture keyword, which tells the switch to capture the traffic for the IDSM. Notice that traffic matching any permit statements that do not use the capture keyword is simply forwarded and not also passed to the IDSM for analysis. Any traffic that is denied by the VACL is dropped and is also not passed to the IDSM.

Using VACLs to capture traffic for IDS analysis overcomes limitations of SPAN, which include the following:

Selective Traffic Monitoring With SPAN, *all* traffic sent, received, or sent and received is mirrored to the IDS sensor. SPAN provides no mechanism whereby you can selectively mirror certain types of traffic based on layer 3 or 4 parameters of the traffic. VACLs allow you to selectively capture traffic— only permitted traffic is forwarded to the IDS sensor. This is important because the IDSM can process only 100Mbps of traffic, and using SPAN with a set of source ports whose bandwidth sum exceeds the bandwidth of the destination port means some traffic may be missed by the sensor. By using VACLs, you can selectively filter only certain types of traffic, allowing you to control the amount of traffic the IDS sensor must analyze.

TIP

If a Cisco Secure IDS sensor detects it is dropping packets due to monitoring interface oversubscription, it generates an alarm that has a signature ID of 993 (the missed packet alarm). The thresholds that trigger this alarm are configurable.

SPAN Session Limitations   Because the Catalyst 6000/6500 switch has SPAN session limits, you may be restricted with your IDS monitoring capabilities if you use SPAN. For example, you might install two IDSMs into a single Catalyst 6000/6500 switch, because you need to monitor 200Mbps of traffic. Assuming you are mirroring received traffic for both sessions, you have reached the SPAN session limits of the switch. You might also have a network probe that requires a SPAN session to capture traffic for network performance analysis. If you want to capture received traffic on the probe, you cannot do so, because your SPAN session limits have been reached. You do not need to worry about SPAN session limitations when using VACLs.

INSTALLING AND CONFIGURING THE CATALYST 6000 IDSM

Now that you understand the architecture of the IDSM, you are ready to install it. Once you have physically installed the IDSM, you must perform the initial IDSM configuration and configure traffic-capture parameters. Finally, you can verify the configuration.

Physically Installing the IDSM

The IDSM is an integrated component of the Catalyst 6000/6500 switch; however, your switch must meet certain requirements to ensure the operation of the IDSM. The following are the requirements of the Catalyst 6000/6500 switch:

- ▶ Catalyst OS 6.1(1) software or higher (no Cisco Catalyst IOS support)

- ▶ Supervisor IA or Supervisor II engine

- ▶ A PFC for the VACL capture feature

- ▶ No crossbar switch fabric module(s) installed (this module enables a 256Gbps backplane)

Part IV

The IDSM can be installed in any free slot on a Catalyst 6000/6500 switch, and it can be installed while the switch is powered on. Make sure you know which slot number you installed the IDSM into, because this number is required for management purposes.

After your IDSM has been physically inserted into the Catalyst switch, and the switch is powered on and operational, you should verify that IDSM is installed correctly. Then you can gain management access to the IDSM and configure the basic IDSM parameters.

Verifying IDSM Installation

After you have installed the IDSM, verify that the Catalyst switch recognizes the module by executing the show module command, as shown here:

```
Switch> (enable) show module
Mod Slot Ports Module-Type          Model            Sub Status
--- ---- ----- -------------------- ---------------- --- ------
1   1    2     1000BaseX Supervisor WS-X6K-SUP1A-2GE yes ok
2   2    1     Intrusion Detection Sys WS-X6381-IDS   no  ok
3   3    48    10/100BaseTX (RJ-45) WS-X6248-RJ-45   no  ok
...
...
```

The show module output shows that the switch can see the IDSM module installed in slot 2. The Status column shows that the IDSM has booted okay and is online.

NOTE
While the IDSM is booting, the Status column of the show module output is set to other.

Gaining Management Access to the IDSM

The IDSM runs a separate operating system independently of the switch, and thus has a separate management interface for configuration. Configuration of the IDSM is CLI-based and can be performed using one of the following methods:

Console   Although the IDSM does not include any external serial ports for console access, it does include an internal console interface that can be accessed using a management session on the switch itself.

Telnet   You can gain CLI access by using Telnet to access the IDSM directly via the IP address assigned to the command-and-control port (port 2) on the IDSM.

If you are configuring a new IDSM, you can initially access the module only by using the console method. To access the IDSM via the console, you must use the `session` command from a switch-management session. You specify the module number of the IDSM in conjunction with the `session` command (for example, if the IDSM is installed in module 2, you would use the `session 2` command). Once you have opened a connection to the IDSM, you will be presented with a login prompt, where you must enter a username and password to gain access to the IDSM CLI. The username is always `ciscoids`, and the default password is set to `attack`. Here is an example of using the `session` command and logging in to the IDSM:

```
Switch> (enable) session 2
Trying IDS-2...

Connected to IDS-2.

Escape character is '^]'.
login: ciscoids
password:
#
```

NOTE
As with any default passwords, you should change the IDSM password imme-diately to avoid system compromise.

Performing Initial Configuration of the IDSM

Now that you have gained administrative access to the IDSM, you are ready to perform the initial configuration of the IDSM using the IDSM setup utility. The goal of this initial configuration is to get your IDSM to a state where it can be managed by a Director platform such as CSPM.

From the CLI # prompt, execute the `setup` command to start the System Configuration Dialog, where you can enter IP addressing and PostOffice configuration. When you first start the System Configuration Dialog, you are presented with the current configuration of the IDSM, as shown here:

```
# setup

    --- System Configuration Dialog ---

At any point you may enter a question mark '?' for help.
Use ctrl-c to abort configuration dialog at any prompt.
Default settings are in square brackets '[]'.

Current Configuration:

Configuration last modified: Never

Sensor:
IP Address:                0.0.0.0
Netmask:                   255.255.255.0
Default Gateway:           Not Set
Host Name:                 Not Set
Host ID:                   Not Set
Host Port:                 45000
Organization Name:         Not Set
Organization ID:           Not Set

Director:
IP Address:                Not Set
Host Name:                 Not Set
Host ID:                   Not Set
Host Port:                 45000
Heart Beat Interval (secs): 5
Organization Name:         Not Set
Organization ID:           Not Set

Direct Telnet access to IDSM: Disabled

Continue with configuration dialog? [yes]:
```

Because the IDSM has just been installed, many of the configuration parameters have not been configured. To start configuration, type **yes**, and then press Enter at the Continue with configuration dialog? prompt. A new screen appears to prompt you for each configuration parameter, as follows:

```
Enter virtual terminal password [<Use Current>]: cisco123
Enter sensor IP address[0.0.0.0]:              192.168.1.22
Enter sensor netmask [255.255.255.0]:          255.255.255.0
Enter sensor default gateway []                192.168.1.1
Enter sensor host name []:                     idsm
Enter sensor host id []:                       22
Enter sensor host post office port [45000]:    45000
Enter sensor organization name []:             cids
Enter sensor organization id []:               100


Enter director IP address []:                  192.168.1.20
Enter director host name []:                   cspm
Enter director host id []:                     20
Enter director host post office port [45000]:  45000
Enter director heart beat interval []:         5
Enter director organization name []:           cids
Enter director organization id []:             100
Enable direct telnet access to IDSM [no]:      yes
Permit:                              192.168.1.0 0.0.0.255
```

These System Configuration Dialog parameters work as follows:

Virtual Terminal Password   Allows you to change the Telnet password (recommended).

Sensor IP Parameters   Allows you to configure the IP address, subnet mask, and default gateway of the IDSM.

Sensor PostOffice Parameters   Allows you to configure the sensor (IDSM) hostname/ID, organization name/ID, and the UDP port used for PostOffice communications (normally, the default setting of 45000). These values must match the sensor object configuration defined on your Director platform.

Part IV

Director PostOffice Parameters   Allows you to configure the Director (for example, CSPM) IP address, hostname/ID, organization name/ID, heartbeat interval (by default, 5 seconds), and UDP port (by default, 45000) used for PostOffice communications. These values must match the configuration of your Director platform.

Virtual Terminal Access   Allows you to enable or disable (default) direct Telnet access to the IDSM. If you enable Telnet access, you can restrict Telnet access to a single host or range of hosts.

Once configuration is complete, you will be presented with a summary of the new configuration. At this point, you should ensure that the new configuration is correct. If it is correct, type **yes** and press Enter at the Apply this configuration? prompt. If you notice a mistake, type **no** and press Enter to cancel any configuration changes. The following example shows how to apply the new configuration:

```
The following configuration was entered:


Sensor
IP Address:           192.168.1.22
Netmask:              255.255.255.0
Default Gateway:      192.168.1.1
Host Name:            idsm
Host ID:              22
Host Port:            45000
Organization Name:    cids
Organization ID:      100


Director
IP Address:           192.168.1.20
Host Name:            cspm
Host ID:              20
Host port:            45000
Heart Beat Interval:  5
Organization Name:    cids
Organization ID:      100
```

```
Use this configuration? [yes]: yes
Configuration Saved.
```

NOTE

After the configuration is saved, the IDSM will automatically reboot. After rebooting, your IDSM is ready to communicate with your Director platform.

Configuring Traffic-Capture Parameters

In the previous section, you configured the IDSM with all the necessary parameters so that it could communicate with a Director platform such as CSPM. You must now configure the Catalyst 6000/6500 switch to place the internal command-and-control port of the IDSM into the correct VLAN, so that communications with the Director can take place. You must also configure the switch to capture and mirror the appropriate traffic to the internal monitoring port of the IDSM, so that the IDSM can analyze traffic for intrusive activity and send alarms to the Director.

As described previously, you can use either SPAN or VACLs for traffic capture. Configuring the traffic-capture parameters entails the following tasks:

- ▶ Assigning the command-and-control port VLAN
- ▶ Configuring traffic-capture SPAN or traffic-capture VACLs
- ▶ Configuring the monitoring port

It is important to note that each of these tasks is performed on the switch, not the IDSM. The configuration of the IDSM described in the previous section is sufficient to allow a Director platform such as CSPM manage the IDSM.

Assigning the Command-and-Control Port VLAN

To allow the IDSM sensor to communicate with the Director platform, you must place the command-and-control port into the appropriate VLAN so that the port is in the correct logical IP subnet. For example, if your IDSM has an IP address of 192.168.1.22 and a default gateway of 192.168.1.1, you should place your IDSM into the same VLAN as the default gateway, ensuring that the IDSM can communicate with the IP network correctly.

Assigning the command-and-control port to a VLAN is performed on the switch (not the IDSM) using the set vlan command:

```
Console>. (enable) set vlan vlan_id module/port
```

For example, if your IDSM is installed in module 2, then your command-and-control port is identified to the switch as port 2/2. To assign the IDSM command-and-control port to VLAN 100, you should configure the switch as follows:

```
Console> (enable) set vlan 100 2/2
VLAN 100 modified.


VLAN  Mod/Ports
____  _____
100   2/2, 3/1
101
```

In this example, port 3/1 represents the default gateway of the IDSM, meaning the IDSM and the default gateway can now communicate via IP. After you have assigned the command-and-control port to the correct VLAN, you should verify IP connectivity to the IDSM from the network by using the ping utility.

Configuring Traffic Capture Using SPAN

As discussed previously, SPAN is the traditional method of mirroring traffic to an IDS sensor in a switched environment. To configure SPAN for traffic capture, you must create a SPAN session, which has the following characteristics:

Set of Source Ports   Defines the source ports from which traffic will be mirrored. This set can include administratively defined physical ports or all the ports from a particular VLAN.

Capture Direction on the Source Ports   Defines the type of traffic you wish to capture from the set of source ports. You can capture traffic received, transmitted, or both received and transmitted. The direction is important, because it influences the maximum number of SPAN sessions you can run on the switch.

A Single Destination Port   Defines the destination port that receives the mirrored traffic from the set of source ports. In an IDSM environment, the destination port is the monitoring port of the IDSM. A single SPAN session can have only a single destination port.

Before configuring SPAN, you must understand your IDS monitoring requirements and plan carefully for each of these parameters. You must bear in mind SPAN session limits, and you must also ensure that you do not oversubscribe the destination port. Once you have defined each of the SPAN session parameters, you are ready to configure SPAN. SPAN is configured from the switch (not the IDSM) using the set span command:

```
Console> (enable) set span {src_ports | src_vlans}
    dst_port [tx | rx | both] create
```

You can specify source ports or source VLANs for the span session, and use the tx, rx, or both keyword to define the direction of traffic that is mirrored. Figure 21.30 shows a sample network topology where we want to mirror traffic on an Internet DMZ segment to the IDSM monitoring port using SPAN.

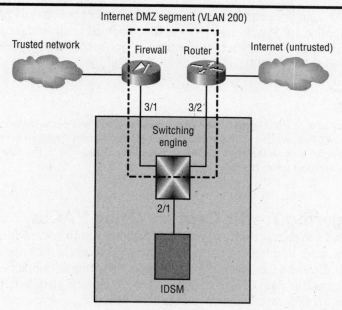

FIGURE 21.30:   A SPAN example

Let's assume in Figure 21.30 that we want to mirror traffic received by each Internet DMZ port to the IDSM monitoring port. To create the SPAN session, you could execute the following command:

```
Console> (enable) set span 3/1-2 2/1 rx create
Enabled monitoring of Port 3/1-2 receive traffic by Port 2/1
```

A more efficient way of configuring the SPAN session would be to mirror any traffic received by ports belonging to the Internet DMZ VLAN. Thus if a port were added to the VLAN in the future, you would not need to reconfigure the SPAN session. The following example demonstrates replacing the previous port-based SPAN configuration with a VLAN-based SPAN configuration:

```
Console> (enable) set span disable
This command WILL disable your span session(s).
Do you want to continue (y/n) [n]?y
Disabled all sessions
Console> (enable) set span 200 2/1 rx create
Enabled monitoring of VLAN 200 receive traffic
   by Port 2/1
```

Because a single destination port cannot have more that one SPAN session applied, all SPAN sessions were first disabled to allow the creation of a new SPAN session that mirrors any traffic received by ports that belong to VLAN 200.

TIP

Instead of destroying the SPAN session, you can omit the create keyword from a new SPAN session configuration. If the destination port specified in the new SPAN session already has a SPAN session associated with it, the new SPAN session overwrites the existing SPAN session.

Configuring Traffic Capture Using VACLs

Using VACLs to mirror traffic to your IDSM allows you to select which traffic you wish to mirror at the layer 3 and layer 4 levels. The use of VACLs requires the Catalyst 6000/6500 Supervisor engine (a line card that contains the main CPU of the switch) to have a PFC installed. If you do not have a PFC installed, you cannot use VACLs.

As the name suggests, VACLs filter traffic at a VLAN level, and each access control entry (ACE) in the VACL allows you to optionally specify a capture option that will mirror any traffic that matches the ACE to a capture port. To configure VACLs, you must perform the following steps:

▶ Create a VACL that defines interesting traffic.

▶ Commit the VACL to PFC memory.

▶ Map the VACL to a VLAN.

▶ Add the IDSM monitoring port to the VACL capture list.

Because VACLs are more complex to configure than SPAN, a full VACL configuration example is included at the end of this section.

Creating a VACL   A VACL is identified by a name and can hold many entries that are known as ACEs. Each ACE defines a particular type of traffic that has certain layer 3 and layer 4 characteristics. To create a VACL, you use the set security acl ip command on the switch (not the IDSM). The syntax of the set security acl ip command depends on which layer 3 or layer 4 characteristics you specify. Here are some examples of VACLs:

```
set security acl ip TEST_VACL1 permit 192.168.1.0
   255.255.255.0 capture
set security acl ip TEST_VACL2 permit ip 10.0.0.0
   255.0.0.0 20.0.0.0 255.0.0.0 capture
set security acl ip TEST_VACL3 permit icmp 10.0.0.0
   255.0.0.0 20.0.0.0 255.0.0.0 echo capture
set security acl ip TEST_VACL3 permit tcp 10.0.0.0
   255.0.0.0 20.0.0.0 255.0.0.0 eq 80 capture
set security acl ip TEST_VACL4 permit udp 10.0.0.0
   255.0.0.0 gt 1024 20.0.0.0 255.0.0.0 eq 53 capture
```

Notice that each VACL ACE includes the capture keyword, which specifies any traffic that matches the VACL ACE should be forwarded to the capture port list. It is crucial to understand that the capture keyword is required to mirror traffic that matches the respective ACE. In the previous example, there are four VACLs:

▶ TEST_VACL1 allows any IP traffic from a source IP address that resides within the 192.168.1.0/24 subnet (such as 192.168.1.0– 192.168.1.255).

▶ TEST_VACL2 allows any IP traffic from a source IP address that resides within the 10.0.0.0/8 subnet destined to the 20.0.0.0/8 subnet.

▶ TEST_VACL3 allows any ICMP traffic from a source IP address that resides within the 10.0.0.0/8 subnet destined to the 20.0.0.0/8 subnet. The VACL also has an ACE that allows any TCP web traffic

Part IV

from a client on the 10.0.0.0/8 subnet to a web server on the 20.0.0.0/8 subnet.

▶ TEST_VACL4 allows any UDP DNS traffic from a DNS client that resides within the 10.0.0.0/8 subnet destined to a DNS server that resides on the 20.0.0.0/8 subnet. The DNS client must also use a source port of greater than 1024.

NOTE

You may notice that TEST_VACL1 does not include the ip keyword. This keyword is not required for strictly IP traffic.

In each VACL, an implicit deny all blocks any other traffic that is not permitted.

Committing the VACL to PFC Memory   Once you have created your VACL, although the VACL is automatically stored in the switch NVRAM, you must manually commit the VACL to the PFC hardware. Doing so loads the VACL into a special memory structure (known as TCAM) on the PFC that allows the PFC to apply the VACL to traffic at wire speed, incurring no performance penalties.

To commit the VACL to hardware, use the commit security acl command from the switch (not the IDSM):

```
Console> (enable) commit security acl vacl_name | all
```

You can commit a specific VACL by specifying the VACL name, or you can commit all VACLs to hardware by specifying the all keyword.

Mapping the VACL to a VLAN   Now that your VACL has been created and committed to hardware, you can apply the VACL to one or more VLANs. By applying the VACL to a VLAN, you immediately begin filtering traffic on the VLAN based on the VACL.

WARNING

Be aware that the primary purpose of a VACL is to filter traffic. When using VACLs for IDS traffic capture, do not forget that a VACL is also filtering traffic. If you just capture specific traffic, rather than filtering it, add a permit ip any any ACE at the end of the VACL to override the implicit deny any any action. By using the capture keyword with specific ACEs above this permit ip any any ACE, you can control which traffic is monitored by the IDS, yet still permit all traffic through the VLAN.

As explained earlier, a single VLAN can have only a single VACL applied per protocol at any time. Because Cisco Secure IDS monitors only IP traffic, each VLAN can have only a single IP VACL applied. However, you can map a VACL to multiple VLANs.

To map a VACL to a VLAN, use the set security acl map command from the switch:

```
Console> (enable) set security acl map vacl_name vlans
```

Adding the IDSM Monitoring Port to the VACL Capture List

When you specify the capture keyword on a VACL ACE, any traffic that matches that ACE is mirrored to the VACL capture list. This is simply a list of ports that received traffic that match any VACL ACEs that include the capture keyword. When an IDSM is present in the system, the monitoring port on the IDSM is automatically configured as the default destination capture port for all captured VACL traffic.

You can add other ports to the capture list by using the set security acl capture-ports command:

```
set security acl capture-ports module/ports
```

A VACL Capture Example   Suppose we have the same sample network topology as shown earlier in Figure 21.30. We wish to monitor only web and mail traffic (HTTP and SMTP) on the Internet DMZ segment, yet still permit other traffic without passing it to the IDSM for analysis. First, we must create a VACL that specifies to capture only web and e-mail traffic, and permits all other traffic without capturing it:

```
Console> (enable) set security acl ip TEST permit tcp
    any any eq 80 capture
TEST editbuffer modified.  Use `commit' command to
    apply changes.
Console> (enable) set security acl ip TEST permit tcp
    any any eq 25 capture
TEST editbuffer modified.  Use `commit' command to
    apply changes.
Console> (enable) set security acl ip TEST permit ip
    any any
TEST editbuffer modified.  Use `commit' command to
    apply changes.
```

Notice that we use the capture keyword at the end of the ACEs that define web and mail traffic, but omit the capture keyword on the permit any any ACE to capture only web and mail traffic.

The next step is to commit the VACL to hardware:

```
Console> (enable) commit security acl TEST
Hardware programming in progress...
ACL TEST is committed to hardware.
```

Now, we must map the VACL to the Internet DMZ VLAN (200), using the set security acl map command:

```
Console> (enable) set security acl map TEST 200
ACL TEST mapped to vlan 1
```

Finally, we must assign the IDSM monitoring port to the VACL capture list. We don't actually need to do this, because the IDSM monitoring port is automatically assigned to the VACL capture list when the IDSM is installed. However, for demonstration purposes, the following shows how to assign the IDSM monitoring port (port 2/1) to the VACL capture list:

```
Console> (enable) set security acl capture-ports 2/1
Successfully set 2/1 to capture ACL traffic.
```

Configuring the Monitoring Port to Control Trunk Traffic

So far, you have learned all the necessary fundamentals to allow a Catalyst IDSM to monitor traffic that passes through a Catalyst 6000/6500 switch. You can apply optional configuration on the monitoring port, which may be required in certain situations. Because the monitoring port is a trunk interface, you may need to control which VLANs are trunked to ensure the port is not oversubscribed.

By default, the monitoring port on the IDSM trunks traffic for *all* VLANs (VLANs 1 through 1024), meaning the port is a member of all VLANs. In scenarios where you use multiple IDSMs in conjunction with VACL traffic capture, the same captured traffic is mirrored to both IDSMs, because a single capture list is used. It is a good idea to limit the VLANs that are trunked on the monitoring port to only those that you wish the IDSM to monitor.

In a multiple-IDSM configuration, you typically use multiple IDSMs because you want to monitor more than 100Mbps of traffic. For example, if your VACL capture traffic may total 200Mbps, you should clear VLANs from each trunk to limit the amount of traffic each IDSM monitors to 100Mbps. Figure 21.31 illustrates this concept.

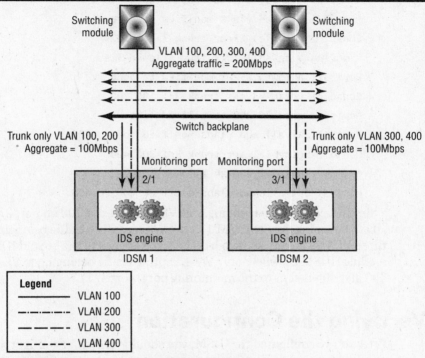

FIGURE 21.31:   A multiple IDSM configuration

In Figure 21.31, each VLAN carries a constant stream of 50Mbps traffic. Thus the total bandwidth aggregate on the backplane is 200Mbps (4×50Mbps), which exceeds the capabilities of a single IDSM. To alleviate this situation, a second IDSM is installed, and the aggregate backplane bandwidth is split into two 100Mbps streams by selectively trunking two VLANs on each IDSM monitoring port trunk. Each IDSM can handle 100Mbps, so all traffic can now be monitored.

To control the VLANs that are trunked to the IDSM port, use the clear trunk command to remove all VLANs from the trunk, and then use the set trunk command to selectively add VLANs to the trunk. All configuration is performed from the switch CLI. The following example

Part IV

shows how you would map the appropriate VLANs in Figure 21.31 to each IDSM monitoring trunk:

```
Console> (enable) clear trunk 2/1 1-1024
Removing Vlan(s) 1-1024 from allowed list.
Port 2/1 allowed vlans modified to none.
Console> (enable) clear trunk 3/1 1-1024
Removing Vlan(s) 1-1024 from allowed list.
Port 3/1 allowed vlans modified to none.
Console> (enable) set trunk 2/1 100,200
Adding vlans 100,200 to allowed list.
Port(s) 2/1 allowed vlans modified to 100,200.
Console> (enable) set trunk 3/1 300,400
Adding vlans 300-400 to allowed list.
Port(s) 3/1 allowed vlans modified to 300,400.
```

In this example, by trunking only VLANs 100 and 200 on port 2/1 (the monitoring port of IDSM 1), only VACL capture traffic belonging to those VLANs is sent to the port. The same applies to the second IDSM module (IDSM 2), where only VACL capture traffic belonging to VLANs 300 and 400 is sent to the monitoring port (port 3/1).

Verifying the Configuration

After you've configured the IDSM, you should verify your configuration to ensure it is correct and does not cause any problems later. You can verify both the switch configuration and the IDSM configuration.

Verifying the Switch Configuration

The Catalyst 6000/6500 switch features show commands that allow you to verify configuration. In relation to supporting the IDSM, the following show commands are useful:

▶ The show config command displays the nondefault system configuration file, which contains any nondefault configuration commands. This information lets you verify that you have configured a particular command.

▶ The show span command displays information about any current SPAN sessions and how they are configured. It allows you to check which source ports/VLANs are associated with a session, the traffic direction that is being monitored, and whether the destination port is correct.

▶ The show security acl command displays all VACLs as they are saved in NVRAM. It allows you to check a VACL to ensure that the correct ACEs have the capture keyword applied, and also to check for any errors.

Verifying the IDSM Configuration

The IDSM operating system also features commands that allow you to verify configuration. These commands must be executed in the diagnostics configuration mode. To enter this mode, type **diag** from the # prompt and press Enter:

```
idsm# diag
idsm(diag)#
```

The (diag) portion of the idsm(diag)# prompt indicates that the IDSM management session is in diagnostics mode. To exit diagnostic mode, type **exit** at the (diag)# prompt and press Enter.

The following commands (entered in diagnostic mode) are useful for verifying the IDSM configuration:

▶ The show configuration command displays current version and configuration information for the IDSM.

▶ The show eventfile command displays the contents of the IDSM alarm log files, which are used when you specify the log action with a signature on the Director platform.

▶ The diag resetcount command resets all IDSM statistics.

NOTE

The clear config command removes all configuration from the IDSM, effectively disabling the IDSM.

Configuring CSPM to Allow Management of the IDSM

You've almost finished the process of getting your Director platform (CSPM) to communicate with the Catalyst IDSM. Your IDSM is ready to

Part IV

capture and analyze traffic, as well as communicate with the Director platform for management and alarm notification purposes. All that is left is for you to create a sensor object that represents the IDSM in the CSPM database, and then upload your first configuration to the IDSM.

The procedure for adding an IDSM sensor to CSPM is almost identical to the procedure used for the Cisco Secure IDS 4200 sensors, described in the "Configuring CSPM for 4200 Series Sensor Management" section earlier in this chapter. The only difference is that you specify a different software version during the configuration process.

To add a new IDSM sensor object, perform the following steps:

1. Ensure you are logged in to Policy Administrator with full rights, and select the Wizards ➤ Add Sensor menu item to begin the Add Sensor Wizard.

2. On the Sensor Identification page, enter the sensor name, IP address, PostOffice parameters, and policy enforcement network service, as shown in Figure 21.32. Click the Next button to proceed.

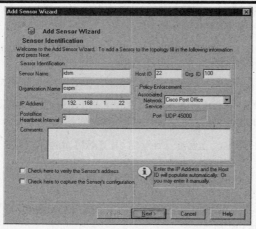

FIGURE 21.32: The Sensor Identification page for an IDSM

3. On the Default Gateway Address page, enter the default gateway IP address and subnet mask, and then click Next.

4. On the Sensor Configuration page, select the appropriate sensor software version, as shown in Figure 21.33. All IDSM modules have an IDSM suffix on the version number. Also select the appropriate signature template to apply to the IDSM.

TIP

If you are unsure of the IDSM software version, execute the show config command from the IDSM CLI to display the current software version.

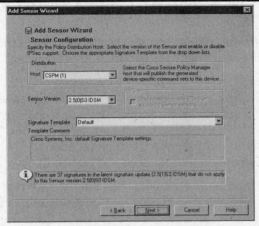

FIGURE 21.33:   The Sensor Configuration page for an IDSM

5. Click the Finish button to confirm the configuration parameters and complete the configuration of the new sensor object.

Now that you have added the IDSM object to the CSPM database, you should save, update, and upload your first configuration to the IDSM. Click the Save and Update buttons on the CSPM toolbar in Policy Administrator to save and update the CSPM database. Next, select the newly created IDSM object in the NTT to display the sensor object properties page; click the Command tab. On the Command page, click the Approve Now button to begin the process of uploading the configuration file to the IDSM.

MAINTAINING THE IDSM

You need to understand how to maintain the IDSM. New signatures are available on a regular basis, and they must be installed on the IDSM to keep its intrusion-detection capabilities up-to-date. Service packs and version upgrades can include fixes for software bugs and new features that extend the capabilities of the IDSM. Another important component of maintaining the IDSM is understanding how to troubleshoot it.

Part IV

However, before you can maintain or troubleshoot the IDSM, you need to understand its filesystem.

Understanding the IDSM Filesystem

The IDSM consists of a single hard disk drive that is split into two separate 4GB partitions:

Application Partition   The *application partition* contains the IDS engine. It is the active partition (partition that is booted) by default.

Maintenance Partition   The *maintenance partition* contains maintenance and diagnostic features that allow you to update the application partition if required. For example, this action would be required if the application partition became corrupted. The maintenance partition has no IDS capabilities.

The application partition is used to update the maintenance partition if required. You do not need to access the maintenance partition to install service packs and signature updates on the IDS engine on the active partition; you can perform these activities from the application partition.

The IDSM can be configured to boot from either partition. If you need to change the partition that you wish the IDSM to boot from, you can use the Catalyst switch (not the IDSM) set boot device command, as follows:

```
Console> (enable) set boot device hdd:partition module
```

The *module* parameter is the slot number in which the IDSM is installed. The *partition* parameter is the partition number to boot from. The application partition has a partition number of 1, and the maintenance partition has a partition number of 2. The following shows an example of setting the boot partition of an IDSM installed in module 2 of a Catalyst switch to the maintenance partition:

```
Console> (enable) set boot device hdd:2 2
```

TIP

If you wish to set the boot device back to its default for a module, execute the clear boot device *mod_num* command. For example, executing the clear boot device 2 command sets the boot device to the default on module 2.

The set boot device command permanently sets the boot partition. For example, if you set the boot partition to be partition 2 (the maintenance partition), the IDSM will always boot to that partition, even after a reboot. To boot to an alternative partition without modifying the default boot behavior, use the reset command, as follows:

```
Console> (enable) reset module hdd:partition
```

Updating IDSM Files and Partitions

All IDSM updates are released in files that can be obtained from the Cisco website with a valid CCO account. Cisco uses a convention for update filenames that identifies the purpose of the file. To update IDSM, you download the correct file type and then install the update.

Downloading the Update

Each IDSM update file uses a common filenaming convention, as illustrated here:

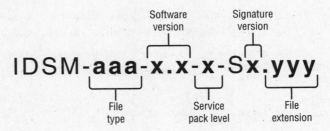

An IDSM update filename has five parts:

- ▶ The file type indicates the type of update. There are four types of updates:

    - ▶ Application (a) files contain an IDS engine application partition image (must be installed from the maintenance partition).

    - ▶ Maintenance (m) files contain an IDS maintenance partition image (must be installed from the application partition).

    - ▶ Service pack (sp) files contain an IDS service pack release with IDS engine bug fixes (can be installed from the application partition).

    - ▶ Signature update (sig) files contain new or updated IDS signatures (can be installed from the application partition).

► The IDSM version indicates the software version the update is designed for or the version the update will bring the existing image up to. The version includes a major release number, followed by a decimal point, and then a minor release number.

► The service pack level indicates the service pack level the update is designed for or the service pack level the update will bring the existing image up to.

► The signature version indicates the signature version the update is designed for or the signature version the update will bring the existing image up to.

► The extension of the file depends on the type of update, as follows:

  ► An .exe file is a self-extracting executable file that is used for signature or service pack upgrades.

  ► A .cab file is a Microsoft CAB format file that is used for IDSM application or maintenance software image files.

  ► A .lst file is a text file that contains a list of the CAB files required for a complete software image file.

  ► A .dat file is a binary file that contains information required for the installation of a CAB software image file.

For example, the update file IDSM-sig-2.5-1-S2a.exe is a signature file (sig) for version 2.5, service pack level 1 of the IDSM sensor software and contains signature version 2a. The IDSM-sp-2.5-1-S0.exe file is a service pack file (sp) for version 2.5, signature version 0 and contains service pack level 1. The IDSM-a-3.0-1-S4.lst file is part of an application image (a). The file contains a list of the required files for the application image installation (as defined by the lst extension). The application image contains IDSM sensor software version 3.0, service pack level 4 and includes signature version 4.

Installing Signature Updates and Service Packs

Installing signature updates and service packs is relatively simple and can be performed from the application partition. You must have an FTP server on your network that contains the appropriate IDSM signature update or service pack. You also must know the IP address, path to the update, and a valid account to log in to the FTP server.

To install a signature update or service pack, first you must gain management access to the IDSM via a console connection from the Catalyst switch (using the session command) or via a direct Telnet connection to the command-and-control port of the IDSM. Once you have gained access to the IDSM module, you should first check the current version of the IDSM module to ensure the new update file is compatible with the current IDSM software version. To do this, execute the show config command:

```
idsm# show config
Using 92258304 out of 200593408 bytes of available memory
!
Using 634650624 out of 2195980288 bytes of available
  disk space
!
Sensor version 3.0(1)S4
!
nr.postofficed      running
nr.fileXferd        running
nr.loggerd          running
nr.packetd          running
nr.sapd             running
nr.managed          running
```

To install a signature update or service pack, you must enter configuration mode on the IDSM by issuing the configure terminal command and pressing Enter. Once you are in configuration mode, use the apply command to download the file from an FTP server and install it:

```
idsm(config)# apply [signatureupdate | servicepack]
    site ftp_site user ftp_user dir ftp_path file ftp_file
```

You use the signatureupdate parameter to specify a signature update file, or you use the servicepack parameter to specify a service pack file. The remaining parameters define the IP address, username, path, and filename on the FTP server.

The following example demonstrates installing a service pack file:

```
idsm# config terminal
idsm(config)# apply servicepack site 192.168.1.20
    user ftpguy dir IDSM file IDSM-sp-2.5-1-S0.exe
```

Part IV

TIP

You can use the `remove [servicepack | signatureupdate]` command to remove the last service pack or signature update installed.

Updating IDSM Partitions

Updating an IDSM partition means the entire application or maintenance partition requires an upgrade. The common reasons for upgrading an IDSM partition include the following:

- ▶ The existing software image has been corrupted.

- ▶ The software image upgrade requires replacement of the current image.

- ▶ The password to access the IDSM has been lost.

TIP

A common cause of software image corruption is the IDSM not being shut down correctly. If you cannot shut down the IDSM via remote management using the IDSM `shutdown` command, push the shutdown button on the IDSM front panel to shut down the IDSM correctly.

When updating an IDSM partition, you must first determine which partition you are updating. You need to know this because you perform the update from the opposite partition; for example, if you need to update the application partition, you must do so from the maintenance partition.

Once you know the partition from which you must run the update, you need to boot into the partition by using the `set boot device` command or the `reset` command (described in the "Understanding the IDSM Filesystem" section earlier in the chapter). Next, you must log in and enter diagnostics mode. In diagnostics mode, use the `ids-installer` command to update the inactive partition:

```
idsm(diag)# ids-installer system /nw /install
/server=ftp_server /user=ftp_user /dir=ftp_path
/prefix=ftp_file
```

The `system` keyword tells the IDSM that a system-level action is being performed. The `/nw` and `/install` keywords specify that an installation is being performed from a network FTP source. The remaining keywords specify the various FTP parameters. For the /prefix keyword, you must specify the .dat file associated with the image upgrade.

The following example demonstrates an application partition IDSM upgrade:

```
Console> (enable) reset 2 hdd:2
This command will reset module 2 and may disconnect
  your telnet session.
Do you want to continue (y/n) [n]? y
Resetting module 2...

Console> (enable) session 2
Trying IDS-2...
Connected to IDS-2.
Escape character is '^]'.
login: ciscoids
password: ******

maintenance# diag
maintenance(diag) ids-installer system /nw /install
  /server=192.168.1.20 /user=ftpguy /dir=IDSM
  /prefix=IDSM-a-2.5-0-S0.dat
maintenance(diag) exit
maintenance# exit

Console> (enable) reset 2
```

NOTE

The previous example assumes an IP address, mask, and default gateway have already been configured on the maintenance partition. If they haven't, you must use the ids-installer net-config command to configure IP parameters, reboot the IDSM, and then proceed with the image update.

In this example, the IDSM is booted into the maintenance partition to allow the application partition to be updated. The update is then applied using the ids-installer command, after which the IDSM is again rebooted. Because the default boot partition has not been changed, the IDSM now boots into the new image on the application partition.

Part IV

Troubleshooting the IDSM

There may be times when your IDSM does not operate correctly or at all, and you need to troubleshoot to determine the problem and resolve it as quickly as possible.

A simple method of quickly determining the state of the IDSM is to examine the LED status color on the front panel of the IDSM. Table 21.2 (earlier in this chapter) shows the meaning of the various colors that may be indicated by the LED.

Using the Catalyst Switch to Troubleshoot

If you are unable to gain management access to your IDSM, you can use the Catalyst switch to perform some basic diagnostics. You can also troubleshoot issues with the IDSM ports. The following commands are useful for verifying that the IDSM is online and functioning:

▶ The show module command displays module status and information. You should see the IDSM displayed in the module list. The Status column gives an indication of the status of the IDSM.

▶ The show port <module_number> command shows information about the IDSM monitoring and command-and-control ports. It allows you to determine if the port is enabled and up, and to check for any port errors.

▶ The reset module hdd:partition command allows you to reboot the IDSM gracefully if it appears to have crashed or gone offline. You can boot into the maintenance partition if you need to repair a damaged application partition.

▶ The show top pkts command allows you to verify the monitoring interface is receiving traffic. Doing so may help you resolve problems related to your IDS not picking up signatures.

Using the IDSM to Troubleshoot

The following IDSM troubleshooting and diagnostic commands are available:

▶ The shutdown command shuts down the IDSM gracefully. Once the IDSM is shut down, you can use the switch set module power down <module_number> and set module power up <module_number> commands to restart the IDSM.

▶ The nrconns command displays the current communications status with the Director platform.

▶ The diag bootresults command shows the last IDSM boot process and if any problems were reported.

▶ The show errorfile command displays error log files for each of the IDS engine processes.

▶ The report systemstatus command allows you to generate an HTML report of the system status and send this report to a remote FTP server.

With the exception of the shutdown command, these commands must be executed from diagnostics mode.

WHAT'S NEXT

In this chapter, you learned about the Cisco Secure IDS sensor platforms: the Cisco Secure IDS 4200 series sensors and the Cisco Catalyst IDSM. First, we discussed sensor deployment, including common locations (Internet, extranet, intranet, and remote-access segments) and common deployment methods (basic, device management, firewall sandwich, and remote installation).

Next, we covered the procedures for installing the IDS 4210 and 4230 sensors. Sensor installation requires physical installation, gaining management access, and performing initial configuration using the sysconfig-sensor utility.

Then, we introduced the IDSM, which is an integrated component of the Catalyst 6000/6500 switch. After describing its features and architecture, we explained how to install and configure the sensor, including how to configure the Catalyst 6000/6500 switch to capture the appropriate traffic and forward it to the IDSM. The IDSM can operate with two types of traffic capture methods: SPAN or VACLs (which require a PFC).

We also covered how to configure CSPM (the Director) so it can communicate with and manage the sensor. Once the installation and configuration of the sensor is complete, you must configure the CSPM host, populating the CPSM database with objects that represent each sensor and the CSPM host itself. After these objects have been saved to the database, CSPM creates device-specific configuration files that can be downloaded to each sensor.

Part IV

Finally, we explained how to maintain and troubleshoot the IDSM. You can update IDSM files and partitions (the application partition or maintenance partition) by downloading and installing update files. You can troubleshoot the IDSM by using switch or IDSM commands.

In Chapter 22, you will learn more about configuring signature files for intrusion detection and how to establish and manage alarms when an intrusion is detected.

Chapter 22

SENSOR CONFIGURATION

I n the previous chapter, you learned how to install and configure a Cisco Secure IDS sensor so that the sensor is ready to begin intrusion detection on the network. You have seen how you need to initially configure each sensor via a local management session, setting IP addressing and PostOffice parameters to allow initial communications with CSPM. This chapter focuses on further configuration tasks that may be required on the sensor object within the CSPM database.

The CSPM database represents each sensor as an object within a network topology tree (NTT). Each sensor object has various parameters you can configure that modify how the sensor interacts with the Director and the rest of the network. This chapter covers the basic sensor parameters, which you will most likely need to configure, as well as advanced sensor parameters, which may be necessary for certain network environments.

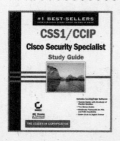

Adapted from *CSS1™/CCIP™: Cisco Security Specialist Study Guide* by Todd Lammle, Tom Lancaster, Eric Quinn, and Justin Menga

ISBN 0-7821-4049-1 $89.99

Part IV

BASIC SENSOR CONFIGURATION

Every Cisco Secure IDS sensor has basic configuration parameters that should be defined to allow the sensor to operate properly. These include sensor identification, internal network, monitoring interface, and log file configuration.

Configuring Sensor Identification

Sensor identification parameters are the most fundamental parameters you must define. These settings determine the unique sensor identification parameters that allow CSPM to communicate with each sensor.

When you first add a sensor object to CSPM using the Add Sensor Wizard, you configure sensor identification settings because they are required to establish communications between CSPM (the Director) and the sensor. The procedure for configuring CSPM using the Add Sensor Wizard was described in Chapter 21, "Installing Cisco Secure Sensors and IDSMs." If you need to verify or make changes to this configuration, open Policy Administrator and click the appropriate sensor object in the NTT. Click the Properties tab in the configuration pane for the sensor object, and then click the Identification tab. Figure 22.1 shows the Properties page for an IDS sensor object called ids-4210 with the Identification tab selected.

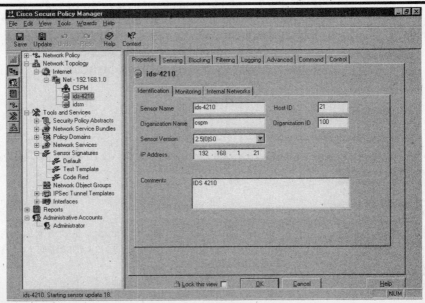

FIGURE 22.1:   The Identification page for a sensor

The Identification page contains the following fields to uniquely identify the sensor:

Sensor Name   This field contains the name of the sensor (ids-4210 in this example).

Host ID   This defines the numeric host ID of the sensor, which is used in PostOffice communications between the Director and sensor, and must match the host ID configured on the sensor.

Organization Name   This field contains the name of the organization to which the sensor belongs.

Organization ID   This defines the numeric organization ID of the sensor. This ID is used in PostOffice communications between the Director and sensor, and it must match the organization ID configured on the sensor.

Sensor Version   This defines the current level of Cisco Secure IDS software running on the sensor. The version is important, because it tells CSPM which signatures and features the sensor supports. The sensor object version information must match the actual version of software running on the sensor. In Figure 22.1, the IDS software version selected is 2.5(0)S0. You can set this to a different version by clicking the drop-down arrow and choosing the appropriate version.

TIP

You can determine the IDS software version running on a 4200 sensor by issuing the nrvers command when logged in to the sensor via console or telnet as the netrangr user. You can determine the IDS software version on a Catalyst 6000 IDSM by issuing the show configuration command from diagnostics mode on the IDSM. If the IDS software version of your sensor does not appear on the list, you must update your CSPM installation by downloading the appropriate update from the Cisco website. You need a CCO login with rights to download this software.

IP Address   This is the IP address of the command-and-control interface on the sensor.

Comments   This field allows you to add comments. You might use this to note anything specific to the sensor, such as the location or primary purpose of the sensor.

Part IV

Configuring Internal Networks

When designing, implementing, and supporting network security systems, one of the key concepts relating to the system is the definition of external networks and internal networks.

An *external network* is normally an untrusted network, and it is a network that is administratively not under your jurisdiction, meaning that you have no means of verifying the network security of the external network.

An *internal network* is normally a trusted network, because you have administrative control over either the entire network or over some portion of the network with other trusted administrators (that is, other staff within your organization) controlling the rest of the network. You can presume the internal network is trusted, assuming the necessary steps to secure your network have been taken.

WARNING

Trust is a dangerous word if used in its absolute form when referring to network security. Always be aware of the attack from the inside. Such an attack is an exploitation of trust and is potentially the most dangerous attack that can occur, due to the lesser security measures that are in place for trusted members of the organization.

Many organizations also create separate networks that provide a buffer, or intermediate zone (also referred to as a demilitarized zone or DMZ), between an external network and the internal network. This zone is under the control of the organization and allows for the organization to place applications and services that required access from external networks. If a system in this zone is breached, the impact to the organization is lessened because the compromised system is not located on the internal network with potential access to business-critical systems and information.

An essential component of any network that has a connection to some external or untrusted network is a firewall, which provides access control for traffic between the external network and internal network. The firewall acts like a border patrol post between each network; it regulates and inspects all traffic coming into one network and going out to another network. Here is an example of a network that contains an internal network and external network, with a firewall interconnecting each of the networks:

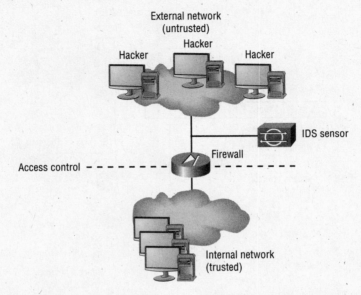

In this example, you can see that most threats are considered to be located on the external system. A firewall and an IDS sensor to monitor traffic are on the external segment.

Cisco Secure IDS sensors allow you to establish which systems are considered internal and which systems are considered external. These definitions are based on IP addressing in the source and destination IP address fields of an IP packet. Each signature always has a source (the system that the intrusive activity originates from) and a destination (the system that the intrusive activity is directed toward). Normally, your internal network is a well-defined set of IP subnets, and the external network consists of everything else. For example, your network might use subnets within the 10.10.0.0/16 address space, so the internal network includes any IP address within 10.10.0.0/16 (10.10.0.0 through 10.10.255.255), and the external network comprises any address outside that address range (192.168.1.1 or 172.16.1.1 and so on).

Part IV

Here is an example of an attack that is originating from an external network and is directed toward an internal network:

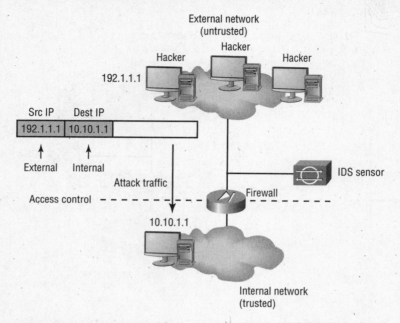

In this example, the source of the attack is considered external (because the source IP address, 192.1.1.1, of the attack traffic is outside the internal network) and the destination of the attack (target system) is considered internal (because the IP address, 10.10.1.1, of the attack traffic is within the internal network).

You can configure Cisco Secure IDS sensors with a set of internal networks (IP addresses), which define the IP addresses of systems considered internal to your network. Doing so allows the sensor to determine whether the source and destination of intrusive activity is internal or external. Any source or destination IP address that falls within the set of configured internal IP addresses is considered internal; any source or destination IP address that falls outside the set of internal IP addresses is considered external. The sensor indicates whether both the source and destination are internal or external in alarms that are generated, which makes it easier to quickly determine where an attack is originating from and which systems are being targeted.

NOTE

The Event Viewer application displays alarms from Cisco Secure IDS sensors in real time. Two of the attributes of an alarm are source location and destination location. These fields contain one of two possible values: IN, which means the source or destination IP address is internal, and OUT, which means the source or destination IP address is external.

By default, no internal networks are defined for each sensor, meaning the source and destination IP addresses of intrusive traffic will be considered external, and any alarms generated will indicate this. To configure the internal networks for a sensor, click the sensor in the NTT, and click the Properties tab in the configuration pane for the sensor object. Then click the Internal Networks tab, shown in Figure 22.2.

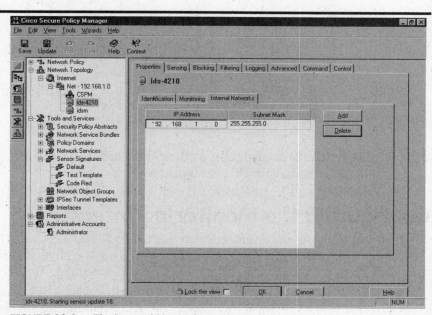

FIGURE 22.2:   The Internal Networks property page

The Internal Networks page contains a table with a list of IP addresses, each with an appropriate subnet mask to define a range of addresses. You can see a single entry in Figure 22.2, which indicates an IP address of 192.168.1.0 and a subnet mask of 255.255.255.0. This entry defines as internal the address range of 192.168.1.0 through 192.168.1.255. IP addresses outside this range are considered external.

Part IV

To add a new entry, click the Add button. To delete an entry, select the entry and click the Delete button. You can modify an existing entry by clicking in any of the octets of the IP address or subnet mask values and entering the appropriate configuration. The following illustrates the process of adding a single host (192.168.100.100) to the list of internal addresses:

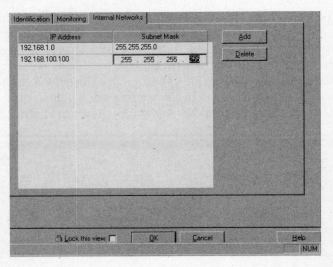

Notice that the example uses a subnet mask of 255.255.255.255, which allows you to add a specific host address to the list.

Configuring the Monitoring Interface

As you've learned in previous chapters, each Cisco Secure IDS sensor (the 4200 series sensors and the Catalyst 6000 IDSM) has two physical network interfaces: the monitoring interface and the command-and-control interface.

When you add a 4200 series sensor to CSPM, by default, CSPM assumes the sensor is a 4230 Ethernet sensor, and sets a monitoring interface within the sensor object based on this. If your sensor is not a 4230 sensor, you must ensure the monitoring interface is configured correctly.

After you have created a sensor object in CSPM, a default sensor interface name is assigned as the monitoring interface. This configuration parameter is called the *packet capture device*, and it is required for the 4200 series family of sensors, because different interface names are used, depending on the sensor model within the 4200 series family. For example, the 4210 sensor has a monitoring interface called /dev/iprb0, and the 4230 has a monitoring interface called /dev/spwr0. These names refer to the Solaris operating system device names that represent the monitoring NIC. Because sensor objects defined within CSPM do not have a field that indicates the actual physical sensor model (for example, IDS-4210 or IDS-4230), you must configure the packet capture device according to the model of the physical sensor for each sensor object.

TIP

You do not need to configure a packet capture device for the Catalyst 6000 IDSM sensor. If the software version of the sensor includes the suffix IDSM, CSPM knows that the sensor is a Catalyst 6000 IDSM and therefore automatically knows the name of the packet capture device, because only one Catalyst 6000 IDSM sensor model exists.

When you add a sensor object for a 4200 series sensor to CSPM, the packet capture device defaults to /dev/spwr0, which is the correct monitoring interface device name for the 4230 sensor. If the sensor is an IDS-4210, you must modify the packet capture device to the correct value (/dev/iprb0); otherwise, the sensor will not monitor traffic.

To configure the packet capture device for a sensor, click the sensor object in the NTT, and then click the Sensing tab in the configuration pane for the sensor object, shown in Figure 22.3.

The Sensing page includes a Packet Capture Device field, and the current value is set to /dev/sprw0. To change the value in this field, click the drop-down arrow and select the appropriate device name. As you can see in Figure 22.3, the Packet Capture Device drop-down list offers the following device names:

▶ /dev/spwr0, for 4220-E (Ethernet) sensors and 4230-FE (Fast Ethernet) sensors

▶ /dev/mtok, for 4220-TR (Token Ring) sensors with NICs not labeled 100/16/4

▶ /dev/mtok36, for 4220-TR (Token Ring) sensors with network interface cards labeled 100/16/4

▶ /dev/ptpci0, for 4230 sensors with FDDI NICs

▶ /dev/iprb0, for 4210 sensors

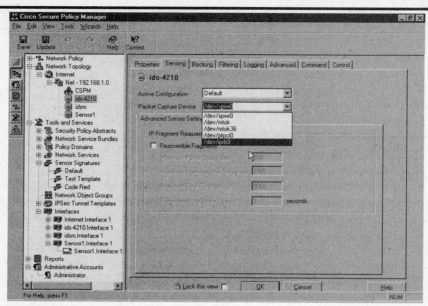

FIGURE 22.3: The Sensing page for a sensor

For the ids-4210 object in Figure 22.3, the Packet Capture Device field must be changed to /dev/iprb0, because the sensor is a 4210 sensor.

Configuring Log Files

Alarms are integral components of the Cisco Secure IDS architecture. An alarm is generated when a Cisco Secure IDS sensor detects intrusive activity (traffic triggering a signature); the alarm is then sent as a message to the Cisco Secure IDS Director platform. The alarm is the real-time notification mechanism used to alert security administrators to intrusive activity on the network.

By default, any alarms sent to a Director have a medium severity or higher. CSPM classifies alarms based on a low, medium, or high severity level. You can optionally configure a sensor to also generate a local log file, which is a flat file that contains alarms of all severity levels, not just alarms that are forwarded to the Director. This means that you can keep a record on your sensors of all events that occur and avoid flooding your Director with low-severity alarms.

If you enable log files on a sensor, it is important to understand how the log files are managed with relation to certain events.

A new log file is created for the following events:

► Sensor IDS services are restarted

► New configuration is uploaded to a sensor

► Log file is 24 hours old

► Log file exceeds a size of 1GB

► Log file has been open for more than one hour

The current log file is located in the /usr/nr/var directory and is called log.*yyyymmddhhmm*, where *yyyymmddhhmm* is the timestamp when the file was created. Any old log files are moved to a directory on the sensor called /usr/nr/var/new, and these files maintain their original name. You can also automatically copy any old (archived) log files to an FTP server on your network. The FTP transfer is triggered by the moving of a log file to the /usr/nr/var/new directory. Figure 22.4 illustrates what happens when alarms are generated and logging is enabled.

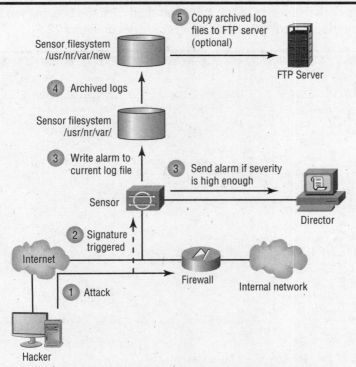

FIGURE 22.4:   Logging locally on a Cisco Secure IDS sensor

Part IV

In Figure 22.4, the following events take place:

1. An attack is launched by a hacker on the Internet.

2. The Cisco Secure IDS sensor captures the traffic, analyzes it, and triggers an attack signature.

3. The alarm is written to the current log file located in the /usr/nr/var directory on the local sensor filesystem. If the alarm is of a sufficient severity, an alarm notification is also sent to the Director.

4. The current log file is archived when events such as a configuration upload or service restart occurs. All archived log files are placed in the /usr/nr/var/new directory.

5. If configured, the sensor monitors the /usr/nr/var/new directory for any new files and copies these files to a remote FTP server.

By default, logging to a local file on a sensor is disabled. To configure logging, click the sensor in the NTT, and then click the Logging tab in the configuration pane for the sensor object, shown in Figure 22.5.

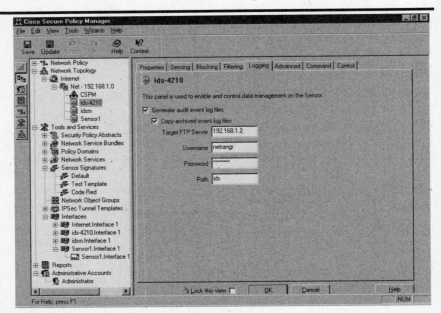

FIGURE 22.5:   The Logging page for a sensor

In Figure 22.5, you must select the Generate Audit Event Log Files option to enable the sensor to generate a local log file. You can also copy archived event logs to an FTP server by enabling the Copy Archived Event Log Files option. When specifying an FTP server, you must specify the IP address or DNS name of the server, an appropriate username and password, and an optional path in which to place the files. In Figure 22.5, an FTP server is configured with address 192.168.1.2, username `netrangr`, password `netrangr` (shown as asterisks for security), and a path of `ids`.

ADVANCED SENSOR CONFIGURATION

In the previous section, you learned about the basic sensor parameters, which you will normally configure for every sensor in your network. Cisco Secure IDS sensors also feature some advanced parameters, which allow you to fine-tune the operation of your sensors. These include packet reassembly and PostOffice settings, as well as the ability to send alarms to multiple destinations.

Configuring Packet Reassembly

Packet reassembly parameters allow you to configure a sensor to reassemble data streams that consist of multiple IP packets, such as IP fragments or multiple TCP packets from a single TCP session. Once reassembly is complete, the sensor can analyze the traffic in its complete form, reducing the chances of missing intrusive activity.

Cisco Secure IDS sensors detect intrusive activity on the network by using signature-based detection (also referred to as misuse detection). A Cisco Secure IDS signature defines a set of rules that uniquely identify a particular type of intrusive activity. In order to understand packet reassembly, you need to understand a bit about signature structure. Signature structure can be defined in one of two ways:

▶ An atomic signature is triggered by information contained within a single packet.

▶ A composite signature is triggered by information contained within multiple packets.

Atomic signatures are easy to understand and detect—a single IP packet is received and inspected, and triggers a signature due to some information contained within the packet. Composite signatures are more complex and much harder to deal with for a sensor. The number of packets in the signature can vary, and the time interval between each packet can vary as well. To add to the complexity of detecting composite signatures, traffic may be sent out of order.

Clearly, composite signatures introduce some issues for IDS, and attackers may use some advanced techniques designed to bypass IDS sensor signature analysis. Cisco Secure IDS sensors can protect against these techniques by using IP fragment reassembly and TCP session reassembly.

IP Fragment Reassembly

IP fragmentation can be used to mask an attack by fragmenting the attack into IP fragments. IP fragments pose a problem not only for IDS sensors, but also for access-control devices such as firewalls and perimeter routers. An IP fragment is normally used to transport an IP datagram that is larger than the maximum transmission unit (MTU) for a network over which the datagram is being sent.

NOTE
The MTU defines the maximum size of a frame or unit of data that can be sent across the network. For example, the MTU of an Ethernet network is 1518 bytes. This MTU defines the Ethernet header and data contents of a frame. Any layer 3 protocol packets carried in Ethernet frames are transported in the data section of the frame. Because the Ethernet header is 18 bytes, the data MTU (or layer 3 MTU) for Ethernet is 1500 bytes (18 + 1500 = 1518 bytes).

When the IP datagram is larger than the MTU, the datagram must be split into fragments that are less than or equal in size to the MTU of the transit network. Figure 22.6 demonstrates the process of fragmenting an IP datagram.

In Figure 22.6, the IP MTU of the Ethernet link between each router is 1500 bytes, and the IP datagram size is 3000 bytes. The following events take place:

1. An IP packet of 3000 bytes is received by Router A. The packet includes an IP header of 20 bytes, a TCP header of 20 bytes, and TCP data of 2960 bytes (the IP data portion is defined as 2980 bytes). Because the next hop router (Router B) is connected by an Ethernet link with an IP MTU of 1500 bytes, Router A must fragment the packet.

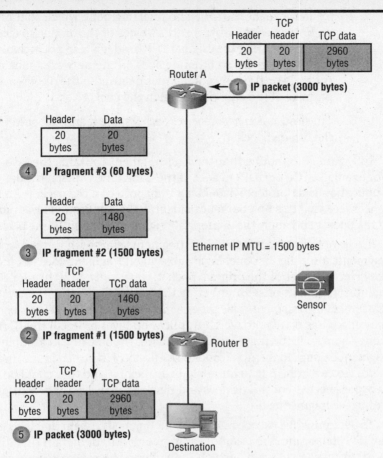

FIGURE 22.6: IP fragmentation

2. Router A fragments the original packet and sends the first fragment, which contains an IP header of 20 bytes, the original TCP header of 20 bytes, and 1460 bytes of the original packet data.

3. Router A sends the second fragment, which contains an IP header of 20 bytes and 1480 bytes of the original packet data. Notice that the original TCP header is not included in this fragment, so other devices on the network (such as firewalls or IDS sensors) cannot determine the upper-layer protocol of the data contained in the packet.

4. Router A sends the third and final fragment, which contains an IP header of 20 bytes and 20 bytes of the original packet data. Notice that the original TCP header is also not included in this fragment, so other devices on the network (such as firewalls or IDS sensors) cannot determine the upper-layer protocol of the data contained in the packet.

5. The destination host receives each fragment and reconstructs the original packet.

In Figure 22.6, notice that the first fragment contains the layer 4 (for example, TCP or UDP) header of the datagram, which indicates the Application-layer protocol data being transported in the packet. An IDS sensor receiving this first packet can identify the Application-layer protocol of the packet and apply the appropriate signature analysis to the packet.

The problems associated with IP fragments start with the subsequent fragments after the first one. Each subsequent fragment does not include the layer 4 header of the original packet; it has only an IP header that includes fragment-offset numbering that helps the destination system reassemble the fragment. This poses a problem for the IDS sensor, because the sensor has no idea to which Application-layer protocol the IP fragment belongs. If the fragment is legitimate, the sensor can assume the fragment belongs to the Application-layer protocol indicated in the first fragment. However, the fragments could be malicious, and they could be used to bypass access-control devices and mask intrusive activity contained within the fragments.

To determine the exact content of an IP fragment stream that is received, the IDS sensor must reassemble a fragmented IP datagram (just like a destination system must), which then allows the sensor to analyze the datagram in full. This process is known as *IP fragment reassembly*, and this feature is supported on the 4200 series sensors and the Catalyst IDSM.

By default, IP fragment reassembly is disabled, meaning an attack that has been fragmented into IP fragments will pass by the sensor undetected. IP fragment reassembly is configured on a per-sensor basis. To configure IP fragment reassembly, click the sensor in the NTT, click the Sensing tab in the configuration pane, and click the Advanced Sensor Settings tab. Figure 22.7 shows the Advanced Sensor Settings page for an IDS sensor object named idsm.

Checking the Reassemble Fragments option on the Advanced Sensor Settings page enables IP fragment reassembly.

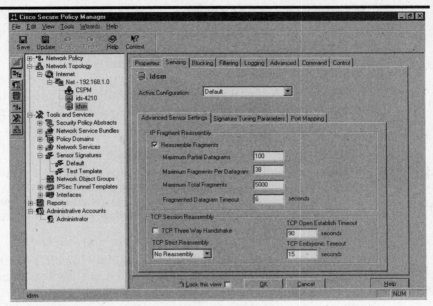

FIGURE 22.7: The Advanced Sensor Settings page

Beneath this option are several settings you can configure for IP fragment reassembly:

Maximum Partial Datagrams This defines the maximum number of partial datagrams that can be in the process of reassembly at any one time. The default value is 100.

Maximum Fragments per Datagram This defines the maximum number of fragments that can exist per datagram. The default value is 38, which means if 39 fragments are received for a single IP datagram, the sensor will discard all fragments and cease signature analysis on the fragmented datagram.

Maximum Total Fragments This defines the maximum number of fragments that can be stored in memory at any one time. This value should be greater than or equal to the product of Maximum Partial Datagrams and Maximum Fragments per Datagram values.

Fragmented Datagram Timeout This defines the maximum amount of time the sensor will spend on reassembling a single datagram. If the timeout is exceeded, the sensor will discard all fragments and cease signature analysis on the fragmented datagram. The default value is 6 seconds.

Part IV

TCP Session Reassembly

In the previous section, you learned that Cisco Secure IDS can protect against the use of IP fragmentation to hide intrusive activity. Another potential threat that can pose a problem to security-monitoring devices is that information sent over TCP sessions can be sent out of sequence. TCP provides automatic resequencing of segments before passing the data contained within each segment up to the Application-layer protocol.

NOTE

Each protocol at the various layers of the OSI model has a different name for the units of data with which the protocol communicates. Ethernet (layer 2) works with *frames*. IP (layer 3) works with *packets*. TCP (layer 4) works with *segments*. A TCP segment includes the TCP header and payload contained within a single IP packet.

Attackers can mask TCP-based intrusive activity from IDS sensors by sending the attack information out of sequence. Out-of-sequence delivery is a problem for IDS sensors when monitoring for composite signatures (signatures that consist of more than one packet). The out-of-sequence monitoring can potentially confuse the IDS sensor and bypass a positive match (false negative) or cause a positive match in error (false positive).

In order for an IDS sensor to correctly inspect TCP packets that are out of sequence, the IDS sensor must cache all TCP packets of a session (much like the process for IP fragments), and then reassemble the information in the correct order before passing the data stream to the IDS engine for analysis. This process is known as *TCP session reassembly*, and this feature is supported on only the Catalyst IDSM sensor.

NOTE

Remember that TCP session reassembly is supported only on the Catalyst IDSM sensor. This feature is not available on the Cisco Secure 4200 series sensors.

By default, TCP session reassembly is disabled, meaning an attack that uses out-of-sequence TCP packets could pass by the sensor undetected. TCP session reassembly is configured on a per-sensor basis. Like the IP fragment reassembly settings, the TCP session reassembly settings are on the Advanced Sensor Settings page, accessed by clicking the sensor in the NTT, clicking the Sensing tab in the configuration pane for the sensor object, and then clicking the Advanced Sensor Settings tab:

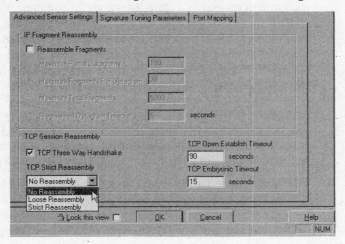

The following configurable options are available for TCP session reassembly:

TCP Strict Reassembly   This defines the method of TCP session reassembly. By default, this field is set to No Reassembly, which means TCP packets are inspected in the order they are received (in effect, TCP session reassembly is disabled). The drop-down list contains two other options. The Loose Reassembly option tells the sensor to reconstruct a TCP data stream on a periodic basis, and then analyze the information even if there are some missing TCP segments. The Strict Reassembly option tells the sensor to reconstruct a TCP data stream on a periodic basis and ensure that all segments from a TCP stream are present. With this option, the sensor waits until all segments are received; if a segment is not received after a certain time limit, the sensor does not inspect the data stream at all.

TCP Three-Way Handshake   If enabled, this option tells the sensor to inspect only TCP sessions that have completed the TCP three-way handshake. All valid TCP connections must establish a connection by first performing the TCP three-way handshake, so if the sensor sees TCP data from a session that

Part IV

has not performed the handshake, the sensor knows the data is invalid and does not analyze it. An attacker could send large amounts of invalid TCP data, which could consume all the IDS sensor resources if analyzed, allowing the attacker to then perform a real attack undetected. When the TCP Three Way Handshake check box is checked, the IDS sensor ignores any invalid TCP data. This configuration option is independent of the TCP Strict Reassembly mode of operation.

TCP Open Establish Timeout   This defines the maximum amount of time, in seconds, the sensor should cache TCP session data for established TCP sessions without receiving any subsequent session data. The default value is 90 seconds.

TCP Embryonic Timeout   This defines the maximum amount of time, in seconds, the sensor should cache TCP session data for half-open TCP sessions without receiving any subsequent session data. A half-open TCP session is a session that has not fully completed the TCP three-way handshake (in other words, the session has been initiated but not fully established). This option protects the IDS sensor from caching too many TCP sessions during a prolonged TCP SYN flood attack. The default value is 15 seconds.

If you plan to enable TCP session reassembly (remember, this feature is supported only on the IDSM sensor), the best TCP Session Reassembly option to use for most environments is the Loose Reassembly option.

The No Reassembly option inspects TCP packets as they arrive, with no consideration for out-of-sequence information. This can generate *false positives* and *false negatives*, so using this option is not recommended.

The Strict Reassembly option will not inspect any data of a session, which has missing TCP packets at all, so this can easily lead to false negatives (missed signature matches).

The Loose Reassembly option tolerates missed TCP packets, so it will reconstruct a TCP session and inspect the session, even if parts of the session are missing. This can sometimes lead to false positives, but the chances of this occurring are much less likely than if no reassembly is used. The Loose Reassembly option also avoids the false negative issues associated with the Strict Reassembly option.

NOTE

False negatives are very dangerous—they are an indication an attack is able to bypass your IDS. Furthermore, you have no indication that an attack has bypassed your IDS. False negatives are synonymous with an invisible man walking past security cameras undetected. False positives are not as danger-ous, because you know that they have occurred. However, false positives lead to complacency and also can overwhelm an alarm log, making it difficult to deci-pher the real alarms. False positives are synonymous with the boy who cried wolf—after a while, you're less likely to believe any positives, even if they are real.

Configuring PostOffice Settings

As you've learned in previous chapters, the Cisco Secure IDS architecture uses the PostOffice protocol to facilitate communication between sensors and Directors. The primary purpose of the PostOffice protocol is to allow configuration and alarm messages to be exchanged between a sensor and Director. The PostOffice protocol also features other communications, which are used to increase the reliability and availability of the Cisco Secure IDS architecture. Two mechanisms that are used by PostOffice to ensure Cisco Secure IDS components are up and running are the heartbeat and watchdog process.

The *PostOffice heartbeat* is a simple message that is generated by default every five seconds, and it is similar in concept to the ICMP ping mechanism. The message queries if the PostOffice on a remote device is up and expects a response from the remote PostOffice confirming this. If no response is received, communications with the device as a whole are assumed to be down, and a Route Down alarm is generated.

Watchdog is a diagnostic process that queries services (or daemons) on a local or remote sensor or Director. If a service is detected that is not running, a Daemon Down alarm is generated, and the watchdog process attempts to restart the service. If the service cannot be started after a con-figurable number of attempts, the service is declared down and a Daemon Unstartable alarm is generated. Note that this alarm does not constitute an entire failure on a remote device, as a Route Down alarm indicates.

You can modify parameters associated with the heartbeat and watchdog features for each sensor object in the CSPM database. These parameters are configured on a per-sensor basis. To configure PostOffice settings, click the sensor in the NTT, click the Advanced tab in the configuration pane for the

Part IV

sensor object, and then click the PostOffice Settings tab. Figure 22.8 shows the PostOffice Settings page for an IDS sensor object named ids-4210.

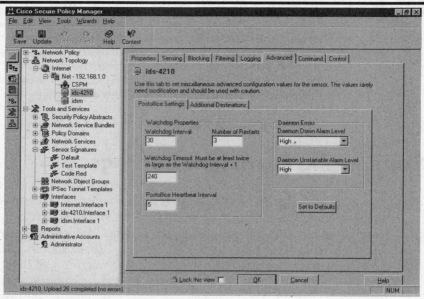

FIGURE 22.8: The PostOffice Settings page for a sensor

You can configure the following options for PostOffice settings:

Watchdog Interval This setting defines the interval, in seconds, at which the watchdog process periodically queries services running on the sensor. By default, this value is 30 seconds.

Watchdog Timeout This setting defines how long, in seconds, the watchdog process should wait for a response to a watchdog query. By default, this value is 240 seconds, and as you can see in Figure 22.8, the configured value must be greater than twice the Watchdog Interval setting plus 1. If a response to a watchdog query is not received within this period, a Daemon Down alarm is generated, and the watchdog process will then attempt to restart the service.

Number of Restarts This setting defines the amount of times the watchdog process attempts to restart a service that has failed (gone into a Daemon Down state). By default, this value is 3 restarts for a 4200 series sensor and 0 restarts for an IDSM.

If a service fails to restart after these attempts, the service is declared down and a Daemon Unstartable alarm is generated.

PostOffice Heartbeat Interval This setting defines how often, in seconds, the PostOffice service on the sensor is queried to check the service is still running. If no response is received, a Route Down alarm is generated. By default, this value is 5 seconds.

Daemon Down Alarm Level This defines the CSPM severity level (low, medium, or high) of a Daemon Down alarm, which is generated if a watchdog query times out waiting for a response. By default, the severity level is set to high.

Daemon Unstartable Alarm Level This defines the CSPM severity level (low, medium, or high) of a Daemon Unstartable alarm, which is generated if the watchdog process cannot restart a failed service within the Number of Restarts value. By default, the severity level is set to high.

You will normally need to modify these settings only if you have a slow network (for example, you might increase the PostOffice interval), or if you wish to alter the severity of the alarms (for example, you might lower the Daemon Down alarm level to medium). If you make changes and then need to restore these parameters to their default values, click the Set to Defaults button.

Working with Multiple Directors

The Cisco Secure IDS architecture allows sensors to send alarms to multiple destinations. This feature can be used to send alarms not only to multiple Directors for alarm management purposes, but also to other services running on a Director or sensor platform.

The service that runs on CSPM (Director) that is responsible for accepting alarms and displaying these alarms in the Event Viewer console is called smid. By default, a sensor object in CSPM is configured to forward alarms to the smid service running on the local CSPM host. You can configure additional destinations for alarms, and you can forward these alarms to different services on the destination system. For example, Cisco Secure IDS Director for UNIX allows you to configure a service called eventd, which you can monitor for new alarms and run user-defined scripts based on those alarms. By configuring a sensor to forward alarms to the Director

Part IV

for UNIX, and configuring the destination service as the eventd service, alarms will be forwarded to this service, and the user-defined scripts can run as intended.

You can modify the list of destinations a sensor sends alarms to by modifying a parameter called Additional Destinations. To configure Additional Destinations, click the sensor in the NTT, click the Advanced tab in the configuration pane for the sensor object, and then click the Additional Destinations tab. Figure 22.9 shows the Additional Destinations page for an IDS sensor object named ids-4210.

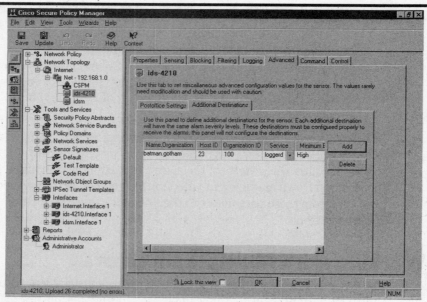

FIGURE 22.9:   The Additional Destinations page for a sensor

The Additional Destinations page contains a table that lists each additional destination. To add a new destination, click the Add button, and a new entry will appear in the destination list table. Click in each field to configure the appropriate parameters, as follows (you'll need to scroll right to see all of the fields):

Name.Organization   This is a text string consisting of the PostOffice name and organization of the destination device. For example, Figure 22.9 shows a destination being added that has the name batman and belongs to the organization gotham.

Host ID   This defines the numeric PostOffice host ID of the destination device. This setting must match the configured host ID on the device.

Organization ID   This defines the numeric PostOffice organization ID of the destination device. This setting must match the configured organization ID on the device.

Service   This defines the service on the destination device to which the alarm is forwarded. The default service is smid, which is the service used on Directors to display alarms. You can also configure eventd (used on Director for UNIX) to trigger custom user-defined scripts.

Minimum Event Level   This defines the minimum severity of an alarm that can be forwarded to the destination. The default setting is Medium.

IP Address   This defines the IP address of the destination device.

Heartbeat Timeout   This defines how often the destination device expects to hear heartbeats from the sensor object being configured. The default setting is 5 seconds.

Port   This defines the UDP port on which the PostOffice service listens on the destination device. The default setting is port 45000.

If you wish to modify an existing destination, click in the field that you wish to modify. To delete a destination, select the destination and click the Delete button.

WHAT'S NEXT

In this chapter, you learned how to configure sensor objects contained in the CSPM database that represents each physical sensor on your network. You also learned how the Cisco Secure IDS architecture allows sensors to send alarms to multiple Directors or sensors on the network.

In the next chapter, our discussion will move from Cisco security to preparing for the Microsoft MCSE exams. The next several chapters provide in-depth information about how to prepare for the security-related portions of Microsoft's premiere certification.

Part IV

Part V
SECURITY-RELATED MCSE HIGHLIGHTS

Chapter 23

Evaluating the Impact of the Security Design on the Technical Environment

We are now going to begin looking at some of the features of the distributed security strategy and how they will impact your existing and planned technical environment.

In this chapter we will analyze the new security features of Windows 2000 and what the impact of each will be on the technical environment. Then we can take that information and put it to use to figure out how existing applications can be enhanced with Windows 2000 security. If parts of the security structure don't quite measure up, they will fall into a separate category that we can deal with later.

Because this process implies massive amounts of change, you know that technical support will be busy (at least until the bugs are worked out of the new system and users become familiar with it); the analysis of the technical support structure will determine if it is ready to handle the load.

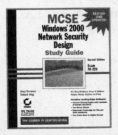

Adapted from *MCSE: Windows® 2000 Network Security Design Study Guide*, Second Edition by Gary Govanus and Robert King

ISBN: 0-7821-2952-8 $59.99

Finally, we will look at the existing and planned network and systems management. Doing so will show us how the security configuration tool can make systems management an easier task.

In Chapter 24, we'll begin the actual design phase by looking at the Windows 2000 security baseline.

Windows 2000 Security Concepts

Let's start with a review of basic security concepts as they relate to the Windows 2000 and XP environment. Because some of the people reading this book may be long-term security professionals, and some may be just beginning in the security field, we should spend some time defining terms. These terms will be helpful when you write your security plan, and they will go a long way toward helping you familiarize yourself with distributed security. In as many cases as possible, we will compare and contrast the NT 4 system with the Windows 2000/XP system or point out how concepts apply to the upcoming migration or upgrade. The following pages introduce various aspects of Windows 2000/XP security, from authentication to domain trusts. Each is covered in greater detail elsewhere in the book.

Authentication and Authorization Model

The most basic foundation of Windows 2000 security is a simple model of authentication and authorization that uses the Microsoft Active Directory service. Unless you select the Automatic Logon choice during the installation of Windows 2000 or XP, each user is required to log on each time they sit down at a workstation by using a unique username and password. *Authentication* identifies the user using these credentials and matches them to a security database. If a valid username and password are detected, the computer makes network connections to services on behalf of the user. Once the user has been identified, the user is *authorized* to access a specific set of network resources based on permissions. Authorization takes place through the mechanism of access control, using *access control lists* (ACLs) that define permissions on filesystems, network file and print shares, and entries in Active Directory.

Domain Model

In Windows 2000, a *domain* is a collection of network objects—such as user accounts, groups, and computers—that share a common directory database with respect to security. A domain identifies a security authority and forms a boundary of security with consistent internal policies and explicit security relationships to other domains.

Migrating Domains to Windows 2000

Before you can migrate Windows NT domains to Windows 2000, you must accomplish certain steps:

1. Complete the design of the Windows 2000 forest.

2. Plan the migration of Windows NT domains to Windows 2000 native domains and deploy new features of Windows 2000 Server.

3. Plan the restructure of the Windows 2000 domains.

If you were to put this process into a flowchart, it would look like Figure 23.1.

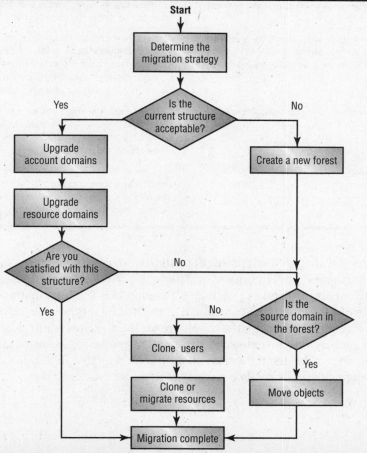

FIGURE 23.1: Domain migration flowchart

When you begin analyzing your current domain environment and looking at migrating to Windows 2000, you want to make sure the migration is as painless as possible. The migration should meet certain goals. Table 23.1 lists these goals as well as the actions you need to take.

TABLE 23.1:   The Path to a Perfect Migration

GOAL	ACTION
Make a seamless transition to Windows 2000, with little or no disruption to the production network.	Make sure you have planned for all eventualities to ensure that users can access their data, resources are available, and applications are accessible during the migration process.
Maintain the current levels of system performance or improve response time.	Because most people dislike change, strive to make sure the users' familiar environment is maintained during and after the migration.
Eliminate network downtime, or increase the average mean time between failures. Minimize the administrative overhead.	Make sure every effort is made to minimize the number of times a member of the IT staff needs to touch a user's computer after the up grade. Keeping the number of user contacts to a minimum means your upgrade was seamless.
Maximize the number of *quick wins*.	Getting a quick win means to have some feature of the new network available at the earliest opportunity so people can see how they will benefit from the upgrade.
Maintain system security.	There should be little or no negative impact on the current security policy. Make sure the security of the network is maintained or is strengthened after the upgrade.

As you analyze your current domain trust structure, your goal should be to migrate the NT domains and move the Windows 2000 domains to native mode as soon as possible. Native mode is the final operational state of a Windows 2000 domain; it is enabled by setting a switch on the user interface. Although the procedure for the switch is relatively simple, the implications are extensive. Switching to native mode means all the domain controllers in the domain have been migrated to Windows 2000. Changing to native mode is a one-way street because once you do it, you can't go back!

DOMAIN MIGRATION CONCEPTS

Domain upgrade is sometimes referred to as *in-place upgrade* or simply *upgrade*. A domain upgrade is the process of upgrading the Primary Domain Controller (PDC) and the Backup Domain Controllers (BDCs) of a Windows NT domain from Windows NT Server to Windows 2000 Server.

Domain restructure is sometimes referred to as *domain consolidation*. A domain restructure is a complete redesign of the domain structure, usually resulting in fewer, larger domains. This choice is for those who are dissatisfied with their current domain structure or who feel they cannot manage an upgrade without serious impact to their production environment.

Upgrade and restructure are not mutually exclusive; some organizations might upgrade first and then restructure, and others might restructure from the start. Both require careful thought and planning before choices are implemented.

Trust Management

A *trust* is a logical relationship established between two domains to allow *pass-through authentication*, in which a trusting domain honors the logon authentications of a trusted domain. In Windows 2000, you will hear the term *transitive trust*. A transitive trust refers to authentication across a chain of trust relationships. In Windows 2000, trust relationships support authentication across domains by using the Kerberos v5 protocol and Windows NT LAN Manager (NTLM) authentication for backward compatibility.

To begin the examination of a domain structure of an enterprise network, look at Figure 23.2. It is fairly indicative of a common multiple master domain design found in many organizations.

As you look at your existing NT domain structure, ask yourself the following questions about each domain:

▶ What purpose does this domain serve? The answer can help you set a priority for the upgrade.

▶ Can this domain be collapsed into another domain, eliminating an administrative center?

▶ How many domain controllers will be needed to manage this domain, and where will they be physically located?

▶ What DNS namespace(s) exists within your organization? (Once domains are named in Windows 2000, they cannot be renamed. You need to know the existing naming conventions and what additional namespaces your organization requires so that you can create a unique namespace for the forest.)

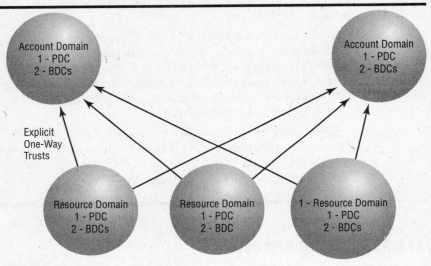

FIGURE 23.2: Common domain design

Upgrading Account Domains to Windows 2000

After you have looked at the logical design of your domains, you can set your upgrade priorities. As you upgrade from NT 4, you can bring the domain into the forest:

▶ Remember the point we just made about forest naming. Make sure the forest namespace is defined just the way you want it. If it is not, the entire forest will need to be restructured just to correct the namespace.

▶ Because the root domain is the first domain in a forest, create it carefully. After the root domain has been created, the name cannot be changed.

▶ When you create other domains, they are referred to as *child domains*. Be careful when adding a child domain. If it is added to the wrong part of the forest, you will have to do extra work to get the domain configuration the way you want it. The amount of work will depend on the number of objects in the misplaced domain.

▸ When you set up policies for the use of groups and ACLs, make sure the policies will not obstruct the way you plan to do things in the future.

Upgrading Resource Domains to Windows 2000

Resource domains were commonly used in Windows NT to hold the computer accounts of resources such as servers and client computers. Resource domains existed primarily to limit the size of the account database. If you are working in a smaller environment, you may not have needed resource domains. In large organizations with thousands of computers, the resources simply overwhelmed the security database. By creating a resource domain, the system administrator, in effect, partitioned the database to make authentication easier and faster. With Windows 2000 this problem no longer exists, so now you have to plan a way to get rid of the resource domains.

NT Limits on the Size of the Account Database   In Windows NT, the maximum size recommended for the Security Accounts Manager (SAM) account database is 40MB. In a domain containing user accounts, security groups, and Windows NT client and server computer accounts, this might equal fewer than 20,000 user accounts. If you worked for a very large company and you wanted to scale an organization with more than this number, user and computer accounts had to be stored in separate domains. In design terminology, that meant account domains were created for user accounts, and resource domains were created for computer accounts. If the resource domain was created as a holding area for servers and computer accounts, they were usually created with explicit one-way trusts to either a single account domain (master domain model) or a number of account domains (multiple-master domain model). With Windows 2000, some of these domains may be eliminated.

Provide Local Administrative Capability   There were times when it was not feasible to carry out administration from one location. In that case, the organization utilized decentralized administration. In a decentralized organization with geographically disparate facilities, it is often desirable to have local personnel authorized to administer resources. After all, what administrator wants to travel potentially hundreds of miles just to add user accounts? To allow this kind of decentralized responsibility in Windows NT systems, it was recommended that resource domains be created with their own administrative structure.

As was the case with scaling beyond SAM size limits, the results were master or multiple-master domain structures with explicit one-way trusts to the account domains in the organization. The administrators in the remote locations were not usually given administrative responsibility over the account domain. In other words, imposing one-way trusts ensured that resource domain administrators had administrative scope only over the resource domain.

NOTE
As part of your upgrade plan, your administrative model must reflect the implications of upgrading a resource domain. If you have already upgraded the account domain, and then you upgrade the resource domain as a child of the account domain, a transitive trust is established between them. For this reason, you need to consider how this transitive trust affects local administration of resources.

If you do not want administrative permissions to extend beyond the resource domain, you might consider other options, which include the following:

Restructuring Resource Domains into Organizational Units
You might redesign your domain structure. You could consider merging your resource domains into the upgraded account domain as Organizational Units (OUs). This option would obviously influence your thinking on the order of domain upgrade.

Upgrading a Resource Domain within the Existing Forest and Using Windows 2000 Delegation of Administration Features   Another approach would have you upgrade your resource domain to be in the same forest as the account domain(s). This way, you would use Windows 2000 delegation of administration features to limit the capabilities of the local administrators. Before you do this, check the administrative groups in the resource domain and remove all administrators who are not administrators in the account domains. If there are only local resource domain administrators, add one or more of your account domain administrators. These administrators will be able to administer the domain while it is being upgraded. As a further precaution, make sure resource domain administrators do not have administrative access to the domain controllers through local computer accounts.

After the PDC is upgraded, you might even create a new domain local group to hold your resource administrators, and use Windows 2000 delegated administration to grant them sufficient privilege to carry out their roles.

Upgrading a Resource Domain as a Tree in a New Forest
Finally, you can upgrade your resource domain and make it a tree in a new forest, linking the tree to the account domain through an explicit one-way trust. Doing so would effectively mirror the structure that existed before the upgrade.

PLANNING A DOMAIN MIGRATION

Suppose your customer has just presented you with a high-level map of the corporate network. The company is medium to large. It is not General Motors, to be sure, but it is not a Mom-and-Pop grocery store, either. It is a national food chain with stores all over the country.

The network map shows the way the distribution points are connected. Each regional distribution point has a master administrative domain with several resource domains. The resource domains are connected to the master domains with one-way trust relationships. The master domains are all linked with two-way trust relationships.

The head of IT complains about the administrative cost of keeping up this system. Dozens of domains are scattered all over the country, and remembering why each one was created is a nightmare. That doesn't include keeping straight what domain trusts what other domain and why.

You take the head of IT on a mental walk through the forest. At least, it *will* be a forest, once the PDC in the central IT department is upgraded to Windows 2000 and the rollout begins.

To be sure, trust management under Windows NT could be a real trial for an administrator, especially when the relationships between the domains are largely undocumented. Windows 2000 has alleviated a lot of this hardship through the introduction of transitivity, OUs, and administrative delegation.

Part V

SECURITY POLICY COMPONENTS

Security policy settings define the security behavior of the system. Through
the use of Group Policy Objects in Active Directory, administrators can
centrally apply explicit security policies to various classes of computers
in the enterprise. For example, Windows 2000 comes with a default Group
Policy Object called Default Domain Controllers Policy that governs the
security behavior of domain controllers. Let's take a look at some of
the components and the way they work together to provide security.

Security Identifiers

Keep in mind that Windows 2000 is built on Windows NT technology.
Because the basis for 2000 is NT, the developers took every precaution to
make sure security would be backward-compatible to the NT security
model. In the Windows NT security model, resources are identified as
security principals. Security principals include objects such as users, groups,
and computers. Each of these objects is uniquely tracked by security identifiers (SIDs). SIDs are domain-unique values, built when the user or group
is created or when the computer is registered with the domain.

When describing a SID, Microsoft says, "The components of a SID
follow a hierarchical convention. A SID contains parts that identify the
revision number, the authority that assigned the SID, the domain, and
a variable number of sub-authority or Relative Identifier (RID) values
that uniquely identify the security principal relative to the issuing authority." That description may sound complex, but let's break it down. Basically,
it says SIDs have built-in pieces. The first piece is the revision number
of the SID. The revision number helps to provide the uniqueness of the
SID. Then there is a piece that identifies which authority assigned the SID
to the object. Obviously, the SID was provided by a PDC. There should
also be a piece of the SID that identifies which domain the controllers
were part of. Finally, the RID is in the SID.

Because these SIDs can be assigned to hundreds of users and hundreds of computers, there has to be a way to ensure that they are unique. That is where the RID comes in. The variable number that uniquely identifies the security principal relative to the issuing authority means that somewhere, some authority gave this computer or user another unique number, just to be sure the previous unique number was really a unique number. Better to be safe than sorry.

NOTE

Keep in mind that some well-known SIDs identify generic groups and users across all systems; the security principals discussed are identified in the context of a domain. These security principals cannot be moved between domains without their SIDs changing. If SIDs are altered in any way, resource access is affected. During an upgrade, however, security principals remain in the same domain in which they were created, so the SIDs identifying the security principals remain unchanged. As a result, resource access is unaffected by upgrade.

Security Configuration and Analysis

Have you ever had the experience of configuring dozens of computers exactly the same way? Sometimes the only way to do that was to click your way through each individual setting, making the appropriate changes in the appropriate spots. This process was very inefficient, and definitely unscientific.

With Windows 2000, you can use the *security configuration and analysis* tool. With this tool, you take a machine that you have configured just the way you want it, and then you compare the security settings to a standard template. Once the comparisons are finished, you can view the results and resolve any discrepancies revealed by the analysis. You can also use the tool to import a security template into a Group Policy Object and apply that security profile to many computers at once. To make your life even easier, Windows 2000 has several predefined security templates to mirror various levels of security and to configure different types of clients and servers on the network.

Data Encryption

Encryption of various types of data is a primary security tool of Windows 2000. Authentication protocols, which are discussed later in this chapter, use encryption to ensure that an attacker cannot intercept and alter usernames and passwords. Sensitive files and applications sent over the network can also be protected by using different types of encryption available in Windows 2000. Data that is stored locally on a kiosk or laptop computer may also be protected against theft by using encryption.

NOTE
For more information about data encryption and cipher technologies, see Chapter 5: "Windows 2000 Security."

Symmetric Key Encryption

Symmetric key encryption is also called *secret key encryption*. It uses the same key to encrypt and decrypt data. It provides rapid processing of data and is used in many forms of data encryption for networks and filesystems.

Public Key Encryption

Public key encryption, also called *asymmetric key encryption*, has two keys: one public and one private. Either key can encrypt data that can only be decrypted by the other key. This technology opens up numerous security strategies and is the basis for several Windows 2000 security features. These features are all dependent on a Public Key Infrastructure (PKI). Such a PKI is necessary in order to support certificates that are used for authentication. Certificates are widely used to log external users on to websites or to use certificate-based applications.

Authentication

Authentication confirms the identity of any user trying to log on to a domain or to access network resources. Windows 2000 authentication enables *single sign-on* to all network resources. With single sign-on, a user can log on to the domain once, using a single password or smart card, and authenticate to any computer in the domain. Authentication for local users in Windows 2000 is usually controlled by using either the Kerberos v5 protocol or the NTLM authentication protocol. Other methods of authentication, such as smart cards and certificates, are not as widely utilized for local users.

Access Control

Once authentication is complete, authorization is implemented through *access control*. When a user attempts to access any resource, a decision must be made whether the action should be permitted or denied. This decision is determined by the permissions associated with the resource. Permission levels are different depending on the resource; in the case of a printer, for example, one permission level allows printing only, whereas a higher permission level allows deleting of print queue documents. To control the access, Windows 2000 uses object-specific access control lists (ACLs). How does this compare with the way NT used to do the same thing?

Authentication and Access Tokens in NT 4

Just as with Windows 2000, *authentication* in NT 4 is the means by which a user is identified to the domain. The user, in effect, is presenting credentials, usually in the form of a username and password. Assuming these credentials are acceptable, the security subsystem creates an access token for the user. The access token includes the primary SID (the SID of the user) as well as the SIDs of all the groups of which the user is a member.

You can think of the user access token as the form of user ID presented to the system. When the user wants to access a resource, the user presents the access token. This is a lot like a key opening a door: If the key fits, the door opens. If the access token fits, the user can access the resource.

Authorization and Security Descriptors

If the object that needs access is not a user, the access token is called a *security descriptor*; it is attached to resources like files or printers. Just like a user access token, a security descriptor contains an ACL. This list consists of access control entries (ACEs). An ACE is made up of a SID as well as an indicator that the security principal is granted or denied some sort of access to the resource. This access would be in the form of permissions such as read, write, and execute. The system then performs an access check verification by simply comparing the SIDs in the access token against the SIDs in the ACL to determine whether to grant or deny requested permissions.

Single Sign-On

Users dislike having to authenticate separately to multiple network servers and applications. A user might have to provide separate passwords to log on to the local computer, to access a file or print server, to send e-mail, to use a database, and so forth. Different servers can demand a change of passwords at different intervals, often with no reuse permitted.

In this case, a typical user might be required to remember half a dozen passwords. Not only is this type of authentication tedious for the user, but at some point, users may begin to write down a list of current passwords. If this happens, a multiple-authentication network can become vulnerable to identity interception.

The *single sign-on* strategy makes a user authenticate once and then permits authenticated sign-on to other network applications and devices. These subsequent authentication events are transparent to the user.

Two-Factor Authentication

Two-factor authentication requires users to present some form of physical object that encodes their identities, plus a password. The most common example of *two-factor authentication* is the automated teller machine (ATM) card that requires a personal identification number or PIN.

Biometric identification is another form of two-factor authentication. A special device scans the user's handprint, thumbprint, iris, retina, or voiceprint, in place of an access card. Then the user enters the equivalent of a password. This approach is expensive, but it makes identity interception and masquerading very difficult.

For business enterprises, the emerging two-factor technology is the *smart card*. This card is not much larger than an ATM card and is physically carried by the user. It contains a chip that stores a digital certificate and the user's private key. The user enters a password or PIN after inserting the card into a card reader at the client computer. Because the private key is carried on a chip in the user's pocket, the private key is very hard for a network intruder to steal.

Digital Signatures and Data Confidentiality

When you talk about ensuring *data integrity*, you are talking about how to protect the data on your network from becoming corrupted. This corruption may come from a malicious attack or just from some accidental modification or deletion. When you are talking about stored data, this means only authorized users can edit, overwrite, or delete the data. For network communication, this means a data packet must contain a *digital signature* so that the recipient computer can detect if the packet has been tampered with. Another application of digital signatures lies in *code authentication.* Code authentication requires that code downloaded from the Internet be signed with a digital signature. In order for this digital signature to be accepted, it must come from a trusted software publisher. You can configure web browsers to avoid running unsigned code. Note that software signing proves that the code is authentic, meaning it has not been tampered with after publication. It does not guarantee that the code is safe to run. You have to decide which software publishers to trust.

Data confidentiality means making sure that only the right people can read or see the data. Using this strategy of data confidentiality, you encrypt data before it passes through the network and decrypt it afterward. This strategy stops data from being read by someone sniffing on the network (data interception). A packet of nonencrypted data that is transmitted across a network can be easily viewed from any computer on the network by using a packet-sniffing program downloaded from the Internet in about 15 minutes or less.

Nonrepudiation

Nonrepudiation means that a data packet cannot be denied by the person sending it. In other words, you can be absolutely certain who sent the packet. There are two parts to nonrepudiation. The first part is to establish that a specific user, who cannot disavow the message, actually sent the message. The second part is to ensure that the message could not have been sent by anyone else who might have been masquerading as the user.

This is another application for the Public Key Infrastructure (PKI). The user's private key is used to place a digital signature on the message. If the recipient can read the message using the sender's public key, then only that specific user and no one else could have sent the message.

Audit Logs

Auditing user account management as well as access to important network resources is an important part of a security policy. Auditing leaves a trail of network operations, showing what was attempted and by whom. Not only does auditing help to detect intrusion, but the logs become legal evidence if the intruder is caught and prosecuted. Finding and deleting or modifying the audit logs poses an additional time-consuming task for the sophisticated intruder, making detection and intervention easier for you.

Part V

NOTE

For more information about enabling auditing in Windows XP, see Chapter 6: "Living with Windows XP Professional Strict Security."

Auditing serves other purposes as well. When kept as a log over a period of months, auditing can be used as a justification for network improvements such as new hardware or new security implementations. Auditing can also be used as a means of tracking bandwidth usage and even keeping track of licensing among server applications.

Physical Security

It should go without saying that critical enterprise network services need to reside in locked rooms. If intruders can sit down at the network server console, they may be able to take control of the network server. If critical network servers are not physically secure, a disgruntled employee can damage your hardware by using something exceptionally accessible, like a cup of coffee!

Your data is also open to physical attack. In this case, anyone with access to Explorer can do serious damage by just indiscriminately using the Delete key. Damage from these kinds of intrusions can result in just as much loss of data and downtime as a more sophisticated, external attack to your network.

Attacks on the network do not have to be sophisticated to be effective. One of the easiest forms of a denial of service attack for someone to master is simply turning off or unplugging a server. Locking up the server will make that harder to accomplish.

User Education

The best defense against a social engineering attack (the kind of attack where an unauthorized user poses as an IT official and asks legitimate users to reveal their user names and passwords) is to educate your users about keeping their passwords confidential and secure. Business policies about distribution of critical information need to be clearly stated. Publish a security policy and require everyone to follow it. One way to educate is by example: Make sure that the IT staff protects their passwords and that they encourage users to protect theirs too.

AMATEUR PASSWORD GUESSING

Suppose you have just entered a customer site for the very first time. The customer has decided that he may want your firm to do a security audit of his network, but he has questioned your salesperson about the company's reputation and how he would know whether you are really any good.

The customer so far seems to be impressed. As a matter of fact, he wants to show you around the company. The first stop is the newly upgraded accounting department. As you walk around, you poke your head into cube after cube, noting all the new computers. As you are about to enter one cube, you notice that C. J. Carpenter is the name on the nameplate. While you are admiring the new computer, the client tells you that this is the cube of an up-and-coming new auditor who specializes in IT matters. As you glance at the monitor, you happen to see a Post-it note with the words "PW-Cardinals" on it. Hmm ... the Cardinals are your favorite baseball team.

When you get back to the client's office, he is talking about how he is not really sure he needs to have a security check run. After all, the 200 users in this company are just like family, and no one would ever do anything to damage the network. As an aside, you begin talking to the client and asking rather generic questions, such as "What kind of policy do you have for logon names?" He proudly boasts that he has come up with a masterstroke: The naming convention is the first letter of the person's first name, the first letter of his middle name, and the first four letters of his last name.

As you continue to talk, you walk over to a conference table and ask if you can use the laptop on the credenza. The client says, "Sure, but it won't do you much good because it isn't logged in." At that point, you smile and log on as CJCARP, with the password Cardinals. You then show the client how you can now go in and rename some very sensitive documents. Needless to say, you get the job.

In most situations, only a full security analysis can highlight deficiencies in a company's network infrastructure. The more careful the planning, the less risk there is of a security hole, but the possibility will always exist. In other words, always perform a full security analysis even after the entire network migration has taken place and is in production.

THE EFFECT OF SECURITY DESIGN ON EXISTING SYSTEMS AND APPLICATIONS

All through this chapter, we have been talking as if the only systems you were going to upgrade would be the server side. What about the client upgrades and the application upgrades? When do these need to be done? Do you need to wait until a domain is upgraded to Windows 2000 before you can upgrade the client? Other questions such as "Why should I upgrade my clients to Windows 2000 or XP?" and "How can I be sure my older applications will coexist with Windows 2000 or XP?" need to be asked when planning upgrades and rollouts. After all, most migrations will not be made onto brand new hardware, but will require that most of the legacy hardware in the company still pull its weight.

Upgrading Client Systems

Just as Windows 2000 Server products are backward-compatible with NT 4 clients, you can use Windows 2000 and XP clients and servers with Active Directory in your existing Windows NT environment. As a matter of fact, if you do upgrade, your life may actually be easier. Table 23.2 lists some of the reasons you may decide to upgrade clients to Windows 2000.

TABLE 23.2:   Features and Benefits of a Simple Client Upgrade

FEATURE OF SIMPLE CLIENT UPGRADE	BENEFIT OF SIMPLE CLIENT UPGRADE
Simplified manageability	Makes use of plug and play. Makes use of the Hardware Wizard with Device Manager. Provides support for Universal Serial Bus (USB). Administration with the Microsoft Management Console. Windows 2000 has a new backup utility.
More advanced setup and troubleshooting tools	For those systems that are working on networks with an Active Directory domain controller and properly configured Group Policy Objects, the automatic application installation allows an administrator to specify a set of applications that are always available to a user or group of users. If a required application is not available when needed, it is automatically installed in the system.

TABLE 23.2 continued: Features and Benefits of a Simple Client Upgrade

FEATURE OF SIMPLE CLIENT UPGRADE	BENEFIT OF SIMPLE CLIENT UPGRADE
Improved filesystem support	NTFS has changed. NTFS 5 enhancements include support for disk quotas and encryption. A defrag utility is also included for NTFS with Windows 2000. Windows 2000 also supports FAT32, in addition to the already-supported FAT system.
Improved application services	Uses the Win32 driver model. Uses DirectX 5. Uses the Windows Scripting Host (WSH).
Improved information sharing and publishing	The Microsoft distributed filesystem (Dfs) for Windows 2000 Server makes it easier for users to find and manage data on the network.
Improved print server services	Provides for easier location of printers through Active Directory.
Increased scalability and availability	Improves symmetric multiprocessor support.
Encrypted data security for laptops or sensitive information	Uses the Encrypting File System (EFS).

Client and Server Interoperability Requirements

It seems that so far we have been talking about the perfect world, where all servers are Windows 2000 and all clients are Windows 2000 Professional or Windows XP Professional. That just doesn't happen much anymore. You will have to consider the extent to which your Windows 2000 system needs to interoperate with both Windows legacy systems and non-Microsoft operating systems. If you plan to maintain a heterogeneous environment that includes network operating systems other than Windows 2000, you need to determine which legacy applications and services must be retained or upgraded to maintain acceptable functionality across all platforms.

What are the interoperability requirements with respect to operating in a heterogeneous environment? We will take a look at the degree to which the migrated environment will need to interoperate with other operating systems like Novell and Unix, as well as other network services.

Important considerations might include:

▶ The need to support pre–Windows 2000 clients, which means you must plan to maintain services such as Windows Internet Name Service (WINS) to support name resolution.

▶ The need to maintain pre–Windows 2000 domains, which means you need to maintain and manage explicit trusts.

▶ The need to interoperate with non-Microsoft operating systems, such as Unix. This could be a reason for rapid migration to enable widespread use of the Kerberos authentication.

▶ The interoperability requirements with respect to the source environment (where you are migrating from).

NOTE
Utilizing Kerberos to interoperate with non-Microsoft operating systems may require some third-party solutions.

This section may not take up a lot of pages, but it is very important. Any time you upgrade or migrate to a new network operating system, you'll find that the developers of the operating system put wizards or utilities in place that will help you move from one environment to another. Although the wizards and utilities are wonderful, the developers can't think of everything. They also can't think of every possible scenario for upgrades. This is another case where testing before rollout or just exploring before rollout will pay *huge* dividends. Few things are worse than having to kludge together a solution in the middle of a major rollout. You probably have scheduled your rollout to take place during downtime (or at least slack time), and although there is certainly a fudge factor, the fudge factor usually won't cover the time needed to redo a legacy operating system!

Application Compatibility

By now you have figured out how you will perform the domain migration. A big question remains: When you upgrade to Windows 2000, will all the business applications still work? Before going any further, this is a good time to make a list of all your strategic applications and then test them. Some important questions you need to ask about your applications include the following:

Will the Application Run on Windows 2000 and XP?
Don't assume that because the application runs on Windows NT, it will run on Windows 2000. If, after testing, the answer to this question is "no," you will have to decide how important the application is to the business. You may have to scrap it, or even scrap the upgrade. The necessity of always thoroughly testing

your applications has also become painfully obvious to users upgrading from Windows 2000 to Windows XP.

Does the Application Need to Run on a BDC?   If the answer is "yes," and the application will not run on Windows 2000, it will be impossible to switch the upgraded domain to native mode.

Do You Have Contacts with Your Application Software Vendors?   If you experience problems running the application on Windows 2000, you need to be aware of how the application vendor plans to provide support for Windows 2000. Again, this is a dangerous area for assumption. Don't assume the vendor will have an application upgrade—check to be sure.

If the Application Was Internally Developed, Do the Company Programmers Have Plans to Develop a Windows 2000 Version?   If the application cannot run on Windows 2000, and there are no plans to upgrade, you are facing the decision of scrapping the application or scrapping the upgrade. The programmers should have a relatively easy time reprogramming the application to the appropriate Windows 2000 application programming interface (API). If the application needs to be scrapped, another can be developed in its place.

What Operating Systems Are Deployed on Your Clients and Servers?   The answer to this question has implications for your migration path. Certain software upgrade paths to Windows 2000 are not supported (for example, from Windows NT 3.5).

NOTE

You may ask just how backward-compatible Windows 2000 is. Well, let's put it this way: You might not want to maintain Windows NT 3.51 servers in your resource domains, because Windows NT 3.51 does not support universal or domain local group membership. If you are running NT 3.51 or earlier, it may be wise to first upgrade to NT 4.0 before making the final switch to 2000.

Knowing the answers to these questions will help you formulate a test plan covering the important test cases. It will also help you develop a project risk assessment. This risk assessment spells out the implications of various applications that are not functioning correctly. If a really important, corporate-wide application isn't going to work in a Windows 2000 environment, that fact could have massive repercussions on any proposed migration. It is obviously important to find out before you begin the rollout, not after.

NOTE

Some application services designed for Windows NT, such as Windows NT Routing and Remote Access Service (RRAS), assume unauthenticated access to user account information. The default security permissions of Active Directory do not allow unauthenticated access to account information. The Active Directory installation wizard gives you the option of configuring Active Directory security for compatibility by granting additional permissions. If you feel that loosening the security of Active Directory to allow the use of RRAS servers would compromise your security policy, you need to upgrade these servers first. If you are using LAN Manager Replication Service to replicate scripts within the domain, then you need to upgrade the server hosting the export directory last.

UPGRADES AND RESTRUCTURING

At this point in the planning process, you will be making the decision to either maintain your current domain relationships and upgrade the PDCs and BDCs or, in many cases, restructure the domain structure to take advantage of the flexibility of Windows 2000. Why would you restructure your entire domain structure just to accommodate a new operating system?

Why Restructure Domains?

The main reason to restructure domains is money. Your company has spent all this money on studies, planning, and analysis to determine that you will upgrade to Windows 2000. As the upgrade planning progresses, your primary responsibility is to make sure you make full use of whatever features Windows 2000 has that your company needs. Here are some of the features that may be applicable:

Greater Scalability   You might have designed your previous Windows NT domain structure around the size limitations of the SAM database, leading you to implement a master or multiple-master domain model. With the improved scalability of Active Directory, you could restructure or collapse your current Windows NT domains into fewer, larger Windows 2000 domains. Windows 2000 domains can scale to millions of user accounts or groups.

Delegation of Administration   We have already talked about resource domains that allow administrative responsibility to be delegated. Windows 2000 OUs can contain any type of security principal, and administration can be delegated as you require.

Finer Granularity of Administration Depending on the scope of the network, your domain map may look like a complex mesh of trusts. Now is the time to consider implementing some of these domains as OUs to simplify administration, or you might simply redesign your domain model to benefit from fewer explicit trusts.

The question to ask now is, when do you upgrade a domain, and when do you restructure your entire network?

The difference between an upgrade and a restructure is simple. With an upgrade, you keep the domain configuration that you have now, and just upgrade the PDC and BDCs of each domain to Windows 2000, while moving the domains into the Windows 2000 forest.

Restructuring says that you are not satisfied with the way the current domain structure is laid out. You may want to merge some domains because their functionality has changed. You may want to eliminate domains and move the users or resources into another domain. In any case, if your needs call for a reconfiguration of your domain architecture, you are looking at restructuring. You should consider the following question when determining whether and how to restructure your domains: Do you need to restructure? You will probably answer "yes" if some or all of the following conditions are true:

- You are happy with much of your domain structure and can carry out a two-phase migration: upgrade to Windows 2000, and then restructure to fix any problems.

- You are unhappy with your current domain structure.

- You feel you cannot manage the migration without impacting your production environment.

When to Restructure Domains

Depending on your migration plan, you might choose to restructure your domains immediately after upgrade, in place of an upgrade, or as a general domain redesign some time in the future. When to restructure depends on the reason you are restructuring:

- If you can solve your migration requirements by doing a two-phase migration, then you need to restructure after upgrade.

▶ If you feel your domain structure cannot be salvaged (for example, if you decide you need to redesign your directory services infrastructure to take advantage of the enhanced capabilities of Active Directory), you need to restructure at the beginning of the migration process.

▶ If you feel you cannot avoid impacting your production environment, you need to restructure at the beginning of the migration process.

An ideal situation would favor the building of a new forest, as described in the "Restructuring Instead of Upgrade" section, but doing so is applicable only in limited circumstances. All of the following options are otherwise recommended equally.

Restructuring After the Upgrade

The most likely time for domain restructure is after an upgrade, as the second phase of migration to Windows 2000. The upgrade has already addressed the less complex migration situations, and the network should be stable.

When you choose to restructure after upgrade, most likely you will be reworking the domain structure to reduce its complexity or just to bring resource domains into the forest in a secure way.

NOTE

It is recommended that if you restructure after completing the upgrade, you should do so before using features such as application deployment or the new Group Policy. If you restructure after some of these features have been used, it can create more difficulties than if the restructure had taken place at the beginning of the migration process.

Restructuring Instead of Upgrade

You might feel that your current domain structure cannot be salvaged (for example, if you need to redesign your directory services infrastructure to take advantage of Active Directory), or that you cannot afford to jeopardize the stability of the current production environment during migration. In either case, the easiest migration path might be to design and build a *pristine forest*: an ideal Windows 2000 forest isolated from the current production environment. Doing so ensures that business can carry on normally during pilot project operation and that the pilot project eventually becomes the production environment.

After you have built the pilot project, you can begin domain restructuring by migrating a small number of users, groups, and resources into the pilot. When this phase has been completed successfully, transition the pilot project into a staged migration to the new environment. Subsequently, make Windows 2000 the production environment, decommission the old domain structure, and redeploy the remaining resources.

Restructuring After the Migration

At this stage, domain restructure takes place as part of a general domain redesign in a pure Windows 2000 environment. This might occur several years down the line, when, for reasons such as organizational change or a corporate acquisition, the current structure becomes inappropriate.

The Implications of Restructuring Domains

After you have determined why and when you need to restructure domains, you must examine the implications of such a restructure. Most of the implications involve the moving of security principals, such as users and groups. However, restructuring a domain may also involve such things as adjusting trust relationships and administrative duties. Note that we do not intend to provide solutions to specific problems here; we're just presenting some of the possible difficulties that might occur.

Moving Security Principals

What makes domain restructure fundamentally possible is the ability to move some of the security principals between domains in Windows 2000. Although you can move some types of security principles, there are a number of implications—for example, how security principals are identified by the system and how access to resources is maintained. Some of these implications can affect how you approach a domain restructuring.

Effect on SIDs and the ACLs   Remember from our discussion of SIDs earlier in the chapter that the SID is partly made up of a domain identifier. This domain-centric nature of SIDs will have the same consequence when you move a security principal, such as a user or a group, between domains. Obviously, if part of the SID identifies the domain and the domain changes, the security principal must be issued a new SID for the account in the new domain.

In the Windows NT security model, the way a user can access resources is affected by the way the operating system looks at the user access token and compares the primary SID of the user, as well as the SIDs of any groups the user is a member of, to the access control list (ACL) on the resource security descriptor. Because the lists of SIDs contained in the ACL have information that can cause access to be granted or denied to the security principals identified by the SIDs, changing the SID will require changing or updating the ACL.

Access to resources could be maintained by adding the new SID for the user to the ACLs on all the resources the user formerly had access to, but this fix would be time-consuming and overly complicated.

Because some security principals can be moved in Windows 2000, entire groups could be moved to the new domain. However, the ACLs referencing the group also reference the group SID, so the resources would have to be repermissioned to refer to the new SID—again, more time-consuming and overly complicated.

Effects on Global Group Membership   Because a global group can only contain members from its own domain, moving a user account to the new domain would cause the new account to be excluded from some of the access to resources in the old location. Assuming appropriate trust relationships exist between the new domain and the resource domain, it would seem that this situation could be fixed in a number of ways.

Also, if the group is moved to another domain, a problem will occur if all the group members are not moved in one fell swoop. So, the group would have to be maintained in the old domain, and a new group would have to be created in the new domain. Resource access would be maintained for the original group and its members, but resources would need to be repermissioned to grant access to the new group. Again, repermissioning would have to continue while the groups existed in both domains.

Because a global group can contain only members from its own domain, when a user is moved between domains, any global groups of which the user is a member must also be moved. This has to occur just to maintain access to resources protected by ACLs that refer to global groups. In addition, if a global group is moved, its members must also be moved:

▶ For each user being moved, all the affected global groups are also moved.

▶ For each group being moved, all of its members are also being moved.

If the source domain is a native mode domain, global groups can also contain other global groups. This means all the members of each nested group and all the global groups that have members in that nested group must be moved. Sounds complicated, doesn't it? Just be sure you know the implications of moving users and groups.

NOTE

This is just an example of what happens when you decide to move a security principal. For further information on the impact of moving principals, check out the *Microsoft Windows 2000 Resource Kit* and the published white papers.

ANALYZING THE TECHNICAL SUPPORT STRUCTURE

How can your help desk adapt to the new environment? As a network administrator, you are faced with a multitude of challenges, not the least of which is delivering an appropriate business computing environment to your user community while maintaining this environment and keeping down the costs associated with it. You have to deliver the right applications and environment for the user to do the job and deliver a level of administrative control to ensure that the quality of service and uptime provided for the enterprise as a whole are high.

To help lower management and support costs, most organizations have three distinct groups of administrators. Each group has its own unique set of management tasks and requirements and the common need for remote management tools and services. We will look at each group in the following sections, as well as the security requirements for each.

Desktop Support Management

The goal of the desktop support management group is to ensure that people have the computing resources they need. This is a challenge because of the multiple desktop configurations that are the norm in each organization. You know how it goes: The IT department sets a *standard* desktop machine that will be rolled out to all new users and all users who require an upgrade. By the time the information gets to Purchasing, it has been changed from "standard" to "suggestion," and you end up with desktops from whatever clone manufacturer has the lowest price on machines designed to run Windows 2000 on any given day.

No matter what the computer type or desktop standard, desktop support management usually involves repetitious work—installing and upgrading applications, moving users, and so forth. Accordingly, desktop support managers are often the front line for finding, troubleshooting, and resolving problems. In addition, because users may be spread across a large physical space, people doing desktop support try to resolve as many problems as possible without actually visiting every desktop. This leads to a demand for management tools that work well remotely. When a desktop visit is unavoidable, it is necessary to have accurate configuration information before the technician arrives.

Network Management

The network management group is responsible for making sure the network is up and running, 24 hours a day, seven days a week. That means providing on-demand bandwidth.

The network support group also has to contend with multiple points of failure. The network design may be perfect, but if a router goes out, things quickly turn rather sour. To make matters worse, it doesn't even have to be your router. Suppose the router belongs to your ISP; if it is the link to your gateway to the outside world, your customers will not care that it was not under your direct control—they just want access. It is now up to you to make sure your ISP's equipment is protected, and that there is some semblance of fault tolerance.

Network management involves two sometimes conflicting goals. The first is to move as much information as possible while maintaining excellent uptime, availability, and security. Second, you must spend the least amount possible on plant costs, maintenance, and support. Even more than data center or desktop management, network management depends on simultaneously monitoring the health of hundreds, thousands, or tens of thousands of network devices. Ideally, tools will predict problems, automatically flag them when they occur, and escalate warning notices if necessary.

Data Center Management

Finally, there is the data center management group. The goal of this team is to make sure the data and the services are available on demand. The service levels must remain consistent, and critical data must be preserved.

Data center managers typically provide application services to large groups of users and are therefore most concerned with overall uptime for applications delivered to users. Because of this focus on providing robust application services to many users, and because those services are usually run from a small number of servers, data center managers tend to be more interested in data integrity, security, and accounting than desktop support managers are. In addition, data center managers typically spend more time on maintenance and upgrades, per server, than desktop managers.

Security Requirements

Users generally do not care what the security implications are—they just want access to the data they are supposed to have access to. At a minimum, it is necessary to provide a single flexible security model that embraces networks, systems, middleware, applications, and user services. The following are some Windows 2000 tools that can make this possible.

Administrators create Group Policy by using the Group Policy MMC snap-in, either as a stand-alone tool or as an extension to the Active Directory Users And Computers tool and the Active Directory Site and Services tool via Manage Group Policy. All Group Policy settings are contained in Group Policy Objects (GPOs) that are associated with Active Directory containers (sites, domains, or OUs), thus using the Active Directory.

Administrators can filter the effects of Group Policy on computers and users by using membership in security groups and setting ACL permissions.

Group Policy requires a source template that is used to create the user interface settings. The Group Policy can use either an MMC extension snap-in to the Group Policy snap-in, or an ASCII file referred to as an administrative template (.adm) file. The .adm file consists of a grouping of categories and subcategories that together define how the options will be displayed through the Group Policy user interface. The file also indicates the Registry locations where changes should be made if a particular selection is made, and also specifies any options or restrictions for the selection. In some cases, a default value will be specified.

ANALYZING EXISTING AND PLANNED NETWORK AND SYSTEMS MANAGEMENT

What kinds of management tools do you have, and what kinds will you need? Windows 2000 has some tools that will help the security teams to better manage the network. They include tools for managing change and configuration, protecting data, managing the users' environment, and helping install and deploy applications.

Change and Configuration Management Tools

When you begin discussing system management, you are usually talking about a very big job. It includes things such as managing configurations and deploying applications. System administrators everywhere are trying to find easy ways to install applications, standardize a desktop, and lock down the desktop configuration.

IntelliMirror

One tool that administrators can use is IntelliMirror. You can use it to mirror users' data, applications, and customized operating system settings to a Windows 2000 Server–based server, using intelligent caching and centralized synchronization. This means that users have access to all their data and applications, even if they are not connected to the network. The user has the peace of mind of knowing that the data is safely maintained on the server, where it can be backed up. IntelliMirror provides users and administrators with the following functionality:

- Managing the users' data
- Assisting with software installation and maintenance
- Managing advertised applications
- Assisting with the management of user settings
- Providing remote operating system installation functionality

User Data Management   As the name *IntelliMirror* suggests, data is mirrored. The data can be mirrored from the local system to the network, or network data can be cached locally. The data can reside on the local laptop or workstation for offline use while a copy of the data resides on the server for protection. In this case, the data does not reside in only one location; it can be configured to follow the user if the user moves to another computer.

Software Installation and Maintenance   Windows 2000 Server has some software installation technologies that have been designed to simplify the installation of applications, as well as updates, repairs, and even uninstalls of applications.

System administrators can use the Software Installation and Maintenance tool that will assign applications to users. When properly configured, all users who need the applications will automatically have the application on their desktops.

Administrators can make available applications that users may not need but may want. In this case, it will be up to the users to decide whether to install the application.

Advertised Applications   When administrators assign an application to users, the application is advertised to users during logon at a workstation. Basically, this process works almost like having the application installed on the local computer. Shortcuts for the application appear in appropriate locations (including the Start menu or the Desktop), and the appropriate Registry entries for the application are added to the local computer registry.

When an application is published rather than assigned, the application is advertised to the Active Directory directory service. In this case, the application has no shortcuts on the user's Desktop or Start menu, and no changes are made to the local computer registry. Published applications are available for users to install by using the Add/Remove Programs Control Panel tool or by clicking a file associated with the application (for example, by clicking a .doc file for Microsoft Word).

User Settings Management   IntelliMirror also includes ways for administrators to manage user and computer settings. With IntelliMirror, user settings are mirrored to the network, and administrators can define specific computing environments for users and computers. Administrators can do the following:

- ▶ Add new users and computers remotely.
- ▶ Define settings for users and computers.
- ▶ Apply changes for users.
- ▶ Restore a user's settings if the user's computer fails.
- ▶ Ensure that a user's Desktop settings follow the user if the user moves to another computer.

Remote Operating System Installation   Another problem that faces network administrators and desktop support personnel is the installation of the operating system. When you are installing a new operating system on a computer, you know you have to allocate a substantial amount of time for the task. It is especially onerous because you know much of the time will be spent waiting. The remote operating system installation allows remote install–capable clients like Net PCs and computers with a Net PC–compatible floppy boot disk to install the operating system files automatically from a Windows 2000 remote install server.

The remote installation process installs an operating system on the local computer's hard disk using a remote source like a CD image on a server. Normally, a workstation that is participating in the remote installation model is set to boot off the local disk. However, the workstation first boots from the network (remotely) to get the operating system installed on the local hard disk. The network boot is initiated either by the BIOS (Basic Input Output System) or by a special boot floppy. In either case, the network boot is controlled by boot code that adheres to the Net PC specification. The preferred BIOS boot model for this environment is one in which the BIOS gives the user a small window prior to booting off the disk, in which a special key-press causes a *service* boot off the network.

In a Net PC–compatible network boot, the boot code uses Dynamic Host Configuration Protocol (DHCP) and Boot Information Negotiation Layer (BINL) to get an IP address for the workstation and to find a Remote Installation Service (RIS) server. Then the boot code uses Trivial File Transfer Protocol (TFTP) to download a boot program from the RIS server. It then transfers control to the boot program.

Security Configuration Manager

Another tool used for change and configuration management is the Security Configuration Manager. System administrators can use the Security Settings extension of the Group Policy MMC snap-in to define security configurations for computers within a Group Policy object. A security configuration consists of the security settings that are applied to each security area supported for the Windows 2000 Professional or Windows 2000 Server.

This security configuration is included within a GPO. The GPO is then applied to computers as part of the group policy enforcement. The Security Settings extension reads a standard security configuration and performs the required operations automatically. These security areas can be configured for computers:

Account Policies   Account policies include computer security settings for the password policy, the account lockout policy, and Kerberos policy in Windows 2000 domains.

Local Policies   Local policies include the security settings for the audit policy, any of the standard user rights assignment, and other security options. The local policies also allow administrators to configure who has local or network access and how local events are audited.

Event Log   The event log controls security settings for the application, security, and system event logs. Administrators can access these logs using the Event Viewer.

Restricted Groups   Computer security settings are included for built-in groups that have certain set standards. Restricted group policies affect the membership of these groups. Examples of restricted groups are local and global groups.

System Services   The system services policies control the configuration settings and security options for system services such as network services, file and print services, telephony and fax services, Internet/intranet services, and so on.

Registry   The Registry policies are used to configure and analyze settings for security descriptors, the ACL, and auditing information for each Registry key.

Filesystem   The filesystem policy is used to configure and analyze settings for security descriptors (including object ownership), the ACL, and auditing information for each object (volume, directory, or file) in the local filesystem.

What's Next

In this chapter, we reviewed some of the security concepts that go along with working with Windows 2000. We used the comparisons between Windows 2000 and NT to lead into a discussion of how to assess the problems or challenges you will have with security when you upgrade existing systems and applications. Next we examined how to decide if you should upgrade or roll out, and, if you roll out, what you will have to do to consolidate domains into a forest.

Chapter 24 gets deeper into security, as we look at establishing baselines and auditing policies.

Chapter 24

DESIGNING SECURITY BASELINES

In the last chapter, we went over some security terms and how some of the Windows 2000 security features work. In this chapter, we will look at how to begin laying out security baselines for many of the resources on your network. We will present the strategies, and you will need to apply them to the specific situation. You will understand this approach clearly as we get into it.

You may wonder why we are not going to lay out for you the required level of security for each resource, or develop a security baseline that includes domain controllers, operations masters, application servers, and file and print servers. The answer is simple: Not only is there no right answer to these questions, but there may be several right answers for each scenario, and each scenario will be unique.

Some aspects of this security planning process may be pretty straightforward. For example, take the case of the operations master. It must be available when a server attempts to join an

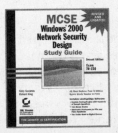

Adapted from *MCSE: Windows® 2000 Network Security Design Study Guide*, Second Edition by Gary Govanus and Robert King

ISBN: 0-7821-2952-8 $59.99

existing tree by creating a new domain. Therefore, you should make sure that operations masters are placed in areas where they are readily accessible by Active Directory.

On the other end of the spectrum are kiosk machines—the stand-alone workstations you see in places like malls and airports. They are important to your security plan because you must lay out your Group Policy to install the exact applications they need to operate.

Distributed Security Strategies

Although designing security for domain controllers, desktop computers, kiosks, and so on may differ in some aspects, the basics are all the same. In this section, we will begin looking at how security affects all the computers in the enterprise, regardless of their role. In Microsoft terms, we are talking about *distributed security*, which refers to the logical security features that operate primarily within the network. Microsoft identifies seven primary security strategies that you should pursue in making the enterprise network secure:

- Authenticate all user access to system resources.

- Apply appropriate access control to all resources.

- Establish appropriate trust relationships between multiple domains. (We covered this topic in depth in Chapter 23, "Evaluating the Impact of the Security Design on the Technical Environment.")

- Set uniform security policies.

- Enable data protection for sensitive data.

- Deploy secure applications.

- Manage security administration.

As you begin to lay out your *network security matrix* (otherwise referred to as your *network security plan*), you should make these seven themes central to the distributed security plan. Because each of these strategies is central to designing a baseline of security for all roles of computers in an enterprise, we will examine them individually. Whenever an area is of interest to a particular type of computer, such as portable systems, we will note it specifically.

Authenticating All User Access

Probably the first tenet of security that everyone learns is, "Make sure the people who need to get into the network can have access and the people who should not have access to the network are blocked (or at least hindered) from entering." So, to provide security for your Windows 2000 network, you must provide access for legitimate users but screen out intruders who are trying to break in. This means you must set up your security features to authenticate all user access to system resources. Authentication strategies set the level of protection against intruders trying to steal identities or impersonate users.

In Windows 2000, authentication for domain users is based on user accounts in Active Directory. Administrators manage these accounts using the Active Directory Users And Computers snap-in to the Microsoft Management Console (MMC). User accounts can be organized into containers called *Organizational Units* (OUs), which reflect the design of your Active Directory namespace. The default location for user accounts is the Users folder of this snap-in. Look at Figure 24.1 to see this demonstrated.

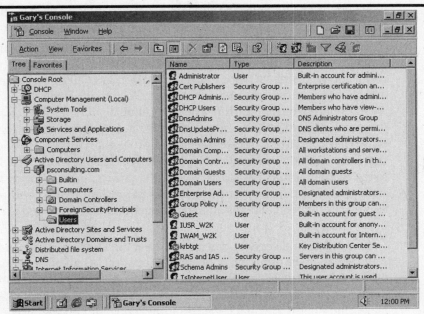

FIGURE 24.1: MMC with OU and Users folder

When someone new joins the company, the administrator creates only a single account for that user, rather than having to create half a dozen or more separate accounts on different servers and application databases. With the domain authentication service integrated with the enterprise directory, that single user account is also a directory entry for global address book information, and a way to provide access to all network services. The user can log on at different client computers or laptops in the domain using only one password.

Windows 2000 automatically supports single sign-on for users within a forest. Domain trust relationships in the forest are transitive or two-way by default, so authentication in one domain is sufficient for referral or pass-through authentication to resources in other domains in the forest. The user logs on at the beginning of a session, after which network security protocols like Kerberos v5, Windows NT LAN Manager (NTLM), and Secure Sockets Layer/Transport Layer Security transparently prove the user's identity to all requested network services.

If your installation needs an even more secure means of authentication, Windows 2000 also supports logging on with *smart cards.* A smart card is an identification card carried by the user that is used instead of a password for interactive logon. It can also be used for remote dial-up network connections and as a place to store public key certificates used for Secure Sockets Layer (SSL) client authentication or secure e-mail.

When you use Active Directory, authentication is not limited to users. Computers and services are also authenticated when they make network connections to other servers. For example, Windows 2000–based servers and client computers connect to their domain's Active Directory for policy information during startup. They authenticate to Active Directory and download computer policy from Active Directory before any user can log on to that computer. Services also must prove their identity to clients that request mutual authentication. In mutual authentication, both parties to the communication have to be assured they are communicating with the right host. Mutual authentication works to prevent an intruder from adding another computer as an impostor between the client and the real network server.

Computers and services can be *trusted for delegation*, which means services can make other network connections "on behalf of" a user without knowing the user's password. The user must already have a mutually authenticated network connection to the service before the service can make a new network connection to another computer for that user. This feature is particularly useful in the context of an Encrypting File System (EFS) running on a file server. To use a service to delegate a network connection, use the Active Directory Users And Computers MMC snap-in.

Then, select the Trust Computer For Delegation check box on the property sheet, as shown in Figure 24.2.

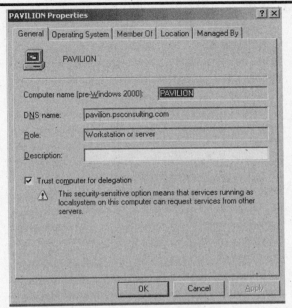

FIGURE 24.2:   Trust Computer For Delegation part of the MMC

Trusting a computer for delegation is a very powerful capability. It is not enabled by default and requires Domain Administrator privileges to enable it for specific computers or service accounts.

NOTE
Computers or accounts that are trusted for delegation need to be under restricted access to prevent introduction of Trojan horse programs that would misuse the capability of making network connections on behalf of users.

Some accounts might be too sensitive to permit delegation, even by a trusted server. You can set individual user accounts so that they cannot be delegated, even if the service is trusted for delegation. To use this feature, go to the Active Directory Users And Computers MMC snap-in and open the property sheet for the account. Look for the Account Is Sensitive And Cannot Be Delegated check box on the Account tab of the property sheet; it is shown in Figure 24.3.

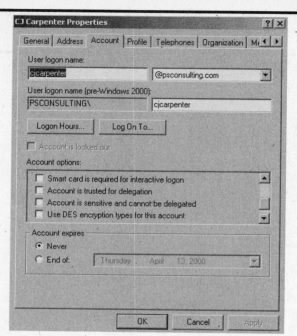

FIGURE 24.3:   The Account tab, including a check box to specify that an account cannot be delegated

Passwords

As you look at the network and put together your security matrix, there are some considerations you should be sure to address. These are the best practices that Microsoft recommends when planning your authentication policies.

The first issue is passwords. A discussion of passwords can be long and tedious. As far as passwords go, you will probably always have some IT professionals who say your users should have long, complex passwords. Others think that passwords, while not useless, are pretty close. We have all seen too many passwords taped to monitors or hidden under keyboards to swear by them as the last line of security.

No matter where you stand, the fact remains that the simplest way to defend against brute force or dictionary password-cracking tools is to establish and enforce long, complex passwords. Windows 2000 lets you set policy to govern the complexity, length, lifetime, and reusability of

Part V

user passwords. By traditional definition, a complex password has 10 or more characters, including upper- and lowercase letters, punctuation, and numerals. An example of a complex password is *CJ,will,be,3,on2,15,01.* Obviously, enforcing this type of complexity may have negative effects on your coworkers' view of you, especially if they don't like having to type in passwords in the first place.

If complex passwords are out of the question and you are still looking for a strong front line of security, there are other options, but all of them are somewhat costly. For example, smart cards provide much stronger authentication than passwords, but they also involve extra overhead. Smart cards require configuration of the Microsoft Certificate Services, smart card reader devices, and the smart cards themselves.

NOTE
Third-party vendors offer a variety of Windows 2000–compatible security products besides smart cards. Many of these products provide two-factor authentication, including *security tokens* and *biometric* accessories. These accessories use extensible features of the Windows 2000 graphical logon user interface to provide alternate methods of user authentication.

So, what is the trick? How do you determine the appropriate password length and what your users will stand? There are some examples you may want to follow.

The Windows 2000 MMC has a section for *security templates.* These are intended to be sample templates for various types of network resources. For example, there are templates for high-security domain controllers and high-security workstations, as well as basic domain controllers and work-stations that have the password functions listed as "not defined."

In the high-security templates, password history is enforced with up to 24 passwords remembered. That means users cannot reuse a password until it has been changed 24 times. As far as how often the user must change the password, the maximum age is 42 days and the minimum age is 2 days. Specifying a minimum age means the creative user cannot simply change her password 25 times in the same day to keep the same password.

In addition, you can enable only passwords that meet complexity requirements. This approach is similar to installing the `Passfilt.dll` implementations in Windows NT 4, SP2, which instituted a password policy with the following requirements:

1. Passwords must be at least six (6) characters long.

2. Passwords must contain characters from at least three (3) of the following four (4) classes:

Description	Example
English uppercase letters	A, B, C, ... Z
English lowercase letters	a, b, c, ... z
Westernized Arabic numerals	0, 1, 2, 3, ... 9
Non-alphanumeric	Special characters, such as punctuation symbols

3. Passwords may not contain your username or any part of your full name.

Finally, passwords may be stored using reversible encryption for all users in the domain.

It comes down to, "How secure do you want to make it?" Before you make decisions that will affect the entire enterprise, it is always best to involve serious levels of management. If you decide to begin instituting the complexity policy, you can bet that you will be a very popular person— your phone will start ringing off the wall with people who want to talk to you. Having a management sponsor will help alleviate this situation.

THE CASE OF THE IMPROPER PASSWORD

It is a normal Monday morning, and you are going about your business. You decide to stop in at a client site and see how an upgrade went that weekend. You had laid the groundwork for the upgrade, but it was up to the staff to pull it all together. You figure a courtesy call wouldn't hurt.

When you come in, you are invited into a meeting that has apparently been going on for a while. As a matter of fact, the discussion has been somewhat heated. The IT manager is trying to get a password policy passed, and the IT staff is fighting the change—not because they don't want a secure network, but because they feel the policy won't do any good. After all, people are people, and they will tape their passwords to the monitor, no matter what you do.

In the middle of the meeting, someone turns to you and asks what should be done. You recognize that each side has a valid point. It is difficult to get users to use passwords that are hard to crack without having them tape the passwords to the monitor. You begin by suggesting that, because it is in its own domain, the IT department

CONTINUED ➡

Part V

should begin the process by requiring secure passwords. You point out that with templates, it is possible to require secure passwords without too much problem. Once the IT department has lived with secure passwords for a month or so, they can begin the sales job necessary to roll them out to the rest of the company.

You also mention that it will be a sales job, and some thought must be put into how to handle it. If the users believe the policy is important, they will be more likely to follow through. Just in case, however, you suggest preparing a demonstration on how easy it is to hack into a short password. You also suggest showing how the security staff will be randomly checking accounts to make sure there is compliance.

Implementing and enforcing a password policy may be the first line of defense against a brute force or mechanical attack. It will also be an effective barrier against most amateur hackers who may have set their sights on your network.

Kerberos Authentication Technology

By the time you have reached this stage of working with Windows 2000, you realize the extent to which Microsoft has taken an enterprise approach with the product. The network infrastructure used to be more fragmented and segmented. Now, the infrastructure can be managed from one location. That's nice for the administrator, but it also means users will be able to access resources in the far-flung reaches of the network. This is done through Kerberos authentication. Although we have already discussed Kerberos briefly in previous chapters, it is a fairly detailed subject that deserves more coverage. In the next several sections, we will discuss this major topic in depth.

The Kerberos authentication protocol is a technology that provides for single sign-on to network resources. Windows 2000 uses the Kerberos v5 protocol to provide single sign-on to network services within a domain, and also to provide services residing in trusted domains. The Kerberos protocol verifies the identity of both the user and the network services, and it provides mutual authentication. What does this mean to the system administrator?

Suppose you have a domain with a user Gary. If Gary is authenticated into that domain and needs to access an application in another domain, the other domain accepts the fact that Gary really is who he says he is, just because he is Kerberos authenticated.

How Kerberos Authentication Works   In the previous example, when Gary enters *domain credentials* (by username and password or smart card logon), Windows 2000 locates an Active Directory server and the Kerberos Key Distribution Center (KDC). The Kerberos KDC issues a *ticket granting ticket* to the user Gary. This is a temporary ticket containing information that identifies the user to network servers. After the initial interactive logon, the first ticket granting ticket is used to request other Kerberos tickets to log on to subsequent network services. This process is complex and involves mutual authentication of the user Gary and the server to one another, but it is completely transparent to the user.

The Kerberos v5 protocol verifies both the identity of the user and the integrity of the session data. This means not only that the user is who he says he is, but also that the session the verification comes from is the actual communication session. In Windows 2000, Kerberos v5 services are installed on each domain controller, and a Kerberos client is installed on each Windows workstation and server. The Kerberos v5 service stores all the encrypted client passwords and identities in the Active Directory. Therefore, a user's initial Kerberos authentication provides the user a single sign-on to enterprise resources, using Active Directory.

Users are enthusiastic about Kerberos, because Kerberos authentication reduces the number of passwords they need to remember. Because users have fewer passwords, they have less reason to write them down, and the risk of identity interception is reduced. In addition, users may have access to more resources. The trust relationships between all the domains in a forest can extend the scope of Kerberos authentication to a wide range of network resources.

Implementing Kerberos   As you design your security matrix, remember that there are no prerequisites for implementing Kerberos authentication. The Kerberos protocol is used pervasively in Windows 2000. Note, however, that there really is no such thing as *implementation*. You do not need to install or initiate Kerberos—it comes ready to go.

However, you can set Kerberos security policy parameters in the Group Policy snap-in to MMC. Within a Group Policy Object (GPO), the Kerberos settings are located under Account Policies. The settings are shown in Figure 24.4.

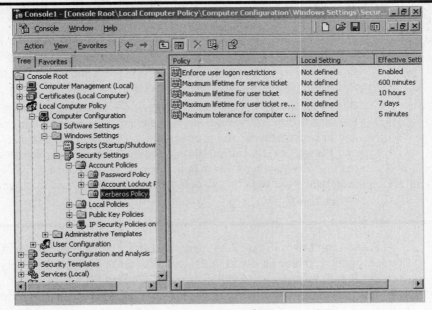

FIGURE 24.4:   Kerberos settings in a Security MMC

GROUP POLICIES: APPLICATION

Group Policies are applied to computer accounts or to user accounts. They are stored in GPOs that can work at the domain level, the site level, or the Organizational Unit (OU) level. Keep in mind when you begin using Group Policies that they only work with Windows 2000 clients; they are not backward compatible with Windows NT or Windows 9x systems.

Windows 2000 still maintains compatibility with the NTLM authentication protocol to support backward compatibility with previous versions of Microsoft operating systems. You can continue to use NTLM for Windows 95, Windows 98, Windows NT 4 Server, and Windows NT 4 Workstation clients. NTLM authentication is also used on Windows 2000 by applications designed for previous versions of Windows NT that specifically request NTLM security.

When are Group Policies applied? It depends on what is defined in the Group Policy. Computer settings are applied when the computer

CONTINUED ➡

starts. User settings are applied when the user logs on. Policies are also applied at various intervals, so leaving a computer on all the time or staying logged on and locking the workstation will not avoid Group Policies—they will still be applied on the fly.

Basically, Group Policies are live as soon as you apply them. Because Group Policies can limit what computers or users can do, and because Group Policies affect all the computers or users in a site, domain, or OU, you should not deploy them without extensive testing. Misapplying a Group Policy can cause chaos on a network. Test these policies in the lab before rolling them out, and roll them out carefully!

As you can see in Figure 24.4, you can use Kerberos security to enforce user logon restrictions. By default, the maximum lifetime for a service ticket is 600 minutes, and the maximum lifetime for a user ticket is 10 hours. Finally, the maximum lifetime for computer clock synchronization is 5 minutes.

NOTE

The maximum lifetime for service tickets is configurable in one-minute increments, and the maximum lifetime for user tickets is configurable in one-hour intervals.

Considerations for Using Kerberos Authentication   If you want to take advantage of the performance improvements and security that Kerberos authentication provides, you might consider using the Kerberos sign-in as the only network logon protocol in your enterprise. The design of the Windows 2000 version of Kerberos implements the Internet Engineering Task Force (IETF) standard version of the Kerberos v5 authentication protocol for supposedly improved cross-platform interoperability. For example, users on Unix systems can use Kerberos credentials to log on to Unix systems and to securely connect to Windows 2000 services for applications that are enabled by Kerberos authentication.

Enterprise networks that already use Kerberos authentication based on Unix realms can create trust relationships with Windows 2000 domains and integrate Windows 2000 authorization for Unix accounts using Kerberos name mapping, with the aid of third-party products.

NOTE

One issue with Windows 2000 is that Windows 2000 Professional computers can receive tickets from Kerberos KDCs running on Windows 2000 servers. At this time, there is a problem getting the certificates from machines that are not KDCs running Windows 2000.

Some aspects of Kerberos may make it difficult to use. For example, when you institute Kerberos, make sure all computers on a Kerberos-authenticated network have their time settings synchronized with a common time service. (Note the time synchronization setting mentioned earlier!) Not only that, but enterprise network communication must keep that time service on all machines within five minutes, or authentication fails. Windows 2000 computers automatically update the current time using the domain controller as a network time service. Domain controllers use the primary domain controller for the domain as the authoritative time service.

NOTE

If you are worried about time zones, don't be. Even if the current time is different on computers within a domain, or across domains, Windows 2000 automatically handles time zone differences to avoid logon problems.

By default, domains in a Windows 2000 tree use transitive trusts. With Kerberos, when using transitive trusts between domains in a forest, the Kerberos service searches for a trust path between the domains to create what is called *across-domain referral*. In large trees, it might be more efficient to establish cross-links of bidirectional (or two-way) trusts between domains where there is a high degree of cross-domain communication. Doing so permits faster authentication by giving the Kerberos protocol *shortcuts* to follow when generating the referral message.

Kerberos authentication uses transparent transitive trusts among domains in a forest, but it cannot authenticate between domains in separate forests. To use a resource in a separate forest, the user has to provide credentials that are valid for logging on to a domain in that forest.

Smart Card Logon

As mentioned earlier, Windows 2000 supports optional smart card authentication. Smart cards provide a very secure means of user authentication, interactive logon, code signing, and secure e-mail. However, deploying and maintaining a smart card program requires additional resources and costs.

How Smart Cards Work   The smart card, which is usually the size of a common credit card, contains a chip that stores the user's private key, logon information, and public key certificate for various purposes. The user inserts the card into a smart card reader attached to the computer. The user then types in a *personal identification number* (PIN) when requested.

Smart cards are designed to provide a form of tamper-resistant authentication through onboard private key storage. The private key stored on the smart card is used in turn to provide other forms of security related to things like digital signatures and encryption.

Smart cards use what is called a *two-factor authentication policy*, which indirectly permits things like data confidentiality, data integrity, and nonrepudiation for multiple applications, including domain logon, secure mail, and secure web access.

Implementing Smart Cards   Smart cards rely on the Public Key Infrastructure (PKI) of Windows 2000. First, you need to implement a PKI; then purchase the smart card equipment. In addition to PKI and the cards themselves, each computer needs a smart card reader. Set up at least one computer as a smart card enrollment station, and authorize at least one user to operate it. This enrollment station does not require special hardware beyond a smart card reader, but the user who operates it needs to be issued an Enrollment Agent certificate.

Considerations for Using Smart Cards   You need an enterprise certification authority rather than a stand-alone or third-party certification authority to support smart card logon to Windows 2000 domains.

Microsoft supports industry standard *Personal Computer/Smart Card* (PC/SC)–compliant smart cards and readers—and if you check the hardware compatibility list, you will see that Windows 2000 provides drivers for commercially available Plug and Play smart card readers. Smart card logon is supported for Windows 2000 Professional, Windows 2000 Server, Windows 2000 Advanced Server systems, and Windows 2000 Data Center.

TIP

Microsoft Windows 2000 does not support non-PC/SC-compliant or non–Plug and Play smart card readers. Some manufacturers provide drivers for non–Plug and Play smart card readers that work with Windows 2000; nevertheless, it is recommended that you purchase only Plug and Play PC/SC-compliant smart card readers that are on the HCL.

Smart cards can be combined with employee card keys and identification badges to support multiple uses per card.

Because cost is always a factor, you should know that the overall cost of administering a smart card program depends on several factors, including:

▶ The number of users who use the smart card program and where they are located.

▶ How you decide to issue smart cards to users. This process should include stringent requirements for verifying user identities. For example, will you require users to simply present a valid personal identification card, or will you require a background investigation? Your policies affect the level of security provided as well as the actual cost. Depending on your industry, some of these decisions may be made for you, by law.

▶ Your practices for users who lose or misplace their smart cards. For example, will you issue temporary smart cards, authorize temporary alternate logon to the network, or make users go home to retrieve their smart cards? Your policies affect how much worker time is lost and how much help desk support is needed.

Your network security deployment plan needs to describe the network logon and authentication methods you use. Include the following information in your security matrix:

▶ Identify the network logon and authentication strategies you want to deploy.

▶ Describe all the smart card deployment considerations you have identified and the issues with each.

▶ Describe the PKI certificate services that are required to support your implementation of smart cards.

Applying Access Control

No matter how users get onto the network, it is what happens once they have been authenticated that counts. This is when they have access to all the resources, and this is when they can do damage.

After a user logs on, the user is authorized to access various network resources, such as file servers and printers that grant permissions to Authenticated Users. As you plan your matrix, you will have to make certain you restrict a user's view of network resources to job-related devices, services, and directories. Doing so limits the damage that an intruder can do by impersonating a legitimate user.

NOTE

Think of this as the domino effect of security. As one security expert put it, "Don't think of it as *if* you will be compromised, just think of it as *when* you will be compromised." In this case, assume the resource has already been accessed and try to figure out what will fall next. Once that has been determined, you can figure out what you can do to protect the resource.

Access to network resources is based on permissions. These permissions serve to identify the users and groups that are allowed to perform specific actions by using specific resources. For example, suppose the Accounting Group has been given read/write permission to access files in the Accounting Reports folder. Meanwhile, the Auditor Group has been granted read-only access to files in the Accounting Reports folder. In this case, the Accounting Group can make changes to the files in the folder, but the Auditor Group can only look at them.

Using an access control list that is associated with each resource enables permissions. You can find the ACL on the Security tab of the property sheet. An ACL is a list of the security groups (and, rarely, the individuals) who have access to that resource. If you look at Figure 24.5, you will see that the group Everyone has the ability to read and execute files, list folder contents, and read the information contained in the TechNet folder.

As you plan your matrix, remember to be democratic. Security groups are the most efficient way to manage permissions. Because you are assigning permissions to large groups, instead of individuals, you don't have to work as hard. Remember that although it is possible to assign permissions to individual users, it's not the recommended way. Also, it really is easier to grant permissions to a group and then add or remove users as members of the group.

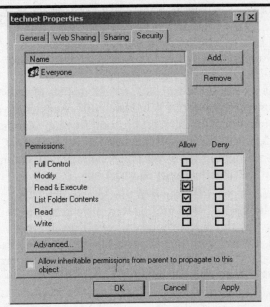

FIGURE 24.5:   Example of the rights given to the group Everyone

Windows 2000 has a security group called Everyone, which appears on network-share ACLs by default when they are created. To restrict access to network shares, you must remove the Everyone group and substitute a more appropriate group or groups. Do not assume that the default permissions for a resource are necessarily appropriate permissions.

Here is an example: When a new share is created, full control permissions are granted by default to the security group called Everyone. Any user authenticated to the domain is in the group called Authenticated Users, which is also a member of Users. Look at what the resource is used for and determine the appropriate permissions. Some resources are public, and others need to be available to specific sets of users. Sometimes a large group has read-only permission to a file or directory, and a smaller group has read/write permission.

Access Control Lists

ACLs describe the groups and individuals who have access to specific objects in Windows 2000. The individuals and security groups are defined in the Active Directory Users And Computers snap-in to the MMC. All types of Windows 2000 objects have associated ACLs, including all Active Directory objects, local NTFS files and folders, the Registry, and printers. The granularity of ACLs is so fine that you can even place security-access restrictions on individual fonts.

Implementing ACLs   Access control lists, which are lists of security groups and users, show up throughout Windows 2000. As part of your security matrix, you must decide which groups best fit your organizational needs. Project teams or business roles may define the groups. You may look to the company organization chart for inspiration, or you may start grouping by location. The flexibility is amazing!

The ACL for an object is generally found in the Security tab of the property sheet. This tab shows the list of groups that have access to this object, plus a summary of the permissions enjoyed by each group. As mentioned earlier, an Advanced button displays the group permissions in detail so that users can use more advanced features for granting permissions, such as defining access inheritance options.

For example, to view the ACL for a printer, click Start ➤ Settings ➤ Control Panel ➤ Printers. Right-click a printer and select Properties. The ACL for that printer is in the Security tab and is shown in Figure 24.6.

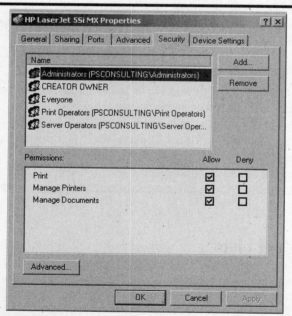

FIGURE 24.6:   Printer ACL

You can do the same thing to see the ACL for a local folder. Simply open My Computer and use Explore to navigate to the folder. Right-click the folder. Point to Properties, and click the Security tab.

NOTE
To view the ACL of an OU in the Active Directory Users And Computers MMC snap-in, you must open the View menu and select Advanced Features. Otherwise, the Security tab is not visible in the Properties dialog box.

Considerations for Using ACLs   Although an ACL usually refers to the Security tab listing for an object, there is another type of ACL—that of the Share tab. Of course, the levels of permissions on this tab differ from NTFS permissions and have several restrictions. To review, share permissions apply only to a resource that is connected to remotely (a local logon will bypass all share permissions). Also, share permissions cannot be applied at the individual file level—they are applied at the folder level and then automatically propagated downward.

Another consideration about using ACLs is that different objects will have different permission levels. The levels for a printer, for example, are print, manage documents, and manage printers, whereas the levels for a file include read, read and execute, and full control, among others. A final note about ACLs is that although they are very flexible, Microsoft has put a limit on the number of access control entries (ACEs) an ACL can have. It's a very large number (1,820), but it still could be a concern in a large enterprise network.

Security Groups

We have mentioned several times in this book that the best way to make sure your users can get access to information is through the use of security groups. Windows 2000 allows you to organize users and other domain objects into groups for easy administration of access permissions. Defining security groups is a major task when you are planning your security matrix.

The Windows 2000 security groups let you assign the same security permissions to large numbers of users in one operation. Doing so ensures consistent security permissions across all members of a group. Using security groups to assign permissions means the ACLs on resources remain fairly static. "Fairly static" means that they are easy to control and audit. Users who need access are added to or removed from the appropriate security groups as needed, and the ACLs change infrequently. It all falls under that principle mentioned earlier: to do unto as many others as possible without doing too much work.

How Security Groups Work   There are two *types* of groups in Windows 2000: security groups and distribution groups. Security groups can have security permissions associated with them and can also be used as mailing lists. Distribution groups are used simply for the creation of mailing lists.

NOTE
No security functions are associated with distribution groups.

When you create a new user, you add the user to existing security groups to completely define the user's permissions and access limits. To get you started defining groups, Windows 2000 comes with several predefined security groups.

Security Group Types   Windows 2000 supports four kinds of security groups, and these groups are set apart by *scope*:

Domain Local Groups   These are best used for granting access rights to resources. Resources can be defined as filesystems or printers that are located on any computer in the domain where common access permissions are required. Domain local groups are also known as *resource groups*. The advantage of using domain local groups to protect resources is that members of the domain local groups can come from both inside the same domain and outside the domain.

Global Groups   These are used for combining users who share a similar resource-access profile based on job function or business role. These permissions can be assigned to global groups in any domain in the forest. In addition, global groups can be made members of domain local and universal groups in any domain in the forest. Typically, organizations use global groups for all groups where membership is expected to change frequently. These groups can have as members only user accounts defined in the same domain as the global group or global groups from the same domain in native mode. Global groups can be nested to allow for overlapping access needs or to scale for very large group structures. The most convenient way to grant access to global groups is by making the global group a member of a domain local group that is granted access permissions to a set of related project resources.

Universal Groups   These are used in larger, multidomain organizations where there is a need to grant access to similar groups of accounts that are defined in multiple domains. Permissions can be assigned to *universal groups* in any domain in the entire forest. It is better to use global groups as members of universal groups to reduce overall replication traffic from changes to universal group membership.

Users can be added to and removed from the corresponding global group within their domains, and a small number of global groups are the direct members of the universal group. Universal groups are easily granted access by making them a member of a domain local group used to grant access permissions to resources. Universal groups are used only in multiple domain trees or forests. A Windows 2000 domain must be in native mode to use universal security groups.

NOTE
Membership in universal groups is included in the global catalog. Membership in global groups is not. Therefore, using global groups for members of universal groups will make them more stable than including individual user accounts (whose membership in groups is more dynamic and numerous, thus causing more global catalog—forest-wide—replication).

Local Groups   These security groups are specific to a computer and are not recognized elsewhere in the domain. If a member server is a file server and hosts 100GB of data on multiple shares, you can use a *local group* for administrative tasks performed directly on that computer or for defining local access permission.

Default Permissions of Security Groups   For member servers and client computers, the default Windows 2000 access control permissions provide different levels of security for the following groups:

Everyone and Users Groups (Normal Users)   Members of these groups do not have broad read/write permission as in Windows NT 4. These users have read-only permission to most parts of the system and read/write permission only in their own profile folders. Users cannot install applications that require modification to system directories, nor can they perform administrative tasks.

Power Users Group   Members of this group have all the access permissions that Users and Power Users had in Windows NT 4. Power Users have read/write permission to other parts of the system in addition to their own profile folders. Power Users can install applications and perform many administrative tasks.

Administrators Group   Members of this group have the same level of rights and permissions as they did for Windows NT 4. In other words, for any right that is defined at a non–domain controller level, a member of this group will have that right. It is the group with the most power, because virtually nothing is beyond members' control.

For servers configured as domain controllers, the default Windows 2000 security groups provide different levels of security for the following groups:

Everyone and Users Groups   Members of these groups do not have broad read/write permission as in Windows NT 4. Normal users have read-only permission to most parts of the system and read/write permission in their own profile folders. Normal users can only access domain controllers over the network—interactive logon to domain controllers is not granted to regular users.

Account Operators, Server Operators, and Print Operators Groups   Members of these groups have the same access permissions as they did in Windows NT 4. As a simple review, account operators have the ability to manage users and group membership, server operators have the rights necessary to manage various aspects of server operation such as system shutdown, and print operators have administrative rights to network printers.

Administrators Group   Members of this group have total control of the system as listed previously for the Administrators group, except with all additional rights that are defined only for a domain controller.

Implementing Security Groups   Security groups are a built-in feature of Active Directory. No special installation or prerequisite is required.

To create new users and place them in security groups, use the Active Directory Users And Computers snap-in of the MMC. Figure 24.7 shows the New Object—Group dialog box.

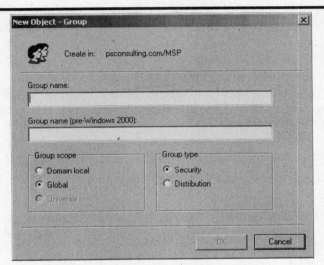

FIGURE 24.7:   New Object—Group dialog box

As you can see, defining the group as Domain Local, Global, or Universal, as well as setting the Group Type as Security or Distribution, is as simple as clicking radio buttons.

Considerations for Using Security Groups   When designing your security matrix and deciding on security groups, a good strategy is for project or resource owners to define their own domain local groups based on required access permissions. This strategy is part of the distributed administrative principles. In this case, you allow the owner or manager of a resource to manage the group memberships—the resource owners or project leads can manage access by updating the appropriate group. In addition, the enterprise administrators don't have to become involved in day-to-day, lower-level decisions.

NOTE

Microsoft says that members of global security groups should have similar job functions. Members of domain local security groups should have similar access needs.

A security group is composed of people with similar jobs or roles in the company. The group is often named after the role, such as the Windows 2000 built-in groups for Account Operators, Administrators, and Backup Operators. Personnel who naturally belong on the same project or department mailing list probably belong in the same security group in Active Directory. As mentioned earlier, these Windows 2000 security groups have a secondary role as mailing lists.

Using groups that correspond to project teams or responsibilities is an effective way to grant access appropriately. For example, everyone in a department usually needs access to the department printers, and the engineers on a software project need access to the common source directories. These are natural groups.

NOTE

The system must determine all of a user's universal and global security group affiliations at logon time. When a user is a member of many groups, there may be some impact on performance while the system determines all the group memberships.

One of the NT security theories that has migrated to Windows 2000 is the idea of *nested groups*. In Windows NT, we put global groups into local groups. In Windows 2000, the technology and the verbiage have been upgraded: Now we use nested groups. You can use nested groups to make it easier to manage group membership for large groups.

For example, a large group might have 5,000 members. It would be very difficult to list every employee of your company individually in a single group. The whole-company group would be easier to administer if it was defined as the group that contains each of your department groups. The department groups could then be nested within the whole-company group.

USING GROUPS FOR BANDWIDTH CONSERVATION

Using departmental groups is especially important if your whole-company group is a universal group. If you are working in an

CONTINUED ➡

Part V

organization that has a single LAN site, you can use universal groups with no performance degradation. However, if your organization has a WAN, you need to consider the impact of frequent changes to universal group membership on replication traffic across links between sites. If a universal group contains only other groups as members, it does not change often, and replication traffic is essentially nothing. A universal group containing thousands of individual users is likely to require frequent updates across multiple WAN links as each change replicates to all global catalog servers in the enterprise. Defining universal groups as groups of groups reduces this network activity.

NOTE

You might find that your Windows 2000 Server implementation does not permit nested groups. Windows 2000 Server initially operates in *mixed mode*, which means that Windows 2000 and Windows NT 4 servers can interoperate in the same network. Mixed mode places some restrictions on security groups. When all domain controllers in the domain have been upgraded to Windows 2000, you can switch to *native mode*. This is a one-way transition that enables advanced features such as nesting of security groups.

There are some other holdovers from the NT 4 days. For example, on a specific computer, the users in the local administrator security group have full rights and permissions for that computer. When a Windows 2000 computer is joined to a domain, the Domain Admins group is added as a member of the local administrator group. Local users of the computer generally do not need to be members of the Administrators group. The full-privilege Administrators group must be used for local administration activities, such as changing the system configuration.

Uniform Security Policies

Uniform security policies allow consistent security settings to be applied and enforced on different classes of computers, where a *class of computer* is something like the domain controller class. Applying such policies is a simple matter of creating an OU in Active Directory, collecting appropriate computer account objects into the OU, and then applying a GPO to the OU. The security policies specified in the Group Policy are then enforced automatically and consistently on all the computers represented by the computer accounts in the OU.

Windows 2000 comes with a selection of default GPOs that are automatically applied to domains and to domain controllers. There is also a selection of security templates representing different levels of security for various types of enterprise computers. These templates can be used to create a Group Policy for a group of computers or to analyze the security settings on a specific computer.

A GPO contains a detailed profile of security permissions that apply primarily to the security settings of a domain or a computer (rather than to users). A single GPO can be applied to all the computers in an OU. Group Policy is applied when the individual computer starts up and is periodically refreshed if changes are made without restarting.

How Group Policy Works

GPOs are associated with domains and OUs (containers) in the Active Directory Users And Computers snap-in to MMC. The permissions granted by the Group Policy are applied to the computers stored in that container. Group Policy can also be applied to sites using the Active Directory Sites And Services snap-in.

Group Policy settings are inherited from parent folders to child folders, which might in turn have their own GPOs. A single container could have more than one GPO assigned to it.

NOTE

For more information on Group Policy precedence and how conflicts are resolved among multiple policy objects, see Windows 2000 Help.

Implementing Group Policy   Group Policy is a feature of the Windows 2000 Active Directory. Active Directory must be installed on a server before you can edit and apply GPOs. As is common with most Windows components, Group Policy settings can be implemented and managed through a variety of means. Perhaps the most widely used is the MMC with the Group Policy snap-in. Once you've chosen the appropriate security settings, the policy can be saved and then applied, or linked to any of three specific levels in the Active Directory schema: the site level, the domain level, and the OU level. After the GPO has been linked to a level, you must complete one more step before the policy will actually affect any security principles within that Active Directory level. That step—filtering—ensures that the appropriate groups and/or users have the read and apply Group Policy permissions set.

Considerations for Using Group Policy   Perhaps the most important consideration when using Group Policy for security purposes is the network infrastructure design. The number and location of OUs and domains, for example, may be adequate given your GPO implementation desires. However, the design of your Active Directory schema may depend heavily on the number and type of GPOs applied. Separate group password policies will require separate domains, for instance, because password policies are not effective at the site or OU level.

Microsoft recommends that the number of GPOs applied be limited, for two reasons. First, doing so limits complexity. Troubleshooting can be very difficult if multiple GPOs (some of which might conflict) are applied to the object in question. Second, the speed of the network can be adversely affected by a large number of GPOs being applied. Another consideration would be the ability to block or force policy inheritance. Although these abilities are powerful and give an administrator great flexibility, their overuse is a common problem in larger networks.

Providing Data Protection for Sensitive Data

Information security strategies are designed to protect data on your servers and client computers. They also must conceal and protect packets traversing insecure networks. That problem is usually apparent, but one danger that occurs may not be so obvious. In this age of the home-based office, the traveling user, and the remote user, your company has a lot of data that is on the road. We have all heard horror stories about laptops being stolen. Although that certainly occurs with regularity, laptops can also be lost. As an IT administrator, your distributed security matrix needs to identify which information must be protected in the event that computer equipment is lost or stolen. You must also realize that some types of network traffic are sensitive or private and need to be protected from network sniffers. This information must also be included in the security matrix.

In terms of users on your enterprise network, access control (discussed earlier) is the primary mechanism to protect sensitive files from unauthorized access. However, because the computers themselves are portable, they are subject to physical theft. Another specific computer role to be aware of is that of the kiosk station. Although not technically portable, it could be physically broken into, and the hard disk could be stolen. Access control is obviously not sufficient to protect the data stored on these computers. To address this problem, Windows 2000 provides the Encrypting File System (EFS).

To make the communication links secure, and to keep network data packets confidential, you can use Internet Protocol Security (IPSec). It works to encrypt network traffic among some or all of your servers. IPSec provides the ability to set up authenticated and encrypted network connections between two computers. For example, you could configure your e-mail server to require secure communication with clients and thereby prevent a packet sniffer from reading e-mail messages between the clients and the server. IPSec is ideal for protecting data from existing applications that were not designed with security in mind.

Network and dial-up connections (remote access) should always protect network data transmitted over the Internet or public phone lines. Remote access uses a virtual private network that uses the Point-to-Point Tunneling Protocol (PPTP) or Layer 2 Tunneling Protocol (L2TP) tunneling protocol over IPSec.

We will look at both EFS and IPSec in the following sections.

Encrypting File System

Windows 2000 EFS lets users encrypt designated files or folders on a local computer for added protection of data stored locally. EFS automatically decrypts the file for use and re-encrypts the file when it is saved. No one can read these files except the user who encrypted the file and an administrator with an EFS File Recovery certificate. Because the encryption mechanism is built into the filesystem, its operation is transparent to the user and extremely difficult to attack.

EFS is particularly useful for protecting data on a computer that might be physically stolen, such as a laptop. You can configure EFS on laptops to ensure that all business information is encrypted in users' document folders. Encryption protects the information even if someone attempts to bypass EFS and uses low-level disk utilities to try to read information.

NOTE

For more information about using EFS in Windows 2000, see Chapter 5.

EFS is intended primarily for protection of user files stored on the disk of the local NTFS filesystem. As you move away from this model (remote drives, multiple users, editing encrypted files), you need to be aware of numerous exceptions and special conditions.

How EFS Works   EFS encrypts a file using a symmetric encryption key unique to each file. Then it encrypts the encryption key as well, using the public key from the file owner's EFS certificate. Because the file owner is the only person with access to the private key, that person is the only one who can decrypt the key, and therefore the file.

To protect against an end-user becoming disgruntled or leaving the organization and keeping the only key, there is a provision for the original encryption key to be encrypted using the public key of an administrator's EFS File Recovery certificate. The private key from that certificate can be used to recover the file in an emergency. It is highly recommended that an organization establish an independent recovery agent.

File encryption provides great security, because even if the file is stolen, it cannot be decrypted without first logging on to the network as the appropriate user. Because it cannot be read, it cannot be surreptitiously modified. EFS addresses an aspect of a policy of data confidentiality.

Implementing EFS   To implement EFS, a PKI must be in place, and at least one administrator must have an EFS File Recovery certificate so the file can be decrypted if anything happens to the original author. The author of the file must have an EFS certificate. The files and folders to be encrypted must be stored on the version of NTFS included with Windows 2000.

Once the PKI has been established, to implement EFS, you open Windows Explorer and right-click a folder or a file. Select Properties; then, on the General tab, click Advanced. Select the Encrypt Contents To Secure Data check box. The contents of the file, or of all the files in the selected folder, are now encrypted until you clear the check box.

Considerations for Using EFS   Once again, before you get excited about using EFS, remember that it is only supported for the version of NTFS used in Windows 2000 (NTFS 5). It does not work with any other filesystem, including previous versions of NTFS.

EFS can also be used to store sensitive data on servers. Doing so will allow for normal data management—otherwise known as backups. The servers must be well protected and must be trusted for delegation. In the case of data saved to a server, EFS services will impersonate the EFS user and make other network connections on the user's behalf when encrypting and decrypting files.

If, for some reason, the user who owns the data loses the key, EFS uses a Data Recovery policy that enables an authorized data recovery agent to decrypt encrypted files. EFS requires at least one *recovery agent*. Recovery agents can use EFS to recover encrypted files if users leave the organization or lose their encryption credentials. You need to plan to deploy the PKI components and issue one or more certificates for EFS data recovery. These certificates should be securely stored offline so they cannot be compromised. Such storage usually involves a safety deposit box, a vault, or a large safe. You don't have to use any other kind of certificate-generation service, because EFS can generate its own certificates for both EFS users and EFS recovery agents.

NOTE

By default, EFS issues EFS *recovery certificates* to the Domain Administrator account as the recovery agent for the domain. For stand-alone computers that are not joined to a domain, EFS issues EFS recovery certificates to the local Administrator user account as the recovery agent for that computer.

Many organizations might want to designate other EFS recovery agents to centrally administer the EFS recovery program. For example, you can create OUs for groups of computers and designate specific recovery agent accounts to manage EFS recovery for specific OUs.

You can deploy Microsoft Certificate Services to issue certificates to EFS recovery agents and EFS users. When certificate services are available online, EFS uses the certificate services to generate EFS certificates.

As you plan your security matrix, be sure to include strategies for EFS and EFS recovery. As an example of EFS strategies, you might include the following kinds of information:

- ▶ Filesystem strategies for both laptops and other computers

- ▶ How EFS recovery agents are to be handled

- ▶ The recommended EFS recovery processes

- ▶ The recommended EFS recovery agent private key management and archive processes

- ▶ Which certificate services are needed to support the EFS recovery certificates

THE CASE OF THE MISSING LAPTOP

It's the day before the company shuts down for its annual 30-day December holiday. You and the rest of the IT team figure that once you get everyone out of the building, you will be able to finish cleaning up the servers and adding hardware to the network in about 7 days, giving you 23 days of vacation.

Your thoughts are interrupted by the appearance of Fred. Fred comes with a signed authorization to check out a laptop. He works for the research and design department and is taking some material home with him to work on over the shutdown. Because the data is highly confidential, you decide to use the Encrypting File System, even though it isn't used much. You encrypt all the appropriate files and make sure Fred can decrypt them and work on them. The system administration team keeps the EFS recovery agents locked in a safe, so you figure you're covered.

Fast-forward 30 days. The shutdown is over. Everyone comes back to work, and because the IT team had to make sure everything was ready, you have been at work since early morning. You find out that Fred is currently meeting with the research and design management team. They have just called for the head of IT and the head of security. Your pager goes off, and the message is to report to the IT manager's office immediately.

Your boss tells you that Fred discovered the borrowed laptop has been stolen. That laptop contained all the plans for the new project—the next great iteration to come out of your company. The boss wanted to talk with you because you checked out the laptop. The only thing that saved the company from being out more than the price of the laptop, your boss continues, was your following procedure and making sure all the critical files were encrypted. You saved the day.

As with most security measures, EFS may slow operations a little, and it certainly is more overhead than usual to implement into a security infrastructure. However, the safety and peace of mind that may come from using it can be invaluable.

IP Security

Windows 2000 incorporates IPSec for data protection of network traffic. IPSec is a suite of protocols that allows secure, encrypted communication between two computers over an insecure network. This communication can include home users dialing into the company's RAS server, or even two computers communicating across an intranet. The encryption is applied at the IP network layer, so it is transparent to most applications that use specific protocols for network communication. IPSec provides end-to-end security, meaning that the IP packets are encrypted by the sending computer, are unreadable en route, and can be decrypted only by the recipient computer. Due to a special algorithm for generating the same shared encryption key at both ends of the connection, the key does not need to be passed over the network.

How IPSec Works   At a high level, here is how IPSec works:

1. An application on Computer A generates outbound packets to send to Computer B across the network. In this case, the network can be anything from a dial-in connection to connections across the Internet.

2. Inside TCP/IP, the IPSec driver compares the outbound packets against IPSec filters, checking to see if the packets need to be secured. The filters are associated with a filter action in IPSec security rules. Many IPSec security rules can be part of one IPSec policy that is assigned to a computer.

3. If a matched filter has to negotiate a security action, Computer A begins security negotiations with Computer B, using a protocol called the *Internet Key Exchange (IKE)*. The two computers exchange identity credentials according to the authentication method specified in the security rule. Authentication methods could be Kerberos authentication, public key certificates, or a pre-shared key value (much like a password). The IKE negotiation establishes two types of agreements, called *Security Associations (SAs)*, between the two computers. One type (called the *phase I IKE SA*) specifies how the two computers trust each other and protects their negotiation. The other type is an agreement about how to protect a particular type of application communication. This consists of two SAs (called *phase II IPSec SAs*) that specify security methods and keys for each direction of communication. IKE automatically creates and refreshes a shared, secret key for each SA. The secret key is created independently at both ends without being transmitted across the network.

4. The IPSec driver on Computer A signs the outgoing packets for integrity, and optionally encrypts them for confidentiality using the methods agreed upon during the negotiation. It transmits the secured packets to Computer B.

NOTE

Firewalls, routers, and servers along the network path from Computer A to Computer B do not require IPSec. They simply pass along the packets in the usual manner.

5. The IPSec driver on Computer B checks the packets for integrity and decrypts their content if necessary. It then transfers the packets to the receiving application.

IPSec provides security against data manipulation, data interception, and replay attacks. As part of your security matrix, IPSec is important to strategies for data confidentiality, data integrity, and nonrepudiation.

Implementing IPSec   The computers in your network need to have an IPSec security policy defined that is appropriate for your network security strategy and for the type of network communication they perform. Computers in the same domain might be organized and have IP security policy applied to the set of computers. Computers in different domains might have complementary IPSec security policies to support secure network communications.

Basic IPSec setup includes several steps. First, the type of traffic that needs security should be identified. The port, protocol, and/or the source or destination IP address for that traffic are discovered and used as filters. Finally, certain service characteristics that match the filters are applied to the traffic.

Considerations for Using IPSec   The overhead that IPSec requires may be enough to push it out of range on your security matrix. Because IPSec provides encryption of both outgoing and incoming packets, there is a cost of additional CPU utilization. This is especially true when the encryption is performed by the operating system. For many installations, the clients and servers may have considerable CPU resources available, so that IPSec encryption will not have a noticeable impact on performance. For servers supporting many simultaneous network connections, or servers that transmit large volumes of data to other servers, the additional cost of encryption is significant. The cost of the hardware and bandwidth capable of carrying the load will be a factor to be considered in your plan.

Another offshoot of this consideration is testing. You will need to test IPSec using simulated network traffic before you deploy it. Testing is also important if you are using a third-party hardware or software product to provide IP security.

NOTE

Windows 2000 provides device interfaces to allow hardware acceleration of IPSec per-packet encryption by intelligent network cards. Network card vendors might provide several versions of client and server cards, and might not support all combinations of IPSec security methods. Be sure to check the product documentation for each card to be sure the card supports the security methods and the number of connections you expect in your deployment.

You can define IPSec policies for each domain or OU. You can also define local IPSec policy on computers that do not have domain IPSec policy assigned to them. You can configure IPSec policies to handle these tasks:

▶ Set the level of authentication that is required between IPSec clients.

▶ Set the lowest security level at which communications are allowed to occur between IPSec clients.

▶ Decide whether to allow or prevent communications with non-IPSec clients.

▶ Require all communications to be encrypted or allow communications in plain text.

So, you should consider using IPSec to provide security if your security matrix calls for the following applications:

▶ Peer-to-peer communications over your organization's intranet

▶ Client-server communications to protect sensitive (confidential) information stored on servers

▶ Remote access (dial-up or virtual private network) communications

▶ Secure router-to-router WAN communications

That takes care of how people can securely access your network, even over an open data communication line. Next we'll discuss accessing secure applications off the network.

Deploying Secure Applications

It is not enough to set up distributed security and then just go back to business as usual. A secure enterprise network also needs software that has been designed with security features in mind. For example, you may have an exceptionally secure network in most regards, but if your most business-sensitive application transmits passwords over the wire in plain text, much of your security could be compromised. A secure environment needs *secure applications*, and secure applications will reside only on a secure applications server.

When evaluating software for your enterprise, look for applications designed with these security-enabled features. Look for integration with single sign-on capabilities for authenticated network connections, and the ability to run properly in secured computer configurations. The software need not require administrator privileges if it is not an administrator tool or utility.

One way to check an application's compliance is to look for the Certified For Microsoft Windows logo. It can be used just as the hardware compatibility list is used for hardware. The *Application Specification for Windows 2000* defines the technical requirements that an application must meet to earn the Certified For Microsoft Windows logo. The document identifies the minimum requirement areas that secure applications must support:

- ▶ Run on secured Windows 2000 servers.

- ▶ Use single sign-on by using the Kerberos authentication for establishing network connections.

- ▶ Use impersonation of the client to support consistent Windows 2000 access control mechanisms using permissions and security groups.

- ▶ Run application services by using service accounts rather than a local system (which has full system privileges).

These requirements are a minimum.

One approach to making sure your users are running "safe" applications is to require that application components be digitally signed. Microsoft *Authenticode*, through Microsoft Internet Explorer, lets users identify who published a software component and verify that no one tampered with it before downloading it from the Internet.

Also, regularly remind users not to run programs directly from e-mail attachments if they are unfamiliar with the sources or if they are not expecting to receive e-mail from the source. This is also a great form of proactive virus protection.

Authenticode and Software Signing

IT people have recognized that software downloaded from the Internet can contain unauthorized programs or viruses that are intended to wreak havoc on the system or even provide access to intruders. As networks become more interconnected, the threat of malicious software and viruses has extended to the intranet.

How Authenticode Works   Microsoft's Authenticode was developed to enable software developers to digitally sign software using a standard X.509 public key certificate. That way, users can verify the publisher of digitally signed software as well as verify that the software has not been tampered with, because the publisher signed the code.

Implementing Authenticode Screening   You can enable Authenticode-based screening of downloaded software in Internet Explorer by choosing the Tools menu ≻ Internet Options ≻ Security tab. Higher levels of security set from this tab screen software components for trusted digital signatures.

The question for the security administrator is whether you can trust your users to increase their levels of security. In each case, increasing the level of security tends to decrease response and functionality. That will probably lead to a minor insurrection when it comes to increasing security. You can bypass the user intervention and take control of these Internet Explorer security settings through Group Policy. Open the Group Policy snap-in to MMC and navigate to the Internet Explorer container. Then, choose Computer Configuration ≻ Administrative Templates ≻ Windows Components ≻ Internet Explorer. Figure 24.8 shows the default template, with nothing altered.

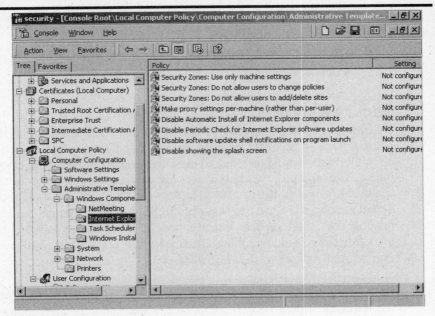

FIGURE 24.8: Default template

Internet Explorer policies permit you to lock down security settings so that users cannot change them, and to require that all downloaded components have trusted signatures.

Considerations for Using Authenticode and Software Signing

When it comes time to set your strategy for software signing in your security matrix, it might include the following information:

▶ Which internal and external groups need the capability of signing software

▶ The strategies for signing software intended for internal distribution

▶ The strategies for signing software intended for external distribution

▶ How the certification authority deployment and trust management strategies should be modified to support the new software signing strategies

▶ Processes and strategies are needed to enroll users as software signers

▶ The education plan that will be implemented to inform users they are not to run unsigned or untrusted components

Secure E-mail

Information comes into your enterprise from a wide variety of digital sources. One of the most popular ways to transfer information is with e-mail. In today's business, e-mail messages containing sensitive personal information and proprietary business information are routinely sent over the intranet or even the Internet. Hackers can easily intercept plain-text e-mail messages. People can easily intercept and modify e-mail messages, or spoof the IP address of an e-mail sender and send false messages. Many of today's secure e-mail solutions are based on the open *Secure/Multipurpose Internet Mail Extensions (S/MIME)* standard.

How Secure E-mail Works   Secure e-mail systems based on S/MIME use industry standard X.509 digital certificates and public key technology to provide e-mail security between senders and recipients of e-mail messages. Secure e-mail systems typically provide the following security functions:

▶ Senders can digitally sign e-mail messages.

▶ Recipients can verify the identity of the message sender and verify that the message has not been tampered with en route.

▶ Senders cannot repudiate signed messages because only the sender has possession of the signing credentials.

▶ Senders can encrypt e-mail messages to provide confidential communications.

▶ Intended recipients can decrypt the message using private credentials, but others cannot decrypt and read the message.

▶ Administrators can centrally store users' private credentials in a secure database. If a user's private credentials are lost or damaged, administrators can retrieve the private credentials necessary to decrypt messages.

Implementing Secure E-mail   The most common method of sending e-mail is the Simple Mail Transfer Protocol (SMTP), and the most common method of receiving e-mail is the POP3 protocol. Although basic authentication may be in place, neither method is inherently secure. There are primarily two methods by which e-mail communication can be made to ensure its integrity and safety.

The first method is indirect, and relies on the security of the channel over which the e-mail is transmitted. The easiest example is the establishment of a VPN using IPSec over the Internet, and then using the channel to transmit secure packets, including e-mail. The second method's exact implementation is beyond the scope of this book, but relies on a client-side e-mail application such as Microsoft Outlook to implement a protocol such as S/MIME as noted earlier.

Considerations for Using Secure E-mail   To address strategies for secure e-mail, consider including the following suggestions in your deployment plan:

- ▶ Make sure the e-mail server and client applications are secure.

- ▶ Make sure to plan for the number of e-mail servers and user groups needing to upgrade or migrate to secure e-mail.

- ▶ Define general policies for using secure e-mail organization-wide.

- ▶ Research and define the encryption technology to be used, including international export restrictions and limitations.

- ▶ Research and define the certificate services needed to support secure e-mail.

- ▶ Set up strict enrollment processes and strategies to enroll users in the secure e-mail program.

- ▶ Set up the key recovery database backup capabilities and recommended backup and restore practices.

- ▶ Set up and define the key recovery capabilities and recommended general recovery practices.

- ▶ Define and publish e-mail policies. Make sure your users know that e-mail is owned and operated by the company, and therefore their mail box may be opened at any time by authorized members of management or the IT staff.

Secure Websites and Communications

The website and the browser have become tools for information exchange both on organizations' intranets and on the Internet. While all this information is being moved, standard web protocols such as HyperText Transfer Protocol (HTTP) provide limited security.

The issue at hand is that websites in general are becoming more sophisticated than the older-style "information kiosk." Today's websites can provide a portal into a company's intranet at even an administrative level, and can be used for private communications such as videoconferencing. Financial transactions are becoming more common on the Web as well, as consumers seem to be more and more willing to purchase items online. Because the web technologies of today allow such connection and flexibility, the security risks of maintaining an Internet presence are continually increasing.

How Secure Websites and Communications Work   You can configure most web servers to provide directory- and file-level security based on usernames and passwords. Or, you can provide web security by programming solutions using the Common Gateway Interface (CGI) or Active Server Pages (ASP). Although these are solutions, they are not great—they have proven to be susceptible to compromise on more than one occasion. Instead, you can use Internet Information Services (IIS), included with Windows 2000 Server. IIS will give you the ability to provide a certain level of security for websites and communications using standards-based secure communications protocols and standard X.509 certificates. You can use IIS to provide the following security for websites and communications:

▶ By using the Secure Sockets Layer (SSL) and Transport Layer Security (TLS) protocols, you can authenticate users and establish secure channels for confidential communications.

▶ If you need secure channels for confidential encrypted financial transactions, you can use the Server Gated Cryptography (SGC) protocol.

▶ You can map user certificates to network user accounts to authenticate users and control user rights and permissions for web resources based on users' possession of valid certificates issued by a trusted certification authority.

Implementing Secure Websites and Communications   The best way for most companies to ensure proper security of a website is to use the IIS software that is included with Windows 2000 Server. IIS is installed using the Windows Components section of the Add/Remove

Programs applet of Control Panel. When in use, IIS supports SSL and TLS, as mentioned earlier. The X.509 standard certificate is also used.

Digital certificates can also be part of the overall security plan. Such certificates can be obtained either through a third-party company such as Verisign or by taking advantage of an internal certificate authority (CA) server from Microsoft.

Considerations for Using Secure Websites and Communications

Consider including the following suggestions in your deployment plan:

▶ Make sure you extend your deployment plan to define the websites and user groups that must be upgraded or migrated to secure websites.

▶ Be sure to lay out your strategies for using SSL or TLS.

▶ See to it that you have defined the strategies for using certificate mapping to control user rights and permissions to website resources.

▶ Make sure you have set up the certification authority deployment needed to support websites.

▶ Document and define the enrollment process and strategies to enroll users in the secure websites program.

SECURE APPLICATIONS

You are just beginning to explore how to hook your company to the Internet and provide Internet mail to everyone in the system. At the present time, the company naming conventions are such that the users' logon name and e-mail name are the same. No problem—that is the way Windows 2000 likes it.

A problem begins to show itself when people send messages to the Everyone group of their departments. You notice that when you look in the properties of the address list, you can suddenly see all the e-mail addresses of all the users in that department. Hmmm... If that e-mail message had been sent outside the company, someone would have had all the logon names for an entire department, whether they knew it or not. That is not a good thing.

In this case, there are a couple of solutions. You can educate the users about the proper use of the blind copy box; doing so will help

CONTINUED ➡

some, but will certainly not alleviate the problem. You can also work on a new e-mail naming standard, so the e-mail address and the logon name are not the same.

Expanding your corporate intranet in any way can compromise security. In this case, simply wanting to incorporate some Internet capabilities may render the current logon naming scheme untrustworthy. Deploying secure applications and securing websites on the Internet may require extra standards that are not already in place in the company.

Managing Administration

Some of the policies in your security plan will involve the daily duties of your IT department staff. Windows 2000 supports delegation of administrative permissions, allowing specific personnel limited rights to administer their own groups. Windows 2000 also supports audit logs of system activity, with a fine degree of detail about which types of events will be logged and in what context.

NOTE
If you are interested in learning more about auditing, be sure to study Chapters 5, 6, and 25.

It is also extremely important that your plan describes how you intend to protect your Domain Administrator accounts from penetration by an intruder. It is recommended that you set up your domain account policies to require all accounts to use a long, complex password that cannot be cracked easily. This policy is common sense, but it needs to be explicitly stated in your plan.

It is not as obvious that security will be compromised if too many people know the administrator password. The administrator of the root domain of a domain tree is also automatically a member of the Schema Administrators group and the Enterprise Administrators group. This is a highly privileged account, via which an intruder can do unlimited damage. Your plan needs to state that access to this account is limited to a very small number of trusted personnel. Think about establishing a long, complex password and then sealing it in an envelope and putting the envelope in a safe. In some cases where PKI is implemented, the CA server is a stand-alone system that is locked away in a secured room.

The Domain Administrator account must be used only for tasks that require administrator privileges. It must never be left logged on and unattended. Encourage your administrator staff to use a second, real-person account for their non-administrative activities (reading e-mail, web browsing, and so on).

Server consoles used for domain administration must be physically secured so that only authorized personnel have access to them. Your security plan should state this and list the personnel who might use the consoles. It is not as obvious that users of the Administrator account must never log on to client computers managed by someone who is not equally trusted. That administrator might introduce other code on the computer that will unknowingly exploit the administrator privileges. There are many hack utilities that trap information being typed so it can be reviewed later.

As you have just seen, the amount of responsibility put on a one-person administrative team under many circumstances would be prohibitive. Also, many IT departments have more than one member. Ideally, all members of the department should have a clear understanding of their personal duties and of the boundaries of their control. Windows 2000 improves on the ability of the head of the department to delegate some of this responsibility while maintaining these ideals as much as possible.

Delegation

The delegation of administrative tasks is a practical necessity in a Windows 2000 enterprise environment. Thanks to the capabilities of Windows 2000, it is common to delegate authority not only to members of the IT group but also to human resources personnel and various managers for tasks related to their duties. Delegation distributes the administrator's workload without granting sweeping privileges to every assistant. This is an expression of the security concept of *principle of least privilege*: that is, granting only the permissions necessary for the task.

Through various means, Windows 2000 allows you to delegate to groups or individuals a prescribed degree of control over a limited set of objects. The only prerequisite is that the appropriate delegation elements (users, groups, GPOs, files, directories, and so forth) must be in place before delegation can be performed. We will look at an important method of delegation, namely the Delegation Of Control Wizard, in more detail in the next chapter.

What's Next

This chapter has been rough; it contains a great deal of material. We looked at several ways you can authenticate all user access to system resources, including mechanisms that involve single sign-on and double verification. That led to the discussion of how to apply appropriate access control to all those resources.

Because Windows 2000 is an enterprise-wide solution, it must have ways to establish appropriate trust relationships between multiple domains. We examined some of these ways for Windows 2000, including Kerberos v5.

Protecting data has always been an issue with any network operating system. Now, using the technology of EFS, sensitive data can be protected within the enterprise network and while that data is being carried on the road. We even discussed ways that files can be decrypted if the owner leaves the company.

One of the problems with security is the ability to replicate it, workstation after workstation. In the past, once you set how you wanted a computer to be protected, there were few methods to push that security out to hundreds of workstations simultaneously. With security policies, you can define how you want something to be handled and then link the GPO to a site, domain, or OU that contains the computer; in other words, every system in the container will have identical settings.

Networks were designed to provide multiple users access to the same resources, both hardware and software. Because hardware is an inanimate object, it is relatively easy to provide security policies that will hold. Software, on the other hand, may not be so easy. You may secure access to the applications, but if there are holes in the code, you may have no way of knowing until it is too late.

Finally, we allayed some fears about the amount of work you will have to do. In a large network, managing security administration is a full-time job for a department. In this chapter, we discussed how to distribute those responsibilities over several users or groups.

In the next chapter, you will take much of what you learned in this chapter and apply it to creating an actual security solution with Windows 2000.

Chapter 25

DESIGNING THE SECURITY SOLUTION

In this chapter, we will talk about a long litany of things that are important but just don't fit well in other categories. We address them here, but you must understand from the start that transition from one topic to another may be a bit abrupt.

Most of these subjects have already been broached. For example, you should already know the basics of how and why to use security groups, so we will just touch on a security strategy for these groups. We'll spend the bulk of this chapter on auditing and how to use it as an effective security strategy.

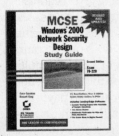

Adapted from *MCSE: Windows® 2000 Network Security Design Study Guide*, Second Edition by Gary Govanus and Robert King

ISBN 0-7821-2952-8 $59.99

AUDIT POLICIES

An *audit policy* is a policy that determines which security events should be reported to the administrator. *Auditing* is the process of tracking the activities of users by recording selected types of events in the security log of a server or workstation.

If you look at these definitions as they apply to Windows 2000, you will see that we are talking about local events. By *local*, we mean that you can turn on auditing for a server and record all the comings and goings of access to a certain file—but you can only do so on that server. To be able to access the information that auditing returns, you must have access to the security log of that server or workstation. Auditing can be turned on for a domain controller, a member server, or a mission-critical workstation.

NOTE

Remember that auditing runs only on the local machine, and is set using local security policy.

Establishing an Audit Policy

Before you implement auditing, you must decide on an auditing policy. An auditing policy simply specifies the categories of security-related events that you wish to audit. As you will see in a few paragraphs, when Windows 2000 and XP are first installed, all auditing categories are turned off. By turning on various auditing event categories, you can implement an auditing policy that suits the security needs of your organization.

If you choose to audit access to objects as part of your audit policy, you must turn on either the *audit directory service access category* (for auditing objects on a domain controller) or the *audit object access category* (for auditing objects on a member server or Windows 2000 Professional system). Once you have turned on the correct object access category, you can use each individual object's properties to specify whether to audit successes or failures for the permissions granted to each group or user. That means you can set up auditing for a file (for example, resume.doc) or a resource (for example, the check printer in the payroll department). For example, auditing may report that a user successfully accessed the file resume.doc, but when they tried to print something on the check printer in payroll, they were unsuccessful. It is important to note that auditing can be considered nonjudgmental—it just tells you that a user accessed a file. You must determine if the user was supposed to do so.

Implementing an Audit Policy

Audit policies are implemented from the Local Security Policy section of Administrative Tools. If you choose Start ➢ Programs ➢ Administrative Tools ➢ Local Security Policy ➢ Local Policies ➢ Audit Policy, you get the screen shown in Figure 25.1.

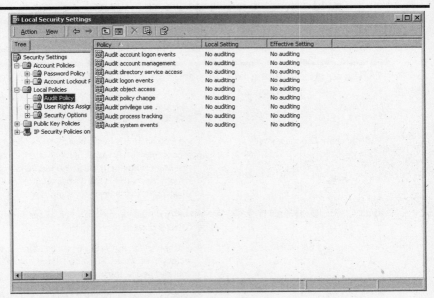

FIGURE 25.1:   Blank audit policies box

As with most things in computing, there are several ways to arrive at this screen. Another way is through the Microsoft Management Console (MMC). To accomplish the task this way, do the following:

1. Click Start, click Run, type **mmc /a**, and then click OK.

2. On the Console menu, choose Add/Remove Snap-in, and then click Add.

3. Under Snap-in, click Group Policy, and then click Add.

4. In Select Group Policy Object, click Local Computer, click Finish, click Close, and then click OK.

5. Select Local Computer Policy ➢ Computer Configuration ➢ Windows Settings ➢ Security Settings ➢ Local Policies ➢ Audit Policy.

6. In the details pane, right-click Audit Object Access, and then click Security.

7. In Local Security Policy Setting, click the options you want, and then click OK.

You can choose to audit a variety of things on this machine. For example, you can audit account logon events, access to Active Directory, or even account management. Table 25.1 shows what each of the auditing events entails.

TABLE 25.1:   Auditing Features and Functions in Windows 2000 and Windows XP

Event	Description
Audit Account Logon Events	Triggered when a logon request is received by a domain controller. An account logon event is recorded on the computer where the account is validated. For a domain logon, this is the domain controller. For a local account, this is the local computer.
Audit Account Management	An entry is made in the log when a user or group account is created or modified.
Audit Directory Service Access	An entry is made in the log when an object in Active Directory is accessed. This audit event needs to be further defined at the object level.
Audit Logon Events	An entry is made in the log when a user logs on or off a computer. A logon event is only located on the computer where the logon actually occurs. This is always the local computer.
Audit Object Access	An entry is made in the log when an object such as a file, directory, or printer is accessed. This can mean a file was opened or someone attempted to print to a printer.
Audit Policy Change	An entry is made in the log when the security options, the user rights, or the audit policies are altered.
Audit Privilege Use	An entry is made in the log when a user right is used to perform a specific action.
Audit Process Tracking	An entry is made in the log when an application performs an action that is being tracked by a programmer.
Audit System Events	An entry is made in the log when an event occurs that matches the system events criteria.

Think of this event section as a portal to the rest of auditing. For example, if you want to audit access to folders and files, you must turn on object access auditing. Basically, by making changes to this page, you open up other auditing opportunities elsewhere on the network. We will look at how to audit the Active Directory and a filesystem in the following sections.

Auditing Active Directory

Auditing the events that happen on a network can be useful, but you can learn other things. Auditing access to objects in ADS can be useful for establishing usage trends or tracking access to certain objects for security reasons. Before you can audit any objects in Active Directory on a domain controller, you must enable auditing of the directory service access by going to Start ➢ Programs ➢ Administrative Tools ➢ Domain Controller Security Policy ➢ Security Settings ➢ Local Policies ➢ Audit Policies. Once there, double-click Audit Directory Service Access to audit the success or failure of directory service access. Once that is done, all the events in Table 25.2 are available.

TABLE 25.2:   Events That Can Be Audited in Active Directory

Event	Description
Full Control	An entry is made in the audit log when any level of access is made to the object.
List Contents	An entry is made in the audit log when the contents of the object are listed.
List Object	An entry is made in the audit log when the object is viewed.
Read All Properties	An entry is made in the audit log when any of the object's properties are read.
Write All Properties	An entry is made in the audit log when any of the object's properties are changed or written to.
Create All Child Objects	An entry is made in the audit log when any child object is created.
Delete All Child Objects	An entry is made in the audit log when any child object is deleted.
Read Permissions	An entry is made in the audit log when the object's permissions are read.
Modify Permissions	An entry is made in the audit log when the object's permissions are modified.
Modify Owner	An entry is made in the audit log when the owner of an object is changed.

Auditing the Filesystem

Auditing filesystem events can help simplify administration and keep track of information on the network. To audit any of these events, you first must enable auditing of the Object Access event. You can set this event to On using the Group Policy Editor. After enabling the auditing for the Object Access event, you can audit the events listed in Table 25.3 to track usage trends or to monitor who is accessing files and folders on your network.

TABLE 25.3:   Auditing Filesystem Events

Event	Description
Open a Folder or Execute a File	An entry is made to the log when a folder is opened or an application is run.
List a Folder or Read Data	An entry is made to the audit log when a file or folder is listed.
Read Attributes	An entry is made to the audit log when just the attributes of a file or folder are read.
Read Extended Attributes	An entry is made to the audit log when the extended attributes of a file or a folder are read.
Create Files or Write Data	An entry is made to the audit log when a file is modified or created.
Create Folders or Append Data	An entry is made to the audit log when a folder is modified or created.
Write Attributes	An entry is made to the audit log when an attribute is modified.
Write Extended Attributes	An entry is made to the audit log when an extended attribute is modified.
Delete Subfolders and Files	An entry is made to the audit log when a file or subfolder in a folder is deleted.
Delete	An entry is made to the audit log when a specific file or folder is deleted.
Read Permissions	An entry is made to the audit log when the permissions of a file or folder are read.
Change Permissions	An entry is made to the audit log when the permissions of a file or folder are modified.
Take Ownership	An entry is made to the audit log when a user takes ownership of a file or folder.
Synchronize	An entry is made to the audit log when a file or folder is synchronized with an offline copy.

Auditing at the file or folder level must be enabled at the file or folder level.

NOTE

Just a reminder: You can only audit a file or a folder if it resides on an NTFS partition.

Follow these steps to set, view, change, or remove auditing for a file or folder:

1. Open Windows Explorer and locate the file or folder you want to audit.

2. Right-click the file or folder, choose Properties, and click the Security tab.

3. Click Advanced and click the Auditing tab.

Best Practices when Auditing

When an item is audited, any time there is an event, it is written to the security log. Because the security log is limited in size, you should carefully select the files and folders to be audited—you don't want the security log to fill up. In addition, auditing requires frequent reads and writes to the hard disk, using resources that otherwise could be used to do important server tasks. Be sure you carefully consider the amount of disk space you are willing to devote to the security log. The maximum size is defined in Event Viewer.

To view the security log:

1. Open Computer Management by choosing Start ➤ Settings ➤ Control Panel. Double-click Administrative Tools and double-click Computer Management.

2. In the console tree, click Event Viewer. Double-click Security Log, and in the details pane, examine the list of audit events.

Microsoft has proposed a best practices list to minimize the risk of security threats. Table 25.4 shows various events that you should audit, as well as the specific security threat the audit event monitors.

To prevent files and subfolders within the tree from inheriting these audit entries, select Apply These Auditing Entries.

TABLE 25.4:   Identifying Potential Network Threats

AUDIT EVENT	POTENTIAL THREAT
Audit for the failure of a logon.	Auditing this event helps you recognize random-password hacks.
Audit for the success of a logon/logoff.	Comparing this information to instances when a user may actually be using the account acts as a check for stolen password break-ins.
Audit for the successful change to user rights, user and group management, security change policies, restart, shutdown, and system events.	This audit helps prevent the misuse of privileges.
Set up a success and failure audit for file-access and object-access events.	This audit checks for improper attempts to access sensitive or restricted files.
Set up an audit for the success and check failure of file-access printers and object-access events.	This audit helps the network support team for improper access to printers.
Set up an audit for the success and failure of write access for program files (.EXE and .DLL extensions). Set up an audit policy for the success and failure of auditing for process tracking. Run suspect programs; examine the security log for unexpected attempts to modify program files or create unexpected processes. Run this audit only when actively monitoring the system log.	This audit helps to keep track of a virus outbreak.

AUDITING THE AUDITORS

As you are pondering the day's list of things to do, the phone rings. The chief financial officer would like to see you.

When you get to the office of the CFO, he looks concerned. In his usual manner, he starts right off: "Someone who was not authorized to be there has apparently hacked into the database and made changes." Now, this gets your attention. As you begin to probe deeper, you find that it is not actually the database that has been

CONTINUED ➡

accessed but an Excel spreadsheet out on the network share. The share was designed to share information between members of the accounting department. The accounting department has undergone some changes in the past few months; several contractors were let go, and several new employees have been added to the company. It is possible someone has been abusing their privileges.

When you ask for specifics, the CFO says it appears some percentages were changed in the file. Because the file is a list of all raises employees will be getting for the next year, the CFO immediately suspects the people whose raises have been increased. You point out that it might be a simple mistake, or it might be someone trying to make you think it was the people involved. You also point out that there are ways of checking, and you begin by setting up auditing on the file and by auditing all the people who will access the file. You ask if any other files might be vulnerable, and you set up auditing on those as well. Now it is time to keep watch and check access to the files. The CFO has copies of the files on his local drive so he can make spot checks to see if they have been altered. In addition, you tell the CFO that when the audit results are in, you will check with him to see if there is any suspicious behavior.

All the security measurements available in Windows 2000, including auditing, are useful only if a "watchdog" system is in place. Without such a system, potential attackers may be able to bypass the network's defense perimeter and do whatever they please.

DELEGATING AUTHORITY AND SECURITY GROUPS

We have covered the topic of administrative delegation a bit in previous chapters, but it is now time to discuss it in detail. There is no better way of delegating authority than by making proper use of Active Directory. Take a look at Figure 25.2: You can see a domain called Minneapolis, and inside that domain are five Organizational Units (OUs).

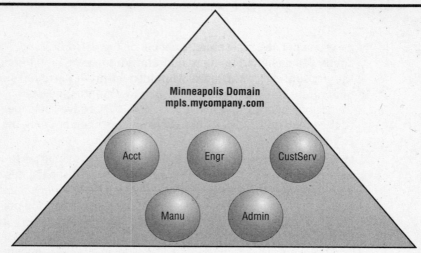

FIGURE 25.2:   Domain model with OUs

NOTE

For a more detailed explanation of OUs and their role in designing an Active Directory infrastructure, see *MCSE: Windows 2000 Directory Services Design Study Guide*, 2nd ed. (Sybex, 2001) by Robert King and Gary Govanus. It goes into great detail about the whys and hows of adding OUs to an Active Directory.

One of the advantages of creating OUs is that they make perfect areas for delegating authority. You can delegate authority down to the lowest level of your organization by creating a tree of OUs within each domain and delegating authority for parts of the OU subtree to other users or groups. You know it is not a good thing to have dozens of people logging into your network with the power of an administrator. By delegating administrative authority, you can eliminate the need to have people with sweeping authority over an entire domain regularly logging on to accounts. Although you will still have an Administrator account and a Domain Admins group with administrative authority over the entire domain, you can reserve them for occasional use by a very limited number of highly trusted administrators.

When you decide how to structure your OUs and in which OUs to put each user, consider the hierarchy of administration. For example, you may want to create an OU tree that enables you to grant to a user the administrative rights for all branches of a single department, such as

an accounting department. Alternatively, you may want to grant administrative rights to a subunit within an OU, such as the accounts payable
unit of an accounting OU. Another possible delegation of administrative
rights would be to grant to an individual the administrative rights for the
accounting OU, but not to any OUs contained within the accounting OU.

Delegating Administration

Because of the size of the Microsoft designated sample network, the
delegation of administrative tasks is a practical necessity in a Windows 2000
enterprise environment. You may have designed a situation where administration was divided along OU lines. That is not the only way it can be
done, however—you don't even have to make administration IT-specific.
If technically savvy people have a reason for needing rights to administer
certain types of objects, you can certainly give them the appropriate
administrative rights. For example, why not delegate authority to human
resources personnel and various others for tasks related to their duties?
With careful planning, you can distribute the administrator's workload
without granting too much power to every assistant. This is way of prac-
ticing the security concept of *principle of least privilege*. In other words,
you can grant the permissions necessary to accomplish their particular
tasks, and no more.

Using various methods in Windows 2000, you can delegate a prescribed
degree of control over a limited set of objects to specific groups or individuals. Just keep in mind that the appropriate Active Directory objects
(users, groups, Group Policy Objects, files, directories, and so forth) must
be in place before the delegation can be performed. Let's take a look at
several of the ways to accomplish these tasks.

Security Groups, Group Policy, and Access Control Lists

These things have been described in previous chapters, so we won't
go into extensive detail here. They help to form the mechanisms for
distributed administration.

Built-in Security Groups   Windows 2000 has a set of built-in security groups that come with permissions in place, already delegated to each
group. Open the Active Directory Users And Computers snap-in to MMC.
Open View ➤ Advanced Features. The predefined security groups are in

the Builtin and Users folders. If you want to directly delegate control of one of these groups, open the property sheet of the group and click the Security tab. Once there, all you have to do is add the group's manager to the ACL and check the appropriate privileges, as shown in Figure 25.3.

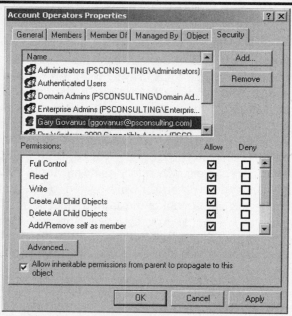

FIGURE 25.3:   MMC showing delegation of control over groups

There are other ways you can handle this process. One of the ways is to use the Delegation of Control Wizard.

Delegation of Control Wizard   Again, go into the Active Directory Sites And Services snap-in to MMC. Click Action and then Delegate Control (see Figure 25.4).

Using the Delegation Wizard to Distribute Administration   This time, begin by opening the Active Directory Users And Computers snap-in to MMC. Right-click an OU and select Delegate Control. The Delegation of Control Wizard sets up user group permissions to administer OUs containing computers and user groups. An example is the delegated right to create new user accounts (see Figure 25.5).

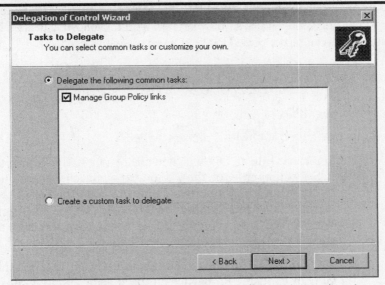

FIGURE 25.4:   MMC showing the Delegation of Control Wizard getting ready to delegate the Manage Group Policy links

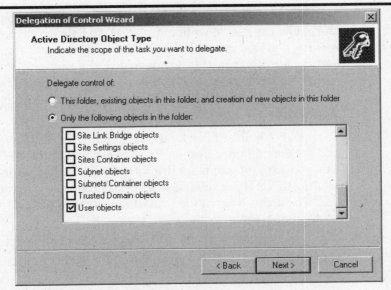

FIGURE 25.5:   MMC for delegation of administration over users

Delegating Control of Group Policy Objects   To delegate administration using Group Policies, you must deal with the following tasks. These
three tasks can be performed together or separately, as needed:

▶ Managing Group Policy links for a site, domain, or OU

▶ Creating Group Policy Objects (GPOs)

▶ Editing GPOs

Let's take a look at how this process works:

1. You can create an OU and then create a new GPO linked to
    it: Select Properties on the OU context menu, click the Group
    Policy tab in the Properties dialog box, and then click the
    New button. After creating the GPO, launch the Delegation
    Wizard. The Delegation Wizard provides a clear sequence of
    steps for delegating specific functionality.

2. You can also directly access the security settings for the
    GPO by choosing Properties on the specific GPO's context
    menu and then clicking the Security tab. Add your non-
    administrator user to the list of users for whom security is
    defined.

3. You can give your user Full Control—Allow privilege. Full Con-
    trol allows the user to write to the GPO, and also to change
    security permissions on the GPO. To prevent this user from
    setting security, you may decide to give the user only the
    Write—Allow permission. If you decide the user should be
    exempt from the application of this policy, you can clear the
    Apply Group Policy—Allow privilege.

4. To simplify administration for the user, launch the MMC and
    add the Group Policy snap-in. Browse for and add the GPO
    that you are configuring for delegation. After properly con-
    figuring this MMC session, save the session and give it to the
    user. The user can now utilize and administer their GPO with
    no additional setup.

Because we keep talking about Group Policies and the Group Policy
MMC snap-in, this is a good time to examine Group Policies in more
depth.

ORGANIZATION AND DELEGATION

It has not been a great day. You have just come from a Windows 2000 planning meeting, where you were chosen as the fortunate person who gets to decide how to group people together for your domain. In most cases this wouldn't sound like a difficult task, but your company has 3,000 people working in this domain. Other than the people who work on your floor, and maybe some folks who eat lunch at the same time you do, you have no clue who most of these people are. The CIO has tasked you with "using the capabilities of Windows 2000 to the utmost to create groups that make sense within the organization."

Just as you are getting your hands around this concept, it is time to go to another meeting. This one is a full-blown production, announcing a reorganization of some new teams. At this second meeting, you notice that all of senior management is on the stage, and you are impressed. When the meeting kicks off, you realize that what is happening here will have a direct impact on your life. They begin by introducing the executive vice presidents, who introduce their vice presidents. Each vice president then announces the team leaders who will be their direct reports. It is made clear that each of the team leads will pick their people, and some people will be on several different teams. As you begin to think what a problem this might be for you, you glance down at the handout and notice the list of team leaders. Suddenly, a light comes on. These people are doing all the picking and choosing anyway; you can just create groups that match the teams, and give the team leaders the ability to figure out what people go where. That approach will surely simplify your life. At that point, you truly begin to appreciate the phrase "using the capabilities of Windows 2000 to the utmost" and the delegation of authority.

Delegation of authority in Windows 2000 is almost a necessity when domains are scaled to a large number of users. This delegation capability was among the chief reasons Microsoft introduced the Active Directory structure, including OUs.

IMPLEMENTING GROUP POLICY SECURITY SETTINGS

By this stage, you know that implementing a Group Policy consists of creating a new GPO (or modifying an existing one), enabling appropriate settings within the object, and then linking the GPO to an OU, site, or domain that contains computers or users in the domain.

Let's look at a sample OU and its associated Group Policy. Doing so will give you a feel for the nine security policy settings.

Start by opening the Active Directory Users And Computers MMC snap-in, and right-click the Domain Controllers OU. Open the property sheet and click the Group Policy tab. Select the Default Domain Controllers Policy and click Edit. Doing so opens the Group Policy snap-in to MMC. In this module, navigate to the Security Settings container by choosing Computer Configuration ≻ Windows Settings ≻ Security Settings. Your screen should now look like Figure 25.6.

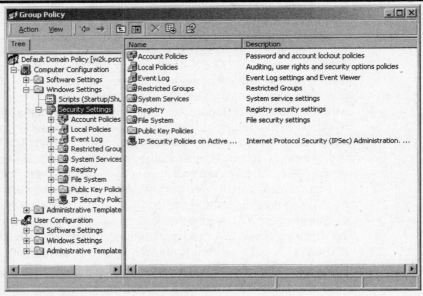

FIGURE 25.6:   Security Settings Group Policy

Under Security Settings are nine security policy subsettings:

- ▶ Account Policies
- ▶ Local Policies
- ▶ Event Log
- ▶ Restricted Groups
- ▶ System Services

- Registry
- File System
- Public Key Policies
- IPSec Security Policies on Active Directory

NOTE
Some of these policy areas can be applied domain-wide only. Account policies, for example, are applied to all the user accounts in the specific domain. That means you cannot define different account policies for different OUs in the same domain. If two groups of users need different password policies, you will need to put the groups into two separate domains.

Of the security policy areas, account policies and public key policies are domain-wide. The other policies can be specified at the OU level. We'll now look at each of the nine settings in more detail. Some of the areas, such as account policies, are much more detailed than others. Therefore, we'll take a deeper look at those areas.

Account Policies

Table 25.5 shows the scope of the account policies and what they can do. They are generally concerned with rules associated with a user's account, and not other settings such as user rights and desktop restrictions. An important note here: Remember that account policies cannot be implemented by creating a GPO and then linking it to a particular domain. This process will only take the policy and apply it to every local machine in the domain. Because users in a domain environment do not authenticate to a local machine, the policy will be of no value. In order for account policies to be applied appropriately, you must use the Domain Security Policy administrative tool.

NOTE
The policies you choose affect the level of help desk support required for users as well as the vulnerability of your network to security breaches and attacks. For example, specifying a restrictive account lockout policy increases the potential for denial of service attacks, and setting a restrictive password policy results in increased help desk calls from users who cannot log on to the network. In addition, specifying a restrictive password policy can actually reduce the security of the network. For example, if you require passwords longer than seven characters, most users have difficulty remembering them. They might write their passwords down and leave them where an intruder can easily find them.

TABLE 25.5: Account Policies

POLICY	DESCRIPTION
Password policy	With a password policy, you can set parameters such as the minimum length of a user's password. You can also define how long a user can use the same password by setting the maximum password age. If you are working in a highly secure environment, make sure you require complex passwords. Doing so will help prevent users from reusing the same password or a simple variation of their password.
Account lockout policy	To protect your network against brute force attacks, where someone tries the same logon name and different passwords over and over again, you can force users to be locked out after a specified number of failed logon attempts. Not only that, but you can specify the amount of time accounts are locked.
Kerberos authentication policy	You can also modify the default Kerberos settings for each domain in your network, if you desire. Such changes would include things like setting the maximum lifetime of a user ticket.

Local Computer Policies

The second category of security settings we will look at is local computer policies. Table 25.6 summarizes tweaks you can make to these policies. From a security standpoint, all of these areas are significant. Audit policy is used to track events on Windows 2000 and XP systems, as we discussed previously, and is an integral part of a good security infrastructure. User rights are designed to give administrators the ability to grant or restrict various system privileges, such as adding device drivers and shutting down servers. If these rights are abused in any way, the secure nature of your entire network may be at risk. Other general security options, such as forcing users to log off when their logon hours expire, or not allowing Alt+Ctrl+Del sequences, are important in their own way.

TABLE 25.6: Defining Local Computer Policies

POLICY	DESCRIPTION
Audit policy	By setting the audit policy, Windows 2000 and XP can track a variety of security event types. These event types can be system-wide, such as a user logging on, or more specific, such as a particular user attempting to open and read a specific file. You can have auditing track both successful and unsuccessful attempts.

TABLE 25.6 continued: Defining Local Computer Policies

POLICY	DESCRIPTION
User rights assignment	You can also use local policies to control the rights assigned to user accounts and security groups for local computers. In this case, you can set which users or security groups have rights to perform tasks that may affect your network security. An example would be controlling who can gain access to computers on the network, who can log on locally to a domain controller, or even who can shut a computer down. You can also use policies to define who can back up and restore files or who can take ownership of files.
Security options	The security options policies allow the administrator to control settings that would force users to log off when logon hours expire or prohibit the use of the Alt+Ctrl+Del keys to access the Windows logon dialog. That would force users to use a smart card to log on to the local computer.

Event Log Policies

You can use event log policies to control the settings of the application, system, and security event logs on local computers. For example, you can specify how large logs can grow, how long logs are kept, and how logs are retained.

These settings can be important when you're determining how to archive. The computer generates events for almost everything that happens, including auditing. For example, if an application has an error, then more than likely the error will be reported in the application event log. Similarly, system events relating to Active Directory or services such as DNS are noted in the system event log. All successes and failures related to auditing are listed in the application event log.

You can use Event Viewer to examine each of these logs in detail, but you may find as an administrator that you need larger log files (especially on a complex enterprise network). Also, if your company is fond of keeping detailed records, then you may need to adjust how long those log files are kept. Your archive files may grow quite large, but at least you can spot trouble areas by looking at old log files and noticing trends.

Restricted Group Policies

You can define restricted group policies to let the IT team manage the membership of the built-in Windows 2000–defined groups or the user-defined groups. All of these groups have special rights and permissions. The restricted group policies contain a list of members of specific groups whose membership is defined as part of the security policy. Enforcement of the restricted group policies forcibly sets any computer local group membership to match the membership list settings defined in the policy. If a local computer administrator tries to change the membership, any changes will be overwritten by the policy.

Restricted group policies are generally used to manage membership in the built-in groups. These built-in groups include local groups such as Administrators, Power Users, Print Operators, Account Operators, and Server Operators, as well as global groups such as Domain Admins. You can see that the central IT team may have an interest in making sure only certain users can belong to these groups. If you have other groups that you consider sensitive, you can add them to the restricted groups list, along with their membership list. This way, you enforce the membership of these groups by policy and make sure there will not be local variations on each computer.

System Services Policies

System services policies can be a potential entry point for intruders. If a service is running, it may have a default service account with a default password that can open a door. For example, a number of articles have been written about ways an intruder can try to exploit weaknesses in various web servers to gain access to a computer's operating system or files. To try to prevent this type of access, you can configure system services policies to do the following:

- ▶ Define the startup mode for Windows 2000 services, either manual or automatic—or, if you know the service won't be used, just disable it. This approach can work to your advantage if you configure system services to prevent any unnecessary services from running. Doing so can provide security for special servers like domain controllers, DNS servers, proxy servers, remote access servers, and certification authority servers.

- ▶ Define the exact rights and permissions that are granted to each of the system services when they run. In this case, you configure system services to operate with the minimum rights and permissions needed. Doing so will go a long way toward limiting potential damage that could be caused by intruders who try to exploit the service.

▶ Define security auditing levels for system services. Make sure you specify the exact types of events to be logged for both failed and successful events. In the example of using auditing to protect against a compromised service, refine auditing to monitor for any inappropriate actions taken by running the susceptible services.

Registry Policies

You can use registry policies to configure the security audit policy. Because Windows 2000 can record a range of security event types, this can be a useful way of detecting intrusion. These policies are summarized in Table 25.7.

TABLE 25.7: Defining Registry Policies

POLICY	DESCRIPTION
Security options	In this case, you are controlling security auditing for Registry keys and their subkeys. For example, to make sure that only administrators can change certain information in the Registry, you can use Registry policies to grant administrators full control over Registry keys and their subkeys and to grant read-only permission to other users. You can also use Registry policies to prevent certain users from viewing portions of the Registry.

You can use Registry policies to audit user activity in the Registry of the computer when auditing is enabled. You can specify which users and which user events are logged for both failed and successful events.

Filesystem Policies

Filesystem policies are used to provide data on your network. This includes giving you the ability to control security auditing of files and folders. One way you can use these policies effectively is to make sure that only users with administrator capabilities can modify system files and folders. In this case, you can use filesystem policies to give the administrators full control over these areas and grant just read-only permissions to other users. There may be some areas of the network you don't want users to access at all; in that case, you can use filesystem policies to prevent certain users from even looking at the files or folders.

You can also use filesystem policies to audit the activity of those users who can access files and folders. In this case, you specify which users and which events are logged for both failed and successful events.

Public Key Policies

To add things like a new Encrypted Data Recovery Agent or set up an Automatic Certificate request, you can use the public key policies area of security settings. You can also use this area to manage the list of trusted certification authorities (CAs).

IP Security Policies on Active Directory

The information in the IP Security (IPSec) policies area tells the workstation or the server how to handle a request for IPSec communication. For example, the server may require that any communications between the server and a client be secure, it may permit only secure communications, or it may not even allow secure communications.

If you decide to use IPSec, it is a good idea to make sure these policies are redefined for your implementation. As always, thorough testing before the actual implementation is of the utmost importance.

WORK SMARTER, NOT HARDER, WITH GROUP POLICIES

As the CIO of a company with a major enterprise network, you know that the best thing you can do for the company is to come up with a good plan to delegate authority down to the people who really know the technical side of the network. You are a manager, not a technical person.

You also know that there are things you want out of your Windows 2000 network. In the past, one of the major problems of networking has always been inconsistency. Even when you had "corporate standards," sometimes they weren't met. Other times, the major vendors whose products you decided on changed the products—or worse yet, stopped making the products. In the case of Windows 2000 and security, too many things need to be set on each and every workstation to bring it into compliance with your standards. You are concerned about ensuring that the machines will be rolled out properly and that each setting will be duplicated across the entire domain.

CONTINUED ➡

You call in your most trusted assistant and run the problem by her. She commiserates with you for a while and then remembers Group Policies. She suggests appointing one member of your team to be the Group Policy guru. Giving someone that power and the ability to test Group Policies will be crucial in the very near future.

There is no question that using GPOs and delegating authority may make the difference between a lot of unnecessary work for management and an efficient work environment.

THE PLACEMENT AND INHERITANCE OF SECURITY POLICIES

Security policies are implemented at the site, the domain, or the OU. Because multiple GPOs can be linked to any single site, domain, or OU, multiple security policies can be installed at any level. The policies are applied in a specific order: site, domain, and OU. The nature of security policies under Windows 2000 is that any lower level will inherit its upper levels' security policies by default. Therefore, multiple inherited policies may apply to any level. In addition, due to the hierarchy of the ADS, it is important in troubleshooting to understand what takes priority over what in the likely case of a conflict.

Group Policy Hierarchy

By default, Group Policy is inherited and cumulative, and it affects all computers and users in an Active Directory container. Group Policy is always processed according to the following order: local, site, domain, and OU. By default, remember, if there are conflicting policies, the policy closest to the computer or the user wins. To say it another way, the default inheritance method is to evaluate Group Policy starting with the Active Directory container furthest away from the computer or user object. The Active Directory container closest to the computer or user can override Group Policy set in a higher-level AD container. If there are no conflicts, then the policies are cumulative.

Enforcing and Blocking Policy Options

Options exist that allow you to enforce the Group Policy in a specific GPO so that GPOs in lower-level Active Directory containers are prevented from overriding that policy. For example, if you have defined a specific GPO at the domain level and specified that the GPO be enforced, the policies that the GPO contains apply to all OUs under that domain; that is, the lower-level containers (OUs) cannot override that domain Group Policy.

You can also block inheritance of Group Policy from parent Active Directory containers. For example, if you specify a particular policy for a domain or OU and then mark that policy as having the Block Policy Inheritance property, you prevent policy in higher-level Active Directory containers (such as a higher-level OU or domain) from applying. However, enforced policy options always take precedence.

Block Policy Inheritance can be set only at the domain or OU level. It cannot be set on individual Group Policies. No Override can be set on individual policies.

Defining Group Policy Links for a Site, Domain, or OU

As we have said before, administrators can configure Group Policy for sites, domains, or OUs. You do so using the Active Directory tools and setting properties for the specified site, domain, or OU. The Group Policy tab on the Properties page allows you to specify which GPOs are linked to this site, domain, or OU. This property page stores the user's choices in two Active Directory properties: gPLink and gPOptions. The gPLink property contains the prioritized list of GPOs, and the gPOptions property contains the Block Policy Inheritance policy setting.

Active Directory supports security settings on a per-property basis. This means a non-administrator can be given read and write access to specific properties. In this case, if non-administrators have read and write access to the gPLink and gPOptions properties, they can manage the list of GPOs linked to that site, domain, or OU. To give a user read and write access to these properties, use the Delegation Wizard and select the Manage Group Policy Links predefined task.

DESIGNING AN ENCRYPTING FILE SYSTEM STRATEGY

The Encrypting File System (EFS) is used to secure local files. To review, EFS is part of the Public Key Infrastructure (PKI), so a key is obtained and used to encrypt the file. The decryption key is controlled by the user and by a recovery agent. If someone attempts to attack the file, that person will be unable to open it. If the computer is stolen, the information remains in a secure state. If the end user loses the decryption key, the information remains in a secure state.

In the following sections, we will discuss some important concepts about EFS that we have not previously covered. We will also go into some detail about recovery policies and ideas for implementing EFS in a business situation.

Things to Know about EFS

EFS is one of the most heavily used methods of security for portable computers and kiosk machines. You must keep a few things in mind before implementing it in a production environment, however:

▶ EFS has some built-in protection. For example, EFS does not run if there is no recovery agent certificate. It will, however, designate a recovery agent account by default and generate the necessary certificate. It will do this even if you don't explicitly.

▶ You can use EFS to encrypt or decrypt data on a remote computer, but you cannot use it to encrypt data sent over the network.

▶ Windows 2000 helps prevent some catastrophes in the making. It makes sure you cannot encrypt system files or folders.

▶ You cannot encrypt compressed files and folders until you decompress them, because compression and encryption are mutually exclusive.

▶ Encrypting an entire folder ensures that the temporary copies of encrypted files it contains are also encrypted.

▶ Copying an unencrypted file into an encrypted folder encrypts the file, but moving it into the folder in the same partition leaves the file encrypted or unencrypted, just as it was before you moved the file.

▶ If an already-encrypted file can stay encrypted, then it will, regardless of the destination folder's attributes.

▶ Moving or copying EFS files to another filesystem removes the encryption, but backing them up preserves the encryption. Remember that only NTFS 5 supports EFS.

▶ Other file permissions are unaffected. An administrator, for instance, can still delete a user's EFS file even though the user cannot open it.

EFS and the End User

Users work with encrypted files and folders just as they do with any other files and folders. As long as the EFS user is the same person who encrypted the file or folder, the system automatically decrypts the file or folder when the user accesses it later. However, an intruder is prevented from accessing any encrypted files or folders. To encrypt a file, all the user has to do is go into Windows Explorer and browse to the file. The user highlights the file, right-clicks and chooses Properties, clicks the General tab, clicks the Advanced button, and then sees the screen shown in Figure 25.7.

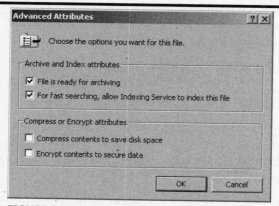

FIGURE 25.7: Encrypting a file

Once the Encrypt Contents to Secure Data check box is selected, the file is encrypted if it is in a folder that holds encrypted files. Folders themselves are not encrypted—only the contents of the files within a folder. Like folders, subfolders are not encrypted; however, they are marked to indicate that they contain encrypted file data. If the folder is not designated to handle encrypted files, the user receives a warning to encrypt the entire folder (see Figure 25.8).

Any file that is saved in an encrypted folder is encrypted by default.

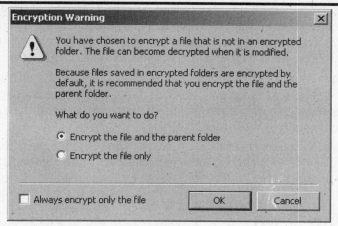

FIGURE 25.8:   Encryption warning

Data Encryption and Decryption

Because the entire encryption/decryption operation is transparent to
the user, you have to figure a lot of work is going on in the background.
Encryption and decryption apply both per file and to an entire folder.
The encryption for a folder is transparent; all the files and subfolders
created in an encrypted folder are automatically encrypted. Each file has
a unique encryption key. The file does not have to be decrypted to use
it—EFS automatically takes care of that for you. EFS will go out and
locate the user's file encryption key from the systems key store and apply it.

Storing Encrypted Files on Remote Servers

You should consider some caveats to file encryption when creating your
file encryption strategy. For example, it is perfectly okay for a user to
store an encrypted file on a remote server. Just because the file is stored
on the remote server, though, is not an indication that there is support
for sharing the file with multiple users. As a matter of fact, storing
encrypted files on a remote server can make them vulnerable to sniffer
attacks. Encrypted data is not encrypted when it is in transit over the
network—only when it is stored on disk. The exception to this rule is if
your system is using IPSec. In that case, IPSec encrypts the data while it
is transported over a TCP/IP network.

Microsoft also suggests that users should never store highly sensitive data on servers where physical security might be at risk. Finally, if there are any Macintosh clients on the network, you may want to think twice about encryption. Encrypted files are not accessible to Macintosh clients.

You must do some other preliminary work before users can encrypt files that will be stored on a remote server. First, that server must be designated as *trusted for delegation*. Doing so allows all users with files on that server to encrypt those files.

To designate a remote server for file encryption, open Active Directory Users And Computers. Highlight the remote server name, right-click, and choose Properties. Then, select the Trusted for Delegation check box.

Recovering Data

The process of data recovery becomes very important when you need to access data that has been encrypted by an employee after the employee leaves, or when the user's private key is lost. When we first heard about EFS in Windows 2000, we thought about all the damage a disgruntled employee could do. Imagine the problems if someone could go to the accounting area and encrypt all the data files so no one could read them! Even if the employee was *not* disgruntled, keys can be lost. What if someone's hard disk failed? Through no fault of their own, they would have lost their file encryption certificate and private key. To protect against this occurrence, Windows provides for a designated recovery agent using a required recovery policy.

Mandatory Recovery Policy

EFS provides for built-in data recovery by enforcing a recovery policy requirement. The requirement is that a recovery policy must be in place before users can encrypt files. The recovery policy provides for a person to be designated as the recovery agent. Again, this is a transparent process. The default recovery policy is automatically put in place when the administrator logs on to the system for the first time (during installation), making the administrator the recovery agent.

The recovery agent account has a special certificate and associated private key that allow data recovery for the scope of influence of the recovery policy. In other words, if you are the recovery agent for the domain, any time someone loses their key or leaves the company without being polite enough to decrypt their files, you will be called on.

NOTE

You need to protect your recovery certificate and private key. If you are the recovery agent, you should be sure to use the Export command from Certificates in MMC to back up the recovery certificate and associated private key to a secure location. After backing up, use Certificates in MMC to delete the recovery certificate from the recovery agent's personal store, not from the recovery policy. When you need to perform a recovery operation for a user, you begin by restoring the recovery certificate and associated private key to the recovery agent's personal store, using the Import command from Certificates in MMC. After recovering the data, you should again delete the recovery certificate from the recovery agent's personal store. You do not have to repeat the export process. Deleting the recovery agent's recovery certificate from the computer and keeping it in a secure location apart from the computer is an additional security measure for the protection of sensitive data. Keeping the recovery certificate on tape or disk and locking the media in a physical safe would be ideal.

The default recovery policy is configured locally for stand-alone computers. For computers that are part of a network, the recovery policy is configured at either the domain, OU, or individual computer level, and applies to all Windows 2000 and XP–based computers within the defined scope of influence. Recovery certificates are issued by a CA and managed using Certificates in MMC.

In a network environment, the domain administrator controls how EFS is implemented for users for all computers in the domain. In a default Windows 2000 installation, when the first domain controller is set up, the domain administrator is the specified recovery agent for the domain. The way the domain administrator configures the recovery policy determines how EFS is implemented for users on their local machines. The domain administrator logs on to the first domain controller to change the recovery policy for the domain.

Types of Recovery Policies

Administrators can define one of three kinds of policies with one or more recovery agents:

No Recovery Policy   When an administrator deletes the recovery policy on the first domain controller, a *no-recovery policy* at the domain level is in effect. Because there is no domain recovery policy, the default local policy on individual computers is used for data recovery. This means local administrators control the recovery of data on their computers.

Empty Recovery Policy When an administrator deletes all recovery agents and their public-key certificates, an *empty recovery policy* is in effect. An empty recovery policy means that no one is a recovery agent, and that users cannot encrypt data on computers within the scope of influence of the recovery policy. The effect of an empty recovery policy is to turn off EFS altogether.

Recovery-Agent Policy When an administrator adds one or more recovery agents, a *recovery-agent policy* is in effect. These agents are responsible for recovering any encrypted data within their scope of administration. This is the most common type of recovery policy.

A variety of recovery options are available. Table 25.8 summarizes them.

TABLE 25.8: Effect of Recovery Policies

RECOVERY POLICY	EFFECT	RECOVERY AGENT	TASKS
Empty recovery policy	EFS cannot be used.	There is no recovery agent.	You will have to delete every recovery agent.
No recovery policy at the domain level	EFS is available on a local computer.	The default recovery agent is set to the administrator of the local computer.	You can delete the recovery policy on first domain controller.
Recovery policy configured with designated recovery agent(s)	EFS is available locally.	The default recovery agent is set to the domain administrator.	This is the default configuration in a network environment.

NOTE

Because the Windows 2000 security subsystem handles enforcing, replicating, and caching the recovery policy, users can implement file encryption on a system that is temporarily offline, such as a portable computer. This process is similar to logging on to their domain account using cached credentials.

Modifying the Recovery Policy

To modify the default recovery policy for a domain, you must log on to the first domain controller as an administrator. Then, start the Group Policy MMC through the Active Directory Users And Computers snap-in, right-click the domain whose recovery policy you wish to change, and choose Properties. Click the recovery policy you wish to change and click Edit. In the console tree, click Encrypted Data Recovery Agents. Finally, right-click the details pane and click the appropriate action you wish to take.

Best Practices When Using EFS

As you plan your EFS policy, remember that you have the option to disable EFS if you feel it will not benefit your enterprise. You can (and should) designate alternate recovery agent accounts, just in case. You should also make sure that you protect the recovery keys from misuse. Just for safety's sake, make sure you keep archives of obsolete recovery agent certificates and private keys.

Disabling EFS for a Set of Computers

If you want to disable EFS for a domain, OU, or stand-alone computer, you can do so by simply applying an empty Encrypted Data Recovery Agents policy setting. Until Encrypted Data Recovery Agents settings are configured and applied through Group Policy, there is no policy, and EFS uses the default recovery agents. However, EFS must use the recovery agents that are listed in the Encrypted Data Recovery Agents Group Policy. If the policy that is applied is empty, there is no recovery agent, and therefore EFS does not operate.

Designating Alternate Recovery Agents

You can configure Encrypted Data Recovery Agents policy to designate alternative recovery agents. For example, you may want to distribute the administrative workload in your organization, so you can designate alternative EFS recovery accounts for categories of computers grouped by OUs. You might also configure Encrypted Data Recovery Agents settings for portable computers so that they use the same recovery agent certificates when they are connected to the domain and when they are operated as stand-alone computers.

Securing Recovery Keys

Because recovery keys can be misused to decrypt and read files that have been encrypted by EFS users, it is recommended that you provide additional security for private keys for recovery. The first step in providing security for recovery keys is to disable default recovery accounts by exporting the recovery agent certificate and the private key to a secure medium and to select the option to remove the private key from the computer. When the recovery certificate and key are exported, the key is removed from the computer. You then store the exported certificate and key in a secure location to be used later for file recovery operations. Securing private keys for recovery ensures that nobody can misuse the recovery agent account to read encrypted files. This is especially important for mobile computers or other computers that are at high risk of falling into the wrong hands.

Maintaining Archives of Recovery Keys

For EFS encrypted files, the recovery agent information is refreshed every time the filesystem performs an operation on the file (for example, when the file is opened, moved, or copied). However, if an encrypted file isn't used for a long time, the recovery agents can expire. To make sure encrypted files that have not been accessed for a long period of time can be recovered, you should maintain backups of the recovery agent certificates and all the private keys. To create the backup, simply export the certificate and its private key to a secure medium like a floppy disk or a Zip disk and then store the disk in a safe location. A safe location should be something like a safe or safety deposit box, preferably off site. When you export the private keys, you must provide a secret password for granting access to the exported key. The secret key is then stored in an encrypted format to protect its confidentiality.

What happens if you have to recover some files that have expired recovery agent information? In that case, import the appropriate expired recovery agent certificate and private key from the backup to a recovery account on a local computer and then perform the recovery.

Tips for Using EFS

Now that you have seen the best practices, here are a few tips on how to use EFS:

- ▶ Make sure you encrypt the entire folder where you save most of your documents. Doing so will ensure that your personal documents are encrypted by default.

- ▶ Take the precaution of encrypting your Temp folder. That way, all the temporary files on your computer are automatically encrypted.

▶ Be sure to take the precaution of encrypting folders rather than individual files. That way, when a program creates temporary files during editing, they are encrypted.

▶ Remember: To make archives, you can use the Export command from the Certificates snap-in to back up the file encryption certificate and associated private key on a floppy disk. Make sure you keep the backup in a secure location such as a safe or safety deposit box.

DESIGNING YOUR SECURITY PLAN

This section falls under the best practices part of the Group Policy security setting implementation. Suggestions include the following (in this order):

▶ When you lay out your Active Directory, create OUs that will contain computers that have similar roles in your network.

▶ Create another OU that will be specific to application servers.

▶ Create an OU that can contain all your client computers.

▶ Apply to each of these OUs a single GPO that can implement consistent security settings.

NOTE

The number-one rule in using Group Policies is to test. Limit the number of administrators who can edit GPOs, and limit inheritance modifications, filtering, and loopbacks. It is also a very good idea to limit the number of GPOs that apply to any site, domain, or OU.

Microsoft also recommends that you keep the number of GPOs that apply to users and computers to a minimum. Because the user and computer GPOs must be downloaded to a computer at logon time, having multiple GPOs increases computer startup and user logon time. Also, applying multiple GPOs can create policy conflicts that are difficult to troubleshoot.

In general, Group Policy can be passed down from parent to child sites, domains, and OUs. If you have assigned a specific Group Policy to a high-level parent, that Group Policy applies to all OUs beneath the parent, including the user and computer objects in each container. If you have multiple GPOs, trying to figure out which one is causing a problem can be difficult.

It is time now to lay out your network security deployment plan. This plan needs to itemize all the important policy choices in each policy category. When you create your plan, be sure to cover the following details:

▶ Specify the Group Policy settings that you want to change from the default settings, and how they will be changed.

▶ Be sure to describe all the issues that may be related to changing the settings for the Group Policy. This description will assist the help desk by giving them a heads-up about potential problems.

▶ Be sure to document any special security requirements and also how you configured Group Policy to meet them.

Deployment Planning Checklist

When you are developing your deployment plan, it's helpful to have a checklist to refer to. The following could serve as a guide:

▶ Decide which security risks affect your network. List all risks and provide enough detail to clarify the problems.

▶ Fill in enough background information to help your readers understand the issues.

▶ Describe the security strategies you are employing to deal with the risks.

▶ Decide who needs to use strong authentication for interactive or remote access login.

▶ Make sure all network access is authenticated through domain accounts.

▶ Define the complexity, length, and lifetime of passwords for domain user accounts; determine the best way to convey these requirements to your users. Inform staff of the company's policy prohibiting transmission of plain-text passwords. Enable single sign-on or protect password transmission.

▶ If strong authentication is indicated, deploy public key security for smart card logon.

▶ With reference to broad security access to enterprise-wide resources, describe the top-level security groups you plan on using (probably enterprise universal groups).

▶ Describe your strategy for providing necessary remote access; convey your plan to those who need to know, and include details such as connection methods.

▶ Identify how your company uses groups and establishes conventions for group names and how group types are used.

▶ Describe how your access control policies support consistent use of security groups.

▶ Define procedures for creating new groups and decide who is responsible for managing the groups.

▶ Determine which existing domains belong in the forest, and which domains use external trust relationships.

▶ Describe your domains, domain trees, and forests, and describe the trust relationships between them.

▶ Identify which servers are likely to carry sensitive data and therefore need network data protection to prevent eavesdropping.

▶ Outline your policy for identification and management of sensitive data.

▶ Describe how IPSec will be used for protecting data or sensitive applications in remote access situations.

▶ If EFS is part of the plan, describe the data recovery policy involved, and define the role of the recovery agent in your company. Describe how you will implement a data recovery process, and be sure it works.

▶ If you are using IPSec, identify how it will be used in your network and explain the performance implications.

▶ Define domain-wide account policies and tell your users what they are.

▶ List the local security policy requirements and Group Policy settings for all system categories: desktops, file servers, print servers, and mail servers.

- Identify application servers where security templates can simplify the management of security settings. Consider managing them through Group Policy.

- For systems that will get an upgrade from NT 4 instead of a clean installation, describe an effective security template.

- For different classes of computers, use security templates to describe the intended security level.

- Plan testing to verify that existing applications will run properly under the newly implemented security design.

- List any additional applications needed to meet security objectives.

- Describe the security level required for downloaded code.

- Deploy code signing for all publicly distributed software that has been developed within the organization.

- State the policies regarding security of the Administrator account and the administration consoles.

- Identify your policies regarding auditing, including staffing.

- Describe any situations where you might delegate administrative control for specific tasks.

What's Next

In this chapter, we looked at the way an IT department can use audit policies to determine who accesses what on the network. Whether it is a file, an application, or a resource, you can track who accesses it. In addition, you can set up several audit policies to check who accesses the network and how they get in.

The next section touched on how to delegate authority. One popular concept is the idea of letting team leads manage the team group. IT security sets up a group and gives it all the permissions it needs, but the team lead takes care of adding or removing members from the group. The fact that several tools are available to help with the delegation of administration is a plus, too.

Next, we discussed security groups, how to implement them, and how to best use the default groups. We looked at how to design and configure security policies and where to place them within the forest so that you get the most bang for your buck.

Finally, we looked at how to manage your users and the Encrypting File System. We pointed out several built-in safety features and how best to use them.

Throughout this book, you have been introduced to many Sybex authors covering a variety of subjects. This book serves as an introduction to the concepts of security for each OS, and each concept is covered in even greater detail in the source books listed at the beginning of each chapter. For more information about additional Sybex books, refer to www.sybex.com.

Glossary of Networking Terms

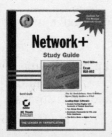

Adapted from the *Network+™ Study Guide,* Third Edition
by David Groth

ISBN 0-7821-4014-9 $49.99

10Base2 Ethernet   An implementation of Ethernet that specifies a 10Mbps signaling rate, baseband signaling, and coaxial cable with a maximum segment length of 185 meters.

10BaseFL   An implementation of Ethernet that specifies a 10Mbps signaling rate, baseband signaling, and fiber-optic cabling.

10BaseT   An implementation of Ethernet that specifies a 10Mbps signaling rate, baseband signaling, and twisted-pair cabling.

100BaseVG   Star topology using round-robin for allowing systems to transmit data on the network.

100VG (Voice Grade)   IEEE 802.12 standard for 100BaseVG networks.

100VGAnyLAN   A networking technology that runs 100Mb Ethernet over regular (Cat 3) phone lines. It hasn't gained the industry acceptance that 100BaseT has. *See also* AnyLAN.

A

access control list (ACL)   List of rights that an object has to resources in the network. Also a type of firewall. In this case, the lists reside on a router and determine which machines can use the router and in what direction.

ACK   *See* acknowledgment.

acknowledgment (ACK)   A message confirming that the data packet was received. This occurs at the Transport layer of the OSI model.

ACL   *See* access control list.

Active Directory   The replacement for NT Directory Service (NTDS) that is included with Windows 2000. It acts similarly to NDS (Novell Directory Services) because it is a true X.500-based directory service.

active hub   A hub that is powered and actively regenerates any signal that is received. *See also* hub.

active monitor   Used in Token Ring networks, a process that prevents data frames from roaming the ring unchecked. If the frame passes the active monitor too many times, it is removed from the ring. Also ensures that a token is always circulating the ring.

adapter   Technically, the peripheral hardware that installs into your computer or the software that defines how the computer talks to that hardware.

address   Designation to allow PCs to be known by a name or number to other PCs. Addressing allows a PC to transmit data directly to another PC by using its address (IP or MAC).

address record   Part of a DNS table that maps an IP address to a domain name. Also known as an A (or host) record.

ad hoc RF network   A network created when two RF-capable devices are brought within transmission range of each other. A common example is hand-held PDAs beaming data to each other.

ADSL   *See* asymmetrical digital subscriber line.

alias record   *See* CNAME record.

antivirus   A category of software that uses various methods to eliminate viruses in a computer. It typically also protects against future infection. *See also* virus.

AnyLAN   Another name for 100VGAnyLAN created in 802.12. *See also* 100VGAnyLAN.

Application layer   The seventh layer of the OSI model, which deals with how applications access the network and describes application functionality, such as file transfer, messaging, and so on.

ARCnet   The Attached Resource Computer Network, which was developed by Datapoint Corporation in the late 1970s as one of the first baseband networks. It can use either a physical star or bus topology.

ARP table   A table used by the ARP protocol. Contains a list of known TCP/IP addresses and their associated MAC addresses. The table is cached in memory so that ARP lookups do not have to be performed for frequently accessed TCP/IP and MAC addresses. *See also* media access control, Transmission Control Protocol/Internet Protocol.

asymmetrical digital subscriber line (ADSL)   An implementation of DSL where the upload and download speeds are different. *See also* digital subscriber line.

Asynchronous Transfer Mode (ATM)   A connection-oriented network architecture based on broadband ISDN technology that uses constant size 53-byte cells instead of packets. Because cells don't change size, they are switched much faster and more efficiently than packets across a network.

ATM   *See* Asynchronous Transfer Mode.

Attachment Unit Interface (AUI) port   Port on some NICs that allows connecting the NIC to different media types by using an external transceiver.

B

backbone   The part of most networks that connects multiple segments together to form a LAN. The backbone usually has higher speed than the segments. *See also* segment, local area network.

Backup Domain Controller (BDC)   Computer on a Windows NT network that has a copy of the SAM database for fault tolerance and performance enhancement purposes. *See also* Security Accounts Manager.

backup plan   Term used to describe a company's strategy to make copies of and restore its data in case of an emergency.

backup window   The amount of time that an administrator has available to perform a complete, successful backup.

bandwidth   In network communications, the amount of data that can be sent across a wire in a given time. Each communication that passes along the wire decreases the amount of available bandwidth.

baseband   A transmission technique in which the signal uses the entire bandwidth of a transmission medium.

baseline   A category of network documentation that indicates how the network normally runs. It includes such information as network statistics, server utilization trends, and processor performance statistics.

bearer channel (B channel)   The channels in an ISDN line that carry data. Each bearer channel typically has a bandwidth of 64Kbps.

blackout   *See* power blackout.

blank   These are often referred to as slot covers. If a PC card is removed, there will be an opening in the computer case. This will allow dirt and dust to enter the computer and prevent it from being cooled properly. Some computer cases have the blanks as part of the case, and they must be broken off from the case before a bus slot may be used to insert a PC card into it.

BNC connector   Tubular connectors most commonly used with coaxial cable.

bonding   A procedure where two ISDN B channels are joined together to provide greater bandwidth.

bounded media   A network medium that is used at the Physical layer where the signal travels over a cable of some kind.

bridge   A network device, operating at the Data Link layer, that logically separates a single network into segments, but lets the two segments appear to be one network to higher layer protocols.

broadband   A network transmission method in which a single transmission medium is divided so that multiple signals can travel across the same medium simultaneously.

broadcast address   A special network address that refers to all users on the network. For example, the TCP/IP address 255.255.255.255 is the broadcast address. Any packets sent to that address will be sent to everyone on that LAN.

brouter   A device that combines the functionality of a bridge and a router, but can't be distinctly classified as either.

brownout   *See* power brownout.

bus   Pathways in a PC that allow data and signals to be transmitted between the PC components. Types of buses include ISA and PCI.

bus topology   A topology where the cable and signals run in a straight line from one end of the network to the other.

C

cable   A physical transmission medium that has a central conductor of wire or fiber surrounded by a plastic jacket.

cable map   General network documentation indicating each cable's source and destination as well as where each network cable runs.

cable tester   A special instrument that is used to test the integrity of LAN cables. *See also* time-domain reflectometer.

carrier   Signal at a frequency that is chosen to carry data. Addition of data to the frequency is modulation and the removal of data from the frequency is demodulation. This is used on analog devices like modems.

Carrier Sense Multiple Access/Collision Avoidance (CSMA/CA)   A media access method that sends a request to send (RTS) packet and waits to receive a clear to send (CTS) packet before sending. Once the CTS is received, the sender sends the packet of information.

Carrier Sense Multiple Access/Collision Detection (CSMA/CD)   A media access method that first senses whether there is a signal on the wire, indicating that someone is transmitting currently. If no one else is transmitting, it attempts a transmission and listens for someone else trying to transmit at the same time. If this happens, both senders back off and don't transmit again until some specified period of time has passed. *See also* collision.

categories   Different grades of cables that determine how much protection is offered against interference from outside the cable. Category 1 allows voice data only. Category 2 allows data transmissions up to 4Mbps. Category 3 allows data transmissions up to 10Mbps. Category 4 allows data transmissions up to 16Mbps. Category 5 allows data transmissions up to 100Mbps.

cell   Similar to a packet or frame, except that the ATM cell does not always contain the destination or source addressing information. It also does not contain higher-level addressing or packet control information.

central office   The office in any metropolitan or rural area that contains the telephone switching equipment for that area. The central office connects all users in that area to each other as well as to the rest of the PSTN. *See also* Public Switched Telephone Network.

Channel Service Unit (CSU)   Generally used with a T1 Internet line, it is used to terminate the connection from the T1 provider. The CSU is usually part of a CSU/DSU unit. It also provides diagnostics and testing if necessary.

checkpoints   A certain part or time to allow for a restart at the last point that the data was saved.

checksum   A hexadecimal value computed from transmitted data that is used in error-checking routines.

circuit switching   A switching method where a dedicated connection between the sender and receiver is maintained throughout the conversation.

Classless Internetwork Domain Routing (CIDR)   The new routing method used by InterNIC to assign IP addresses. CIDR can be described as a "slash x" network. The x represents the number of bits in the network that InterNIC controls.

client   A client is a part of a client/server network. It is the part where the computing is usually done. In a typical setting, a client will use the server for remote storage, backups, or security such as a firewall.

client/server network   A server-centric network in which all resources are stored on a file server and processing power is distributed among workstations and the file server.

clipper chip   A hardware implementation of the skipjack encryption algorithm.

clustering   A computing technology where many servers work together so that they appear to be one high-powered server. If one server fails, the others in the cluster take over the services provided by the failed server.

CNAME record   A DNS record type that specifies other names for existing hosts. This allows a DNS administrator to assign multiple DNS host names to a single DNS host. Also known as an *alias record*.

coaxial cable   Often referred to as coax. A type of cable used in network wiring. Typical coaxial cable types include RG-58 and RG-62. 10Base2 Ethernet networks use coaxial cable. Coaxial cable is usually shielded.

collision   The error condition that occurs when two stations on a CSMA/CD network transmit data (at the Data Link layer) at the same time. *See also* Carrier Sense Multiple Access/Collision Detection.

collision light   A light on a NIC or hub that indicates when a collision has occurred.

concentrator   *See* hub.

connectionless   Communications between two hosts that have no previous session established for synchronizing sent data. The data is not acknowledged at the receiving end. This can allow for data loss.

connectionless services   *See* connectionless, connectionless transport protocol.

connectionless transport protocol   A transport protocol, such as UDP, that does not create a virtual connection between sending and receiving stations. *See also* User Datagram Protocol.

connection-oriented   Communications between two hosts that have a previous session established for synchronizing sent data. The data is acknowledged by the receiving PC. This allows for guaranteed delivery of data between PCs.

connection-oriented transport protocol   A transport protocol that uses acknowledgments and responses to establish a virtual connection between sending and receiving stations. TCP is a connection-oriented protocol. *See also* Transmission Control Protocol.

controller   Part of a PC that allows connectivity to peripheral devices. A disk controller allows the PC to be connected to a hard disk. A network controller allows a PC to be connected to a network. A keyboard controller is used to connect a keyboard to the PC.

Control Panel   A special window inside Microsoft Windows operating systems (Windows 95 and above) that has icons for all of the configurable options for the system.

core OS   The core component, or kernel, of NetWare.

cost   A value given to a route between PCs or subnets to determine which route may be best. The word *hop* is sometimes used to refer to the number of routers between two PCs or subnets. *See also* hop.

country codes   The two-letter abbreviations for countries, used in the DNS hierarchy. *See also* Domain Name Service.

CRC   *See* cyclical redundancy check.

crossover cable   The troubleshooting tool used in Ethernet UTP installations to test communications between two stations, bypassing the hub. *See also* unshielded twisted-pair cable.

crosstalk   A type of interference that occurs when two LAN cables run close to each other. If one cable is carrying a signal and the other isn't, the one carrying a signal will induce a "ghost" signal (crosstalk) in the other cable.

CSMA/CA   *See* Carrier Sense Multiple Access/Collision Avoidance.

CSMA/CD   *See* Carrier Sense Multiple Access/Collision Detection.

cyclical redundancy check (CRC)   An error-checking method in data communications that runs a formula against data before transmissions. The sending station then appends the resultant value (called a checksum) to the data and sends it. The receiving station uses the same formula on the data. If the receiving station doesn't get the same checksum result for the calculation, it considers the transmission invalid, rejects the frame, and asks for a retransmission.

D

datagram   A unit of data smaller than a packet.

Data Link layer   The second layer of the OSI model. It describes the logical topology of a network, which is the way that packets move throughout a network. It also describes the method of media access. *See also* Open Systems Interconnect.

data packet   A unit of data sent over a network. A packet includes a header, addressing information, and the data itself. A packet is treated as a single unit as it is sent from device to device. Also known as a *datagram*.

Data Service Unit (DSU)   It transmits data through a Channel Service Unit (CSU) and is almost always a part of a single device referred to as a CSU/DSU.

D channel   *See* delta channel.

default gateway   The router that all packets are sent to when the workstation doesn't know where the destination station is or when it can't find the destination station on the local segment.

delta channel (D channel)   A channel on an ISDN line used for link management. *See also* Integrated Services Digital Network.

demarcation point (demarc)   The point on any telephone installation where the telephone lines from the central office enter the customer's premises.

denial of service (DoS) attack   Type of hack that prevents any users—even legitimate ones—from using the system.

destination port number   The address of the PC to which data is being sent from a sending PC. The port portion allows for the demultiplexing of data to be sent to a specific application.

DHCP   *See* Dynamic Host Configuration Protocol.

dialogs   Communications between two PCs.

digital subscriber line (DSL)   A digital WAN technology that brings high-speed digital networking to homes and businesses over POTS. There are many types, including HDSL (high-speed DSL) and VDSL (very high bit-rate DSL). *See also* plain old telephone service, asymmetrical digital subscriber line.

directory   A network database that contains a listing of all network resources, such as users, printers, groups, and so on.

directory service   A network service that provides access to a central database of information, which contains detailed information about the resources available on a network.

disaster recovery   The procedure by which data is recovered after a disaster.

disk striping   Technology that enables writing data to multiple disks simultaneously in small portions called stripes. These stripes maximize use by having all of the read/write heads working constantly. Different data is stored on each disk and is not automatically duplicated (this means that disk striping in and of itself does not provide fault tolerance).

distance vector routing protocol   A route discovery method in which each router, using broadcasts, tells every other router what networks and routes it knows about and the distance to them.

DIX   Another name for a 15-pin AUI connector or a DB-15 connector.

DNS   *See* Domain Name Service.

DNS server   Any server that performs DNS host name–to–IP address resolution. *See also* Domain Name Service, Internet Protocol.

DNS zone   An area in the DNS hierarchy that is managed as a single unit. *See also* Domain Name Service.

DoD Networking Model   A four-layer conceptual model describing how communications should take place between computer systems. The four layers are Process/Application, Host-to-Host, Internet, and Network Access.

domain   A group of networked Windows computers that share a single SAM database. *See also* Security Accounts Manager.

Domain Name Service (DNS)   The network service used in TCP/IP networks that translates host names to IP addresses. *See also* Transmission Control Protocol/Internet Protocol.

dotted decimal   Notation used by TCP/IP to designate an IP address. The notation is made up of 32 bits (4 bytes), each byte separated by a decimal. The range of numbers for each octet is 0–255. The leftmost octet contains the high-order bits and the rightmost octet contains the low-order bits.

DSL   *See* digital subscriber line.

D-type connector   The first type of networking connector, the D-type connector, is used to connect many peripherals to a PC. A D-type connector is characterized by its shape. Turned on its side, it looks like the letter *D* and contains rows of pins (male) or sockets (female). AUI connectors are examples.

dual-attached stations (DAS)   Stations on an FDDI network that are attached to both cables for connection redundancy and fault tolerance.

dumb terminal   A keyboard and monitor that send keystrokes to a central processing computer (typically a mainframe or minicomputer) that returns screen displays to the monitor. The unit has no processing power of its own, hence the moniker "dumb."

duplexed hard drives   Two hard drives to which identical information is written simultaneously. A dedicated controller card controls each drive. Used for fault tolerance.

duplicate server   Two servers that are identical for use in clustering.

dynamically allocated port   TCP/IP port used by an application when needed. The port is not constantly used.

dynamic ARP table entries   *See* dynamic entry.

dynamic entry   An entry made in the ARP table whenever an ARP request is made by the Windows TCP/IP stack and the MAC address is not found in the ARP table. The ARP request is broadcast on the local segment. When the MAC address of the requested IP address is found, that information is added to the ARP table. *See also* Internet Protocol, media access control, Transmission Control Protocol/Internet Protocol.

Dynamic Host Configuration Protocol (DHCP)   A protocol used on a TCP/IP network to send client configuration data, including TCP/IP address, default gateway, subnet mask, and DNS configuration, to clients. *See also* default gateway, Domain Name Service, subnet mask, Transmission Control Protocol/Internet Protocol.

dynamic packet filtering   A type of firewall used to accept or reject packets based on the contents of the packets.

dynamic routing   The use of route discovery protocols to talk to other routers and find out what networks they are attached to. Routers that use dynamic routing send out special packets to request updates of the other routers on the network as well as to send their own updates.

dynamic state list   *See* dynamic routing.

E

EEPROM   *See* electrically erasable programmable read-only memory.

electrically erasable programmable read-only memory (EEPROM)   A special integrated circuit on expansion cards that allows data to be stored on the chip. If necessary, the data can be erased by a special configuration program. Typically used to store hardware configuration data for expansion cards.

electromagnetic interference (EMI)   The interference that can occur during transmissions over copper cable because of electromagnetic energy outside the cable. The result is degradation of the signal.

electronic mail (e-mail)   An application that allows people to send messages via their computers on the same network or over the Internet.

electrostatic discharge (ESD)   A problem that exists when two items with dissimilar static electrical charges are brought together. The static electrical charges jump to the item with fewer electrical charges, causing ESD, which can damage computer components.

e-mail   *See* electronic mail.

EMI   *See* electromagnetic interference.

encoding   The process of translating data into signals that can be transmitted on a transmission medium.

encryption key   The string of alphanumeric characters used to decrypt encrypted data.

endpoint   The two ends of a connection for transmitting data. One end is the receiver, and the other is the sender.

ESD   *See* electrostatic discharge.

Ethernet   A shared-media network architecture. It operates at the Physical and Data Link layers of the OSI model. As the media access method, it uses baseband signaling over either a bus or a star topology with CSMA/CD. The cabling used in Ethernet networks can be coax, twisted-pair, or fiber-optic. *See also* Carrier Sense Multiple Access/Collision Detection, Open Systems Interconnect.

Ethernet address   *See* MAC address.

expansion slot   A slot on the computer's bus into which expansion cards are plugged to expand the functionality of the computer (for example, using a NIC to add the computer to a network). *See also* network interface card.

extended AppleTalk network   An AppleTalk network segment that is assigned a 16-bit range of numbers rather than a single 16-bit number.

F

failover device   A device that comes online when another fails.

failover server   A hot site backup system in which the failover server is connected to the primary server. A heartbeat is sent from the primary server to the backup server. If the heartbeat stops, the failover system starts and takes over. Thus, the system doesn't go down even if the primary server is not running.

Fast Ethernet   The general category name given to 100Mbps Ethernet technologies.

fault-resistant network   A network that will be up and running at least 99 percent of the time or that is down less than 8 hours a year.

fault-tolerant network   A network that can recover from minor errors.

FDDI   *See* Fiber Distributed Data Interface.

Fiber Channel   A type of server-to-storage system connection that uses fiber-optic connectors.

Fiber Distributed Data Interface (FDDI)   A network topology that uses fiber-optic cable as a transmission medium and dual, counterrotating rings to provide data delivery and fault tolerance.

fiber-optic   A type of network cable that uses a central glass or plastic core surrounded by a plastic coating.

file server   A server specialized in holding and distributing files.

File Transfer Protocol (FTP)   A TCP/IP protocol and software that permit the transferring of files between computer systems. Because FTP has been implemented on numerous types of computer systems, files can be transferred between disparate computer systems (for example, a personal computer and a minicomputer). *See also* Transmission Control Protocol/Internet Protocol.

firewall   A combination of hardware and software that protects a network from attack by hackers who could gain access through public networks, including the Internet.

FQDN   *See* Fully Qualified Domain Name.

frame relay   A WAN technology that transmits packets over a WAN using packet switching. *See also* packet switching.

frequency division multiplexing (FDM)   A multiplexing technique whereby the different signals are sent across multiple frequencies.

FTP   *See* File Transfer Protocol.

FTP proxy   A server that uploads and downloads files from a server on behalf of a workstation.

full backup   A backup that copies all data to the archive medium.

Fully Qualified Domain Name (FQDN)   An address that uses both the host name (workstation name) and the domain name.

G

gateway   The hardware and software needed to connect two disparate network environments so that communications can occur.

global group   A type of group in Windows NT that is used network-wide. Members can be from anywhere in the network, and rights can be assigned to any resource in the network.

ground loop   A condition that occurs when a signal cycles through a common ground connection between two devices, causing EMI interference. *See also* electromagnetic interference.

H

hardware address   A Data Link layer address assigned to every NIC at the MAC sublayer. The address is in the format xx:xx:xx:xx:xx:xx; each xx is a two-digit hexadecimal number. *See also* media access control, network interface card.

hardware loopback   Connects the transmission pins directly to the receiving pins, allowing diagnostic software to test if a NIC can successfully transmit and receive. *See also* network interface card.

heartbeat   The data transmissions between two servers in a cluster to detect when one fails. When the standby server detects no heartbeats from the main server, it comes online and takes control of the responsibilities of the main server. This allows for all services to remain online and accessible.

hop   One pass through a router. *See also* cost, router.

hop count   As a packet travels over a network through multiple routers, each router will increment this field in the packet by one as it crosses the router. It is used to limit the number of routers a packet can cross on the way to its destination.

host   Any network device with a TCP/IP network address. *See also* Transmission Control Protocol/Internet Protocol.

Host-to-Host layer   A layer in the DoD model that corresponds to the Transport layer of the OSI model. *See also* DoD Networking Model, Open Systems Interconnect.

HTML   *See* Hypertext Markup Language.

HTTP   *See* Hypertext Transfer Protocol.

hub   A Physical layer device that serves as a central connection point for several network devices. A hub repeats the signals it receives on one port to all other ports. *See also* active hub.

Hypertext Markup Language (HTML)   A set of codes used to format text and graphics that will be displayed in a browser. The codes define how data will be displayed.

Hypertext Transfer Protocol (HTTP)   The protocol used for communication between a web server and a web browser.

I

IBM data connector   A proprietary data connector created by IBM. This connector is unique because there isn't a male version and female version; any IBM connector can connect with another IBM connector and lock together.

ICMP   *See* Internet Control Message Protocol.

IEEE   *See* Institute of Electrical and Electronics Engineers, Inc.

IEEE 802.x standards   The IEEE standards for LAN and MAN networking.

IEEE 802.1 LAN/MAN Management   Standard that specifies LAN/MAN network management and internetworking.

IEEE 802.2 Logical Link Control   Standard that specifies the operation of the logical link control (LLC) sublayer of the Data Link layer of the OSI model. The LLC sublayer provides an interface between the MAC sublayer and the Network layer. *See also* media access control, Open Systems Interconnect.

IEEE 802.3 CSMA/CD Networking   Standard that specifies a network that uses Ethernet technology and a CSMA/CD network access method. *See also* Carrier Sense Multiple Access/Collision Detection.

IEEE 802.4 Token Bus   Standard that specifies a physical and logical bus topology that uses coaxial or fiber-optic cable and the token-passing media access method.

IEEE 802.5 Token Ring   Specifies a logical ring, physical star, and token-passing media access method based on IBM's Token Ring.

IEEE 802.6 Distributed Queue Dual Bus (DQDB) Metropolitan Area Network   Provides a definition and criteria for a DQDB metropolitan area network (MAN).

IEEE 802.7 Broadband Local Area Networks   Standard for broadband cabling technology.

IEEE 802.8 Fiber-Optic LANs and MANs   A standard containing guidelines for the use of fiber optics on networks, which includes FDDI and Ethernet over fiber-optic cable. *See also* Ethernet, Fiber Distributed Data Interface.

IEEE 802.9 Integrated Services (IS) LAN Interface   A standard containing guidelines for the integration of voice and data over the same cable.

IEEE 802.10 LAN/MAN Security   A series of guidelines dealing with various aspects of network security.

IEEE 802.11 Wireless LAN   Defines standards for implementing wireless technologies such as infrared and spread-spectrum radio.

IEEE 802.12 Demand Priority Access Method   Defines a standard that combines the concepts of Ethernet and ATM. *See also* Asynchronous Transfer Mode, Ethernet.

IETF   *See* Internet Engineering Task Force.

Institute of Electrical and Electronics Engineers, Inc. (IEEE)   An international organization that sets standards for various electrical and electronics issues.

Integrated Services Digital Network (ISDN)   A telecommunications standard that is used to digitally send voice, data, and video signals over the same lines. *See also* delta channel.

intelligent hub   A hub that can make some intelligent decisions about network traffic flow and can provide network traffic statistics to network administrators.

internal bridge   A bridge created by placing two NICs in a computer.

internal modem   A modem that is a regular PC card that is inserted into the bus slot. These modems are inside the PC.

International Organization for Standardization (ISO)   The standards organization that developed the OSI model. This model provides a guideline for how communications occur between computers.

Internet   A global network made up of a large number of individual networks interconnected through the use of public telephone lines and TCP/IP protocols. *See also* Transmission Control Protocol/Internet Protocol.

Internet Architecture Board (IAB)   The committee that oversees management of the Internet. It is made up of two subcommittees: the Internet Engineering Task Force (IETF) and the Internet Research Task Force (IRTF). *See also* Internet Engineering Task Force, Internet Research Task Force.

Internet Control Message Protocol (ICMP)   A message and management protocol for TCP/IP. The Ping utility uses ICMP. *See also* Ping, Transmission Control Protocol/Internet Protocol.

Internet Engineering Task Force (IETF)   An international organization that works under the Internet Architecture Board to establish standards and protocols relating to the Internet. *See also* Internet Architecture Board.

Internet Protocol (IP)   The protocol in the TCP/IP protocol suite responsible for network addressing and routing. *See also* Transmission Control Protocol/ Internet Protocol.

Internet Research Task Force (IRTF)   An international organization that works under the Internet Architecture Board to research new Internet technologies. *See also* Internet Architecture Board.

Internet service provider (ISP)   A company that provides direct access to the Internet for home and business computer users.

internetwork   A network that is internal to a company and is private.

Internetwork Packet eXchange (IPX)   A connectionless, routable network protocol based on the Xerox XNS architecture. It is the default protocol for versions of NetWare before NetWare 5. It operates at the Network layer of the OSI model and is responsible for addressing and routing packets to workstations or servers on other networks. *See also* Open Systems Interconnect.

inverse multiplexing   The network technology that allows one signal to be split across multiple transmission lines at the transmission source and combined at the receiving end.

IP   *See* Internet Protocol.

IP address   An address used by the Internet Protocol that identifies the device's location on the network.

ipconfig   A Windows NT utility used to display that machine's current configuration.

IP proxy   All communications look as if they originated from a proxy server because the IP address of the user making a request is hidden. Also known as *Network Address Translation (NAT)*.

IP spoofing   A hacker trying to gain access to a network by pretending his or her machine has the same network address as the internal network.

IPX   *See* Internetwork Packet eXchange.

IPX network address   A number that represents an entire network. All servers on the network must use the same external network number.

ISDN   *See* Integrated Services Digital Network.

ISDN terminal adapter   The device used on ISDN networks to connect a local network (or single machine) to an ISDN network. It provides power to the line as well as translates data from the LAN or individual computer for transmission on the ISDN line. *See also* Integrated Services Digital Network.

ISP   *See* Internet service provider.

J

Java   A programming language, developed by Sun Microsystems, that is used to write programs that will run on any platform that has a Java Virtual Machine installed.

Java Virtual Machine (JVM)   Software, developed by Sun Microsystems, that creates a virtual Java computer on which Java programs can run. A programmer writes a program once without having to recompile or rewrite the program for all platforms.

jumper   A small connector (cap or plug) that connects pins. This creates a circuit that indicates a setting to a device.

JVM   *See* Java Virtual Machine.

K

kernel   The core component of any operating system that handles the functions of memory management, hardware interaction, and program execution.

key   A folder in the Windows Registry that contains subkeys and values, or a value with an algorithm to encrypt and decrypt data.

L

LAN   *See* local area network.

LAN driver   The interface between the NetWare kernel and the NIC installed in the server. Also a general category of drivers used to enable communications between an operating system and a NIC. *See also* network interface card.

Large Internet Packet (LIP)   A technology used by the IPX protocol so that IPX can use the largest possible packet size during a transmission. *See also* Internetwork Packet eXchange.

laser printer   A printer that uses a laser to form an image on a photo-sensitive drum. The image is then developed with toner and transferred to paper. Finally, a heated drum fuses toner particles onto the paper.

Layer 2 Switch   A switching hub that operates at the Data Link layer and builds a table of the MAC addresses of all the connected stations. *See also* media access control.

Layer 3 Switch   Functioning at the Network layer, a switch that performs the multiport, virtual LAN, data pipelining functions of a standard Layer 2 Switch, but it can perform basic routing functions between virtual LANs.

LCP   *See* Link Control Protocol.

line conditioner   A device used to protect against power surges and spikes. Line conditioners use several electronic methods to clean all power coming into the line conditioner.

line noise   Any extraneous signal on a power line that is not part of the power feed.

line voltage   The voltage, supplied from the power company, that comes out at the outlets.

Link Control Protocol (LCP)   The protocol used to establish, configure, and test the link between a client and PPP host. *See also* Point-to-Point Protocol.

link light   A small light-emitting diode (LED) that is found on both the NIC and the hub. It is usually green and labeled "Link" or something similar. A link light indicates that the NIC and the hub are making a Data Link layer connection. *See also* hub, network interface card.

link state route discovery   A route discovery method that transmits special packets (Link State Packets, or LSPs) that contain information about the networks to which the router is connected.

link state routing   A type of routing that broadcasts its entire routing tables only at startup and possibly at infrequently scheduled intervals. Aside from that, the router only sends messages to other routers when changes are made to the router's routing table.

link state routing protocol   A routing table protocol where the router sends out limited information, such as updates to its routing tables, to its neighbors only.

Link Support Layer (LSL)   Part of the Novell client software that acts as sort of a switchboard between the Open Datalink Interface (ODI) LAN drivers and the various transport protocols.

Linux   A version of Unix, developed by Linus Torvalds. Runs on Intel-based PCs and is generally free. *See also* Unix.

LIP   *See* Large Internet Packet.

local area network (LAN)   A network that is restricted to a single building, group of buildings, or even a single room. A LAN can have one or more servers.

local groups   Groups created on individual servers. Rights can be assigned only to local resources.

local loop   The part of the PSTN that goes from the central office to the demarcation point at the customer's premises. *See also* central office, demarcation point, Public Switched Telephone Network.

log file   A file that keeps a running list of all errors and notices, the time and date they occurred, and any other pertinent information.

logical bus topology   Type of topology in which the signal travels the distance of the cable and is received by all stations on the backbone. *See also* backbone.

logical link control (LLC)   A sublayer of the Data Link layer. Provides an interface between the MAC sublayer and the Network layer. *See also* media access control, topology.

logical network addressing   The addressing scheme used by protocols at the Network layer.

logical parallel port   Port used by the CAPTURE command to redirect a workstation printer port to a network print queue. The logical port has no relation to the port to which the printer is actually attached or to the physical port. *See also* physical parallel port.

logical port address   A value that is used at the Transport layer to differentiate between the upper-layer services.

logical ring topology   A network topology in which all network signals travel from one station to another, being read and forwarded by each station.

logical topology   Describes the way the information flows. The types of logical topologies are the same as the physical topologies, except that the flow of information, rather than the physical arrangement, specifies the type of topology.

LSL   *See* Link Support Layer.

M

MAC   *See* media access control.

MAC address   The address that is either assigned to a network card or burned into the NIC. This is how PCs keep track of one another and keep each other separate.

mail exchange (MX) record   A DNS record type that specifies the DNS host name of the mail server for a particular domain name.

MAU   *See* Multistation Access Unit.

media access   The process of vying for transmission time on the network media.

media access control (MAC)   A sublayer of the Data Link layer that controls the way multiple devices use the same media channel. It controls which devices can transmit and when they can transmit.

media converter   A networking device that converts from one network media type to another. For example, converting from an AUI port to an RJ-45 connector for 10BaseT.

member server   A computer that has Windows NT server installed but doesn't have a copy of the SAM database. *See also* Security Accounts Manager.

mesh topology   A network topology where there is a connection from each station to every other station in the network.

modem   A communication device that converts digital computer signals into analog tones for transmission over the PSTN and converts them back to digital upon reception. The word "modem" is an acronym for "modulator/demodulator."

multiple-server clustering   A system in which multiple servers run continuously, each providing backup and production services at the same time. (Expensive servers, therefore, are not sitting around as designated "backup" servers, used only when an emergency arises.) If a server fails, another just takes over, without any interruption of service.

multiplexing   A technology that combines multiple signals into one signal for transmission over a slow medium. *See also* frequency division multiplexing, inverse multiplexing.

multipoint RF network   An RF network consisting of multiple stations, each with transmitters and receivers. This type of network also requires an RF bridge as a central sending and receiving point.

Multistation Access Unit (MAU)   The central device in Token Ring networks that acts as the connection point for all stations and facilitates the formation of the ring.

N

name resolution   The process of translating (resolving) logical host names to network addresses.

NAT   Acronym that means Network Address Translation. *See* IP proxy.

National Computing Security Center (NCSC)   The agency that developed the Trusted Computer System Evaluation Criteria (TCSEC) and the Trusted Network Interpretation Environmental Guideline (TNIEG).

National Security Agency (NSA)   The U.S. government agency responsible for protecting U.S. communications and producing foreign intelligence information. It was established by presidential directive in 1952 as a separately organized agency within the Department of Defense (DoD).

nbtstat (NetBIOS over TCP/IP statistics)   The Windows TCP/IP utility that is used to display NetBIOS over TCP/IP statistics. *See also* network basic input/output system, Transmission Control Protocol/Internet Protocol.

NCP   *See* NetWare Core Protocol.

NCSC   *See* National Computing Security Center.

NDPS   *See* Novell Distributed Print Services.

NDS   *See* Novell Directory Services.

NDS tree   A logical representation of a network's resources. Resources are represented by objects in the tree. The tree is often designed after a company's functional structure. Objects can represent organizations, departments, users, servers, printers, and other resources. *See also* Novell Directory Services.

nearline site   When two buildings can almost be seen from one another. Obstructions in between are few.

NetBEUI   *See* NetBIOS Extended User Interface.

NetBIOS   *See* network basic input/output system.

NetBIOS Extended User Interface (NetBEUI)   Transport protocol based on the NetBIOS protocol that has datagram support and support for connectionless transmission. NetBEUI is a protocol that is native to Microsoft networks and is mainly for use by small businesses. It is a nonroutable protocol that cannot pass over a router, but does pass over a bridge since it operates at the Data Link layer. *See also* network basic input/output system.

NetBIOS name   The unique name used to identify and address a computer using NetBEUI.

netstat   A utility used to determine which TCP/IP connections—inbound or outbound—the computer has. It also allows the user to view packet statistics, such as how many packets have been sent and received. *See also* Transmission Control Protocol/Internet Protocol.

NetWare   The network operating system made by Novell.

NetWare 3.x   The version series of NetWare that supported multiple, cross-platform clients with fairly minimal hardware requirements. It used a database called the bindery to keep track of users and groups and was administered with several DOS, menu-based utilities (such as SYSCON, PCONSOLE, and FILER).

NetWare 4.x   The version series of NetWare that includes NDS. *See also* Novell Directory Services.

NetWare 5.x   The version series of NetWare that includes a multiprocessing kernel. It also includes a five-user version of Oracle 8, a relational database, and the ability to use TCP/IP in its pure form.

NetWare Administrator   The utility used to administer NetWare versions 4.*x* and later by making changes to the NDS Directory. It is the only administrative utility needed to modify NDS objects and their properties. *See also* Novell Directory Services.

NetWare Core Protocol (NCP)   The upper-layer NetWare protocol that functions on top of IPX and provides NetWare resource access to workstations. *See also* Internet Packet eXchange.

NetWare Link State Protocol (NLSP)   Protocol that gathers routing information based on the link state routing method. Its precursor is the Routing Information Protocol (RIP). NLSP is a more efficient routing protocol than RIP. *See also* link state routing.

NetWare Loadable Module (NLM)   A component used to provide a NetWare server with additional services and functionality. Unneeded services can be unloaded, thus conserving memory.

network   A group of devices connected by some means for the purpose of sharing information or resources.

Network Address Translation (NAT)   *See* IP proxy.

network attached storage   Storage, such as hard drives, attached to a network for the purpose of storing data for clients on the network. Network attached storage is commonly used for backing up data.

network basic input/output system (NetBIOS)   A Session layer protocol that opens communication sessions for applications that want to communicate on a network.

network-centric   Refers to network operating systems that use directory services to maintain information about the entire network.

Network File System (NFS)   A protocol that enables users to access files on remote computers as if the files were local.

network interface card (NIC)   Physical device that connects computers and other network equipment to the transmission medium.

Network layer   This third layer of the OSI model is responsible for logical addressing and translating logical names into physical addresses. This layer also controls the routing of data from source to destination as well as the building and dismantling of packets. *See also* Open Systems Interconnect.

network media   The physical cables that link computers in a network; also known as *physical media*.

network operating system (NOS)   The software that runs on a network server and offers file, print, application, and other services to clients.

network software diagnostics   Software tools, either Protocol Analyzers or Performance Monitoring Tools, used to troubleshoot network problems.

Network Support Encyclopedia (NSEPro)   *See* Novell Support Connection.

NFS   *See* Network File System.

NIC   *See* network interface card.

NIC diagnostics   Software utilities that verify the NIC is functioning correctly and test every aspect of NIC operation. *See also* network interface card.

NIC driver   *See* LAN driver.

NLM   *See* NetWare Loadable Module.

NLSP   *See* NetWare Link State Protocol.

non-unicast packet   A packet that is not sent directly from one workstation to another.

NOS   *See* network operating system.

Novell Directory Services (NDS)   A NetWare service that provides access to a global, hierarchical directory database of network entities that can be centrally managed.

Novell Distributed Print Services (NDPS)   A printing system designed by Novell that uses NDS to install and manage printers. NDPS supports automatic network printer installation, automatic distribution of client printer drivers, and centralized printer management without the use of print queues.

Novell Support Connection   Novell's database of technical information documents, files, patches, fixes, NetWare Application Notes, Novell lab bulletins, Novell professional developer bulletins, answers to frequently asked questions, and more. The database is available from Novell and is updated quarterly.

NSA   *See* National Security Agency.

N-series connector Used with Thinnet and Thicknet cabling that is a male/female screw and barrel connector.

nslookup Allows you to query a name server to see which IP address a name resolves to.

NT Directory Services (NTDS) System of domains and trusts for a Windows NT Server network.

NTDS *See* NT Directory Services.

O

object The item that represents some network entity in NDS. *See also* Novell Directory Services.

octet Refers to eight bits; one-fourth of an IP address.

ODI *See* Open Datalink Interface.

OE (operator error) When the error is not software or hardware related, it may be a problem with the user not knowing how to operate the software or hardware. OE can be a serious problem.

offline The general name for the condition when some piece of electronic or computer equipment is unavailable or inoperable.

Open Datalink Interface (ODI) A driver specification, developed by Novell, that enables a single workstation to communicate transparently with several different protocol stacks, using a single NIC and a single NIC driver.

OpenLinux A version of the Linux network operating system developed by Caldera.

Open Systems Interconnect (OSI) A model defined by the ISO to categorize the process of communication between computers in terms of seven layers. The seven layers are Application, Presentation, Session, Transport, Network, Data Link, and Physical. *See also* International Organization for Standardization.

OSI *See* Open Systems Interconnect.

oversampling Method of synchronous bit synchronization in which the receiver samples the signal at a much faster rate than the data rate. This permits the use of an encoding method that does not add clocking transitions.

overvoltage threshold   The level of overvoltage that will trip the circuit breaker in a surge protector.

P

packet   The basic division of data sent over a network.

packet filtering   A firewall technology that accepts or rejects packets based on their content.

packet switching   The process of breaking messages into packets at the sending router for easier transmission over a WAN. *See also* frame relay.

passive detection   A type of intruder detection that logs all network events to a file for an administrator to view later.

passive hub   A hub that simply makes physical and electrical connections between all connected stations. Generally speaking, these hubs are not powered.

password history   List of passwords that have already been used.

patch   Software that fixes a problem with an existing program or operating system.

patch cable   A central wiring point for multiple devices on a UTP network. *See also* unshielded twisted-pair cable.

patch panel   A central wiring point, containing no electronic circuits, for multiple devices on a UTP network. Generally, patch panels are in server rooms or located near switches or hubs to provide an easy means of patching over wall jacks or hardware.

PDC   *See* Primary Domain Controller.

peer-to-peer network   Computers hooked together that have no centralized authority. Each computer is equal and can act as both a server and a workstation.

peripheral   Any device that can be attached to the computer to expand its capabilities.

permanent virtual circuit (PVC)   A technology used by frame relay that allows virtual data communications (circuits) to be set up between sender and receiver over a packet-switched network.

PGP *See* Pretty Good Privacy.

physical address *See* MAC address.

physical bus topology A network that uses one network cable that runs from one end of the network to the other. Workstations connect at various points along this cable.

Physical layer The first layer of the OSI model that controls the functional interface. *See also* Open Systems Interconnect.

physical media *See* network media.

physical mesh topology A network configuration in which each device has multiple connections. These multiple connections provide redundant connections.

physical parallel port A port on the back of a computer that allows a printer to be connected with a parallel cable.

physical port An opening on a network device that allows a cable of some kind to be connected. Ports allow devices to be connected to each other with cables.

physical ring topology A network topology that is set up in a circular fashion. Data travels around the ring in one direction, and each device on the ring acts as a repeater to keep the signal strong as it travels. Each device incorporates a receiver for the incoming signal and a transmitter to send the data on to the next device in the ring. The network is dependent on the ability of the signal to travel around the ring.

physical star topology Describes a network in which a cable runs from each network entity to a central device called a hub. The hub allows all devices to communicate as if they were directly connected. *See also* hub.

physical topology The physical layout of a network, such as bus, star, ring, or mesh.

Ping A TCP/IP utility used to test whether another host is reachable. An ICMP request is sent to the host, who responds with a reply if it is reachable. The request times out if the host is not reachable.

Ping of Death A large ICMP packet sent to overflow the remote host's buffer. This usually causes the remote host to reboot or hang.

plain old telephone service (POTS)   Another name for the Public Switched Telephone Network (PSTN). *See* asymmetrical digital subscriber line, digital subscriber line, Public Switched Telephone Network.

plenum-rated coating   Coaxial cable coating that does not produce toxic gas when burned.

point-to-point   Network communication in which two devices have exclusive access to a network medium. For example, a printer connected to only one workstation would be using a point-to-point connection.

Point-to-Point Protocol (PPP)   The protocol used with dial-up connections to the Internet. Its functions include error control, security, dynamic IP addressing, and support for multiple protocols.

Point-to-Point Tunneling Protocol (PPTP)   A protocol that allows the creation of virtual private networks (VPNs), which allow users to access a server on a corporate network over a secure, direct connection via the Internet. *See also* virtual private network.

polling   A media access control method that uses a central device called a controller that polls each device in turn and asks if it has data to transmit.

POP3   *See* Post Office Protocol version 3.

port   Some kind of opening that allows network data to pass through. *See also* physical port.

Post Office Protocol version 3 (POP3)   The protocol used to download e-mail from an SMTP e-mail server to a network client. *See also* Simple Mail Transfer Protocol.

POTS   *See* plain old telephone service.

power blackout   A total loss of power that may last for only a few seconds or as long as several hours.

power brownout   Power drops below normal levels for several seconds or longer.

power overage   Too much power is coming into the computer. *See also* power spike, power surge.

power sag   A lower power condition where the power drops below normal levels for a few seconds, then returns to normal levels.

power spike   The power level rises above normal for less than a second and drops back to normal.

power surge   The power level rises above normal and stays there for longer than a second or two.

power underage   The power level drops below the standard level. *See also* power sag.

PPP   *See* Point-to-Point Protocol.

PPTP   *See* Point-to-Point Tunneling Protocol.

Presentation layer   The sixth layer of the OSI model; responsible for formatting data exchange such as graphic commands and conversion of character sets. Also responsible for data compression, data encryption, and data stream redirection. *See also* Open Systems Interconnect.

Pretty Good Privacy (PGP)   A shareware implementation of RSA encryption. *See also* RSA Data Security, Inc.

Primary Domain Controller (PDC)   An NT server that contains a master copy of the SAM database. This database contains all usernames, passwords, and access control lists for a Windows NT domain. *See also* Security Accounts Manager.

print server   A centralized device that controls and manages all network printers. The print server can be hardware, software, or a combination of both. Some print servers are actually built into the network printer NICs. *See also* network interface card.

print services   The network services that manage and control printing on a network, allowing multiple and simultaneous access to printers.

private key   A technology in which both the sender and the receiver have the same key. A single key is used to encrypt and decrypt all messages. *See also* public key.

private network   The part of a network that lies behind a firewall and is not "seen" on the Internet. *See also* firewall.

protocol   A predefined set of rules that dictates how computers or devices communicate and exchange data on the network.

protocol analyzer   A software and hardware troubleshooting tool that is used to decode protocol information to try to determine the source of a network problem and to establish baselines.

protocol suite   The set of rules a computer uses to communicate with other computers.

proxy   A type of firewall that prevents direct communication between a client and a host by acting as an intermediary. *See also* firewall.

proxy cache server   An implementation of a web proxy. The server receives an HTTP request from a web browser and makes the request on behalf of the sending workstation. When the response comes, the proxy cache server caches a copy of the response locally. The next time someone makes a request for the same web page or Internet information, the proxy cache server can fulfill the request out of the cache instead of having to retrieve the resource from the Web.

proxy server   A type of server that makes a single Internet connection and services requests on behalf of many users.

PSTN   *See* Public Switched Telephone Network.

public   For use by everyone.

public key   A technology that uses two keys to facilitate communication, a public key and a private key. The public key is used to encrypt a message to a receiver. *See also* private key.

public network   The part of a network on the outside of a firewall that is exposed to the public. *See also* firewall.

Public Switched Telephone Network (PSTN)   This is the U.S. public telephone network. It is also called the plain old telephone service (POTS). *See also* central office.

punchdown tool   A hand tool used to terminate twisted-pair wires on a wall jack or patch panel.

PVC   *See* permanent virtual circuit.

Q

QoS   *See* Quality of Service.

quad decimal   Four sets of octets separated by a decimal point; an IP address.

Quality of Service (QoS)   Data prioritization at the Network layer of the OSI model. Results in guaranteed throughput rates. *See also* Open Systems Interconnect.

R

radio frequency interference (RFI)   Interference on copper cabling systems caused by radio frequencies.

RAID   *See* Redundant Array of Independent (or Inexpensive) Disks.

RAID levels   The different types of RAID, such as RAID 0, RAID 1, etc.

README file   A file that the manufacturer includes with software to give the installer information that came too late to make it into the software manuals. It's usually a last-minute addition that includes tips on installing the software, possible incompatibilities, and any known installation problems that might have been found right before the product was shipped.

reduced instruction set computing (RISC)   Computer architecture in which the computer executes small, general-purpose instructions very rapidly.

Redundant Array of Independent (or Inexpensive) Disks (RAID)   A configuration of multiple hard disks used to provide fault tolerance should a disk fail. Different levels of RAID exist, depending on the amount and type of fault tolerance provided.

regeneration process   Process in which signals are read, amplified, and repeated on the network to reduce signal degradation, which results in longer overall possible length of the network.

remote access protocol   Any networking protocol that is used to gain access to a network over public communication links.

remote access server   A computer that has one or more modems installed to enable remote connections to the network.

repeater   A Physical layer device that amplifies the signals it receives on one port and resends or repeats them on another. A repeater is used to extend the maximum length of a network segment.

replication   The process of copying directory information to other servers to keep them all synchronized.

RFI   *See* radio frequency interference.

RG-58   The type designation for the coaxial cable used in thin Ethernet (10Base2). It has a 50ohm impedance rating and uses BNC connectors.

RG-62   The type designation for the coaxial cable used in ARCnet networks. It has a 93ohm impedance and uses BNC connectors.

ring topology   A network topology where each computer in the network is connected to exactly two other computers. With ring topology, a single break in the ring brings the entire network down.

RIP   *See* Router Information Protocol.

RISC   *See* reduced instruction set computing.

RJ (Registered Jack) connector   A modular connection mechanism that allows for as many as eight copper wires (four pairs). RJ connectors are most commonly used for telephone (such as the RJ-11) and network adaptors (such as RJ-45).

roaming profiles   Profiles downloaded from a server at each login. When a user logs out at the end of the session, changes are made and remembered for the next time the user logs in.

route   The path to get to the destination from a source.

route cost   How many router hops there are between source and destination in an internetwork. *See also* hop, router.

router   A device that connects two networks and allows packets to be transmitted and received between them. A router determines the best path for data packets from source to destination. *See also* hop.

Router Information Protocol (RIP)   A distance-vector route discovery protocol used by IPX. It uses hops and ticks to determine the cost for a particular route. *See also* Internet Packet eXchange.

routing   A function of the Network layer that involves moving data throughout a network. Data passes through several network segments using routers that can select the path the data takes. *See also* router.

routing table   A table that contains information about the locations of other routers on the network and their distance from the current router.

RSA Data Security, Inc.   A commercial company that produces encryption software. RSA stands for Rivest, Shamir, and Adleman, the founders of the company.

S

sag *See* power sag.

SAM *See* Security Accounts Manager.

Secure Hypertext Transfer Protocol (S-HTTP) A protocol used for secure communications between a web server and a web browser.

Security Accounts Manager (SAM) A database within Windows NT that contains information about all users and groups and their associated rights and settings within a Windows NT domain. *See also* Backup Domain Controller.

security log Log file used in Windows NT to keep track of security events specified by the domain's Audit policy.

security policy Rules set in place by a company to ensure the security of a network. This may include how often a password must be changed or how many characters a password should be.

segment A unit of data smaller than a packet. Also refers to a portion of a larger network (a network can consist of multiple network segments). *See also* backbone.

self-powered A device that has its own power.

Sequenced Packet eXchange (SPX) A connection-oriented protocol that is part of the IPX protocol suite. It operates at the Transport layer of the OSI model. It initiates the connection between the sender and receiver, transmits the data, and then terminates the connection. *See also* Internet Packet eXchange, Open Systems Interconnect.

sequence number A number used to determine the order in which parts of a packet are to be reassembled after the packet has been split into sections.

Serial Line Internet Protocol (SLIP) A protocol that permits the sending of IP packets over a serial connection.

server A computer that provides resources to the clients on the network.

server and client configuration A network in which the resources are located on a server for use by the clients.

server-centric A network design model that uses a central server to contain all data as well as control security.

service   Services add functionality to the network by providing resources or doing tasks for other computers. In Windows 9*x*, services include file and printer sharing for Microsoft or Novell networks.

service accounts   Accounts created on a server for users to perform special services, such as backup operators, account operators, and server operators.

Session layer   The fifth layer of the OSI model, it determines how two computers establish, use, and end a session. Security authentication and network naming functions required for applications occur here. The Session layer establishes, maintains, and breaks dialogs between two stations. *See also* Open Systems Interconnect.

share-level security   In a network that uses share-level security, instead of assigning rights to network resources to users, passwords are assigned to individual files or other network resources (such as printers). These passwords are then given to all users that need access to these resources. All resources are visible from anywhere in the network, and any user who knows the password for a particular network resource can make changes to it.

shell   Unix interfaces that are based solely upon command prompts. There is no graphical interface.

shielded   When cabling has extra wrapping to protect it from stray electrical or radio signals. Shielded cabling is more expensive than unshielded.

shielded twisted-pair cable (STP)   A type of cabling that includes pairs of copper conductors, twisted around each other, inside a metal or foil shield. This type of medium can support faster speeds than unshielded wiring.

S-HTTP   *See* Secure Hypertext Transfer Protocol.

signal   Transmission from one PC to another. This could be a notification to start a session or end a session.

signal encoding   The process whereby a protocol at the Physical layer receives information from the upper layers and translates all the data into signals that can be transmitted on a transmission medium.

signaling method   The process of transmitting data across the medium. Two types of signaling are digital and analog.

Simple Mail Transfer Protocol (SMTP)   A program that looks for mail on SMTP servers and sends it along the network to its destination at another SMTP server.

Simple Network Management Protocol (SNMP)   The management protocol created for sending information about the health of the network to network management consoles.

single-attached stations (SAS)   Stations on an FDDI network that are attached to only one of the cables. They are less fault tolerant than dual-attached stations.

skipjack   An encryption algorithm developed as a possible replacement for Data Encryption Standard (DES) that is classified by the National Security Agency (NSA). Not much is known about this encryption algorithm except that it uses an 80-bit key.

SLIP   *See* Serial Line Internet Protocol.

SMTP   *See* Simple Mail Transfer Protocol.

SNMP   *See* Simple Network Management Protocol.

socket   A combination of a port address and an IP address.

SONET (Synchronous Optical Network)   A standard in the U.S. that defines a base data rate of 51.84Mbps; multiples of this rate are known as optical carrier (OC) levels, such as OC-3, OC-12, etc.

source address   The address of the station that sent a packet, usually found in the source area of a packet header.

source port number   The address of the PC that is sending data to a receiving PC. The port portion allows for multiplexing of data to be sent from a specific application.

splitter   Any device that electrically duplicates one signal into two.

SPS   *See* Standby Power Supply.

SPX   *See* Sequenced Packet eXchange.

Standby Power Supply (SPS)   A power backup device that has power going directly to the protected equipment. A sensor monitors the power. When a loss is detected, the computer is switched over to the battery. Thus, a loss of power might occur (typically for less than a second).

star topology   A network topology where all devices on the network have a direct connection to every other device on the network. These networks are rare except in very small settings due to the huge amount of cabling required to add a new device.

state table   A firewall security method that monitors the states of all connections through the firewall.

static ARP table entries   Entry in the ARP table that is manually added by a user when a PC will be accessed often. This will speed up the process of communicating with the PC since the IP-to-MAC address will not have to be resolved.

static routing   A method of routing packets where the router's routing is updated manually by the network administrator instead of automatically by a route discovery protocol.

straight tip (ST)   A type of fiber-optic cable connector that uses a mechanism similar to the BNC connectors used by Thinnet. This is the most popular fiber-optic connector currently in use.

subnet mask   A group of selected bits that identify a subnetwork within a TCP/IP network. *See also* Transmission Control Protocol/Internet Protocol.

subnetting   The process of dividing a single IP address range into multiple address ranges.

subnetwork   A network that is part of another network. The connection is made through a gateway, bridge, or router.

subnetwork address   A part of the 32-bit IPv4 address that designates the address of the subnetwork.

subscriber connector (SC)   A type of fiber-optic connector. These connectors are square shaped and have release mechanisms to prevent the cable from accidentally being unplugged.

supernetting   The process of combining multiple IP address ranges into a single IP network.

surge protector   A device that contains a special electronic circuit that monitors the incoming voltage level and then trips a circuit breaker when an overvoltage reaches a certain level called the overvoltage threshold.

surge suppressors   *See* surge protector.

switched   A network that has multiple routes to get from a source to a destination. This allows for higher speeds.

symmetrical keys   When the same key is used to encrypt and decrypt data.

SYN flood   A denial of service attack in which the hacker sends a barrage of SYN packets. The receiving station tries to respond to each SYN request for a connection, thereby tying up all the resources. All incoming connections are rejected until all current connections can be established.

T

TCP   *See* Transmission Control Protocol.

TCP/IP   *See* Transmission Control Protocol/Internet Protocol.

TDMA   *See* Time Division Multiple Access.

TDR   *See* time-domain reflectometer.

telephony server   A computer that functions as a smart answering machine for the network. It can also perform call center and call routing functions.

Telnet   A protocol that functions at the Application layer of the OSI model, providing terminal emulation capabilities. *See also* Open Systems Interconnect.

template   A set of guidelines that you can apply to every new user account created.

terminal emulator   A program that enables a PC to act as a terminal for a mainframe or a Unix system.

terminator   A device that prevents a signal from bouncing off the end of th network cable, which would cause interference with other signals.

test accounts   An account set up by an administrator to confirm the basi functionality of a newly installed application, for example. The test accoun equal rights to accounts that will use the new functionality. It is importan use test accounts instead of administrator accounts to test new functiona an administrator account is used, problems related to user rights may n fest themselves because administrator accounts typically have right network resources.

TFTP   *See* Trivial File Transfer Protocol.

Thick Ethernet (Thicknet)   A type of Ethernet that uses thick co and supports a maximum transmission distance of 500 meters. Al 10Base5.

Thin Ethernet (Thinnet)   A type of Ethernet that uses RG-58 cable and 10Base2.

Time Division Multiple Access (TDMA)   A method to divide individual channels in broadband communications into separate time slots, allowing more data to be carried at the same time. It is also possible to use TDMA in baseband communications.

time-domain reflectometer (TDR)   A tool that sends out a signal and measures how much time it takes to return. It is used to find short or open circuits. Also called a *cable tester*.

Time to Live (TTL)   A field in IP packets that indicates how many routers the packet can still cross (hops it can still make) before it is discarded. TTL is also used in ARP tables to indicate how long an entry should remain in the table.

token   The special packet of data that is passed around the network in a Token Ring network. *See* Token Ring network.

oken passing   A media access method in which a token (data packet) is sed around the ring in an orderly fashion from one device to the next. A ion can transmit only when it has the token. If it doesn't have the token, it transmit. The token continues around the network until the original sender s the token again. If the token has more data to send, the process repeats. e original sender modifies the token to indicate that the token is free for e to use.

network   A network based on a physical star, logical ring topo- data is passed along the ring until it finds its intended receiver. packet can be passed along the ring at a time. If the data packet e ring without being claimed, it is returned to the sender.

A small electronic device used to test network cables for breaks that sends an electronic signal down one set of UTP wires. Used *See also* tone locator, unshielded twisted-pair cable.

ice used to test network cables for breaks and other ense the signal sent by the tone generator and emit a etected in a particular set of wires.

d/or logical layout of the transmission media speci- l layers of the OSI model. *See also* Open Systems

Trace Router   *See* tracert.

tracert   The TCP/IP Trace Route command-line utility that shows the user every router interface a TCP/IP packet passes through on its way to a destination. *See also* Transmission Control Protocol/Internet Protocol.

trailer   A section of a data packet that contains error-checking information.

transceiver   The part of any network interface that transmits and receives network signals.

transient   A high-voltage burst of current.

transmission   Sending of packets from the PC to the network cable.

Transmission Control Protocol (TCP)   The protocol found at the Host-to-Host layer of the DoD model. This protocol breaks data packets into segments, numbers them, and sends them in random order. The receiving computer reassembles the data so that the information is readable for the user. In the process, the sender and the receiver confirm that all data has been received; if not, it is re-sent. This is a connection-oriented protocol. *See also* connection-oriented transport protocol.

Transmission Control Protocol/Internet Protocol (TCP/IP)   The protocol suite developed by the DoD in conjunction with the Internet. It was designed as an internetworking protocol suite that could route information around network failures. Today it is the de facto standard for communications on the Internet.

transmission media   Physical cables and/or wireless technology across which computers are able to communicate.

Transport layer   The fourth layer of the OSI model, it is responsible for checking that the data packet created in the Session layer was received error free. If necessary, it also changes the length of messages for transport up or down the remaining layers. *See also* Open Systems Interconnect.

Trivial File Transfer Protocol (TFTP)   A protocol similar to FTP that does not provide the security or error-checking features of FTP. *See also* File Transfer Protocol.

trunk lines   The telephone lines that form the backbone of a telephone network for a company. These lines connect the telephone(s) to the telephone company and to the PSTN. *See also* Public Switched Telephone Network.

T-series connections   A series of digital connections leased from the telephone company. Each T-series connection is rated with a number based on speed. T1 and T3 are the most popular.

TTL   *See* Time to Live.

twisted-pair cable   A type of network transmission medium that contains pairs of color-coded, insulated copper wires that are twisted around each other. A twisted-pair cable consists of one or more twisted pairs in a common jacket.

type   A DOS command that displays the contents of a file. Also, short for *data type*.

U

UDP   *See* User Datagram Protocol.

Uniform Resource Locator (URL)   A URL is one way of identifying a document on the Internet. It consists of the protocol that is used to access the document and the domain name or IP address of the host that holds the document, for example, http://www.sybek.com.

uninterruptible power supply (UPS)   A natural line conditioner that uses a battery and power inverter to run the computer equipment that plugs into it. The battery charger continuously charges the battery. The battery charger is the only thing that runs off line voltage. During a power problem, the battery charger stops operating, and the equipment continues to run off the battery.

Unix   A 32-bit, multitasking operating system developed in the 1960s for use on mainframes and minicomputers.

unshielded   When cabling has little protection of wrapping to protect it from stray electrical or radio signals. Unshielded cabling is less expensive than shielded.

unshielded twisted-pair cable (UTP)   Twisted-pair cable consisting of a number of twisted pairs of copper wire with a simple plastic casing. Because no shielding is used in this cable, it is very susceptible to EMI, RFI, and other types of interference. *See also* crossover cable, electromagnetic interference, radio frequency interference.

upgrade   To increase an aspect of a PC, for example, by upgrading the RAM (increasing the RAM), upgrading the CPU (changing the current CPU for a faster CPU), etc.

UPS   *See* uninterruptible power supply.

uptime   The amount of time a particular computer or network component has been functional.

URL   *See* Uniform Resource Locator.

user   The person who is using a computer or network.

User Datagram Protocol (UDP)   Protocol at the Host-to-Host layer of the DoD model, which corresponds to the Transport layer of the OSI model. Packets are divided into segments, given numbers, sent randomly, and put back together at the receiving end. This is a connectionless protocol. *See also* connectionless transport protocol, Open Systems Interconnect.

user-level security   A type of network in which user accounts can read, write, change, and take ownership of files. Rights are assigned to user accounts, and each user knows only his or her own username and password, which makes this the preferred method for securing files.

V

vampire tap   A connection used with Thicknet to attach a station to the main cable. It is called a vampire tap because it has a tooth that "bites" through the insulation to make the physical connection.

virtual COM   Serial port that is used as if it were a serial port, but the actual serial port interface does not exist.

Virtual LAN (VLAN)   Allows users on different switch ports to participate in their own network separate from, but still connected to, the other stations on the same or connected switch.

virtual private network (VPN)   Using the public Internet as a backbone for a private interconnection (network) between locations.

virus   A program intended to damage a computer system. Sophisticated viruses encrypt and hide in a computer and may not appear until the user performs a certain action or until a certain date. *See also* antivirus.

virus engine   The core program that runs the virus-scanning process.

volume   Loudness of a sound, or the portion of a hard disk that functions as if it were a separate hard disk.

VPN   *See* virtual private network.

W

WAN   *See* wide area network.

web proxy   A type of proxy that is used to act on behalf of a web client or web server.

web server   A server that holds and delivers web pages and other web content using the HTTP protocol. *See also* Hypertext Transfer Protocol.

wide area network (WAN)   A network that crosses local, regional, and international boundaries.

Windows Internet Name Service (WINS)   A Windows NT service that dynamically associates the NetBIOS name of a host with a domain name. *See also* network basic input/output system.

Windows NT   A network operating system developed by Microsoft that uses that same graphical interface as the Desktop environment, Windows 95/98.

Windows NT 3.51   The version of Windows NT based on the "look and feel" of Windows 3.x. *See also* Windows NT.

Windows NT 4   The version of Windows NT based on the "look and feel" of Windows 95/98. *See also* Windows NT.

Windows NT Service   A type of Windows program (a file with either an .EXE or a .DLL extension) that is loaded automatically by the server or manually by the administrator.

winipcfg   The IP configuration utility for Windows 95/98 that allows you to view the current TCP/IP configuration of a workstation.

WinNuke   A Windows-based attack that affects only computers running Windows NT 3.51 or 4. It is caused by the way that the Windows NT TCP/IP stack handles bad data in the TCP header. Instead of returning an error code or rejecting the bad data, it sends NT to the Blue Screen of Death (BSOD). Figuratively speaking, the attack nukes the computer.

WINS *See* Windows Internet Name Service.

wire crimper Used for attaching ends onto different types of network cables by a process known as crimping. Crimping involves using pressure to press some kind of metal teeth into the inner conductors of a cable.

wireless access point (WAP) A wireless bridge used in a multipoint RF network.

wireless bridge Performs all the functions of a regular bridge but uses RF instead of cables to transmit signals.

workgroup A specific group of users or network devices, organized by job function or proximity to shared resources.

workstation A computer that is not a server but is on a network. Generally a workstation is used to do work, while a server is used to store data or perform a network function. In the most simple terms, a workstation is a computer that is not a server.

World Wide Web (WWW) A collection of HTTP servers running on the Internet. They support the use of documents formatted with HTML. *See also* Hypertext Markup Language, Hypertext Transfer Protocol.

worms Similar to a virus. Worms, however, propagate themselves over a network. *See also* virus.

WWW *See* World Wide Web.

X

X Window A graphical user interface (GUI) developed for use with the various flavors of Unix.

INDEX

Note to the reader: Throughout this index **boldfaced** page numbers indicate primary discussions of a topic. *Italicized* page numbers indicate illustrations.

H

ABOUT THE CONTRIBUTORS

S ome of the best—and best-selling—Sybex authors have contributed chapters fr their books to *Security Complete*, Second Edition.

Chris Brenton is the author of several Sybex books, including *Mastering Cisco Routers*. He is a network consultant specializing in implementing network securi and troubleshooting multiprotocol environments.

James E. Gaskin is President of Gaskin Computer Services, a Dallas-area network cc sulting and integration company. He regularly teaches NetWare-related workshop at NetWorld+Interop. His other books include *Novell's Guide to Integrating Unix and NetWare Networks* and *Mastering NetWare 6*.

Gary Govanus MCSE, MCT, and Master CNI, is the president of PS Consulting Servic Inc. in Minneapolis, Minnesota. He has over 20 year's experience in the IT industry, an currently works as an independent instructor. He is the author of *Server+ Study Guide*.

Ramón J. Hontañón has over 10 years of UNIX, TCP/IP internetworking, and information security experience. He is widely published in *Network* and *SysAdmin* magazines, and authored *Linux Security*.

Cameron Hunt is a network consultant and trainer. He co-authored *Active Defense A Comprehensive Guide to Network Security*.

Robert King MCT, MCNI, has over 10 year's experience teaching and working with Microsoft technologies. He is also the author of *Mastering Active Directory*.

Todd Lammle is a world-renowned Cisco authority with over 15 year's experience with LANs and WANs. He is President of GlobalNet Systems, a network integratior and training firm based in Colorado. He is the author of *CCNA: Cisco Certified Network Associate Study Guide*.

Tom Lancaster, CCIE #8829, CNX# 1105, is a consultant with IBM Global Service He has written over 100 technical articles and frequently teaches classes and speak: at web seminars.

Justin Menga, CCIE #6640, MCSE+I, CCSE, is a Network Solutions Architect in tl wireless and e-infrastructure practice for Compaq Computer New Zealand.

Mark Minasi is a much sought-after speaker at conferences. His firm, MR&D, ha taught tens of thousands of people to design and run NT networks. Some of the book he has authored include *Mastering Windows XP Professional*, *Mastering Windows 200(Server*, and *The Complete PC Upgrade and Maintenance Guide*.

Eric Quinn, CCSI, CSS1, CCNP + Voice, is an Arizona-based instructor and securit consultant.

Roderick W. Smith is a Linux networking expert and the author of several book including *Linux Samba Server Administration* and *Linux+ Study Guide*.

Matthew Strebe is a free-range consultant and owner of Netropolis, a network integration firm specializing in high-speed networking and Windows NT. His book: include *Network Security JumpStart*, *Windows 2000 Server 24seven*, and *From Serf Surfer: Becoming a Network Consultant*.

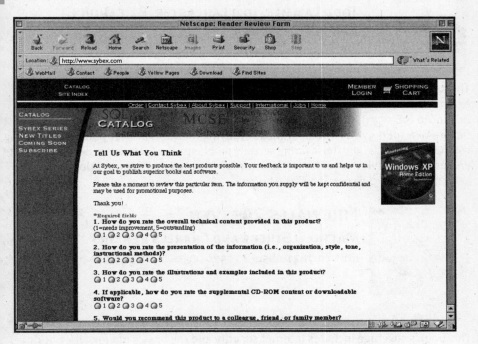

Your feedback is critical to our efforts to provide you with the best books and software on the market. Tell us what you think about the products you've purchased. It's simple:

1. Go to the Sybex website.
2. Find your book by typing the ISBN number or title into the Search field.
3. Click on the book title when it appears.
4. Click **Submit a Review.**
5. Fill out the questionnaire and comments.
6. Click **Submit.**

With your feedback, we can continue to publish the highest quality computer books and software products that today's busy IT professionals deserve.

www.sybex.com

SYBEX Inc. • 1151 Marina Village Parkway, Alameda, CA 94501 • 510-523-8233

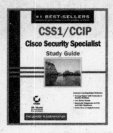

CSS1™/CCIP™: Cisco Security Specialist Study Guide

Todd Lammle, Tom Lancaster, Eric Quinn, and Justin Menga

ISBN: 0-7821-4049-1   1,200 pages   US $89.99

This book is a thorough guide that saves you money! Covers all four Cisco security exams: Managing Cisco Network Security (640-442), Cisco Secure PIX Firewall Advanced (9E0-571), Cisco Secure Intrusion Detection System (9E0-572), and Cisco Secure VPN (9E0-570). Perfect for those studying for the exams, IT personnel working with Cisco products, and those facing security problems. The CD includes pre-assessment exams, bonus review questions, flashcards, sample adaptive questions, and a searchable electronic version of the book.

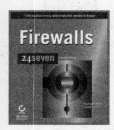

Firewalls 24seven™

Matthew Strebe and Charles Perkins

ISBN: 0-7821-4054-8   576 pages   US $49.99

This book's coverage includes Internet security and the basics of firewalls, hacking prevention technologies, and Unix and Windows environments. Updated for current firewall technologies and devices, the book also includes new information on security administration, virus scanning and protection, VPNs and remote access, and creating a security policy.